Yao & Artusio's

Anesthesiology

Problem-Oriented Patient Management

FOURTH EDITION

Yao & Artusio's

Anesthesiology

Problem-Oriented Patient Management

FOURTH EDITION

Editor

Fun-Sun F. Yao, M.D.

Associate Professor of Clinical Anesthesiology
Cornell University Medical College
Attending Anesthesiologist
The New York Hospital
New York, New York

WITH 40 CONTRIBUTORS

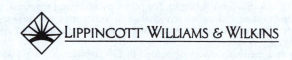

LIPPINCOTT WILLIAMS & WILKINS

Philadelphia • New York

Acquisitions Editor: R. Craig Percy
Developmental Editor: Ellen DiFrancesco
Manufacturing Manager: Dennis Teston
Production Manager: Robert Pancotti
Production Editor: Christina Zingone
Cover Designer: Kevin Kall
Indexer: Dorothy Hoffman
Compositor: Maryland Composition
Printer: R.R. Donnelley-Crawfordsville

Printed in the United States of America

9 8 7 6 5 4 3 2

Library of Congress Cataloging-in-Publication Data

Yao & Artusio's anesthesiology : problem-oriented patient management /
    [edited by] Fun-Sun F. Yao. — 4th ed.
        p.   cm.
    Rev. ed. of: Anesthesiology / [edited by] Fun-Sun F. Yao, Joseph
F. Artusio, Jr. c1993.
    Includes bibliographical references and index.
    ISBN 0-397-58759-7
    1. Anesthesia—Case studies.   2. Anesthesiology—Examinations,
questions, etc.   I. Yao, Fun-Sun F., 1942–   II. Artusio, Joseph
Francis, 1917–   .   III. Title: Anesthesiology.
    [DNLM: 1. Anesthesia—examination questions.   WO 218.2 Y25   1998]
RD82.45.A54   1998
617.96'—DC21
DNLM/DLC
for Library of Congress

This book is dedicated

to

Joseph F. Artusio Jr., M.D.

who

has taught me

not only

to be a good anesthesiologist

but also

to become a better person.

Contents

Contributing Authors

Isaac Azar, M.D.
Professor of Anesthesiology
Albert Einstein College of Medicine
Vice Chairman of Anesthesiology
Director of Pain Management
Beth Israel Medical Center
1st Avenue at 16th Street
New York, New York 10003

Robert F. Bedford, M.D.
Professor of Anesthesiology
University of South Florida
Attending Anesthesiologist
James A. Haley Veterans Hospital
13000 Bruce B. Downs Boulevard
Tampa, Florida 33612

Su-Pen Bobby Chang, M.D.
Assistant Professor of Anesthesiology
Cornell University Medical College
Assistant Attending Anesthesiologist
The New York Hospital
525 East 68th Street
New York, New York 10021

Davy C.H. Cheng, M.D., M.Sc., F.R.C.P.C.
Associate Professor of Anaesthesia
University of Toronto
Deputy Anaesthetist-in-Chief
The Toronto Hospital
200 Elizabeth Street
Toronto, Ontario
Canada M5G 2C4

Samyadev Datta, M.D., F.R.C.A.
Instructor in Anesthesiology
Cornell University Medical College
Assistant Attending Anesthesiologist
Memorial Sloan-Kettering Cancer Center
1275 York Avenue
New York, New York 10021

Miles Dinner, M.D.
Associate Professor of Clinical Anesthesiology
  and Pediatrics
Cornell University Medical College
Associate Attending Anesthesiologist and
  Pediatrician
The New York Hospital
525 East 68th Street
New York, New York 10021

Rita Donovan, C.R.N.A., B.S.N.
Clinical/Didactic Instructor of Anesthesia
State University of New York Health Science
  Center at Brooklyn
Nurse Anesthetist
Kings County Hospital Center
451 Clarkson Avenue
Brooklyn, New York 11203

Jill Fong, B.A., M.D.
Assistant Professor of Anesthesiology
Cornell University Medical College
Assistant Attending Anesthesiologist
The New York Hospital
525 East 68th Street
New York, New York 10021

Farida Gadalla, M.D., M.B. Ch.B.
Associate Professor of Clinical Anesthesiology
Cornell University Medical College
Attending Anesthesiologist
The New York Hospital
525 East 68th Street
New York, New York 10021

Matthew C. Gomillion, M.D.
Assistant Professor of Anesthesiology
Cornell University Medical College
Associate Attending Anesthesiologist
The New York Hospital
525 East 68th Street
New York, New York 10021

Alexander W. Gotta, M.D.
Professor of Anesthesiology
State University of New York Health Science
    Center at Brooklyn
Chief of Service, Anesthesiology
Kings County Hospital Center
457 Clarkson Avenue, Box B
Brooklyn, New York 11203

Gregg S. Hartman, M.D.
Associate Professor of Clinical Anesthesiology
Cornell University Medical College
Associate Attending Anesthesiologist
The New York Hospital
525 East 68th Street
New York, New York 10021

Paul M. Heerdt, M.D., Ph.D.
Associate Professor of Anesthesiology
Cornell University Medical College
Associate Attending Anesthesiologist
The New York Hospital
525 East 68th Street
New York, New York 10021

Subhash Jain, M.D.
Associate Professor of Clinical Anesthesiology
Cornell University Medical College
Attending Anesthesiologist
Chief, Pain Service
Memorial Sloan-Kettering Cancer Center
1275 York Avenue
New York, New York 10021

Robert E. Kelly, M.D.
Associate Professor of Clinical Anesthesiology
Cornell University Medical College
Attending Anesthesiologist
The New York Hospital
525 East 68th Street
New York, New York 10021

Gregory E. Kerr, M.D.
Assistant Professor of Anesthesiology
Cornell University Medical College
Assistant Attending Anesthesiologist
The New York Hospital
525 East 68th Street
New York, New York 10021

Alan D. Kestenbaum, M.D.
Assistant Professor of Anesthesiology
Cornell University Medical College
Associate Attending Anesthesiologist
The New York Hospital
525 East 68th Street
New York, New York 10021

Howard D. Koff, M.D.
Assistant Professor of Anesthesiology
Cornell University Medical College
Associate Attending Anesthesiologist
The New York Hospital
525 East 68th Street
New York, New York 10021

Theresa T. Kudlak, M.D., M.A., B.A.
Attending Anesthesiologist
Maine Medical Center
22 Bramhall Street
Portland, Maine 04102-3175

Cynthia A. Lien, M.D.
Associate Professor of Anesthesiology
Cornell University Medical College
Associate Attending Anesthesiologist
The New York Hospital
525 East 68th Street
New York, New York 10021

Patricia Fogarty Mack, M.D.
Assistant Professor of Anesthesiology
Cornell University Medical College
Assistant Attending Anesthesiologist
The New York Hospital
525 East 68th Street
New York, New York 10021

Vinod Malhotra, M.B., B.S., M.D.
Professor of Clinical Anesthesiology
Cornell University Medical College
Attending Anesthesiologist
Clinical Director of Operating Rooms
The New York Hospital
525 East 68th Street
New York, New York 10021

Elon H. Mehr, M.D.
Assistant Professor of Anesthesiology
Cornell University Medical College
Associate Attending Anesthesiologist
The New York Hospital
525 East 68th Street
New York, New York 10021

Mindy Lyn Nestampower, M.D.
Fellow in Anesthesiology
Memorial Sloan-Kettering Cancer Center
1275 York Avenue
New York, New York 10021

Jeffrey Y.F. Ngeow, M.D., M.B., B.S.
Clinical Associate Professor of Anesthesiology
Cornell University Medical College
Attending Anesthesiologist
Hospital for Special Surgery
535 East 70th Street
New York, New York 10021

Dana L. Oster, M.D.
Assistant Professor of Anesthesiology
Cornell University Medical College
Assistant Attending Anesthesiologist
The New York Hospital
525 East 68th Street
New York, New York 10021

Onofrio Patafio, M.D.
Assistant Professor of Anesthesiology
Cornell University Medical College
Associate Attending Anesthesiologist
The New York Hospital
525 East 68th Street
New York, New York 10021

Howard L. Rosner, M.D.
Associate Professor of Clinical Anesthesiology
Cornell University Medical College
Associate Attending Anesthesiologist
The New York Hospital
525 East 68th Street
New York, New York 10021

Lori A. Rubin, M.D.
Assistant Professor of Anesthesiology
Cornell University Medical College
Associate Attending Anesthesiologist
The New York Hospital
525 East 68th Street
New York, New York 10021

John J. Savarese, M.D.
Professor and Chairman of Anesthesiology
Cornell University Medical College
Anesthesiologist-in-Chief
The New York Hospital
525 East 68th Street
New York, New York 10021

Edwina Sia-Kho, M.D.
Assistant Professor of Clinical Anesthesiology
Cornell University Medical College
Attending Anesthesiologist
The New York Hospital
525 East 68th Street
New York, New York 10021

Ralph L. Slepian, M.D.
Assistant Professor of Anesthesiology
Cornell University Medical College
Associate Attending Anesthesiologist
The New York Hospital
525 East 68th Street
New York, New York 10021

Colleen A. Sullivan, M.B. Ch.B.
Clinical Professor of Anesthesiology
State University of New York Health Science
   Center at Brooklyn
450 Clarkson Avenue
Brooklyn, New York 11203

Stephen J. Thomas, M.D.
Professor and Vice Chairman of Anesthesiology
Cornell University Medical College
Attending Anesthesiologist
The New York Hospital
525 East 68th Street
New York, New York 10021

Joseph Tjan, M.D.
Assistant Professor of Anesthesiology
Cornell University Medical College
Assistant Attending Anesthesiologist
The New York Hospital
525 East 68th Street
New York, New York 10021

Marjorie J. Topkins, M.D.
Professor Emeritus of Clinical Anesthesiology
Cornell University Medical College
Attending Anesthesiologist
The New York Hospital
525 East 68th Street
New York, New York 10021

Alan Van Proznak, A.B., M.D.
Professor of Anesthesiology and Pharmacology
Cornell University Medical College
Attending Anesthesiologist
The New York Hospital
525 East 68th Street
New York, New York 10021

Judith Weingram, M.D.
Assistant Professor of Anesthesiology
Cornell University Medical College
Attending Anesthesiologist
The New York Hospital
525 East 68th Street
New York, New York 10021

Doreen L. Wray Roth, M.D.
Assistant Professor of Anesthesiology
Cornell University Medical College
Associate Attending Anesthesiologist
The New York Hospital
525 East 68th Street
New York, New York 10021

Fun-Sun F. Yao, M.D.
Associate Professor of Clinical Anesthesiology
Cornell University Medical College
Attending Anesthesiologist
The New York Hospital
525 East 68th Street
New York, New York 10021

Victor M. Zayas, M.D.
Clinical Assistant Professor of Anesthesiology and
   Pediatrics
Cornell University Medical College
Associate Attending Anesthesiologist and
   Pediatrician
Hospital for Special Surgery
535 East 70th Street
New York, New York 10021

Preface

Important advances in surgical procedures and the clinical practice of anesthesiology have prompted the production of a new edition of this text. The book has been published in four languages: English, German, Japanese, and Chinese. The remarkable popularity of the first three editions in the anesthesiology community, both here and abroad, encouraged us to update and expand its subject matter. The fourth edition is written to further improve anesthesia management for sophisticated surgery.

As with our previous editions, *Yao & Artusio's Anesthesiology: Problem-Oriented Patient Management* was written to present a group of important clinical entities covering the most critical anesthetic problems. It is intended to provide logical and scientific fundamentals for individualized patient management.

In this fourth edition, *Yao & Artusio's Anesthesiology* is organized by organ systems into nine sections consisting of 57 chapters. Each chapter begins with a brief case presentation, followed by essential problems of each disease covering four areas: 1) pathophysiology and differential diagnosis, 2) preoperative evaluation and preparation, 3) intraoperative management, and 4) postoperative anesthetic management. The book is designed to stress anesthetic problems and to give the anesthesiologist the opportunity to organize his or her own ideas of patient care. A reasonable answer, with updated references, follows each question.

To maintain the fresh quality of the textbook, approximately one third of the fourth edition consists of new chapters or contributions by new authors. We have added 11 new chapters: lung transplantation, heart transplantation and subsequent noncardiac surgery, transposition of the great arteries, ischemic heart disease and noncardiac surgery, cancer pain, cerebral aneurysm, laparoscopic surgery, nerve blocks of the lower extremity, airway trauma, cervical mass in infancy, and magnetic resonance imaging.

The text originally reflected the clinical experience of the Department of Anesthesiology at Cornell University Medical College The New York Hospital. In this edition, experts from other prestigious institutions have contributed their valuable opinions to make this book more universally acceptable. The material in the book is prepared for the education of the resident and the practicing anesthesiologist; it also serves as a review source for the continuing education of the anesthesiologist. The question-and-answer format, combined with current references, enhances its educational value.

Acknowledgments

I wish to express my personal gratitude to the individual contributors. This book would not have been possible without their hard work and dedication. I particularly thank Joseph F. Artusio, Jr., M.D., who is my mentor and the co-editor of the previous three editions. In honor of his contributions to the development and the advances of modern anesthesiology and with his permission, Dr. Artusio's name is part of the book's title. I am grateful to Irusia R. Kocka for her editorial assistance. I would also like to thank Kenya Diaz for her help with typing. In addition, I am especially indebted to John J. Savarese, M.D. for his constructive advice and support. Above all, my deepest appreciation goes to my family, Tong-Yi, Ning-Yen, Jean-Kuan and especially to my dear compassionate wife Baw-Chyr Peggy Yao. Her understanding, patience, and encouragement made this book possible.

The Respiratory System

1

Asthma—Chronic Obstructive Pulmonary Disease (COPD)

Fun-Sun F. Yao

A 45-year-old man with cholelithiasis was scheduled for cholecystectomy. He had a long history of asthma and developed dyspnea with only moderate exertion. He slept on two pillows. There was no peripheral edema. Arterial blood gases showed the following: pH, 7.36; P_{CO_2}, 60 mm Hg; P_{O_2}, 70 mm Hg; CO_2 content, 36 mEq/liter.

A. Medical Disease and Differential Diagnosis

1. What differential diagnosis is compatible with these symptoms?
2. How would you distinguish obstructive lung disease from restrictive lung disease by spirometry?
3. Define normal lung volumes and lung capacities and their normal values in the average adult male.
4. What are flow-volume loops? Draw flow-volume loops in a normal subject, in a patient with COPD, and in a patient with restrictive lung disease.
5. Define closing capacity and closing volume. What is the normal value of closing volume?
6. What are the effects of age and posture on functional residual capacity (FRC) and closing capacity (CC)?
7. What are the effects of anesthesia on FRC and CC?
8. Why is the FRC important in oxygenation?
9. Are there methods to measure FRC and closing volume?
10. Are there any other pulmonary function tests?
11. Define lung compliance, chest wall compliance, and total compliance. What are their interrelations and their normal values?
12. Give the equations for shunt (QS/QT) and dead space/tidal volume (VD/VT). What are their normal values?
13. Interpret the following arterial blood gases: pH, 7.36; P_{CO_2}, 60 mm Hg; P_{O_2}, 70 mm Hg; CO_2 content, 36 mEq/liter.
14. What is normal PaO_2 if F_IO_2 is 1.0?
15. What are the common physiologic causes of hypoxemia?
16. What is the prevalence of asthma?
17. What is the etiology of asthma?
18. Discuss the pathogenesis of asthma.
19. What are the predisposing factors of asthmatic attacks?
20. What is the universal finding in arterial blood gases during asthmatic attacks—hypoxemia or CO_2 retention?
21. What changes are seen in spirometry, lung volumes, and lung capacities during an asthmatic attack?

B. Preoperative Evaluation and Preparation

1. What preoperative workup would you order?
2. Would you order any special preoperative preparations for asthmatic patients with chronic obstructive lung disease?
3. How long would you postpone elective surgery if the patient had a recent upper respiratory infection (URI)?
4. What medicines would you expect the patient to have taken in the past or be taking at the present time?
5. Would you order preoperative steroid preparation? Why?
6. What is the onset of action of intravenous steroid therapy in asthma?
7. What are the effects of cimetidine on asthmatic patients?
8. How would you premedicate the patient? Why?

C. Intraoperative Management

1. What are the disadvantages of administering atropine to the asthmatic patient?
2. If the patient had a severe asthmatic attack in the operating room before the induction of anesthesia, would you put the patient to sleep or postpone the surgery?
3. The patient did not have an asthmatic attack in the operating room. How would you induce anesthesia?
4. Why would you use methohexital instead of thiopental?
5. Would you use propofol, etomidate, or ketamine for induction?
6. Would you use lidocaine for intubation?
7. If this is emergency surgery and rapid-sequence induction is indicated, how would you induce anesthesia in this patient?
8. What is your choice of agents for maintenance of anesthesia? Why?
9. What are the mechanisms of halothane that produce bronchodilation?
10. Why would you choose an inhalational instead of an intravenous technique?
11. Is regional anesthesia better than general anesthesia in this situation?
12. Which muscle relaxants would you use? Why?
13. In the middle of surgery, the patient developed a severe wheezing attack. How do you manage it?
14. How would you give beta-2 agonists? What problems may arise when isoproterenol is given during halothane anesthesia? What is its mechanism of action on asthma?
15. How would you administer aminophylline? How does aminophylline relieve bronchospasm? What is the mechanism of action? What are the therapeutic blood levels of aminophylline? What are the toxic effects of aminophylline?
16. If the patient does not respond to the above treatment and becomes cyanotic, what would you do?
17. What are the differential diagnoses of intraoperative bronchospasm?
18. The asthmatic attack was finally relieved and the operation was completed. The patient was found to be hypoventilating. What are the common causes of hypoventilation? Would you like to reverse the muscle relaxant?

D. Postoperative Management

1. Would you extubate the asthmatic patient while he was deeply anesthestized?
2. When the patient cannot be extubated early in the recovery room, how would you keep the endotracheal tube in place without causing bronchoconstriction?

3. In asthmatic patients, are narcotics contraindicated for postoperative pain control?
4. The patient was breathing well and was extubated. How much oxygen would you give to this asthmatic patient with COPD in the recovery room?

A. Medical Disease and Differential Diagnosis

A.1. What differential diagnosis is compatible with these symptoms?

The differential diagnosis of wheezing and dyspnea includes bronchial asthma, acute left ventricular failure (cardiac asthma), upper airway obstruction by tumor or laryngeal edema, endobronchial disease such as foreign body aspiration, neoplasms, bronchial stenosis, carcinoid tumors, recurrent pulmonary emboli, chronic bronchitis, eosinophilic pneumonias, chemical pneumonias, and occasionally polyarteritis. To differentiate asthma from other diseases with wheezing and dyspnea is usually not difficult. The triad of dyspnea, coughing, and wheezing, in addition to a history of periodic attacks, is quite characteristic. A personal or family history of allergic diseases is valuable contributory evidence. A patient with long-standing asthma may develop chronic obstructive lung disease and suffer from exertional dyspnea and orthopnea. Cardiac asthma is a misnomer and refers to acute left ventricular failure. Although the primary lesion is cardiac, the disease manifests itself in the lungs. The symptoms and signs may mimic bronchial asthma, but the findings of moist basilar rales, gallop rhythms, blood-tinged sputum, peripheral edema, and a history of heart disease allow the appropriate diagnosis to be reached.

Fauci AS, Braunwald E, Isselbacher KJ et al (Eds): Harrison's Principles of Internal Medicine, 14th ed, p 1423. New York, McGraw-Hill, 1998

Rakel RE (ed): Saunders Manual of Medical Practice, pp 117–119. Philadelphia, WB Saunders, 1996

A.2. How would you distinguish obstructive lung disease from restrictive lung disease by spirometry?

Table 1-1 summarizes the distinctions between the two types of lung diseases. In restrictive lung disease (e.g., pulmonary fibrosis and ankylosing spondylitis) the forced vital capacity (FVC) is low because of limited expansion of the lungs or chest wall. However, the forced expiratory volume at 1 second (FEV$_1$) is often not reduced proportionately, because airway resistance is normal. Thus, the FEV$_1$/FVC percentage is normal or high.

In obstructive lung disease (e.g., emphysema) the FEV$_1$/FVC is grossly reduced

Table 1-1. Difference of Obstructive and Restrictive Lung Diseases

	OBSTRUCTIVE	RESTRICTIVE
VC	N or ↓	↓
TLC	N or ↑	↓
RV	↑	↓
FEV$_1$/FVC	↓	N or ↑
MMEFR	↓	N
MBC	↓	N

N = normal; ↑ = increased; ↓ = decreased

because the airway resistance is high. Maximum breathing capacity (MBC) and maximal midexpiratory flow rate (MMEFR) are reduced early in small airway obstruction. MMEFR is also called $FEF_{25-75\%}$. MMEFR is obtained by dividing the volume between 75% and 25% of the vital capacity (VC) by the corresponding elapsed time. Unlike FEV_1, MMEFR is independent of patient effort.

Normally, FEV_1 is >80% of FVC and VC should be >80% of predicted value. The predicted values depend on body size, age, and sex. The total lung capacity (TLC) is increased in obstructive lung disease and decreased in restrictive lung disease. However, TLC cannot be obtained by routine screening spirometry. Normal MBC is >125 liters/min and normal MMEFR is >300 liters/min.

Barash PG, Cullen BF, Stoelting RK (eds): Clinical Anesthesia, 3rd ed, pp 764–765. Philadelphia, Lippincott-Raven, 1997

Crapo RO: Pulmonary function testing. N Engl J Med 331:25–30, 1994

Fauci AS, Braunwald E, Isselbacher KJ et al (eds): Harrison's Principles of Internal Medicine, 14th ed, pp 1410–1412. New York, McGraw-Hill, 1998

A.3. Define normal lung volumes and lung capacities and their normal values in the average adult male.

There are four basic "volumes" and four derived "capacities" which are combinations of these volumes (Fig. 1-1).

Tidal volume (VT) is the volume of air inhaled or exhaled during normal breathing. Normal VT is 500 ml.

Inspiratory reserve volume (IRV) is the maximal volume of gas that can be inhaled following a normal inspiration while at rest. Normal IRV is 3000 ml.

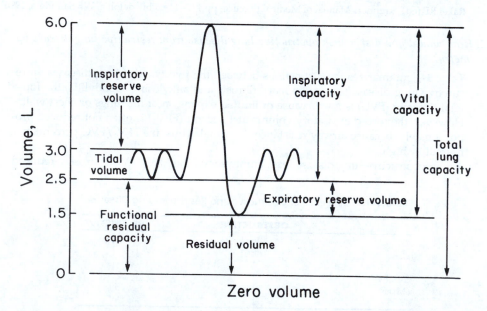

Figure 1-1.   *Lung volumes and lung capacities.*

Expiratory reserve volume (ERV) is the maximal volume of gas that can be exhaled following a normal expiration. Normal ERV is 1000 ml.

Residual volume (RV) is the volume of gas remaining in the lungs after a forced exhalation. Normal RV is 1500 ml.

Vital capacity (VC) is the maximal amount of gas that can be exhaled after a maximum inhalation. The vital capacity is the sum of VT, ERV, and IRV. Normal VC is 4500 ml.

Inspiratory capacity (IC) is the maximal amount of gas that can be inhaled from the resting expiratory position after a normal exhalation. It is the sum of VT and IRV. Normal IC is 3500 ml.

Functional residual capacity (FRC) is the remaining lung volume at the end of a normal quiet expiration. It is the sum of RV and ERV. Normal FRC is 2500 ml.

Total lung capacity (TLC) is the lung volume at the end of a maximal inspiration. It is the sum of VC and RV. Normal TLC is 6000 ml.

Nunn JF: Nunn's Applied Respiratory Physiology, 4th ed, pp 49–52. Boston, Butterworth-Heinemann, 1993

A.4. What are flow-volume loops? Draw flow-volume loops in a normal subject, in a patient with COPD, and in a patient with restrictive lung disease.

Flow-volume loops provide a graphic analysis of flow at various lung volumes. Both flow and volume are plotted simultaneously on an X-Y recorder as subjects inspire fully to total lung capacity (TLC) and then perform a forced vital capacity (FVC) maneuver. This is immediately followed by a maximal inhalation as fast as possible back to TLC (Fig. 1-2). The entire inspiratory portion of the loop and the expiratory

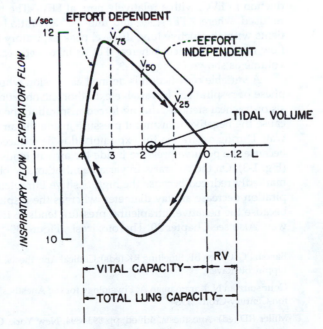

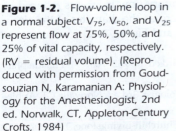

Figure 1-2. Flow-volume loop in a normal subject. $\dot{V}_{75}$, $\dot{V}_{50}$, and $\dot{V}_{25}$ represent flow at 75%, 50%, and 25% of vital capacity, respectively. (RV = residual volume). (Reproduced with permission from Goudsouzian N, Karamanian A: Physiology for the Anesthesiologist, 2nd ed. Norwalk, CT, Appleton-Century Crofts, 1984)

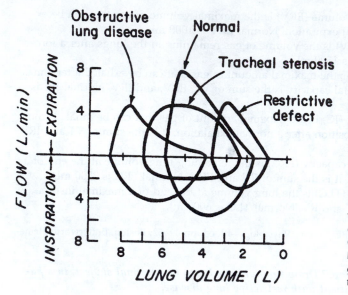

Figure 1-3. Flow-volume loops relative to lung volumes in a normal subject, a patient with COPD, a patient with fixed obstruction (tracheal stenosis), and in a patient with pulmonary fibrosis (restrictive defect). Note the concave expiratory form in the patient with COPD and the flat inspiratory curve in the patient with a fixed obstruction. (Reproduced with permission from Goudsouzian N, Karamanian A: Physiology for the Anesthesiologist, 2nd ed. Norwalk, CT, Appleton-Century Crofts, 1984)

curve near TLC are highly effort dependent, whereas the expiratory flow at 75% to 25% of vital capacity (VC) is effort independent. The ratio of expiratory flow to inspiratory flow at 50% of VC (mid-VC flow ratio) normally is about 1.0. This ratio is particularly useful in identifying the presence of upper airway obstruction. In patients with restrictive lung disease such as pulmonary fibrosis and scoliosis, there is a reduction in FVC, with a relatively normal FEV_1. The total lung capacity is markedly reduced, whereas $FEF_{25-75\%}$ and mid-VC flow ratio is usually normal (Fig. 1-3). In patients with obstructive lung disease, peak expiratory flow rate, $FEF_{25-75\%}$ and mid-VC flow ratio are reduced, whereas TLC is increased secondary to increase in residual volume as shown in Figure 1-3.

A variable obstruction is defined as a lesion whose influence varies with the phase of respiration. In variable extrathoracic obstructions such as vocal cord paralysis or tracheal stenosis, during forced inspiration the respiratory flow is reduced because the negative transmural pressure inside the airway tends to collapse the airway. During expiration the expiratory flow is reduced far less and may be normal because the positive pressure inside the airway tends to decrease the obstruction (Fig. 1-3). On the contrary, in variable intrathoracic obstruction, the expiratory flow is markedly reduced because the high positive intrapleural pressures during forced expiration decrease airway diameter, whereas the inspiratory flow is far less reduced because the negative intrapleural pressure tends to increase the diameter of the airway. Also see Chapter 30, Thyrotoxicosis, Figure 30-1 and Figure 30-2.

Barash PG, Cullen BF, Stoelting RK (eds): Clinical Anesthesia, 3rd ed, pp 762–763, 771. Philadelphia, Lippincott-Raven, 1997

Goudsouzian N, Karamanian A: Physiology for the Anesthesiologist, 3rd ed. Norwalk, CT, Appleton-Century-Crofts, 1984

Miller RD (ed): Anesthesia, 4th ed, pp 893–894. New York, Churchill-Livingstone, 1994

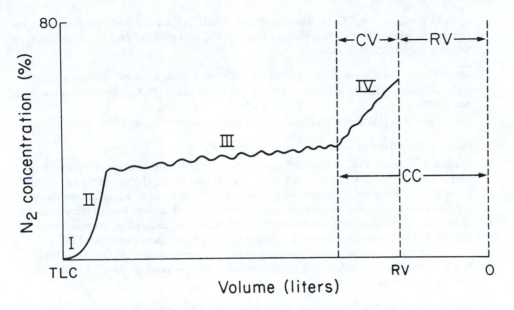

Figure 1-4.   Closing volume measurement by single-breath nitrogen test.

A.5. Define closing capacity and closing volume. What is the normal value of closing volume?

Closing capacity (CC) is the lung volume at which the small airways in the dependent parts of the lung begin to close. Closing capacity is the sum of closing volume and residual volume. Closing volume (CV) is the gas volume expelled during phase IV of the single-breath nitrogen test; it denotes the lung volume from the beginning of airway closure to the end of maximal expiration. Therefore, CV = CC − RV (Fig. 1-4).

In normal young people, the closing volume is approximately 10% of the vital capacity, or 400 to 500 ml. The closing volume and the closing capacity increase with age. The closing volume is increased in patients with small-airway disease and in chronic smokers.

Buist AS: The single-breath nitrogen test. N Engl J Med 293:438, 1975

Editorial: Closing volume. Lancet 2:908, October 1972

Nunn JF: Nunn's Applied Respiratory Physiology, 4th ed, pp 49–52. Boston, Butterworth-Heinemann, 1993

A.6. What are the effects of age and posture on functional residual capacity (FRC) and closing capacity (CC)?

FRC is either independent of age in adults or increases very slightly with increasing age. CC, however, increases with age. Normally, CC becomes equal to the FRC at the age of 66 in the upright position and at the age of 44 in the supine position.

FRC increases approximately 30% by changing from the supine position to the upright position. The CC, on the other hand, is independent of body position. It is important to remember that the effects of age on CC and posture on FRC determine whether airway closure exists.

Miller RD (ed): Anesthesia, 4th ed, pp 593–594, 2151. New York, Churchill Livingstone, 1994

Nunn JF: Nunn's Applied Respiratory Physiology, 4th ed, pp 53–55. Boston, Butterworth-Heinemann, 1993

Rehder K, Marsh HM, Rodarte JR et al: Airway closure. Anesthesiology 47:40, 1977

A.7. What are the effects of anesthesia on FRC and CC?

During anesthesia, FRC is reduced approximately 20% with spontaneous breathing and about 16% with artificial ventilation. This is due to the change in thoracic cage muscle tone. After the induction of general anesthesia, there is a loss of inspiratory tone and an appearance of end-expiratory tone in the abdominal expiratory muscles at the end of exhalation. The end-expiratory tone in the abdominal muscles increases intraabdominal pressure, forces the diaphragm cephalad, and decreases FRC.

Closing capacity was previously reported to be unchanged during anesthesia, but later studies concluded that closing capacity has reduced in parallel with FRC during anesthesia.

Bergman NA, Tien YK: Contribution of the closure of pulmonary units to impaired oxygenation during anesthesia. Anesthesiology 59:395, 1983

Gilmour I, Burnham M, Craig DB: Closing capacity measurements during general anesthesia. Anesthesiology 45:477, 1976

Juno P, Marsh HM, Knopp TJ et al: Closing capacity in awake and anesthetized-paralyzed man. J Appl Physiol 44:238, 1978

Nunn JF: Nunn's Applied Respiratory Physiology, 4th ed, pp 393–397. Boston, Butterworth-Heinemann, 1993

A.8. Why is the FRC important in oxygenation?

First, when the FRC is decreased to below closing capacity (CC), airways close in the dependent parts of the lung during certain periods of normal tidal ventilation. Airway closure results in shunting of pulmonary blood flow through the unventilated alveoli. Therefore, QS/QT is increased and arterial oxygenation is decreased. Second, pulmonary circulation and alveolar gas exchange are continuous during both inspiratory and expiratory phases of respiration. Whether or not there is airway closure, blood oxygenation during the expiratory phase is mainly dependent on the remaining lung volume, which is FRC. Therefore, when the FRC is high, blood oxygenation is better and there is more time for oxygenation before hypoxemia occurs during apnea. FRC is decreased in the supine position during general anesthesia and in the adult respiratory distress syndrome. Positive end-expiratory pressure (PEEP) increases FRC and decreases airway closure.

Nunn JF: Nunn's Applied Respiratory Physiology, 4th ed, pp 52–54. Boston, Butterworth-Heinemann, 1993

A.9. Are there methods to measure FRC and closing volume?

FRC may be measured by helium dilution, nitrogen washout, and body plethysmography. Closing volume may be determined by two techniques, the single-breath nitrogen test (residual gas technique) and the bolus technique with an inert tracer gas such as helium, xenon, or argon.

Buist AS: The single-breath nitrogen test. N Engl J Med 293:438, 1975

Nunn JF: Nunn's Applied Respiratory Physiology, 4th ed, pp 60, 88–89. Boston, Butterworth-Heinemann, 1993

A.10. Are there any other pulmonary function tests?

Arterial blood gases, chest x-ray film, computed tomography (CT) scan, magnetic resonance imaging (MRI), radioisotope lung scan, ventilation/perfusion study, diffusion capacity, QS/QT, VD/VT, compliance.

Fauci AS, Braunwald E, Isselbacher KJ et al (eds): Harrison's Principles of Internal Medicine, 14th ed, pp 1410–1419. New York, McGraw-Hill, 1998

Nunn JF: Nunn's Applied Respiratory Physiology, 4th ed, pp 55, 187, 217. Boston, Butterworth-Heinemann, 1993

A.11. Define lung compliance, chest wall compliance, and total compliance. What are their interrelations and their normal values?

Lung compliance is the change in lung volume by per unit change in alveolar/intrathoracic pressure gradient. The normal value is 200 ml/cm H_2O in the upright position. Chest wall compliance is the change in lung volume by per unit change in ambient/intrathoracic pressure gradient. Its normal value is 200 ml/cm H_2O. Total compliance is the change in lung volume by per unit change in alveolar/ambient pressure gradient. Its normal value is 100 ml/cm H_2O.

$$\frac{1}{\text{Lung compliance}} + \frac{1}{\text{Chest wall compliance}} = \frac{1}{\text{Total compliance}}$$

Nunn JF: Nunn's Applied Respiratory Physiology, 4th ed, pp 47–49. Boston, Butterworth-Heinemann, 1993

A.12. Give the equations for QS/QT and VD/VT. What are their normal values?

$$QS/QT = \frac{CcO_2 - CaO_2}{CcO_2 - C\bar{v}O_2} \qquad VD/VT = \frac{PaCO_2 - P\bar{E}CO_2}{PaCO_2}$$

Normal QS/QT is 4% to 5% and VD/VT is about 0.3.

Nunn JF: Nunn's Applied Respiratory Physiology, 4th ed, pp 171–172, 178–180. Boston, Butterworth-Heinemann, 1993

A.13. Interpret the following arterial blood gases: pH, 7.36; P_{CO_2}, 60 mm Hg; P_{O_2}, 70 mm Hg; CO_2 content, 36 mEq/liter.

The F_IO_2 is essential to evaluate PaO_2. We assume the blood is taken while the patient is breathing room air. The blood gases show respiratory acidosis, compensated by metabolic alkalosis, and mild hypoxemia. The blood gases are compatible with chronic obstructive lung disease.

A.14. What is normal PaO_2 if F_IO_2 is 1.0?

If F_IO_2 is 1.0, normal PaO_2 should be 500 mm Hg to 600 mm Hg. To estimate the normal PaO_2 at different values of F_IO_2, we may assume that every 10% oxygen increases 50 to 60 mm Hg of PaO_2. If the F_IO_2 is 0.4, we expect the normal PaO_2 to be 200 to 240 mm Hg.

Nunn JF: Nunn's Applied Respiratory Physiology, 5th ed, pp 257–260. Boston, Butterworth-Heinemann, 1993

Shapiro BA, Harrison RA, Cane RD, Walton JR: Clinical Application of Blood Gases, 4th ed, pp 82–83. Chicago, Year Book Medical Publishers, 1989

A.15. What are the common physiologic causes of hypoxemia?

From the shunt equation, arterial oxygen content is related to the change in pulmonary capillary oxygen content, venous oxygen content, and venous admixture. It is easier to classify hypoxemia into the following three categories:

Decreased Pulmonary Capillary Oxygen Tension
- Hypoventilation
- Low F_IO_2
- Ventilation/perfusion abnormalities from pulmonary parenchymal change
- Diffusion abnormality (rare)

Increased Shunting, Either Intrapulmonary or Cardiac
Reduced Venous Oxygen Content
- Congestive heart failure—low cardiac output
- Increased metabolism—fever, hyperthyroidism, shivering
- Decreased arterial oxygen content—anemia

Fauci AS, Braunwald E, Isselbacher KJ et al (eds): Harrison's Principles of Internal Medicine, 14th ed, pp 1415–1417. New York, McGraw-Hill, 1998

Nunn JF: Nunn's Applied Respiratory Physiology, 4th ed, pp 256–257. Boston, Butterworth-Heinemann, 1993

Shapiro BA, Harrison RA, Cane RD, Walton JR: Clinical Application of Blood Gases, 4th ed, pp 71–72. Chicago, Year Book Medical Publishers, 1989

A.16. What is the prevalence of asthma?

Approximately 5% of adults and 7% to 10% of children in the United States and Australia have asthma. It occurs at all ages but is predominant in early life. About one-half of the patients develop asthma before age 10 and another third before age 40. In childhood, there is a 2:1 male/female preponderance, which equalizes by age 30.

Fauci AS, Braunwald E, Isselbacher KJ et al (eds): Harrison's Principles of Internal Medicine, 14th ed, p 1420. New York, McGraw-Hill, 1998

A.17. What is the etiology of asthma?

Asthma is a heterogeneous disease. It is difficult to define its etiology. The common denominator that underlies the asthmatic diathesis is a nonspecific hyperirritability of the tracheobronchial tree. Clinically, asthma is classified into two groups, allergic (extrinsic) and idiosyncratic (intrinsic). Allergic asthma is usually associated with a personal or a family history of allergic diseases, positive skin reactions to extracts of airborne antigens, and increased levels of IgE in the serum. Immunologic mechanisms appear to be causally related to 25% to 35% of all cases and contributory in another one-third. Idiosyncratic asthma cannot be classified on the basis of immunologic mechanisms. It is probably due to abnormality of the parasympathetic nervous system. Bronchospasm is provoked when certain agents stimulate tracheobronchial receptors.

Adelroth E, Morris MM, Hargreave FE et al: Airway responsiveness to leukotriene, C4 & D4 and to methacholine in patients with asthma and normal controls. N Engl J Med 315:480–484, 1986

Fauci AS, Braunwald E, Isselbacher KJ et al (eds): Harrison's Principles of Internal Medicine, 14th ed, p 1420. New York, McGraw-Hill, 1998

A.18. Discuss the pathogenesis of asthma.

The common denominator underlying the asthmatic diathesis is a nonspecific hyperirritability of the tracheobronchial tree. The basic mechanism of the airway hyperirritability remains unknown. The most popular hypothesis at present is that of airway inflammation. Even when asthmatics are in remission, bronchial biopsy reveals infiltration by inflammatory cells and epithelial shedding from the mucosa. Following exposure to an initiating stimulus, mast cells, eosinophils, and macrophages can be activated to release a variety of mediators which lead to contraction of airway smooth muscle, vascular congestion, increased capillary permeability (airways edema), and thick tenacious secretions, thereby evoking an intense inflammatory reaction (Fig. 1-5). The net result is an increase in airway resistance, decreased forced ex-

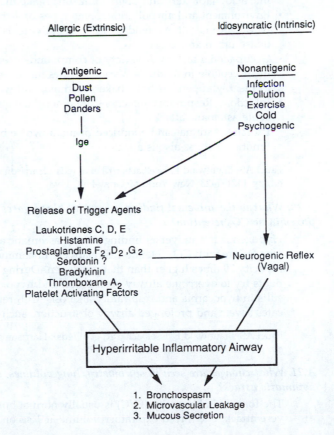

Figure 1-5. The pathogenesis of bronchial asthma.

piratory volumes and flow rates, hyperinflation of the lungs and thorax, increased work of breathing, alterations in respiratory muscle function, mismatched ventilation/perfusion, and altered blood gases.

Chung KF: Role of inflammation in the hyperactivity of the airways in asthma. Thorax 41:657–662, 1986

Djukanvic R, Roche WR, Wilson JW et al: State of the art: Mucosal inflammation in asthma. Am Rev Respir Dis 142:434–457, 1990

Fauci AS, Braunwald E, Isselbacher KJ et al (eds): Harrison's Principles of Internal Medicine, 14th ed, pp 1420–1422. New York, McGraw-Hill, 1998

O'Byrne PM, Hargreave FE, Kirby JG: Airway inflammation and hyperresponsiveness. Am Rev Respir Dis 136:535–537, 1987

A.19. What are the predisposing factors of asthmatic attacks?

- Allergens. Airborne allergens are the most common.
- Pharmacologic stimuli. The drugs most commonly associated with the induction of acute asthmatic attacks are aspirin, coloring agents such as tartrazine, beta-adrenergic antagonists, and sulfiting agents. Aspirin and other nonsteroidal anti-inflammatory agents such as indomethacin, mefenamic acid, ibuprofen, fenoprofen, flufenamic acid, naproxen, and phenylbutazone make the asthma worse.
- Environment and air pollution. Some types of asthma, such as Tokyo-Yokohama or New Orleans asthma, tend to occur in individuals who live in heavy-industrial or dense urban areas.
- Occupational factors. A variety of compounds used in industry can cause asthma in susceptible individuals. Various names have been applied to this condition, such as meat wrappers' asthma, bakers' asthma, and woodworkers' asthma.
- Infections. Respiratory infections are among the most common stimuli that evoke acute asthmatic attacks.
- Exercise. Asthma can be induced or made worse by physical exertion.
- Emotional stress also is a factor.

Fauci AS, Braunwald E, Isselbacher KJ et al (eds): Harrison's Principles of Internal Medicine, 14th ed, pp 1421–1423. New York, McGraw-Hill, 1998

A.20. What is the universal finding in arterial blood gases during asthmatic attacks—hypoxemia or CO_2 retention?

Hypoxemia is a universal finding during asthmatic attacks. However, frank ventilatory failure with CO_2 retention is relatively uncommon because CO_2 has a diffusion capacity 20 times higher than that of oxygen. During acute asthmatic attacks, most patients try to overcome airway obstruction and hypoxia by hyperventilation. This results in hypocarbia and respiratory alkalosis. CO_2 retention is a late finding and indicates severe and prolonged airway obstruction, such as in status asthmaticus.

Fauci AS, Braunwald E, Isselbacher KJ et al (eds): Harrison's Principles of Internal Medicine, 14th ed, p 1422. New York, McGraw-Hill, 1998

A.21. What changes are seen in spirometry, lung volumes, and lung capacities during an asthmatic attack?

The forced vital capacity (FVC) is usually normal but may be decreased during a severe attack. The forced expiratory volume at 1 second (FEV_1) is sharply reduced, usually to less than50% of FVC. The maximum midexpiratory flow rate and maximal breathing capacity are sharply reduced as well. Residual volume is markedly increased, while expiratory reserve volume is moderately decreased. Therefore, functional residual capacity and total lung capacity are increased.

Fauci AS, Braunwald E, Isselbacher KJ et al (eds): Harrison's Principles of Internal Medicine, 14th ed, p 1422. New York, McGraw-Hill, 1998

Gold MI, Han YH, Helrich M: Pulmonary mechanics and blood gas tensions during anesthesia in asthmatics. Anesthesiology 27:216, 1966

Kingston HGG, Hirshman CA: Perioperative management of the patient with asthma. Anesth Analg 63:844, 1984

B. Preoperative Evaluation and Preparation

B.1. What preoperative workup would you order?

In addition to routine tests such as complete blood count, serum electrolytes, urinalysis, ECG, and coagulation screening, special attention should be paid to cardiopulmonary function, chest x-ray film, pulmonary function tests, including response to bronchodilator, and baseline arterial blood gases. A history of allergy and symptoms and signs of cardiac or respiratory failure must be checked carefully.

B.2. Would you order any special preoperative preparations for asthmatic patients with chronic obstructive lung disease?

Yes. The preoperative preparation should include the following:

- Eradication of acute and chronic infection with appropriate antibiotics.
- Relief of bronchial spasm with a bronchodilator.
- Chest physiotherapy to improve sputum clearance and bronchial drainage.
- Reversal of uncompensated or borderline *cor pulmonale* with diuretics, digitalis, improved oxygenation, and correction of acidemia by more efficient ventilation.
- Correction of dehydration and electrolyte imbalance.
- Familiarization with respiratory therapy equipment likely to be used in the postoperative period.
- Cessation of smoking, if possible for 2 months, to improve mucociliary clearance and decrease sputum production.
- Abstinence from smoking for at least 12 hours to reduce carboxyhemoglobin levels, resulting in improvement of blood oxygen content and increasing the release of oxygen in hemoglobin.
- Continuation of prophylactic cromolyn inhalation up to the time of surgery to prevent the degranulation of mast cells and the subsequent release of chemical mediators responsible for bronchoconstriction.
- Initiation of a tapered steroid therapy in the week prior to surgery for patients with ongoing wheezing and scheduled elective surgery.

Barash PG, Cullen BF, Stoelting RK (eds): Clinical Anesthesia, 3rd ed, p 765. Philadelphia, Lippincott-Raven, 1997

Bishop MJ: Bronchospasm, avoiding an anesthetic disaster. ASA Refresher Courses in Anesthesiology 19:15–27, 1991

Heironimus TW III: The anesthetic management of the pulmonary cripple. ASA Refresher Courses in Anesthesiology 3:92–93, 1975

Hirshman CA: Anesthesia and bronchospastic disease. ASA Refresher Courses in Anesthesiology 13:89, 1985

Marsh HM: Anesthesia for patients with chronic pulmonary disease. ASA Refresher Courses in Anesthesiology 12:133, 1984

B.3. How long would you postpone elective surgery if the patient had a recent upper respiratory infection (URI)?

Respiratory infections are the most common stimuli that evoke acute exacerbations of asthma. The airway responsiveness of even normal subjects to nonspecific stimuli is transiently increased after a viral infection. Increased airway responsiveness can last from 2 to 8 weeks after the infection in both normals and asthmatics. Recently Cohen and Cameron reported that if a child had a URI and had endotracheal anesthesia, the risk of a respiratory complication increased 11-fold. In addition, Tait and Knight found that laryngospasm and bronchospasm were significantly increased even in normal children 2 weeks after a URI. Therefore, it has been recommended to wait 2 to 3 weeks after clinical recovery from a URI in asthmatics even if clinical symptoms are not present.

Bishop MJ: Bronchospasm, avoiding an anesthetic disaster. ASA Refresher Courses in Anesthesiology 19:15–27, 1991

Cohen MM, Cameron CB: Should you cancel the operation when a child has an upper respiratory infection? Anesth Analg 72:282–288, 1991

Fauci AS, Braunwald E, Isselbacher KJ et al (eds): Harrison's Principles of Internal Medicine, 14th ed, p 1422. New York, McGraw-Hill, 1998

Tait AR, Knight PR: Intraoperative respiratory complications in patients with upper respiratory tract infections. Can J Anaesth 34:300–303, 1987

B.4. What medicines would you expect the patient to have taken in the past or be taking at the present time?

The asthmatic patient might take bronchodilators such as methylxanthines and sympathomimetics. Special attention is required if the patient has taken systemic glucocorticoids. Recently, aerosol therapy has become quite popular because it provides optimal local therapeutic effects and minimizes the systemic side-effects. A variety of relatively selective beta-2 agonists (albuterol, fenoterol, terbutaline, and bitolterol), anticholinergic bronchodilators (ipratropium bromide and methylatropine nitrate), mast cell stabilizer (cromolyn), and various steroids are now available as aerosols and are frequently able to control most chronic asthma.

Fauci AS, Braunwald E, Isselbacher KJ et al (eds): Harrison's Principles of Internal Medicine, 14th ed, pp 1423–1425. New York, McGraw-Hill, 1998

Newhouse MT, Dolovich MB, Eng P: Control of asthma by aerosols. N Engl J Med 315:870, 1986

Rakel RE (ed): Saunders Manual of Medical Practice, pp 117–119. Philadelphia, WB Saunders, 1996

B.5. Would you order preoperative steroid preparation? Why?

It is recommended that preoperative glucocorticoid replacement therapy be given to all patients with known or suspected adrenal insufficiency. Patients who have been treated with high-dose glucocorticoids within the previous year should also be assumed to have an unknown element of adrenocortical suppression that should be treated with full replacement therapy. The human adrenal glands normally secrete approximately 30 mg of hydrocortisone (cortisol) per day under baseline conditions; however, under stress up to 200 to 500 mg a day may be secreted. It is reasonable to replace 300 mg of hydrocortisone per day during perioperative periods. The night before surgery, 100 mg of hydrocortisone acetate may be given intramuscularly. In addition, a 100-mg dose of hydrocortisone phosphate is given intravenously before induction and during operation. Postoperatively, hydrocortisone phosphate, 100 mg IV, is given every 8 hours for 48 hours and then the steroid therapy is tapered. The biologic half-life of hydrocortisone is 8 to 12 hours. If the patient had <1 week of systemic steroid therapy >6 months previously and there are no signs of adrenal insufficiency, routine steroid preparation is not advised. However, intravenous steroid preparations should be available in the operating room in case intractable hypotension from adrenal insufficiency occurs during surgery.

The increasing emphasis on reactive airways as an inflammatory disease has led to greater appreciation of the importance of steroids in controlling the incidence of attacks and in aborting acute attacks. It has been recommended that systemic steroid preparation be used preoperatively in patients with moderate to severe asthma and a history of requiring steroids in the past. One day of high dose steroids should not significantly affect wound healing. In the face of ongoing wheezing and scheduled elective surgery, a steroid course in the week(s) prior to surgery may be useful. The concern that steroids will increase the rate of wound-healing problems or of infection are not well-founded. A recent study of asthmatics treated with steroids preoperatively found no increase in the incidence of wound infections or wound-healing problems.

Bishop MJ: Bronchospasm, avoiding an anesthetic disaster. ASA Refresher Courses in Anesthesiology 19:15–27, 1991

Kabalin CS, Yarnold PR, Grammer LC: Low complication rate of corticosteroid-treated asthmatics undergoing surgical procedures. Arch Intern Med 155:1379–1384, 1995

Katz J, Benumof J, Kadis LB (eds): Anesthesia and Uncommon Diseases, Pathophysiologic and Clinical Correlations, 3rd ed, pp 274–275. Philadelphia, WB Saunders, 1990

Sheffer AL: Expert panel on the management of asthma. J Allergy Clin Immunol 88:425–534, 1991

Vandam LD (ed): To make the patient ready for anesthesia. Medical Care of the Surgical Patient, 2nd ed, p 258. Menlo Park, CA, Addison-Wesley, 1984

B.6. What is the onset of action of intravenous steroid therapy in asthma?

The bronchial effects of intravenous steroids are not immediate and may not be seen for 6 hours or more after the initial administration. When severe bronchospasm is not resolving despite intense optimal bronchodilator therapy, intravenous corticosteroid administration is indicated. A loading dose of hydrocortisone, 4 mg/kg, is given to achieve plasma cortisol levels above 100 μg/dl, followed by 3 mg/kg every 6 hours.

Fauci AS, Braunwald E, Isselbacher KJ et al (eds): Harrison's Principles of Internal Medicine, 14th ed, p 1424. New York, McGraw-Hill, 1998

Parker SD, Brown RH, Darowski MJ, Hirshman CA: Time related decrease in airway reactivity by corticosteroids (abstract). Anesthesiology 71:A1077, 1989

B.7. What are the effects of cimetidine on asthmatic patients?

Cimetidine is an H_2-receptor antagonist. Nathan and associates found that histamine mediates bronchoconstriction through the H_1-receptor (blocked by chlorpheniramine), while bronchodilation is mediated by H_2-receptor agonism (blocked by cimetidine). H_2-receptors are thought to be responsible for inhibitory feedback control of mediator release. Cimetidine may potentiate histamine H_1-receptor bronchoconstrictions. It should be avoided in asthmatic patients. Cimetidine also slows clearing of theophylline by inhibiting microsomal metabolism. Therefore, theophylline dosage should be decreased to avoid toxicity.

Miller RD (ed): Anesthesia, 4th ed, pp 1452–1454. New York, Churchill Livingstone, 1994

Nathan R, Segall N, Schocket A: A comparison of the actions of H_1 and H_2 antihistamines on histamine-induced bronchoconstriction and cutaneous wheal response in asthmatic patients. J Allergy Clin Immunol 67:171, 1981

B.8. How would you premedicate the patient? Why?

There are no good controlled studies of premedication use in asthmatic patients. The asthmatic patient may be premedicated with atropine and diphenhydramine alone or in combination with droperidol. Atropine is an anticholinergic drug. It decreases airway resistance, diminishes secretion-initiated airway reactivity, and probably prevents bronchospasm and bradycardia from vagal reflex following intubation. Diphenhydramine is an H_1-receptor blocking drug. It inhibits histamine-mediated bronchoconstriction and possesses a sedative effect. Droperidol decreases airway resistance by its alpha-adrenergic blockade. The sedative effects of droperidol and diphenhydramine may prevent bronchospasm induced by psychological stress. Hydroxyzine hydrochloride (Vistaril) is a frequently used alternative because of its sedative, antihistaminic, and bronchodilating effects.

Inhaled or systemic steroids may be given to patients with moderate to severe asthma to decrease the incidence of attacks.

Inhaled beta-2 agonists, cromolyn, or steroids should be continued up to the time of surgery.

Aviado DM: Regulation of bronchomotor tone during anesthesia. Anesthesiology 42:68–80, 1975

Bishop MJ: Bronchospasm, avoiding an anesthetic disaster. ASA Refresher Courses in Anesthesiology 19:15–27, 1991

Editorial views: Clinical epilog on bronchomotor tone. Anesthesiology 42:1–3, 1975

Vandam LD (ed): To make the patient ready for anesthesia. Medical Care of the Surgical Patient, 2nd ed, p 258. Menlo Park, CA, Addison-Wesley, 1984

C. Intraoperative Management

C.1. What are the disadvantages of administering atropine to the asthmatic patient?

Some physicians consider atropine relatively contraindicated because it causes drying of secretions, further plugging, and perhaps the initiation of a severe attack of asthma. This assumption has proven to be more theoretical than real in the reasonably well-managed asthmatic patient.

Editorial views: Clinical epilog on bronchomotor tone. Anesthesiology 42:1–3, 1975

Gal TJ: Bronchospasm: Physiological and pharmacological insights. International Anesthesia Research Society Review Course Lectures, pp 1–6, 1991

C.2. If the patient had a severe asthmatic attack in the operating room before the induction of anesthesia, would you put the patient to sleep or postpone the surgery?

First of all, medical treatment should be given to relieve the asthmatic attack. Elective surgery should be postponed and the patient should be reevaluated carefully and better prepared preoperatively. If this is emergency surgery such as acute appendicitis, the operation can be performed after the asthmatic attack is terminated with medical treatment. During surgery the medical treatment should be continued.

C.3. The patient did not have an asthmatic attack in the operating room. How would you induce anesthesia?

The principles of anesthetic management for the asthmatic patient are threefold—to block airway reflexes before laryngoscopy and intubation, to relax airway smooth muscle, and to prevent release of biochemical mediators. Methohexital is used for induction. Then oxygen and a potent inhalation agent, such as halothane, enflurane, or isoflurane, is administered by mask to achieve adequate depth of anesthesia before endotracheal intubation following injection of succinylcholine. Topical endotracheal spray of 80 to 120 mg of lidocaine through LTA kit may be used before intubation to suppress the cough reflex induced by intubation, but the introduction of lidocaine itself may cause cough reflex when the depth of anesthesia is light.

C.4. Why would you use methohexital instead of thiopental?

Hirshman and associates, using human-skin mast cell preparations, demonstrated histamine release by thiopental and thiamylal, but not by methohexital and pentobarbital. Thiopental and thiamylal are thiobarbiturates, while methohexital and pentobarbital are oxybarbiturates. This suggests that the sulfur atom is important in barbiturate-induced histamine release. Moreover, they further found that thiobarbiturates, but not oxybarbiturates, constricted guinea pig tracheas and that this constriction was mediated by thromboxane. Therefore, methohexital may be preferred as the induction agent in patients showing extreme sensitivity to histamine (asthmatics) or increased histamine releasability (atopics). However, thiopental itself does not cause bronchospasm. Because it provides only a light plane of anesthesia, airway instrumentation under thiopental anesthesia alone may trigger bronchospasm. Therefore, clinically, both barbiturates have been used successfully in the asthmatic patient, provided that an adequate depth of anesthesia is achieved before stimulating the airway.

Bishop MJ: Bronchospasm: Successful Management. ASA Annual Refresher Course Lectures no. 272, 1997

Converse JG, Smotrilla MM: Anesthesia and the asthmatic. Anesth Analg 40:336, 1961

Curry C, Lenox WC, Spannhake EW, Hirshman CA: Contractile responses of guinea pig trachea to oxybarbiturates and thiobarbiturates. Anesthesiology 75:679–683, 1991

Editorial views: Anaphylactoid reactions and histamine release by barbiturate induction agents: Clinical relevance and pathomechanisms. Anesthesiology 63:351, 1985

Hirshman CA, Edelstein RA, Ebertz JM et al: Thiobarbiturate-induced histamine release. Anesthesiology 63:353, 1985

C.5. Would you use propofol, etomidate, or ketamine for induction?

Propofol may be the induction agent of choice for the patient with reactive airway who was hemodynamically stable. A recent report found that induction of asthmatics with 2.5 mg/kg of propofol resulted in a significantly lower incidence of wheezing following tracheal intubation when compared with induction with 5 mg/kg thiopental or thiamylal, or 1.75 mg/kg methohexital. The incidence of wheezing was none (0/17), 45% (23/67), and 26% in patients who received propofol, a thiobarbiturate, and oxybarbituate, respectively. Another study found that in unselected patients, propofol resulted in a significantly lower respiratory resistance following tracheal intubation than did induction with thiopental or etomidate.

Etomidate does not depress myocardial function. Therefore, it provides hemodynamic stability in critically ill patients. Although it was advertised as an ideal agent for asthmatic patients, there has been little evidence to support the claim except that etomidate does not release histamine. A recent study suggests that neither etomidate nor thiopental prevents wheezing following intubation, as opposed to the marked protection afforded by propofol.

Ketamine produces bronchodilation both directly and via release of catecholamines. In an actively wheezing patient, it is the induction agent of choice, especially when hemodynamics are unstable.

Bishop MJ: Bronchospasm: Successful Management. ASA Annual Refresher Course Lectures no. 272, 1997

Eames WO, Rooke GA, Wu RS, Bishop MJ: Comparison of the effects of etomidate, propofol, and thiopental on respiratory resistance following tracheal intubation. Anesthesiology 84:1307–1311, 1996

Pizov R, Brown RH, Weis YS et al: Wheezing during induction of general anesthsia in patients with and without asthma. A randomized, blind trial. Anesthesiology 82:1111–1116, 1995

C.6. Would you use lidocaine for intubation?

Intravenous lidocaine, 1 mg/kg, may be given 1 to 2 minutes before intubation to prevent reflex-induced bronchospasm. Topical endotracheal spray of lidocaine has to be used cautiously because it may provoke reflex bronchoconstriction if adequate depth of anesthesia has not been achieved. Lidocaine infusion, 1 to 2 mg/kg/h, may be used in cardiac or elderly COPD patients whose airways need more anesthesia than their cardiovascular system can tolerate.

Hirshman CA: Anesthesia and bronchospastic disease. ASA Refresher Courses in Anesthesiology 13:81–95, 1985

McAlpine LG, Thomson NC: Lidocaine-induced bronchoconstriction in asthmatic patients. Relation to histamine airway responsiveness and effect of preservative. Chest 96:1012–1015, 1989

C.7. If this is emergency surgery and rapid-sequence induction is indicated, how would you induce anesthesia in this patient?

All the precautions to prevent aspiration of gastric contents and asthmatic attack have to be considered simultaneously. Rapid-sequence induction and tracheal intubation using propofol, thiopental or methohexital, and succinylcholine are necessary to prevent aspiration, but light anesthesia may precipitate severe bronchospasm.

Ketamine, 2 mg/kg, may be the induction agent of choice in noncardiac asthmatic patients, because ketamine increases catecholamine release with resultant bronchodilation.

In asthmatic patients who have ischemic heart disease, we give a moderate dose of fentanyl (5 µg/kg) 2 to 3 minutes before the administration of methohexital (1.5

mg/kg) to suppress airway reflexes and prevent tachycardia and hypertension caused by intubation.

Intravenous lidocaine (1 to 2 mg/kg), given immediately before the administration of ketamine or fentanyl and succinylcholine, is a useful adjunct drug to prevent reflex bronchospasm, especially in an emergency situation when deep anesthesia cannot be achieved before intubation.

A full stomach should be emptied by a functioning nasogastric tube. The patient should be denitrogenated with 100% oxygen by mask. Pancuronium or vecuronium, 1 mg, should be given 3 minutes before administration of succinylcholine.

If the patient has a wheezing attack before anesthesia, a loading dose of aminophylline may be given to relieve bronchospasm, followed by a continuous intravenous infusion of aminophylline. Inhalation of sympathomimetics such as albuterol may be used as the first-line therapy for acute asthmatic attack.

Bishop MJ: Bronchospasm, avoiding an anesthetic disaster. ASA Refresher Courses in Anesthesiology 19:15–27, 1991

Gal TJ: Bronchospasm: Physiological and pharmacological insights. International Anesthesia Research Society Review Course Lectures, pp 1–6, 1991

Kingston HGG, Hirshman CA: Perioperative management of the patient with asthma. Anesth Analg 63:844, 1984

Martin DE, Rosenberg H, Aukburg SJ et al: Low-dose fentanyl blunts circulatory responses to tracheal intubation. Anesth Analg 61:680, 1982

C.8. What is your choice of agents for maintenance of anesthesia? Why?

We use inhalational agents such as halothane, enflurane, and isoflurane with nitrous oxide and oxygen. Halothane, enflurane, and isoflurane are potent direct bronchodilators. They are more efficacious in reducing bronchomotor tone than are diethyl ether, ketamine, and flaxene, all of which produce a release of adrenal medullary catecholamines that is not totally dose dependent. Enflurane and isoflurane are preferable to halothane, because halothane sensitizes the myocardium to arrhythmic effects of circulating catecholamines more than enflurane and isoflurane. However, some authorities prefer halothane and sevoflurane to isoflurane and desflurane because the latter anesthetics have a pungent odor that can cause airway irritation. The inhaled anesthetics inhibit chemically induced tracheal contractions in the order halothane>enflurane≥isoflurane>sevoflurane.

Barash PG, Cullen BF, Stoelting RK (eds): Clinical Anesthesia, 3rd ed, p 367. Philadelphia, Lippincott-Raven, 1997

Editorial views: Clinical epilog on bronchomotor tone. Anesthesiology 42:1–3, 1975

Gal TJ: Bronchospasm: Physiological and pharmacological insights. International Anesthesia Research Society Review Course Lectures, pp 1–6, 1991

Hirschman CA: Anesthesia and bronchospastic disease. ASA Refresher Courses in Anesthesiology 13:81, 1985

Yamakage M, Kohro S, Kawamata T et al: Inhibitory effects of four inhaled anesthetics in canine tracheal smooth muscle contraction and intracellular Ca^{2+} concentration. Anesth Analg 77:67, 1993

C.9. What are the mechanisms of halothane that produce bronchodilation?

The major component of bronchodilation elicited by halothane is mediated through beta-adrenergic receptor stimulation, which is decreased by beta-blocking agents. The beta-agonistic effect works through two intracellular mechanisms. The first mechanism is direct relaxation of bronchial musculature mediated by an increase in intracellular cyclic 3,5-adenosine monophosphate (cAMP). Increased cAMP may bind free calcium within bronchial myoplasm and thus promote relaxation by a negative-feedback mechanism. The second mechanism may arise from the first, inasmuch as elevated levels of cAMP seem to impede antigen-antibody mediated enzyme production and release of histamine from leukocytes. However, a recent study by Hirshman and associates suggests that the mechanism of action involves the depression of airway reflexes as well as direct effects on airway smooth muscle.

Aviado DM: Regulation of bronchomotor tone during anesthesia. Anesthesiology 42:68–80, 1975

Editorial views: Clinical epilog on bronchomotor tone. Anesthesiology 42:1–3, 1975

Hirshman CA, Edelstein G, Peetz S et al: Mechanism of action of inhalational anesthesia on airways. Anesthesiology 56:107, 1982

C.10. Why would you choose an inhalational instead of an intravenous technique?

First, inhalational agents such as halothane, enflurane, and isoflurane have dose-related direct bronchodilator effect. Ketamine has an indirect bronchodilator effect, which is not dose related and not predictable. Large doses of morphine produce bronchoconstriction because morphine increases central vagal tone and releases histamine. Droperidol has an alpha-blocking effect that may relieve bronchospasm induced by alpha stimulation. Meperidine was shown to have a spasmolytic effect in asthmatic patients, but not in experimental dogs. Fentanyl does not have a significant effect on bronchial tone. Second, cholinesterase inhibitors can induce bronchospasm. Inhalational agents potentiate muscle relaxants; therefore, lower doses of relaxants are needed for surgery. The use of cholinesterase inhibitors to reverse the effect of muscle relaxants may be avoided or decreased.

Aviado DM: Regulation of bronchomotor tone during anesthesia. Anesthesiology 42:68–80, 1975

Bishop MJ: Bronchospasm: Successful Management. ASA Annual Refresher Course Lectures no. 272, 1997

Editorial views: Clinical epilog on bronchomotor tone. Anesthesiology 42:1–3, 1975

Gal TJ: Bronchospasm: Physiological and pharmacological insights. International Anesthesia Research Society Review Course Lectures, pp 1–6, 1991

Kingston HGG, Hirshman CA: Perioperative management of the patient with asthma. Anesth Analg 63:844, 1984

C.11. Is regional anesthesia better than general anesthesia in this situation?

This issue is controversial. The use of regional anesthesia avoids the possibility of bronchospasm that may be induced by endotracheal tube stimulation. However, respiratory complications were reported to be quite common (83%) in patients undergoing intraperitoneal surgery who had relatively high spinal anesthesia (T6–T4). Low spinal, epidural, and caudal anesthesia for surgery of the perineum, lower extremities, and pelvic extraperitoneal organs resulted in fewer respiratory complications than did general anesthesia. A study of patients with asthma demonstrated no differences between those anesthetized with high epidurals (T2–T4) and those undergoing general anesthesia with ketamine and isoflurane.

Endotracheal general anesthesia is advantageous because it provides a controlled airway to deliver the desirable oxygen concentration, but the endotracheal tube may also induce bronchospasm during light anesthesia.

Bishop MJ: Bronchospasm: Successful Management. ASA Annual Refresher Course Lectures no. 272, 1997

Gold MI, Helrich M: A study of the complications related to anesthesia in asthmatic patients. Anesth Analg 42:283–293, 1963

Ramanathan J, Osborne B, Sibai B: Epidural anesthesia in asthmatic patients. Anesth Analg 70: S317–318, 1990

C.12. *Which muscle relaxants would you use? Why?*

Muscle relaxants that cause histamine release should be avoided (Table 1-2). Pancuronium, rocuronium, cisatracurium, and vecuronium are the preferred relaxants because the histamine released is insignificant. Vecuronium, rocuronium, and cisatracurium may be better choices of relaxant because of their intermediate action durations, allowing early recovery without reversal with an anticholinesterase, which may precipitate bronchospasm. D-tubocurarine can cause bronchospasm by histamine release. Metocurine and succinylcholine also cause histamine release, but to a lesser extent. Gallamine has minimal histamine release, but has been reported to cause bronchospasm in patients. Atracurium, mivacurium, and doxacurium in high doses increase histamine release. Therefore, they are not the relaxants of choice.

Basta SJ: Modulation of histamine release by neuromuscular blocking drugs. Curr Opin Anesth 5:572, 1992

Caldwell JE, Lau M, Fisher DM: Atracurium versus vecuronium in asthmatic patients. A blinded, randomized comparison of adverse events. Anesthesiology 83:985–991, 1995

Mehr EH, Hirshman CA, Lindeman KS: Mechanism of action of atracurium on airways. Anesthesiology 76:448–454, 1992

Miller RD (ed): Anesthesia, 4th ed, pp 441–444. New York, Churchill Livingstone, 1994

Table 1-2. Histamine Release from Nondepolarizing Muscle Relaxants

MUSCLE RELAXANT	HISTAMINE RELEASE[a]
Benzylisoquinolinium compounds	
d-Tubocurarine	0.6
Metocurine	2.0
Doxacurium	>4.0
Mivacurium	3.0
Atracurium	2.5
Cisatracurium	None
Steroidal Compounds	
Pancuronium	None
Vecuronium	None
Pipecuronium	None
Rocuronium	None
Others	
Alcuronium	None
Gallamine	None

[a] Definition: number of multiples of the ED_{95} for neuromuscular blockade required to produce histamine release.

C.13. In the middle of surgery, the patient developed a severe wheezing attack. How do you manage it?

First, deepen the level of anesthesia and increase F_IO_2. Remember that the patient is under anesthesia and surgery. Therefore, medical intervention, such as aminophylline administration, is not the first choice of treatment. The most common cause of asthmatic attack during surgery is inadequate anesthesia. The asthmatic patient has an extremely sensitive tracheobronchial tree. When the level of anesthesia is too light, he may develop bucking, straining, or coughing due to the foreign body (endotracheal tube) in his trachea, and go on to bronchospasm. First of all, the blood pressure is taken to make sure it is normal or high. Then anesthesia is deepened by increasing the concentration of inhalational agents, such as halothane, enflurane, or isoflurane, which are direct bronchodilators as well. An incremental dose of ketamine may be a quick way of maintaining blood pressure, rapidly deepening anesthesia, achieving bronchodilation, and avoiding the problem of delivering an inhaled anesthetic to a patient with poor ventilation. At the same time, oxygenation can be improved by increasing the oxygen concentration and decreasing the nitrous oxide. The patient should be continuously ventilated with a volume-cycled ventilator.

Second, relieve mechanical stimulation. Pass a catheter through the endotracheal tube to suction secretions and to determine whether there is any obstruction or kinking of the tube. The cuff of the endotracheal tube can be deflated, the tube moved back 1 to 2 cm, and the cuff reinflated. Occasionally the endotracheal tube slips down and stimulates the carina of the trachea, causing severe bronchospasm during light anesthesia. Surgical stimulation, such as traction on the mesentery, intestine, or stomach, should be stopped temporarily, since it causes vagal reflex and can cause bronchospasm.

Third, medical intervention is necessary if the above treatment cannot break the bronchospasm or anesthesia cannot be increased because of hypotension. The cornerstone of the treatment of the intraoperative bronchospasm is inhalation of beta-2 agonists such as albuterol, which induce further bronchodilation even in the presence of adequate inhalational anesthesia. Beta-2 agonists produce more rapid and effective bronchodilation than intravenous aminophylline. However, recommended therapy has also included intravenous aminophylline. When severe bronchospasm is not resolving despite intense optimal bronchodilation therapy, intravenous corticosteroid is indicated (see question B.5.).

Fourth, bring in an ICU ventilator. Anesthesia ventilators are not designed for patients with high airway resistance. It is impossible to deliver adequate alveolar ventilation because the anesthesia circuit has too much compressible volume (tubing compliance) and the anesthesia ventilator does not have enough driving power. An ICU ventilator can generate inspiratory pressures as high as 120 cm H_2O. With low tubing compliance, little ventilation is wasted into the circuit. High inspiratory flow rate allows for shorter inspiratory time with adequate time for expiration and lower auto-PEEP. The major disadvantage of an ICU ventilator is its inability to use inhalation anesthetics. However, the Siemens 900D anesthesia machine incorporates an ICU-type ventilator with vaporizers and oxygen mixers. It may be ideal for this situation.

Barnes PJ: A new approach to the treatment of asthma. N Engl J Med 321:1517–1527, 1989

Bishop MJ: Bronchospasm, avoiding an anesthetic disaster. ASA Refresher Courses in Anesthesiology 19:15–27, 1991

Bishop MJ: Bronchospasm: Successful Management. ASA Annual Refresher Course Lectures no. 272, 1997

Gal TJ: Bronchospasm: Physiological and pharmacological insights. International Anesthesia Research Society Review Course Lectures, pp 1–6, 1991

Tobias JD, Hirshman CA: Attenuation of histamine-induced airway constriction by albuterol during halothane anesthesia. Anesthesiology 72:105–110, 1990

C.14. How would you give beta-2 agonists? What problems may arise when isoproterenol is given during halothane anesthesia? What is its mechanism of action on asthma?

In the past it was fashionable to treat episodes of severe asthma with intravenous sympathomimetics such as isoproterenol. This approach no longer appears justifiable. Isoproterenol infusions can induce ventricular arrhythmias during halothane anesthesia. In addition, isoproterenol infusion can clearly cause myocardial damage, and even the beta-2 selective agents such as terbutaline and albuterol when given intravenously offer no advantages over the inhaled route.

Beta-2 agonists such as albuterol, terbutaline, fenoterol, and pirbuterol may be administered via metered dose inhaler (MDI) adapters or small-volume jet nebulizers to the anesthetic circuit. Because MDI adapters are not very efficient in the intubated patient, more than two puffs are needed to break acute bronchospasms.

Adrenergic stimulants produce bronchodilation through action on beta-adrenergic receptors. Beta-agonists increase intracellular cAMP by activating adenyl cyclase, which produces cAMP from adenosine triphosphate (ATP). Increased cAMP promotes bronchial relaxation and inhibits the release of mediators from mast cells (see Fig. 1-4).

Barnes PJ: A new approach to the treatment of asthma. N Engl J Med 321:1517–1527, 1989

Bishop MJ: Bronchospasm, avoiding an anesthetic disaster. ASA Refresher Courses in Anesthesiology 19:15–27, 1991

Fauci AS, Braunwald E, Isselbacher KJ et al (eds): Harrison's Principles of Internal Medicine, 14th ed, pp 1423–1424. New York, McGraw-Hill, 1998

Gal TJ: Bronchospasm: Physiological and pharmacological insights. International Anesthesia Research Society Review Course Lectures, pp 1–6, 1991

C.15. How would you administer aminophylline? How does aminophylline relieve bronchospasm? What is the mechanism of action? What are the therapeutic blood levels of aminophylline? What are the toxic effects of aminophylline?

The usual intravenous loading dose is 6.0 mg/kg given slowly, followed by a continuous infusion of 1.0 mg/kg/h for smokers, 0.5 mg/kg/h for nonsmokers, and 0.3 mg/kg/h for severely ill patients, such as those with congestive heart failure, pneumonia, and liver disease. Maintenance doses must also be reduced to 0.3 mg/kg/h for patients taking cimetidine, which interferes with hepatic microsomal enzymes.

It was formerly thought that aminophylline increases intracellular cyclic AMP (cAMP) through inhibition of the enzyme phosphodiesterase (PDE), which inactivates cyclic AMP (Fig. 1-6). However, the available evidence does not support this concept. The therapeutic plasma levels of aminophylline range from 10 to 20 µg/ml. The common side-effects of aminophylline include nervousness, nausea, vomiting, anorexia, and headache; cardiac arrhythmias and seizures occur with high plasma levels.

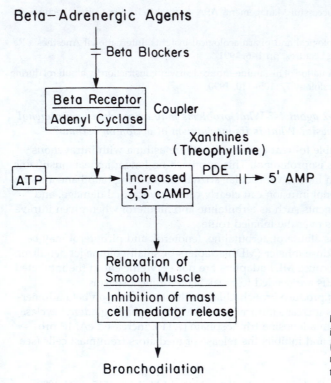

Beta–Adrenergic Agents

Figure 1-6. Cyclic AMP pathways involved in bronchdilator action. (Hirshman C: Airway reactivity in humans: Anesthetic implications. Anesthesiology 58:170, 1983)

The use of aminophylline in the therapy of bronchospasm appears to be declining because of its narrow therapeutic-toxic window and its relatively weak bronchodilating effect. In addition, aminophylline does not add to the bronchodilating efficacy of inhaled halothane.

Fauci AS, Braunwald E, Isselbacher KJ et al (eds): Harrison's Principles of Internal Medicine, 14th ed, p 1424. New York, McGraw-Hill, 1998

Hirshman CA: Airway reactivity in humans: Anesthetic implications. Anesthesiology 58:170, 1983

Tobias JD, Kubos KL, Hirshman CA: Aminophylline does not attenuate histamine-induced airway constriction during halothane anesthesia. Anesthesiology 71:723–729, 1989

C.16. If the patient does not respond to the above treatment and becomes cyanotic, what would you do?

The values of arterial blood gases should be determined immediately. In a severe, prolonged asthmatic attack, there will be combined respiratory and metabolic acidosis due to CO_2 retention and lactic acidosis from tissue hypoxia. $NaHCO_3$ should be given to correct the acidosis, because aminophylline and beta-agonists are not effective in severe acidosis. At the same time, bronchodilator therapy should be continued or increased. Consultation with senior staff or physician in pulmonary medicine may be necessary.

Kampschulte S, March J, Safar P: Simplified physiologic management of status asthmaticus in children. Crit Care Med 1:69–74, 1973

C.17. What are the differential diagnoses of intraoperative bronchospasm?

The causes of wheezing and increased airway pressure include the following:
- Kinked endotracheal tube
- Solidified secretions or blood
- Pulmonary edema
- Tension pneumothorax
- Aspiration pneumonitis
- Pulmonary embolism
- Endobronchial intubation
- Persistent coughing and straining
- Negative pressure expiration

Bishop MJ: Bronchospasm, avoiding an anesthetic disaster. ASA Refresher Courses in Anesthesiology 19:15–27, 1991

Gal TJ: Bronchospasm: Physiological and pharmacological insights. International Anesthesia Research Society Review Course Lectures, pp 1–6, 1991

C.18. The asthmatic attack was finally relieved and the operation was completed. The patient was found to be hypoventilating. What are the common causes of hypoventilation? Would you like to reverse the muscle relaxant?

The following are common causes of apnea or hypoventilation at the end of surgery:
- Respiratory center depression by inhalational anesthetics, narcotics, or hyperventilation
- Peripheral blockade by muscle relaxants

Since the patient is a severe asthmatic, it is better to avoid the use of an anticholinesterase, such as neostigmine, to reverse a nondepolarizing relaxant. Neostigmine may trigger bronchospasm by a cholinergic mechanism. Although atropine given simultaneously with neostigmine may prevent bronchospasm, the action duration of neostigmine is longer than that of atropine. If reversal is required, it appears prudent to administer larger than customary doses of glycopyrolate (more than0.5 mg) or atropine (more than1.0 mg) to minimize the possibility of bronchospasm. It is advisable to use inhalation agents to potentiate relaxants and to use smaller amounts of relaxants for surgery. If spontaneous respiration is not adequate, artificial ventilation should be continued.

Editorial views: Clinical epilog on bronchomotor tone. Anesthesiology 42:1–3, 1975

Gal TJ: Bronchospasm: Physiological and pharmacological insights. International Anesthesia Research Society Review Course Lectures, pp 1–6, 1991

D. Postoperative Management

D.1. Would you extubate the asthmatic patient while he was deeply anesthestized?

In order to avoid bronchospasm triggered by coughing and bucking due to laryngeal and pharyngeal reflexes during emergence and extubation, patients may be extubated at surgical (deep) levels of anesthesia. However, the risks of aspiration, airway

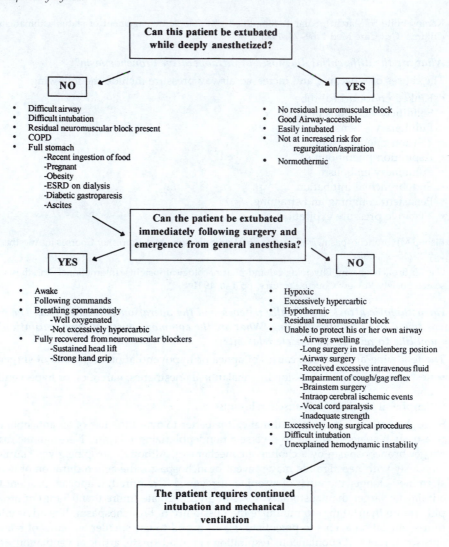

Figure 1-7.   A systemic approach to emergence and extubation.

obstruction, and hypoventilation should be weighed against its benefits. With a history of severe COPD, chronic hypoxemia, and CO_2 retention, the patient was not a good candidate for extubation while deeply anesthetized. A systematic approach for emergence and extubation is illustrated in Fig 1-7. However, the guidelines do not include all possible patient/surgical/anesthetic conditions. Certainly the practitioner's clinical judgment is of utmost importance in the decision as to whether or not to extubate the patient.

Lien CA, Koff H, Malhotra V, Gadalla F: Emergence and extubation: A systemic approach. Anesth Analg 85:1177, 1997

Miller KH, Harkin CP, Bailey PL: Postoperative tracheal extubation. Anesth Analg 80:148–172, 1995

D.2. When the patient cannot be extubated early in the recovery room, how would you keep the endotracheal tube in place without causing bronchoconstriction?

Loading doses of lidocaine or aminophylline followed by continuous infusion, as described in the answers to questions C.6. and C.15., may be administered intravenously to prevent bronchoconstriction induced by stimulation of the endotracheal tube.

D.3. In asthmatic patients, are narcotics contraindicated for postoperative pain control?

Narcotics should be used very carefully because prolonged respiratory depression may further compromise the airway. Morphine is avoided because of possible histamine release and increased central vagal tone, which may cause bronchospasm. Meperidine may be a better choice for postoperative analgesia because of its spasmolytic action. Narcotics should be titrated carefully to control pain and not depress respiration. Poor pain control may compromise respiration because of splinting of the thoracic cage and decreased ability to cough. Paravertebral or intercostal nerve blocks, epidural analgesia, or transcutaneous electrical nerve stimulation (TENS) may be used to control postoperative pain without depressing respiration.

Aviado DM: Regulation of bronchomotor tone during anesthesia. Anesthesiology 42:77, 1975

Marsh HM: Anesthesia for patients with chronic pulmonary disease. ASA Refresher Courses in Anesthesiology 12:133, 1984

D.4. The patient was breathing well and was extubated. How much oxygen would you give to this asthmatic patient with COPD in the recovery room?

Forty percent oxygen by mask is usually used postoperatively in the recovery room. However, for patients with COPD the hypoxic drive might be taken away by increased F_IO_2. It is important to watch the patient's respiration very carefully during oxygen therapy. Venturi masks with F_IO_2 of 0.24 to 0.4 may be used for patients with COPD. It should be emphasized that high oxygen concentration should be used in the presence of hypoxemia. Hypoventilation can be assisted or controlled by artificial ventilation.

Heironimus TW III: The anesthesic management of the pulmonary cripple. ASA Refresher Courses in Anesthesiology 3:97, 1975

Shapiro BA, Kacmarek RM, Cane RD et al (eds): Clinical Application of Respiratory Care, 4th ed, p 421. St. Louis, Mosby-Year Book, 1991

2 Bronchoscopy and Thoracotomy

Fun-Sun F. Yao

A 60-year-old man has suffered from cough, hemoptysis, and weight loss for 2 months. He has smoked one pack of cigarettes per day for 40 years. Chest x-ray film showed left lower lobe infiltrate. The infiltrate did not respond to antibiotic therapy. He was scheduled for fiberoptic bronchoscopy and thoracotomy for possible lobectomy or pneumonectomy.

A. Medical Disease and Differential Diagnosis

1. What is your tentative diagnosis?
2. How many types of bronchogenic carcinoma are there?
3. What are the uncommon metabolic manifestations of bronchogenic carcinoma?
4. How would you diagnose bronchogenic carcinoma?
5. The patient has a long history of cigarette smoking. What does this mean to you?

B. Preoperative Evaluation and Preparation

1. How would you evaluate the patient preoperatively?
2. What are the pulmonary function guidelines that indicate high risk of morbidity and mortality in major general surgery?
3. How do you know the patient can tolerate lobectomy or pneumonectomy?
4. How would you premedicate the patient? Why?

C. Intraoperative Management

1. How would you monitor the patient?
2. What kind of anesthesia would you give for fiberoptic bronchoscopy?
3. How many types of bronchoscopes are there?
4. Are there other anesthetic techniques for bronchoscopy?
5. After bronchoscopy, the surgeon decided to perform a thoracotomy. How would you maintain the anesthesia?
6. Why was the muscle jumping during electrocautery and cutting even after a paralyzing dose of *d*-tubocurarine was given? How would you prevent muscle twitching during electrocautery?
7. The patient was put in the lateral decubitus position for thoracotomy. Describe the circulatory and respiratory effects of the lateral position in the anesthetized and paralyzed patient.
8. Would you control respiration or let the patient breathe spontaneously? Why?
9. Would you consider one-lung anesthesia for left lower lobectomy? Why?
10. What are the indications for one-lung anesthesia?
11. How could you achieve one-lung anesthesia if it is indicated?
12. Could you use double-lumen endotracheal tubes in pediatric patients?
13. What are the contraindications to the use of double-lumen endotracheal tubes?

30

14. Would you use a right- or left-sided double-lumen tube?
15. How do you know that the tube is in the proper position?
16. How do you identify the right and the left mainstem bronchi during fiberoptic bronchoscopy?
17. How many types of bronchial blockers are available? What are the advantages and disadvantages of bronchial blockers?
18. What are the advantages of the Univent bronchial blocker tube?
19. What are the limitations to the use of the Univent bronchial blocker tube and solutions to the limitations?
20. How would you monitor arterial oxygenation continuously during one-lung anesthesia? What is the mechanism of oximetry?
21. What is hypoxic pulmonary vasoconstriction (HPV)?
22. What are the effects of anesthetics on hypoxic pulmonary vasoconstriction (HPV) and their clinical implications?
23. Describe the blood flow distribution during two-lung ventilation in the upright, supine, and lateral decubitus positions.
24. Discuss pulmonary blood flow distribution, shunt flow, and PaO_2 ($F_IO_2 = 1.0$) during one-lung ventilation.
25. During one-lung anesthesia, the following arterial blood gases were noted: pH, 7.10; Pco_2, 86 mm Hg; Po_2, 90 mm Hg; CO_2, 24 mEq/liter. What would you do?
26. How could you improve oxygenation during one-lung anesthesia?
27. Are there any advantages or disadvantages of high-frequency positive pressure ventilation (HFPPV) for thoracotomy?
28. Left lower lobectomy was performed. Would you extubate the patient or leave the patient on the respirator at the end of the procedure?

D. Postoperative Management

1. What are the immediate life-threatening complications that follow lobectomy or pneumonectomy?
2. How would you prevent postoperative atelectasis? Would you order intermittent positive pressure breathing (IPPB) or incentive spirometry?
3. Why is it important to control postoperative pain? How would you control it?
4. Discuss the alternative methods of postoperative pain control.

A. Medical Disease and Differential Diagnosis

A.1. What is your tentative diagnosis?

Any pulmonary infiltrate not responding to antibiotic therapy should suggest carcinoma. The differential diagnosis of atypical pneumonia includes mycoplasmas, mycobacteria, fungi, Q fever, psittacosis, adenovirus, influenzal pneumonia, and pulmonary infarction. Sputum cytology, sputum culture, skin test, and biopsy are necessary to make a definite diagnosis.

Fauci AS, Braunwald E, Isselbacher KJ et al (eds): Harrison's Principles of Internal Medicine, 14th ed, pp 554–555. New York, McGraw-Hill, 1998

Rakel RE (ed): Saunders Manual of Medical Practice, pp 174–175. Philadelphia, WB Saunders, 1996

A.2. How many types of bronchogenic carcinoma are there?

According to the World Health Organization classification, the principal histologic types include the following:

- Epidermoid (squamous) carcinoma
- Small (oat) cell carcinoma (including fusiform, polygonal, lymphocyte-like, and others)
- Adenocarcinoma (including acinar, papillary, and bronchioloalveolar)
- Large cell carcinoma (including solid tumors with and without mucin and giant cell and clear cell tumors)
- Combined epidermoid and adenocarcinomas
- Carcinoid tumors
- Bronchial gland tumors (including cylindromas and mucoepidermoid tumors)
- Papillary tumors of the surface epithelium
- "Mixed" tumors and carcinosarcomas
- Sarcomas
- Unclassified
- Mesotheliomas (including localized and diffuse)
- Melanomas

The first four major cell types make up 95% of all primary lung neoplasma. In general, small cell carcinoma has spread beyond the bounds of resectional surgery at the time of presentation and is primarily managed with chemotherapy with or without radiotherapy. The 5-year survival after curative resection is <1%. In contrast, non-small cell cancers found to be localized at the time of presentation should be considered for a curative attempt with either surgery or radiotherapy. The 5-year survival after surgery is 27% to 37%.

Fauci AS, Braunwald E, Isselbacher KJ et al (eds): Harrison's Principles of Internal Medicine, 14th ed, pp 552–556. New York, McGraw-Hill, 1998

A.3. What are the uncommon metabolic manifestations of bronchogenic carcinoma?

The recognized metabolic manifestations are symptoms that resemble those of myasthenia gravis; peripheral neuritis involving both motor and sensory components; Cushing's syndrome; carcinoid syndrome; hypercalcemia and hypophosphatemia resulting from ectopic parathyroid hormone or PTH-related peptide by epidermoid cancer; hypokalemia due to ectopic secretion of ACTH by small cell cancer; and hyponatremia due to inappropriate excessive secretion of antidiuretic hormone or possibly atrial natriuretic factor by small cell cancer.

Fauci AS, Braunwald E, Isselbacher KJ et al (eds): Harrison's Principles of Internal Medicine, 14th ed, p 555. New York, McGraw-Hill, 1998

A.4. How would you diagnose bronchogenic carcinoma?

The symptoms of nonproductive cough, hemoptysis, and the unresolved lung infiltrate suggest carcinoma. However, some laboratory tests are needed to confirm the diagnosis. They include sputum cytology, bronchoscopy and brush biopsy, biopsy of palpable nodes in the neck or axilla, mediastinoscopy, needle aspiration biopsy, and exploratory thoracotomy biopsy. Prior to thoracotomy, a search should be made for metastases that would contraindicate surgery.

Fauci AS, Braunwald E, Isselbacher KJ et al (eds): Harrison's Principles of Internal Medicine, 14th ed, pp 555–557. New York, McGraw-Hill, 1998

Rakel RE (ed): Saunders Manual of Medical Practice, pp 174–175. Philadelphia, WB Saunders, 1996

A.5. The patient has a long history of cigarette smoking. What does this mean to you?

The patient may develop chronic bronchitis and emphysema from cigarette smoking. He may also develop cor pulmonale and pulmonary hypertension from long-standing pulmonary disorders. Preexisting pulmonary and cardiac disorders increase operative risk and postoperative complications. Heavy smokers have an increased closing volume that may cause postoperative atelectasis.

Miller RD (ed): Anesthesia, 4th ed, pp 900, 957–961. New York, Churchill Livingstone, 1994

Tisi GM: Preoperative evaluation of pulmonary function: Validity, indications, and benefits. Am Rev Respir Dis 119:293, 1979

B. Preoperative Evaluation and Preparation

B.1. How would you evaluate the patient preoperatively?

All preoperative evaluations should include a complete systemic history, physical examination, and laboratory tests. Special attention should be paid to the respiratory and circulatory function in this patient. A history of smoking, cough, sputum production or dyspnea are hallmarks of respiratory disease. Assessment of exercise tolerance, such as climbing stairs, can anticipate the patient's response to the stress of anesthesia and surgery.

A physical examination should include the character of respiration and any signs of right ventricular failure and pulmonary hypertension, such as right ventricular heave, palpable pulmonary artery pulsation, hepatojugular reflux, distended jugular veins, and peripheral edema. Laboratory tests should include the following:

Routine Tests
- ECG, chest x-ray film, complete blood count, prothrombin time, partial thromboplastin time, urinalysis, electrolytes, BUN, creatinine, and blood sugar

Pulmonary Function Tests
- Arterial blood gases
- Spirometry, including forced vital capacity (FVC), forced expiratory volume in the first second (FEV_1), and maximum breathing capacity (MBC)
- Diffusion capacity
- Residual volume and total lung volume
- Xenon scanning
- Pulmonary artery pressure with unilateral balloon occlusion

Benumof JL: Anesthesia for Thoracic Surgery, 2nd ed, pp 152–210. Philadelphia, WB Saunders, 1995

Miller RD (ed): Anesthesia, 4th ed, pp 1664–1670. New York, Churchill Livingstone, 1994

B.2. What are the pulmonary function guidelines that indicate high risk of morbidity and mortality in major general surgery?

Spirometry
- FVC <50% of predicted
- FEV_1 <50% of FVC or 2 liters

- MBC <50% of predicted or 50 liter/minute
- Diffusion capacity <50% of predicted
- Residual volume/total lung volume >50%

Arterial Blood Gases

- Arterial P_{CO_2} > 45 mm Hg
- Arterial P_{O_2} < 50 mm Hg

Pulmonary Vasculature

- Pulmonary artery pressure during unilateral occlusion >30 mm Hg

Benumof JL: Anesthesia for Thoracic Surgery, 2nd ed, pp 188–189. Philadelphia, WB Saunders, 1995

Miller RD (ed): Anesthesia, 4th ed, pp 898–899, 1666–1667. New York, Churchill Livingstone, 1994

Tisi GM: Preoperative evaluation of pulmonary function: Validity, indications, and benefits. Am Rev Respir Dis 119:293, 1979

B.3. How do you know the patient can tolerate lobectomy or pneumonectomy?

The patient should be evaluated carefully, especially his cardiopulmonary status. The above mentioned pulmonary function tests should be performed; of particular importance are differential xenon scanning and unilateral pulmonary artery pressure measurement.

If pulmonary function tests suggest that a patient will be at high risk for major extrathoracic surgery, then he should be considered unsuitable for major thoracic surgery. The minimal pulmonary function test criteria for various-sized pulmonary resections are listed in Table 2-1. If differential xenon scan suggests that the pulmonary resection will remove "useful" lung, the surgical procedure will be less acceptable than it would be if it were designed to remove the "bad part" of the lung. If the scans reveal gross abnormalities throughout the lung fields, then any pulmonary surgery will entail a high risk. If the mean pulmonary artery pressure during unilateral pulmonary artery occlusion exceeds 22 mm Hg, the patient can be considered as being at risk for resection. If the pulmonary artery pressure in the "good" lung rises to above 35 mm Hg on exercise, then the resection is contraindicated.

Benumof JL: Anesthesia for Thoracic Surgery, 2nd ed, pp 178–189. Philadelphia, WB Saunders, 1995

Miller RD (ed): Anesthesia, 4th ed, pp 1666–1667. New York, Churchill Livingstone, 1994

Table 2-1.   Minimal Pulmonary Function Test Criteria for Various-Sized Pulmonary Resections

TEST	UNIT	NORMAL	PNEUMONECTOMY	LOBECTOMY	BIOPSY OR SEGMENTAL
MBC	Liters/minute	>100	>70	40–70	40
MBC	Percentage predicted	100	>55	>40	>35
FEV_1	Liters	>2	>2	>1	>0.6
FEV_1	Percentage predicted	>100	>55	40–50	>40
$FEV_{25-75\%}$	Liters	2	>1.6	>0.6–1.6	>0.6

MBC, maximum breathing capacity; FEV_1, forced expiratory volume in first second; $FEV_{25-75\%}$, forced expiratory volume from 25% to 75% of forced vital capacity.
(Reprinted with permission from Miller RD: Anesthesia, 4th ed, p 1667. New York, Churchill Livingstone, 1994)

B.4. How would you premedicate the patient? Why?

Atropine, 0.4 mg, and pentobarbital, 100 to 150 mg, or diazepam, 10 mg, are given for premedication. Atropine is given to eliminate excessive airway secretions and possibly to prevent bradycardia induced by intubation. Pentobarbital is an intermediate-acting barbiturate sedative to eliminate anxiety. Diazepam, a benzodiazepine, is used for amnesic and anxiolytic effects. It can be given orally 1 hour before surgery. Narcotics or heavy sedation should be avoided because of respiratory depression.

C. Intraoperative Management

C.1. How would you monitor the patient

Circulatory Monitoring
- Electrocardiogram to monitor heart rate, rhythm, and ischemia, using simultaneous leads II and V_5
- Blood pressure cuff
- Arterial line, if frequent determinations of blood gases, one-lung ventilation, or serious cardiac problems are anticipated
- Central venous pressure, to evaluate circulatory volume and cardiac performance
- Swan-Ganz catheter, only when there is documented left ventricular dysfunction, severe pulmonary hypertension, or cor pulmonale
- Intake and output
- Capillary refill

Respiratory Monitoring
- Esophageal stethoscope or precordial stethoscope over the dependent lung
- Inspired oxygen concentration
- End-tidal CO_2
- Arterial blood gases, when indicated
- Airway pressure
- Pulse oximeter

Temperature

Urine Output
- To evaluate circulatory and renal function
Neuromuscular blockade by peripheral nerve stimulator

C.2. What kind of anesthesia would you give for fiberoptic bronchoscopy?

Since bronchoscopy is followed by thoracotomy, I recommend general anesthesia for both procedures. Anesthesia is induced with thiopental sodium, deepened with oxygen and an inhalation agent such as isoflurane, enflurane, or halothane. Endotracheal intubation is facilitated with succinylcholine. Prior to intubation, 2 ml of 4% lidocaine is sprayed to the larynx and tracheobronchial tree by means of the LTA kit to prevent bucking and coughing during intubation and bronchoscopy. Anesthesia is maintained with oxygen and a potent inhalation agent to maintain adequate oxygenation during bronchoscopy. The fiberoptic bronchoscope can be introduced by means of a swivel adapter into the endotracheal tube, and ventilation can be assisted or controlled during bronchoscopy.

C.3. How many types of bronchoscope are there?

There are three types of bronchoscopes in current use: flexible fiberoptic, rigid ventilating, and rigid venturi (Sanders injector).

The fiberoptic bronchoscope is often used in the sedated patient under local anesthesia. This bronchoscope can be used with endotracheal intubation while the patient is under general anesthesia. The patient can be ventilated through a swivel adapter.

The rigid ventilating bronchoscope has a side-arm adapter that can be attached to the anesthesia machine. A variable air leak usually exists around the bronchoscope, so high flow rates of inspired gases are needed.

The rigid venturi-effect bronchoscope relies on an intermittent (10–12/min) high pressure oxygen jet to entrain air and insufflate the lungs with an air-oxygen mixture. The jet is delivered through a reducing valve into a 16- or 18-gauge needle inside and parallel to the lumen of the bronchoscope. The major disadvantage of this bronchoscope is lack of control of the inspired oxygen concentration.

Benumof JL: Anesthesia for Thoracic Surgery, 2nd ed, pp 492–495. Philadelphia, WB Saunders, 1995

Schwartz SI (ed): Principles of Surgery, 6th ed, p 709. New York, McGraw-Hill, 1994

C.4. Are there other anesthetic techniques for bronchoscopy?

There are five anesthetic techniques for bronchoscopy. They can be used separately or in combination.

Local Anesthesia with Intravenous Sedation
Local anesthesia is accomplished by lidocaine spray through a nebulizer with a long nozzle or an LTA kit under direct laryngoscopy, or a bilateral superior laryngeal nerve block, or a transtracheal block. Intravenous sedation is supplemented with 2.5-mg increments of diazepam or 0.5-mg increments of midazolam, until the patient is calm and cooperative but not obtunded and obstructed.

General Anesthesia with an Inhalation Agent, Sevoflurane, Desflurane
Halothane is the agent of choice. Isoflurane and enflurane can also be used smoothly and successfully. Only oxygen and a potent inhalation agent are used to provide a high oxygen concentration. Respiration may be assisted or controlled. Succinylcholine, mivacurium or atracurium drip may be used for muscle relaxation.

Balanced General Anesthesia with Nitrous Oxide, Oxygen, Thiopental Sodium, Narcotics, and Succinylcholine Drip
This technique is useful only for short procedures by experienced surgeons. Hypoxemia may ensue because nitrous oxide decreases the inspired oxygen concentration and alveolar hypoventilation is not unusual during the procedure.

Apneic Oxygenation
Following preoxygenation and induction of anesthesia with thiopental sodium, the patient is paralyzed, and oxygen is insufflated by a small catheter placed above the carina, or through the side arm of a rigid bronchoscope, or through a swivel adapter to the endotracheal tube. The period of apnea should be limited to <5 minutes because carbon dioxide accumulates at a rate of 3 to 6 mm Hg/min, and thus, respiratory acidosis and cardiac arrhythmias may ensue.

General Anesthesia with High Frequency Positive Pressure Ventilation (HFPPV)
A ventilatory frequency of 60/min and a relative insufflation time of 22% of the venti-

latory cycle are used. By using HFPPV and a pneumatic valve principle, it is possible to ventilate the patient safely through an open bronchoscope.

Benumof JL: Anesthesia for Thoracic Surgery, 2nd ed, pp 491–504. Philadelphia, WB Saunders, 1995

Eriksson I, Sjostrand U: Effects of high frequency positive-pressure ventilation (HFPPV) and general anesthesia on intrapulmonary gas distribution in patients undergoing diagnostic bronchoscopy. Anesth Analg 59:585–593, 1980

Kaplan JA (ed): Thoracic Anesthesia, 2nd ed, pp 328–337. New York, Churchill Livingstone, 1991

C.5. After bronchoscopy, the surgeon decided to perform a thoracotomy. How would you maintain the anesthesia?

I would maintain anesthesia with a potent inhalation agent such as isoflurane, enflurane, or halothane. Nitrous oxide may be added to decrease the concentration of a halogenated agent. Oxygen concentration should be kept at 50% or more to minimize the risk of hypoxemia from compression and packing of the nondependent lung. A pulse oximeter is used to monitor arterial oxygenation and adjust inspired oxygen concentration. A nondepolarizing muscle relaxant, such as vecuronium, atracurium, cisatracurium, *d*-tubocurarine, or pancuronium, is given to facilitate surgical exposure.

Boldt J, Müller M, Uphus D et al: Cardiorespiratory changes in patients undergoing pulmonary resection using different anesthetic management techniques. J Cardiothorac Vasc Anesth 10:854–859, 1996

Reid CW, Slinger PD, Lewis S: A comparison of the effects of propofol-alfentanil versus isoflurane anesthesia on arterial oxygenation during one-lung ventilation. J Cardiothorac Vasc Anesth 10:860–863, 1996

C.6. Why was the muscle jumping during electrocautery and cutting even after a paralyzing dose of d-tubocurarine was given? How would you prevent muscle twitching during electrocautery?

D-tubocurarine is a nondepolarizing relaxant that blocks neuromuscular transmission at the neuromuscular junction. It cannot block direct muscle stimulation. Succinylcholine is a depolarizing relaxant that keeps the muscle depolarized and not responding to direct muscle stimulation.

Hardman JG, Limbird LE, Molinoff PB (eds): Goodman and Gilman's The Pharmacological Basis of Therapeutics, 9th ed, pp 182–184. New York, Macmillan, 1996

C.7. The patient was put in the lateral decubitus position for thoracotomy. Describe the circulatory and respiratory effects of the lateral position in the anesthetized and paralyzed patient.

Circulatory Effect
Pooling of blood in the dependent half of the body can result in decreased venous return and a subsequent fall in cardiac output. This effect is intensified by raising the kidney bar or hyperextending the table.

Respiratory Effects
• The lateral position causes mechanical interference with chest movement and, therefore, limitation of lung expansion.

- Mismatching of ventilation and perfusion in the lateral position is another effect. The lower lung is compressed by the mediastinum and abdominal contents. If the patient is awake, the lower diaphragm is able to contract more efficiently during spontaneous respiration and preferential ventilation to the lower lung matches the increased perfusion by gravity. In the patient who is anesthetized, with or without paralysis, most ventilation is preferentially switched from the lower lung to the upper lung. This preferential ventilation of the upper lung, coupled with the greater perfusion of the lower lung, results in an increased degree of mismatching of ventilation and perfusion.

The ventilation/perfusion ratio increases in the upper lung, resulting in an increased physiologic dead space and CO_2 retention. The ventilation/perfusion ratio decreases in the lower lung, resulting in an increased intrapulmonary shunt and hypoxemia. The application of positive end-expiratory pressure to both lungs restores ventilation to the lower lung.

Benumof JL: Anesthesia for Thoracic Surgery, 2nd ed, pp 125–130. Philadelphia, WB Saunders, 1995

Kaplan JA (ed): Thoracic Anesthesia, 2nd ed, pp 197–202. New York, Churchill Livingstone, 1991

Rehder K, Hatch DJ, Sessler AD et al: The function of each lung of anesthetized and paralyzed man during mechanical ventilation. Anesthesiology 37:16, 1972

C.8. Would you control respiration or let the patient breathe spontaneously? Why?

Controlled positive pressure ventilation is the only practical way to provide adequate ventilation during thoracotomy. Spontaneous breathing is usually inadequate because of depressed ventilation from anesthesia and muscle relaxants. Moreover, spontaneous respiration in the open-chest patient with lateral position causes mediastinal shift and paradoxical respiration. During inspiration, negative pressure in the intact lower hemithorax causes the mediastinum to move downward. During expiration, relative positive pressure in the intact lower hemithorax causes the mediastinum to move upward. During inspiration, movement of air into the open hemithorax and movement of gas from the exposed lung into the intact lung cause collapse of the exposed lung. During expiration, the reverse occurs, and the exposed lung expands.

Benumof JL: Anesthesia for Thoracic Surgery, 2nd ed, pp 124–125. Philadelphia, WB Saunders, 1995

Kaplan JA (ed): Thoracic Anesthesia, 2nd ed, pp 203–204. New York, Churchill Livingstone, 1991

Tarhan S, Mofitt EA: Principles of thoracic anesthesia. Surg Clin North Am 53:813, 1973

C.9. Would you consider one-lung anesthesia for left lower lobectomy? Why?

I would consider one-lung anesthesia only if the surgeon requested it. Left lower lobectomy does not routinely require collapse of the lung on the operative side; it can be done easily with regular two-lung anesthesia. However, one-lung anesthesia still significantly aids surgical exposure and eliminates the need for the surgeon to retract, compress, and pack away the operative lung. Although one-lung anesthesia may provide better operating conditions for a surgeon, there are certain disadvantages and complications associated with one-lung anesthesia and the use of double-lumen endotracheal tubes. A large and variable alveolar-to-arterial oxygen pressure difference (P [A-a] O$_2$) is a necessary consequence, because there is continued perfusion to the nondependent, nonventilated lung, creating an increase in transpulmonary shunt.

The increased P (A-a) O$_2$ often results in systemic hypoxemia. Severe hypoxemia and hypercarbia may be caused by incorrect positioning of double-lumen tubes. Other complications include traumatic laryngitis and traumatic tracheobronchial rupture.

Benumof JL: Anesthesia for Thoracic Surgery, 2nd ed, p 331. Philadelphia, WB Saunders, 1995

Miller RD (ed): Anesthesia, 4th ed, pp 1689–1690. New York, Churchill Livingstone, 1994

C.10. What are the indications for one-lung anesthesia?

Absolute Indications
- Isolation from spillage or contamination
  - Infection—bronchiectasis and lung abscess
  - Massive hemorrhage
- To control the distribution of ventilation
  - Bronchopleural fistula
  - Bronchopleural cutaneous fistula
  - Giant unilateral lung cyst or bulla
  - Tracheobronchial tree disruption
  - Surgical opening of major conducting airway
  - Life-threatening hypoxemia due to unilateral lung disease
  - Unilateral bronchopulmonary lavage
  - Pulmonary alveolar proteinosis

Relative Indications
- Facilitation of surgical exposure—high priority
  - Thoracic aortic aneurysm
  - Pneumonectomy
  - Upper lobectomy
  - Mediastinal exposure
  - Thoracoscopy
  - Pulmonary resection via median sternotomy
- Facilitation of surgical exposure—low priority
  - Esophageal resection
  - Middle and lower lobectomies and segmental resection
  - Procedures on the thoracic spine
- Post cardiopulmonary bypass status after removal of totally occluding chronic unilateral pulmonary emboli
- Severe hypoxemia due to unilateral lung disease

The advantages of one-lung anesthesia should be weighed against its disadvantages.

Benumof JL: Anesthesia for Thoracic Surgery, 2nd ed, p 331. Philadelphia, WB Saunders, 1995

Miller RD (ed): Anesthesia, 3rd ed, pp 1689–1690. New York, Churchill Livingstone, 1994

C.11. *How could you achieve one-lung anesthesia if it is indicated?*

There are three techniques available for providing one-lung anesthesia: bronchial blockers, endobronchial tubes, and double-lumen endotracheal tubes. Currently, the Robertshaw, Carlens, and White (right-sided Carlens) and disposable polyvinylchloride (PVC) double-lumen tubes are most commonly used. They allow simultaneous ventilation of both lungs, as well as selective ventilation of either lung.

Benumof JL: Anesthesia for Thoracic Surgery, 2nd ed, pp 334–339. Philadelphia, WB Saunders, 1995

Miller RD (ed): Anesthesia, 3rd ed, pp 1690–1692. New York, Churchill Livingstone, 1994

C.12. *Could you use double-lumen endotracheal tubes in pediatric patients?*

No. Children's tracheas are too small to allow passage of double-lumen endotracheal tubes. The Robertshaw tubes come in three sizes: small, medium, and large, which correspond to internal diameters of 8 mm, 9.5 mm, and 11 mm, respectively. The Carlens and White tubes are available in four sizes: 35, 37, 39, and 41 French catheter gauge (size in French = 3.14 × external diameter or 4 × internal diameter + 2). The smallest size of the disposable double-lumen tube is 28 French.

Benumof JL: Anesthesia for Thoracic Surgery, 2nd ed, pp 338–339. Philadelphia, WB Saunders, 1995

Kaplan JA (ed): Thoracic Anesthesia, 2nd ed, p 378. New York, Churchill Livingstone, 1991

Miller RD (ed): Anesthesia, 4th ed, pp 1690–1692. New York, Churchill Livingstone, 1994

C.13. *What are the contraindications to the use of double-lumen endotracheal tubes?*

Because insertion of the tube is either difficult or dangerous, double-lumen endotracheal tubes are relatively contraindicated in the following situations:

- Patients with a full stomach (risk of aspiration).
- Patients with a lesion (airway stricture, endoluminal tumor) that is present somewhere along the pathway of the tube and thus could be traumatized.
- Small patients for whom a 35-French tube is too large to fit comfortably through the larynx and a 28-French tube is considered too small.
- Patients whose upper airway anatomy precludes safe insertion of the tube (recessed jaw, prominent teeth, bull neck, anterior larynx).
- Extremely critically ill patients who have a single-lumen tube already in place and who cannot tolerate being taken off mechanical ventilation and PEEP for a short period of time. However, under these circumstances, it is still possible to achieve one-lung ventilation by using an endobronchial blocker or endobronchial tube in a mainstem bronchus.

Benumof JL: Anesthesia for Thoracic Surgery, 2nd ed, p 370. Philadelphia, WB Saunders, 1995

Miller RD (ed): Anesthesia, 4th ed, pp 1690, 1700. New York, Churchill Livingstone, 1994

C.14. *Would you use a right- or left-sided double-lumen tube?*

I would use a left-sided double-lumen tube (DLT) if the surgery is performed on the right lung. Even when the surgery is on the left lung, I still use a left-sided DLT for most cases because the margin of safety in positioning a right-sided DLT is much less than that for a left-sided DLT. The length of the left mainstem bronchus (approximately 50 to 55 mm) is much longer than that of the right mainstem bronchus (approximately 15 to 20 mm). The right-sided DLT may block the right upper lobe when the tube is in too far or the endobronchial cuff blocks the right upper lobe. In addition, the right-sided tube may block the left lung when the tube is out too far and the endobronchial cuff blocks the tracheal carina. A right-sided DLT is indicated when a left-sided DLT is contraindicated, such as when there is a large exophytic lesion on the left mainstem bronchus, there is a tight left mainstem bronchus stenosis, or the left mainstem bronchus is distorted by an adjacent tumor.

Benumof JL: Anesthesia for Thoracic Surgery, 2nd ed, pp 339–341. Philadelphia, WB Saunders, 1995

Miller RD (ed): Anesthesia, 4th ed, p 1692. New York, Churchill Livingstone, 1994

C.15. How do you know that the tube is in the proper position?

The position of the DLT may be checked by listening to the breath sounds of each lung while clamping each lumen of the DLT. If the breath sounds are unclear, as in patients with emphysema, a fiberoptic bronchoscope may be used to make sure that the tracheal opening is 1 to 2 cm above the tracheal carina, the upper surface of the blue left endobronchial cuff is just below the tracheal carina, and the left lumen goes off to the left side. This is to ensure that the left lumen tip does not obstruct the left upper lobe.

Benumof JL: Anesthesia for Thoracic Surgery, 2nd ed, pp 344–345, 352. Philadelphia, WB Saunders, 1995

Miller RD (ed): Anesthesia, 4th ed, pp 1696–1697. New York, Churchill Livingstone, 1994

C.16. How do you identify the right and the left mainstem bronchi during fiberoptic bronchoscopy?

During bronchoscopy, the tracheal cartilaginous rings are anterior and the tracheal membrane is posterior. Therefore, the right and the left can be oriented by the relationship of the mainstem bronchi to the anterior cartilaginous ring and the posterior membrane (Fig. 2-1). In addition, the right bronchial carina is visible at the level of the tracheal carina.

Benumof JL: Anesthesia for Thoracic Surgery, 2nd ed, pp 23–24, 372. Philadelphia, WB Saunders, 1995

Miller RD (ed): Anesthesia, 4th ed, p 1701. New York, Churchill Livingstone, 1994

C.17. How many types of bronchial blocker are available? What are the advantages and disadvantages of bronchial blockers?

The bronchial blocker most often used for adults is a Fogarty occlusion catheter with a 3-ml balloon. Other devices include gauze tampons, Magill balloon-tipped luminal blocker, Foley catheter, and Univent tube. The Univent tube is a single-lumen tube (7.0-mm internal diameter) that has a small lumen along the anterior concave side of the tube, which contains a small hollow lumen catheter that has a cuff at the end of it.

Bronchial blockers are relatively simple and inexpensive and can be used in children and adults who cannot take even the smallest double-lumen tubes (28 French).

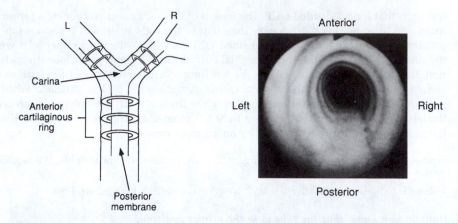

Figure 2-1. The orientation of the right and the left mainstem bronchus during bronchoscopy. (Reprinted with permission from Ovassapin A: Fiberoptic Airway Endoscopy in Anesthesia and Critical Care, p 62. New York, Raven Press, 1990)

The other advantage of bronchial blockers is that there is no need to change endotracheal tubes for postoperative mechanical ventilation.

The disadvantages of bronchial blockers compared with double-lumen tubes include the following:

- Inability to suction
- Inability to ventilate the lung distal to the blocker
- Increased placement time
- Definite need for a fiberoptic or rigid bronchoscope to position
- Obstruction of trachea and contamination of both lungs if the bronchial blocker backs out into the trachea

Kaplan JA (ed): Thoracic Anesthesia, 2nd ed, pp 372–374. New York, Churchill Livingstone, 1991

Miller RD (ed): Anesthesia, 4th ed, pp 1700–1703. New York, Churchill Livingstone, 1994

C.18. What are the advantages of the Univent bronchial blocker tube?

The advantages of the Univent bronchial blocker tube system relative to a double-lumen tube and other bronchial blockers are as follows:

- Easier to insert and properly position
- Can be properly positioned during continuous ventilation and in the lateral decubitus position
- No need to change the tube for postoperative mechanical ventilation
- No need to change the tube intraoperatively when turning from the supine to the prone position
- Selective blockade of some lobes of each lung
- Possible to apply nonventilated operative lung continuous positive airway pressure (CPAP).

Benumof JL: Anesthesia for Thoracic Surgery, 2nd ed, pp 373–374. Philadelphia, WB Saunders, 1995

C.19. What are the limitations to the use of the Univent bronchial blocker tube and solutions to the limitations?

The limitations and solutions are as follows:

- Slow inflation time due to the small lumen of the bronchial blocker, which can be corrected by
  - Deflating bronchial blocker cuff and administering a positive pressure breath through the main single lumen
  - Administering carefully one short high-pressure (20 to 30 psi) jet ventilation
- Slow deflation time due to the small lumen of the bronchial blocker, which can be corrected by
  - Deflating bronchial blocker cuff and compressing and evacuating the lung through the main single lumen
  - Applying suction to bronchial blocker lumen
- Blockage of bronchial blocker lumen by blood and/or pus because of small lumen, which can be corrected by
  - Suction with high pressure and breaking with a wire stylet
- High-pressure cuff when intracuff volume is >2 ml, which can be corrected by
  - Using a just-seal volume of air to inflate the bronchial blocker cuff
- Intraoperative leak around the bronchial blocker cuff, which can be corrected by
  - Making sure that bronchial blocker cuff is subcarinal
  - Increasing inflation volume
  - Rearranging surgical field

Benumof JL: Anesthesia for Thoracic Surgery, 2nd ed, pp 374–376. Philadelphia, WB Saunders, 1995

Miller RD (ed): Anesthesia, 4th ed, pp 1702–1703. New York, Churchill Livingstone, 1994

C.20. How would you monitor arterial oxygenation continuously during one-lung anesthesia? What is the mechanism of oximetry?

Continuous assessment of arterial oxygenation can be achieved noninvasively by a pulse oximeter. Because there is continuous perfusion to the nondependent, nonventilated lung, one-lung ventilation increases transpulmonary shunt to 20% to 30%. The result is systemic hypoxemia. Meanwhile, severe hypoxemia and hypercarbia may be caused by incorrect positioning of double-lumen tubes.

Pulse oximetry uses spectrophotoelectric oximetric principles to determine oxygen saturation. It is similar to classical oximetry in that discrete wavelengths of light are used to measure optical density of hemoglobin. Pulse oximeters are essentially multiple wavelength pleythysmographs. The pulse amplitude detected is a function of the arterial distention, hemoglobin oxygen saturation of the inflow of arterial blood, and wavelength of light. In order to determine the arterial hemoglobin oxygen saturation, the oximeter measures the ratio of the pulse amplitude of red light (660 nm) to the pulse amplitude of infrared light (940 nm). Because the detected pulsatile waveform is produced solely from arterial blood, Beer's law and the amplitude at each wavelength allow exact beat-to-beat continuous calculation of arterial hemoglobin oxygen saturation with no interference from surrounding venous blood, skin, connective tissue, or bone. Because pulse oximetry uses light absorption changes pro duced by arterial pulsations, any event that significantly reduces vascular pulsations will reduce the instrument's ability to calculate saturation. Adequate finger pulsation generally is lost with hypothermia of a few degrees, hypotension (mean blood pressure <50 mm Hg), and infusion of vasoconstrictive drugs. Meanwhile, the presence of dyshemoglobinemias (carboxyhemoglobin, methemoglobin, sulfhemoglobin) also may affect the oximeter accuracy.

Other methods of monitoring arterial oxygenation continuously include transcutaneous oxygen tension ($PtcO_2$) and arterial oxygen tension using an indwelling oxygen electrode. $PtcO_2$ requires special site preparation, airtight probe mantling, and a potentially harmful local heat source to induce arterialization. Moreover, $PtcO_2$ fails to perfectly reflect true arterial oxygenation. An indwelling arterial oxygen electrode is inserted into the arterial line and may increase the incidence of thromboembolism.

Brodsky JB, Shulman MS, Swan M et al: Pulse oximetry during one-lung ventilation. Anesthesiology 63:212–214, 1985

Kagle DM, Alexander CM, Berko RS et al: Evaluation of the Omeda 3700 pulse oximeter: Steady-state and transient response characteristics. Anesthesiology 66:376–380, 1987

Tremper KK, Barker SJ: Pulse oximetry. Anesthesiology 70:98–108, 1989

C.21. What is hypoxic pulmonary vasoconstriction (HPV)?

Alveolar hypoxia, whether caused by a low F_IO_2, hypoventilation, or atelectasis, causes pulmonary vasoconstriction. The phenomenon is called hypoxic pulmonary vasoconstriction (HPV). The selective increase of vascular resistance in the hypoxic lung diverts blood away from the hypoxic lung to the better-ventilated normoxic lung. The diversion of blood flow decreases the amount of shunt flow that can occur throughout the hypoxic lung. Therefore, the regional HPV response is an autoregulatory mechanism to prevent ventilation/perfusion mismatch and improve arterial oxygenation.

Benumof JL: Anesthesia for Thoracic Surgery, 2nd ed, pp 132–135. Philadelphia, WB Saunders, 1995

C.22. What are the effects of anesthetics on hypoxic pulmonary vasoconstriction (HPV) and their clinical implications?

Intravenous anesthetics, such as thiopental, ketamine, morphine, and fentanyl, have no effect on HPV. However, inhalation anesthetics, such as halothane, methoxyflurane, enflurane, and isoflurane, directly inhibit HPV in a dose-related fashion. Isoflurane, 2.4%, depresses HPV response by 50%, while low concentrations of isoflurane (0.5%) have little adverse effect on HPV.

Theoretically, inhibition of HPV increases intrapulmonary shunt and consequently causes hypoxemia. However, Rogers and Benumof have demonstrated that halothane and isoflurane do not decrease PaO_2 during one-lung ventilation in intravenously anesthetized patients. Craig et al recently compared the effects of propofol-alfentanil versus isoflurane anesthesia on arterial oxygenation. Their study did not support the theory that total intravenous anesthesia will decrease the risk of hypoxemia during one-lung ventilation. Clinically, there are a number of important, nonanesthetic drug factors that influence the effect of inhalation anesthetics on shunting and arterial oxygenation during one-lung ventilation.

- The effect of a given increase in shunt on PaO_2 depends on the absolute level of the initial shunt and the inspired oxygen concentration. For example, if the one-lung ventilation shunt without isoflurane is 30% and with isoflurane is 34%, then the decrease in PaO_2 will be very small. In practice, nearly 100% oxygen is used. Even though shunt is increased, PaO_2 usually remains well above 100 mm Hg. The oxygen saturation and oxygen content are hardly changed.
- The secondary effects of inhalation anesthetics may counteract the direct HPV-inhibition effect of the anesthetics. Thus, a decrease in cardiac output, mixed venous-oxygen tension and pulmonary pressure, all of which may accompany deep inhalation anesthesia, would increase nondependent-lung HPV at the same time that inhalation anesthetics were decreasing it.
- The presence of chronic, irreversible disease in the vessels of the nondependent lung may render these vessels incapable of an HPV response.
- The presence of disease in the dependent lung will make the dependent lung less able to accept redistributed blood flow and thereby decrease the HPV effect of the nondependent lung.
- Surgical interference with blood flow to the nondependent lung also decreases the anesthetic effect on HPV of the nondependent lung.

Benumof JL: Anesthesia for Thoracic Surgery, 2nd ed, pp 138–139. Philadelphia, WB Saunders, 1995

Benumof JL: Isoflurane anesthesia and arterial oxygenation during one-lung ventilation. Anesthesiology 64:419 422, 1986

Boldt J, Müller M, Uphus D et al: Cardiorespiratory changes in patients undergoing pulmonary resection using different anesthetic management techniques. J Cardiothorac Vasc Anesth 10: 854–859, 1996

Carlsson AJ, Bindeslev L, Hedenstierna G: Hypoxia-induced pulmonary vasoconstriction in the human lung. The effect of isoflurane anesthesia. Anesthesiology 66:312–316, 1987

Domino KB, Borowec L, Alexander CM et al: Influence of isoflurane on hypoxic pulmonary vasoconstriction in dogs. Anesthesiology 64:423–428, 1986

Reid CW, Slinger PD, Lewis S: A comparison of the effects of propofol-alfentanil versus isoflurane anesthesia on arterial oxygenation during one-lung ventilation. J Cardiothorac Vasc Anesth 10:860–863, 1996

Rogers SN, Benumof JL: Halothane and isoflurane do not decrease PaO_2 during one-lung ventilation in intravenously anesthetized patients. Anesth Analg 64:946–954, 1985

C.23. Describe the blood flow distribution during two-lung ventilation in the upright, supine, and lateral decubitus positions.

In both the upright and supine positions, the right lung receives 55% of the total blood flow, while the left lung receives the remaining 45%. Gravity causes a vertical gradient in the distribution of blood flow in the lateral decubitus position. Therefore, blood flow to the dependent lung is significantly greater than blood flow to the nondependent lung. When the right lung is nondependent, it receives only 45% of the total blood flow; the dependent left lung receives the remaining 55%. When the left lung is nondependent, it receives only 35% of the total blood flow, while the dependent right lung receives the remaining 65%. Therefore, the average blood flow of the nondependent lung is approximately 40% of the total blood flow, while that of the dependent lung is approximately the remaining 60%.

Benumof JL: Anesthesia for Thoracic Surgery, 2nd ed, pp 125–126. Philadelphia, WB Saunders, 1995

Rehder K, Wenthe FM, Sessler AD: Function of each lung during mechanical ventilation with ZEEP and with PEEP in man anesthetized with thiopental-meperidine. Anesthesiology 39:597–606, 1973

Walff KE, Aulin I: The regional lung function in the lateral decubitus position during anesthesia and operations. Acta Anesthesiol Scand 16:195–205, 1972

C.24. Discuss pulmonary blood flow distribution, shunt flow, and PaO_2 (F_IO_2 = 1.0) during one-lung ventilation.

When the nondependent lung is nonventilated (made atelectatic), HPV in the nondependent lung will increase nondependent lung pulmonary vascular resistance and decrease nondependent lung blood flow. In the absence of any complicating factors, a single-lung HPV response should decrease the blood flow to that lung by 50%. Consequently, the nondependent lung should be able to reduce its blood flow from 40% to 20% of total blood flow, and the nondependent/dependent lung blood flow ratio during one-lung ventilation should be 20%:80%.

All of the blood flow to the nonventilated nondependent lung is shunt flow, and therefore one-lung ventilation creates an obligatory right-to-left transpulmonary shunt flow that was not present during two-lung ventilation. If no shunt existed during two-lung ventilation conditions (ignoring the normal 1% to 3% shunt flow due to the bronchial, pleural, and thebesian circulation), then we would expect the ideal total shunt flow during one-lung ventilation to be a minimal 20% of total blood flow. PaO_2 with fractional inspired O_2 concentration (F_IO_2) equal to 1 should be approximately 280 mm Hg if hemodynamic and metabolic states are normal. Clinically, PaO_2 (F_IO_2 = 1) ranges from 150 to 250 mm Hg.

Benumof JL: Anesthesia for Thoracic Surgery, 2nd ed, pp 132–135. Philadelphia, WB Saunders, 1995

Benumof JL: Isoflurane anesthesia and arterial oxygenation during one-lung ventilation. Anesthesiology 64:419–422, 1986

Marshall BE, Marshall C: Continuity of response to hypoxic pulmonary vasoconstriction. J Appl Physiol 59:189–196, 1980

C.25. During one-lung anesthesia, the following arterial blood gases were noted: pH, 7.10; P_{CO_2}, 86 mm Hg; P_{O_2}, 90 mm Hg; CO_2, 24 mEq/liter. What would you do?

The blood gases showed severe acute respiratory acidosis from alveolar hypoventilation. Because the minute volume of the respirator was >90 to 100 ml/kg, alveolar hypoventilation probably resulted from malposition of the double-lumen tube, which increased airway resistance and hence peak inspiratory pressure. Consequently, a large portion of tidal volume was lost in the respirator bellows and anesthesia circuit tubes. The tubing compliance ranges from 4 to 8 ml/cm H_2O. If inspiratory pressure is 60 cm H_2O, 240 to 480 ml of tidal volume is lost to expand the anesthesia tubings. When the double-lumen tube was pushed too far into the bronchus with both cuffs inflated in the bronchus, or the endobronchial opening was pulled back to the trachea with both cuffs inflated in the trachea, the dependent lung was not ventilated. When the nondependent lung was clamped, neither lung was ventilated. PaO_2 was maintained by mass movement oxygenation (apneic oxygenation).

Cuffs of double-lumen tubes should be deflated and two-lung ventilation should be resumed to correct respiratory acidosis. Then the double-lumen tube should be repositioned and preferably confirmed by fiberoptic bronchoscopy.

Increased pulmonary shunt may cause severe hypoxemia, but not significant increase in $PaCO_2$, since $PvCO_2$ is only 7 mm Hg higher than $PaCO_2$.

C.26. How could you improve oxygenation during one-lung anesthesia?

The following sequence could be done to improve oxygenation:

- Use the highest oxygen concentrations.
- Maintain two-lung anesthesia as long as possible.
- Use a moderate tidal volume of 10 ml/kg to ventilate the dependent lung because a higher tidal volume may increase dependent lung airway pressure and pulmonary vascular resistance and thereby increase nondependent lung blood flow and a lower tidal volume may promote dependent lung atelectasis.
- Set the respiratory rate to achieve $PaCO_2$ at 40 mm Hg because hypocapnia may inhibit HPV in the nondependent lung and hyperventilation may increase airway pressure, hence increasing pulmonary vascular resistance in the dependent lung.
- Check the position of the double-lumen tube with a fiberoptic bronchoscope to ensure that the orifice of the right or the left upper lobe is not occluded.
- Use differential lung CPAP/PEEP search:
  - Add 5 cm H_2O of CPAP to the nondependent lung during the deflation phase of a large tidal volume breath to overcome critical opening pressure in the atelectatic lung.
  - Apply 5 cm H_2O of PEEP to the dependent lung.
  - Increase nondependent lung CPAP to 10 cm H_2O while the dependent lung is maintained at 5 cm H_2O of PEEP.
  - Increase dependent lung PEEP to 10 cm H_2O to match the nondependent lung CPAP. The above differential lung CPAP/PEEP search is conducted in this way to find the optimal (best) end-expiratory pressure for each lung and minimum QS/QT for the patient as a whole.
- Use two-lung ventilation intermittently if severe hypoxia is still present.
- Clamp the pulmonary artery to the nondependent lung temporarily.

Benumof JL: Anesthesia for pulmonary surgery. ASA Refresher Courses in Anesthesiology 18:19–31, 1990

Benumof JL: Anesthesia for pulmonary surgery. ASA Refresher Course Lectures No. 225, 1991

Benumof JL: Anesthesia for Thoracic Surgery, 2nd ed, pp 408–428. Philadelphia, WB Saunders, 1995

Capan LM, Turndorf H, Patel C et al: Optimization of arterial oxygenation during one-lung anesthesia. Anesth Analg 59:847–851, 1980

Katz JA, Laverne RG, Fairley B et al: Pulmonary oxygen exchange during endobronchial anesthesia: Effect of tidal volume and PEEP. Anesthesiology 56:164–171, 1982

Miller RD (ed): Anesthesia, 3rd ed, p 1565. New York, Churchill Livingstone, 1990

C.27. Are there any advantages or disadvantages of high-frequency positive pressure ventilation (HFPPV) for thoracotomy?

During volume-controlled HFPPV with a fixed frequency of 60/min and a relative insufflation time of 22%, the exposed lung is moderately expanded and exhibits only minor movements during insufflation. Repeated blood gas analyses during surgery show normocarbia and good oxygenation, even during compression of the exposed lung. After compression, the lung can readily be reexpanded with the aid of a brief period of positive end-expiratory pressure. Thus, even relatively low intrapulmonary pressures during volume-controlled HFPPV without PEEP are adequate to keep the open-chest lung expanded during thoracotomy. This creates optimal conditions for the surgeons.

Glenski and associates studied high frequency ventilation (HFV) during thoracic surgery. HFV at an oscillatory frequency of 3 Hz and a delivered gas volume of 1.3 to 1.9 ml/kg provided adequate pulmonary gas exchange and excellent surgical conditions for peripheral lung procedures. However, during HFV, surgical conditions were unsatisfactory for mediastinal or major airway procedures. They did not recommend HFV as a routine procedure for thoracic surgery because they believed the disadvantages of HFV outweighed the advantages. The disadvantages of HFV are as follows:

- Monitoring heart and breath sounds with an esophageal stethoscope is difficult during HFV.
- The adequacy of ventilation cannot be judged from the motion of the chest or lung.
- The use of anesthetic gases is high.
- Assessment of lung volume is difficult.

Benumof JL: Anesthesia for Thoracic Surgery, 2nd ed, pp 433–448. Philadelphia, WB Saunders, 1995

Glenski JA, Crawford M, Rehder K: High-frequency, small-volume ventilation during thoracic surgery. Anesthesiology 64:211–214, 1986

Malina JR, Nordstrom SG, Sjostrand UH et al: Clinical evaluation of high frequency positive-pressure ventilation (HFPPV) in patients scheduled for open-chest surgery. Anesth Analg 60:324–330, 1981

Miller RD (ed): Anesthesia, 4th ed, pp 1715–1716. New York, Churchill Livingstone, 1994

C.28. *Left lower lobectomy was performed. Would you extubate the patient or leave the patient on the respirator at the end of the procedure?*

It is our practice to have an awake, comfortable, extubated patient at the end of the procedure. However, if the patient cannot maintain adequate oxygenation and ventilation, mechanical ventilation is indicated. Extubation avoids the potential hazards of postoperative positive pressure ventilation on fresh bronchial stump suture lines. It is important to reexpand both the collapsed upper lung and the compressed lower lung before closing the chest to prevent atelectasis.

Miller RD (ed): Anesthesia, 4th ed, pp 1719–1720. New York, Churchill Livingstone, 1994

D. Postoperative Management

D.1. *What are the immediate life-threatening complications that follow lobectomy or pneumonectomy?*

The serious complications include massive hemorrhage caused by loosening of a ligature from a pulmonary vessel; bronchopleural fistula from blowout of a bronchial stump; herniation of the heart following radical pneumonectomy by the intrapericardial approach; pulmonary torsion due to increased mobility of a lobe; acute right-sided heart failure following pulmonary resection; right-to-left shunting across a patent foramen ovale due to increased pulmonary vascular resistance and right ventricular pressure; injuries of phrenic, vagus, and recurrent laryngeal nerves during radical hilar dissection or excision of mediastinal tumors; and acute respiratory insufficiency.

Benumof JL: Anesthesia for Thoracic Surgery, 2nd ed, pp 696–715. Philadelphia, WB Saunders, 1995

Miller RD (ed): Anesthesia, 4th ed, pp 1717–1719. New York, Churchill Livingstone, 1994

D.2. How would you prevent postoperative atelectasis? Would you order intermittent positive pressure breathing (IPPB) or incentive spirometry?

Before the chest is closed, both the collapsed upper lung and the compressed lower lung must be reexpanded by deep positive pressure breaths. Chest tubes have to be positioned properly and connected to constant negative pressure suction (about 15 to 20 cm H_2O).

Postoperatively, the following are recommended: chest physiotherapy, including incentive spirometry, deep breathing, encouragement to cough; mobilization of secretions; early ambulation; and proper pain control. We recommend incentive spirometry instead of IPPB for post-lobectomy patients. The ideal respiratory maneuver is one in which a high alveolar-inflating pressure is sustained for a relatively long period of time, and this can be achieved only with a large inhaled volume. A high inhaled volume can be achieved passively by proper IPPB or actively by incentive spirometry. Recently, IPPB lost its popularity, because, as usually performed, the inflating volume is not measured and the tidal volume is limited by the peak airway pressure. In addition, the use of IPPB may lead to cross-contamination from the equipment, pneumothorax or blowout of a bronchial stump from high airway pressure, and decreased cardiac output by decreasing the venous return to the heart. Moreover, the cost of using IPPB is ten times that of using incentive spirometry.

Benumof JL: Anesthesia for Thoracic Surgery, 2nd ed, pp 746–747. Philadelphia, WB Saunders, 1995

Miller RD (ed): Anesthesia, 4th ed, pp 1721–1724. New York, Churchill Livingstone, 1994

D.3. Why is it important to control postoperative pain? How would you control it?

Postoperative pain control is important not only for patient comfort but also to minimize pulmonary complications by enabling the patient to breathe deeply without splinting, to cough, and to ambulate. Systemic administration of narcotics is employed most often to control postoperative pain. We titrate small doses of morphine in 2-mg increments to achieve adequate pain relief and avoid excessive sedation and respiratory depression. The titration of narcotic dosages can also be achieved by a patient-controlled analgesia (PCA) device. Recently, epidural analgesia with narcotics and/or local anesthetics has been widely used. A lumbar or thoracic epidural catheter is routinely placed before the induction of general anesthesia and checked for proper position by using a small dose of local anesthetic. A loading dose of fentanyl, 1 to 2 µg/kg, in 15 ml of saline solution is administered approximately 30 minutes before the end of surgery. Then continuous infusion of fentanyl, 1 to 2 μg/kg/h, is started in the recovery room.

Benumof JL: Anesthesia for Thoracic Surgery, 2nd ed, pp 756–770. Philadelphia, WB Saunders, 1995

Miller RD (ed): Anesthesia, 4th ed, pp 1722–1724. New York, Churchill Livingstone, 1994

D.4. Discuss the alternative methods of postoperative pain control.

The alternative methods of pain control include intercostal or paravertebral nerve block, interpleural regional analgesia, epidural analgesia with local anesthetics, transcutaneous electrical nerve stimulation (TENS), cryoanalgesia, and intrathecal and epidural narcotics.

Intercostal or Paravertebral Nerve Block

Intercostal or paravertebral nerve blocks with long-acting local anesthetics such as bupivacaine are often used to control postoperative pain after thoracotomy. These blocks are usually done by the surgeon intraoperatively under direct vision to avoid pneumothorax and incidental dural puncture. The blocks are placed to the intercostal nerves at the level of the incision and two or three interspaces above and below this level. Catheters that can be injected postoperatively when pain occurs may be placed in the appropriate intercostal grooves at the time of thoracotomy closure.

Interpleural Regional Analgesia

This is the percutaneous introduction of a catheter (usually an epidural catheter) into the thoracic cage between the parietal and visceral pleura. Bupivacaine, 0.25% to 0.5%, with epinephrine is most commonly used. Analgesia is thought to occur as a result of (1) diffusion of local anesthetic through the parietal pleura and the innermost intercostal muscle to reach the intercostal nerves where the blockage occurs, (2) blockage of the intrathoracic sympathetic chain, and (3) direct action of local anesthetic on nerve endings within the pleura. However, the results of treating pain caused by thoracotomy have been disappointing because of the loss of anesthetic via thoracotomy drainage, the presence of extravasated blood and tissue fluid in the pleural space, and possibly sequestration and channeling of the flow of local anesthetic by the restricted motion of an operated lung. Recently, multiple catheters were introduced to achieve more even distribution of local anesthetic over the pleura and the quality of interpleural analgesia was improved.

Epidural Analgesia with Local Anesthetics

Thoracic or lumbar epidural analgesia may be achieved by a single injection or continuous infusion of 0.25% bupivacaine. Potential complications of this technique include hypotension from sympathetic blockade, inadvertent dural puncture, trauma to the spinal cord, and intravascular injection of local anesthetics with resultant cardiovascular and central nervous system toxicity.

Transcutaneous Electrical Nerve Stimulation

The advantages of TENS include low cost, ease of application, and lack of undesirable side-effects. However, TENS has a weak analgesic effect. It is generally reserved for adjunctive use with narcotics to relieve postthoracotomy pain.

Cryoanalgesia

Cryoanalgesia is a relatively new technique. Extremely long-lasting (3 to 4 weeks) intercostal nerve block is obtained by intercostal nerve freezing with a cryoprobe. Two 30-second freeze cycles, separated by a 5-second thaw period, are applied to each of the nerves selected. However, recent experience with one 30-second freeze exposure has resulted in no loss of postoperative pain control with a significantly reduced period of numbness (from 3.0 months to 1.2 months). Since cryoanalgesia has been shown to reliably and effectively relieve pain and to allow significant improvements in postoperative pulmonary function, it may be a treatment of choice in thoracic pain situations that are expected to last a long time (e.g., pain from chest trauma) and to limit respiratory function significantly.

Intrathecal and Epidural Narcotics

Single intrathecal injection of morphine has been successfully used preoperatively or intraoperatively to provide postoperative pain relief for 18 to 24 hours. However, it appears to be associated with an increased incidence of severe late respiratory depression (4% to 7% compared with <1% for epidural administration). Therefore, epidural narcotics have generally replaced intrathecal narcotics. The advantages of epidural narcotics include selective blockade of spinal pain without sympathetic blockade or loss of motor function, and greater predictability of pain relief over that provided by parenteral narcotics.

Epidural and intrathecal narcotics block the presynaptic and postsynaptic neuron cells of the substantia gelatinosa of the spinal cord by passive diffusion across the dura into the cerebrospinal fluid. The lipophilic narcotics, such as fentanyl, methadone, and meperidine, in doses of 0.1 mg, 5 mg, and 30 to 100 mg, respectively, have a relatively short onset of action of <12 minutes. They provide complete pain relief in 20 to 30 minutes and have a duration of action of 6 to 7 hours.

In contrast, a lipophobic narcotic, such as morphine, in a 5-mg dose has a relatively slow onset of action of 15 to 30 minutes; provides maximal pain relief in 40 to 60 minutes; and has a duration of action of >12 hours. Since the thoracic epidural approach has risks of dural puncture and spinal cord damage, the lumbar epidural route with a slightly higher dose of morphine and adequate diluent volume has been suggested.

The most serious complications of epidural narcotics are early and late respiratory depression. The other side-effects include urinary retention, pruritus, and nausea and vomiting. The narcotic antagonist, naloxone, can reverse all the above side-effects. However, the use of naloxone can reverse the analgesic effect as well, so it must be used cautiously.

Ali J, Yaffe CS, Serrette C: The effect of transcutaneous electric nerve stimulation in treatment of postoperative pain. Surgery 89:507–512, 1981

Benumof JL: Anesthesia for Thoracic Surgery, 2nd ed, pp 756–770. Philadelphia, WB Saunders, 1995

Cousins MJ, Mather LE, Wilson PR: Intrathecal and epidural administration of opioid analgesic. Anesthesiology 61:276, 1984

deLeon-Casa Sola OA, Lema MJ: Postoperative epidural opioid analgesia. What are the choices? Anesth Analg 83:867–875, 1996

Delilkan AE, Lee LK, Yong NK et al: Postoperative intercostal nerve block analgesia versus narcotic analgesia. Anaesthesia 28:561, 1973

Ferrante FM, Chan VWS, Arthur R et al: Interpleural analgesia after thoracotomy. Anesth Analg 72:105–109, 1991

James EL, Kolberg HL, Iwen GW et al: Epidural analgesia for post-thoracotomy patients. J Thorac Cardiovasc Surg 82:898, 1981

Kaplan JA, Miller ED Jr, Gallagher EG Jr: Postoperative analgesia for thoracotomy patients. Anesth Analg 54:773, 1975

Kavanagh BP, Katz J, Sandler AN: Pain control after thoracic surgery. A review of current techniques. Anesthesiology 81:737–759, 1994

Liu S, Carpenter RL, Neal JM: Epidural anesthesia and analgesia. Their role in postoperative outcome. Anesthesiology 82:1474–1506, 1995

Maiwand MO, Makey AR, Rees A: Cryoanalgesia after thoracotomy: Improvement of technique and review of 600 cases. J Thorac Cardiovasc Surg 92:291, 1986

Miller RD (ed): Anesthesia, 4th ed, pp 1722–1724. New York, Churchill Livingstone, 1994

Aspiration Pneumonitis and Acute Respiratory Failure

3

Fun-Sun F. Yao

A 20-year-old full-term pregnant woman was rushed to the operating room for emergency cesarean section because of fetal distress. After rapid induction with thiopental and succinylcholine, the patient vomited and aspirated.

A. Management of Aspiration

1. What would you do right away?
2. What is Mendelson's syndrome?
3. What is the critical pH value of aspirate to cause Mendelson's syndrome? What is the definition of the term "at risk" for aspiration?
4. Would you give prophylactic antibiotics to the patient? Why or why not?
5. Would you give steroid therapy? Why or why not?
6. Would you irrigate the bronchial tree with bicarbonate or saline solution?
7. How would you prevent aspiration during emergency surgery?

B. Oxygen Therapy

The patient was extubated in the recovery room. Chest x-ray films showed questionable mottled density. She was sent back to her floor. Six hours later, she was found dyspneic and cyanotic. Arterial blood gases showed pH 7.46; P_{CO_2}, 30 mm Hg, P_{O_2}, 55 mm Hg, HCO_3^- 20 mEq/liter on room air.

1. Interpret the blood gases.
2. What is adult respiratory distress syndrome (ARDS) and what is its pathogenesis?
3. What are the common causes of ARDS?
4. What oxygen therapy would you order?
5. How many liters of air are entrained into a venturi mask or venturi humidifier when 1 liter of oxygen is used to deliver 50% oxygen?
6. Are there other ways to give oxygen?
7. Is it possible to give 100% F_IO_2 to the patient through a face mask?

C. Mechanical Ventilation

The patient did not improve after receiving 50% oxygen through face mask. Arterial blood gases showed pH, 7.25; P_{CO_2}, 50 mm Hg; P_{O_2}, 55 mm Hg; CO_2 content, 22 mEq/liter. Respiratory rate was 40/min.

1. What would you do now?
2. What are the criteria for mechanical ventilation?
3. What kind of ventilator would you order?
4. What are the advantages and disadvantages of pressure-cycled ventilators?

5. What are the advantages and disadvantages of volume-cycled or volume-limited ventilators?
6. How would you set the volume-cycled ventilator?
7. Would you set sigh volume? How much? How often?
8. How do you know the ventilator settings are right?
9. What are the effects of intermittent positive pressure ventilation (IPPV) on the cardiovascular system?
10. What are the complications of mechanical ventilation?
11. What are the disadvantages of hyperventilation?
12. How do you normalize $PaCO_2$?

D. Continuous Positive Pressure Ventilation

The patient did not improve clinically. The arterial blood gases on F_IO_2 0.7 showed pH 7.30; Pco_2, 40 mm Hg; Po_2, 57 mm Hg; CO_2 content, 18 mEq/liter.

1. What would you do to improve the oxygenation?
2. What are the major factors governing oxygen toxicity?
3. What is the mechanism of oxygen toxicity?
4. What is the pathology of pulmonary oxygen toxicity?
5. How do you improve oxygenation without increasing F_IO_2?
6. What are your criteria to start PEEP?
7. What are PEEP, CPAP, CPPV, EPAP, IPAP, and ZEEP?
8. How does PEEP improve arterial oxygenation?
9. What are prophylactic, conventional, and high PEEP?
10. What is best PEEP or optimal PEEP?
11. How would you monitor the level of PEEP?
12. What are the cardiovascular effects of PEEP?
13. How would you correct hypotension during mechanical ventilation with PEEP?
14. What are the complications of CPPV?
15. What is pressure support ventilation (PSV)? Discuss its advantages.
16. What is airway pressure release ventilation (APRV)? What are the advantages of APRV?
17. What is extended mandatory minute ventilation (EMMV)?
18. What is pressure control ventilation (PCV)?
19. What is inverse-ratio ventilation (IRV)?

E. Weaning from Ventilatory Support

The patient's condition improved after respiratory support with 20 cm H_2O PEEP. Arterial blood gases showed pH 7.45; Pco_2, 35 mm Hg; Po_2, 150 mm Hg; F_IO_2 0.75.

1. What would you do now? Lower F_IO_2 or lower PEEP?
2. The patient continued to improve. When would you consider weaning the patient from the respirator? Discuss the criteria for weaning.
3. How would you wean the patient from the respirator?
4. What are IMV, IAV, and IDV?
5. What are the advantages and disadvantages of IMV over controlled or assisted ventilation?

F. Special Techniques of Respiratory Support

1. **What is differential or selective PEEP? What are the indications?**
2. **What are the indications and contraindications for extracorporeal membrane oxygenation (ECMO)? How many ways can ECMO be used? What are the results of ECMO?**
3. **What is HFPPV? What are the characteristics of HFPPV?**
4. **What are the frequencies used in high frequency ventilation (HFV)? How are they classified?**
5. **What are the indications and precautions for high frequency ventilation?**
6. **What is nitric oxide? What is the role of inhaled nitric oxide in the treatment of ARDS?**

A. Management of Aspiration

A.1. What would you do right away?

Rapidly tilt the operating table to a 30° head-down position to have the larynx at a higher level than the pharynx and to allow gastric content to drain to the outside. Suction the mouth and pharynx as rapidly as possible. Endotracheal intubation should be done immediately, and the cuff should be inflated to prevent further aspiration. Quickly suction through the endotracheal tube before administering 100% oxygen by positive pressure ventilation. This is to prevent pushing aspirated material beyond your reach. Suction should be brief to avoid cardiac arrest from hypoxia. Give 100% oxygen both before and after suctioning. Once the patient is intubated and suctioned, the table can be straightened and surgery should be continued to save the fetus.

A nasogastric tube should be inserted to empty the stomach. The *p*H of the gastric content should be determined. Tracheobronchial aspirate is collected for culture and sensitivity test. Auscultation of the chest will determine if there are diminished breathing sounds, wheezing, rales, and rhonchi. Beta-2 agonists such as albuterol or terbutaline may be administered via metered dose inhaler adapters to the anesthetic circuit to relieve bronchospasm.

The earliest and most reliable sign of aspiration is hypoxemia, which follows aspiration of even the mildest and most benign aspirate. Therefore, analysis of arterial blood gases should be taken to determine the severity of hypoxemia. Early application of positive end-expiratory pressure (PEEP) is recommended to improve pulmonary function.

Abouleish E, Grenvik A: Vomiting, regurgitation, and aspiration in obstetrics. Pa Med 77:45–58, 1974

Barash PG, Cullen BF, Stoelting RK (eds): Clinical Anesthesia, 3rd ed, pp 1293–1294. Philadelphia, Lippincott-Raven, 1997

Katz J, Benumof JL, Kadis LB (eds): Anesthesia and Uncommon Diseases, 3rd ed, p 480. Philadelphia, WB Saunders, 1990

A.2. What is Mendelson's syndrome?

Acute chemical aspiration pneumonitis was first described by Mendelson in 1946. The triphasic sequence of immediate respiratory distress with bronchospasm, cyanosis, tachycardia, and dyspnea followed by partial recovery and a final phase of gradual return of respiratory dysfunction is characteristic of Mendelson's syndrome. No signs of mediastinal shift are seen, but chest x-ray films usually show irregular mottled densities. This syndrome is due to the irritative action of gastric hydrochloric acid that produces bronchiolar spasm and a peribronchiolar exudate and congestive action.

Mendelson CC: The aspiration of stomach contents into the lungs during obstetric anesthesia. Am J Obstet Gynecol 52:191–205, 1946

A.3. What is the critical pH value of aspirate to cause Mendelson's syndrome? What is the definition of the term "at risk" for aspiration?

The critical *p*H value is 2.5. Above *p*H 2.5 the response is similar to that of distilled water. Maximum pulmonary damage is achieved at an aspirate *p*H of 1.5. A patient is thought to be at risk when there is >25 ml (0.4 ml/kg) of gastric contents and the *p*H of the gastric contents is <2.5.

Barash PG, Cullen BF, Stoelting RK (eds): Clinical Anesthesia, 3rd ed, p 1294. Philadelphia, Lippincott-Raven, 1997

Miller RD (ed): Anesthesia, 4th ed, p 1441. New York, Churchill Livingstone, 1994

Teabeault JR: Aspiration of gastric contents: Experimental study. Am J Pathol 28:51–67, 1952

A.4. Would you give prophylactic antibiotics to the patient? Why or why not?

We usually do not give prophylactic antibiotics to the patient unless there are signs of infection such as fever, leukocytosis, and positive cultures. The initial aspirate, excluding feculent aspirate, is usually sterile and remains so for the first 24 hours. Thereafter, cultures demonstrate gram-positive or gram-negative superinfection or both, usually with *Escherichia, Klebsiella Staphylococcus, Pseudomonas,* and *Bacterioides,* or anaerobes. No prophylactic antibiotic has been shown to improve mortality or reduce secondary infection rates. It is important to take cultures as soon as possible after aspiration and thereafter as clinically indicated. The antibiotic therapy is given according to the sensitivity test. Prophylactic use of broad-spectrum antibiotics may develop drug-resistant bacterial and fungal superinfection, too. However, if there is a possibility of intestinal obstruction, antimicrobial drugs, such as penicillin plus an aminoglycoside, are sometimes administered without waiting for evidence of progressive pulmonary infection. They can be discontinued if there is no laboratory or clinical evidence of infection.

Barash PG, Cullen BF, Stoelting RK (eds): Clinical Anesthesia, 3rd ed, p 1295. Philadelphia, Lippincott-Raven, 1997

Miller RD (ed): Anesthesia, 4th ed, p 1458. New York, Churchill Livingstone, 1994

A.5. Would you give steroid therapy? Why or why not?

The value of systemic corticosteroids is controversial. The immediate use of corticosteroids has been advocated because of their effect in reducing inflammation and in stabilizing lysosomal membranes. In addition, they prevent pulmonary cellular damage by protecting type II alveolar pneumocytes and preventing agglutination of leukocytes and platelets.

In experimental studies, the effectiveness of corticosteroid therapy appeared to be related to the *p*H of aspirates. When the *p*H of the aspirate was in the narrow range of 1.5 to 2.5, corticosteroid therapy was beneficial in treating acid-aspiration pneumonitis. Dexamethasone 0.08 mg/kg every 6 hours decreased pulmonary water content significantly starting at 24 hours, with return to the normal range by 72 hours. When the *p*H of the aspirate was <1.5, the pulmonary parenchymal damage was maximal. Therefore, the steroid therapy was not effective. When the *p*H of the aspirate was above 2.5, the response was similar to that of water. Therefore, steroids are not necessary.

In a double-blind controlled clinical trial, corticosteroids hastened recovery in young drug-overdose patients with mild to moderate aspiration pneumonitis but did not improve mortality or morbidity. Corticosteroids may reduce the patient's resistance to infection and interfere with normal healing mechanisms; therefore, we do not routinely recommend corticosteroids for patients with aspiration pneumonitis.

Barash PG, Cullen BF, Stoelting RK (eds): Clinical Anesthesia, 3rd ed, pp 1294–1295. Philadelphia, Lippincott-Raven, 1997

Bernard GR, Luce JM, Sprung CL et al: High-dose corticosteroids in patients with the adult respiratory distress syndrome. N Engl J Med 317:1565–1570, 1987

Downs JB, Chapman RL Jr, Modell JH et al: An evaluation of steroid therapy in aspiration pneumonitis. Anesthesiology 40:129–135, 1974

Dudley WR, Marshall BE: Steroid treatment for acid-aspiration pneumonitis. Anesthesiology 40:136–141, 1974

Miller RD (ed): Anesthesia, 4th ed, p 1458. New York, Churchill Livingstone, 1994

Sukumaran M, Granada MJ, Berger HW et al: Evaluation of corticosteroid treatment in aspiration of gastric contents: A controlled clinical trial. Mt Sinai J Med 47:335–340, 1980

A.6. *Would you irrigate the bronchial tree with bicarbonate or saline solution?*

No. In acid-aspiration pneumonitis, Bannister and associates demonstrated that pulmonary lesions were aggravated by irrigation with sodium bicarbonate, normal saline, and sodium hydroxide. This was explained on the basis that (1) the large volume of fluid served to push the hydrochloric acid deeper into the lungs; (2) mixing of the acid and treatment solution was impossible because of the minute size of the interface; (3) hydrochloric acid probably causes damage within a very short time; (4) if equal volumes of hydrochloric acid (e.g., with a *p*H of 1.6) and sodium chloride are mixed together, the *p*H only increases to 1.8; and (5) neutralization of hydrochloric acid with sodium bicarbonate produces heat, and a thermal burn of the bronchial mucosa may occur.

Bronchial irrigation is indicated only in the obstructive type of aspiration. Five to ten milliliters of normal saline are instilled into the tracheobronchial tree, followed immediately by suction. It is preceded and followed by oxygenation. The sequence is repeated until the aspirate fluid is clear.

Bannister WK, Sattilaro AJ, Otis RD: Therapeutic aspects of aspiration pneumonitis in experimental animals. Anesthesiology 22:440–443, 1961

Miller RD (ed): Anesthesia, 4th ed, p 1458. New York, Churchill Livingstone, 1994

A.7. *How would you prevent aspiration during emergency surgery?*

An ounce of prevention is worth a pound of cure. The following principles of preoperative preparation are of extreme importance:

- Administration of nothing by mouth
- Application of gastric decompression by a wide-bore nasogastric tube
- Use of regional anesthesia whenever possible
- Preoperative administration of a clear antacid, such as 30 ml of 0.3 M sodium citrate
- Premedication with anticholinergic agents, such as atropine or glycopyrrolate
- Administration of metoclopramide to stimulate gastric emptying and to increase lower esophageal sphincter tone
- Preoperative administration of an H_2-receptor antagonist such as cimetidine or ranitidine to decrease further secretion of additional acid
- Use of awake intubation whenever possible
- Pretreatment with 3 mg of *d*-tubocurarine or 1 mg of pancuronium to prevent or attenuate fasciculations caused by succinylcholine
- Use of rapid-sequence induction and intubation without positive-pressure ventilation before intubation
- Application of cricoid compression to control regurgitation of gastric contents
- Extubation only when the patient is fully awake

Barash PG, Cullen BF, Stoelting RK (eds): Clinical Anesthesia, 3rd ed, pp 590, 922, 1143–1144. Philadelphia, Lippincott-Raven, 1997

Miller RD (ed): Anesthesia, 4th ed, pp 1447–1456. New York, Churchill Livingstone, 1994

B. Oxygen Therapy

The patient was extubated in the recovery room. Chest x-ray films showed questionable mottled density. She was sent back to her floor. Six hours later, she was found dyspneic and cyanotic. Arterial blood gases showed pH 7.46; P_{CO_2}, 30 mm Hg; P_{O_2}, 55 mm Hg; HCO_3^-, 20 mEq/liter on room air.

B.1. Interpret the blood gases.

pH 7.46 means mild alkalosis. P_{CO_2}, 30 mm Hg means alveolar hyperventilation to compensate for hypoxemia. P_{O_2}, 55 mm Hg on room air means moderate hypoxemia due to aspiration pneumonitis. P_{CO_2} of 30 mm Hg alone normally increases the pH to 7.50. Now the pH is 7.46. It means there is mild metabolic acidosis. HCO_3^- 20 mEq/liter correlates with mild metabolic acidosis due to hypoxemia.

B.2. What is adult respiratory distress syndrome (ARDS) and what is its pathogenesis?

ARDS is a term given to a disorder resulting from diffuse injury to the alveolar capillary membranes. It encompasses a clinical syndrome that was previously labeled "post-traumatic pulmonary insufficiency," "Da Nang lung," "shock lung," "stiff lung syndrome," "wet lung," and "congestive atelectasis." It can follow almost any injury. Although the onset may be acute, there is usually a latent period of hours or days during which respiratory damage is minimal or slowly progressing. Then, progressive, severe respiratory failure develops, and usually advances rapidly to the point of requiring tracheal intubation, mechanical ventilation, and use of positive end-expiratory pressure (PEEP). The physiologic changes are characterized by hypoxemia, reduced functional residual capacity and compliance, increased intrapulmonary shunting, and radiologically, by pulmonary interstitial infiltrate.

The pathogenesis of ARDS involves activation of the plasma complement system. Activation of the complement cascade through the alternative pathway by endotoxin or lipopolysaccharides results in the production of C_5a complement. C_5a complement causes microvascular occlusion and pulmonary granulocyte aggregation and embolization. The granulocytes adhere to the pulmonary capillary endothelial walls and release toxic oxygen, free radicals, and proteases. The resultant damage to the endothelium leads to capillary leakage and pulmonary interstitial edema, ultimately producing terminal airway and alveolar edema and collapse. However, studies have shown limitations of the complement-neutrophil theory. Complement activation does not necessarily correlate with the development or severity of ARDS. ARDS can develop in patients with neutropenia, and pulmonary sequestration of neutrophils may not produce lung injury. As a result, the complement-neutrophil theory of ARDS has been expanded to include central roles for additional humoral mediators (such as endotoxin, tumor necrosis factor, interleukins, thromboxane) and cellular mediators (the macrophage-monocyte system, for instance). The lung in ARDS is now viewed as one of the organs involved in the multiple-organ system dysfunction that occurs as a result of the systemic inflammatory response syndrome. Increased mediator levels are found in bronchoalveolar lavage fluid from patients with ARDS.

Barash PG, Cullen BF, Stoelting RK (eds): Clinical Anesthesia, 3rd ed, pp 1371–1372. Philadelphia, Lippincott-Raven, 1997

Collina JA: The acute respiratory distress syndrome. Adv Surg 11:171, 1977

Pearl RG: New therapies to manage adult respiratory distress syndrome, including nitric oxide. ASA Refresher Courses in Anesthesiology 23:177–187, 1995

Yeston N: Complement-induced respiratory dysfunction: A story. Curr Rev Respir Ther 6:83, 1984

B.3. What are the common causes of ARDS?

The common causes of ARDS include multiple trauma, massive blood transfusion, septic shock, fat or air embolism, disseminated intravascular coagulation, aspiration pneumonitis, fluid overload, burns, smoke or gas inhalation, and viral and mycobacterial pneumonia. The following conditions are also associated with ARDS: acute renal failure, oxygen toxicity, drug overdose, radiation, immunosuppression, neurogenic pulmonary edema, acute vasculitis, pancreatitis, postcardioversion, postcardiopulmonary bypass, and Goodpasture's syndrome.

Barash PG, Cullen BF, Stoelting RK (eds): Clinical Anesthesia, 3rd ed, p 1372. Philadelphia, Lippincott-Raven, 1997

Fauci AS, Braunwald E, Isselbacher KJ et al (eds): Harrison's Principles of Internal Medicine, 14th ed, p 1484. New York, McGraw-Hill, 1998

B.4. What oxygen therapy would you order?

We run oxygen at 10 to 15 liters/min through a venturi humidifier to deliver 50% oxygen with mist to the patient. It is important to specify a high oxygen flow rate in order to satisfy the patient's inspiratory flow rate.

The F_IO_2 depends on the patient's inspiratory flow rate and the flow rate and the concentration of delivered oxygen. The inspiratory flow rate is usually 30 to 40 liters/min. If the delivered flow rate is lower than the inspiratory flow rate, air will be breathed into mix with the delivered oxygen and the F_IO_2 will be lowered.

If the patient is cooperative and not at further risk of aspiration, up to 10 to 15 cm H_2O continuous positive airway pressure (CPAP) can be administered by means of a tightly fitting face mask with high oxygen flow and a reservoir bag.

B.5. How many liters of air are entrained into a venturi mask or venturi humidifier when 1 liter of oxygen is used to deliver 50% oxygen?

1.67 liters of air are entrained. It is important to remember that air contains 20% oxygen. Let V_A be the volume of air, V_O the volume of oxygen. The total oxygen delivered from 100% oxygen and entrained air is equal to the oxygen in the mixed air and oxygen. Therefore, the total oxygen delivered $= V_O \times 100\% + V_A \times 20\% = (V_O + V_A) \times F_IO_2$. Solving the equation,

$$V_O + 0.2V_A = V_O \times F_IO_2 + V_A \times F_IO_2.$$

The equation can be rearranged thus:

$$V_O - V_O \times F_IO_2 = V_A \times F_IO_2 - 0.2V_A$$
$$V_O(1 - F_IO_2) = V_A(F_IO_2 - 0.2)$$

Therefore, $V_O:V_A = (F_IO_2 - 0.2):(1 - F_IO_2)$

when $F_IO_2 = 0.5$

$$V_O:V_A = (0.5 - 0.2):(1 - 0.5)$$
$$V_O:V_A = 0.3:0.5 = 3:5 = 1:1.67$$

Let oxygen flow rate be 1 liter/min. When F_IO_2 is set at 0.3, 0.4, 0.5, and 0.6, the air entrained will be 7, 3, 1.67, and 1 liter/min, respectively.

Gibson RL et al: Actual tracheal oxygen concentrations with commonly used oxygen equipment. Anesthesiology 44:71–73, 1976

Nakamara Y, Jebson P: Inspired oxygen concentrations using a humidifier/tracheostomy T-piece system. Br J Anesth 44:61–65, 1961

Shapiro BA, Kacmarek RM, Cane RD et al (eds): Clinical Application of Respiratory Care, 4th ed, p 126. St. Louis, Mosby-Year Book, 1991

B.6. Are there other ways to give oxygen?

Oxygen may be administered through a face mask, nasal catheter, nasal cannula, face hood, face tent, face mask with a reservoir bag, venturi mask, and a T-piece for the endotracheal tube.

Shapiro BA, Kacmarek RM, Cane RD et al (eds): Clinical Application of Respiratory Care, 4th ed, pp 124–132. St. Louis, Mosby-Year Book, 1991

B.7. Is it possible to give 100% F_IO_2 to the patient through a face mask?

The wall oxygen meter can only deliver oxygen up to 10 to 15 liters/min. It is not enough to satisfy normal inspiratory flow rate, which is usually 30 to 40 liters/min. (Inspiratory flow rate is different from minute volume.) Therefore, air has to be breathed in to mix with oxygen to meet the inspiratory flow rate. Usually, the oxygen mask can deliver only 40% to 50% oxygen to the airway. If a high concentration of oxygen is needed, a nonrebreathing face mask with reservoir bag and one-way valve has to be used. Clinically, it is not used very often, because mechanical ventilation is usually indicated when high concentrations of oxygen are needed.

Shapiro BA, Kacmarek RM, Cane RD et al (eds): Clinical Application of Respiratory Care, 4th ed, p 125. St. Louis, Mosby-Year Book, 1991

C. Mechanical Ventilation

The patient did not improve after receiving 50% oxygen through face mask. Arterial blood gases showed *p*H 7.25; P_{CO_2}, 50 mm Hg; P_{O_2}, 55 mm Hg; CO_2 content, 22 mEq/liter. Respiratory rate was 40/min.

C.1. What would you do now?

The patient should be intubated and mechanical ventilation should be started.

C.2. What are the criteria for mechanical ventilation?

The physiologic criteria for mechanical ventilation are as follows:

Mechanics
- Respiratory rate of >35/min
- Vital capacity of <15 ml/kg
- Inspiratory force <25 cm H_2O

Oxygenation
- PaO_2 <70 mm Hg on mask oxygen
- P (A-a) DO_2 >350 mm Hg on 100% F_IO_2 or QS/QT >20%

Ventilation
- $PaCO_2$ >55 mm Hg, except in patients with chronic hypercarbia
- VD/VT >0.60

The trend of values is of utmost importance. The numerical guidelines should not be followed to the exclusion of clinical judgment.

Pontoppidan H, Geffin B, Lowenstein E: Acute respiratory failure in the adult. N Engl J Med 287:743–751, 1972

Shapiro BA, Kacmarek RM, Cane RD et al (eds): Clinical Application of Respiratory Care, 4th ed, pp 283–286. St. Louis, Mosby-Year Book, 1991

C.3. What kind of ventilator would you order?

I recommend using a volume-cycled ventilator, such as the Bennett MA-1, MA-2, Bennett MA-2+2, Puritan Bennett 7200, Bourns-Bear 5, Engstrom, Siemens-Servo, or Ohio 560.

C.4. What are the advantages and disadvantages of pressure-cycled ventilators?

The pressure-cycled or pressure-limited ventilators deliver gas until a preset pressure has been reached, at which point inspiration stops and passive expiration starts. The advantages are that these ventilators can compensate for mild leakage in the system and deliver the same amount of gas to the patient, provided the compliance is not changed. Also, the instruments are smaller and cheaper than volume-cycled ventilators. The main disadvantage is that the tidal volume varies with the patient's total compliance. When airway resistance increases, tidal volume decreases, resulting in hypoventilation. Therefore, frequent measurement of the expired tidal volume is necessary. Moreover, most pressure-cycled ventilators lack the sufficient flow and pressure capabilities necessary to ventilate critically ill patients. Therefore, they are generally used for IPPB therapy and short-term ventilatory support in the postanesthetic recovery room or emergency room.

Miller RD (ed): Anesthesia, 4th ed, pp 2413–2414. New York, Churchill Livingstone, 1994

C.5. What are the advantages and disadvantages of volume-cycled or volume-limited ventilators?

The volume-cycled ventilators deliver a preset volume of inflation gas regardless of the pressure required to do so. The main advantage is that the tidal volume does not change with total pulmonary compliance or airway resistance. The disadvantages are that there is no compensation for leaks in the system and airway pressure may reach very high levels when the resistance is high. There is usually a pressure limit control to prevent excessive airway pressure. But this device will not maintain delivery of a constant tidal volume to the patient.

Miller RD (ed): Anesthesia, 4th ed, p 2409. New York, Churchill Livingstone, 1994

C.6. How would you set the volume-cycled ventilator?

It is most important to set tidal volume, respiratory rate, inspiratory flow rate, and F_IO_2. Normal tidal volume is 7 ml/kg of body weight. For patients with respiratory failure, the tidal volume is usually set at 10 to 12 ml/kg of body weight because of increased physiologic dead space (VD/VT). Respiratory rate is usually set at 10 to 15/min. Inspiratory flow rate is usually set at 30 to 40 liters/min. Slow inspiratory flow rate allows more even distribution of inspired gas but may compromise venous return because of prolonged inspiratory phase. F_IO_2 is set at 50% to 60% oxygen. The settings are changed according to blood gases.

The high airway pressure limit is set at 10 to 20 cm H_2O above the patient's normal peak airway pressure to prevent barotrauma owing to sudden increase in resistance. The safety alarm system can be set by low inspiratory airway pressure and/or low exhaled tidal volume to detect leak or disconnection of the ventilator. Usually, the low limit of exhaled tidal volume is set at 100 to 200 ml below the preselected tidal volume; the low limit of inspiratory pressure is set at 10 to 15 cm below the patient's usual peak inspiratory pressure.

Benumof JL: Anesthesia for Thoracic Surgery, 2nd ed, pp 721–723. Philadelphia, WB Saunders, 1995

C.7. Would you set sigh volume? How much? How often?

When tidal volume is >10 ml/kg, it is not necessary to set sigh volume. Normal tidal volume, 7 ml/kg, needs occasional sighs to prevent atelectasis. Sigh volume is usually set at twice the tidal volume and 3 to 6/h. Periodic sighs have been replaced by the use of large tidal volumes because of a lack of demonstrated clinical efficacy and frequent intolerance by awake patients. Moreover, periodic sighs are not necessary whenever PEEP is applied.

Pontoppidan H, Laver MB, Geffin B: Acute respiratory failure in the surgical patient. Advances in Surgery, Vol 4. Chicago, Year Book Medical Publishers, 1970

Wilson RS: Techniques of ventilatory control: Indications and complications. ASA Refresher Courses in Anesthesiology 13:221–232, 1985

C.8. How do you know the ventilator settings are right?

Arterial blood gas determinations and clinical evaluation of the patient's condition are the only ways to tell whether the settings are right or not.

C.9. What are the effects of intermittent positive pressure ventilation (IPPV) on the cardiovascular system?

The hemodynamic consequences of both spontaneous and positive-pressure ventilation may be profound and may have opposite effects on cardiovascular stability in different patient populations. Thus, no firm rules apply as to the specific response that will be seen in all patients and under all conditions. Some generalities, however, are probably reasonable. In patients with markedly increased work of breathing, hypervolemia, or impaired LV pump function, the institution of mechanical ventilatory support can be life-saving because of its ability to support the cardiovascular system, independent of any beneficial effects that mechanical ventilation may have on gas exchange. In patients with decreased pulmonary elastic recoil, increased pulmonary vascular resistance, hypovolemic, or airflow obstruction, the institution of mechanical ventilatory support may induce cardiovascular instability, which, if not corrected, can lead to total cardiovascular collapse.

The initiation of IPPV is associated with a decrease in cardiac output and in arterial blood pressure in patients without significant lung consolidation. Cardiac output and stroke volume decrease as the peak airway pressure increases. There is also a fall in cardiac output with increasing inspiratory-to-expiratory ratios. IPPV increases intrathoracic pressure, resulting in decreased venous return and cardiac output. Patients with normal lungs behave differently from patients with significant cardiopulmonary disease. When pulmonary compliance decreases, the transmission of airway pressure to intrathoracic pressure decreases. Patients with more rigid lungs can tolerate higher airway pressures.

IPPV decreases transmural pulmonary artery pressure as well. There is no change in pulmonary vascular resistance. The systemic vascular resistance increases slightly when IPPV is begun. The fall in cardiac output during IPPV is rarely of any clinical significance because it is compensated by an increase in peripheral vascular resistance in nonanesthetized patients. When patients are hypovolemic, the decrease in blood pressure can be significant.

Pinsky MP: Cardiovascular effects of ventilatory support and withdrawal. Anesth Analg 79:567–576, 1995

Shapiro BA, Kacmarek RM, Cane RD et al (eds): Clinical Application of Respiratory Care, pp 285–286. St. Louis, Mosby-Year Book, 1991

C.10. What are the complications of mechanical ventilation?

Physiologic Complications
- Decreased cardiac output owing to increased intrathoracic pressure
- Respiratory alkalosis from hyperventilation
- Increased venous admixture (QS/QT) from prolonged low tidal volume ventilation

Pulmonary Complications
- Infection
- Barotrauma-pneumothorax, mediastinal, interstitial, and subcutaneous emphysema in 10% to 15% of adults
- Oxygen toxicity if the inspired oxygen concentration is >60%
- Atelectasis caused by immobilization, ineffective humidification, and low tidal volume ventilation

Complications from Endotracheal Intubation
- Problems with tubes—bronchial intubation, kinking or obstruction, leaking cuffs
- Nasal damage from nasal intubation—nose bleeding, fractured turbinates, septal perforation, partial loss of alae nasae, nasal synechiae
- Laryngeal damage—edema, vocal cord paresis and granulomata, laryngotracheal membranes, subglottic fibrotic stenosis
- Tracheal damage—tracheal erosion, tracheoesophageal fistula, tracheomalacia, tracheal stenosis
- Complications from mechanical device malfunction

Benumof JL: Anesthesia for Thoracic Surgery, 2nd ed, pp 748–750. Philadelphia, WB Saunders, 1995

Pinsky MP: Cardiovascular effects of ventilatory support and withdrawal. Anesth Analg 79:567–576, 1995

Shapiro BA, Kacmarek RM, Cane RD et al (eds): Clinical Application of Respiratory Care, 4th ed, pp 376–383. St. Louis, Mosby-Year Book, 1991

C.11. What are the disadvantages of hyperventilation?

- Decreased cardiac output owing to increased intrathoracic pressure and decreased sympathetic stimulation and catecholamine release from hypocarbia
- Respiratory alkalosis
- Left shift of oxygen dissociation curve and increased oxygen affinity to hemoglobin
- Decreased cerebral blood flow, decreasing 2% to 4% by every mm Hg decrease in $PaCO_2$ when $PaCO_2$ ranges from 20 to 80 mm Hg
- Hypokalemia and cardiac arrhythmias from alkalosis
- Decreased ionized calcium and tetany from alkalosis
- Decreased PaO_2
- Increased oxygen consumption

Breivik H, Grenvik A, Millen E et al: Normalizing low arterial CO_2 tension during mechanical ventilation. Chest 63:525–531, 1973

Miller RD (ed): Anesthesia, 4th ed, pp 1393–1394. New York, Churchill Livingstone, 1994

C.12. How do you normalize $PaCO_2$?

- Decrease the rate or tidal volume of the ventilator or both.
- Add mechanical dead space to the ventilator tubing.
- Add 1% to 3% CO_2 mixture to the inspired gases.
- Use intermittent mandatory ventilation (IMV).

Breivik H, Grenvik A, Millen E et al: Normalizing low arterial CO_2 tension during mechanical ventilation. Chest 63:525–531, 1973

D. Continuous Positive Pressure Ventilation

The patient did not improve clinically. The arterial blood gases on F_IO_2 0.7 showed *p*H 7.30; P_{CO_2}, 40 mm Hg; P_{O_2}, 57 mm Hg; CO_2 content, 18 mEq/liter.

D.1. What would you do to improve the oxygenation?

PaO_2 may be improved by increasing the F_IO_2 or applying positive end-expiratory pressure (PEEP). Diuresis may improve oxygenation if there is interstitial or frank pulmonary edema.

D.2. What are the major factors governing oxygen toxicity?

Oxygen toxicity is governed by the oxygen partial pressure during exposure, the duration of exposure, and the susceptibility of the individual to pulmonary oxygen injury. The degree of toxicity is related to the partial pressure, but not to the percentage of oxygen inspired, as shown by toleration of 100% oxygen for 2 to 4 weeks at a tension of 250 mm Hg during U.S. space flights. Systemic oxygen toxicity is related to arterial oxygen tension, whereas pulmonary oxygen toxicity depends on alveolar oxygen tension. Retrolental fibroplasia (retinopathy of prematurity) in the premature neonate has been reported after exposure to PaO_2 of >80 to 150 mm Hg for a few hours. Pulmonary toxicity can develop after prolonged exposure to oxygen at concentrations between 0.5 and 1.0 atmospheres. It must be emphasized that generally the adult patient can tolerate one atmosphere of oxygen partial pressure for at least 24 hours. Moreover, there is no evidence that clinically relevant pulmonary oxygen toxicity occurs in humans at inspired partial pressures below 0.5 atmosphere. Moreover, no patients should ever experience life-threatening levels of hypoxemia in order to avoid possible oxygen toxicity.

Barash PG, Cullen BF, Stoelting RK (eds): Clinical Anesthesia, 3rd ed, pp 1111–1112. Philadelphia, Lippincott-Raven, 1997

Deneke SM, Fanburg BL: Normobaric oxygen toxicity of the lung. N Engl J Med 303:76–86, 1980

Frank L, Massaro D: Oxygen toxicity. Am J Med 69:117, 1980

Miller RD (ed): Anesthesia, 4th ed, p 614. New York, Churchill Livingstone, 1994

Nunn JF: Nunn's Applied Respiratory Physiology, 4th ed, pp 542–554. Oxford, Butterworth-Heinemann, 1993

Shapiro BA, Kacmarek RM, Cane RD et al (eds): Clinical Application of Respiratory Care, 4th ed, pp 148–149. St Louis, Mosby-Year Book, 1991

Winter PM: Pulmonary oxygen toxicity. ASA Refresher Courses in Anesthesiology 2:163–177, 1974

D.3. What is the mechanism of oxygen toxicity?

The so-called free radical theory of oxygen toxicity proposed in the early 1960s has garnered a great deal of recent experimental support and is now accepted as the most probable molecular-level explanation for oxygen toxicity. Various highly reactive and potentially cytotoxic free radical products of oxygen are generated metabolically in the cell. These short-lived O_2 metabolites, including superoxide anion (O_2^-), hydroxyl radical (OH), hydrogen peroxide (H_2O_2), and singlet oxygen (O_2), have been shown to be capable of effects such as inactivation of sulfhydryl enzymes, interaction with and disruption of DNA, and peroxidation of unsaturated membrane lipids with resultant loss of membrane integrity. The cell is also equipped with an array of antioxidant defenses, including the enzymes superoxide dismutase (SOD), catalase, glutathione peroxidase, vitamin E, and ascorbate. Under hyperoxia, the intracellular generation and influx of free radicals is believed to increase markedly and may overwhelm the detoxifying capacity of the normal complement of antioxidant defenses, with resultant cytotoxicity.

Frank L, Massaro D: The lung and oxygen toxicity. Arch Intern Med 139:347–350, 1979

Freeman BA, Crapo JD: Free radicals and tissue injury. Lab Invest 47:412, 1982

Nunn JF: Nunn's Applied Respiratory Physiology, 4th ed, pp 542–554. Oxford, Butterworth-Heinemann, 1993

Shapiro BA, Kacmarek RM, Cane RD et al (eds): Clinical Application of Respiratory Care, 4th ed, pp 148–149. St. Louis, Mosby-Year Book, 1991

D.4. What is the pathology of pulmonary oxygen toxicity?

The pathology of oxygen toxicity is nonspecific and consists of atelectasis, edema, alveolar hemorrhage, inflammation, fibrin deposition, and thickening and hyalinization of alveolar membranes. There are exudative and proliferative phases. Capillary endothelium is damaged early and plasma leaks into interstitial and alveolar spaces. Pulmonary surfactant may be altered. Type I alveolar lining cells are injured early and bronchiolar and tracheal ciliated cells can be damaged by 80% to 100% oxygen. Resolution of exudative changes, hyperplasia of alveolar type II cells, fibroplastic proliferation, and interstitial fibrosis occur with recovery or with the development of tolerance to oxygen. Total resolution is possible if the initial hyperoxia is not overwhelming.

Deneke SM, Fanbarg BL: Normobaric oxygen toxicity of the lung. N Engl J Med 303:76–86, 1980

Nunn JF: Nunn's Applied Respiratory Physiology, 4th ed, pp 542–554. Oxford, Butterworth-Heinemann, 1993

D.5. How do you improve oxygenation without increasing F_IO_2?

Positive end-expiratory pressure (PEEP) may be applied to improve oxygenation. Diuretic therapy may be used to decrease interstitial pulmonary edema and improve oxygenation.

D.6. What are your criteria to start PEEP?

If PaO_2 is <60 mm Hg with F_IO_2 of 0.50 or more, PEEP is indicated. However, since 5 to 10 cm H_2O PEEP has little or no clinically detrimental effect on cardiovascular function while improving arterial oxygenation, there is little contraindication for PEEP therapy.

Shapiro BA, Kacmarek RM, Cane RD et al (eds): Clinical Application of Respiratory Care, 4th ed, p 356. St. Louis, Mosby-Year Book, 1991

D.7. What are PEEP, CPAP, CPPV, EPAP, IPAP, and ZEEP?

PEEP refers to positive end-expiratory pressure. CPAP denotes continuous positive airway pressure. CPPV signifies continuous positive pressure ventilation. EPAP means expiratory positive airway pressure. IPAP stands for inspiratory airway pressure. ZEEP denotes zero end-expiratory pressure. The terminology is not standardized. In order to understand the literature, it is important to know the airway pressure patterns during inspiration and expiration. Respiration may be categorized into the following three types: spontaneous breathing (SB); mechanical ventilation (MV); and intermittent mandatory ventilation (IMV), which is the combination of SB and MV. Mechanical ventilation with IPAP and ZEEP is called intermittent positive pressure ventilation (IPPV). Mechanical ventilation with PEEP is equal to CPPV. Therefore, CPPV = IPPV + PEEP. Both CPPV and CPAP have positive airway pressure during both inspiratory and expiratory phases (IPAP + EPAP). CPPV is usually used with mechanical ventilation, whereas CPAP is usually used with spontaneous breathing. PEEP is often referred to as CPPV. However, "spontaneous PEEP" has been used to describe a different respiratory pattern. In spontaneous PEEP, the inspiratory airway pressure can be positive, zero, or negative, depending on the inspiratory efforts and the level of PEEP. When PEEP is low and inspiratory effort is strong, the inspiratory airway pressure tends to reach levels below zero. PEEP or EPAP only describes the airway pressure during expiration and is not equivalent to CPAP or CPPV. The different airway pressure patterns are shown in Figure 3-1.

Ashbough DG et al: Continuous positive-pressure breathing (CPPV) in adult respiratory distress syndrome. J Thorac Cardiovasc Surg 57:31–41, 1969

Gillick JS: Spontaneous positive end-expiratory pressure (SPEEP). Anesth Analg 56:627–632, 1977

Gregory GA et al: Treatment of the idiopathic respiratory distress syndrome with continuous positive airway pressure. N Engl J Med 284:1333–1340, 1971

Shapiro BA, Cane RD, Harrison RA: Positive end-expiratory pressure therapy in adults with special reference to acute lung injury: A review of the literature and suggested clinical correlations. Crit Care Med 12:127–141, 1984

Shapiro BA, Kacmarek RM, Cane RD et al (eds): Clinical Application of Respiratory Care, 4th ed, pp 304, 336. St. Louis, Mosby-Year Book, 1991

D.8. How does PEEP improve arterial oxygenation?

The mechanism is related to an increase in the functional residual capacity (FRC) and redistribution of extravascular lung water. The FRC expands linearly with increases in the end-expiratory pressure, usually at a rate of 400 cc or more for each 5 cm H_2O end-expiratory pressure. This increase in FRC represents alveoli that remain open and available for gas exchange during all phases of the respiratory cycle. The increase in FRC improves the relationship between FRC and closing capacity and therefore decreases intrapulmonary shunt or venous admixture.

PEEP therapy changes the distribution of interstitial lung water but does not di-

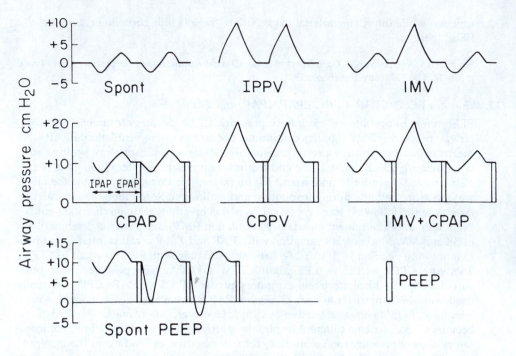

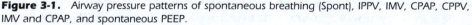

Figure 3-1. Airway pressure patterns of spontaneous breathing (Spont), IPPV, IMV, CPAP, CPPV, IMV and CPAP, and spontaneous PEEP.

rectly decrease lung water. PEEP facilitates the movement of water from the less compliant interstitial spaces (between the alveolar epithelium and capillary endothelium, where gas exchange occurs) to the more compliant interstitial spaces (toward the peribronchial and hilar areas). This redistribution of interstitial lung water improves oxygen diffusion across the alveolar-capillary membrane, resulting in increased arterial oxygenation.

Abbound N, Rehder K, Rodarte JR et al: Lung volume and closing capacity with continuous positive airway pressure. Anesthesiology 42:138–142, 1975

Benumof JL: Anesthesia for Thoracic Surgery, 2nd ed, pp 724–725. Philadelphia, WB Saunders, 1995

Miller WC, Rice DL, Unger KM et al: Effect of PEEP on lung water content in experimental noncardiogenic pulmonary edema. Crit Care Med 9:7, 1981

Pare PD, Warriner B, Baile M et al: Redistribution of pulmonary extravascular water with positive and expiratory pressure in canine pulmonary edema. Am Rev Respir Dis 127:590, 1983

Pinsky MP: Cardiovascular effects of ventilatory support and withdrawal. Anesth Analg 79:567–576, 1995

Shapiro BA, Kacmarek RM, Cane RD et al (eds): Clinical Application of Respiratory Care, 4th ed, pp 335–340. St. Louis, Mosby-Year Book, 1991

D.9. What are prophylactic, conventional, and high PEEP?

The ranges of PEEP can be divided into the following three groups:

- Prophylactic PEEP—1 to 5 cm H_2O, used to increase FRC to more than closing capacity, to prevent atelectasis and decrease shunting
- Conventional PEEP—6 to 20 cm H_2O, indicated if PaO_2 is <60 mm Hg with F_IO_2 >50%
- High PEEP—over 20 cm H_2O, used in extreme hypoxemia when there is no response to conventional PEEP

D.10. What is best PEEP or optimal PEEP?

Best *conventional* PEEP was described by Suter and associates in 1975. The best PEEP is defined as the level of PEEP with the highest oxygen transport, which is the product of cardiac output and oxygen content. This PEEP correlates with the highest total respiratory compliance, the highest mixed venous oxygen tension, and the lowest VD/VT (Fig. 3-2). Arterial oxygen tension and intrapulmonary shunt are not good indicators of the best conventional PEEP. They continue to improve even after this level has been reached. Oxygen transport decreases after the best PEEP is reached, because the cardiac output decreases.

Optimal *high* PEEP was described by Civetta in 1975. It is defined as the level of PEEP with the lowest intrapulmonary shunt and without compromising cardiac output. The PEEP used in Civetta's report is so-called high or super PEEP, over 25 cm H_2O, while the PEEP in Suter's article is conventional PEEP, ranging from 5 to 20 cm H_2O. However, the concept of best or optimal PEEP has evolved over the years. Recently, the end point for PEEP application is the lowest level of PEEP that provides an adequate PaO_2 on an F_IO_2 of <0.5. Increasing PEEP beyond this level to obtain optimal values for various other end points, such as the production of maximum oxygen transport, maximum static pulmonary compliance, shunt <15% to 20%, minimal arterial end-tidal CO_2 gradient, decreased mixed venous oxygen tension, and minimal F_IO_2 will not be clinically helpful and may be harmful.

Albert RK: Least PEEP: Primum non nocere. Chest 87:2–3, 1985

Benumof JL: Anesthesia for Thoracic Surgery, 2nd ed, p 725. Philadelphia, WB Saunders, 1995

Carrol GC, Tuman KJ, Braverman B et al: Minimal positive end-expiratory pressure (PEEP) may be best PEEP. Chest 93:1020–1025, 1988

Civetta JM, Barnes TA, Smith LO: Optimal PEEP and intermittent mandatory ventilation in the treatment of acute respiratory failure. Respiratory Care 20:551–557, 1975

Suter PM, Fairley HB, Isenberg MD: Optimum end-expiratory airway pressure in patients with acute pulmonary failure. N Engl J Med 292:284–288, 1975

D.11. How would you monitor the level of PEEP?

The level of PEEP needed depends on the severity of pulmonary injury and the response of the individual patient. It is important to titrate the levels of PEEP individually to lower the F_IO_2 to below 50%. PEEP is progressively added in 2.5 to 5.0 cm H_2O increments until the PaO_2 is relatively normal for the patient or at least above 60 mm Hg with an F_IO_2 <0.5. When low levels of PEEP (< 10 cm H_2O) are used, PaO_2, total respiratory compliance, $P\bar{v}O_2$, $(A-a)DO_2$, and QS/QT have to be monitored. When high levels of PEEP are used, cardiac output measurement is necessary

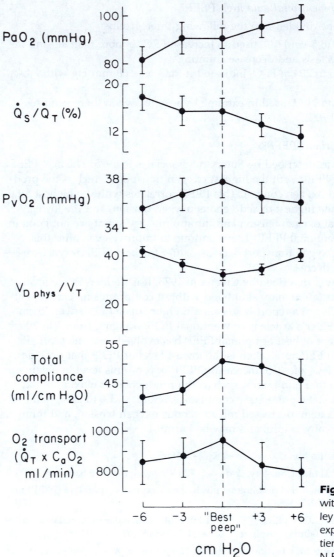

Figure 3-2. Best PEEP. (Modified with permission from Suter PM, Fairley HB, Isenberg MD: Optimal end-expiratory airway pressure in patients with acute pulmonary failure. N Engl J Med 292:284–288, 1975)

because excessive PEEP decreases cardiac output. Moreover, PEEP should be increased and decreased in increments. The evaluation of cardiac and pulmonary effects may be accomplished within a short time period (as early as 5 minutes) after a change in PEEP level.

Benumof JL: Anesthesia for Thoracic Surgery 2nd ed, p 725. Philadelphia, WB Saunders, 1995

Shapiro BA, Kacmarek RM, Cane RD et al (eds): Clinical Application of Respiratory Care, 4th ed, pp 351–354. St. Louis, Mosby-Year Book, 1991

D.12. What are the cardiovascular effects of PEEP?

The cardiovascular effects of PEEP depend on the severity of respiratory failure, the level of PEEP, the intravascular volume, the contractility of the heart, and the pulmonary vasculature. In normal subjects without respiratory failure, PEEP decreases cardiac output mainly because of increased intrathoracic pressure resulting in decreased venous return. PEEP also causes pulmonary parenchymal overdistention, which makes the lung come in close contact with the left ventricle, changing compliance and interfering with ventricular function. In addition, PEEP increases pulmonary pressure and resistance, resulting in right ventricular dilatation, which causes intraventricular septum shift into the left ventricle. The leftward septal shift decreases left ventricular diastolic filling, resulting in decreased stroke volume and cardiac output. In addition, unilateral pulmonary hyperinflation may cause neural reflex, resulting in a decreased cardiac output and heart rate. Moreover, humoral depression of myocardial contractility may also be a factor.

In persons with respiratory failure, PEEP, up to optimal levels, usually increases or does not change cardiac output because of an increase in oxygenation with resultant improvement of cardiac performance. Cardiac output falls when PEEP exceeds the individual's optimal PEEP. Hypovolemia increases hypotension during PEEP therapy.

In patients with underlying left ventricular failure and filling pressure >18 mm Hg, PEEP may increase cardiac output by increasing coronary arterial oxygen content, augmenting systolic function, or reducing venous return. The decreased venous return may produce a shift in the Starling curve to filling pressures associated with better myocardial function.

Benumof JL: Anesthesia for Thoracic Surgery, 2nd ed, pp 725–729. Philadelphia, WB Saunders, 1995

Pinsky MP: Cardiovascular effects of ventilatory support and withdrawal. Anesth Analg 79:567–576, 1995

Robotham JL, Lixfeld W, Holland L et al: The effects of positive end-expiratory pressure on right and left ventricular performance. Am Rev Respir Dis 121:677–683, 1980

D.13. How would you correct hypotension during mechanical ventilation with PEEP?

Hypovolemia has to be corrected first. When the patient is normovolemic, hypotension and low cardiac output from PEEP may be corrected by either expansion of the blood volume or infusion of dopamine. When there is some degree of cardiac failure, hypervolemia can be dangerous. Therefore, dopamine is preferred in cardiac patients. However, dopamine produces a substantial increase in pulmonary shunt.

Berk JL, Hagen JF, Tongirk, Maly GI: The use of dopamine to correct the reduced cardiac output resulting from positive end-expiratory pressure: A two-edged sword. Crit Care Med 5:269–271, 1977

Quist J, Pontoppidan H, Wilson RS et al: Hemodynamic responses to mechanical ventilation with PEEP: The effect of hypervolemia. Anesthesiology 42:45–55, 1975

D.14. What are the complications of CPPV?

CPPV has the same complications as IPPV. Because of higher mean and peak airway pressures with CPPV, the incidences of barotrauma and hypotension are greater with

CPPV. IPPV increases urinary output and decreases plasma antidiuretic hormone (ADH). CPPV decreases urinary output and increases plasma ADH.

Baratz RA, Philbin DM, Patterson RW: Plasma antidiuretic hormone and urinary output during continuous positive-pressure breathing in dogs. Anesthesiology 34:510–513, 1971

Hedley-Whyte J, Burgess GE, Feeley TW et al: Applied Physiology of Respiratory Care, pp 23–26. Boston, Little, Brown, 1976

Shapiro BA, Kacmarek RM, Cane RD et al (eds): Clinical Application of Respiratory Care, 4th ed, pp 376–383. St. Louis, Mosby-Year Book, 1991

D.15. *What is pressure support ventilation (PSV)? Discuss its advantages.*

Pressure support ventilation is pressure-limited, flow-controlled, positive pressure ventilation during which each spontaneous inspiratory effort is assisted by mechanically maintaining a predetermined inspiratory pressure plateau throughout inspiration. PSV can be used for patients who are breathing completely spontaneously or who are being supported with IMV; it can also be used for patients receiving CPAP.

PSV, which is an adjunct form of ventilatory support, is controlled with a microprocessor incorporated into the mechanical ventilator's circuit. When the patient makes the initial inspiratory effort, the slight negative pressure change is detected by a very sensitive pressure transducer, and application of a constant support pressure is begun. Pressure is applied continuously throughout inspiration at the value selected by the operator. The airway pressure curves of pressure support ventilation are shown in Figure 3-3.

The advantages of PSV are as follows:

- Achieving larger tidal volumes with lower airway pressures
- Decreasing work of breathing
- Improving spontaneous breathing patterns, including decreased respiratory rate, longer expiratory phase, and better synchrony with mechanical ventilation
- Promoting weaning from mechanical ventilation because of decreased respiratory muscle fatigue

Unfortunately, to date there are few clinical studies documenting the efficacy of PSV, although theoretical advantages and safety of the mode in appropriately monitored patients support its use.

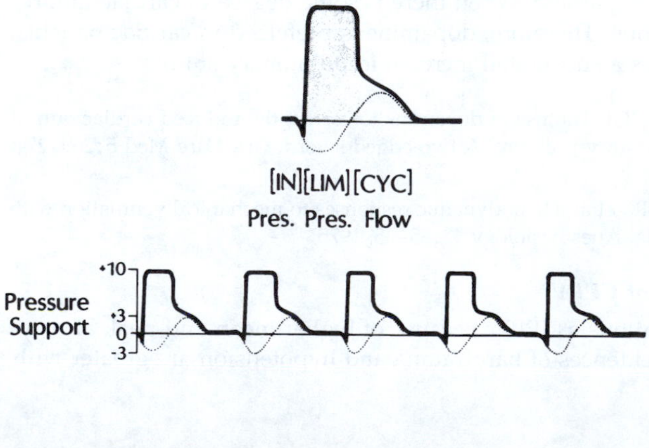

Figure 3-3. Airway pressure tracings of pressure support ventilation (solid line) and spontaneous ventilation (dotted line). IN = initiation; LIM = limit; CYC = cycle. (Reprinted with permission from Shapiro BA, Kacmarek RM, Cane RD et al: Clinical Application of Respiratory Care, 4th ed, p 317. St. Louis, Mosby-Year Book, 1991)

Barash PG, Cullen BF, Stoelting RK (eds): Clinical Anesthesia, 3rd ed, p 1374. Philadelphia, Lippin-cott-Raven, 1997

Benumof JL: Anesthesia for Thoracic Surgery, 2nd ed, pp 741–742. Philadelphia, WB Saunders, 1995

Shapiro BA, Kacmarek RM, Cane RD et al (eds): Clinical Application of Respiratory Care, 4th ed, pp 313–316. St. Louis, Mosby-Year Book, 1991

D.16. What is airway pressure release ventilation (APRV)? What are the advantages of APRV?

Airway pressure release ventilation is a new ventilatory support technique designed to augment alveolar ventilation in patients who require ventilatory assistance despite reduction of ventilatory work with CPAP. The APRV system includes a CPAP circuit in which inflation airway pressure is maintained above ambient pressure with the use of a threshold resistor valve and either a high gas flow or a pressurized volume reservoir. A release valve is situated in the expiratory limb of the CPAP circuit to allow rapid decrease in airway pressure (release pressure). The release valve must have extremely low resistance to allow an adequate emptying of the lungs during pressure release. The release valve is driven by a timing device that allows adjustment of the extent, length, and frequency of pressure release. The airway pressure curves of APRV are shown in Figure 3-4.

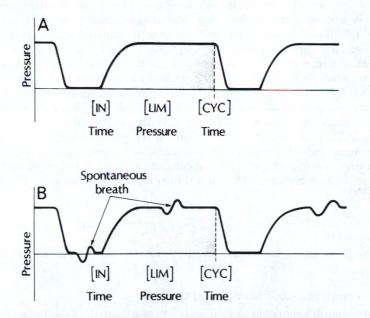

Figure 3-4. APRV airway pressure curves. A represents APRV without spontaneous breathing efforts. B represents APRV with spontaneous breaths. IN = initiation; LIM = limit; CYC = cycle. (Reprinted with permission from Shapiro BA, Kacmarek RM, Cane RD et al: Clinical Application of Respiratory Care, 4th ed, p 319. St. Louis: Mosby-Year Book, 1991)

The APRV technique is utilized to produce an inversed I:E ratio of 4:1 or 5:1. The lung volume at end-inspiration will be primarily determined by the inflation pressure and the pulmonary compliance. The end-exhalation lung volume will be determined by lung compliance, airway resistance, release time, and the gradient between the inflation and release preset pressures.

The advantages of APRV include the following:

- Delivering mechanical breaths to ventilate the lungs without increasing airway pressure excessively
- Delivering the required CPAP level without depressing cardiac output
- Allowing unrestricted spontaneous ventilation
- Having the advantages of IMV without the risk of high airway pressure

Barash PG, Cullen BF, Stoelting RK (eds): Clinical Anesthesia, 3rd ed, pp 1374–1375. Philadelphia, Lippincott-Raven, 1997

Benumof JL: Anesthesia for Thoracic Surgery, 2nd ed, pp 743–744. Philadelphia, WB Saunders, 1995

Shapiro BA, Kacmarek RM, Cane RD et al (eds): Clinical Application of Respiratory Care, 4th ed, pp 316–319. St. Louis, Mosby-Year Book, 1991

D.17. *What is extended mandatory minute ventilation (EMMV)?*

EMMV provides a preset minute volume of gas either from a positive pressure breath or from spontaneous breathing. The airway pressure waveform is similar to that of IMV (Fig. 3-5). The clinician determines the minimal accepted minute volume and selects the appropriate rate and tidal volume. The advantage is that the patient is guaranteed a minimal minute ventilation regardless of the patient's own spontaneous effort or drive. As the patient's ability to breathe spontaneously improves, less assisted ventilation is provided and the weaning process becomes automatic. However, there are two main disadvantages. First, it is difficult to estimate the right value of minute volume because it varies greatly according to the patient's dead space ventilation and CO_2 level. Second, minute volume is composed of both ventilatory rate and tidal volume. Indeed, the patient may accomplish the preset minute volume value by shallow hyperventilation, which is not clinically acceptable and might signify impending respiratory catastrophe. Thus, it is difficult to see the practicality of EMMV at this stage.

Barash PG, Cullen BF, Stoelting RK (eds): Clinical Anesthesia, 3rd ed, p 1374. Philadelphia, Lippincott-Raven, 1997

Benumof JL: Anesthesia for Thoracic Surgery, 2nd ed, pp 744–745. Philadelphia, WB Saunders, 1995

D.18. *What is pressure control ventilation (PCV)?*

Pressure control ventilation is a patient- or time-triggered, pressure-limited, time-cycled mode of ventilatory support (Fig. 3-5). It is characterized by a rapid rise to peak pressure afforded by a decelerating inspiratory flow pattern. A pressure-controlled breath can be delivered in intermittent mandatory ventilation or assist mechanical ventilation instead of volume-oriented breaths, or in conjunction with pressure support ventilation. During PCV, the peak airway pressure is maintained throughout in-

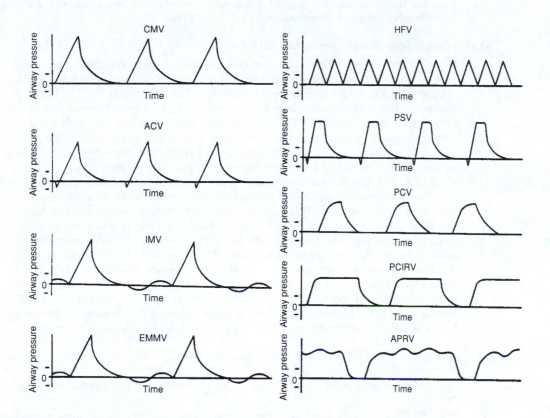

Figure 3-5. Airway pressure waveforms. CMV = controlled mechanical ventilation; ACV = assist control ventilation; IMV = intermittent mandatory ventilation; EMMV = extended mandatory minute ventilation; HFV = high-frequency ventilation; PSV = pressure support ventilation; PCV = pressure control ventilation; PCIRV = pressure control inverse ratio ventilation; APRV = airway pressure release ventilation. (Reprinted with permission from Barash PG, Cullen BF, Stoelting RK [eds]: Clinical Anesthesia, 3rd ed, p 1375. Philadelphia, Lippincott-Raven, 1997)

spiration, allowing inflation of all lung units to a degree that depends primarily on compliance. Thus lung units that are not inflated during conventional volume-controlled ventilation (VCV) may be inflated during PCV, a process called alveolar recruitment. These recruited lung units are maintained open by the addition of an appropriate level of PEEP. The combination of a low-level PEEP and a moderate but constant level of inspiratory pressure during PCV increases mean airway pressure at a lower peak pressure than occurs during VCV. The major disadvantage of pressure control ventilation is that tidal volume varies as compliance and resistance of the airways change.

Barash PG, Cullen BF, Stoelting RK (eds): Clinical Anesthesia, 3rd ed, p 1375. Philadelphia, Lippincott-Raven, 1997

Pearl RG: New therapies to manage adult respiratory distress syndrome, including nitric oxide. ASA Refresher Courses in Anesthesiology 23:177–187, 1995

D.19. What is inverse-ratio ventilation (IRV)?

In spontaneous breathing and conventional mechanical ventilation, the expiratory time is longer than the inspiratory time, whereas in inverse-ratio ventilation, the inspiratory time is longer than the expiratory time. The I:E ratio is >1:1 in IRV. Inflation of the lungs, therefore, proceeds at a lower mean inspiratory flow. Like conventional mechanical ventilation, IRV may be either volume or pressure preset, but it is usually pressure preset. Pressure control inverse ratio ventilation (PC-IRV) is a time-triggered, pressure-limited, time-cycled mode of ventilation characterized by a decelerating inspiratory flow pattern, square wave air pressure pattern, and I:E ratio of ≥1:1 (Fig. 3-5). The potential advantage of this mode of ventilation is the recruitment of collapsed alveoli by prolonged inspiratory times, which allow alveolar units with slow time constants to fill. This improves both oxygenation and ventilation. Many studies have suggested that PC-IRV may produce better oxygenation and carbon dioxide elimination than does conventional VCV. However, PC-IRV commonly results in the development of intrinsic or auto-PEEP (dynamic hyperinflation) due to the short expiratory times used. Thus total PEEP (the sum of intrinsic PEEP plus applied PEEP) is frequently increased during PC-IRV and may be responsible for the improvement in oxygenation. The potential hazard is the development of auto-PEEP with consequent high airway pressure. Another potential disadvantage is the need of heavy sedation or paralysis to allow the patient to tolerate the long inspiration.

Barash PG, Cullen BF, Stoelting RK (eds): Clinical Anesthesia, 3rd ed, p 1375. Philadelphia, Lippincott-Raven, 1997

Benumof JL: Anesthesia for Thoracic Surgery, 2nd ed, pp 742–743. Philadelphia, WB Saunders, 1995

Pearl RG: New therapies to manage adult respiratory distress syndrome, including nitric oxide. ASA Refresher Courses in Anesthesiology 23:177–187, 1995

E. Weaning from Ventilatory Support

The patient's condition improved after respiratory support with 20 cm H_2O PEEP. Arterial blood gases showed pH 7.45; Pco_2, 35 mm Hg; Po_2, 150 mm Hg; F_IO_2 0.75.

E.1. What would you do now? Lower F_IO_2 or lower PEEP?

Because PaO_2 is 150 mm Hg, F_IO_2 should be lowered gradually to prevent oxygen toxicity. When F_IO_2 is lowered to <0.5 or 0.6, PEEP level should be lowered gradually to avoid increased barotrauma and decreased cardiac output associated with excessive PEEP. The suggested criteria to lower PEEP level are a stable, nonseptic patient; $PaO_2/F_IO_2 > 200$ mm Hg; effective compliance > 25 ml/cm H_2O; $(A-a)DO_2 < 200$ mm Hg at F_IO_2 0.5. PEEP should not be decreased by >5 cm H_2O during a trial. At least 6 hours should elapse before undertaking a further attempt at lowering the PEEP level.

Benumof JL: Anesthesia for Thoracic Surgery, 2nd ed, p 724. Philadelphia, WB Saunders, 1995

Luterman A, Hororvitz JH, Carrico CJ et al: Withdrawal from PEEP. Surgery 39:328–332, 1978

Shapiro BA, Kacmarek RM, Cane RD et al (eds): Clinical Application of Respiratory Care, 4th ed, pp 296–302. St. Louis, Mosby-Year Book, 1991

E.2. The patient continued to improve. When would you consider weaning the patient from the respirator? Discuss the criteria for weaning.

The criteria for discontinuance of mechanical ventilation are essentially the converse of the criteria for the institution of mechanical support and are as follows:

- Clear consciousness with adequate gag and cough reflex
- Cardiovascular stability
- Stable metabolic state without hypothermia, hyperpyrexia, metabolic acidosis, or alkalosis
- Adequate pulmonary function

Mechanics
- A vital capacity of >10 ml/kg or more than twice the normal tidal volume
- A maximum inspiratory force of at least -20 to -30 cm H_2O

Oxygenation
- $PaO_2 > 80$ mm Hg with F_IO_2 0.4
- $(A-a)DO_2 < 300$ mm Hg with F_IO_2 1.0
- $QS/QT < 15\%$

Ventilation
- $PaCO_2 < 45$ mm Hg
- $VD/VT < 0.6$

Benumof JL: Anesthesia for Thoracic Surgery, 2nd ed, pp 738–740. Philadelphia, WB Saunders, 1995

Shapiro BA, Kacmarek RM, Cane RD et al (eds): Clinical Application of Respiratory Care, 4th ed, pp 296–302. St. Louis, Mosby-Year Book, 1991

E.3. How would you wean the patient from the respirator?

There are two common methods for weaning the patient from the respirator—the conventional T-piece technique and the intermittent mandatory ventilation technique.

Conventional T-Piece Technique
When the patient meets the criteria for weaning, a T-piece adapter and heated nebulizer are connected to the patient's endotracheal tube. The patient should be in a semi-sitting or sitting position. The inspired oxygen concentration is set at a level 5% to 10% higher than the patient was receiving during mechanical ventilation. The vital signs and cardiac rhythm are monitored carefully every 5 to 10 minutes. Arterial blood gases are determined 15 minutes after weaning is begun and then every hour. The patient who tolerates the T-piece very well is extubated after 2 to 4 hours. Oxygen is then administered through a face mask with a heated nebulizer, at the same inspired oxygen concentration as during the T-piece trial.

Intermittent Mandatory Ventilation Technique
Weaning is accomplished by a gradual decrease in the IMV rate that the ventilator delivers, allowing the patient slowly to take over spontaneous ventilation. This system allows the patient to breathe spontaneously between the preset mechanical venti-

lation. This system assures intermittent hyperinflation of the lung. IMV has been reported to be helpful in weaning when conventional methods have failed.

Spontaneous PEEP can be applied to both weaning techniques. PEEP is especially useful in patients in whom rapid alveolar collapse and hypoxemia develop during weaning. Five cm H_2O PEEP during weaning minimizes alveolar collapse and improves the relationship between the closing capacity and functional residual capacity.

There are several other methods of weaning. These include progressively decreasing the level of pressure support, increasing periods of time on a T-piece, and increasing the trigger threshold of the assist-control mode. There is no evidence that any one of the techniques of partial support is inherently better than the others.

Benumof JL: Anesthesia for Thoracic Surgery, 2nd ed, pp 738–740. Philadelphia, WB Saunders, 1995

Feeley TW, Hedley-Whyte J: Weaning from controlled ventilation and supplemental oxygen. N Engl J Med 292:903–906, 1975

Shapiro BA, Kacmarek RM, Cane RD et al (eds): Clinical Application of Respiratory Care, 4th ed, pp 296–302. St. Louis, Mosby-Year Book, 1991

E.4. What are IMV, IAV, and IDV?

IMV refers to intermittent mandatory ventilation. IMV comprises breaths controlled by the ventilator as well as breaths supplied spontaneously by the patient (Fig. 3-1). The same inspired oxygen concentration is used for both forms of ventilation. The air-oxygen mixture is led to a reservoir bag and connected to the ventilator tubing by a one-way valve immediately before the humidifier. Although IMV was originally introduced as a weaning technique, it is now used by some groups as a primary means of ventilatory support, especially in combination with high levels of PEEP, throughout the entire course of a patient's illness. Because the ventilator cycles are independent of the patient's breathing phase, airway and intrapleural pressure may increase when IMV inflations come at the end of spontaneous inhalation.

IAV stands for intermittent assisted ventilation, which is also called synchronized IMV (SIMV). Each mechanical ventilation is triggered by the patient. Both IMV and IAV rates are set by the operator.

IDV means intermittent demand ventilation. Each mechanical ventilation is triggered by the patient as in IAV. The operator sets the IDV/spontaneous breathing ratio rather than the IDV rate. Therefore, the total IDV rate varies with the spontaneous breathing rate.

Benumof JL: Anesthesia for Thoracic Surgery, 2nd ed, pp 738–740. Philadelphia, WB Saunders, 1995

Kaplan JA (ed): Thoracic Anesthesia, 2nd ed, pp 665–666. New York, Churchill Livingstone, 1991

E.5. What are the advantages and disadvantages of IMV over controlled or assisted ventilation?

The advantages of IMV are as follows:

- There is selective application of mechanical support in accord with the individual patient's need.
- It is more comfortable for the patient. There is less need for sedatives or narcotics.

- There is a higher cardiac output because intrathoracic pressure is lower.
- There is decreased incidence of barotrauma because airway pressure is lower.
- There is less discoordination on spontaneous breathing because the respiratory center is activated and the patient uses his respiratory muscles.
- There is less psychological dependence on the ventilator.

The disadvantages of IMV are as follows:

- The risk of CO_2 retention is greater because IMV does not respond to increased ventilatory demand.
- The work of breathing is increased.
- There is a possibility of respiratory muscle fatigue.
- Weaning may be prolonged if the IMV rate is decreased too slowly.
- Cardiac decompression occurs more frequently during weaning from mechanical ventilation.

Shapiro BA, Kacmarek RM, Cane RD et al (eds): Clinical Application of Respiratory Care, 4th ed, pp 311–312. St. Louis, Mosby-Year Book, 1991

Wilson RS: Techniques of ventilatory control: Indications and complications. ASA Refresher Courses in Anesthesiology 13:221–232, 1985

F. Special Techniques of Respiratory Support

F.1. What is differential or selective PEEP? What are the indications?

By using a double-lumen endobronchial tube, both lungs can be ventilated simultaneously and separately with different levels of PEEP to each lung. Two ventilators have to be synchronized by a controller to prevent mediastinal movement and cardiovascular instability. A modified circuit has been described by Power and associates to permit independent ventilation from a single ventilator. Selective PEEP is indicated when there is a severe unilateral pulmonary disorder, such as pneumonia or atelectasis, because certain PEEP levels may be too high for the normal lung and too low for the pathologic lung. The second indication for selective PEEP is bilateral basilar disease. Reversal of atelectasis and improvement in ventilation/perfusion ratio in both lungs can be achieved by placing the patient in the lateral decubitus position, ventilating each lung separately and applying PEEP to only the dependent lung. Three additional specific indications for selective lung ventilation are bronchiopleural fistula, massive refractory unilateral atelectasis and excessive air trapping (causing hypotension) in a remaining emphysematous lung after single-lung transplantation.

Benumof JL: Anesthesia for Thoracic Surgery, 2nd ed, pp 729–733. Philadelphia, WB Saunders, 1995

Power DJ, Eross B, Grenvik A: Differential lung ventilation with PEEP in the treatment of unilateral pneumonia. Crit Care Med 5:170–172, 1977

Trew GF, Warren BR, Potter WA: Differential ventilation of the lungs in man. Crit Care Med 4:112, 1976

F.2. What are the indications and contraindications for extracorporeal membrane oxygenation (ECMO)? How many ways can ECMO be used? What are the results of EMCO?

ECMO should be used for patients in severe acute respiratory failure with reversible lung disease, who are dying of severe hypoxemia despite maximal conventional ventilatory care as defined here (tracheal intubation, mechanical ventilation with 10 to 15 cm H_2O PEEP, diuresis, chest physical therapy, antibiotics, normothermia or mild hypothermia, sedation, paralysis, and increased oxygen concentration). National Institutes of Health indications are as follows: a $PaO_2 < 50$ mm Hg for > 2 hours with F_IO_2 of 1.0 and conventional PEEP; and a $PaO_2 < 50$ mm Hg for > 12 hours with F_IO_2 of >0.6 and conventional PEEP. Active bleeding is the only absolute contraindication to use of the artificial lung. There are three routes for ECMO—venovenous perfusion from the inferior vena cava by way of the femoral vein to the oxygenator and then to the superior vena cava; venoarterial perfusion from the femoral vein to the oxygenator and then to the femoral artery; and venovenous arterial perfusion from the femoral vein to the oxygenator and then to both the internal jugular vein and the femoral artery.

A collaborative study on ECMO has been completed under the auspices of the National Heart, Lung, and Blood Institute of the National Institutes of Health. The results of this controlled study were as follows:

- Compared with the control group of conventional respiratory therapy, ECMO did not improve mortality (90%), the predominant cause of death still being progressive respiratory failure.
- ECMO did not affect the progress of disease (or lung pathology in those patients who died) any differently than conventional respiratory therapy.
- Although ECMO is an effective means of short-term life support, its clinical application for the treatment of acute respiratory distress syndrome is not appropriate or economically justified.

However, data analyzed from a national registry series of 715 neonatal ECMO patients (1980 to 1987) demonstrated an overall survival of 81%, which, in earlier series, had been the overall mortality rate with conventional therapy. As neonatal ECMO has evolved, entry criteria have been used, and experience with ECMO technology has been shown to improve survival. ECMO is now a proven support modality for neonatal respiratory failure that is due to several causes, such as meconium aspiration syndrome, persistent pulmonary hypertension of the newborn, congenital diaphragmatic hernia, and infant respiratory distress syndrome.

Barash PG, Cullen BF, Stoelting RK (eds): Clinical Anesthesia, 3rd ed, pp 1092–1093, 1104. Philadelphia, Lippincott-Raven, 1997

Extracorporeal support for respiratory insufficiency. A collaborative study. National Heart, Lung, and Blood Institute: US Dept Health, Education & Welfare, 1979

F.3. What is HFPPV? What are the characteristics of HFPPV?

High-frequency ventilation (HFV) was originally used as a technique to provide adequate oxygenation and alveolar ventilation for rigid bronchoscopy and laryngeal surgery. Since that time, the literature is replete with clinical applications of HFV. HFPPV signifies high frequency positive pressure ventilation. The major characteristics of the ventilatory pattern of volume-controlled HFPPV are as follows:

- A ventilatory frequency of about 60 to 100/min and an inspiration-expiration ratio of <0.3
- Smaller tidal volumes and therefore lower maximal and mean airway and transpulmonary pressures, yet a higher FRC than in conventional IPPV/CPPV

- Positive intratracheal and negative intrapleural pressures throughout the ventilatory cycle
- Less circulatory interference than in IPPV/CPPV
- Reflex suppression of spontaneous respiratory rhythmicity during normoventilation
- Decelerating inspiratory flow without an end-inspiratory plateau
- More efficient pulmonary gas distribution than in IPPV/CPPV

Barash PG, Cullen BF, Stoelting RK (eds): Clinical Anesthesia, 3rd ed, p 1375. Philadelphia, Lippincott-Raven, 1997

Shapiro BA, Kacmarek RM, Cane RD et al (eds): Clinical Application of Respiratory Care, 4th ed, pp 319–322. St. Louis, Mosby-Year Book, 1991

Sjostrand U: High frequency positive-pressure ventilation (HFPPV): A review. Crit Care Med 8:345–364, 1980

F.4. What are the frequencies used in high frequency ventilation (HFV)? How are they classified?

HFV is a generic term encompassing any form of mechanical ventilation operating at a frequency at least 4 times higher than the natural breathing frequency of the subject being ventilated. Smith categorized HFV in three groups:

- High frequency positive pressure ventilation (HFPPV), 60 to 110/min
- High frequency jet ventilation (HFJV), 110 to 400/min
- High frequency oscillatory ventilation (HFOV), 400 to 2400/min

Froese summarized HFV into five groups as shown in Figure 3-6.

HFPPV was first introduced by Sjostrand in Sweden. It is administered with a very low compliant ventilator with high gas flow rates. This produces a flow profile with rapid upstroke to a high peak flow rate, followed by a passive expiration. Because it is a closed circuit, there is no entrainment of additional gas during inspiration. The frequency of HFPPV is 60 to 110/min.

HFJV delivers a small tidal volume at a high flow rate by means of a narrow orifice at an adjustable drive pressure, rate, and inspiratory time or I:E ratio. Gas is regulated by a solenoid or fluidic mechanism. Since jet flow is delivered to a small-lumen tube, entrainment occurs owing to subambient pressure created at the distal end of a cannula. Exhalation occurs around the tube or through another lumen and is passive. Frequencies are commonly 100 to 200/min, occasionally up to 400/min.

HIFI (or HFFI) refers to high frequency flow interrupters. They are closely related to jet ventilators. Gas from a high pressure source is "chopped" into pulses by a rotating ball valve and directed into the lung. The frequencies are usually 100 to 200/min in adults and 300 to 1200/min in infants.

CHFV means combined high frequency ventilation. Combined approaches usually superimpose some form of HFV onto back-up conventional mechanical ventilation. The reported combinations vary considerably, with the slow component ranging from 1 to 60/min, and the fast component being delivered at 100 to 3000/min.

HFOV is delivered by an oscillator-type ventilator consisting of a rotary-driven piston to produce to-and-fro movement of gas within the airway. Unlike all the other modalities, during HFOV both inspiratory and expiratory flows are actively driven by the ventilator. Ventilator rates of 300 to 2400/min have been used.

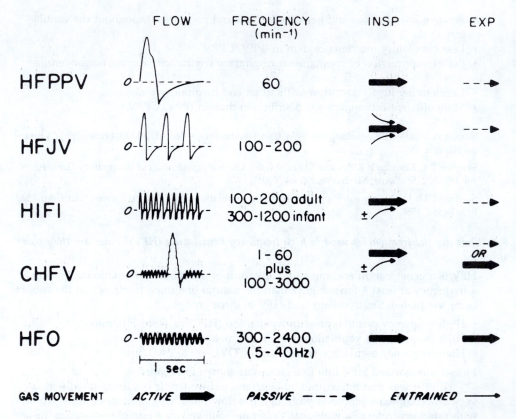

Figure 3-6. *Summary of features of several commonly encountered high-frequency modalities. See text for details. (Reprinted with permission from Froese AB: High-frequency ventilation: Uses and abuses. ASA Refresher Courses in Anesthesiology 14:127–138, 1986)*

Barash PG, Cullen BF, Stoelting RK (eds): Clinical Anesthesia, 3rd ed, p 1375. Philadelphia, Lippincott-Raven, 1997

Butler WJ, Bohn DJ, Bryan AC et al: Ventilation by high frequency oscillation in humans. Anesth Analg 59:577–584, 1980

Carlon GC, Kahn RC, Howland WS et al: Clinical experience with high frequency jet ventilation. Crit Care Med 9:1–6, 1981

El-Baz N, Faber LP, Doolas A: Combined high frequency ventilation for management of terminal respiratory failure: A new technique. Anesth Analg 62:39–49, 1983

Froese AB: High frequency ventilation: Uses and abuses. ASA Refresher Courses in Anesthesiology 14:127–138, 1986

Shapiro BA, Kacmarek RM, Cane RD et al (eds): Clinical Application of Respiratory Care, 4th ed, pp 319–322. St. Louis, Mosby-Year Book, 1991

Smith RB: Ventilation at high respiratory frequencies. Anaesthesia 37:1011, 1983

F.5. What are the indications and precautions for high frequency ventilation?

The indications for HFV include the following:

- Respiratory failure with bronchopleural fistula, tracheoesophageal or bronchoeso-phageal fistula, barotrauma, pulmonary fibrosis, and pulmonary hemorrhage, be-cause of low airway pressure with HFV.
- Anesthesia for special procedures, such as bronchoscopy, laryngoscopy, tracheal re-construction over a T-tube, and laser resection of a bronchial lesion, because HFV uses a small cannula for ventilation, leaving adequate room for surgeons to op-erate.
- Anesthesia for open thoracic surgery because of a moderately expanded lung and minimal respiratory movement with HFV.
- Improving oxygenation in adult and infant respiratory distress syndrome when hy-poxemia persists in spite of maximal conventional ventilatory support.
- Enhancement of CO_2 elimination when conventional mechanical ventilation has been unable to support adequate CO_2 elimination despite multiple adjustments of ventilator settings in situations such as persistent fetal circulation in the neonate. HFV could prove advantageous in achieving a respiratory alkalosis by hyperventi-lation at low peak and mean airway pressures.

The precautions with HFV include the following:

- HFV must never be used in a situation where expiratory outflow of gas from the lung is impeded. Under such circumstances, lethal barotrauma can occur.
- HFV should never be used with inadequate humidification, because serious tra-cheal injury may happen.
- HFV system pressure should be accurately and appropriately sampled and moni-tored in order to drive an automatic shut-off mechanism, so that gas entry into the lungs can be terminated immediately if an overpressure situation occurs.
- HFV should never be used without adequate training.

Benumof JL: Anesthesia for Thoracic Surgery, 2nd ed, pp 433–448. Philadelphia, WB Saunders, 1995

Borg U, Eriksson I, Sjostrand U: High frequency positive pressure ventilation (HFPPV): A review based upon its use during bronchoscopy and for laryngoscopy and microlaryngeal surgery under general anesthesia. Anesth Analg 59:594–603, 1980

Carlon GC, Howland WS, Ray C et al: High frequency jet ventilation. A prospective randomized evaluation. Chest 84:551–559, 1983

Carlon GC, Kahn RC, Howland WS et al: Clinical experience with high frequency jet ventilation. Crit Care Med 9:1–6, 1981

El-Baz N, Holinger L, El-Ganzouri A et al: High frequency positive-pressure ventilation for tracheal reconstruction supported by tracheal T-tube. Anesth Analg 61:796–800, 1982

Froese AB: High frequency ventilation: Uses and abuses. ASA Refresher Courses in Anesthesiology 14:127–138, 1986

Kaplan JA (ed): Thoracic Anesthesia, 2nd ed, pp 672–676. New York, Churchill Livingstone, 1991

Malina JR, Nordstrom SG, Sjostrand UH et al: Clinical evaluation of high frequency positive-pressure ventilation in patients scheduled for open-chest surgery. Anesth Analg 60:324–330, 1981

Shapiro BA, Kacmarek RM, Cane RD et al (eds): Clinical Application of Respiratory Care, 4th ed, pp 319–322. St. Louis, Mosby-Year Book, 1991

F.6. What is nitric oxide? What is the role of inhaled nitric oxide in the treatment of ARDS?

In 1987, endothelium-derived relaxing factor was identified as nitric oxide (NO). Nitric oxide produced by the endothelium diffuses into vascular smooth muscle where NO activates soluble guanylate cyclase. The subsequent increase in intracellular cyclic guanosine monophosphate (GMP) causes smooth muscle vasodilation. Endothelium-independent nitrovasodilators such as nitroglycerin and nitroprusside also act via guanylate cylcase activation by directly releasing NO.

Inhaled NO is a selective pulmonary vasodilator. NO is not effective during systemic administration because it is rapidly inactivated by hemoglobin. Therefore, inhaled NO may diffuse from the alveoli to pulmonary vascular smooth muscle and produce pulmonary vasodilation without systemic vasodilatation because any NO that diffuses into blood will be inactivated by hemoglobin. Inhaled NO has been shown to be effective in treating primary pulmonary hypertension, and decreasing pulmonary hypertension and improving oxygenation after mitral valve replacement and in the newborn with persistent pulmonary hypertension.

Pulmonary hypertension and hypoxemia universally occur in ARDS. Pulmonary hypertension in ARDS may be due to active vasoconstriction from local alveolar hypoxic pulmonary vasoconstriction and other vasoconstrictor mediators. Hypoxemia in ARDS is due to ventilation perfusion mismatch, intrapulmonary shunting, or anatomic shunting. Intravenous pulmonary vasodilator therapy with agents such as nitroglycerin, nitroprusside, prostaglandin E, prostacyclin, and nifedipine produces small reduction in pulmonary artery pressure but large reduction in systemic blood pressure and arterial oxygenation. The adverse effect on oxygenation is primarily due to reversal of hypoxic pulmonary vasoconstriction. On the contrary, inhaled NO can decrease pulmonary hypertension and improve oxygenation in patients with ARDS because inhaled NO is distributed according to ventilation so that the associated vasodilatation increases blood flow to well-ventilated alveoli.

Rossaint et al published the first major report of the use of inhaled NO in patients with ARDS. They found that inhaled NO (5 to 20 ppm) effectively decreased pulmonary hypertension and improved oxygenation. In a subsequent study, they showed that inhaled concentrations of only 60 to 250 parts per billion (ppb) could increase PaO_2 by 30%. These concentrations had little or no effect on pulmonary artery pressure. The other major study by Bigatello et al demonstrated that inhaled NO produced dose-related decreases in pulmonary artery pressure with 50% of the maximal effect occurring at 5 ppm. Inhaled NO also increased oxygenation, but dose-response effects could not be demonstrated.

Inhaled NO has been effective on ARDS in combination with other therapies. The combination of inhaled NO (5 to 10 ppm) and almitrine bismesylate, a potentiator of hypoxic pulmonary vasoconstrictor, had additive effects on improving oxygenation in ARDS and simultaneously decreased pulmonary hypertension.

However, an important unsolved issue is the potential pulmonary toxicity of inhaled NO. Toxicity may be due either to NO itself or its reactive metabolic NO_2. Nitric oxide can combine with superoxide anion to produce peroxynitrite anion, which is a powerful oxidizing agent. Therefore, it is unclear whether inhaled NO will exacerbate lung injury in ARDS. In addition, NO_2 toxicity may occur during inhaled NO therapy. The effects of NO and NO_2 on repair versus fibrosis in injured lung and on pulmonary host defenses are unknown. Therefore, the effects of inhaled NO on outcome in patients with ARDS are not predictable.

Recently, Dcering et al studied intravenous phenylephrine, 50 to 200 μg/min, titrated to a 20% increase in mean arterial pressure; inhaled NO, 40 ppm; and the combination of phenylephrine and NO. They found that phenylephrine alone can improve PaO_2 in patients with ARDS. In phenylephrine-responsive patients, phenylephrine augments the improvement in PaO_2 seen with inhaled NO. These results may reflect selective enhancement of hypoxic pulmonary vasoconstriction by phenylephrine, which complements selective vasodilation by inhaled NO.

Bigatello LM, Hurford WE, Kacmarek RM, et al: Prolonged inhalation of low concentrations of nitric oxide in patients with severe adult respiratory distress syndrome. Effect on pulmonary hemodynamics and oxygenation. Anesthesiology 80:761–770, 1994

Dcering EB, Hanson CW III, Reily DJ et al: Improvement in oxygenation by phenylephrine and nitric oxide in patients with adult respiratory distress syndrome. Anesthesiology 87:18–25, 1997

Gerlach H, Pappert D, Lewandowski K et al: Long-term inhalation with evaluated low doses of nitric oxide for selective improvement of oxygenation in patients with adult respiratory distress syndrome. Intens Care Med 19:443–449, 1993

Pearl RG: New therapies to manage adult respiratory distress syndrome, including nitric oxide. ASA Refresher Courses in Anesthesiology 23:177–187, 1995

Rossaint R, Falke KJ, Lopez F et al: Inhaled nitric oxide for the adult respiratory disease syndrome. N Engl J Med 328:399–405, 1993

Zwissler B, Welte M, Habler O et al: Effects of inhaled prostacyclin as compared with inhaled nitric oxide in a canine model of pulmonary microembolism and oleic acid edema. J Cardiothorac Vasc Anesth 9:634–640, 1995

4 Tracheoesophageal Fistula

Marjorie J. Topkins

A 12-hour-old neonate born after 37 weeks of gestation and weighing 2200 grams had frothing about the nose and mouth. The infant regurgitated the first feeding almost immediately. Coughing and cyanosis were associated with the regurgitation.

A. Medical Disease and Differential Diagnosis

1. What is the working diagnosis?
2. What information is needed to confirm the diagnosis? What information is obtained from each of the following?
   - Radiopaque catheter
   - Barium swallow or instillation
   - Chest x-ray film
   - Flat plate of the abdomen
3. Classify tracheoesophageal (TE) fistula or atresia.
4. What other congenital anomalies are associated with TE fistula or atresia?
5. What is the embryology of TE fistula?

B. Preoperative Evaluation and Preparation

1. What problems concern you and what laboratory data do you need to evaluate these problems?
2. Discuss the risk classification of infants with TE fistula or atresia according to Waterston or Calverley. What are the implications for this infant? Does this classification still hold?
3. Discuss fluid replacement for this infant.
4. What is the role of antibiotics preoperatively or postoperatively?
5. Discuss the role of gastrostomy in the management of TE fistula.
6. What premedication is indicated in this patient?

C. Intraoperative Management

1. Discuss the problems associated with transportation of this infant to the operating room.
2. What type of monitoring would you use for this case?
3. What emergency drugs should be available?
4. Discuss the problems of induction and intubation. Where would you place the endotracheal tube in relation to the fistula?
5. In what position would surgery be performed? How would this affect the management of the patient?
6. What problems can be anticipated during surgery? What anesthetic agent would you

86

use? How can a stable mediastinum be accomplished? Is there a role for muscle relaxants?

D. Postoperative Management

1. **When can this infant be extubated?**
2. **What are the dangers of hypothermia?**
3. **What are the complications seen following tracheoesophageal fistula repair?**
4. **Discuss the management of postoperative pneumonia or atelectasis. Are these anesthetic complications?**

A. Medical Disease and Differential Diagnosis

A.1. What is the working diagnosis?

The presence of frothing about the nose and mouth suggests tracheoesophageal pathology.

A history of polyhydramnios in the mother, supplied by the obstetrician, should
alert the physician to the possibility of tracheoesophageal pathology or other gastrointestinal atresias. Whether or not a catheter passes easily into the stomach is important. In some institutions it is standard practice to pass a catheter into the stomach at
birth, increasing the likelihood of early diagnosis. This is important to prevent pulmonary complications that can occur from feeding or reflux. Early diagnosis offers the
surgeon and anesthesiologist the opportunity to operate on the neonate before pulmonary complications occur.

Motoyama EK, Davis PJ (eds): Smith's Anesthesia for Infants and Children, 6th ed, pp 464–465.
St. Louis, CV Mosby, 1996

Schwartz SI (ed): Principles of Surgery, 6th ed, pp 1690–1693. New York, McGraw Hill, 1994

*A.2. What information is needed to confirm the diagnosis? What information is obtained
from each of the following?*

- *Radiopaque catheter*
- *Barium swallow or instillation*
- *Chest x-ray film*
- *Flat plate of the abdomen*

A radiopaque catheter passed into the esophagus stops abruptly at 10 to 12 cm or
less from the nares. An x-ray film will show the curled catheter in the upper pouch.
A small amount of water-soluble contrast may be used; however, it is better to avoid
this method for fear that either the contrast will be aspirated into the lung from over-
flow or material will enter the lung through a fistulous tract. If contrast is necessary,
a small amount of barium diluted in saline may be safer than water-soluble contrast,
which is hyperosmolar and if aspirated could damage the respiratory mucosa. A
chest x-ray will determine the presence of pneumonia, especially of the right upper
lobe, and may give some information concerning associated cardiac lesions. A flat
plate of the abdomen will show the presence or absence of air in the gastrointestinal
tract. Fewer than 2% of patients have common TE fistula with no gas in the gastroin-

testinal (GI) tract. The absence of air is pathognomonic for esophageal atresia, though not necessarily associated with a fistula. The presence of air does not rule out atresia. Air may enter the GI tract through a fistula between the trachea and a lower esophageal segment. This is present in the Type C (Gross Classification), the most commonly seen type of TE fistula.

Cook DR, Marcy JH (eds): Neonatal Anesthesia, pp l68–169. Pasadena, Appleton Davies, 1988

DeVries PA, Shapiro SR: Complications of Pediatric Surgery, p 115. New York, John Wiley, 1982

Gregory GA (ed): Pediatric Anesthesia, 3rd ed, p 439. New York, Churchill Livingston, 1994

Schwartz SI (ed): Principles of Surgery, 6th ed, pp l690–1693. New York, McGraw Hill, 1994

A.3. Classify tracheoesophageal (TE) fistula or atresia.

Gross enumerated five types of atresia with or without fistula (Fig. 4-1):

- Type A—esophageal atresia with no fistula
- Type B—esophageal atresia, the upper segment communicating with the trachea
- Type C—esophageal atresia with a blind upper pouch and the lower segment communicating with the trachea
- Type D—esophageal atresia with both upper and lower segments communicating with the trachea
- Type E—no atresia present but a communication exists between the esophagus and the trachea, the so-called H type, or more precisely the N type, since the tracheal opening is usually more cephalad than the esophageal opening.

The most common type is C, a blind upper pouch and a lower fistulous segment, accounting for almost 87% of all cases. Atresia alone, Type A, accounts for approximately 8% of cases. Type E, the H or N type, accounts for 4% to 5%. This type is frequently missed, and the diagnosis is not made until frequent pulmonary problems present, often months after birth. A triad of symptoms should suggest this anomaly: choking when feeding, gaseous distention, and recurrent pneumonia. The other two types, Type B and Type D account for fewer than 1% each.

Gross RE: The Surgery of Infancy and Childhood, p 76. Philadelphia, WB Saunders, 1953

Schwartz SI (ed): Principles of Surgery, 6th ed, p l691. New York, McGraw Hill, 1994

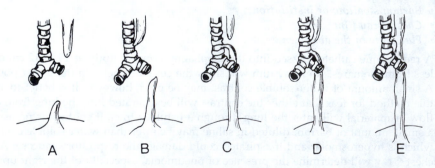

Figure 4-1. Gross's classification of esophageal atresia and tracheoesophageal fistula. (Reprinted with permission from Gregory GA [ed]: Pediatric Anesthesia, 2nd ed, p 921. New York, Churchill Livingstone, 1989)

A.4. What other congenital anomalies are associated with TE fistula or atresia?

Associated anomalies occur in approximately 30% to 50% of atresia in reported large series. The most common are cardiovascular, genitourinary, imperforate anus and other intestinal atresias, and neurologic and orthopedic anomalies. VATER is an acronym for a group of associated defects identified by Quan and Smith, which include vascular and vertebral defects, anal atresia and other GI atresias, tracheoesophageal fistulae, and renal and radial anomalies. The more common cardiac anomalies include ventricular septal defect, coarctation of the aorta, tetralogy of Fallot, and atrial septal defect. Patent ductus was seen frequently in one series. The incidence of cardiac anomalies associated with TE fistula is approximately 14% and as high as 24% in one series. Approximately one-half of the patients with TE fistula have some other congenital anomaly.

The majority of these anomalies should not defer the aggressive treatment of the TE fistula. However, ductal dependent cardiac anomalies may require the use of prostaglandin E_1 to maintain patency of the ductus. Failing this, a palliative shunt may be required before repair of the TE fistula is undertaken. In nonductal dependent cardiac lesions, repair or ligation of the TE fistula takes precedence.

Motoyama EK, Davis PJ (eds): Smith's Anesthesia for Infants and Children, 6th ed, pp 464–465. St. Louis, CV Mosby, 1996

Quan L, Smith DW: The VATER association, vertebral defects, anal atresia, TE fistula with esophageal atresia, radial and renal dysplasia; A spectrum of associated defects. J Pediatr 82:104, 1973

Spitz L: Current Opinions in Pediatrics 5:347–352, 1993

Spitz L, Kiely EM, Morecroft JA, Drake DP: Oesophageal atresia: At risk groups for the 1990s. J Pediatr Surg 29:723–725, 1994

Stroedel WE et al: Esophageal atresia. Arch Surg 114:523–527, 1979

A.5. What is the embryology of TE fistula?

The esophagus is developed from the first part of the primitive gut, the upper part of the esophagus from the pregastric segment, and the lower part of the esophagus from the pregastric segments. As the neck differentiates and the heart, lungs and stomach move caudal, the esophagus elongates rapidly. Vacuoles appear in the epithelium to form a lumen by the eighth week. By the fourth week, the laryngotracheal groove develops to become the larynx, trachea, and primordia of the lungs. Two furrows develop along the sides of the respiratory primordia and move inward, separating the respiratory portion from the esophagus. Tracheoesophageal fistula results from an imperfect division of the foregut into the anterior larynx and trachea and the posterior esophagus.

Stehling LC, Zauder HL (eds): Anesthetic Implications of Congenital Anomalies in Children, pp 90–91. New York, Appleton-Century-Croft, 1980

B. Preoperative Evaluation and Preparation

B.1. What problems concern you and what laboratory data do you need to evaluate these problems?

Infants who have tracheoesophageal fistula may have pneumonia or atelectasis secondary to aspiration of secretions that cannot be swallowed, or to reflux from the stomach through the fistula. To evaluate this condition, a chest x-ray film is mandatory. This infant was admitted early and the diagnosis was made promptly. Therefore, extensive pulmonary complications are not expected. If the diagnosis is delayed, aspiration pneumonia and atelectasis, with or without bacterial pneumonia, may result in sepsis, shunting, hypoxia, and hypercarbia. Metabolic acidosis, secondary to dehydration, may be added to the already existing respiratory acidosis.

Blood gases may be helpful in differentiation of acidosis. A complete blood count and urinalysis are needed. Type and cross match in anticipation of surgery should also be carried out at this time. Most deaths or serious complications occur in infants with other congenital anomalies, especially cardiac anomalies. If cyanosis is prominent, it could be due to cardiac anomalies or to respiratory complications secondary to the TE fistula, with atelectasis, gastric distention, and elevation of the diaphragm. The absence of obvious pulmonary complications should alert the physician to the possible existence of congenital heart disease. Prematurity adds an increased risk if associated with severe anomalies. A complete physical examination is essential, as well as the pre- and perinatal maternal history.

Once the diagnosis is made, the infant is placed in the head up–face down position. The upper pouch is placed on continuous or intermittent suction using a sump pump. If atelectasis or pneumonia is a prominent feature, endotracheal intubation with ventilatory support may be required. Care must be taken not to overdistend the stomach, which could rupture. Gastrostomy may be required if distention of the stomach prevents adequate ventilation.

Calverley PK, Johnston AE: The anesthetic management of tracheoesophageal fistula: A review of ten year's experience. Can Anaesth Soc J 19:270–282, 1972

Cook DR, Marcy JH (eds): Neonatal Anesthesia, pp 168–172. Pasadena, Appleton Davies, 1988

Gregory GA (ed): Pediatric Anesthesia, 3rd ed, pp 438–439. New York, Churchill Livingstone, 1994

Katz J, Steward DJ (eds): Anesthesia and Uncommon Pediatric Diseases, 2nd ed, p 110. New York, WB Saunders, 1993

B.2. Discuss the risk classification of infants with TE fistula or atresia according to Waterston or Calverley. What are the implications for this infant? Does this classification still hold?

The classification according to the criteria of Waterston includes five groups.

- Group A—birth weight > 2500 grams and well
- Group B_1—birth weight 1800 to 2500 grams and well
- Group B_2—higher birth weight (>2500 grams), moderate pneumonia and congenital anomaly
- Group C_1—birth weight < 1800 grams
- Group C_2—higher birth weight and severe pneumonia and severe congenital anomaly

Waterston concluded from his study that infants classified in group A could be operated on immediately with definitive correction undertaken. Those infants in groups B_1 and B_2 could safely undergo a staged repair. Groups C_1 and C_2 presented the greatest challenge, and surgery should be delayed in these cases. In Calverley's 10-year report, 100% of groups A, B_1, and B_2 survived. The survival rates were 22% in group C_1 and 59% in group C_2. On the basis of this classification, our infant weighing 2200 grams and with an early diagnosis, has an excellent chance of survival, assuming there is no severe congenital anomaly. Distinction should be made between infants who are premature and those who are small for gestational age. The premature are at greater risk than those who are small for gestational age. In addition to the TE fistula, they have a higher incidence of respiratory distress syndrome; immature organ systems, especially the liver and lungs; and a decreased resistance to infection. The small for gestational age may be hypoglycemic or hypocalcemic or may have meconium aspiration complicating the pulmonary problems associated with TE fistula.

This classification served the surgeons, anesthesiologists, and pediatricians well when evaluating a particular patient. However, recent articles indicate that overall survival in a two-decade analysis of morbidity and mortality was 95%. Outcome was independent of birth weight. The major cause of death was cardiac, with sleep apnea, renal failure, and unknown causes together accounting for half the cardiac rate. The roles played by neonatologists, neonatal anesthesia, and sophisticated ventilatory support now available in the OR and ICU, in addition to improved surgical technique, early treatment of associated congenital anomalies, and aggressive treatment of reflux in improving survival rates is acknowledged and appear to make the Waterston classification less valuable in predicting outcome in the face of improvements made over the last 25 years. The general opinion from a number of papers is that prematurity by itself does not significantly affect outcome and the preexistence of severe congenital anomalies and/or severe pulmonary complications prior to surgery are the principal causes of perioperative morbidity and mortality. In almost all series, cardiac anomalies were the most common and were responsible for the majority of the deaths.

A new classification referred to as the Montreal classification by the authors from Montreal include just two groups, a high-risk group with life-threatening anomalies or both a major anomaly and ventilator dependence, and a low-risk group that includes all other patients.

Calverley RK, Johnstone AE: The anaesthetic management of tracheoesophageal fistula: A review of ten years' experience. Can Anaesth Soc J 19:270–282, 1972

Engum SPA, Grosfeld JL, West KW et al: Analysis of morbidity and mortality in 127 cases of esophageal atresia and/or tracheoesophageal fistula over two decades. Arch Surg 130:502–508, 1995

Gott DW, Brereton RJ: Success and failure with neonatal tracheoesophageal anomalies. Br J Surg 78:834–837, 1991

Poenaru D, Laberge JM, Neilson IR, Gutterman FM: A new prognostic classification for esophageal atresia. Surg 113: 426–432, 1993

Spitz L, Kiely EM, Morecroft JA, Drake DP: Oesophageal atresia: At risk groups for the 1990s. J Pediatr Surg 29:723–725, 1994

Waterston DJ, Bonham-Carter RE et al: Oesophageal atresia: Tracheoesophageal fistula. A study of survival in 218 infants. Lancet 1:819, 1962

B.3. *Discuss fluid replacement for this infant.*

Unless dehydration is obvious, which should not be the case in this infant, fluid replacement should be conservative. Approximately 4 ml/kg/h should be sufficient, with allowances for suction and gastric drainage and blood loss. Because of the high incidence of congenital cardiac disease (15% to 24%) associated with TE fistula, special care is required to prevent fluid overload. The diagnosis of congenital cardiac disease cannot always be made early and should remain suspect until ruled out. A solution of dextrose 5% in $\frac{1}{4}$ strength normal saline, may be used at the rates suggested above. The use of a halter pump or similar device will prevent administration of excessive fluid. When administering intravenous drugs or anesthetics the site of administration should be as close to the entry site of the infusion as possible. To ensure that the medication reaches the patient, small measured flush volumes may be used and should be calculated in the total volume of fluid administered.

Dierdorf SF, Krishna G: Anesthetic management of neonatal surgical emergencies. Anesth Analg 60:204–215, 1981

Gregory GA (ed): Pediatric Anesthesia, 3rd ed, pp 440–441. New York, Churchill Livingstone, 1994

Motoyama EK, Davis PJ (eds): Smith's Anesthesia for infants and Children, 6th ed, p 454. St. Louis CV Mosby, 1996

B.4. What is the role of antibiotics preoperatively or postoperatively?

It is standard practice to use preoperative antibiotics to control pulmonary infection. Specifically, a broad spectrum antibiotic is used. Postoperatively, antibiotics are used for the same purpose. In addition, antibiotics are used to control infection if there is anastomotic leak. This is one of the more common surgical complications. The presence of chemical pneumonitis secondary to reflux is more serious and may require in addition to antibiotics, aggressive pulmonary toilet and ventilatory support.

Motoyama EK, Davis PJ (eds): Smith's Anesthesia for Infants and Children, 6th ed, p 464. St. Louis, CV Mosby, 1996

Schwartz SI (ed): Principles of Surgery, 6th ed, p 1691. New York, McGraw-Hill, 1994

B.5. Discuss the role of gastrostomy in the management of TE fistula.

Gastrostomy may be performed as a first step. The presence of a functioning gastrostomy will decrease the possibility of gastric distention and prevent reflux of gastric contents into the lungs. It is necessary for proper nutrition, particularly in the postoperative period. If gastrostomy is not undertaken as a first step, it will be performed during the definitive repair, for all the above-mentioned reasons. In some cases, as in acute distention of the stomach with elevation and immobilization of the diaphragm, gastrostomy may be a life-saving maneuver. In the critically ill infant it is the first step undertaken in a staged repair, which is followed at a later date by ligation of the fistula. Still later, when the overall status of the infant has improved sufficiently, the esophageal atresia will be repaired. If surgery is delayed and a gastrostomy is not performed, total prenatal nutrition can be employed successfully. However, the gastrostomy may interfere with ventilation. If the resistance to air passage is greater in the lungs than in the stomach, airflow will be preferentially directed toward the stomach. This can be prevented by placing the gastrostomy catheter under water seal of approximately 20 cm H_2O. During surgery, and especially during induction of anesthesia, it may be necessary to totally or partially clamp the gastrostomy tube, if maintenance of ventilation is difficult.

Katz J, Steward DJ (eds): Anesthesia and Uncommon Pediatric Diseases, 2nd ed, pp 1001–1010. New York, WB Saunders, 1993

B.6. What premedication is indicated in this patient?

Atropine is indicated to decrease secretions and to prevent the bradycardia associated with halothane anesthesia. Bradycardia may occur during surgery with traction on the hilum or on the vagus during mobilization of the esophagus. The dose of atropine has been variously given as 0.01 to 0.03 mg/kg intramuscularly with a minimum dose of 0.1 mg. Sedation is not required preoperatively but antibiotics should be given preoperatively and postoperatively to prevent or control pulmonary infection.

Calverley RK, Johnston AE: The anesthetic management of tracheoesophageal fistula: A review of ten years' experience. Can Anaesth Soc J 19:272–280, 1972

Motoyama EK, Davis PJ (eds): Smith's Anesthesia for Infants and Children, 6th ed, p 450. St. Louis, CV Mosby, 1996

Stehling LC, Zander HL (eds): Anesthetic Implications of Congenital Anomalies in Children, p 74. New York, Appleton-Century-Croft, 1980

C. Intraoperative Management

C.1. Discuss the problems of transport of this infant to the operating room.

Every effort must be made to prevent or control the aspiration of secretions from the blind upper pouch, which may cause atelectasis or pneumonia and to prevent reflux of gastric contents through the fistula into the trachea and lungs. The chemical pneumonia produced from this reflux can be serious. For this reason the blind upper pouch is maintained on suction as established in the preoperative period. Since infants are obligate nasal breathers, the suction catheter should be passed via the mouth rather than the nose. Maintaining the 45° head up–face down position used in the preoperative period will further help in preventing aspiration. The infant should not be transported to the operating room until all preparations for that infant have been completed. This includes the warming of the room to 25°C.

Katz J, Steward DJ (eds): Anesthesia and Uncommon Pediatric Diseases, 2nd ed, pp 101–111. New York, WB Saunders, 1993

Koop CE et al: Esophageal atresia and tracheoesophageal fistula: Supportive measures that affect survival. Pediatrics 54:558, 1974

Motoyama EK, Davis PJ (eds): Smith's Anesthesia for Infants and Children, 6th ed, p 464. St. Louis, CV Mosby, 1996

C.2. What type of monitoring would you use for this case?

An ECG for rate and rhythm and a reliable blood pressure monitor are mandatory. In children with complicated cardiac lesions an intraarterial cannula will permit frequent blood gas sampling as well as blood pressure monitoring. A precordial stethoscope used over the precordium during induction or the gastrostomy and under the left scapula during the thoracotomy will monitor both respiratory and cardiac rates and quality. It will also detect the presence of secretions. An esophageal stethoscope is not indicated because of the danger of perforating the blind upper pouch. Pulse oximetry and end-tidal CO_2 monitoring are standard.

Hypothermia can be dangerous. Temperature must be monitored throughout the procedure. The anesthesiologist must be careful to maintain normothermia by using overhead heaters if available, a thermal mattress, warm operating rooms, a Baer Hugger or similar device. Fluids and blood should be warmed prior to administration. Blood loss should be measured accurately by weighing sponges promptly and collecting suction in small graduated containers. Humidification of the inspired gases will help to maintain normothermia and prevent inspiration of mucus and plug formation. Urine output should be measured and serial hematocrits may be helpful.

Chalon J, Patel C, Ali M: Humidity and the anesthetized patient. Anesthesiology 50:195, 1979

Gregory GA (ed): Pediatric Anesthesia, 3rd ed, p 439. New York, Churchill Livingstone, 1994

Motoyama EK, Davis PJ (eds): Smith's Anesthesia for Infants and Children, 6th ed, p 466. St. Louis, CV Mosby, 1996.

Rashad KF, Benson DW: The role of humidity in the prevention of hypothermia in infants and children. Anesth Analg 46:712, 1967

C.3. What emergency drugs should be available?

- Atropine diluted to 0.04 mg/ml. Give 3 to 4 ml or 0.12 to 0.16 mg.
- Calcium chloride, 20 mg/kg
- Epinephrine, 1 mg/ml diluted to 0.1 mg/ml. Give 0.1 ml/kg
- Phenylephrine 0.1 to 1 µg/kg

Atropine is given for bradycardia, to remove any vagal component. Calcium and epinephrine are used as isotropic agents. Phenylephrine is use to produce peripheral vasoconstriction.

C.4. Discuss the problems of induction and intubation. Where would you place the endotracheal tube in relation to the fistula?

During induction, gastric distention and immobilization of the diaphragm (causing severe respiratory embarrassment) is always a potential problem. Bradycardia and severe cardiac depression have been reported secondary to gastric dilatation in cases of TE fistula. For this reason, spontaneous respiration is preferred to assisted or controlled respiration during induction or until the fistula has been ligated. Frequently the infant can be intubated while awake after preoxygenation, but a struggling infant can regurgitate from the stomach into the trachea by way of the distal fistulous tract. If a prior gastrostomy has been performed, the anesthetic gases may pass out of the lungs into the stomach. Partial clamping of the gastrostomy tube may be necessary.

The endotracheal tube should be large enough to permit easy suctioning and a small leak is recommended by many anesthesiologists. This will also prevent gastric distention when assisted or controlled ventilation is employed. Salem has advocated using an endotracheal tube without a Murphy eye, placed first into the right mainstem bronchus and then withdrawn until breath sounds are heard bilaterally but not over the stomach. The endotracheal tube is place with the bevel facing anteriorly. The tracheal opening of the fistula is thereby blocked by the endotracheal tube. This supposes that the opening of the fistula is above the cairn and posterior in the membranous portion of the trachea. This is not a substitute for a gastrostomy.

Another technique involves passing the endotracheal tube beyond the fistulous opening until the fistula is ligated, at which time the tube is withdrawn to ensure ventilation of both lungs. In this case using an endotracheal tube with a Murphy eye will ensure adequate ventilation of the left lung even if the endotracheal tube enters the right mainstem bronchus.

If a gastrostomy has been performed previously, it will permit decompression of the stomach and will decrease the problem of distention and reflux. Secretions from an infected right upper lobe can enter the trachea or endotracheal tube and must be removed.

Still another method of dealing with the fistula involves the use of a Fogarty balloon catheter inserted into the fistula most commonly located in the posterior membranous portion of the trachea. This is done under fiberoptic control prior to intubation and prevents overdistention or loss of anesthetic gases. One complication of its use is that the catheter can slip back into the trachea. The infant then becomes difficult to ventilate, and the situation can be confused with surgical kinking of the trachea (see question C.5.). A skilled pediatric endoscopist is needed for this technique.

Berry FA (ed): Anesthetic Management of Difficult and Routine Pediatric Patients, 2nd ed, pp 149–150. New York, Churchill Livingston, 1990

Block EC, Filston HC: A thin fiberoptic bronchoscope as an aid to occlusion of the fistula in infants with tracheoesophageal fistula. Anesth Analg 67:791–793, 1988

Healy TEJ, Cohen PJ (eds): Wylie and Churchill-Davidson's A Practice of Anaesthesiology, 6th ed, p 642. London, Edward Arnold, 1995

Reeves ST, Bun N, Smith CD: Is it time to reevaluate the airway management of tracheoesophageal fistula? Anesth Analg 81:866–869, 1995

C.5. In what position would surgery be performed? How would this affect the management of the patient?

Gastrostomy is performed in the 45° head-up position, but the definitive repair requires that the infant be placed in the left lateral position, and the thoracotomy performed under the right scapula in the fourth or fifth interspace. Approximately 5% of patients with TE fistula have a right aortic arch, which can complicate the repair in this position. A left thoracotomy repair is generally required in these cases.

In the left lateral position, secretions from the right upper lobe in particular can be a problem, draining into the trachea and the dependent lung. Frequent suctioning may be needed to prevent obstruction of the endotracheal tube by these secretions or by blood. Traction on the upper lung is common during surgery and may kink the bronchus of the dependent lung. A stethoscope placed in the dependent axilla will aid in the diagnosis of airway obstruction caused by blood, mucus, purulent drainage, or kinking. This is an early warning signal, preceding changes in the pulse oximeter reading.

Berry FA (ed): Anesthetic Management of Difficult and Routine Pediatric Patients, 2nd ed, p 149. New York, Churchill Livingstone, 1990

Calverley RK, Johnston AE: The anesthetic management of tracheoesophageal fistula:. A review of ten years' experience. Can Anaesth Soc J 19: 270, 1972

Katz J, Steward DJ (eds): Anesthesia and Uncommon Pediatric Diseases, 2nd ed, pp 110–111. Philadelphia, WB Saunders, 1993

C.6. What problems can be anticipated during surgery? What anesthetic agent would you use? How can a stable mediastinum be accomplished? Is there a role for muscle relaxants?

Some of the problems have been discussed before. Prior to surgery the infant breathes spontaneously to avoid overdistention of the stomach. When the chest has been opened, respirations are gently assisted until the fistula has been ligated. During repair of the esophagus, an absolutely stable mediastinum is essential for a good result. A nondepolarizing muscle relaxant can be used for muscle relaxation. Controlled ventilation is used, and a small amount of continuous positive airway pressure (CPAP) may be needed to maintain mediastinal stability.

Endobronchial intubation can occur at any time during the procedure and must be corrected. Blood or mucus can obstruct the endotracheal tube and must be suctioned. Surgical manipulation can obstruct the endotracheal tube or the trachea itself. Bradycardia can occur from traction and requires treatment with atropine in doses of 0.01 to 0.02 mg/kg. Frequent expansion of the collapsed or retracted lung is advocated by some anesthesiologists. This and any other maneuver that may affect the surgical field must be done in consultation with the surgeon so that it does not interfere with the repair. A degree of trespass may be necessary to accomplish the surgery.

No specific anesthetic agent is required or prohibited. The use of nitrous oxide as part of the anesthetic regimen will decrease the inspired oxygen concentration, thereby avoiding the hyperoxia associated with retinopathy and retrolental fibroplasia in the premature infant. It is recommended to keep arterial oxygen saturation between 90% and 95% to prevent oxygen toxicity in the premature infant.

Gregory GA (ed): Pediatric Anesthesia, 3rd ed, pp 440–441. New York, Churchill Livingstone, 1994

Katz, J, Steward DJ (eds): Anesthesia and Uncommon Pediatric Diseases, 2nd ed, p 111. Philadelphia, WB Saunders, 1993

Motoyama EK, Davis PJ (eds): Smith's Anesthesia for Infants and Children, 6th ed, pp 465–466. St. Louis, CV Mosby, 1996

D. Postoperative Management

D.1. When can this infant be extubated?

If a nondepolarizing muscle relaxant has been used, and the infant is normothermic, and there are no serious pulmonary problems, the relaxant can be reversed. The anesthetic agent should be discontinued early enough to permit spontaneous respiration. Most patients, and our patient in particular, with an early diagnosis and no pulmonary complications, can be extubated at the end of surgery. The endotracheal tube should be suctioned and the lungs inflated with oxygen prior to extubation. Care is taken to avoid stress on the suture line. During surgery a catheter may be passed from above over which the repair of the esophagus is accomplished. This catheter is used to measure the depth of the repair. The catheter is withdrawn on completion of the repair to a point above the suture line. This is measured on the catheter and recorded. All catheters are marked at this point and no suctioning beyond this depth should be done. If pulmonary complications are present, postoperative mechanical ventilation may be needed. When mechanical ventilation has been employed, it is recommended to extubate when intermittent mandatory ventilation has been discontinued, the PaO_2 is > 50 mm Hg and $PaCO_2$ is < 50 mm Hg on an F_IO_2 of 50%.

In those infants with respiratory distress syndrome (RDS) in whom only a gastrostomy is performed without ligation of the fistula, mechanical ventilation may result in life-threatening air leaks. This can be managed by placing the gastrostomy tube under 20 to 25 cm H_2O or by passing a balloon Fogarty catheter retrograde via the distal esophageal segment to occlude the fistula.

Gregory GA (ed): Pediatric Anesthesia, 3rd ed, pp 441–442. New York, Churchill Livingstone, 1994

Karl HW: Control of life-threatening air leaks after gastrostomy in an infant with respiratory distress syndrome and tracheoesophageal fistula. Anesthesia 62:670–672, 1985

Motoyama EK, Davis PJ (eds): Smith's Anesthesia for Infants and Children, 6th ed, p 450. St. Louis, CV Mosby, 1996

Sosio M, Amoroso M: Respiratory insufficiency after gastrostomy prior to tracheoesophageal fistula repair. Anesth Analg 64:748–750, 1985

Stehling LC, Zauder HL (eds): Anesthetic Implications of Congenital Anomalies in Children, pp 94–95. New York, Appleton-Century-Croft, 1980

D.2. What are the dangers of hypothermia?

Hypothermia can affect the physical characteristics of inhalation anesthetics as well as the pharmacokinetics and pharmacodynamics of intravenous agents. Hypothermia lowers MAC of inhalation anesthestics; increases tissue solubility; and decreases requirements of nondepolarizing muscle relaxants, barbiturates, and narcotics. Metabolism may double during light anesthesia. If set core temperature is not maintained by passive techniques, apnea, overdose, hypoventilation, and metabolic acidosis occur. During active rewarming, if nonshivering thermogenesis is unable to meet physiologic demand and maintain core temperature the result is the same. Light anesthesia increases metabolism in response to hypothermia. Norepinephrine release results in peripheral and pulmonary vasoconstriction with an increase in right-to-left shunting, acidosis, hypoxemia, and anaerobic metabolism.

Motoyama EK, Davis PJ (eds): Smith's Anesthesia for Infants and Children, 6th ed, pp 145–151. St. Louis, CV Mosby, 1996

D.3. What are the complications seen following tracheoesophageal fistula repair?

Complications can be divided into two categories:

- Complications that existed prior to surgery, such as continuing pneumonia, and problems related to other congenital anomalies, especially those involving the cardiovascular system
- Complications that occur as a result of surgery, such as pneumothorax, atelectasis, anastomotic leaks, esophageal stricture, subcutaneous emphysema, recurrent laryngeal nerve injury, recurrent fistula, and tracheomalacia. A late finding of impaired pulmonary function has been documented.

The principal causes of death are pulmonary complications, associated anomalies, and anastomotic leaks. In one series minor anastomotic leaks occurred in 18% of cases. Spitz, reporting a 10-year analysis of 303 patients, indicated an overall survival rate of 86.5%. There were associated anomalies in 51.8%, of which cardiac anomalies accounted for 24.4% and the majority of deaths. Esophageal stricture or dysmotility and recurrent upper and lower respiratory infection occur in 35% to 75% of cases. Tracheomalacia occurs in about 25% of patients with tracheoesophageal fistula. Another series indicates that 65% to 75% of patients had some abnormality of the trachea in either the muscle or the cartilage. The normal horseshoe shape of the cartilage was lost. The condition can be mild, moderate, or severe. In the severe form, the patient may present with life-threatening cyanotic and apnea attacks after surgical repair. The differential diagnosis includes esophageal stricture with aspiration, recurrent or secondary fistula, gastroesophageal reflux, and anastomotic leak. Cardiac and neurogenic causes must be ruled out. The diagnosis is make by lateral chest x-ray and confirmed by bronchoscopy. In severe cases of tracheomalacia, tracheopexy is indicated. Endoscopic fibrin sealant has been used to treat recurrent fistulae.

Pulmonary function tests were abnormal in 50% of a group of patients following repair of tracheoesophageal fistula or atresia. Thirty-six percent of this group demonstrated restrictive disease; 12%, obstructive disease; and the remainder (2%), mixed.

Benjamin B, Cohen D, Glasson M: Tracheomalacia in association with congenital tracheoesophageal fistula. Surg 79:504,1976

Conroy PT, Bennett NR: Management of tracheomalacia in association with congenital tracheoesophageal fistula. Br J Anaesth 59:1313–1317, 1987

Hicks LM, Nansfield PB: Esophageal atresia and tracheoesophageal fistula. J Thorac Cardiovasc Surg 81:358–363,1981

Motoyama EK, Davis PJ (eds): Smith's Anesthesia for Infants and Children, 6th ed, p 466. St. Louis, CV Mosby, 1996

Redo SF: Principles of Surgery in the First Six Months of Life, pp 66–69. Hagerstown, Harper & Row, 1976

Robertson DF, Mobaireik K, Davis GM, Coates AL: Late pulmonary function following repair of tracheoesophageal fistula or atresia. Pediatr Pulmonol 20:21-26, 1995

Walloo MP, Emery JL: The trachea in children with tracheoesophageal fistula. Histopath 3:329, 1979

Wiseman NE: Endoscopic fibrin sealant for recurrent fistula. J Pediatr Surg 30:1236–1237, 1995

D.4. Discuss the management of postoperative pneumonia or atelectasis. Are these anesthetic complications?

Pulmonary complications are treated with antibiotics, suctioning, high humidity, chest physiotherapy, and the promotion of crying. These are probably not anesthetic complications, but are the result of traction on the lung during surgery or preexisting infection from reflux or aspiration. Care must be taken at the end of surgery to reinflate the lungs and suction the trachea adequately. When the anastomosis is complete, a catheter previously placed through the defect is removed to a point just above the anastomosis. The length of the catheter at this point is marked and recorded before being removed completely. No suctioning should be deeper than that mark.

If atelectasis develops in a previously extubated infant, the child is reintubated, suctioned, and ventilated; after this the child may be extubated. Hyperextension of the head and neck will place stress on the anastomosis and must be avoided. It may be necessary for the infant to remain intubated and mechanically ventilated. Under these circumstances the position of the endotracheal tube is critical. The endotracheal tube must not extend to the anastomotic site.

Gregory GA (ed): Pediatric Anesthesia, 3rd ed, pp 441–442. New York, Churchill Livingstone, 1994

Katz J, Steward DJ (eds): Anesthesia and Uncommon Pediatric Diseases, 2nd ed, p 111. Philadelphia, WB Saunders, 1993

Redo SF: Principles of Surgery in the First Six Months of Life, pp 66–67. Hagerstown, MD, Harper & Row, 1976

5 Congenital Diaphragmatic Hernia

Fun-Sun F. Yao
John J. Savarese

A full-term male baby was born with respiratory distress and cyanosis. Physical examination showed barrel chest and scaphoid abdomen. The breath sounds were absent in the left chest; the heart sounds were best heard in the right chest. Labored respiration, nasal flaring, and sternal retraction were found. The baby weighed 2800 g. Blood pressure was 60/30 mm Hg; heart rate, 160/min; respiration, 70/min; temperature, 36°C. Arterial blood gases on room air showed pH, 7.20; P_{CO_2}, 55 mm Hg; P_{O_2}, 35 mm Hg; CO_2 content, 19 mEq/liter.

A. Medical Disease and Differential Diagnosis

1. What differential diagnoses are compatible with these signs and symptoms?
2. Describe the incidence and classification of congenital diaphragmatic hernia (CDH).
3. What are the causes of hypoxemia in patients with CDH?
4. Why do varying degrees of pulmonary hypoplasia usually accompany CDH? How do they affect the prognosis?
5. How do you assess the severity of pulmonary hypoplasia?
6. Discuss persistent pulmonary hypertension in the patient with CDH.
7. How do you make a diagnosis of right-to-left shunting through the ductus arteriosus or patent foramen ovale?
8. What other congenital anomalies are usually associated with CDH?

B. Preoperative Evaluation and Preparation

1. How would you interpret the following arterial blood gases: pH, 7.20; P_{CO_2}, 55 mm Hg; P_{O_2}, 35 mm Hg; CO_2 content, 19 mEq/liter? How would you correct them?
2. What immediate treatment should be given to improve the newborn's respiratory status preoperatively?
3. Should CDH be repaired urgently once the diagnosis is made and confirmed?
4. How would you treat pulmonary hypertension and improve oxygenation?
5. What are the effects of nitric oxide (NO) on pulmonary and systemic circulation?
6. How is extracorporeal membrane oxygenation (ECMO) established?
7. What are the advantages of ECMO?
8. What are the indications and contraindications to ECMO?
9. When is the optimal time to repair CDH?
10. What other measures should you take to prepare the patient for surgery?
11. How would you premedicate this patient?

C. Intraoperative Management

1. What monitors would you use for this neonate during surgery?
2. How would you induce and maintain anesthesia?

3. Would you use nitrous oxide for anesthesia? Why?
4. Would you use 100% oxygen during anesthesia?
5. How would you ventilate the patient?
6. How would you maintain the neonate's body temperature?
7. The surgeon returned the intrathoracic stomach and intestine to the peritoneal cavity and the ipsilateral lung was found to be hypoplastic and collapsed. The resident anesthesiologist tried to expand the collapsed lung manually with positive airway pressure. Five minutes after the abdomen was closed, the blood pressure suddenly dropped from 70/40 to 30/20 mm Hg, the heart rate from 150 to 80/min, and the pulse oximeter from 95% down to 60% saturation. What would you do immediately?
8. Discuss fluid therapy in this patient.
9. At the conclusion of surgery, would you extubate the patient in the operating room?

D. Postoperative Management

1. What postoperative problems would you expect in this patient? What is the mortality rate in patients with CDH?
2. The neonate's blood gases improved right after surgery. However, 3 hours later, severe hypoxemia recurred in spite of ventilatory support with high inspired oxygen concentration. What are the possible causes? How should this patient be treated?

A. Medical Disease and Differential Diagnosis

A.1. What differential diagnoses are compatible with these signs and symptoms?

Congenital cardiopulmonary anomalies should be considered whenever cyanosis and respiratory distress are present. Scaphoid abdomen, barrel chest, bowel sounds in the chest, and the shift of heart sounds to the right suggest the diagnosis of congenital diaphragmatic hernia. To confirm the diagnosis, a chest x-ray should be done to demonstrate gas-filled loops of bowel and probably the spleen or liver in the chest. The lung on the side of the hernia is compressed into the hilum, and the mediastinum is shifted to the opposite chest. If in doubt, radiopaque dye may be injected through a nasogastric tube to delineate the stomach and intestine in the chest.

Barash PG, Stoelting RK (eds): Clinical Anesthesia, 3rd ed, pp 1103–1105. Philadelphia, Lippincott-Raven, 1997

Behrman RE, Kliegman RM, Arvin AM (eds): Nelson Textbook of Pediatrics, 15th ed, pp 1161–1164. Philadelphia, WB Saunders, 1996

Gregory GA (ed): Pediatric Anesthesia, 3rd ed, p 433. New York, Churchill Livingstone, 1994

A.2. Describe the incidence and classification of congenital diaphragmatic hernia (CDH).

The incidence of CDH is estimated to be 1 in 600 to 18,000 births; the average is 1 in 5000 live births. The male to female ratio is 2:1, and the left diaphragm is more frequently involved than the right (5:1).

The diaphragm is embryonically formed from the fusion of several components; therefore, a number of developmental defects may occur, resulting in herniation of abdominal contents into the chest. Embryologically, two fundamental types of defect may occur:

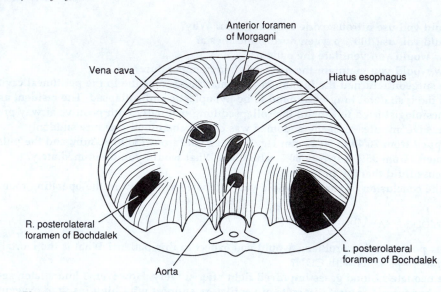

Figure 5-1. Potential sites of congenital diaphragmatic hernia.

- Complete or partial absence of the diaphragm
- Failure of complete muscularization

Embryologic classification is not convenient clinically. A practical classification is used based on the anatomic location of the defects in the diaphragm:

- Absent diaphragm—very rare
- Diaphragmatic hernia (Fig. 5-1)
  - Posterolateral (Bochdalek)—80%
  - Anterior (Morgagni)—2%
  - Paraesophageal—15% to 20%
- Eventration—very rare

Barash PG, Stoelting RK (eds): Clinical Anesthesia, 3rd ed, pp 1103–1105. Philadelphia, Lippincott-Raven, 1997

Behrman RE, Kliegman RM, Arvin AM (eds): Nelson Textbook of Pediatrics, 15th ed, pp 1161–1164. Philadelphia, WB Saunders, 1996

Dierdorf SF, Krishna G: Anesthetic management of neonatal surgical emergencies. Anesth Analg 60:204–214, 1981

Gregory GA (ed): Pediatric Anesthesia, 3rd ed, pp 431–432. New York, Churchill Livingstone, 1994

A.3. What are the causes of hypoxemia in patients with CDH?

The causes of hypoxemia are as follows:

- Atelectasis due to compression of the developed lung by the herniated abdominal organs
- Primary pulmonary hypoplasia with a decrease in number of alveoli and bronchial generations, and abnormal pulmonary vasculature due to a disruption of normal

development of the lung tissue, secondary to the crowding of the herniated abdominal organs in the thorax

- Persistent pulmonary hypertension (PPH) increasing right-to-left shunting through a patent foramen ovale and ductus arteriosus

Behrman RE, Kliegman RM, Arvin AM (eds): Nelson Textbook of Pediatrics, 15th ed, pp 1161–1164. Philadelphia, WB Saunders, 1996

Gregory GA (ed): Pediatric Anesthesia, 3rd ed, pp 432–443. New York, Churchill Livingstone, 1994

Miller RD (ed): Anesthesia, 4th ed, p 2087. New York, Churchill Livingstone, 1994

Stoelting RK, Dierdorf SF, McCammon RL (eds): Anesthesia and Co-Existing Disease, 3rd ed, pp 591–592. New York, Churchill Livingstone, 1993

A.4. Why do varying degrees of pulmonary hypoplasia usually accompany CDH? How do they affect the prognosis?

Embryologic development of the diaphragm, gut, heart, and lungs takes place at about the same time, and abnormal development of one organ affects development of the others. Normally, pleural and peritoneal cavities are separated by the diaphragm during the 8th to 10th week of gestation. At about the same time the gut physiologically herniates into the yolk stalk, but then returns to the peritoneal cavity. The pleuroperitoneal canals progressively narrow and are finally closed by the 10th week. CDH may result either from the early return of the midgut to the peritoneal cavity or from delayed closure of the pleuroperitoneal canal.

The lung is also undergoing development at this time. Alveolar buds begin to differentiate by the 6th week; airways develop during the 10th to 12th week. Bronchial branching continues until the 16th week of gestation. Alveolar multiplication continues until 8 years of age.

The degree of pulmonary hypoplasia is related to the timing of the herniation of abdominal organs into the pleural cavity. The earlier the herniation, the more severe the pulmonary hypoplasia. Hypoplasia of the left ventricle may also occur, resulting in cardiac insufficiency. The degree of pulmonary hypoplasia determines the prognosis of CDH. Severe bilateral hypoplasia predicts high mortality. With unilateral hypoplasia, the patient may survive with aggressive therapy. When pulmonary hypoplasia is insignificant, the prognosis is excellent.

Behrman RE, Kliegman RM, Arvin AM (eds): Nelson Textbook of Pediatrics, 15th ed, pp 1161–1164. Philadelphia, WB Saunders, 1996

Berdon WE, Baker DH, Amoury R: The role of pulmonary hypoplasia in the prognosis of newborn infants with diaphragmatic hernia and eventration. Am J Roentgenol 103:413–421, 1968

Gregory GA (ed): Pediatric Anesthesia, 3rd ed, pp 431–432. New York, Churchill Livingstone, 1994

A.5. How do you assess the severity of pulmonary hypoplasia?

The severity of pulmonary hypoplasia is assessed by the intrapulmonary shunt QS/QT or the alveolar-arterial oxygen gradient (A–a) DO_2. An (A–a) DO_2 of >500 mm Hg when breathing 100% oxygen is predictive of nonsurvival, and an (A–a) DO_2 of <400 mm Hg is predictive of survival; an (A–a) DO_2 between 400 and 500 mm Hg represents a zone of uncertain prognosis.

The severity of pulmonary hypoplasia may also be evaluated more aggressively by cardiac catheterization and pulmonary angiogram to define the size and branching pattern of the pulmonary arteries. Patients with severe pulmonary hypoplasia usually have a fixed right-to-left shunting at the level of ductus arteriosus or patent foramen ovale caused by a supra systemic pulmonary hypertension. Pulmonary angiography demonstrates a small diameter of affected pulmonary artery compared to the main pulmonary artery. The postductal PaO_2 never rises above 60 mm Hg in non-survivors.

Harrington J, Raphaely RC, Downes JJ: Relationship of alveolar-arterial oxygen tension difference in diaphragmatic hernia of the newborn. Anesthesiology 56:473, 1982

Vacanti JP, Crone RK, Murphy JD et al: The pulmonary hemodynamic response to perioperative anesthesia in the treatment of high-risk infants with congenital diaphragmatic hernia. J Pediatr Surg 19:672–679, 1984

A.6. Discuss persistent pulmonary hypertension in the patient with CDH.

Pulmonary hypertension is one of the major causes of hypoxemia in CDH. It was previously called persistent fetal circulation, but this is a misnomer because the fetal circulation is characterized by the presence of the placenta, which is no longer present. It causes right-to-left shunting of desaturated venous blood at the level of the atrium and the ductus arteriosus. Varying degrees of hypoxemia, hypercarbia, and acidosis cause high pulmonary vascular resistance and pressure. Increased pulmonary vascular resistance and pressure also result from a hypoplastic lung. The pulmonary vasculature is abnormal, with a decrease in volume and marked increase in muscular mass in the arterioles. When pulmonary artery pressures are higher than systemic pressure, right-to-left shunting occurs across the ductus, resulting in higher PaO_2 in the upper extremities than in the lower extremities. When right ventricular failure (precipitated by pulmonary hypertension, progressive hypoxemia, and acidosis or by closure of the ductus) increases right atrial pressure to a level higher than left atrial pressure, right-to-left atrial shunting ensues, producing further hypoxemia. Left ventricular failure from hypoxemia and acidosis induces systemic hypotension, resulting in increased ductal shunting and hypoxemia. A vicious cycle is established (Fig. 5-2). Unless pulmonary artery pressure is decreased, progressive hypoxia and death may ensue.

Barash PG, Stoelting RK (eds): Clinical Anesthesia, 3rd ed, pp 1091–1092. Philadelphia, Lippincott-Raven, 1997

Behrman RE, Kliegman RM, Arvin AM (eds): Nelson Textbook of Pediatrics, 15th ed, pp 1161–1164. Philadelphia, WB Saunders, 1996

Gregory GA (ed): Pediatric Anesthesia, 3rd ed, pp 432. New York, Churchill Livingstone, 1994

A.7. How do you make a diagnosis of right-to-left shunting through the ductus arteriosus or patent foramen ovale?

If shunting occurs through the ductus arteriosus, the preductal PaO_2 is at least 15 to 20 mm Hg higher than postductal value. A right-to-left shunt of 20% is considered "normal" for a newborn infant. If shunting occurs through the patent foramen ovale, the preductal PaO_2 is below the value predicted for 20% shunt. When the degree of preductal shunting is severe, detection of ductal shunting is impossible. Echocardiography with color Doppler, cardiac catheterization, and pulmonary angiography will confirm the diagnosis.

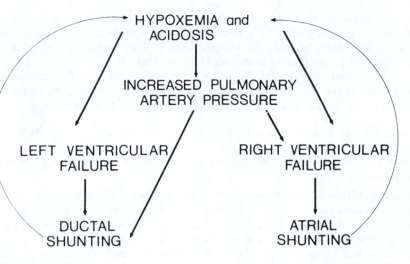

Figure 5-2. Mechanism of right-to-left shunting with persistent fetal circulation. (Reprinted with permission from Gregory GA [ed]: Pediatric Anesthesia, 2nd ed, p 911. New York: Churchill Livingstone, 1989)

Gregory GA (ed): Pediatric Anesthesia, 3rd ed, p 474. New York, Churchill Livingstone, 1994

Nelson NM, Prod'Hom LS, Cherry RB et al: Pulmonary function in the newborn infant: The alveolar-arterial oxygen gradient. J Appl Physiol 18:534, 1963

Stoelting RK, Dierdorf SF, McCammon RL (eds): Anesthesia and Co-Existing Disease, 4th ed, pp 591–592. New York, Churchill Livingstone, 1993

A.8. What other congenital anomalies are usually associated with CDH?

The incidence of other congenital anomalies in newborns with CDH is as follows:

- Cardiovascular system—13% to 23%, e.g., atrial septal defect, ventricular septal defect, coarctation of aorta, tetralogy of Fallot
- Central nervous system—28%, e.g., spina bifida, hydrocephalus, acephalus
- Gastrointestinal system—20%, e.g., malrotation, atresia
- Genitourinary system—15%, e.g., hypospadias

David TJ, Illingworth CA: Diaphragmatic hernia in the southwest of England. J Med Genet 13:253, 1976

B. Preoperative Evaluation and Preparation

B.1. How would you interpret the following arterial blood gases: pH, 7.20; P_{CO_2}, 55 mm Hg; P_{O_2}, 35 mm Hg; CO_2 content, 19 mEq/liter? How would you correct them?

The blood gases showed mixed respiratory and metabolic acidosis and severe hypoxemia. Severe hypoxemia is caused by the pulmonary pathologies and persistent pulmonary hypertension. Hypoxemia stimulates respiratory chemoreceptors and causes hyperventilation, resulting in respiratory alkalosis initially. However, if hypoxemia is not corrected, the patient will become exhausted and CO_2 retention ensues. Meanwhile, severe pulmonary hypoplasia may cause CO_2 retention, too. Severe hypoxemia induces anaerobic metabolism, resulting in lactic acidosis. Systemic hypotension, caused by kinking of major blood vessels, particularly those of the liver, decreases tissue perfusion, and further contributes to lactic acidosis.

Hypoxemia and respiratory acidosis should be treated with mechanical ventilation and oxygen therapy. Metabolic acidosis should be corrected by administration of sodium bicarbonate and improvement of circulation with fluid therapy.

Miller RD (ed): Anesthesia, 4th ed, p 2457. New York, Churchill Livingstone, 1994

B.2. What immediate treatment should be given to improve the newborn's respiratory status preoperatively?

Immediate intervention should include decompression of the stomach with an orogastric or nasogastric tube and administration of supplemental oxygen by mask. Positive pressure ventilation by mask should be avoided to prevent distention of the intrathoracic stomach, which will further compress the lung and compromise respiration. If cyanosis and hypoxemia persist, awake intubation should be done to facilitate mechanical ventilation. Positive airway pressure during mechanical ventilation should not exceed 25 to 30 cm H_2O to reduce the risk of tension pneumothorax. Although pneumothorax can happen on either side, it occurs more frequently on the contralateral side of the hernia because the pressure needed to expand the hypoplastic lung is higher than that required to rupture the normal lung.

Behrman RE, Kliegman RM, Arvin AM (eds): Nelson Textbook of Pediatrics, 15th ed, pp 1161–1164. Philadelphia, WB Saunders, 1996

Gregory GA (ed): Pediatric Anesthesia, 3rd ed, pp 433–434. New York, Churchill Livingstone, 1994

Stoelting RK, Dierdorf SF, McCammon RL (eds): Anesthesia and Co-Existing Disease, 3rd ed, pp 591–592. New York, Churchill Livingstone, 1993

B.3. Should CDH be repaired urgently once the diagnosis is made and confirmed?

In the past, CDH was considered a surgical emergency, in the belief that the herniated contents caused lung collapse and respiratory failure. However, recognition of the role of pulmonary hypertension in addition to pulmonary hypoplasia and the effects of surgical repair on pulmonary function prompted critical reevaluation of that strategy. It is now clear that lung compression by the herniated viscera is a minor factor in the cardiopulmonary compromise compared with the pulmonary hypertension and hypoplasia. The consensus today is to delay surgery and concentrate on medical stabilization. The goal of preoperative therapy is to reverse the persistent pulmonary hypertension (PPH) that results in right-to-left shunting across the patent foramen ovale and the ductus arterious. Improvement in the infant's status is apparent by improved oxygenation and ventilation. Doppler echocardiography may be used to confirm the decreased pulmonary vascular resistance. The time it takes to stabilize the condition varies from 24 to 48 hours in infants with only mild pulmonary hypertension and hypoplasia up until 7 to 10 days in neonates with severe pulmonary hypertension and hypoplasia.

Barash PG, Stoelting RK (eds): Clinical Anesthesia, 3rd ed, pp 1091–1092. Philadelphia, Lippincott-Raven, 1997

Behrman RE, Kliegman RM, Arvin AM (eds): Nelson Textbook of Pediatrics, 15th ed, pp 1161–1164. Philadelphia, WB Saunders, 1996

Charlton AJ: The management of congenital diaphragmatic hernia without ECMO. Paediatr Anaesth 3:201, 1993

Gregory GA (ed): Pediatric Anesthesia, 3rd ed, pp 433–434. New York, Churchill Livingstone, 1994

Haugen SE, Linker D, Eik-Nes et al: Congenital diaphragmatic hernia: Determination of the optimal time for operation by echocardiographic monitoring of the pulmonary arterial pressure. J Pediatr Surg 26:560,1991

B.4. How would you treat persistent pulmonary hypertension and improve oxygenation?

Pulmonary vascular resistance is greatly increased in the hypoplastic lung, and blood flow is minimal because of medial hyperplasia of pulmonary arterioles. When further aggravated by hypoxemia, acidosis, decreased F_IO_2, or sudden changes in pulmonary blood volume, pulmonary vasoconstriction increases and fetal circulation persists. The treatment of pulmonary hypertension includes the following measures in sequence:

- Continue general anesthesia in the intensive care unit, using fentanyl 3 $\mu g/kg/h$ and pancuronium 0.1 mg/kg/h to blunt the autonomically mediated cardiovascular response (pulmonary vasoconstriction) to stimulation.
- Minimize endotracheal suctioning to avoid even transient hypoxemia or decrease in F_IO_2.
- Hyperventilate the neonate with low tidal volume and high respiratory rate 60 to 120/min) to pH 7.55 to 7.60. Respiratory alkalosis is the most consistently effective therapeutic modality to achieve pulmonary vasodilation.
- Moderately restrict fluid to 2 to 4 ml/kg/h.
- Administer pharmacologic vasodilators if the above measures fail to control pulmonary hypertension. Morphine, prednisolone, chlorpromazine, phentolamine, acetylcholine, bradykinin, tolazoline, prostaglandin E_1, prostaglandin D_2, and inhaled nitric oxide have been tried with some success.
- Ligate the patent ductus arteriosus (PDA) to prevent shunting. This is theoretically possible, but practically has been associated with sudden right ventricular failure.
- Support with extracorporeal membrane oxygenation (ECMO) if pharmacologic intervention fails. ECMO has been associated with a 50% to 65% survival rate.

Gregory GA (ed): Pediatric Anesthesia, 3rd ed, pp 433–434. New York, Churchill Livingstone, 1994

Vacanti JP, Crone RK, Murphy JD et al: The pulmonary hemodynamic response to perioperative anesthesia in the treatment of high-risk infants with congenital diaphragmatic hernia. J Pediatr Surg 19:672–679, 1984

B.5. What are the effects of nitric oxide (NO) on pulmonary and systemic circulation?

Nitric oxide is thought to be an endothelium-derived relaxant factor (EDRF). Inhaled NO is unique in that it is a selective pulmonary vasodilator and has no effect on systemic circulation because it is inactivated immediately on exposure to hemoglobin. Clinical studies are limited but have shown some improvement in oxygenation in neonates with PPH exposed to 20 to 80 ppm NO. Nitric oxide has been reported to be ineffective before ECMO therapy in those CDH patients with pulmonary hypoplasia. After ECMO followed by surgery, NO was effective in improving oxygenation.

Behrman RE, Kliegman RM, Arvin AM (eds): Nelson Textbook of Pediatrics, 15th ed, pp 1161–1164. Philadelphia, WB Saunders, 1996

Charlton AJ: The management of congenital diaphragmatic hernia without ECMO. Paediatr Anaesth 3:201, 1993

Gregory GA (ed): Pediatric Anesthesia, 3rd ed, pp 433–434. New York, Churchill Livingstone, 1994

B.6. How is extracorporeal membrane oxygenation (ECMO) established?

Venovenous or venoarterial bypass is used. Venovenous bypass is established with a single cannula through the internal jugular vein, with blood removed from and infused into the right atrium via separate ports. Venoarterial bypass is used preferentially by some centers because it provides the cardiac support that is often needed. The right atrium is cannulated via the internal jugular vein and the aortic arch through the right common carotid artery.

Schwartz SE (ed): Principles of Surgery, 6th ed, p 1687. New York, McGraw-Hill, 1994

B.7. What are the advantages of ECMO?

The theoretical advantages are as follows:

- Diversion of as much as 80% of cardiac output from the right atrium into the extracorporeal circuit immediately reduces or eliminates right-to-left shunting through the foramen ovale or ductus arteriosus.
- Right ventricular work is decreased because of reduced pulmonary blood flow and pressure.
- Pulmonary vasoconstriction is reduced because hypoxemia and acidosis are corrected by ECMO. Improved systemic oxygenation and reduced ductal blood flow may lead to spontaneous closure of the ductus arteriosus.
- The hypoplastic lung is allowed to grow rapidly and alveolar size is increased.
- The incidence of bronchopulmonary dysplasia is reduced since F_IO_2 and airway pressure are lowered by ECMO.

Gregory GA (ed): Pediatric Anesthesia, 3rd ed, pp 435–437. New York, Churchill Livingstone, 1994

B.8. What are the indications and contraindications to ECMO?

Patients with severe hypoxemia and pulmonary hypertension who do not respond to maximal conventional respiratory and pharmacologic intervention are indicated for ECMO. However, ECMO is associated with serious complications of intracranial and pulmonary hemorrhage.

The contraindications to ECMO include the following:

- Gestational age <35 weeks
- Weight <2000 g
- Preexisting intracranial hemorrhage
- Congenital or neurologic abnormalities incompatible with good outcome
- >1 week of aggressive respiratory therapy
- Congenital heart disease

Dilley RE, Zwischenberger JB, Andrews AF et al: Intracranial hemorrhage during extracorporeal membrane oxygenator in neonates. Pediatrics 78:699, 1986

Redmond CR, Goldsmith JP, Sharp MJ et al: Extracorporeal membrane oxygenation for neonates. J La State Med Soc 138:40, 1986

B.9. When is the optimal time to repair CDH?

The baby is maintained on ECMO until the pulmonary hypertension is reversed and improvement in lung function is evident. Doppler echocardiography may be used to confirm the reverse of persistent pulmonary hypertension. This is usually seen within 7 to 10 days, but in some infants is not apparent for up to 3 weeks. Newborns who do not demonstrate significant improvement over this time have pulmonary hypoplasia that will not benefit from further extracorporeal life support. Timing of repair of the CDH on ECMO is controversial. Some centers prefer early repair to allow a greater duration of postrepair ECMO, whereas many centers defer repair until the infant has demonstrated the ability to tolerate weaning from ECMO support.

Behrman RE, Kliegman RM, Arvin AM (eds): Nelson Textbook of Pediatrics, 15th ed, pp 1161–1164. Philadelphia, WB Saunders, 1996

Gregory GA (ed): Pediatric Anesthesia, 3rd ed, pp 433–434. New York, Churchill Livingstone, 1994

Haugen SE, Linker D, Eik-Nes et al: Congenital diaphragmatic hernia: Determination of the optimal time for operation by echocardiographic monitoring of the pulmonary arterial pressure. J Pediatr Surg 26:560, 1991

B.10. What other measures should you take to prepare the patient for surgery?

The patient should be examined carefully for the presence and severity of associated congenital anomalies as described in question A.8. Those patients with congenital heart disease in addition to CDH have significantly increased mortality.

Hypothermia should be prevented and corrected, since hypothermia can increase oxygen consumption and result in further hypoxemia and acidosis. The neonate should be maintained in a neutral thermal environment of 30° to 40°C.

Laboratory studies should include arterial blood gases, complete blood count, electrolytes, blood sugar, blood type, and crossmatch for blood products.

Venous access should be ready prior to surgery. Peripheral veins in the upper extremities are preferred because reduction of the hernia often increases abdominal pressure and partially obstructs the inferior vena cava, making lower extremity veins less reliable. Neck veins are avoided in case ECMO is required.

B.11. How would you premedicate this patient?

No premedication should be given to the neonate with CDH. The newborn does not have any anxiety, and sedatives may just further depress the already compromised cardiopulmonary function.

C. Intraoperative Management

C.1. What monitors would you use for this neonate during surgery?

Respiratory
- Precordial and esophageal stethoscope
- Pulse oximeter, both above and below nipple for preductal and postductal oxygen saturation

- Capnometer or mass spectrometer
- Inspiratory pressure gauge
- Inspiratory oxygen concentration
- Arterial blood gases

Cardiovascular
- ECG
- Doppler blood pressure device
- Precordial stethoscope
- Arterial line—right radial artery for preductal PaO_2
- Central venous pressure line for evaluating volume status and right ventricular performance

Thermoregulatory
- Esophageal or rectal temperature probe

C.2. How would you induce and maintain anesthesia?

If the neonate has not been intubated, awake intubation should be done after preoxygenation. However, if the neonate is too vigorous for awake intubation, he can be intubated without a muscle relaxant after breathing halothane and oxygen spontaneously. Positive pressure ventilation should be avoided before intubation to prevent gastric distention and further compromise of respiration.

The choice of anesthetics depends on the severity of cardiovascular dysfunction. Patients in shock and severe hypoxemia may tolerate only oxygen and a nondepolarizing relaxant such as pancuronium or vecuronium. If blood pressure is adequate and stable, halothane or fentanyl in addition to a muscle relaxant, often pancuronium, may be titrated to maintain anesthesia. Fentanyl and pancuronium may be continued postoperatively to control ventilation and minimize hormonal response to stress, which may increase pulmonary hypertension.

Barash PG, Stoelting RK (eds): Clinical Anesthesia, 3rd ed, pp 1091–1092. Philadelphia, Lippincott-Raven, 1997

Dierdorf SF, Krichna G: Anesthetic management of neonatal surgical emergencies. Anesth Analg 60:204–214, 1981

Gregory GA (ed): Pediatric Anesthesia, 3rd ed, p 435. New York, Churchill Livingstone, 1994

Vacanti JP, Crone RK, Murphy JD et al: The pulmonary hemodynamic response to perioperative anesthesia in the treatment of high-risk infants with congenital diaphragmatic hernia. J Pediatr Surg 19:672–679, 1984

C.3. Would you use nitrous oxide for anesthesia? Why?

No. Nitrous oxide should not be used in patients with CDH before hernia reduction and abdominal closure. Because nitrous oxide has higher diffusion capacity than nitrogen (35:1), the amount of nitrous oxide diffused from blood to the gut is much more than the amount of nitrogen diffused from the gut to the blood. Therefore, nitrous oxide may distend the intrathoracic gut and compress the functioning lung tissue, further compromising pulmonary function. Moreover, a distended gut may cause difficulty in abdominal closure and may increase abdominal pressure, compressing the inferior vena cava and resulting in hypotension.

Barash PG, Stoelting RK (eds): Clinical Anesthesia, 3rd ed, pp 1091–1092. Philadelphia, Lippincott-Raven, 1997

Eger El II, Saidman LJ: Hazards of nitrous oxide anesthesia in bowel obstruction and pneumothorax. Anesthesiology 26:61, 1975

Fink R: Diffusion anoxia. Anesthesiology 16:511–519, 1955

Gregory GA (ed): Pediatric Anesthesia, 3rd ed, p 435. New York, Churchill Livingstone, 1994

C.4. Would you use 100% oxygen during anesthesia?

Selection of the appropriate inspired concentration of oxygen depends on the severity of pulmonary dysfunction. Retrolental fibroplasia is a potential danger during neonatal anesthesia. Current guidelines suggest that infants are at risk for retrolental fibroplasia until 44 to 50 weeks of gestational age. However, hypoxia causes pulmonary vasoconstriction and pulmonary hypertension which may increase right-to-left shunting of desaturated blood at preductal or ductal level. Therefore, air or nitrogen is added to oxygen if the PaO_2 on 100% oxygen is > 90 to 100 mm Hg. PaO_2 should be optimally kept at 80 to 100 mm Hg or the arterial oxygen saturation between 95% to 98%.

Dierdorf SF, Krishna G: Anesthetic management of neonatal surgical emergencies. Anesth Analg 60:204–214, 1981

Gregory GA (ed): Pediatric Anesthesia, 3rd ed, p 435. New York, Churchill Livingstone, 1994

C.5. How would you ventilate the patient?

Ventilation is controlled either manually or by a respirator. Small tidal volumes should be used to keep the airway pressure below 20 to 30 cm H_2O in order to prevent contralateral pneumothorax. High respiratory rates (60 to 120 breaths/min) should be adjusted to achieve hyperventilation to $PaCO_2$ between 25 to 30 mm Hg in order to lower pulmonary vascular resistance and minimize right-to-left shunting through the ductus arteriosus.

Bray RJ: Congenital diaphragmatic hernia. Anesthesia 34:567, 1979

Gregory GA (ed): Pediatric Anesthesia, 3rd ed, p 435. New York, Churchill Livingstone, 1994

C.6. How would you maintain the neonate's body temperature?

The neonate is particularly susceptible to heat loss because of a large surface to volume ratio, lack of insulating fat, and a naturally flaccid and open posture. Body temperature should be monitored carefully and maintained at normal. The following steps are used to maintain body temperature:

- Warm the operating room to 80°F (27°C).
- Use radiant warming lamps and a heating blanket.
- Warm and humidify inspired gases.
- Warm transfused blood and intravenous fluid to 37°C.

Dierdorf SF, Krishna G: Anesthetic management of neonatal surgical emergencies. Anesth Analg 60:204–214, 1981

Gregory GA (ed): Pediatric Anesthesia, 3rd ed, p 435. New York, Churchill Livingstone, 1994

C.7. The surgeon returned the intrathoracic stomach and intestine to the peritoneal cavity and the ipsilateral lung was found to be hypoplastic and collapsed. The resident anesthesiologist tried to expand the collapsed lung manually with positive airway pressure. Five minutes after the abdomen was closed, the blood pressure suddenly dropped from 70/40 to 30/20 mm Hg, the heart rate from 150 to 80/min, and the pulse oximeter from 95% down to 60% saturation. What would you do immediately?

Any sudden deterioration in blood pressure, heart rate, oxygen saturation, or pulmonary compliance is suggestive of tension pneumothorax. Auscultation of the chest, especially the contralateral side, should be done immediately. If absent or diminished breath sounds confirm the diagnosis, a chest tube should be inserted right away. A large-bore intravenous catheter with needle may be inserted to release the tension pneumothorax if a chest tube is not immediately available.

The tension pneumothorax is usually on the contralateral side since the high airway pressure required to inflate the hypoplastic lung may rupture the normal alveoli on the contralateral side, resulting in pneumothorax. Moreover, the ipsilateral chest usually already has a chest tube after surgery.

If there is no pneumothorax or deterioration is not improved after insertion of a chest tube, inferior vena cava compression (causing decreased venous return and decreased cardiac output) should be considered. The peritoneal cavity is often underdeveloped and unable to fully accommodate the returned abdominal organs, which increases the intraabdominal pressure. In this circumstance, the abdominal wound should be opened to relieve the compression on the vena cava and diaphragm. A Silastic patch may be used to cover the abdominal defect temporarily, and the defect will be closed at a later time.

Gregory GA (ed): Pediatric Anesthesia, 3rd ed, p 435. New York, Churchill Livingstone, 1994

Schwartz SI, Shires GT, Spencer FC (eds): Principles of Surgery, 6th ed, pp 1686–1687. New York, McGraw-Hill, 1994

C.8. Discuss fluid therapy in this patient.

Fluid therapy should be aimed to correct the preoperative deficit, provide maintenance fluid, and replace intraoperative evaporative, third space, and blood losses.

Kidneys are 80% to 90% mature by 1 month of age. Before that time, the infant cannot tolerate the extremes of renal stress. Neonates are obligate sodium losers; therefore, exogenous sodium should be supplied. In addition, neonates have decreased glycogen storage and are prone to hypoglycemia after brief periods of starvation. Therefore, glucose should also be provided. However, hyperglycemia may predispose the patient to intracranial hemorrhage and should be avoided. Preoperative fluid deficit may be evaluated by careful history taking, signs and symptoms of dehydration, urine output, and central venous pressure (CVP) monitoring. Maintenance fluids consisting of 5% dextrose in one-fourth to one-half-strength saline are given at 4 ml/kg/h. Intraoperative evaporative and third space losses are replaced with Ringer's lactate or saline at approximately 8 to 10 ml/kg/h. Each milliliter of blood loss is replaced with 3 ml of Ringer's lactate or 1 ml of 5% albumin in saline. Blood pressure, heart rate, urine output, CVP, hematocrit, and sodium and glucose levels are monitored to follow the fluid therapy.

Dierdorf SF, Krishna G: Anesthetic management of neonatal surgical emergencies. Anesth Analg 60:204–214, 1981

Gregory GA (ed): Pediatric Anesthesia, 3rd ed, p 435. New York, Churchill Livingstone, 1994

C.9. At the conclusion of surgery, would you extubate the patient in the operating room?

No. The patient should not be extubated in the operating room since varying degrees of pulmonary dysfunction are always present postoperatively. The endotracheal tube should be left in place and the baby should be transported to the intensive care unit for further postoperative care.

D. Postoperative Management

D.1. What postoperative problems would you expect in this patient? What is the mortality rate in patients with CDH?

The postoperative course is often characterized by a "honeymoon" period of rapid improvement, followed by sudden deterioration with profound arterial hypoxemia, hypercapnia, and acidosis.

The mortality in patients with CDH varies from 30% to 60%. The factors affecting the mortality include the following:

- Pulmonary hypoplasia
- Associated congenital defects—cardiovascular and central nervous systems
- Inadequate preoperative preparation—hypothermia, acidosis, shock, and tension pneumothorax
- Ineffective postoperative management—hemorrhage, tension pneumothorax, inferior vena cava compression, persistent fetal circulation, and excessive suction on chest tube.

Behrman RE, Kliegman RM, Arvin AM (eds): Nelson Textbook of Pediatrics, 15th ed, pp 1161–1164. Philadelphia, WB Saunders, 1996

Vacanti JP, Crone RK, Murphy JD et al: The pulmonary hemodynamic response to perioperative anesthesia in the treatment of high-risk infants with congenital diaphragmatic hernia. J Pediatr Surg 19:672–679, 1984

Waldschmidt J, vonLengerke HG, Berlien P: Causes of death in operated neonates with diaphragmatic defects. Prog Pediatr Surg 13:239, 1979

D.2. The neonate's blood gases improved right after surgery. However, 3 hours later, severe hypoxemia recurred in spite of ventilatory support with high inspired oxygen concentration. What are the possible causes? How should the patient be treated?

As discussed earlier, a tension pneumothorax should be considered and treated if it exists. In the absence of a tension pneumothorax, persistent hypoxemia suggests persistent pulmonary hypertension with right-to-left shunting of venous blood. Recurrent pulmonary hypertension carries a high mortality. ECMO support should be continued or reestablished if already discontinued before surgery. If the infant can not be weaned from ECMO after repair, options include discontinuing support or experimental therapies such as nitric oxide or single-lung transplantation. High frequency jet ventilation and oscillatory ventilation have had limited success in patients with CDH.

Behrman RE, Kliegman RM, Arvin AM (eds): Nelson Textbook of Pediatrics, 15th ed, pp 1161–1164. Philadelphia, WB Saunders, 1996

Gregory GA (ed): Pediatric Anesthesia, 3rd ed, pp 435–437. New York, Churchill Livingstone, 1989

Lung Transplantation

6

Paul M. Heerdt

A 52-year-old male with progressively worsening dyspnea on exertion, limitation of daily activity despite supplemental oxygen, and radiographic and spirometric evidence of severe obstructive pulmonary disease was scheduled for single lung transplantation. History was remarkable for a 30 pack/year smoking history (although none for 10 years) and mild hypertension.

A. Medical Disease and Differential Diagnosis

1. What were the expected manifestations of severe obstructive pulmonary disease in this patient, and why was he a transplant candidate?
2. What other end-stage lung diseases can also be treated with transplantation?
3. How many lung transplants have been performed?
4. What are the selection criteria for recipients?
5. How is the decision made to transplant one or both lungs, and does this influence preoperative management?
6. How does a single lung transplant differ technically from a double lung transplant?

B. Preoperative Evaluation and Preparation

1. What preoperative evaluation is desirable?
2. How would you premedicate this patient?
3. What vascular access is required?
4. Is preoperative epidural catheter placement advantageous?

C. Intraoperative Management

1. What special equipment is necessary?
2. How would you monitor this patient?
3. How would you induce anesthesia in this patient?
4. How would you ventilate this patient? What kind of endotracheal tube would you use?
5. How does the physiology of single lung ventilation influence the procedure?
6. Should volatile anesthetics be avoided during single lung ventilation?
7. At what specific points in the procedure are problems anticipated?
8. What are the problems associated with the lateral position?
9. How does single lung ventilation affect cardiopulmonary function? What are the problems of single lung ventilation in this patient? How would you treat them?
10. How would you deal with problems related to clamping of the pulmonary artery?
11. What hemodynamic alterations would you expect during graft implantation and reperfusion? How would you correct them?

115

12. Should fluid administration be restricted, and are blood products commonly required?
13. Would you extubate the patient upon conclusion of the procedure?

D. Postoperative Management

1. How is postoperative ventilation managed, and for how long is it required?
2. What are the common postoperative problems that may necessitate additional anesthesia and surgery?
3. What special precautions should be taken when a lung transplant recipient requires general anesthesia for subsequent nonpulmonary surgery?
4. Does lung transplantation work in the long run?
5. Are there surgical alternatives to lung transplantation?

A. Medical Disease and Differential Diagnosis

A.1. What were the expected manifestations of severe obstructive pulmonary disease in this patient, and why was he a transplant candidate?

This patient suffered from increased airway resistance, reduced expiratory flow rates, and high residual lung volumes. Chronic obstructive pulmonary disease (COPD) (often secondary to smoking), alpha-1-antitrypsin deficiency, and cystic fibrosis are the most common obstructive disorders in adults undergoing lung transplantation. At one time, concerns about mediastinal displacement and profound ventilation/perfusion ($\dot{V}/\dot{Q}$) mismatch secondary to hyperinflation of the remaining native lung prevented surgeons from attempting single lung transplantation for emphysema. However, clinical experience has demonstrated that many emphysemic patients can be successfully treated by single lung transplantation. Due to the severe shortage of organs for transplant, single lung procedures are desirable whenever possible.

Cooper JD: Current status of lung transplantation. Transplant Proc 23:2107–2114, 1991

Low DE, Trulock EP, Kaiser LR et al: Morbidity, mortality, and early results of single versus bilateral lung transplantation for emphysema. J Thorac Cardiovasc Surg 103:1119–1126, 1992

A.2. What other end-stage lung diseases can also be treated with transplantation?

The first successful (i.e., patient left the hospital) single lung transplant was performed in 1983 for idiopathic pulmonary fibrosis. Since that time, the procedure has been applied to patients suffering from a variety of end-stage pulmonary diseases (Table 6-1). In general, the underlying disease processes produce lung dysfunction that can be broadly characterized as obstructive, restrictive, infectious, or vascular in nature. At the present time, approximately 20% of the single lung transplants performed have been for restrictive lung disease such as idiopathic pulmonary fibrosis. Reflecting a loss of lung parenchymal elasticity and compliance, end-stage restrictive disease is characterized by profoundly reduced lung volumes and diffusing capacity, but relative preservation of ventilatory flow rates. Comparison of flow-volume loops representing obstructive and restrictive disease are shown in Figure 6-1. The underlying disease process also tends to obliterate pulmonary microvasculature, thus chronically increasing vascular resistance, producing pulmonary hypertension and predis-

Table 6-1. Lung Transplants Categorized by Disease

DIAGNOSIS	PERCENT OF TOTAL
COPD	30
Idiopathic pulmonary fibrosis	16
Cystic fibrosis	15
Alpha-1-antitrypsin deficiency	12
Primary pulmonary hypertension	8
Bronchiectasis	3
Eisenmenger's syndrome	3
Retransplant	3
Bronchiolitis obliterans	2
Leiomyomatosis	2
Sarcoidosis	2
Other	6

(Reprinted with permission from St. Louis International Lung Transplant Registry)

posing to cor pulmonale. Most patients with restrictive disease are good candidates for a single lung transplant since the stiff, vasoconstricted native lung will receive relatively little ventilation and perfusion and can thus usually be left without compromising the transplanted lung.

Infectious lung disease such as cystic fibrosis is the most frequent indication for lung transplantation in patients <18 years of age. Characterized by chronic infection and the production of copious purulent secretions, cystic fibrosis patients primarily exhibit functional abnormalities that are obstructive in nature with increased airway reactivity. Under most circumstances, residual volumes and functional residual capacity are increased and bronchodilators have little effect on expiratory flow rates. Due to potential infectious cross-contamination of the transplanted lung, chronic infec-

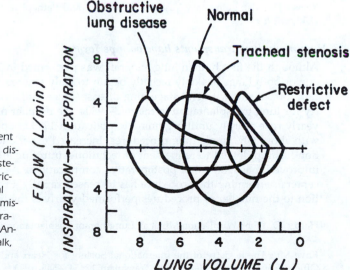

Figure 6-1. Representative tracings of flow-volume loops from a normal subject, a patient with parenchymal obstructive disease, a patient with tracheal stenosis, and a patient with restrictive disease from parenchymal fibrosis. (Reproduced with permission from Goudsouzian N, Karamanian A: Physiology for the Anesthesiologist, 2nd ed. Norwalk, CT, Appleton-Century-Crofts, 1984)

tious disease represents a contraindication to single lung transplantation. However, single lung transplantation with contralateral pneumonectomy has been performed and suggested as an alternative solution.

Pulmonary vascular disease with severe pulmonary hypertension and right ventricular dysfunction has also emerged as an indication for transplantation. Pathologically, severe pulmonary arterial hypertension can result from idiopathic proximal vascular processes (primary pulmonary hypertension) or secondary to chronically increased pulmonary blood flow or pulmonary venous hypertension. Pulmonary hypertension may precipitate chronic hypoxemia if it is associated with an intracardiac defect that allows for development of a right-to-left shunt. Since a native lung can usually be left intact without compromising a transplanted lung (which will receive the majority of blood flow), some patients with pulmonary vascular disease may be reasonable candidates for single lung transplantation, with concurrent repair of any cardiac anomalies. Although some studies have indicated remarkable improvement in survival and New York Heart Association (NYHA) class following single lung transplantation in patients with pulmonary hypertension, other investigation has not provided similar results.

Bando K, Keenan RJ, Paradis IL et al: Impact of pulmonary hypertension on outcome after single-lung transplantation. Ann Thorac Surg 58:1336–1342, 1994

Hinson KFW: Diffuse pulmonary fibrosis. Hum Pathol 1:825–847, 1970

Kaye MP: The Registry of the International Society for Heart and Lung Transplantation: Tenth Official Report–1993. J Heart Lung Transplant 12:541–548, 1993

Pasque MK, Kaiser LR, Dresler CM et al: Single lung transplantation for pulmonary hypertension: Technical aspects and immediate hemodynamic results. J Thorac Cardiovasc Surg 130:475–482, 1992

Shennib H, Massard G, Gauthier R et al: Single lung transplantation for cystic fibrosis: Is it an option? J Heart Lung Transplant 12:288–293, 1993

Voelkel NF, Weir EK: Etiologic mechanisms in primary pulmonary hypertension, in Weir EK, Reeves JT (eds): Pulmonary Vascular Physiology and Pathophysiology, pp 513–539. New York, Dekker, 1989

A.3. How many lung transplants have been performed?

Although the first human lung allograft was performed in 1963, transplantation of one or both lungs has only recently begun to truly emerge as a viable therapeutic option for patients with end-stage lung disease. Since initiation of an international registry for lung transplantation in the mid-1980s, the number of procedures reported yearly rose sharply until beginning to plateau in 1993 at approximately 400/year, with about 60% single lung procedures. Increased experience with lung transplantation has rapidly led to refinement of technique, introduction of new procedures, and improved management of postoperative complications. Accordingly, the number of centers performing the procedure has increased rapidly. Presently, the primary limitation to the number of procedures performed yearly is the limited donor supply.

Hardy JD, Webb WR, Dalton ML et al: Lung homotransplantation in man. JAMA 186:1065–1074, 1963

Kaye MP: The Registry of the International Society for Heart and Lung Transplantation: Tenth Official Report–1993. J Heart Lung Transplant 12:541–548, 1993

A.4. What are the selection criteria for recipients?

As with many of the facets of the surgical procedure itself, selection criteria for lung recipients have also undergone considerable evolution, particularly as more institutions initiate transplant programs. In general, patients with severe end-stage lung disease are considered candidates for transplantation when their life expectancy is 18 months or less, they have minimal disease of other organ systems, and they are mentally and psychologically capable of following strict regimens for rehabilitation and immunosuppressive therapy. In contrast to criteria formulated when lung transplantation was in its infancy, concomitant steroid therapy, previous intrathoracic surgery, mechanical ventilation, and right ventricular failure are no longer considered absolute contraindications.

Bracken CA, Gurkowski MA, Naples JJ: Lung transplantation: Historical perspective, current concepts, and anesthetic management. J Cardiothorac Vasc Anesth 11:220–241, 1997

Triantafillou AN, Heerdt PM: Lung transplantation. Int Anesthesiol Clin 29:87–109, 1991

A.5. How is the decision made to transplant one or both lungs, and does this influence preoperative management?

Whenever possible, single lung transplantation is performed due to the extreme shortage of donor organs. The only absolute contraindication to single lung transplantation is a situation such as infectious lung disease where leaving the native lung could endanger long-term viability of the transplanted lung. As noted above, it was once thought that severe emphysema was a contraindication to single lung transplantation due to the probability of mediastinal shift and marked ventilation mismatch between the highly dispensable native lung and the graft. However, this consideration has turned out to be of only modest physiologic importance in most single lung recipients with obstructive disease. From a practical standpoint, the decision to perform a single or bilateral lung transplant has little impact on preoperative management since both procedures necessitate the same level of preparation.

Cooper JD: Current status of lung transplantation. Transplant Proc 23:2107–2114, 1991

A.6. How does a single lung transplant differ technically from double lung transplant?

It is extremely important that anesthesiologists be broadly familiar with the surgical methods since manipulation of the heart and lungs at specific points during the transplant can produce marked cardiopulmonary disturbances. Ideally, the anesthesiologist will anticipate these changes and adapt the anesthetic management accordingly. Descriptions of the detailed technical aspects of lung transplantation are readily available.

Single lung transplantation is usually performed in lateral decubitus position via a thorocotomy incision, often with the upper leg and pelvis angled to allow groin exposure for potential femoral cannulation and cardiopulmonary bypass. In contrast, bilateral lung transplantation is usually performed with the patient supine via a clamshell incision (bilateral thorocotomies and transverse sternotomy). For both single and bilateral lung transplantation, intermittent single lung ventilation is required during dissection of the native lung to be removed and implantation of the graft. Once stable single lung ventilation is established, dissection of the lung to be transplanted is initiated with isolation of the pulmonary artery (PA). To assess the cardiopulmonary response to diverting the entire cardiac output through one lung, progressive occlusion of the vessel is first performed manually; if well tolerated, the vessel is then clamped and stapled. After ligation of the PA, the pneumonectomy is completed. Implantation of the graft begins with anastomosis of the airway. At some institutions, the bronchial anastomosis is wrapped with an omental pedicle, previously mobilized through a small abdominal incision, in an effort to improve blood supply to the airway and promote healing. Other institutions now routinely use a telescoping bronchial anastomosis, which appears to remove the need for omental wrapping. The PA branch is then connected, followed by anastomosis of a cuff of the left atrium containing the pulmonary veins. The implanted lung is then partially inflated, air removed from the left atrial cuff and pulmonary veins, and circulation to the organ restored. In patients presenting for single lung transplant with chronic, progressive pulmonary hypertension of primary or secondary etiology, the right ventricle has often been seriously compromised and may have little contractile reserve. To avoid additional right ventricular stress, it is the practice at many institutions to institute partial normothermic cardiopulmonary bypass during single lung transplant for primary pulmonary hypertension, or in patients with severe pulmonary hypertension and right ventricular dysfunction secondary to restrictive or obstructive disease. Cannulation is typically via the femoral artery and the right atrium, unless simultaneous correction of an intracardiac defect is planned. In such patients, conventional aortic and single- or double-stage atrial cannulation is performed. Implantation of the lung is otherwise performed in the same fashion as described above.

Double lung transplantation was first described by the Toronto Lung Transplant Group in the mid-1980s as en-bloc implantation of both lungs simultaneously. The procedure is performed via a median sternotomy using hypothermic cardiopulmonary bypass, cardioplegic cardiac arrest, and single tracheal (or double bronchial) anastomosis of the trachea and main PA. However, although the procedure initially produced some encouraging results, considerable limitations related to its technical complexity, morbidity, mortality, and application to many patients with end-stage lung disease soon became apparent. Not surprisingly, application of the procedure declined sharply and has now been largely replaced by the bilateral sequential implantation technique, which does not require hypothermic cardiopulmonary bypass. Introduced in 1990, bilateral lung transplantation has become the surgical procedure of choice when replacement of both lungs is necessary. As noted above, in contrast to single lung transplant, bilateral lung transplantation procedures are performed in the supine position. Technically the procedure involves bilateral anterior thoracotomies which extend from the mid-axillary lines to meet in the center through a transverse sternotomy. In general, the procedure can be regarded as having two phases. First, the most severely compromised lung (as determined by preoperative $\dot{V}/\dot{Q}$ scanning) is removed during ventilation of the good contralateral lung. Removal and implantation of the second lung is then performed. Frequently, the contralateral incision is not made until after implantation, ventilation, and reperfusion of the first lung due to the fact that cardiopulmonary stability is often better maintained if both hemithoraces are not opened simultaneously at the beginning of the procedure. Two reasons for this enhanced stability have been postulated. First, mechanical ventilation of an emphysematous lung without the confines of the chest wall may promote gas trapping and cardiac compression, and second, air leaks created during dissection may further compromise ventilation. The second lung is then removed and transplanted during ventilation of the new lung alone.

Egan TM, Kaiser LR, Cooper JD: Lung transplantation. Curr Probl Surg 26:673–752, 1989

Kaiser LR, Cooper JD: Adult lung transplantation, in Flye MW (ed): Atlas of Organ Transplantation, pp 296–312. Philadelphia, WB Saunders, 1995

Pasque MK, Cooper JD, Kaiser LK et al: An improved technique for bilateral single lung transplantation: Rationale and clinical experience. Ann Thorac Surg 49:785–789, 1990

B. Preoperative Evaluation and Preparation

B.1. What preoperative evaluation is desirable?

At most centers, an extensive physical examination, psychological evaluation, and numerous tests of cardiopulmonary function will have been performed prior to acceptance into the transplant program. This facilitates the preanesthetic evaluation, which ideally is performed when the patient is first accepted into the transplant program. Familiarity with pulmonary function tests, ventilation/perfusion scan results, heart catheterization and echocardiographic data (including performance of intracardiac shunts), exercise tolerance, oxygen use, and dependence on continuous pulmonary vasodilator infusion (i.e., prostacyclin) is beneficial for formulating an anesthetic plan.

Morrison DL, Maurer JR, Grossman RF: Preoperative assessment for lung transplantation. Clin Chest Med 11:207–215, 1990

Triantafillou AN, Heerdt PM: Lung Transplantation. Int Anesthesiol Clin Summer 29:87–109, 1991

B.2. How would you premedicate this patient?

As with all critically ill patients, considerations regarding preoperative sedation are governed primarily by the functional limitations imposed by the underlying disease. Since deterioration of respiratory and/or cardiac function between the preoperative evaluation and eventual transplantation is not unusual, careful reassessment of the patient's general condition and current arterial blood gas data is warranted before administering premedication. When indicated, parenteral sedation is usually chosen due to insufficient time to effectively administer oral anxiolytics. Midazolam alone or in combination with diphenhydramine (potentially protecting the lung against drug-induced histamine release) is often sufficient. Clinically, most patients with end-stage restrictive, obstructive, or infectious lung disease are tachypneic while breathing room air and cannot be aggressively sedated. In contrast, patients with primary pulmonary hypertension and no intracardiac defect often appear reasonably normal and will benefit from sedation due to the potential for stress-related increases in pulmonary vascular resistance. Alternatively, patients with pulmonary hypertension and significant right-to-left intracardiac shunting (i.e., Eisenmenger's physiology) are often cyanotic despite oxygen supplementation and may not tolerate sedation well.

Bracken CA, Gurkowski MA, Naples JJ: Lung transplantation: Historical perspective, current concepts, and anesthetic management. J Cardiothorac Vasc Anesth 11:220–221, 1997

Heerdt PM, Triantafillou AN: Anesthesia for lung transplantation, in Flye MW (ed): Atlas of Organ Transplantation, pp 313–318. Philadelphia, WB Saunders, 1995

B.3. What vascular access is required?

In patients with chronic infectious lung disease or a history of previous intrathoracic procedures, two large-bore intravenous catheters (preferably placed in the wrist or forearm since the arms may be flexed during the procedure) are advisable due to the potential for brisk blood loss during dissection of pulmonary adhesions. Meticulous removal of air from venous infusion lines should be performed, particularly in patents with known or suspected right-to-left shunts. At many institutions, cannulation of a femoral artery instead of a radial artery is performed under local anesthesia in the operating room due to the fact that radial arterial pressures may become damped during the procedure secondary to positioning of the arms.

B.4. Is preoperative epidural catheter placement advantageous?

Pain control after lung transplantation can be critical in facilitating patient extubation and rehabilitation. Both lumbar and thoracic epidural catheters have been used for postoperative pain management. At many institutions, catheters are placed immediately before the procedure in most patients despite the possibility of anticoagulation and cardiopulmonary bypass during the transplant procedure. This practice is supported by data indicating no adverse sequelae to preoperatively placed epidural catheters, including patients who required emergent heparinization and cardiopulmonary bypass. Obvious exception to this approach are patients anticoagulated preoperatively, or those in whom cardiopulmonary bypass is planned. Delaying placement of the epidural catheter until the postoperative period may actually increase the potential risk of complications due to the fact that both hemodilution and immunosuppression tend to promote a coagulopathy.

Body S, Fanciullo G, Ferrante M et al: Thoracic epidural analgesia after lung transplant. Anesthesiology 81(3A):1285, 1994

Triantafillou AN, Heerdt PM: Lung transplantation. Int Anesthesiol Clin 29:87–109, 1991

Triantafillou AN, Heerdt PM, Hogue CW et al: Epidural vs. intravenous morphine for postoperative pain management after lung transplantation. Anesthesiology 77(3A):A857, 1992

C. Intraoperative Management

C.1. What special equipment is necessary?

Items advantageous for lung transplantation procedures include an anesthesia ventilator capable of delivering a wide range of I:E ratios and respiratory rates, a jet ventilator, a CPAP apparatus, and a cardiopulmonary bypass machine on standby. Additionally, having a sterile circuit for the anesthesia machine and sterile tubing for the jet ventilator in the room is useful should the distal airway become disrupted or the endobronchial tube damaged, necessitating direct bronchial intubation or jet ventilation on the surgical field.

C.2. How would you monitor this patient?

Intraoperatively, hemodynamic and respiratory changes are often acute and profound, thus extensive monitoring is imperative. In addition to the electrocardiogram, arterial blood pressure and peripheral arterial oxygen saturation, pulmonary artery (PA) catheter placement is routine for lung transplantation procedures due to the profound changes in pulmonary and systemic hemodynamics that often occur both during and after lung transplantation. In patients undergoing single lung transplant, PA catheters often migrate to the operative side after the patient has been placed in the lateral position even when radiographically confirmed to be positioned in the nonoperative lung. Thus, the surgeon should be reminded to palpate the pulmonary artery and withdraw the catheter if necessary before cross-clamping the vessel. PA catheters capable of measuring right ventricular ejection fraction and mixed venous oxygen saturation have been widely used, often in combination with two-dimensional transesophageal echocardiography (2D-TEE), to quickly assess right ventricular performance. Both of these monitoring methods can be helpful for management of lung transplantation. However, TEE visualization of the right ventricle in laterally positioned emphysemic patients is often poor, and thermodilution measurements of cardiac output and ejection fraction may be distorted by the tricuspid regurgitation that frequently accompanies pulmonary hypertension. In addition to cardiovascular monitoring, continuous measurement of pulmonary mechanics by side-stream spirometry may represent a valuable tool in early detection of reperfusion injury and graft dysfunction.

Bardoczky GI, De Franquen P, Engleman E, Capello M: Continuous monitoring of pulmonary mechanics with the side-stream spirometer during lung transplantation. J Cardiothorac Vasc Anesth 6:731–734, 1992

Konstam MA, Salem DN, Imner JM et al: Vasodilator effect on right ventricular function in congestive heart failure and pulmonary hypertension. Am J Cardiol 54:132–136, 1984

Triantafillou AN, Heerdt PM: Lung Transplantation. Int Anesthesiol Clin 29:87–109, 1991

C.3. *How would you induce anesthesia in this patient?*

As with induction of anesthesia in any critically ill patient, multiple techniques have been safely used in patients undergoing lung transplantation. The only general rule is that induction be relatively gradual since abrupt withdrawal of sympathetic tone in these patients with high catecholamine "drive" can result in severe cardiovascular compromise, particularly during the transition from spontaneous to mechanical ventilation. For this reason, dosing an epidural catheter with local anesthetic prior to induction of anesthesia can be problematic. Since effective alveolar ventilation and nitrogen washout is poor in the patient with severe obstructive lung disease and high residual volumes, prolonged (i.e., 15 to 20 minutes) preoxygenation is worthwhile followed by a rapidly-acting induction agent to shorten the excitement stage, expedite airway management, and prevent opiate-induced truncal rigidity. Thiopental, etomidate, and ketamine have all been used safely, but specific properties of each drug in the setting of the patient's underlying disease should be considered. Thiopental, for example, may not be desirable in patients with bronchospasm or pulmonary hypertension due to a propensity for histamine release. Alternatively, the sympathomimetic properties of ketamine may preclude use in the presence of pulmonary hypertension, while its bronchodilating effects may be beneficial in patients with bronchospasm. After administration of the hypnotic, either fentanyl (10 to 15 mg/kg) or sufentanil (1 to 2 mg/kg) has been commonly used along with either succinlycholine or a nondepolarizing muscle relaxant to complete induction. Benzodiazepines, scopolamine, and/or volatile anesthetic agents are frequently administered after induction to promote amnesia and, in the case of volatile agents, promote bronchodilation.

Conacher ID: Isolated lung transplantation: A review of problems and guide to anesthesia. Br J Anaesth 61:468–474, 1989

Gayes JM, Giron L, Nissen MD, Plut D: Anesthetic considerations for patients undergoing double-lung transplantation. J Cardiothorac Vasc Anesth 4:486–498, 1990

Raffin L, Cherqui MM, Sperandio M et al: Anesthesia for bilateral lung transplantation without cardiopulmonary bypass: Initial experience and review of intraoperative problems. J Cardiothor Vasc Anesth 6:409–417, 1992

Thomas B, Slegel LC: Anesthetic and postoperative management of single-lung transplantation. J Cardiothorac Vasc Anesth 5:266–267, 1991

C.4. How would you ventilate this patient? What kind of endotracheal tube would you use?

Following induction, the trachea is usually intubated with a left endobronchial double-lumen tube for both single lung transplant and bilateral lung transplantation. Use of a single-lumen endotracheal tube in combination with either an external or internal bronchial blocking catheter has been described, but does not appear to be clearly superior to the left endobronchial tube for most procedures. Furthermore, an endobronchial tube allows for differential lung ventilation if required in the postoperative period. One exception to this approach has been in patients with cystic fibrosis who exhibit thick, tenacious secretions that are difficult to suction via the small lumen suction catheters necessary for double-lumen tubes. In these patients, it is often helpful to first place a large single-lumen tube and perform extensive bronchoscopic-directed bronchial lavage and suctioning prior to placement of the double-lumen tube.

The transition from spontaneous to mechanical ventilation invariably produces hemodynamic alteration due to acute changes in intrathoracic pressure and chest-wall compliance. With obstructive lung disease, mechanical ventilation magnifies air trapping leading to "pulmonary tamponade." Adjustment of the ventilatory pattern accordingly (i.e., an I:E ratio of 1:5 or greater with moderate tidal volumes) often lessens circulatory compromise. With restrictive disease, higher inflation pressures and positive end-expiratory pressure are often required. In both obstructive and restrictive patients, optimal balance of ventilation with hemodynamic stability often necessitates tolerating a degree of hypercapnia. Often a brief period of apnea followed by careful hand ventilation will alone restore cardiovascular stability. In patients with pulmonary hypertension, mechanical ventilation usually produces less cardiovascular disturbance if caution is exercised not to increase pulmonary vascular resistance, (e.g., from hypoxia, hypercarbia, or lung hyperinflation).

Since lung recipients have little pulmonary reserve, ventilation with 100% O_2 is commonly used intraoperatively. Although this approach is somewhat controversial, there are few data to suggest acute oxygen toxicity to a transplanted lung. High PaO_2 may also directly promote pulmonary vasodilation and thus be beneficial in reducing right ventricular afterload.

Raffin L, Cherqui MM, Sperandio M et al: Anesthesia for bilateral lung transplantation without cardiopulmonary bypass: Initial experience and review of intraoperative problems. J Cardiothorac Vasc Anesth 6:409–417, 1992

Scheller MS, Kriett JM, Smith CM, Jamieson SW: Airway management during anesthesia for double-lung transplantation using a single-lumen endotracheal tube with an enclosed bronchial blocker. J Cardiothorac Vasc Anesth 6:204–207, 1992

Weir EK, Reeves JT (eds): Pulmonary Vascular Physiology and Pathophysiology, pp 241–290. New York, Dekker, 1989

C.5. How does the physiology of single lung ventilation influence the procedure?

In laterally positioned patients, gravity helps redistribute blood away from the non-ventilated lung during single lung ventilation and lessen intrapulmonary shunt. In patients in the supine position, this benefit is obviously lost and single lung ventilation may not be well tolerated. In general, due to large residual lung volumes that will be slowly filled with a high concentration of oxygen content during the initial stages of the procedure, lung recipients with severe obstructive lung disease may initially maintain oxygenation for the first 10 to 15 minutes of single lung ventilation. However, rapid arterial desaturation may then occur once a substantial portion of the residual volume is absorbed. Alternatively, patients with restrictive lung disease and a low functional residual capacity may rapidly exhibit both hypoxia and hypercarbia. Multiple steps can be taken to improve oxygenation including insufflation of oxygen or continuous positive airway pressure (CPAP) to the nonventilated lung, broncho-scopic-guided suctioning of the ventilated lung, careful manipulation of the ventilatory pattern, and positive end-expiratory pressure (PEEP) to the ventilated lung. Differential PEEP/CPAP should be done cautionsly, however, since increased airway pressure in the ventilated lung can divert blood toward the nonventilated side. In some patients, intermittent ventilation of the operative lung may have to be performed prior to pneumonectomy. In general, oxygenation improves following the clamping of the pulmonary artery supplying the nonventilated lung.

DeMajo WAP: Anesthetic technique for single lung transplantation, in Cooper JC, Novitzky D (eds): The Transplantation and Replacement of Thoracic Organs, pp 555–562. Boston, Kliuwer Academic Publishers, 1990.

Triantafillou AN, Heerdt PM: Lung Transplantation. Int Anesthesiol Clin 29(3):87–109, 1991

C.6. Should volatile anesthetics be avoided during single lung ventilation?

Due to experimental evidence demonstrating inhibition of hypoxic vasoconstriction by the volatile anesthetic agents, some authors have suggested that these drugs be avoided in the anesthetic management of patients with end-stage lung disease requiring single lung ventilation. However, true clinical significance of these experimental observations remains somewhat controversial. From a clinical standpoint, commonly used doses of isoflurane (i.e., end-tidal concentrations of 1.0 or less) have not been empirically associated with worsening of intrapulmonary shunt and hypoxia. Thus, isoflurane remains widely used in these patients and may actually benefit some lung recipients due to bronchodilating properties (also see Chapter 2, question C.22.)

Benumof JL: Anesthesia for one-lung ventilation (reply to letter). Anesthesiology 69:631, 1988

Bjertnaes J, Hauge A, Torgrinson T: The pulmonary vasoconstrictor response to hypoxia: The hypoxia sensitive site studied with a volatile inhibitor. Acta Physiol Scand 109:447–462, 1980

Marshall BE: Anesthesia for one-lung ventilation (letter). Anesthesiology 69:630–631, 1988

Raffin L, Cherqui MM, Sperandio M et al: Anesthesia for bilateral lung transplantation without cardiopulmonary bypass: Initial experience and review of intraoperative problems. J Cardiothorac Vasc Anesth 6:409–417, 1992

C.7. At what specific points in the procedure are problems anticipated?

- Lateral positioning
- Single lung ventilation
- Clamping of the pulmonary artery
- Graft implantation
- Graft reperfusion

C.8. What are the problems associated with the lateral position?

Single lung transplant is usually performed in lateral decubitus position, often with the upper leg and pelvis angled to allow groin exposure for potential femoral cannulation and cardiopulmonary bypass. Not surprisingly, position-related changes in venous return coupled with compression of the dependent lung by the mediastinum and diaphragm may promote systemic hypotension and ventilation/perfusion mismatch. Furthermore, pulmonary arterial pressure usually tends to rise following lateral positioning, probably due to gravity-induced shifts in pulmonary blood flow distribution, vascular congestion, and increased vascular resistance.

C.9. How does single lung ventilation affect cardiopulmonary function? What are the problems of single lung ventilation in this patient? How would you treat them?

Isolated ventilation of the dependent lung is often accompanied by a marked, acute increase in peak inspiratory pressure and a subsequent gradual, progressive rise in pulmonary arterial pressure. As noted above, due to the beneficial effect of gravity on redistributing blood away from the nondependent, nonventilated lung, single lung ventilation is often tolerated better from a respiratory standpoint by patients undergoing single lung transplant in the lateral position than those undergoing bilateral lung transplantation in the supine position. Close monitoring of right ventricular performance during conversion to single lung ventilation is extremely important due to the increase in afterload produced by hypoxic vasoconstriction and redistribution of blood flow. If the right ventricle becomes hypokinetic and distended, or ejection fraction falls, ventilation may have to be altered to minimize airway pressure. If right ventricular performance does not improve or persistent hypoxemia and/or hypercarbia results, heparinization and cardiopulmonary bypass may be required. Some advocate infusion of catecholamines, phosphodiesterase inhibitors, and/or pulmonary vasodilators such as prostaglandin E_1 (PGE$_1$) prior to initiating single lung ventilation in an effort to support the right ventricle and lessen the impact of acutely increased afterload. Interestingly, marked exacerbation of intrapulmonary shunt does not appear to occur with low to moderate doses of PGE$_1$, and thus systemic hypotension can be used as the dosing end-point.

Heerdt PM, Weiss CI: Prostaglandin E_1 and intrapulmonary shunt in cardiac surgical patients with pulmonary hypertension. Ann Thorac Surg 49:463–465, 1990

Triantafillou AN, Pasque MK, Huddleston CB et al: Predictors, frequency, and indications for cardiopulmonary bypass during lung transplantation in adults. Ann Thorac Surg 57:1248–1251, 1994

C.10. How would you deal with problems related to clamping of the pulmonary artery?

To assess the cardiopulmonary response to diverting the entire cardiac output through one lung, progressive occlusion of the vessel is first performed manually. If occlusion is well tolerated, the vessel is then clamped and stapled. If occlusion is poorly tolerated, the vessel is unclamped and a pulmonary vasodilator and/or positive inotrope infusion begun. Some authors advocate the routine infusion of dopamine at this point in lung transplantation procedures. If severe respiratory or cardiovascular derangements persist following reclamping of the vessel despite pharmacologic intervention, heparin is administered and cardiopulmonary bypass instituted to avoid profound hypoxia or right ventricular (RV) failure. However, for most patients undergoing single lung transplant, hypoxemia during single lung ventilation and after PA clamping is rarely a problem and RV performance can be adequately maintained.

C.11. What hemodynamic alterations would you expect during graft implantation and reperfusion? How would you correct them?

During the process of performing the vascular and bronchial anastomoses, major disturbances on cardiac filling and rhythm can be produced. While often transient, systemic hypotension and pulmonary hypertension can ensue. Following reperfusion and subsequent ventilation of the new lung, PA pressures and arterial blood gases should be closely followed. Pulmonary arterial pressure usually falls following reperfusion of the donor organ. If a substantial decrease is not observed, potential causes include anastomotic problems with the atrial cuff or the pulmonary artery, or early reperfusion injury of the donor organ. Assessment of the pulmonary arterial and venous flow pattern by TEE can sometimes be of benefit in evaluating adequacy of the anastomoses. On occasion reperfusion of the first lung is followed by a rapid, progressive increase in PA pressure, often coupled with increased inspiratory pressure, hypoxia, hypotension, and pulmonary edema. This acute, potentially catastrophic event necessitates adjustment of ventilation, addition of positive end-expiratory pressure, and increased pharmacologic support. Should hemodynamic and ventilatory derangements be refractory to treatment, cardiopulmonary bypass may be required. It has been postulated that reperfusion of an organ after lengthy ischemia may directly cause tissue damage or unmask injury sustained during the ischemic period.

Egan TM, Kaiser LR, Cooper JD: Lung transplantation. Curr Probl Surg 26:673–756, 1989

Horgan MJ, Lum H, Malik AB: Pulmonary edema after pulmonary artery occlusion and reperfusion. Am Rev Respir Dis 140:1421–1428, 1989

Sarsam MA, Yonan NA, Beton D et al: Early pulmonary vein thrombosis after single lung transplantation. J Heart Lung Transplant 12:17–19, 1993

C.12. Should fluid administration be restricted, and are blood products commonly required?

The amount of crystalloid that can be safely administered intraoperatively without adversely affecting the graft appears to be widely variable. Although all efforts should be made to minimize fluid infusion intraoperatively, many patients undergoing lung transplantation require large amounts of fluid in order to maintain hemodynamic stability. Not uncommonly, central venous and pulmonary capillary wedge pressures of 3 to 5 mm Hg immediately following a transplant are evident despite infusion of large amounts of crystalloid and colloid, and only moderate blood loss. A recent review of fluid management during 215 lung transplants performed without cardiopulmonary bypass revealed that intraoperative crystalloid administration varied widely (4 to 32 ml/kg/h) with a mean of 13 ± 6 ml/kg/h. Using the PaO_2/F_iO_2 ratio on arrival in the ICU and time to extubation as indices of early graft function and initial outcome, respectively, this study showed no correlation between the amount of fluids administered and either of these indices.

Prior to development of the bilateral lung transplantation procedure without cardiopulmonary bypass, patients with a history of surgery involving the lung or pleura, or chronic infectious lung disease were not deemed acceptable candidates for lung transplantation because of the anticipated excessive bleeding associated with dissecting a scarred lung in an anticoagulated patient. Now, without the uniform requirement for heparinization, such patients are generally regarded as operative candidates. As with other surgical procedures where hemorrhage is anticipated, continuous infusion of aprotinin has been proposed to reduce intraoperative bleeding during surgical procedures in patients with cystic fibrosis or a history of previous intrathoracic surgery. To date, however, data to support this practice are lacking. If blood products are to be administered, it is important for the anesthesiologist to be familiar with whether or not the patient has antibodies to cytomegalovirus (CMV) and to closely check blood products to confirm that they coincide with the patient's status.

Janssens M, Joris J, David JL et al: High-dose aprotinin reduces blood loss in patients undergoing total hip replacement surgery. Anesthesiology 80:23–29, 1994

Karanikolas MS, Triantafillou AN, Pond CG et al: Outcome of lung transplantation in relation to fluid administration. Anesthesiology 81(3A):A1465, 1994

C.13 Would you extubate the patient upon conclusion of the procedure?

Due to the cardiopulmonary insult associated with the procedure, large postoperative volume shifts, hypothermia, and the frequent need for postoperative bronchoscopy, lung transplant recipients are not generally extubated immediately after the procedure. Accordingly, unless intraoperative events (i.e., hyperinflation of the remaining intact lung) suggest that postoperative differential lung ventilation will be required, or functional issues such as profound oropharyngeal edema or difficult intubation are present, the double-lumen tube is exchanged for a single-lumen tube. In many patients, the endotracheal tube change can be facilitated by use of an exchange catheter. However, great care should be taken in not advancing the catheter too far and damaging the graft. It is often beneficial to perform fiberoptic bronchoscopy to examine bronchial anastomoses and aggressively suction secretions or blood following replacement of the double-lumen tube with a single-lumen endotracheal tube.

D. Postoperative Management

D.1. How is postoperative ventilation managed, and for how long is it required?

Following most procedures, the F_iO_2 can be rapidly reduced and weaning from the ventilator begun as soon as the patient is warm and stable. An exception to this approach is the patient who has undergone single lung transplant for pulmonary hypertension. Due to a propensity for episodes of cardiopulmonary instability during the first 48 to 72 hours postoperatively, it is usually advantageous to keep these patients sedated, paralyzed, and ventilated during this period.

Postoperatively, $\dot{V}/\dot{Q}$ mismatch and intrapulmonary shunt are often more pronounced following single lung transplant than bilateral lung transplantation. Not surprisingly, patients with restrictive disease usually display the best pulmonary function following single lung transplant since the graft receives the majority of both ventilation and perfusion. Alternatively, following single lung transplant in emphysemic patients, the remaining native lung often receives a substantial portion of the tidal volume; while in patients with pulmonary hypertension, the native lung continues to be ventilated but receives very little blood flow. Postural changes in arterial oxygen saturation are often prominent in single lung transplant recipients. In general, patients who received a single lung for pulmonary hypertension or emphysema display better postoperative pulmonary function with the transplant side up, whereas the opposite may be true in certain patients with restrictive lung disease. The precise etiology of this response is unclear, but probably reflects positional variation in ventilation/perfusion matching.

Triantafillou AN, Heerdt PM: Lung Transplantation. Int Anesthesiol Clin 29:87–109, 1991

D.2. What are the common postoperative problems that may necessitate additional anesthesia and surgery?

Unfortunately, postoperative infection remains the leading cause of death in the postoperative period (Table 6-2), with the majority of fatal infections either viral or fungal. In general, early complications include bleeding, technical problems with vascular or bronchial anastomoses, and profound reperfusion injury with graft failure necessitating retransplantation, while late complications include airway dehiscence and chronic rejection necessitating retransplantation. Multiple fiberoptic and/or rigid bronchoscopic procedures are common because many patients require tracheal/bronchial dilatation, laser therapy, or placement of endobronchial stents.

Maurer JR, Tullis DE, Grossman RF, Vellend H, Winton TL, Patterson GA: Infectious complications following isolated lung transplantation. Chest 101:1056–1059, 1992

Cooper JD: Current status of lung transplantation. Transpl Proc 23:2107–2114, 1991

Table 6-2. Causes of Death Following Lung Transplantation

CAUSE (% TOTAL) ≤ 90 DAYS	CAUSE (% TOTAL) ≥ 90 DAYS
Non-CMV infection (27)	Bronchiolitis obliterans/rejection (29)
Primary organ failure (12)	Non-CMV infection (25)
Heart failure (9)	Malignancy (6)
Hemorrhage (7)	Respiratory failure (5)
Multiorgan failure (6)	CMV (5)
Airway dehiscence (5)	Hemorrhage (4)
Rejection (5)	Multiorgan failure (3)
CMV (5)	Heart failure (2)
Other (23)	Other (22)

CMV, cytomegalovirus.
(Reprinted with permission from St. Louis International Lung Transplant Registry)

D.3. What special precautions should be taken when a lung transplant recipient requires general anesthesia for subsequent nonpulmonary surgery?

In general, the post–lung transplantation patient can be treated like any other ill, immunocompromised patient. Recipients have subsequently undergone a variety of surgical procedures unrelated to their pulmonary disease following lung transplantation, and have presented few anesthetic problems. Not surprisingly, differences in the compliance and expiratory flow rates of a native and transplanted lung following single lung transplant for emphysema can result in alterations in intraoperative capnography. This phenomenon has been described as producing a biphasic pattern of carbon dioxide exhalation with the first peak reflecting exhalation from the transplanted lung and the second peak exhalation from the native lung.

Cerza RA: Cardiopulmonary bypass in a post-lung transplant patient. J Cardiothorac Vasc Anesth 10:384–386, 1996

Williams EL, Jellish WS, Modica PA et al: Capnography in a patient after single lung transplantation. Anesthesiology 74:621–622, 1991

D.4. Does lung transplantation work in the long run?

Increased experience and improved techniques have made lung transplantation a realistic option for many patients. However, the procedure is not without substantial risk, and a favorable outcome is by no means assured. Actuarial survival of procedures reported to an international registry since lung transplantation became widely applied in the late 1980s is shown in Table 6-3. Clearly there is room for improvement. However, these statistics reflect the combined experience of numerous centers around the world including many with new programs. In well-established centers with extensive experience, survival rates are substantially better than those reflected in the compiled data. Causes of death following lung transplantation generally can be categorized as short term (within 90 days of the procedure) and long term (more than 90 days after the procedure), which are shown in Table 6-2. Notable is the high incidence of rejection and malignancy in patients who survive over 90 days.

D.5. Are there any surgical alternatives to lung transplantation?

Some patients with severe emphysema who are not deemed transplant candidates may be benefited by a procedure known as pulmonary volume reduction surgery or reduction pneumoplasty. Performed either via a median sternotomy or bilateral thoracoscopy, the goal of volume reduction is to remove up to 30% of the patient's most severely compromised lung tissue. Postoperatively, this allows the patient's previously hyperexpanded chest wall and depressed diaphragm to resume more normal

Table 6-3.   Actuarial Survival of Lung Transplant Recipients

	1 YEAR	2 YEAR	3 YEAR	4 YEAR
All transplants	71%	63%	57%	51%
Single	71%	62%	56%	49%
Bilateral	73%	66%	59%	55%
En-bloc double	62%	55%	49%	45%

(Reprinted with permission from St. Louis International Lung Transplant Registry)

shape, thus improving chest wall mechanics and eventually pulmonary function. However, beneficial effects of the procedure are not immediately evident, usually requiring 1 to 2 months. Furthermore, whether the improvement in pulmonary function is sufficient to warrant the risk of the procedure remains controversial.

Cooper JD, Trulock EP, Triantafillou AN et al: Bilateral pneumectomy (volume reduction) for chronic obstructive pulmonary disease. J Thorac Cardiovasc Surg 109:106–119, 1995

Sciurba FC, Rogers RM, Keenan RJ et al: Improvement in pulmonary function and elastic recoil after lung-reduction surgery for diffuse emphysema. N Engl J Med 334:1095–1099, 1996

The Cardiovascular System

II

Ischemic Heart Disease and Coronary Artery Bypass Grafting

7

Fun-Sun F. Yao

A 57-year-old man with triple coronary artery disease was scheduled for coronary artery bypass grafting (CABG). He had a myocardial infarction 7 months ago. He was taking nitroglycerin, digoxin, propranolol, isosorbide dinitrate (Isordil), and nifedipine. His blood pressure was 120/80 mm Hg and his heart rate 60/min.

A. Medical Disease and Differential Diagnosis

1. What is triple-vessel coronary artery disease (CAD)? Name the branches of the coronary arteries.
2. What are the indications for coronary artery bypass grafting?
3. What is percutaneous transluminal coronary angioplasty? Discuss its indications, contraindications, and results.
4. What are the results of coronary artery bypass surgery?

B. Preoperative Evaluation and Preparation

1. Would you discontinue digoxin? Why? What is its half-life?
2. Would you discontinue propranolol? Why? What is its half-life?
3. If the patient who is on propranolol develops hypotension intraoperatively, how would you manage it?
4. What is nifedipine? How does it work?
5. What preoperative tests would you order?
6. How do you evaluate the patient's left ventricular function?
7. What are the three major determinants of myocardial oxygen consumption? How are they measured clinically?
8. What are the rate pressure product (RPP) and the triple index (TI)?
9. What factors determine myocardial oxygen supply?
10. How would you premedicate the patient? Why?

C. Intraoperative Management

C. I. Before Cardiopulmonary Bypass

1. How do you monitor the patient?
2. What is Allen's test?
3. Why do you need both esophageal and rectal temperatures?
4. How do you know that the Swan-Ganz catheter is in the right ventricle (RV) or pulmonary artery (PA)?
5. What is normal pulmonary capillary wedge pressure (PCWP)?
6. Is it necessary to monitor pulmonary artery pressure for coronary artery operations?

7. What are the complications of Swan-Ganz catheterization?
8. What are the hemodynamic consequences of myocardial ischemia? How can you detect myocardial ischemia? Is PCWP a sensitive indicator of myocardial ischemia?
9. How would you monitor ECG? Why V_5? If you do not have precordial leads in your ECG machine, how can you monitor the left ventricle?
10. Discuss the principles and clinical applications of intraoperative transesophageal two-dimensional echocardiography.
11. How would you induce anesthesia?
12. How would you maintain anesthesia?
13. What is the better anesthetic agent for this operation—an inhalation or intravenous agent?
14. What are the cardiovascular effects of halothane, enflurane, isoflurane, desflurane, sevoflurane, morphine, and fentanyl?
15. Is isoflurane dangerous for the patient with coronary artery disease?
16. What is the cardiovascular effect of nitrous oxide?
17. What kind of muscle relaxant would you use? Why?
18. If ST-segment depression is seen during surgery, how would you treat it? What is the relationship between perioperative myocardial ischemia and postoperative myocardial infarction?
19. Would you use prophylactic nitroglycerin during coronary artery bypass grafting (CABG) to prevent intraoperative myocardial ischemia or perioperative myocardial infarction?
20. How would you correct hypertension?
21. How would you treat hypotension?
22. What are the indications for intravenous propranolol or esmolol during surgery? How much would you give? What are the relative contraindications?
23. How would you correct increased PCWP?
24. During sternal splitting, would you do something?
25. Would you monitor PCWP continuously? Why?
26. Discuss autologous transfusion and blood conservation for cardiac surgery.

C. II. During Cardiopulmonary Bypass (CPB)

1. What anticoagulant would you give before CPB? How much would you give? What is its mechanism?
2. What is the half-life of heparin? How is it eliminated?
3. How do you monitor heparin dosage? What is the ACT test?
4. What is total cardiopulmonary bypass? What is partial bypass?
5. What is the purpose of venting the left ventricle? How can it be done?
6. How many types of oxygenators are there? What are the advantages of each type?
7. What kind of priming solution would you use? How much priming solution would you use? Would you prime with blood or not? Why?
8. What are the advantages and disadvantages of hemodilution?
9. What kind of pumps do you use? Are they pulsatile or not?
10. How do you monitor the patient during CPB?
11. How much blood pressure would you keep during CPB? Why?
12. How would you treat hypotension during CPB?
13. How would you treat hypertension (a mean arterial pressure of over 100 mm Hg)?

14. How do you prepare an intravenous infusion of sodium nitroprusside, phentolamine, and nitroglycerin? What are the usual doses? Which do you prefer to use?
15. How much pump flow would you maintain during CPB?
16. How would you adjust the pump flow during hypothermia?
17. How would you adjust the pump flow during hemodilution?
18. What are the advantages of hypothermia? Does hypothermia offer neuroprotection?
19. How does blood viscosity change during hypothermia and hemodilution?
20. What are the main causes of death associated with accidental hypothermia?
21. Would you give anesthesia during CPB? Why?
22. Would you give muscle relaxants during CPB? How is the action of muscle relaxant affected during CPB?
23. How do you know the patient is well perfused during CPB?
24. How much gas flow would you use for the oxygenator? What kind of gas would you use? Why?
25. What are the disadvantages of low $PaCO_2$ during CPB?
26. The arterial blood gases and electrolytes during CPB are pH, 7.36; $PaCO_2$, 42 mm Hg; PaO_2, 449 mm Hg; CO_2 content, 24 mEq/liter; Na, 128 mEq/liter; K, 5.8 mEq/liter; Ht, 20%. The patient's temperature is 27°C. At what temperature are blood gases measured? How would you correct the blood gases according to patient's body temperature? Would you treat the arterial blood gases at 37°C or at patient's body temperature?
27. If the blood level of the oxygenator is low, what would you replace it with? Blood or balanced salt solution?
28. How do you know the fluid balance during CPB?
29. How would you preserve the myocardium during CPB?
30. What is the cardioplegic solution? How much would you use?
31. For how long a period can the aorta be cross-clamped?
32. Why does urine become pink after 2 hours of CPB? What is the renal threshold for plasma hemoglobin?
33. At what temperature can the patient be weaned from CPB?
34. Why does it take longer to rewarm than to cool the patient by the pump oxygenator?
35. How would you defibrillate the heart internally during CPB?
36. Why is calcium chloride usually administered right before the patient comes off the pump?
37. If the heart rate is 40/min, what should you do?
38. How does the blood sugar level change during CPB? Why? Does hyperglycemia increase neurologic complications during CPB?
39. What are the effects of CPB on platelet and coagulation factors?

C. III. After Cardiopulmonary Bypass

1. How would you reverse heparin? How much protamine would you use?
2. What is the action mechanism of protamine?
3. What are the complications of too much protamine?
4. Why did the patient develop hypotension after protamine was administered? How do you treat and prevent this condition?
5. What are the indications for intraaortic balloon pump (IABP)?
6. What are the principles of IABP?
7. What are the complications of IABP?

8. Can pulmonary artery wedge pressure (PAWP) represent left ventricular end-diastolic volume (LVEDV) after coronary artery bypass grafting?

D. Postoperative Management

1. What are the postoperative complications?
2. Would you reverse the muscle relaxants? Why?
3. When will you wean the patient from the respirator?
4. What criteria would you use in deciding when to wean the patient from the respirator?

A. Medical Disease and Differential Diagnosis

A.1. What is triple-vessel coronary artery disease (CAD)? Name the branches of the coronary arteries.

Triple-vessel CAD usually involves the following:

- The right coronary artery (RCA)
- The left anterior descending branch (LAD)
- The left circumflex branch (CFX)

The branches of coronary arteries are shown in Figure 7-1. The sinus node is supplied by the RCA in about 50% to 60% of human beings and by the left circumflex ar-

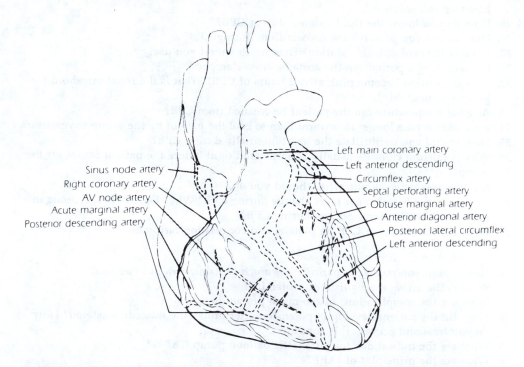

Left main coronary artery
Left anterior descending
Circumflex artery
Septal perforating artery
Obtuse marginal artery
Anterior diagonal artery
Posterior lateral circumflex
Left anterior descending

Sinus node artery
Right coronary artery
AV node artery
Acute marginal artery
Posterior descending artery

Figure 7-1. Branches of the coronary arteries.

tery in the remaining 40% to 50%. The atrioventricular (AV) node is provided by the RCA in 85% to 90% of human beings and by the left circumflex artery in the remaining 10% to 15%. The most common arteries for coronary bypass grafting are left anterior descending, obtuse marginal, and posterior descending arteries.

Braunwald E (ed): Heart Disease, a Textbook of Cardiovascular Medicine, 5th ed, pp 247–253. Philadelphia, WB Saunders, 1997

A.2. What are the indications for coronary artery bypass grafting?

The indications for CABG consist of the need for improvement of the quality or quantity of life. Patients whose angina is not controlled by medical treatment or who have unacceptable side-effects with such management should be considered for coronary revascularization.

Percutaneous transluminal coronary angioplasty (PTCA) is currently accepted as the initial procedure of choice in selected patients with obstructive coronary artery disease. Since its introduction in 1978, PTCA has redefined the candidates for elective surgical myocardial revascularization. Patients with proximal discrete coronary artery stenosis are being referred for PTCA. The candidates who are not suitable for PTCA are usually referred for CABG. The candidates for CABG are usually older patients with more diffuse coronary artery disease and decreased left ventricular function. The following are indications for CABG:

- Unstable angina pectoris or episodes of prolonged myocardial ischemia
- Unacceptable angina pectoris, despite optimal medical therapy
- Repeated episodes of myocardial ischemia following myocardial infarction
- Prinzmetal's angina (variant angina) with coronary artery obstruction
- High-grade left main coronary artery obstruction, triple- or double-vessel obstruction, or proximal left anterior descending artery obstruction
- Acute myocardial infarction, cardiogenic shock, intractable ventricular arrhythmias
- Stable angina pectoris that interferes with desired life style

Braunwald E (ed): Heart Disease, a Textbook of Cardiovascular Medicine, 5th ed, pp 1321–1322, 1329–1330. Philadelphia, WB Saunders, 1997

A.3. What is percutaneous transluminal coronary angioplasty? Discuss its indications, contraindications, and results.

Percutaneous transluminal coronary angioplasty (PTCA) has developed rapidly since its introduction by Gruentzig in 1977. It is now an acceptable method of treating selected patients who have angina pectoris. This technique involves the passage of a small (3F) catheter into the involved coronary artery and through the stenosis. With the balloon portion of the catheter straddling the stenosis, inflations are performed that result in enlargement of the stenotic lumen. The luminal widening is achieved by a controlled injury involving, to a varying degree, plaque compression, intimal fissures, and medial stretching.

The indications for PTCA have changed during the recent past. With the presently available technology, PTCA is considered a therapeutic option in any individual with disabling ischemic symptoms despite good medical therapy, and focal obstructive coronary disease regardless of cause. The indications for PTCA are as follows:

- Isolated discrete proximal single-vessel disease
- Proximal double-vessel disease
- Postcoronary artery bypass grafting with new stenotic lesions or stenosis at distal anastomoses
- Restenosis following PTCA
- Contraindications to CABG
- Coronary stenosis following cardiac transplantation
- Occluded vessels of <6 months in duration and <15 mm in length
- Poststreptokinase therapy for revascularization

PTCA is contraindicated in the following:

- Left main coronary artery disease in which the distal vessels are not protected by at least one completely patent bypass graft
- Multivessel disease with severe diffuse atherosclerosis
- Absence of significant obstructing lesion
- Absence of a formal cardiac surgical program within the institution

The results of PTCA are as follows: The primary success rate is about 90%. The restenosis rate is about 30% 6 months after the procedure. Dilatation is again performed with a 90% success rate. The artery tends to remain patent after the second angioplasty.

Braunwald E (ed): Heart Disease, a Textbook of Cardiovascular Medicine, 5th ed, pp 1313–1316. Philadelphia, WB Saunders, 1997

Hurst JW (ed): The Heart, 8th ed, pp 1041–1043, 2132–2137. New York, McGraw-Hill, 1994

A.4. What are the results of coronary artery bypass surgery?

Kuan and associates reported a perioperative myocardial infarction rate of 4% to 6%. The overall operative mortality rate of CABG at major medical centers is about 1%. Reoperation is associated with a higher operative mortality, about 2% to 3%. Rahimtoola and associates studied the status of patients who had coronary bypass surgery for unstable angina 10 years previously. The 1-month mortality rate was 1.8%. The 5-year survival rate was 92%, and the 10-year survival rate was 83%. Coronary bypass surgery was repeated at a rate of 1% to 2% per year; 81% of patients were angina-free or had only mild angina. Loop and associates found that the 10-year survival rate among the group receiving the internal mammary artery graft, as compared with the group receiving the vein grafts (exclusive of hospital deaths), was 93.4% versus 88% for those with one-vessel disease; 90.0% versus 79.5% for those with two-vessel disease; and 82.6% versus 71.0% for those with three-vessel disease. At the end of the first 10 postoperative years, the patency of internal mammary artery grafts is 85% to 95%, while the patency of saphenous vein grafts is only 38% to 45%.

A systematic overview of the seven randomized trials that compared coronary bypass surgery with medical therapy between 1972 and 1984 yielded 2649 patients. Patients undergoing CABG had a significantly lower mortality at 5, 7, and 10 years, but by 10 years 41% of the patients initially randomized to medical therapy had undergone CABG. Thus coronary bypass surgery prolongs survival in patients with significant left main coronary artery disease irrespective of symptoms, in patients with multivessel disease and impaired left ventricular function, and in patients with three-vessel disease that includes the proximal left anterior descending coronary artery (irrespective of left ventricular function). Surgical therapy also has been demonstrated to prolong life in patients with two-vessel disease and left ventricular dysfunction, particularly in those with a critical stenosis of the proximal left anterior descending coronary artery. Although no study has documented a survival benefit with surgical treatment in patients with single-vessel disease, there is some evidence that such patients who have impaired left ventricular function have a poor long-term survival rate. Such patients with angina and/or evidence of ischemia at a low or moderate level of exercise, especially those with obstruction of the proximal left anterior descending coronary artery, may benefit from coronary revascularization by either angioplasty or bypass surgery.

Braunwald E (ed): Heart Disease, a Textbook of Cardiovascular Medicine, 5th ed, pp 1323–1331. Philadelphia, WB Saunders, 1997

Kuan P, Bernstein SB, Ellestad MH: Coronary artery bypass surgery morbidity. J Am Coll Cardiol 3:1391, 1984

Loop FD, Lytle BW, Cosgrove DM et al: Influence of the internal mammary artery graft on 10-year survival and other cardiac events. N Engl J Med 314:1–6, 1986

Lytle BW, Loop FD, Cosgrove DM et al: Long-term (5 to 12 years) serial studies of internal mammary artery and saphenous vein coronary bypass grafts. J Thorac Cardiovasc Surg 89:248–258, 1985

Rahimtoola SH, Nanley D, Grunckemeier G et al: Ten-year survival after coronary bypass surgery. N Engl J Med 308:676, 1983

B. Preoperative Evaluation and Preparation

B.1. Would you discontinue digoxin? Why? What is its half-life?

In order to prevent digitalis intoxication after cardiopulmonary bypass (CPB), digitalis preparations are usually discontinued one half-life (1.5 to 1.7 days for digoxin, 5 to 7 days for digitoxin) before surgery. Digitalis intoxication is quite possible, especially after CPB when acid-base and electrolytes are abnormal. If the patient is in congestive heart failure (CHF) and digitalis dependent, digitalis is continued until the night before surgery. However, the predisposing factors to digitalis intoxication, especially hypopotassemia and hypercalcemia, have to be prevented.

Kaplan J (ed): Cardiac Anesthesia, 3rd ed, p 567. New York, Grune & Stratton, 1993

B.2. Would you discontinue propranolol? Why? What is its half-life?

Propranolol should be continued not only up until surgery, but probably throughout the perioperative period. Propranolol is generally continued up until the time of surgery. In patients with unstable angina, sudden withdrawal of propranolol may produce an exacerbation of symptoms and may precipitate acute myocardial infarction. The dose of propranolol need not be reduced before surgery to avoid bradycardia, hypotension, or difficulty in weaning from cardiopulmonary bypass. The half-life of oral propranolol is 3.4 to 6 hours. Propranolol disappears from the plasma and atria within 24 to 48 hours after discontinuing doses of 30 to 240 mg/day. Shand and Keats have shown that with a 0.5-mg dose of propranolol IV, blood levels as high as 50 ng/ml are obtained, but rapidly drop off to unmeasurable levels within 5 to 10 minutes. There has been no myocardial depression seen with these small intravenous doses.

Kaplan J (ed): Cardiac Anesthesia, 3rd ed, p 566. Philadelphia, WB Saunders, 1993

Mangano DT (ed): Preoperative Cardiac Assessment, pp 143–147. Philadelphia, JB Lippincott, 1990

Nies AS, Shand DG: Clinical pharmacology of propranolol. Circulation 52:6, 1975

Slogoff S, Keats AS, Ott E: Preoperative propranolol therapy and aortocoronary bypass operation. JAMA 240:1487, 1978

B.3. If the patient who is on propranolol develops hypotension intraoperatively, how would you manage it?

The specific antagonists for propranolol are not the first choice. The more common causes of intraoperative hypotension, such as hypovolemia, deep anesthesia, and surgical manipulation, should be corrected first. In rare instances, it is necessary to administer atropine for bradycardia or isoproterenol, glucagon, calcium, or digitalis to counteract the beta-blockade. Cardiogenic hypotension is usually associated with high pulmonary capillary wedge pressure (PCWP) and low blood pressure.

Kaplan J (ed): Cardiac Anesthesia, 3rd ed, pp 191–192. Philadelphia, WB Saunders, 1993

B.4. What is nifedipine? How does it work?

Nifedipine is a calcium channel blocker. The commonly used calcium channel blockers in the United States are nifedipine, verapamil, and diltiazem hydrochloride. The nine calcium channel blockers that have been approved for clinical use in the United States have diverse chemical structures. Five classes of compounds have been examined: phenylalkylamines, dihydropyridines, benzothiazepines, diphenylpiperazines, and a diarylaminopropylamine. At present, verapamil (a phenylalkylamine); diltiazem (a benzothiazepine); nicardipine, nifedipine, isradipine, amlodipine, felodipine, and nimodipine (dihydropyridines); and bepridil (a diarylaminopropylamine ether) are approved for clinical use in the United States. They inhibit excitation—contraction coupling of myocardial and smooth muscle by blocking calcium influx at cellular membranes. This results in decreased myocardial contractility and in vasodilation. Therefore, myocardial oxygen consumption is decreased. Calcium channel blockers are effective for the treatment of variant angina (Prinzmetal's angina), angina pectoris, and possibly acute myocardial infarction. (See also Chapter 18, question A.11.)

Although nitrates and beta-adrenergic blockers are effective for angina, the calcium channel blockers are longer acting and may be used in the presence of chronic obstructive pulmonary disease and asthma. Calcium also plays a key role in cardiac electrical activity. The electrical activity of the sinoatrial (SA) and atrioventricular (AV) nodal cells are especially dependent on the calcium or "slow" current, whereas the rest of the specialized conduction system is more dependent on the sodium or "fast" current. Verapamil has a more profound influence on the calcium current of the SA and AV nodes. This drug has been most useful in the treatment of supraventricular tachyarrhythmias, which are often caused by reentry through the AV node. In contrast, nifedipine has less influence on the SA node and no effect on AV conduction time. Therefore, nifedipine might be used where further suppression of AV conduction is undesirable. The relative cardiovascular effects of calcium channel blockers are shown in Table 7-1. Verapamil was found to profoundly depress the cardiovascu-

Table 7-1. Relative Cardiovascular Effects of Calcium Channel Blockers

	VERAPAMIL	DILTIAZEM	NIFEDIPINE
Antiarrhythmic	+ + +	+ +	–
Cardiac depression	+ +	+	+
Vasodilation	+	+ +	+ + +
Tachycardia	–	–	+ +

lar system during high concentrations of halothane, enflurane, or isoflurane anesthesia. However, because of a tendency for increased incidence of sinus arrest and bradycardia and more hemodynamic depression during enflurane anesthesia, Rogers and associates concluded that intravenous verapamil is better tolerated during low-dose isoflurane and halothane anesthesia than during comparable concentrations of enflurane anesthesia.

Chelly JE, Rogers K, Hysing ES et al: Cardiovascular effects of and interaction between calcium-blocking drugs and anesthetics in chronically instrumented dogs. I. Verapamil and halothane. Anesthesiology 64:560–567, 1986

Hardman JG, Limbird LE, Molinoff PB et al (eds): Goodman and Gilman's The Pharmacological Basis of Therapeutics, 9th ed, pp 767–769. New York, McGraw-Hill, 1996

Kapur PA: Calcium channel blockers. ASA Refresher Courses in Anesthesiology 17:137–153, 1989

Rogers K, Hysing ES, Merin RG et al: Cardiovascular effects of and interaction between calcium-blocking drugs and anesthetics in chronically instrumented dogs. II. Verapamil, enflurane and isoflurane. Anesthesiology 64:568–575, 1986

B.5. What preoperative tests would you order?

In addition to the routine systemic examinations of all organ systems, special attention should be paid to circulatory functions.

- Renal function—urinalysis, BUN, creatinine
- Hepatic function—bilirubin, albumin/globulin, alkaline phosphatase, SGOT, SGPT
- Pulmonary function—baseline arterial blood gases, spirometry as indicated, chest x-ray film
- Hematologic function—complete blood count, PT, PTT, platelets
- Metabolism—electrolytes and blood sugar
- Cardiovascular function—resting and exercise ECG, cardiac catheterization and coronary angiography, left ventricular function, location and severity of coronary occlusion, and echocardiography

B.6. How do you evaluate the patient's left ventricular function?

- By the history of myocardial infarction and angina
- By symptoms and signs of left ventricular failure, dyspnea, nocturnal orthopnea, pitting edema
- Cardiac catheterization and angiography
  - Ejection fraction (normal 65%)
  - Left ventricular end-diastolic pressure (LVEDP) or PCWP (normal 6 to 15 mm Hg)
  - Left ventricular wall motion—akinesia, hypokinesia, or dyskinesia
  - Cardiac index (normal 3 liters/min/m^2)
- End-systolic pressure volume relationship (ESPVR) from multiple pressure-volume loops

(See also Chapter 8, question A.3.)

Braunwald E (ed): Heart Disease, a Textbook of Cardiovascular Medicine, 5th ed, pp 427–438. Philadelphia, WB Saunders, 1997

B.7. What are the three major determinants of myocardial oxygen consumption? How are they measured clinically?

The three major determinants are myocardial wall tension, contractility, and heart rate.

Myocardial Wall Tension Is Measured by:
- Preload—left ventricular end-diastolic volume, LVEDP, left atrial pressure, or PCWP
- Afterload—systolic ventricular pressure or systolic blood pressure if there is no aortic stenosis

Contractility Is Measured by:
- Invasive technique—maximal velocity of contraction (Vmax), dp/dt (pressure time indices of ventricle), or left ventricular end-systolic pressure/volume ratio
- Noninvasive technique—preejection period (PEP)/left ventricular ejection time (LVET), ventricular wall motion by echocardiography

Heart Rate

Braunwald E (ed): Heart Disease, a Textbook of Cardiovascular Medicine, 5th ed, pp 1161–1162. Philadelphia, WB Saunders, 1997

B.8. What are the rate pressure product (RPP) and the triple index (TI)?

$$\text{RPP} = \text{systolic blood pressure (SBP)} \times \text{heart rate (HR)}$$

$$\text{TI} = \text{SBP} \times \text{HR} \times \text{PCWP}$$

Both RPP and TI are used to measure myocardial oxygen demand. Angina threshold depends on the severity of coronary artery occlusion. Angina threshold of RPP usually ranges from 15,000 to 20,000 mm Hg/min. A high RPP or TI indicates a potential danger of myocardial ischemia, but a normal or low RPP and TI do not rule out ischemia. Patients with tachycardia and hypotension may have a normal RPP, but both tachycardia (increasing O_2 demand, decreasing O_2 supply) and hypotension (decreasing O_2 supply) may cause myocardial ischemia. Precordial lead V_5 ECG and angina (awake patients) are more important monitors for ischemia. Most important is to keep all three factors (SBP, HR, PCWP) as close as possible to their normal values. It is usually recommended to keep RPP below 12,000 and TI below 150,000.

The RPP has been shown to be a useful measure of myocardial oxygen demand (MVO_2) in awake patients, but direct comparisons of MVO_2 in anesthetized patients has shown an unreliable correlation.

Barash PG, Kopriva CJ: The rate pressure product in clinical anesthesia—boon or bane? Anesth Analg 59:229–231, 1980

Leung JM, O'Kelly BF, Mangano DT, SPI group: Relationship of regional wall motion abnormalities to hemodynamic indices of myocardial oxygen supply and demand in patients undergoing CABG surgery. Anesthesiology 73:802–814, 1990

Urban MK, Gordon MA, Harris SN et al: Intraoperative hemodynamic changes are not good indicators of myocardial ischemia. Anesth Analg 76:942–949, 1992

B.9. What factors determine myocardial oxygen supply?

Myocardial oxygen supply = coronary blood flow $\times$ arterial oxygen content

$$\text{Coronary blood flow} = \frac{\text{coronary perfusion pressure}}{\text{resistance}}$$

Coronary blood flow depends on the following:

- Aortic diastolic pressure (DP)
- Left ventricular end-diastolic pressure (LVEDP)
- Patency of coronary arteries
- Coronary vascular tone

Arterial O_2 content is determined by the following equation:

$$CaO_2 = 1.34 \times Hb \times O_2 \text{ saturation} + 0.0031 \times PaO_2$$

Barash PG: Monitoring myocardial oxygen balance: Physiologic basis and clinical application. ASA Refresher Courses in Anesthesiology 13:21–32, 1985

Braunwald E (ed): Heart Disease, a Textbook of Cardiovascular Medicine, 5th ed, pp 1163–1174. Philadelphia, WB Saunders, 1997

B.10. How would you premedicate the patient? Why?

The patient should be well sedated to prevent anxiety, which may precipitate angina. We usually give diazepam, 5 to 10 mg orally, or lorazepam, 1 to 2 mg orally, 1 hour before surgery. Two inches of nitroglycerin paste (Nitropaste) are applied prophylactically to the chest wall.

Even though atropine or scopolamine is not contraindicated, atropine is not given at the New York Hospital–Cornell Medical Center because of the possibility of tachycardia, which will increase O_2 demand.

All antianginal and antihypertensive drugs are continued up to the time of surgery.

C. Intraoperative Management

C. I. Before Cardiopulmonary Bypass

C. I-1. How do you monitor the patient?

- ECG—simultaneous leads V_5 and II, multiple-lead ST-segment analysis if available
- Arterial line for BP and arterial blood gases
- Swan-Ganz catheter—PCWP, PAD, hemodynamic study
- CVP line—if the patient has good left ventricular function and no problems are expected
- Urine output
- Temperature—esophageal and rectal, or bladder
- Laboratory—arterial blood gases, electrolytes, hematocrit, activated coagulation time (ACT), and PvO_2
- Oxygen analyzer for inspired gas mixture
- End-tidal CO_2 analyzer
- Pulse oximeter for arterial oxygenation
- Transesophageal echocardiography if available and indicated

C. I-2. What is Allen's test?

Allen's test is used to detect collateral ulnar circulation. The radial and ulnar arteries are occluded by the examiner's hands. The patient is then asked to make a tight fist to empty blood from the hand. The hand is held above the heart level to help venous drainage. If the patient is under anesthesia, the blood in the hand may be drained by a third person squeezing the hand. Then the hand is opened slowly and put down to the heart level. Only the ulnar compression is released. The flush of the hand is watched.

- Normal— <7 seconds
- Borderline— 7 to 15 seconds
- Abnormal— >15 seconds

A modified Allen's test may be done with a Doppler detector or pulsimeter. Allen's test results are abnormal in approximately 3% of young healthy individuals. Slogoff and associates studied the complications following radial artery cannulation in 1699 cardiovascular surgical patients. They concluded that in the absence of peripheral vascular disease, Allen's test is not a predictor of ischemia of the hand during or after radial artery cannulation and that radial artery cannulation is a low-risk, high-benefit monitoring technique that deserves wide clinical use. However, in the current litigious setting and in the face of some evidence to the contrary, it is probably prudent to continue to perform Allen's test.

Cederholm I, Sorensen J, Carlsson C: Thrombosis following percutaneous radial artery cannulation. Acta Anaesthesiol Scand 30:227, 1986

Miller RD (ed): Anesthesia, 4th ed, pp 1169–1170. New York, Churchill Livingstone, 1994

Slogoff S, Keats AS, Arlund C: On the safety of radial artery cannulation. Anesthesiology 59:42, 1983

C. I-3. Why do you need both esophageal and rectal temperatures?

During cooling and rewarming, there is uneven distribution of body temperature. Esophageal temperature represents core temperature; rectal temperature represents peripheral temperature. During cooling and rewarming using the pump-oxygenator, esophageal temperature changes rapidly, whereas the rectal temperature changes slowly. During surface cooling or warming, the rectal temperature changes quickly, while the esophageal temperature changes slowly. In order to estimate the average temperature and to achieve even distribution of body temperature, it is necessary to record both esophageal and rectal temperatures.

However, bladder temperature monitoring through a Foley catheter is quite convenient and popular; it reflects the body temperature between esophageal and rectal temperature.

Ravlee GP, Davis RF, Utley JR: Cardiopulmonary Bypass, Principles and Practice, pp 150, 592–595. Baltimore, Williams & Wilkins, 1993

Kaplan J (ed): Cardiac Anesthesia, 3rd ed, p 709. Philadelphia, WB Saunders, 1993

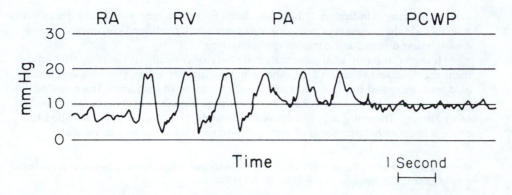

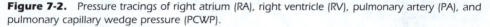

Figure 7-2. Pressure tracings of right atrium (RA), right ventricle (RV), pulmonary artery (PA), and pulmonary capillary wedge pressure (PCWP).

C. I-4. How do you know that the Swan-Ganz catheter is in the right ventricle (RV) or pulmonary artery (PA)?

There are three main differences in the pressure tracings, as shown in Figure 7-2.

Diastolic Pressure Is Higher in PA than in RV
- PA pressure: 20 to 25/5 to 10 mm Hg
- RV pressure: 20 to 25/0 to 5 mm Hg

Pressure Contour
- PA pressure tracing has diacritic notch from closure of pulmonary valve.
- RV pressure tracing has plateau and sharp drop in early diastole.

In the late diastolic phase, PA pressure is going down while the RV pressure is going up because of ventricular filling.

C. I-5. What is normal pulmonary capillary wedge pressure (PCWP)?

- Normal—4 to 12 mm Hg
- Borderline—13 to 17 mm Hg
- Heart failure—over 18 mm Hg

Braunwald E (ed): Heart Disease, a Textbook of Cardiovascular Medicine, 5th ed, pp 188–189. Philadelphia, WB Saunders, 1997

C. I-6. Is it necessary to monitor pulmonary artery pressure for coronary artery operations?

The indication to monitor pulmonary artery pressure depends on the left ventricular function. Patients may be divided into two categories on the basis of left ventricular function. For patients who have good left ventricular function (ejection fractions >0.5 and good ventricular wall motion), the central venous pressure (CVP) correlates well with the pulmonary capillary wedge pressure (PCWP); therefore, pulmonary pressure monitoring may not be necessary for this group of patients. On the other hand, for patients with poor left ventricular function (ejection fractions <0.4 or ventricular dyssynergy), the CVP does not correlate with the PCWP; therefore, pulmonary pressure monitoring is indicated. Other indications for monitoring pulmonary artery pressure include the presence of pulmonary hypertension, combined coronary stenoses and valvular disease, and complex cardiac lesions.

However, recently in an observational study of critically ill patients, after adjustment for treatment selection bias, monitoring pulmonary artery pressure was associated with increased mortality and increased utilization of resources. The cause of this apparent lack of benefit is unclear. The result of this analysis should be confirmed in other studies. These findings justify reconsideration of a randomized controlled trial of right heart catheterization and may guide patient selection for such a study.

Connors AF, Speroff T, Dawson NV et al: The effectiveness of right heart catheterization in initial care of critically ill patients. JAMA 276:889–897, 1996

Editorial views: To (PA) catheterize or not to (PA) catheterize; That is the question. Anesthesiology 53:361–363, 1980

Mangano DT: Monitoring pulmonary arterial pressure in coronary-artery disease. Anesthesiology 53:364–369, 1980

C. I-7. What are the complications of Swan-Ganz catheterization?

From Venopuncture Sites (as for CVP)
- Common complications:
  - Infection—sepsis
  - Hematoma
  - Air embolism
  - Thrombosis
  - Catheter shearing and embolization
- Subclavian approach:
  - Pneumothorax
  - Hemothorax
  - Hydrothorax
- Internal jugular approach:
  - Pneumothorax
  - Neck hematoma from puncture of carotid artery
  - Possible vagus nerve injury and brachial plexus injury
  - Thoracic duct perforation from left side approach

The basilar or cephalic vein approach has fewer complications, but the failure rate is higher.

From Swan-Ganz Catheter
Arrhythmias 1.5% to 11%, complete heart block, thromboemboli, pulmonary infarction from continuous wedging, massive hemorrhage from perforation of PA or RA, failure to wedge, hemoptysis, intracardiac knotting, balloon rupture, endocardial thrombi, and tricuspid valve injury.

Barash PG, Cullen BF, Stoelting RK (eds): Clinical Anesthesia, 3rd ed, pp 632–633. Philadelphia, Lippincott-Raven, 1997

Miller RD (ed): Anesthesia, 4th ed, pp 1184–1185. New York, Churchill Livingstone, 1994

C. I-8. What are the hemodynamic consequences of myocardial ischemia? How can you detect myocardial ischemia? Is PCWP a sensitive indicator of myocardial ischemia?

For four decades following Tennant and Wiggers' classic observation on the effects of coronary occlusion on myocardial contraction, it was believed that transient severe ischemia caused either irreversible cardiac injury—that is, infarction—or prompt recovery. However, in the 1970s it became clear that after a brief episode of severe ischemia, prolonged myocardial dysfunction with gradual return of contractile activity occurred, a condition termed myocardial stunning. Alternatively, severe chronic ischemia can result in diminished contractile performance such as chronic regional wall motion abnormalities (hibernation).

Acute myocardial ischemia affects systolic and diastolic pump function. Systolic dysfunction is usually manifest before alterations in diastolic function. The immediate impact on ventricular compliance is related to the etiology of the ischemic event. Decreased myocardial oxygen supply is initially accompanied by an increase in compliance. In contrast, increased myocardial oxygen demand is associated with an immediate loss of ventricular compliance (e.g., the ventricle becomes stiffer). Thus, the ventricle requires a higher filling pressure (end diastolic pressure [EDP]) to maintain a given stroke volume. A cascade of events occur that may include wall motion abnormalities, dysrhythmias, and conduction block. An 80% reduction of coronary blood flow causes akinesis, while a 95% decrease causes dyskinesis. If the ischemia becomes severe, the rise in EDP will lead to pulmonary edema (Fig. 7-3).

Although a number of sensitive techniques are available for detection of ischemia—such as magnetic resonance spectroscopy, radio-labeled lactate determinations, or direct measurement of end-diastolic pressure—they are impractical. The most popular and accepted sign of ischemia is ECG ST-segment changes. The ECG criteria for ischemia are horizontal or down-sloping ST-segment depression at least 0.1 mV at 0.06 second from J-point, up-sloping ST-segment depression at least 0.2 mV at 0.08 second from J-point, and ST-segment elevation at least 0.15 mV (1 mV = 10 mm). Other ECG signs of ischemia include inverted T waves and a new onset of arrhythmias or conduction abnormalities.

Regional wall motion abnormalities (RWMA), detected with two-dimensional echocardiography, have been shown to be the earliest and most sensitive sign of myocardial ischemia. A 25% decrease in coronary blood flow produced RWMA without ECG changes, while a 50% decrease was required to cause ECG signs of ischemia. In patients with coronary artery disease, during exercise, RWMA occurred after 30 seconds, while ECG changes did not occur until after 90 seconds. Smith and associates found that RWMA was four times more sensitive than ST-segment change on the ECG in detecting intraoperative ischemia. Moreover, ST changes cannot be analyzed when the patient has conduction disturbance such as bundle-branch block or ventricularly paced rhythms. They found that patients experiencing persistent RWMA were more likely to have myocardial infarction than those having only transient changes. No patient without a new wall motion abnormality had myocardial infarction. Hopefully, a smaller and more affordable echocardiography machine will be available in the near future. Although transesophageal echocardiography (TEE) is the most sensitive monitor for myocardial ischemia, a recent study by Eisenberg et al concludes that routine monitoring for myocardial ischemia with TEE or 12-lead ECG during noncardiac surgery appears to have little incremental clinical value over preoperative

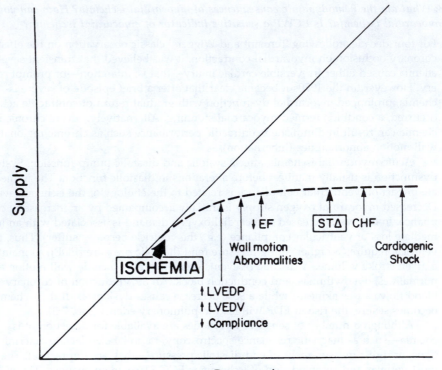

Figure 7-3. Hemodynamic consequences of myocardial ischemia. Ischemia occurs when demand exceeds supply. (LVEDP, left ventricular end-diastolic pressure; LVEDV, left ventricular end-diastolic volume; EF, ejection fraction; ST, segment changes; CHF, congestive heart failure). (Reprinted with permission from Barash PG: Monitoring myocardial oxygen balance: Physiologic basis and clinical application. ASA Refresher Courses in Anesthesiology 13:24, 1985)

clinical data and two-lead ECG monitoring in identifying patients at high risk for perioperative ischemic outcome.

Measurement of pulmonary capillary wedge pressure (PCWP) has been suggested as an early and sensitive indicator of ischemia, to be used when the ECG is nondiagnostic. Although acute increases in PCWP or development of V waves may reflect ischemia, the absence of a change in PCWP does not ensure the absence of ischemia. Haggmark et al reported that the sensitivity, specificity, and predictive value (positive and negative) of PCWP abnormalities for ischemia ranged between 40% and 60%. In CABG patients, Lieberman et al also found a low positive predictive value (24%) but a higher negative predictive value (85%); however, the PCWP was no better than central venous pressure measurement, except in patients with moderate to severe preoperative ventricular dysfunction. Leung et al found that 61% of TEE wall-motion abnormalities in CABG patients occurred without significant changes (>20% of control) in heart rate, systolic arterial pressure, or pulmonary artery pressure. Only

10% of episodes were accompanied by 5 mm Hg or greater changes in pulmonary artery pressure. Roizen et al found that 11 out of 12 patients developed TEE wall-motion abnormalities when the aorta was cross-clamped above the supraceliac artery, but that PCWP remained normal ($\leq$12 mm Hg) in 10 out of 12, with only 2 out of 12 having transient increases. Therefore, these studies question the value of pulmonary artery catheterization and monitoring for detection of intraoperative ischemia.

Barash PG: Monitoring myocardial ischemia: A sequential clinical approach. ASA Annual Refresher Course Lectures No. 112, 1996

Barash PG: Monitoring myocardial oxygen balance: Physiologic basis and clinical application. ASA Refresher Courses in Anesthesiology 13:21–32, 1985

Haggmark S, Hohner P, Ostman M et al: Comparison of hemodynamic, electrocardiographic, mechanical, and metabolic indicators of intraoperative myocardial ischemia in vascular surgical patients with coronary artery disease. Anesthesiology 70:19–25, 1989

Kaplan JA, Wells PH: Early diagnosis of myocardial ischemia using the pulmonary artery catheter. Anesth Analg 60:789–793, 1981

Leung J, O'Kelly B, Browner W et al: Are regional wall motion abnormalities detected by transesophageal echocardiography triggered by acute changes in supply and demand? (abstract). Anesthesiology 69:A801, 1988

Lieberman RW, Orkin FK, Jobes DR et al: Hemodynamic predictors of myocardial ischemia during halothane anesthesia for coronary artery revascularization. Anesthesiology 59:36–41, 1983

Mangano DT: Perioperative cardiac morbidity. Anesthesiology 72:153–184, 1990

Roizen MF, Beaupre PN, Alpert RA et al: Monitoring with two-dimensional transesophageal echocardiography: Comparison of myocardial function in patients undergoing supraceliac, suprarenal-infraceliac, or infrarenal aortic occlusion. J Vasc Surg 1:300–305, 1984

Smith JS, Cahalan MK, Benefiel DJ et al: Intraoperative detection of myocardial ischemia in high-risk patients: Electrocardiography versus two-dimensional transesophageal echocardiography. Circulation 72:1015–1021, 1985

Tennant R, Wiggers CJ: The effect of coronary occlusion on myocardial contraction. Am J Physiol 112:351–361, 1935

C. I-9. *How would you monitor ECG? Why V_5? If you do not have precordial leads in your ECG machine, how can you monitor the left ventricle?*

Multiple-lead ECG monitoring provides the best clinically available method of detecting perioperative ischemia. Based primarily on results obtained from exercise treadmill testing, combined ECG leads II and V_5, which can detect 96% of ischemic events, are suggested optimal leads for detecting intraoperative myocardial ischemia. However, London et al recently found that the standard combination of leads II and V_5 was only 80% sensitive, whereas combining leads V_4 and V_5 increased sensitivity to 90% in patients with known or suspected coronary artery disease undergoing noncardiac surgery with general anesthesia. The sensitivity increased to 96% by combining leads II, V_4, and V_5. If only one lead can be displayed, V_5 should be used because lead V_5 has the greatest sensitivity, 75% intraoperatively and 89% during exercise treadmill testing. See also Chapter 18, question C.3.

Blackburn H, Katigbak R: What ECG leads to take after exercise. Am Heart J 67:184–185, 1964

London MJ, Hollenberg M, Wong MG et al: Intraoperative myocardial ischemia: Localization by continuous 12-lead electrocardiography. Anesthesiology 69:232–241, 1988

C. I-10. Discuss the principles and clinical applications of intraoperative transesophageal two-dimensional echocardiography.

Transesophageal echocardiography (TEE) is a well-established technique to visualize cardiac anatomy and function. Echocardiography is based on fundamental ultrasonic principles. Ultrasound is defined as sound above the upper threshold of human hearing (20,000 Hz). The ultrasound waves (1 to 7 MHz) are created by striking an appropriate piezoelectric crystal with alternating electric current of 500 to 1500 pulses per second. A short burst or pulse of high-frequency, low-intensity sound is then emitted and directed through the human body to detect boundaries between structures of different acoustic impedance. The ultrasound wave is partially reflected at the boundary of different acoustic impedance, a property that is primarily determined by the slight difference in density between different tissues. This technique is termed *pulsed-reflected ultrasound*. The transmission of pulsed-reflected ultrasound through the heart, with detection of the returning echoes detailing the position and movement of cardiac acoustic interfaces, is termed *cardiac ultrasound* or *echocardiography*. The difference between the M-mode and two-dimensional techniques is that the M-mode ultrasonic beam is aimed in one direction and therefore depicts only one dimension of the target structure in an image that does not resemble cardiac structure, whereas the two-dimensional beam sweeps in an arc to give a panoramic view of the heart that results in cross-sectional images that are anatomically recognizable.

Doppler echocardiography provides an alternative method for imaging blood flow by applying Doppler frequency shift analysis to echoes reflected by the moving red blood cells. The Doppler principle states that the frequency of ultrasound reflected by a moving target (red blood cells) is different from the frequency of the emitted ultrasound. The shift in frequency is proportional to the speed of the moving target (red blood cells). Color-coded Doppler flow imaging (color Doppler) simultaneously presents real-time images of intracardiac flow and structure in two dimensions: continuous color maps of flow superimposed on monochromatic cross-sectional echocardiograms. Color Doppler greatly improves the evaluation of valvular function and intracardiac shunts.

The clinical applications of intraoperative echocardiography are as follows:

- *Monitoring Left Ventricular Filling and Ejection*
  When left ventricular short-axis cross-section is monitored at the midpapillary muscle, TEE provides the anesthesiologist with a direct, quantitative method to assess left ventricular preload and ejection in real time to guide the administration of fluids and inotropes.
- *Ischemic Heart Disease*
  Regional wall motion abnormalities, such as hypokinesia, akinesia, and dyskinesia, are the earliest signs of myocardial ischemia, as discussed in question C.I-8. Measurements of systolic wall thickening, another excellent sign of myocardial ischemia, are not reproducible because of a difficulty in delineating the epicardial border accurately in 2-D echocardiography.
- *Valvular Heart Disease*
  Air embolism
  In the left atrium, left ventricle, and aorta, air embolism can be detected by TEE during open-heart surgery. Therefore, TEE can be used to help the surgeon more extensively evacuate air bubbles from the left heart before the heart ejects blood and air into the systemic circulation.

- *Valvular Regurgitation*
  Valvular regurgitation can be determined intraoperatively by color Doppler echocardiography immediately after conservative valve repair, annuloplasty, commissurotomy, or valve replacement.
- *Congenital Heart Disease*
  TEE technique will allow a more aggressive approach to complex cardiac reconstructions because the surgeon will have the ability to visualize the heart and evaluate adequacy of the surgical repair immediately after the operative procedure.
- *Thoracic Aorta*
  TEE can accurately diagnose thoracic aortic aneuryms, dissection, disruption, and atheromatosis. At the New York Hospital–Cornell Medical Center, we routinely use TEE for patients over 65 years of age to screen severe atheromatosis of aortic arch and descending aorta. Epiaortic echocardiography is performed to identify ascending aorta and arch if severe atheromatosis is found in the descending aorta or arch. Severe atheromatosis of thoracic aorta is an independent predictor of postoperative neurologic outcome. The atheroma is graded as follows: Grade I, normal to mild intimal thickening; Grade II, severe intimal thickening; Grade III, atheroma protruding <5 mm into the lumen; Grade IV, atheroma protruding >5 mm; and Grade V, atheroma with a mobile component.
- *Cardiac Tumors*
  Atrial myxoma can be easily diagnosed by TEE. Pre- and postoperative TEE with contrast can assess the presence and severity of mitral regurgitation secondary to valve damage from ball-valve effect of the myxoma.
- *Other Cardiac Lesions*
  Hypertrophic obstructive cardiomyopathy (idiopathic hypertrophic subaortic stenosis) can be identified with the development of systolic anterior motion of the mitral valve (SAM). Cardiac tamponade by pericardial effusion or hematoma can be detected for preoperative differential diagnosis.
- *Neurosurgery*
  TEE was found to be the most sensitive monitor to detect venous air embolism during sitting position neurosurgery. Patent foramen ovale and paradoxical air embolism can be detected by TEE.

Cahalan MK: Transesophageal echocardiography: Should I be using it? ASA Refresher Courses in Anesthesiology 18:69–84, 1990

Clements FM, de Bruijn NP: Perioperative evaluation of regional wall motion by transesophageal two-dimensional echocardiography. Anesth Analg 66:249–261, 1987

Clements FM, de Bruijn NP: Transesophageal Echocardiography, pp 11–20, 32–33, 82–95, 98–110. Boston, Little, Brown, 1991

Feigenbaum H: Echocardiography, 5th ed, pp 1–32, 514. Philadelphia, Lea & Febiger, 1994

Glenski JA, Cucchiara RF, Michenfelder JD: Transesophageal echocardiography and transcutaneous O_2 and CO_2 monitoring for detection of venous air embolism. Anesthesiology 64:541, 1986

Muhiudeen IA, Roberson DA, Silverman NH et al: Intraoperative echocardiography for evaluation of congenital heart defects in infants and children. Anesthesiology 76:165–172, 1992

C. I-11. How would you induce anesthesia?

A smooth induction is essential to prevent hypotension, hypertension, and tachycardia. Different techniques may be used to achieve a smooth induction. For patients with good left ventricular function, anesthesia is induced with fentanyl, 5 to 10 μg/ kg, and thiopental, 1 to 2 mg/kg. The patient is ventilated by mask with 100% oxygen. After administration of succinylcholine, 1 mg/kg, the patient is intubated. If a potent inhalation agent is to be used for maintenance, anesthesia is induced with thiopental, 4 mg/kg, and deepened with 2.0% enflurane or isoflurane for 3 to 5 minutes. When adequately anesthetized, the patient is given succinylcholine and intubated. In our experiences, hypertension and tachycardia frequently developed after endotracheal intubation when the same concentrations of isoflurane instead of enflurane were used to deepen anesthesia. For patients with poor left ventricular function, potent inhalation agents such as enflurane, isoflurane, and halothane are avoided during induction and maintenance of anesthesia. See also Chapter 14, question C.6. for other measures to prevent tachycardia and hypertension at the time of intubation.

Martin DE, Rosenberg H, Aukburg SJ et al: Low-dose fentanyl blunts circulatory responses to tracheal intubation. Anesth Analg 61:680–684, 1982

C. I-12. How would you maintain anesthesia?

Again, smooth anesthesia is essential to achieve a balance between myocardial oxygen demand and supply. Different agents and techniques may be used to accomplish the same goal. I personally prefer neuroleptic technique with a moderate dose of fentanyl-droperidol-N_2O-O_2 for maintenance of anesthesia. After the patient is intubated, a mixture of 60% nitrous oxide and 40% oxygen is administered to keep the patient unconscious.

The depth of anesthesia must be titrated to meet the requirements of the varying intensities of surgical stimulation. Skin incision and sternal splitting are very painful. But the strongest stimulation is usually from sternal retraction with the self-retaining retractor. Fentanyl, 5 μg (0.1 ml)/kg, is given right before the skin incision. Droperidol, 0.1 ml (0.25 mg)/kg, is titrated in after the skin incision to keep systolic blood pressure around 100 to 120 mm Hg. Another dose of fentanyl 5 μg/kg is given before sternotomy. Then fentanyl, 5 μg/kg, is given every 30 to 60 minutes to maintain anesthesia. Very high doses of fentanyl or sufentanil, with or without droperidol, and oxygen without nitrous oxide, have been successfully used for cardiac anesthesia. Diazepam or midazolam is administered to achieve unconsciousness and amnesia if droperidol is not used. I prefer droperidol because of its alpha-blocking effects, which can easily control hypertension when combined with a moderate dose of fentanyl. Meanwhile, we believe mild cardiac depression from nitrous oxide may decrease the cardiac oxygen demand in a way similar to the effect of propranolol. The possibility of oxygen toxicity from the use of 100% oxygen should also be kept in mind. Nitrous oxide is not used after cardiopulmonary bypass, because it will increase potential air embolism in the bypass grafts, coronary circulation, and probably systemic circulation.

Quintin L, Whalley DG, Wynards JE et al: Oxygen-high-dose fentanyl-droperidol anesthesia for aortocoronary bypass surgery. Anesth Analg 60:412–416, 1981

Stanley TH, Philbin DM, Coggins CH: Fentanyl-oxygen anesthesia for coronary artery surgery: Cardiovascular and antidiuretic hormone responses. Can Anaesth Soc J 26:168–172, 1979

C. I-13. What is the better anesthetic agent for this operation—an inhalation or intravenous agent?

The choice of anesthetic agents is still debatable. Both inhalation and intravenous agents have been used successfully. They both have advantages and disadvantages. Understanding the cardiovascular effects of each anesthetic agent and careful titration of each drug will improve the balance between myocardial oxygen demand and supply. Early detection and appropriate control of the major determinants of myocardial oxygen consumption (BP, HR, PCWP) are mandatory if myocardial ischemia is to be avoided.

Recently, three large-scale outcome studies of patients undergoing CABG surgery reported that anesthetic choice did not affect incidence of perioperative morbidity and mortality.

Lowenstein E: Anesthetic considerations in coronary-artery disease. ASA Refresher Courses in Anesthesiology 4:51–64, 1976

Merin RG, Verdoaw PD, de Jong JW et al: Myocardial functional and metabolic responses to ischemia in swine during halothane and fentanyl anesthesia. Anesthesiology 56:84–92, 1982

Slogoff S, Keats AS: Randomized trial of primary anesthetic agents on outcome of coronary artery bypass surgery. Anesthesiology 70:179–188, 1989

Slogoff S, Keats AS, Dear WE et al: Steal-prone coronary anatomy and myocardial ischemia associated with four primary anesthetic agents in humans. Anesth Analg 72:22–27, 1991

Tuman KJ, McCarthy RJ, Spiess BD et al: Does choice of anesthetic agent significantly affect outcome after coronary artery surgery? Anesthesiology 70:189–198, 1989

C.I-14. What are the cardiovascular effects of halothane, enflurane, isoflurane, desflurane, sevoflurane, morphine, and fentanyl?

In general, halothane, enflurane, isoflurane, desflurane, and sevoflurane produce a dose-related depression in ventricular function and vascular tonus. Halothane sensitizes the heart to catecholamine much more than enflurane, isoflurane, desflurane, and sevoflurane. Isoflurane and desflurane depress cardiac output to a lesser degree than does halothane or enflurane secondary to their greater vasodilating capacity. The heart rate changes least with halothane and increases most with desflurane. Isoflurane may cause tachycardia; the mechanism is unclear. Most studies suggest that halothane, enflurane, and isoflurane decrease coronary vascular resistance. Of these, isoflurane is the most potent coronary vasodilator.

All of the potent drugs decrease arterial pressure in a dose-related manner. The mechanism of the decrease in blood pressure includes vasodilation, decreased cardiac output due to myocardial depression, and decreased sympathetic nervous system tone. With halothane, decreased cardiac output is the predominant cause. Halothane also increases venous compliance, and in patients who have high sympathetic tone, such as those with heart failure, halothane decreases systemic vascular resistance. Enflurane causes both vasodilation and decreased myocardial contractility. With isoflurane and desflurane a low peripheral resistance is the major cause of hypotension. Evidence of the relatively greater myocardial depression with halothane and enflurane is the greater increase in right atrial pressure seen with these drugs than with isoflurane.

Narcotics such as morphine and fentanyl at their clinical dose have minimal car-

diovascular effects. Both may cause bradycardia. Neither sensitizes the heart to catecholamine or depresses myocardial function. The cardiovascular effects of morphine
depend on the dose used. Large doses of morphine sulfate have reportedly caused
myocardial lactate production and reduction in coronary blood flow in animals.
Sethna found that morphine sulfate, 0.25 mg/kg IV, did not produce a global myocardial ischemia in patients with coronary artery disease. High doses of morphine, 1
mg/kg, produce a significant decrease in arterial blood pressure and systemic vascular resistance accompanied by an average 750% increase in plasma histamine. On the
other hand, high doses of fentanyl, 50 μg/kg, do not produce any significant changes
in blood pressure, vascular resistance, and plasma histamine levels.

Barash PG, Cullen BF, Stoelting RK (eds): Clinical Anesthesia, 3rd ed, pp 367–369. Philadelphia,
Lippincott-Raven, 1997

Kaplan JA (ed): Cardiac Anesthesia, 3rd ed, pp 450–451, 481–483, 608–612. Philadelphia, WB Saunders, 1993

Malan TP, DiNardo JA, Isner RJ et al: Cardiovascular effects of sevoflurane compared with those
of isoflurane in volunteers. Anesthesiology 83:918–928, 1995

Sethna DH, Moffitt EA, Gray RJ et al: Cardiovascular effects of morphine in patients with coronary
artery disease. Anesth Analg 61:109–114, 1982

C. I-15. Is isoflurane dangerous for the patient with coronary artery disease?

In patients with coronary artery disease, the use of isoflurane is still controversial.
Reiz and associates reported that 1% isoflurane induced coronary vasodilation that
was not related to normal autoregulation and that both decreased coronary perfusion
pressure (systemic hypotension), and redistribution of myocardial blood flow (coronary steal) may contribute to development of regional myocardial ischemia. Another
Reiz study, using 1.5 MAC isoflurane-nitrous oxide anesthesia, concluded that isoflurane may cause coronary steal with myocardial ischemia in patients with coronary artery disease (CAD). However, Smith and associates reported that the substitution of
0.5% to 1.12% isoflurane for 85 μg/kg of fentanyl did not result in an increased incidence of myocardial ischemia, as seen by ST-segment or segmental wall-motion
changes in patients with CAD. Moreover, Tarnow and associates demonstrated that
0.5% isoflurane with 50% nitrous oxide improved the tolerance to pacing-induced
myocardial ischemia in patients with significant CAD. Recently, two large-scale prospective outcome studies by Slogoff et al and Turman et al could find no evidence
that the incidence of ischemia was increased by isoflurane in patients with CAD
undergoing CABG surgery. Furthermore, this finding held true even for patients
with steal-prone coronary anatomy in the studies by Slogoff et al, Pulley et al, and
Leung et al.

Several animal studies further confused this issue. Priebe proved that isoflurane
was a myocardial depressant and a potent coronary vasodilator in the dog. Sill and
associates demonstrated that high concentrations of isoflurane (1.5% and 2.5%) dilated intramyocardial arterioles rather than epicardial coronary arteries in the intact
dog. Buffington and associates reported that isoflurane (1.2% to 1.5%) produced a decrease in collateral flow and a decrement in collateral zone contraction while enhancing flow in the normally perfused zone. They concluded that isoflurane was an arteriolar vasodilator and hence produced coronary steal in dogs with chronic coronary
occlusion. On the contrary, Cason and associates found that in the dog, isoflurane or

halothane at 0.5% MAC and 1.5 MAC had little effect on coronary vascular resistance, and ischemia was precipitated by tachycardia or hypotension rather than by coronary steal. Moreover, Davis and Frank demonstrated that isoflurane decreased myocardial infarct size after left anterior descending coronary artery occlusion in dogs. In addition, Gilbert and associates reported greater coronary reserve in swine anesthetized with isoflurane versus halothane at 0.5 to 2.0 MAC. Recently, Hartman and associates demonstrated that adenosine but not isoflurane redistributed blood flow away from collateral-dependent myocardium in the presence of a coronary steal-prone anatomy in the chronically instrumented dog. They further found that reductions in myocardial perfusion during isoflurane anesthesia depend on systemic arterial pressure and that isoflurane did not produce coronary steal in this model of multivessel coronary artery disease. Furthermore, Cheng and associates found that neither isoflurane nor halothane as the sole anesthetic in clinical concentrations caused significant coronary vasodilation or coronary steal from 55 to 30 mm Hg coronary perfusion pressure in a swine model of chronic coronary occlusion with collateral development.

On the basis of recent animal and recent clinical studies, we can conclude that isoflurane in clinical concentrations may be used safely in patients with coronary artery disease provided that hypotension and tachycardia are avoided.

Barash PG, Cullen BF, Stoelting RK (eds): Clinical Anesthesia, 3rd ed, pp 369–370. Philadelphia, Lippincott-Raven, 1997

Becker LC: Is isoflurane dangerous for the patient with coronary artery disease? Anesthesiology 66:259–261, 1987

Buffington CW, Romson JL, Levine A et al: Isoflurane induces coronary steal in canine model of chronic coronary occlusion. Anesthesiology 66:280–292, 1987

Cason BA, Verrier E, London MJ et al: Effects of isoflurane and halothane on coronary vascular resistance and collateral blood flow. Anesthesiology 63:A15, 1985

Cheng DCH, Moyers JR, Knutson RM et al: Dose-response relationship of isoflurane and halothane versus coronary perfusion pressures. Effects on flow redistribution in a collateralized chronic swine model. Anesthesiology 76:113–122, 1992

Davis RF, Frank LP: Isoflurane decreases myocardial infarct size after left anterior descending coronary artery occlusion in dogs. Anesthesiology 63:A12, 1985

Gilbert M, Roberts SL, Blomberg RW et al: Greater coronary reserve in swine anesthetized with isoflurane versus halothane. Anesthesiology 63:A15, 1985

Hartman JC, Kampine JP, Schmeling WT et al: Steal-prone coronary circulation in chronically instrumented dogs: Isoflurane versus adenosine. Anesthesiology 74:744–756, 1991

Leung JM, Goehner P, O'Kelly BF et al: Isoflurane anesthesia and myocardial ischemia: Comparative risk versus sufentanil anesthesia in patients undergoing coronary artery bypass graft surgery. Anesthesiology 74:838–847, 1991

Lillehaug SL, Tinker JH: Why do "pure" vasodilators cause coronary steal when anesthetics don't (or seldom do)? (editorial). Anesth Analg 73:681–682, 1991

Merin RG: Is anesthesia beneficial for the ischemia heart? III. Editorial views. Anesthesiology 64:137–140, 1986

Priebe HJ: Differential effects of isoflurane on regional right and left ventricular performances and on coronary, systemic, and pulmonary hemodynamics in the dog. Anesthesiology 66:262–272, 1987

Priebe H, Foëx P: Isoflurane causes regional myocardial dysfunction in dogs with critical coronary artery stenoses. Anesthesiology 66:293–300, 1987

Pulley DD, Kirvassilis GV, Kelermenos N et al: Regional and global myocardial circulatory and metabolic effects of isoflurane and halothane in patients with steal-prone coronary anatomy. Anesthesiology 75:756–766, 1991

Reiz S, Balfors E, Sorensen MB et al: Isoflurane: A powerful coronary vasodilator in patients with coronary artery disease. Anesthesiology 59:91–97, 1983

Reiz S, Ostman M: Regional coronary hemodynamics during isoflurane-nitrous oxide anesthesia in patients with ischemic heart disease. Anesth Analg 64:570–576, 1985

Slogoff S, Keats AS: Randomized trial of primary anesthetic agents on outcome of coronary artery bypass operations. Anesthesiology 70:179–188, 1989

Slogoff S, Keats AS, Dear WE et al: Steal-prone coronary anatomy and myocardial ischemia associated with four primary anesthetic agents in humans. Anesth Analg 72:22–27, 1991

Smith JS, Cahalan MK, Benefiel DJ et al: Fentanyl versus fentanyl and isoflurane in patients with impaired left ventricular function. Anesthesiology 63:A18, 1985

Tarnow J, Markschies-Hornung A, Schulte-Sasseu U: Isoflurane improves the tolerance to pacing-induced myocardial ischemia. Anesthesiology 64:147–156, 1986

Turman KJ, McCarthy RJ, Spiess BD et al: Does choice of anesthetic agent significantly affect outcome after coronary artery surgery? Anesthesiology 70:189–198, 1989

C. I-16. What is the cardiovascular effect of nitrous oxide?

Nitrous oxide is a weak central nervous system depressant. It has been generally considered to have minimal effects on other organ systems. Nitrous oxide has significant cardiovascular effects that may be depressant or stimulatory depending on the anesthetics with which it is used. When high-dose fentanyl is used during coronary surgery, the effects of N_2O depend on the patient's cardiac function. Following the administration of 50% N_2O, there are no significant changes in any of the hemodynamic parameters in patients with normal left ventricular function (LVEDP <15 mm Hg). On the contrary, there is a significant decrease in cardiac index and stroke volume index in patients with left ventricular dysfunction (LVEDP >15 mm Hg). When added to other inhalation anesthetics, N_2O increases arterial pressure and systemic vascular resistance, suggesting that it has a vasoconstrictive action. Nitrous oxide increases pulmonary vascular resistance in patients with mitral stenosis and pulmonary hypertension.

The pulmonary vascular effects of nitrous oxide are also variable. Patients with elevated pulmonary artery pressure may have further increases when nitrous oxide is added. Konstadt et al did not corroborate these findings in patients with mitral valvular disease. A study in infants failed to show further increases of pulmonary vascular resistance with the addition of nitrous oxide. It is of interest that the decrease in pulmonary vascular resistance with isoflurane is less than the decrease in systemic vascular resistance.

The contribution of nitrous oxide to myocardial ischemia is controversial. Philbin and associates suggested that addition of nitrous oxide to anesthesia with high-dose fentanyl, 100 μg/kg followed by 1 μg/kg/min, or sufentanil, 30 μg/kg followed by 0.3 μg/kg/min, can produce clinically unapparent regional myocardial ischemia in the areas supplied by stenotic coronary arteries of dogs. However, using two-dimensional transesophageal echocardiography, nitrous oxide added to low-dose fentanyl,

15 µg/kg followed by 0.2 µg/kg/min, or high-dose sufentanil, 20 µg/kg, did not cause myocardial ischemia in patients with CAD.

Clinically, nitrous oxide may be used before cardiopulmonary bypass if high-dose narcotics are not used and hypotension does not occur. However, after cardiopulmonary bypass, nitrous oxide should be avoided because of the possibility of expanding air bubbles in the coronary and cerebral circulation.

Balasaraswathi K, Kumar P, Rao TLK et al: Left ventricular end-diastolic pressure (LVEDP) as an index for nitrous oxide use during coronary artery surgery. Anesthesiology 55:708–709, 1981

Barash PG, Cullen BF, Stoelting RK (eds): Clinical Anesthesia, 3rd ed, pp 368. Philadelphia, Lippincott-Raven, 1997

Cahalan MK, Prakash O, Rulf EN et al: Addition of nitrous oxide to fentanyl anesthesia does not induce myocardial ischemia in patients with ischemic heart disease. Anesthesiology 67:925–929, 1987

Hamilton WK: Con: Nitrous oxide should be used in patients with coronary artery disease. Cardiothorac Vasc Anesth 5:90–91, 1991

Messina AG, Yao FS, Canning H et al: The effect of nitrous oxide on left ventricular pump performance and contractility with coronary artery disease: effect of preoperative ejection fraction. Anesth Analg 77:954–962, 1993

Nathan HJ: Pro: Nitrous oxide should not be used in patients with coronary artery disease. Cardiothorac Vasc Anesth 5:87–89, 1991

Philbin DM, Foëx P, Drummond G et al: Postsystolic shortening of canine left ventricle supplied by a stenotic coronary artery when nitrous oxide is added in the presence of narcotics. Anesthesiology 62:166–174, 1985

Slavik JR, Lamantia KR, Kopriva CJ et al: Does N_2O cause regional wall motion abnormalities in patients with CAD? An evaluation by 2-D transesophageal echocardiography. Anesthesiology 65: A515, 1986

C. I-17. What kind of muscle relaxant would you use? Why?

We usually use pancuronium. When full paralyzing doses are given in a bolus, *d*-tubocurarine tends to produce bradycardia and hypotension from ganglionic blockade and histamine release, whereas pancuronium and gallamine generally produce tachycardia and hypertension caused by vagolytic effect and norepinephrine released from cardiac sympathetic nerves. *D*-tubocurarine may be given in increments of 6 mg every 5 to 10 minutes until patients are fully paralyzed (0.3 mg/kg). Blood pressure and heart rate are usually not changed by this small dose and slow injection rate. Pancuronium is a better choice if hypotension (BP <80 mm Hg systolically) and bradycardia (HR <50/min) are present. Theoretically, pancuronium may increase myocardial O_2 consumption caused by tachycardia and hypertension. However, pancuronium is the most commonly used muscle relaxant for CABG. In practice, most patients with CAD take beta-adrenergic blocking agents, which can decrease the vagolytic effect of pancuronium. Also, the bradycardia associated with the popular narcotic anesthetic techniques can attenuate the tachycardia induced by pancuronium. Vecuronium and cisatracurium have no major cardiovascular effects, but their intermediate duration of action necessitates frequent administration of the relaxant. Pipecuronium and doxacurium are two new long-acting, nondepolarizing muscle relaxants. They seem to have no hemodynamic side-effects associated with neuromuscular blockade. They can be used in large bolus doses.

Fleming N: Con: The choice of muscle relaxants is not important in cardiac surgery. J Cardiothorac Vas Anesth 9:772–774, 1995

Hudson RJ, Thomson IR: Pro: The choice of muscle relaxants is important in cardiac surgery. J Cardiothorac Vasc Anesth 9:768–771, 1995

C. I-18. If ST-segment depression is seen during surgery, how would you treat it? What is the relationship between perioperative myocardial ischemia and postoperative myocardial infarction?

ST-segment depression indicates myocardial ischemia, either from increased O_2 demand or decreased O_2 supply. The treatment includes the following:

- Increase O_2 supply—Correct hypotension and hypoxemia.
- Decrease O_2 demand—Correct hypertension, tachycardia, and increased PCWP or CVP by deepening anesthesia or by using vasodilators and propranolol. All the major determinants have to be considered and corrected to their normal levels.

Gerson and associates (in experimental dogs) found that elevation of ST segments induced by occlusion of the coronary artery was more limited with halothane than with a combination of nitroprusside and propranolol. The more favorable effect of halothane was explained by its effects on coronary vascular reserve and the known effect of nitroprusside to reduce myocardial blood flow to ischemic myocardium.

If there are no obvious changes in blood pressure, heart rate, and pulmonary wedge pressure, nitroglycerin is indicated for coronary spasm. Nitroglycerin may be given by intravenous drip. Sublingual nifedipine or intravenous nicardipine may be given to relieve coronary spasm.

Slogoff and Keats reported that perioperative myocardial ischemia occurred in 37% of all patients undergoing CABG. They proved that perioperative myocardial infarction was almost three times as frequent in patients with ischemia (6.9%) compared with patients without ischemia (2.5%). Intraoperative tachycardia was associated with a higher incidence of myocardial ischemia and infarction. However, Knight et al demonstrated that 42% of CABG patients had preoperative episodes of myocardial ischemia, 87% of which were clinically silent. They further found that anesthesia and surgery did not worsen the preoperative ischemic pattern. Furthermore, Slogoff and Keats in another study postulated that approximately 90% of new myocardial ischemia observed during anesthesia was the manifestation of silent ischemia observed in the patient before the operation and only 10% was related to anesthetic management. Therefore, the relationship between intraoperative ischemia and postoperative outcome is still unsolved.

Gerson JI, Hickey RF, Bainton CR: Treatment of myocardial ischemia with halothane or nitroprusside-propranolol. Anesth Analg 61:10–14, 1982

Hardman JG, Limbird LE, Molinoff PB et al (eds): Goodman and Gilman's the Pharmacological Basis of Therapeutics, 9th ed, pp 767–769. New York, McGraw-Hill, 1996

Hill AB, Bowley CJ, Nahrwold ML et al: Intranasal administration of nitroglycerin. Anesthesiology 54:346–348, 1981

Knight AA, Hollenberg M, London MJ et al: Perioperative myocardial ischemia: Importance of the preoperative ischemia pattern. Anesthesiology 68:681–688, 1988

Mangano DT: Perioperative cardiac morbidity. Anesthesiology 72:153–184, 1990

Slogoff S, Keats AS: Does perioperative myocardial ischemia lead to postoperative myocardial infarction. Anesthesiology 62:107–114, 1985

Slogoff S, Keats AS: Randomized trial of anesthetic agents on outcome of coronary artery bypass operations. Anesthesiology 69:179–188, 1989

C. I-19. Would you use prophylactic nitroglycerin during coronary artery bypass grafting (CABG) to prevent intraoperative myocardial ischemia or perioperative myocardial infarction?

No. It has been reported that prophylactic administration of nitroglycerin, 0.5 or 1.0 mg/kg/min, during fentanyl anesthesia in patients undergoing CABG did not prevent myocardial ischemia or reduce the incidence of perioperative myocardial infarction.

Barash PG, Cullen BF, Stoelting RK (eds): Clinical Anesthesia, 3rd ed, p 689. Philadelphia, Lippincott-Raven, 1997

Gallagher JD, Moore RA, Jose AB et al: Prophylactic nitroglycerin infusion during coronary artery bypass surgery. Anesthesiology 64:785–789, 1986

Thomson IR, Mutch WAC, Culligan JD: Failure of intravenous nitroglycerin to prevent myocardial ischemia during fentanyl-pancuronium anesthesia. Anesthesiology 61:385–393, 1984

C.I-20. How would you correct hypertension?

$$\text{Blood pressure} = \text{blood flow} \times \text{resistance}$$

Hypertension is usually due to inadequate depth of anesthesia. Occasionally it is due to fluid overloading. The treatment of hypertension includes the following:

- Deepen the anesthesia. Inhalation agents, such as halothane, enflurane, and isoflurane are more effective than narcotics because of their vasodilator effect.
- Vasodilators—when inhalation agents are not used.
  - Sodium nitroprusside produces more arteriolar dilation than venodilation.
    Dose—10 to 100 µg/min IV drip titration
  - Nitroglycerin produces more venodilation than arteriolar dilation.
    Dose—20 to 200 µg/min IV drip titration

See also Chapter 14, question C.10.

Gerson JI, Allen FB, Seltzer JL et al: Arterial and venous dilation by nitroprusside and nitroglycerin—Is there a difference? Anesth Analg 61:256–260, 1982

Kaplan J (ed): Cardiac Anesthesia, 3rd ed, pp 1177–1178. Philadelphia, WB Saunders, 1993

C. I-21. How would you treat hypotension?

Hypotension is usually caused by hypovolemia, deep anesthesia, bradycardia, or congestive heart failure (CHF). The treatments are as follows:

- Increase fluid infusion and put the patient in head-down position when CVP or PCWP is low.
- Lighten the level of anesthesia or use a vasoconstrictor—phenylephrine, 0.1 mg IV increments, to correct vasodilation produced by anesthesia.
- Atropine, 0.2 to 2.0 mg, for bradycardia, or isoproterenol, 1 mg/100 ml D_5W IV drip titration.

- Treat CHF when PCWP is high:
  - Lighten the level of anesthesia.
  - Restrict fluids.
  - Diuretics—furosemide (Lasix) 20 to 40 mg IV.
  - Inotropes
    - $CaCl_2$ (0.5–1.0 g).
    - Epinephrine—2 to 8 μg/min IV drip.
    - Dobutamine or dopamine—5 to 20 μg/kg/min IV drip.
    - Amrinone—0.75 to 1.5 mg/kg, then 5 to 10 μg/kg/min IV drip, or
    - Milrinone 0.05 mg/kg, then 0.5 to 0.7 μg/kg/min IV drip.
    - Norepinephrine if peripheral vascular resistance is low.
  - IABP (intraaortic balloon pump).

C. I-22. What are the indications for intravenous propranolol or esmolol during surgery? How much would you give? What are the relative contraindications?

Indications
- ST-segment depression associated with tachycardia; no response to deepening the level of anesthesia
- Supraventricular tachycardia over 120/min
- Recurrent ventricular arrhythmias

Contraindications
- Congestive heart failure
- Asthma, chronic obstructive pulmonary disease

However, esmolol is cardioselective and appears to have little effect on bronchial or vascular tone at doses that decrease heart rate in humans. It has been used successfully in low doses in patients with asthma. Esmolol is metabolized rapidly in the blood by an esterase located in the erythrocyte cytoplasm. Esmolol is a short-acting beta-blocker with an elimination half-life of 9 minutes and a pharmacologic half-life of 10 to 20 minutes.

Dosage—Propranolol, 0.25-mg increments every 1 to 2 minutes—total dose 2 to 3 mg
Esmolol, 10-mg increments up to 0.5 mg/kg followed by 50 to 300 μg/kg/min IV drip.

Barash PG, Cullen BF, Stoelting RK (eds): Clinical Anesthesia, 3rd ed, p 294. Philadelphia, Lippincott-Raven, 1997

Kaplan J (ed): Cardiac Anesthesia, 3rd ed, pp 191–192. Philadelphia, WB Saunders, 1993

C. I-23. How would you correct increased PCWP?

It is important to treat the patient as a whole. All monitors have to be considered together, not only one single parameter. Increased PCWP is usually due to a light level of anesthesia or congestive heart failure (CHF). Combining the readings of PCWP and blood pressure will produce a differential diagnosis.

Inadequate Anesthesia—increased PCWP with hypertension
- Deepen the level of anesthesia with inhalation agents, such as isoflurane, halothane, or enflurane, which also have a vasodilator effect.
- Give a vasodilator. Nitroglycerin is a better venodilator than nitroprusside.

CHF—increased PCWP with hypotension and low cardiac output
- Lighten the level of anesthesia.
- Restrict fluids.
- Use vasodilators.
- Give diuretics.
- Use inotropes.

Kaplan J (ed): Cardiac Anesthesia, 3rd ed, pp 615–616. New York, Grune & Stratton, 1993

C. I-24. During sternal splitting, would you do something?

Stop ventilation and deflate the lungs to prevent lung injury from the electric saw.

C. I-25. Would you monitor PCWP continuously? Why?

No, If the Swan-Ganz catheter balloon is inflated continuously, pulmonary infarction distal to the occlusion may ensue. Usually pulmonary artery diastolic pressure (PADP) is monitored continuously because PADP is very close to PCWP.

Barash PG, Cullen BF, Stoelting RK (eds): Clinical Anesthesia, 3rd ed, pp 630–633. Philadelphia, Lippincott-Raven, 1997

C. I-26. Discuss autologous transfusion and blood conservation for cardiac surgery.

Autologous transfusion is the collection and reinfusion of the patient's own blood or blood components. The realization that homologous blood is responsible for transmission of AIDS, hepatitis, transfusion reaction, and autosensitization has led to increased interest in autologous transfusion and blood conservation. There are several options for autologous transfusion: preoperative autologous blood donation, intraoperative normovolemic hemodilution, intraoperative plasmapheresis, and perioperative blood salvage.

Preoperative Autologous Blood Donation
Donations are appropriate for properly selected patients with stable coronary artery disease, stable valvular disease, and congenital heart disease. The risk of blood donation may be higher for patients with unstable angina or severe aortic stenosis; these patients are usually not considered good candidates for autologous blood donation. The patient should have a hemoglobin of >11 g/dl to donate blood.

The optimal donation period begins 4 to 6 weeks prior to surgery, and the last donation is usually collected no later than 72 hours before surgery.

Intraoperative Normovolemic Hemodilution
This is the removal of blood through an arterial or venous catheter immediately after induction of anesthesia, prior to cardiopulmonary bypass or the administration of heparin. Depending on the patient's size and hematocrit, 500 to 1000 ml of blood is collected into blood bags containing CPDA-1 anticoagulant and is kept at room temperature.

This blood is spared the rigors of CPB, including hemolysis, platelet destruction, and clotting factor degradation. The autologous blood is transfused after reversal of the heparin with protamine. It has been demonstrated that the effect of one unit of fresh whole blood on platelet aggregation after cardiopulmonary bypass is at least equal, if not superior, to the effect of 8 to 10 stored platelet units. However, if the patient's hematocrit is below 33% or the hemoglobin is below 11 g/dl, normovolemic hemodilution is not recommended because further decreasing the oxygen-carrying capacity may worsen myocardial ischemia. In addition, hemodilution during CPB will further decrease hematocrit to levels that require homologous blood transfusion. Normovolemic hemodilution should be performed cautiously in patients with critical left main coronary stenosis since sudden cardiac arrest has been observed during the procedure.

Intraoperative Plasmapheresis

Coagulopathy associated with hypothermia, shock, cardiopulmonary bypass, multiple transfusions, and the blood salvage technique, which removes clotting factors and platelets, often necessitates use of fresh-frozen plasma and platelet packs to control postoperative bleeding and clotting problems. Recently a plasma-collection system has been developed to salvage up to 1000 ml of platelet-rich plasma before cardiopulmonary bypass. This technique does not cause hemodilution; therefore, it can be utilized in all patients, including those with anemia. The platelet-rich plasma can be stored at room temperature until transfused, usually after protamine reversal of the heparin. It is recommended that the collected product be placed on a rocker until infusion and that the *p*H be held constant.

Perioperative Blood Salvage

This is the collection and reinfusion of blood lost during and immediately after surgery. The posttransfusion survival of perioperatively salvaged red cells has been shown to be comparable to that of allogeneic red cells. At the conclusion of cardiopulmonary bypass, all blood remaining in the oxygenator and bypass circuits should be salvaged and, if needed, infused. Blood salvaged intraoperatively may be transfused directly (unwashed) or processed (washed) prior to infusion. Commercially available equipment exists for each option. Blood collected by intraoperative salvage represents an excellent source of red-cell support. However, salvaged blood is deficient in coagulation factors and platelets.

Postoperative blood salvage is another technique of autologous blood transfusion utilizing blood lost following surgery. Blood salvaged following cardiac surgery is generally collected from mediastinal and chest drains and transfused without washing. Since it is usually defibrinated, it does not require anticoagulation prior to transfusion. Although dilute, the blood is sterile and contains viable red cells.

Barash PG, Cullen BF, Stoelting RK (eds): Clinical Anesthesia, 3rd ed, p 199. Philadelphia, Lippincott-Raven, 1997

Del Rossi AJ, Cernaianu AC, Vertrees RA et al: Platelet-rich plasma reduces postoperative blood loss after cardiopulmonary bypass. J Thorac Cardiovasc Surg 100:281–286, 1990

Giordano GF Sr, Giordano GF Jr, Rivers SL et al: Determinants of homologous blood usage utilizing autologous platelet-rich plasma in cardiac operations. Ann Thorac Surg 47:897–902, 1989

Gravlee GP, Davis RF, Utley JR: Cardiopulmonary Bypass, Principles and Practice, pp 107–117. Baltimore, Williams & Wilkins, 1993

Lavee J, Martinowitz U, Mohr R et al: The effect of transfusion of fresh whole blood versus platelet concentrates after cardiac operations. J Thorac Cardiovasc Surg 97:204–212, 1989

Tawes RL Jr, Sydorak GR, Duvall TB et al: The plasma collection system: A new concept in autotransfusion. Ann Vasc Surg 3:304–306, 1989

Transfusion Alert, Use of Autologous Blood, NIH publication #89-3038, September 1989

C. II. During Cardiopulmonary Bypass (CPB)

C. II-1. What anticoagulant would you give before CPB? How much would you give? What is its mechanism?

Heparin has been used conventionally in doses of 300 (200 to 400) units/kg of body weight, assuming an initial concentration of at least 2 to 4 units/ml of whole blood. Empirically, after 2 hours of the initial dose, subsequent doses of 1 mg/kg are given for each additional hour of bypass. Because there is marked individual variation, heparin doses are best monitored by the celite-activated coagulation time (ACT) test.

Heparin acts indirectly by means of a plasma cofactor. The heparin cofactor, or antithrombin III, is an alpha$_2$-globulin and a protease inhibitor that neutralizes several activated clotting factors: XIIa, kallikrein, XIa, IXa, Xa, IIa, and XIIIa. Antithrombin III forms irreversible complexes with thrombin (IIa) and, as a result, both proteins are inactivated. Inhibition of thrombin and factor Xa accounts for most of the anticoagulant effect of heparin. Heparin increases the rates of the thrombin-antithrombin reaction at least 1000-fold by serving as a catalytic template to which both the inhibitor and the protease bind.

Gravlee GP, Davis RF, Utley JR: Cardiopulmonary Bypass, Principles and Practice, pp 345–348. Baltimore, Williams & Wilkins, 1993

Hardman JG, Limbird LE, Molinoff PB et al (eds): Goodman and Gilman's The Pharmacological Basis of Therapeutics, 9th ed, pp 1344–1345. New York, Mc Graw-Hill, 1996

C. II-2. What is the half-life of heparin? How is it eliminated?

The biologic half-life of heparin varies with dosages and temperature. It has a remarkable individual variation. The average half-life is approximately 100 minutes in normothermic man for the initial doses of 300 units, increasing with higher doses and decreasing temperature. When 100, 400, or 800 units of heparin is given intravenously, the approximate half-life is 1, 2.5, and 5 hours respectively.

Heparin appears to be cleared and degraded primarily by the reticuloendothelial system; a small amount of undegraded heparin also appears in the urine.

Gravlee GP, Davis RF, Utley JR: Cardiopulmonary Bypass, Principles and Practice, pp 344–345. Baltimore, Williams & Wilkins, 1993

Hardman JG, Limbird LE, Molinoff PB et al (eds): Goodman and Gilman's The Pharmacological Basis of Therapeutics, 9th ed, p 1345. New York, McGraw-Hill, 1996

C. II-3. How do you monitor heparin dosage? What is the ACT test?

Heparin therapy can be assessed by the PTT, heparin assay, heparin-protamine titration, and the ACT test. The most convenient and practical method used to monitor heparin therapy in the operating room is the celite-activated coagulation time (ACT) test. There is a very good correlation among the ACT, plasma heparin units, and thrombin time. After central venous injection of a heparin bolus, the onset of maximal ACT prolongation in the radial artery blood sample occurs within 1 minute. Previous work suggested that heparin action peaks 10 to 20 minutes after administration, but this finding probably represented an artifact from other factors prolonging the ACT such as hemodilution and hypothermia. Two ml of blood are put into a test tube containing celite to activate coagulation. Then the tube is kept at 37°C and clot formation is watched for ACT. The normal control value of ACT is 105 to 167 seconds. A baseline value is determined before the administration of heparin, and the test is repeated 3 to 5 minutes after heparin is given and at intervals of 30 to 60 minutes thereafter. With the dose of heparin in milligrams per kilogram on the vertical axis and ACT in seconds on the horizontal axis, a dose-response curve can be plotted. ACT values are maintained at at least twice control value and not <300 seconds during normothermia and >400 seconds during hypothermia below 30°C. At the New York Hospital–Cornell Medical Center, we keep the ACT above 480 seconds.

Bull MH, Huse WM, Bull BS: Evaluation of tests used to monitor heparin therapy during extracorporeal circulation. Anesthesiology 43:346–353, 1975

Ellison N, Jobes DR (eds): Effective Hemostasis in Cardiac Surgery, pp 1–8. Philadelphia, JB Lippincott, 1988

Gravlee GP, Davis RF, Utley JR: Cardiopulmonary Bypass, Principles and Practice, pp 343–364. Baltimore, Williams & Wilkins, 1993

C. II-4. What is total cardiopulmonary bypass? What is partial bypass?

Total bypass indicates that all the venous return from superior and inferior venae cavae, and the coronary sinus is drained to the oxygenator, and no blood is pumped by the right ventricle to the lungs. The pulmonary artery and systemic pressure tracings become nonpulsatile. Partial bypass means that some of the blood return is still pumped by both right and left ventricles. Some venous blood is drained to the oxygenator and pumped back to the arterial side. Femoral-femoral bypass is one example.

Gravlee GP, Davis RF, Utley JR: Cardiopulmonary Bypass, Principles and Practice, pp 578, 768. Baltimore, Williams & Wilkins, 1993

C. II-5. What is the purpose of venting the left ventricle? How can it be done?

Even though all the venous return is bypassed from the right ventricle, 2% to 5% of cardiac output is draining to the left ventricle. This is the physiologic shunt from the bronchial, thebesian, and pleural veins. Other sources of blood flow to the left heart during CPB include aortic regurgitation from aortic insufficiency and extracardiac left-to-right shunts such as patent ductus arteriosus and Blalock-Taussig, Waterston, and Potts shunts. The left ventricular sump drain prevents overdistention of the left ventricle, which may cause post-pump heart failure. A suction needle inserted proximal to the aortic cross-clamp may serve the same purpose.

Venting of the left ventricle can be accomplished by inserting a catheter to the following sites:

- Aortic root such as cardioplegia cannula for CABG
- Junction of the right superior pulmonary vein and the left atrium and advancing through the left atrium and mitral valve into the left ventricle
- Apex of the left ventricle
- Pulmonary artery or the left atrium only

Gravlee GP, Davis RF, Utley JR: Cardiopulmonary Bypass, Principles and Practice, pp 76–78. Baltimore, Williams & Wilkins, 1993

C. II-6. How many types of oxygenators are there? What are the advantages of each type?

There are two basic types of oxygenators in terms of their interface with blood.

Direct Gas Interface
- Disc
- Vertical screen
- Bubble

Without Gas Interface
- Membrane—solid or microporous
- Fluid—fluid using fluorocarbon liquid

The disc and screen oxygenators are not disposable and have proven to be somewhat difficult to clean, prepare, and resterilize.

The bubble oxygenator has the advantages of simplicity, disposability, and relatively low cost. It is the most popular oxygenator used at the present time.

The disadvantages of gas interface oxygenators include the following:

- Protein denaturation
- Increased fragility of cells
- Susceptibility to hemolysis
- Denaturation of platelet membrane materials resulting in platelet aggregation, clumping
- Formation of air embolism
- Large priming volume
- Variable reservoir level resulting in potential shifts of blood volume between intracorporeal and extracorporeal circuit

The membrane oxygenator has become more popular, economical, and efficient, and less traumatic to blood. Its advantages include the following:

- Less trauma to blood components
- No deforming stage
- Less complement activation
- Independent control of oxygen and carbon dioxide exchange
- Use of air-oxygen mixture without the risk of gaseous microemboli

However, the advantage of a membrane oxygenator for a short perfusion (<2 hours) is unclear, although lower plasma hemoglobin levels are present using membrane oxygenators.

The disadvantages of membrane oxygenators include the following:

- Expense
- Potential difficulty in eliminating all bubbles during priming
- Moderately large priming volume

The major differences in changes of clotting factors between the bubble and membrane oxygenators become apparent after 4 to 6 hours of extracorporeal circulation (ECC).

Gravlee GP, Davis RF, Utley JR: Cardiopulmonary Bypass, Principles and Practice, pp 46–51. Baltimore, Williams & Wilkins, 1993

Wagner JA: Oxygenator anatomy and function. J Cardiothorac Vasc Anesth 11:175–281, 1997

Kaplan J (ed): Cardiac Anesthesia, 3rd ed, pp 999–1001. Philadelphia, WB Saunders, 1993

C. II-7. What kind of priming solution would you use? How much priming solution would you use? Would you prime with blood or not? Why?

The usual priming solution for adults at the New York Hospital–Cornell Medical Center includes 2000 ml of balanced salt solution (Normosol) and 200 ml of 20% mannitol. The priming volumes vary with the size of the oxygenators used and the tubing volume; most oxygenators for adult patients have priming volumes of 500 to 1000 ml. In general, blood is added to the oxygenator if the patient is markedly anemic (pre-pump hematocrit below 30%) or if the priming volume is large in relation to the patient's blood volume, such as in pediatric patients. In order to maintain oxygen carrying capacity, we try to keep hematocrit levels above 18% to 20%. Mannitol has long been used as an osmotic diuretic in situations where hemolysis or diminished renal function is expected. Mannitol has been found to decrease the incidence of renal failure during hypotension by promoting osmotic diuresis and increasing renal blood flow by decreasing renal vascular resistance. Heparin, 3000 to 10,000 units, is added to the prime depending on the size of the prime volume. This allows heparin to be distributed over the thrombogenic surfaces of the CPB circuit.

Gravlee GP, Davis RF, Utley JR: Cardiopulmonary Bypass, Principles and Practice, pp 132–134, 418. Baltimore, Williams & Wilkins, 1993

Kaplan J (ed): Cardiac Anesthesia, 3rd ed, pp 930–931. Philadelphia, WB Saunders, 1993

C. II-8. What are the advantages and disadvantages of hemodilution?

Advantages of Hemodilution
- An increase in microcirculation due to a decreasing blood viscosity
- Decreased metabolic acidosis
- Increased urine output
- Reduced blood demands
- Reduced incidence of hepatitis, AIDS, or reactions from blood transfusions
- Reduced postoperative blood loss

Disadvantages of Hemodilution
- Decreased oxygen carrying capacity
- Postoperative extracellular fluid overload
- Possible pulmonary edema
- Hypotension from decreased viscosity and peripheral resistance
- Decreased concentration of calcium, magnesium, phosphate, and zinc

DiNardo JA, Schwartz MJ (eds): Anesthesia for Cardiac Surgery, p 226. Norwalk, CT, Appleton & Lange, 1990

Gravlee GP, Davis RF, Utley JR: Cardiopulmonary Bypass, Principles and Practice, pp 124–132. Baltimore, Williams & Wilkins, 1993

Verska JJ, Ludington LG, Brewer LA: A comparative study of cardiopulmonary bypass with nonblood and blood prime. Ann Thorac Surg 18:72–80, 1974

C. II-9. What kind of pumps do you use? Are they pulsatile or not?

There are three types of pumps available for modern CPB machines: the double-headed nonocclusive roller pump, the centrifugal blood pump, and the ventricular-type pneumatic or hydraulic pump. Only the first two types are in common use.

The roller pump is the most commonly used pump. It is driven by a load-independent motor. Once the pump speed is set, it will continue the forward displacement of the same blood volume even if the resistance is increased by kinking or clamping the arterial line. This will result in the rupture of connections between sections of tubing. Some centers use pressure gauges on the arterial inflow line to avoid this type of disaster.

The centrifugal pump is a kinetic pump that operates on the constrained vortex principle. Blood is driven through the pump by centrifugal forces generated by a vortex in the pump. The advantages of centrifugal pumps are as follows:

- Less trauma to blood components than the roller pump.
- Less risk of increasing arterial line pressure because blood flow decreases when line resistance is increased.
- Inflow responsiveness. If a large quantity of air is introduced into the pump, cohesive forces will no longer exist between layers of blood and pumping will stop.
- Less risk of micro-air embolism because small, low-density air bubbles are trapped in the center of the vortex.

Ventricular-type pumps, while potentially more powerful, are rather cumbersome and have not been well accepted. This type of pump is mainly used for pulsatile bypass.

The first two types of pumps are nonpulsatile. The pulsatile pumps are commercially available now. Methods available to generate pulsatile flow include an indwelling intraaortic balloon pump, an extracorporeal balloon, ventricular-type pumps, Keele pump, Polystan pulsatile pump, modified roller pumps, and modified centrifugal pumps. Some studies indicate that with prolonged perfusion, pulsatile flow appears to be more physiologic and superb for organ function; however, scientists are less certain that it is an important factor during short-term bypass. The differences between the two modes and a benefit for pulsatile perfusion are most clearly manifested in identifiable high-risk patient groups.

Gravlee GP, Davis RF, Utley JR: Cardiopulmonary Bypass, Principles and Practice, pp 67–71. Baltimore, Williams & Wilkins, 1993

Hornick P, Taylor K: Pulsatile and nonpulsatile perfusion: The continuing controversy. J Cardiothorac Vasc Anesth 11:310–315, 1997

C. II-10. How do you monitor the patient during CPB?

Clinical Monitoring
- Mean arterial blood pressure should be kept between 50 and 100 mm Hg to maintain tissue perfusion.
- Pulmonary artery pressure should be low or zero to prevent overdistention of the left ventricle.
- Central venous pressure should be low or zero to make sure there is no obstruction to venous return from the head.
- Pump-flow rate should be adequate for tissue perfusion and oxygenation.

- Urine output should be maintained above 1 ml/kg/h by adequate perfusion.
- ECG.
- EEG is used in patients in whom cerebral problems may occur.
- Both rectal and esophageal temperatures are recorded.
- The level of anesthesia should be maintained.
- Pupillary size should remain normal and equal.
- Transcranial Doppler (TCD) and/or TEE may be used to detect aortic and cerebral embolism.

Laboratory Monitoring at Least Once Every Hour
- Arterial blood gases—kept at normal range.
- Venous PO_2 should be 40 to 45 mm Hg.
- Hematocrit maintained between 20% and 30%.
- Electrolytes Na^+, K^+, ionized Ca^{++}.
- ACT measured each hour and maintained above 400 to 480 seconds.
- Blood sugar probably should be kept below 250 mg/dl.

Gravlee GP, Davis RF, Utley JR: Cardiopulmonary Bypass, Principles and Practice, pp 578–600. Baltimore, Williams & Wilkins, 1993

Kaplan J (ed): Cardiac Anesthesia, 3rd ed, pp 922–926. Philadelphia, WB Saunders, 1993

C. II-11. How much blood pressure would you keep during CPB? Why?

Controversy continues over what constitutes adequate pressures while the patient is on bypass. The mean arterial pressure (MAP) is usually maintained at approximately 50 to 100 mm Hg to ensure adequate tissue perfusion. Blood pressure depends on cardiac output (pump flow) and total peripheral resistance. We believe that adequate cardiac output (pump flow) is more important for tissue perfusion than blood pressure.

During hypothermia cardioplegia, higher pressures (mean blood pressure >70 mm Hg) are often avoided because of increased noncoronary collateral blood flow into the heart through the pericardium and pulmonary venous drainage. Such collateral flow of relatively warm blood tends to wash the colder cardioplegic solution out of the heart and decreases the hypothermic protection against myocardial ischemia.

The range of cerebrovascular autoregulation during hypothermia is controversial. Although pooled data from clinical studies indicate a lower autoregulatory threshold of 20 to 30 mm Hg in patients without cerebrovascular disease or preexisting hypertension, other studies suggest a pressure-dependent cerebral circulation when mean arterial pressure is <50 mm Hg. Until prospective studies clearly define the autoregulatory threshold under various clinical conditions, blood pressure of <50 mm Hg should be regarded as potential physiologic trespass, which may compromise cerebral circulation. In patients with cerebrovascular disease or hypertension, higher perfusion pressure is recommended.

We recently studied 248 patients randomized to either low MAP (50 to 70 mm Hg) or high MAP (80 to 100 mm Hg) during CPB and found an across-the-board improvement in combined cardiac and neurologic outcome with high MAP. However, when the TEE results from these patients were analyzed, patients at low risk for cerebral embolization (normal to mild aortic atherosclerosis) had no significant effect of MAP group on neurologic outcome. Patients at high risk (severe aortic atherosclorsis) randomized to higher MAP had a significantly lower risk of neurologic outcome. Other recent data suggest that MAP during CPB is not a primary predictor of cognitive decline or stroke following cardiac surgery. However, there was an association among hypotension (area <50 mm Hg), age, and decline in spatial and figural memory. Therefore, we recommend maintenance of high MAP during CPB in patients with increased risk of neurologic outcome such as history of CVA or TIA, hypertension, carotid stenosis, advanced age, and severe aortic atherosclerosis detected by TEE.

Feddersen K, Aren C, Nilsson NJ, Radegran K: Cerebral blood flow and metabolism during cardiopulmonary bypass with special reference to effects of hypotension induced by prostacyclin. Ann Thorac Surg 41:395, 1986

Gold JP, Charlson ME, Williams-Russo P et al: Improvement of outcomes after coronary artery bypass: A randomized trial comparing intraoperative high versus low mean arterial pressure. J Thorac Cardiovasc Surg 110:1302–1311, 1995

Govier AV, Reves JG, McKay RD et al: Factors and their influence on regional cerebral blood flow during nonpulsatile cardiopulmonary bypass. Ann Thorac Surg 38:592, 1984

Gravlee GP, Davis RF, Utley JR: Cardiopulmonary Bypass, Principles and Practice, pp 579–587. Baltimore, Williams & Wilkins, 1993

Hartman GS, Yao F, Bruefach M et al: Cardiopulmonary bypass at high pressure reduces stroke incidence in patients with TEE diagnosed severe aortic atheromatous disease. Anesthesiology 83:A141, 1995

Murkin JM, Farrar JK, Tweed A et al: Cerebral autoregulation and flow/metabolism coupling during cardiopulmonary bypass: The influence of $PaCO_2$. Anesth Analg 66:825, 1987

Newman MF, Kramer DC, Croughwell ND et al: Differential age effects of mean arterial pressure and rewarding cognitive dysfunction after cardiac surgery. Anesth Analg 81:236–242, 1995

C. II-12. How would you treat hypotension during CPB?

Mean arterial pressure = cardiac output × total peripheral resistance
   (MAP)   (CO)   (TPR)

Hypotension may be caused by low cardiac output or low peripheral resistance. First, cardiac output should be corrected by increasing the pump-flow rate. Then, if the cardiac output is adequate, peripheral resistance can be raised by giving vasopressors. We use the primarily alpha-adrenergic vasopressor phenylephrine in increments of 0.5 mg to raise the MAP to 50 mm Hg. According to Poiseuille's law, low TPR usually is due to decreased viscosity or increased vascular diameter (vasodilation). During CPB using blood-free priming solutions, total viscosity is reduced by hemodilation even though plasma viscosity is increased by hypothermia. A short period of hypotension with a MAP of approximately 30 to 40 mm Hg is usually seen in the first 5 to 10 minutes of bypass. It is due to the following causes:

- Inadequate pump flow at the beginning of bypass
- Hypoxic vasodilation from initial perfusion with blood-free primes carrying no oxygen
- Vasodilation from vasoactive materials released because of the initial reaction of the serum proteins, blood cells, and platelets with the foreign surfaces of the heart-lung machine
- Decreased plasma levels of catecholamines by hemodilution
- Infusion of cardioplegic solution, which contains nitroglycerin

Balasaraswathi K, Glisson SN, El-Etr AA et al: Effect of priming volume on serum catecholamine during cardiopulmonary bypass. Can Anaes Soc J 27:135–139, 1980

Kaplan J (ed): Cardiac Anesthesia, 3rd ed, pp 934–935. Philadelphia, WB Saunders, 1993

C. II-13. How would you treat hypertension (a mean arterial pressure of over 100 mm Hg)?

Hypertension during bypass is usually the result of inadequate depth of anesthesia, which causes increased catecholamine output and increased vascular resistance. Pump-flow rate should not be reduced to lower the pressure. Low pump flow may cause tissue hypoxia even though blood pressure is high. The most effective treatment involves administering an inhalation agent such as halothane, enflurane, or isoflurane through the vaporizer in the heart-lung machine. Intravenous agents, such as sodium thiopental, diazepam, midazolam, droperidol, and large doses of narcotics may be used, but they are frequently not effective and have to be supplemented with vasodilator drugs. One may use nitroprusside, nitroglycerin, phentolamine, or chlorpromazine.

Stanley TH, Berman L, Green O et al: Plasma catecholamine and cortisol responses to fentanyl-oxygen anesthesia for coronary-artery operations. Anesthesiology 53:250–253, 1980

Tarhan S (ed): Anesthesia and Coronary Artery Surgery, p 143. Chicago, Year Book Medical Publishers, 1986

C. II-14. How do you prepare an intravenous infusion of sodium nitroprusside, phentolamine, and nitroglycerin? What are the usual doses? Which do you prefer to use?

Intravenous solutions may be prepared by adding 10 to 20 mg of the above vasodilators to 100 ml of 5% dextrose in water to make a concentration of 100 to 200 μg/ml. The usual doses are 1 to 10 μg/kg/min determined by careful titration. We prefer nitroglycerin infusion. Sodium nitroprusside dilates both arterial and venous smooth muscle. It is very effective in reducing both preload and afterload. It may cause cyanide and thiocyanate toxicity. Because intramyocardial arteriolar vasodilation occurs, intracoronary steal may happen. The solution has to be covered with aluminum foil to prevent decomposition from exposure to light. In addition to alpha-adrenergic blockage, phentolamine has a vasodilating action on vascular smooth muscle not mediated by adrenergic receptors. It also has a beta-stimulating action and may cause arrhythmias. Nitroglycerin primarily causes venodilation, resulting in reduction of preload and myocardial oxygen consumption. At larger doses and by the intravenous route, it has mild arteriolar dilation and reduces afterload. It has no known toxicity and does not produce intracoronary steal because it dilates epicardial arteries. It may redistribute blood flow to the subendocardium and increase collateral circulation through the myocardium.

Barash PG, Cullen BF, Stoelting RK (eds): Clinical Anesthesia, 3rd ed, pp 301–302, 732. Philadelphia, Lippincott-Raven, 1997

Gerson JI, Allen FB, Seltzer JL et al: Arterial and venous dilation by nitroprusside and nitroglycerin—Is there a difference? Anesth Analg 61:256–260, 1982

C. II-15. How much pump flow would you maintain during CPB?

The pump blood flow is equivalent to cardiac output and to supply tissue oxygenation. The normal average cardiac output for adults is 70 ml/kg/min or 3.1 liters/

min/m^2. Because of higher metabolism, pediatric patients need higher flow rates for each unit of body weight. Usually 70% of normal cardiac output is enough to maintain tissue oxygenation. When body surface is used, both pediatric and adult patients require about the same pump flow, 2.2 to 3.1 liters/min/m^2. In summary, at normothermia and normal hemoglobin levels, the pump flow is as follows:

Adults   50 to 70 ml/kg/min
                      or
               2.2 to 3.1 liters/min/m^2

Children   100 to 150 ml/kg/min
                      or
               2.2 to 3.1 liters/min/m^2

However, some perfusion teams use low-flow (40 ml/kg/min), low-pressure (around 40 mm Hg) bypass quite successfully. This technique has the advantages of less bleeding through collaterals back into the heart, less trauma to blood cells and platelets, and lower fluid requirements, but it also has the potential for inadequate perfusion. Clinically, hypothermia and hemodilution are used. Therefore, pump blood flow should be adjusted accordingly to match the oxygen supply with demand.

DiNardo JA, Schwartz MJ (eds): Anesthesia for Cardiac Surgery, p 231. Norwalk, CT, Appleton & Lange, 1990

Gravlee GP, Davis RF, Utley JR: Cardiopulmonary Bypass, Principles and Practice, pp 565–566. Baltimore, Williams & Wilkins, 1993

Kolkka R, Hilberman M: Neurological dysfunction following cardiac operation with low flow, low pressure cardiopulmonary bypass. J Thorac Cardiovasc Surg 79:432–437, 1980

Lake CL: Cardiovascular Anesthesia, pp 321–322. New York, Springer-Verlag, 1985

Pierce C II: Extracorporeal Circulation for Open-Heart Surgery, pp 6–8. Springfield, Charles C Thomas, 1969

C. II-16. *How would you adjust the pump flow during hypothermia?*

Hypothermia decreases oxygen consumption. Therefore, the pump flow may be decreased proportionally if the blood oxygen content does not change. The oxygen consumptions at different body temperatures are listed below.

Temperature	°C	37	32	30	28	25	20	10
Oxygen consumption	%	100	60	50	40	25–30	20	10

The pump flow at 30°C is 50% of the flow at 37°C (50 to 70 ml/kg/min). Therefore, a pump flow of 25 to 35 ml/kg/min is adequate for adults at 30°C without hemodilution. During profound hypothermia (10° to 20°C) the patients usually can tolerate total circulatory arrest without pump support for about 60 to 90 minutes. The decrease in metabolism during hypothermia is not a linear process. From 37°C to 30°C, the metabolism decreases about 7% by each degree centigrade. Below 30°C decrease in metabolism slows down. Usually every 7° to 8°C decrease in temperature reduces oxygen consumption by 50%. Clinically, it has been demonstrated that pump flows as low as 30 ml/kg/min or 1.2 liters/min/m^2 will not compromise whole-body oxygen delivery when moderate systemic hypothermia is employed.

Blair E: Clinical Hypothermia, p 88. New York, McGraw-Hill, 1964

Hickey RF, Hoar PF: Whole-body oxygen consumption during low flow hypothermic cardiopulmonary bypass. J Thorac Cardiovasc Surg 86:903–906, 1983

C. II-17. How would you adjust the pump flow during hemodilution?

Oxygen delivery = cardiac output × arterial oxygen content

Arterial oxygen content = 1.34 × Hb × O_2 saturation + 0.003 × PaO_2

Hemodilution reduces hemoglobin concentration and hence decreases oxygen content. In order to deliver the same amount of oxygen, the pump flow has to be increased accordingly during hemodilution. For example, if the hematocrit is diluted from 40% to 20% during CPB, the pump flow has to be increased by the factor 40/20. Clinically, both hypothermia and hemodilution are applied simultaneously, so that the adjustment has to be done at the same time. For example, the pump flow for adults at a temperature of 30°C and a hematocrit of 25% will be as follows:

50 to 70 ml/kg/min × 50% × 40/25 = 40 to 56 ml/kg/min

C. II-18. What are the advantages of hypothermia? Does hypothermia offer neuroprotection?

Hypothermia decreases oxygen consumption and helps to preserve tissue function during hypoxic or ischemic insult. Pump flow may be decreased during CPB with hypothermia.

Hypothermia has been shown to confer significant protection in the setting of transient, but not permanent, ischemia. The mechanism is unclear at this time. Reduction in cerebral metabolic rate is believed to be less important compared with the effect of hypothermia on the release of excitatory neurotransmitters, catecholamines, or other mediators of cellular injury. It is for this reason that mild hypothermia (33° to 35°C) provides significant neuroprotection.

The effect of hypothermia during CPB on postoperative cognitive or neurologic function remains controversial. Animal models show profound reduction in infarct size and release of excitatory amino acid with minimal levels of hypothermia. However, clinical studies comparing normothermic and moderately hypothermic CPB have yielded conflicting stroke results and no evidence of protection from cognitive decline. This may relate to differences in normothermia. Many groups allow temperature to drift during normothermic CPB with temperature reaching 34°C or below. Mclean in a recent study of this type showed no difference in cognitive or neurologic outcome between warm and moderately hypothermic groups. In actuality, this is a study of mild versus moderate hypothermia confirming the experimental animal data that as little as 2° to 3°C of hypothermia markedly reduces excitatory amino acid release and neurologic injury compared to normothermia. The single large study comparing true normothermia with hypothermia during CPB showed a significantly greater incidence of focal neurologic injury in the warm group, supporting the role of hypothermia in neuroprotection. In addition, recent data showed that minimum CPB temperatures >35°C increased the incidence of perioperative stroke approximately fourfold (4.5% vs. 1.2%).

Gravlee GP, Davis RF, Utley JR: Cardiopulmonary Bypass, Principles and Practice, pp 150, 556–557. Baltimore, Williams & Wilkins, 1993

Mclean RF, Wong BI: Normothermic versus hypothermic cardiopulmonary bypass: Central nervous system outcomes. J Cardiothoracic Vasc Anesth 10:45–53, 1996

C. II-19. How does blood viscosity change during hypothermia and hemodilution?

Blood viscosity varies inversely with temperature; a 2% increase occurs for every 1°C decrease in temperature. With a hematocrit of 40%, a decrease in temperature from 37° to 27°C increases viscosity by approximately 25%. Hemodilution with balanced salt solution will decrease blood viscosity. Decreasing the hematocrit from 40% to 20% at 27°C decreases viscosity by approximately 40%. It has been recommended that the hematocrit be adjusted to the same numerical value as the core body temperature in °C if blood viscosity is to be kept approximately constant.

DiNardo JA, Schwartz MJ (eds): Anesthesia for Cardiac Surgery, p 226. Norwalk, CT, Appleton & Lange, 1990

Gravlee GP, Davis RF, Utley JR: Cardiopulmonary Bypass, Principles and Practice, p 127. Baltimore, Williams & Wilkins, 1993

C. II-20. What are the main causes of death associated with accidental hypothermia?

Ventricular fibrillation and asystole are the major rhythm disturbances leading to cardiac arrest in hypothermia. In humans externally cooled for cardiac surgery, ventricular fibrillation generally occurs at 23°C and asystole at 20°C. However, asystole and ventricular fibrillation have been reported at 21° to 28°C. Respiratory arrest usually accompanies cardiac arrest during accidental hypothermia.

Southwick FS, Dalglish PH: Recovery after prolonged asystolic cardiac arrest in profound hypothermia. JAMA 243:1250–1253, 1980

C. II-21. Would you give anesthesia during CPB? Why?

Yes. Anesthesia is maintained with intermittent administration of intravenous barbiturates or benzodiazepines, narcotic or inhalation agents to achieve unconsciousness and analgesia, to control blood pressure, and to prevent shivering. Intravenous agents are diluted by the priming solution during CPB. Meanwhile, hypothermia itself produces anesthesia and prolongs the action duration of intravenous agents by decreasing hepatic metabolism and urinary excretion. I prefer the use of thiopental to keep the patient unconscious because it has been demonstrated that thiopental in sufficient doses can reduce neuropsychiatric complications after cardiopulmonary bypass. However, Zaiden and associates recently found no evidence of neurologic benefit with similarly administered thiopental infusion in patients undergoing CABG with hypothermia and filtered membrane oxygenators. Moreover, Nussmeier in her recent study reported that subclinical neuropsychologic dysfunction was not mitigated by thiopental. Thus, barbiturates may be of benefit for temporary focal lesions (gas emboli from bypass pump or open chamber) if metabolic suppression is not being achieved by hypothermia.

DiNardo JA, Schwartz MJ (eds): Anesthesia for Cardiac Surgery, pp 236–237. Norwalk, CT, Appleton & Lange, 1990

Gravlee GP, Davis RF, Utley JR: Cardiopulmonary Bypass, Principles and Practice, pp 600–601. Baltimore, Williams & Wilkins, 1993

Nussmeier NA, Arland C, Slogoff S: Neuropsychiatric complications after cardiopulmonary bypass: Cerebral protection by a barbiturate. Anesthesiology 64:165–170, 1986

Nussmeier NA, Fish KJ: Neuropsychological dysfunction after cardiopulmonary bypass: A comparison of two institutions. J Cardiothorac Vasc Anesth 5:584–588, 1991

Zaiden JR, Klochany A, Martin WM et al: Effect of thiopental on neurologic outcome following coronary artery bypass grafting. Anesthesiology 74:406–411, 1991

C. II-22. Would you give muscle relaxants during CPB? How is the action of muscle relaxant affected during CPB?

Yes. Muscle relaxants are given to prevent diaphragmatic movement that interferes with surgery and to prevent shivering during hypothermia. Shivering may increase oxygen consumption to as high as 486% of normal. The effect of a muscle relaxant is altered by both hypothermia and hemodilution. The plasma concentration of muscle relaxants is diluted by the priming solution. Therefore, more relaxant is required to maintain the same degree of relaxation. Hypothermia was originally reported to decrease the effect of nondepolarizing relaxants, because decreased cholinesterase enzyme activity during hypothermia resulted in more acetylcholine accumulation to compete with the nondepolarizing relaxant. Contrary to the earlier reports, it is now established that less *d*-tubocurarine, atracurium, vecuronium, or pancuronium is needed to maintain muscle relaxation during hypothermia because hypothermia reduces renal and biliary excretions of both *d*-tubocurarine and pancuronium. Ham and associates reported that hypothermia in man does not affect *d*-tubocurarine pharmacokinetics or the sensitivity of the neuromuscular junction to *d*-tubocurarine. Hypothermia does prolong the onset of paralysis. Moreover, hypothermic cardiopulmonary bypass *per se* facilitates neuromuscular transmission at the electrochemical level, yet compromises mechanical contractility. Modifications of partial neuromuscular blockade by hypothermic bypass are the result of muscle relaxation enhancing or interfering with the impact of hypothermia on normal neuromuscular transmission. The best way to monitor muscle relaxation is by using a peripheral nerve stimulator.

Buzello W, Pollmaecher T, Schluermann D et al: The influence of hypothermia cardiopulmonary bypass on neuromuscular transmission in the absence of muscle relaxants. Anesthesiology 4:279–281, 1986

Buzello W, Schluermann D, Schindler M et al: Hyperthermic cardiopulmonary bypass and neuromuscular blockade by pancuronium and vecuronium. Anesthesiology 62:201–204, 1985

DiNardo JA, Schwartz MJ (eds): Anesthesia for Cardiac Surgery, pp 230–231. Norwalk, CT, Appleton & Lange, 1990

Gravlee GP, Davis RF, Utley JR: Cardiopulmonary Bypass, Principles and Practice, pp 212, 216. Baltimore, Williams & Wilkins, 1993

Ham J, Stanski DR, Newfield P et al: Pharmacokinetics and dynamics of *d*-tubocurarine during hypothermia in humans. Anesthesiology 55:631–635, 1981

C. II-23. How do you know the patient is well perfused during CPB?

If the perfusion pressure is maintained between 50 mm Hg and 100 mm Hg, and the pump-flow rate is adequately maintained according to the degree of hypothermia and hemodilution, there should be adequate urine output, >1 ml/kg/h, no metabolic acidosis, and normal mixed venous oxygen tension of 40 to 45 mm Hg.

Kaplan J (ed): Cardiac Anesthesia, 3rd ed, pp 905–906. New York, Grune & Stratton, 1993

C. II-24. How much gas flow would you use for the oxygenator? What kind of gas would you use? Why?

Normal alveolar ventilation is 4 liters/min and pulmonary circulation is 5 liters/min. The $\dot{V}/\dot{Q}$ ratio is 0.8. The oxygenator is not as efficient as human lungs. We usually start with 2 liters of gas for each liter of pump-flow rate, and then adjust the gas-flow rate according to blood $PaCO_2$ and PaO_2. The gas flow may be decreased if the $PaCO_2$ is low and the PaO_2 is too high. The ratio may be increased if the $PaCO_2$ is over 40 mm Hg or the PaO_2 is under 100 mm Hg. In the past we used a mixture of 99% oxygen and 1% carbon dioxide for the bubble oxygenator. Because of low CO_2 production during hypothermia, high CO_2 elimination from high gas flow, and high CO_2 diffusion capacity, 1% CO_2 was added to oxygen to prevent severe hypocapnia. Since membrane oxygenators are used routinely, oxygen-air mixtures rather than 100% oxygen have been used. In a bubble oxygenator bubbles containing nitrogen may be slowly absorbed into the systemic circulation, increasing the risk of gaseous microemboli. In a membrane oxygenator this risk does not exist. Meanwhile, air-oxygen mixtures allow better control of oxygen tension during CPB. Since we use alpha-stat regulation for acid-base management, it is not necessary to add CO_2 to the ventilating gas during hypothermia to elevate PCO_2 and decrease the pH.

DiNardo JA, Schwartz MJ (eds): Anesthesia for Cardiac Surgery, pp 223, 232. Norwalk, CT, Appleton & Lange, 1990

C. II-25. What are the disadvantages of low $PaCO_2$ during CPB?

- Cerebral blood flow decreases about 2% to 4% for each mm Hg decrease in $PaCO_2$ when $PaCO_2$ is in the range of 20 mm Hg to 60 mm Hg due to cerebral vasoconstriction.
- Respiratory alkalosis shifts the oxygen dissociation curve to the left, which increases the O_2 affinity to hemoglobin and decreases O_2 release to the tissues.
- Hypokalemia occurs because of the intracellular shift of potassium during alkalosis.
- Alkalosis decreases ionized calcium.

Smith AL, Wollman H: Cerebral blood flow and metabolism: Effects of anesthetic drugs and techniques. Anesthesiology 36:378–400, 1972

C. II-26. The arterial blood gases and electrolytes during CPB are pH, 7.36; $PaCO_2$, 42 mm Hg; PaO_2, 449 mm Hg; CO_2 content, 24 mEq/liter; Na, 128 mEq/liter; K, 5.8 mEq/liter; Ht, 20%. The patient's temperature is 27°C. At what temperature are blood gases measured? How would you correct the blood gases according to patient's body temperature? Would you treat the arterial blood gases at 37°C or at patient's body temperature?

Blood gases are measured at a constant temperature of 37°C. They may be corrected according to body temperature. Each degree centigrade below 37°C increases blood pH by 0.015. If pH is 7.40 at 37°C *in vitro, in vivo* pH will be 7.55 at 27°C body temperature [7.40 + 0.015 × (37 − 27) = 7.55]. The pH increases at lower temperatures,

Table 7-2. Different Hypothermic Acid-Base Regulatory Strategies

STRATEGY	AIM	TOTAL CO$_2$ CONTENT	pH AND PaCO$_2$ MAINTENANCE	INTRACELLULAR STATE	ALPHA-IMIDAZOLE AND BUFFERING	ENZYME STRUCTURE AND FUNCTION	CEREBRAL BLOOD FLOW AND COUPLING	EFFECT ON ISCHEMIC TISSUE
pH-stat	Constant pH	Increases	Normal corrected values	Acidotic (excess H$^+$)	Excess (+) charge Buffering decreased	Altered and activity decreased	Flow close to normothermic ? Flow and metabolism uncoupled	? Lessens hypothermic protection
Alpha-stat	Constant OH$^-$/H$^+$	Constant	Normal uncorrected values	Neutral (H$^-$ = OH$^-$)	Constant net charge Buffering constant	Normal and activity maximal	Flow decreases (appropriate) ? Flow and metabolism coupled	? Allows full hypothermic protection

Reprinted with permission from Tinker JH (ed): Cardiopulmonary Bypass: Current Concepts and Controversies, p 16. Philadelphia, JB Lippincott, 1989.

because of increased Pka and decreased CO_2 tension from increased CO_2 blood solubility during hypothermia. *In vivo* PaO_2 is decreased because of increased oxygen solubility during hypothermia. At the New York Hospital–Cornell Medical Center, we measure blood gases at 37°C and interpret at 37°C without correcting them to body temperature. The normal values of blood gases at 37°C are pH 7.40 ± 0.05, $PaCO_2$ 40 ± 5, PaO2 95 ± 5; we should compare the blood gases at 37°C. During hypothermia, the normal values of blood gases are not the same as those at 37°C. The same blood specimen has different PO_2 values when measured at different temperatures. Yet, the oxygen content remains unchanged. It is easier to calculate the oxygen content at 37°C than at other temperatures where oxygen dissociation curves are shifted.

Optimal management of pH and $PaCO_2$ for patients undergoing hypothermic CPB remains controversial. The two strategies for interpreting blood gases are the pH-stat (temperature-corrected) method and the alpha-stat (temperature-uncorrected) method. The pH-stat strategy aims at keeping constant arterial pH at 7.40 and $PaCO_2$ at 40 mm Hg at any given temperature. A $PaCO_2$ of 60 mm Hg analyzed at 37°C would be equivalent to a $PaCO_2$ of 40 mm Hg if "corrected" for a body temperature of 27°C. The alpha-stat strategy aims at keeping a constant ratio of $[OH^-]:[H^+]$ at about 16:1. This is based on the premise that the pH of blood is regulated to keep the stage of dissociation of imidazole moiety (i.e., the alpha of imidazole) constant. Histidine, which contains the imidazole moiety, is an integral part of the active site of many enzyme systems. The function of enzyme systems has been shown to be optimal when the ratio of $[OH^-]:[H^+]$ is about 16:1. This ratio represents different pH values at different temperatures.

The differences between pH-stat and alpha-stat strategies are listed in Table 7-2. With the pH-stat strategy, the blood gas values are corrected to the patient's temperature; the patient is treated as if he were a hibernating animal. With the alpha-stat strategy, the blood gas values are not corrected regardless of the patient's actual temperature; the patient is treated as if he were a poikilotherm. Studies indicate that myocardial function is better preserved when the alpha-stat strategy is employed. Moreover, maintenance of cerebral blood flow autoregulation appears to remain intact with alpha-stat management, whereas flow becomes pressure dependent with pH-stat management. Therefore, most medical centers use alpha-stat management of blood gases during hypothermic CPB. However, Bashein et al found no difference in neuropsychologic outcome between patients randomized to alpha-stat or pH-stat management.

However, more recent studies have shown less decline in cognitive performance when alpha-stat management is used, especially in cases with prolonged CPB times. This data may support an embolic threshold above which recognizable neurologic injury occurs.

During deep hypothermia cardiac arrest (DHCA) both animal and clinical studies have shown that pH-stat is associated with better neurologic outcome probably because of increased cerebral blood flow which provides better brain cooling and greater cellular oxygen availability. In summary, the majority of recent outcome studies support the utilization of alpha-stat for adult CPB and pH-stat for children under deep hypothermia cardiac arrest.

Bashein G, Townes BD, Nessly ML et al: A randomized study of carbon dioxide management during hypothermic cardiopulmonary bypass. Anesthesiology 72:7–15, 1990

Jonas RA: Hypothermia, circulatory arrest and the paediatric brain. J Cardiothorac Vasc Anesth 10:6–74, 1996

Murkin JM, Farrar JK, Tweed WA et al: Cerebral autoregulation and flow/metabolism coupling during cardiopulmonary bypass: The influence of $PaCO_2$. Anesth Analg 66:825–832, 1987

Murkin JM, MartzKejs, Buchan AM et al: A randomized study of the influence of perfusion technique and pH management strategy in 316 patients undergoing coronary artery bypass surgery. II. Neurologic and cognitive outcomes. J Thorac Cardiovasc Surg 110:349–362, 1995

O'Dwyer C, Prough DS, Johnston WE: Determinants of cerebral perfusion during cardiopulmonary bypass. J Cardiothorac Vasc Anesth 10:54–65, 1996

Prough DS, Rogers AT, Johnston WE: Cardiopulmonary bypass and the brain. International Anesthesia Research Society Review Course Lectures, pp 6–14, 1992

Prough DS, Stump DA, Roy RC et al: Response of cerebral blood flow to phenylephrine infusion during hypothermic cardiopulmonary bypass: Influence of $PaCO_2$. Anesthesiology 64:576–581, 1986

Tallman RD: Acid-base regulation, alpha-stat, and the emperor's new clothes. J Cardiothorac Vasc Anesth 11:282–288, 1997

C. II-27. If the blood level of the oxygenator is low, what would you replace it with? Blood or balanced salt solution?

We try to maintain a hematocrit of at least 18% to 20% during hemodilution. If the hematocrit is below 18% to 20%, blood is given to the oxygenator. If the hematocrit is above 20%, normosol is given to the oxygenator. However, hematocrit values in the range of 15% to 18% appear to be well tolerated clinically.

Gravlee GP, Davis RF, Utley JR: Cardiopulmonary Bypass, Principles and Practice, pp 132–133. Baltimore, Williams & Wilkins, 1993

Hensley FA Jr, Martin DE (eds): The Practice of Cardiac Anesthesia, pp 245–246. Boston, Little, Brown, 1990

C. II-28. How do you know the fluid balance during CPB?

During CPB, all intravenous lines are shut off. The intake includes cardioplegic solution, fluid or blood added to the oxygenator during CPB, and the decreased blood level in the oxygenator. The output includes urine and the increased blood level in the oxygenator.

C. II-29. How would you preserve the myocardium during CPB?

The most popular and effective method of protecting the myocardium is to reduce myocardial oxygen demand by hypothermia and cardioplegia. Hypothermia is induced by a combination of systemic blood cooling by heat exchangers in the oxygenator, local application of cold saline solution or iced slush to the external surface and chambers of the heart (if the heart is open), and infusion of cold cardioplegic solution through the aortic root, venous grafts, retrograde coronary sinus, or coronary ostium to the coronary arterial tree. The myocardial temperature may be decreased to 10° to 15°C.

In addition to inducing hypothermia and cardioplegia, one may take the following measures prior to aortic cross-clamping:

- Avoid tachycardia or increased contractility by discontinuing pacing at rapid rate and discontinuing inotropes if they were utilized.

- Utilize proper venting methods and ensure adequate venous drainage to the pump to avoid ventricular distention, which decreases subendocardial blood supply.
- Prevent and treat ventricular fibrillation, which increases oxygen demand in normothermic myocardium.
- Maintain adequate coronary perfusion pressure of at least 50 mm Hg and >70 mm Hg in the presence of severe coronary disease or left ventricular hypertrophy.

Gravlee GP, Davis RF, Utley JR: Cardiopulmonary Bypass, Principles and Practice, pp 170–206. Baltimore, Williams & Wilkins, 1993

Hensley FA Jr, Martin DE (eds): The Practice of Cardiac Anesthesia, pp 629–632. Boston, Little, Brown, 1990

Jynge P, Hearse DJ, Brainbridge MV: Myocardial protection during ischemic cardiac arrest. J Thorac Cardiovasc Surg 73:848, 1977

C. II-30. What is the cardioplegic solution? How much would you use?

Cardioplegic solution contains mainly high concentrations of potassium (10 to 30 mEq/liter) or magnesium (160 mEq/liter) to relax the heart. Flaccid cardioplegia itself reduces myocardial oxygen consumption and provides optimal conditions for surgery. Bicarbonate or THAM is usually added to raise the *p*H to levels between 7.40 and 7.80 to increase the intracellular shift of potassium and to decrease the metabolic acidosis from ischemia. Steroids, calcium, and procaine may be added to stabilize lysosomal and cell membranes. Glucose and insulin are added to provide energy and improve the intracellular shift of potassium. Nitroglycerin is added to dilate coronary vessels, resulting in better perfusion to the myocardium, including ischemic areas. At the New York Hospital–Cornell Medical Center, for crystalloid cardioplegia we add 20 mEq of potassium chloride and 10 mEq of sodium bicarbonate to 1000 ml of 5% glucose in a 0.225% salt solution, resulting in a final *p*H of 7.83, potassium of 20 mEq/liter, and osmolarity of 380 mOsm/liter.

When blood cardioplegia is used, four parts of bypass blood are mixed with one part of cardioplegic solution. The composition of full-strength solution is as follows: 500 ml of 5% glucose in a 0.225% salt solution, 70 mEq of potassium chloride, 10 mEq of sodium bicarbonate, and 1 mg of nitroglycerin. Blood cardioplegia seems to have several advantages over crystalloid cardioplegia. The heart is arrested while being oxygenated, so that ATP is not depleted before asystole. Repeated infusions provide a source of oxygen and glucose for continued metabolism and ATP repletion. Although little oxygen is released from hemoglobin during hypothermia, enough is probably dissolved in the plasma to sustain metabolism when reinfusion is performed every 30 minutes. Buffering capacity is improved because of the presence of the histidine buffering system present in red cells. Myocardial edema is reduced because of the onconicity of blood. The risk of calcium paradox following ischemia is reduced and functional recovery is improved because of the physiologic calcium concentration provided by blood. The presence of red cell enzyme catalase may scavenge free radicals produced by ischemia. Capillary perfusion is improved and more homogeneous because of the presence of red cells. However, results of clinical studies in which blood cardioplegia was compared with crystalloid cardioplegia either detected no significant difference or showed that blood cardioplegia improved contractility late in the postoperative course. Multiple-dose cardioplegia is required for satisfactory results, whereas single-dose blood cardioplegia results in poor ventricular function.

Intermittent, continuous, or single infusions of cardioplegic solution have been used. Usually 300 to 600 ml of cold cardioplegic solution is needed to paralyze the myocardium and cool the myocardium to 10° to 20°C.

In the case of severe obstructive coronary lesions, antigrade infusion into the aortic root may cause maldistribution of the cardioplegia. Therefore, retrograde infusion through the coronary sinus into the coronary veins may be added to ensure homogeneous distribution of cardioplegia.

In the late 1980s and early 1990s warm cardioplegia with near-systemic normothermia was popular for better myocardial protection. However, one study identified a threefold increase in strokes in the "warm" patients. The technique is no longer popular.

Gravlee GP, Davis RF, Utley JR: Cardiopulmonary Bypass, Principles and Practice, pp 170–191. Baltimore, Williams & Wilkins, 1993

Mclean RF, Wong BI: Normothermic versus hypothermic cardiopulmonary bypass: Central nervous system outcomes. J Cardiothorac Vasc Anesth 10:45–53, 1996

Rao RL, Magovern GJ: Prevention of reperfusional drainage from ischemic myocardium. J Thorac Cardiovasc Surg 91:106–114, 1986

Shapiro N, Kirsh M, Jochim K et al: Comparison of the effect of blood cardioplegia to crystalloid cardioplegia on myocardial contractility in man. J Thorac Cardiovasc Surg 80:647, 1980

C. II-31. For how long a period can the aorta be cross-clamped?

With myocardial hypothermia at 10° to 20°C and cardioplegia, the aorta may be cross-clamped for 60 to 120 minutes without coronary perfusion. The shorter the cross-clamping time is, the better the myocardial function will be. If the cross-clamp time is expected to be prolonged, myocardial hypothermia should be maintained and coronary perfusion through a separate pump should be considered.

Follette D, Fey K, Mulder D et al: Prolonged safe aortic clamping by combining stabilization, multidose cardioplegia, appropriate pH reperfusion. J Thorac Cardiovasc Surg 74:682–694, 1977

C. II-32. Why does urine become pink after 2 hours of CPB? What is the renal threshold for plasma hemoglobin?

Pink urine is a sign of massive hemolysis. Hemolysis is mainly associated with the frothing, violent turbulence, acceleration, and shear forces of negative pressures generated by the suction apparatus and is associated only to a lesser degree with the action of the pumps or with the gas-blood interface effects in the oxygenator. The renal threshold for hemoglobin is 100 to 150 mg/100 ml. It is advisable to maintain a high output of alkaline urine to prevent possible tubular damage from acid hematin crystals, which are converted from hemoglobin.

Gravlee GP, Davis RF, Utley JR: Cardiopulmonary Bypass, Principles and Practice, pp 47, 234. Baltimore, Williams & Wilkins, 1993

Lake CL: Cardiovascular Anesthesia, p 323. New York, Springer-Verlag, 1985

C. II-33. At what temperature can the patient be weaned from CPB?

An esophageal or nasopharyngeal temperature of 37°C and a rectal or bladder temperature at least 35°C must be reached before the patient can come off the pump. After discontinuation of the pump, surface warming should be continued in pediatric patients to prevent hypothermia owing to redistribution of heat in the body. However, in adults the use of warming blankets and warmed humidified airway gases has not been found beneficial in preventing the expected temperature "afterdrop." Usually, esophageal or nasopharyngeal temperature will decrease and rectal or bladder temperature will increase during heat redistribution.

DiNardo JA, Schwartz MJ (eds): Anesthesia for Cardiac Surgery, p 236. Norwalk, CT, Appleton & Lange, 1990

Gravlee GP, Davis RF, Utley JR: Cardiopulmonary Bypass, Principles and Practice, pp 760–761. Baltimore, Williams & Wilkins, 1993

C. II-34. Why does it take longer to rewarm than to cool the patient by the pump oxygenator?

It usually takes 5 to 10 minutes to cool the patient from 37° to 25°C of average body temperature. It takes 20 to 40 minutes to rewarm the patient from 28° to 35°C. The speed of heat exchange by the bloodstream depends on the temperature gradient between venous blood and water in the heat exchanger, the pump blood-flow rate, and the waterflow rate of the heat exchanger. The initial venous blood temperature is 37°C and the water temperature of the heat exchanger is 0° to 4°C during cooling. The temperature gradient is 34° to 37°C. During rewarming, the water temperature is limited to 42°C or less to prevent denaturation and destruction of blood. The temperature gradient is limited to 10°C or less to prevent gas embolism owing to too much of a decrease in gas solubility in the blood with a sharp increase in temperature. The heat exchanger water flow does not differ much during cooling and rewarming. However, the pump blood flow is usually maintained to a very high level during the initial cooling because of low blood pressure in the beginning of cooling. During rewarming, the pump blood flow is frequently maintained at a low level because the blood pressure is usually high and the body temperature is still low. Rewarming may be speeded up by administering inhalation anesthetics or employing vasodilators to decrease vascular resistance and thereby increase pump flow to maintain the same blood pressure. Because the increased vascular resistance is usually due to inadequate anesthesia during rewarming, we prefer inhalation anesthetics to vasodilators in patients with good ventricular function. In cases of poor ventricular function, inhalation agents are avoided because of the potential cardiac depression after CPB.

DiNardo JA, Schwartz MJ (eds): Anesthesia for Cardiac Surgery, p 236. Norwalk, CT, Appleton & Lange, 1990

Gravlee GP, Davis RF, Utley JR: Cardiopulmonary Bypass, Principles and Practice, pp 45, 760–761. Baltimore, Williams & Wilkins, 1993

Stanley TH, Berman L, Green O et al: Plasma catecholamine and cortisol responses to fentanyl-oxygen anesthesia for coronary artery operations. Anesthesiology 53:250–253, 1980

C. II-35. How would you defibrillate the heart internally during CPB?

The heart is defibrillated internally by a DC defibrillator, usually 5 to 10 watt-seconds. If the heart remains in ventricular fibrillation, blood gases, electrolytes, and temperature are rechecked and lidocaine, 1 to 2 mg/kg, is administered before DC defibrillation. Rarely, propranolol and bretylium are added to treat intractable ventricular fibrillation or tachycardia.

Kaplan J (ed): Cardiac Anesthesia, 3rd ed, p 940. Philadelphia, WB Saunders, 1993

C. II-36. Why is calcium chloride usually administered right before the patient comes off the pump?

With hemodilution, the ionized calcium frequently falls to about 1.5 mEq/liter (normal 1.9 to 2.2 mEq/liter or 4.5 to 5.6 mg/dl). Calcium chloride, 0.5 to 1.0 g, is frequently given to increase myocardial contractility and reverse potassium cardioplegia. Calcium increases the inotropic state of the myocardium and induces an increase in systemic vascular resistance that outlasts the inotropic effects. However, some believe that calcium administration is contraindicated at this time because of the compromised calcium hemostasis that accompanies the insult of aortic cross-clamping. Administration of calcium may exacerbate ischemic and reperfusion injury by causing accumulation of intracellular calcium. Beta-blockers, on the other hand, increase intracellular calcium but also promote its reuptake into the sarcoplasmic reticulum and may be more appropriate in this setting. Therefore, use of calcium salts at the conclusion of bypass should be guided by determination of ionized calcium levels. Calcium salts should probably not be given to patients with good ventricular function in the absence of hypocalcemia or hyperkalemia because of the potential detrimental effects of iatrogenic hypercalcemia; whether this is true in patients with ventricular dysfunction is unknown.

DiNardo JA, Schwartz MJ (eds): Anesthesia for Cardiac Surgery, p 240. Norwalk, CT, Appleton & Lange, 1990

Gravlee GP, Davis RF, Utley JR: Cardiopulmonary Bypass, Principles and Practice, pp 525–526, 781. Baltimore, Williams & Wilkins, 1993

C. II-37. If the heart rate is 40/min, what should you do?

Atropine may be administered to treat sinus or nodal bradycardia. Frequently, temporary AV block is found at the end of bypass because of potassium cardioplegia and ischemic insult during aortic cross-clamping. A temporary epicardial pacemaker may be needed if atropine is not effective. Atrial pacing is preferred because of better cardiac output with atrial kick. Ventricular pacing is necessary if there is complete AV block. AV sequential pacing is indicated when ventricular pacing does not provide adequate cardiac output.

Kaplan J (ed): Cardiac Anesthesia, 3rd ed, pp 879–880. New York, Grune & Stratton, 1993

C. II-38. How does the blood sugar level change during CPB? Why? Does hyperglycemia increase neurologic complications during CPB?

Blood sugar levels are elevated during perfusion, possibly indicating a defect in glucose utilization owing to catecholamine inhibition of insulin secretion, or to the direct effect of catecholamine on the catabolism of glycogen to blood glucose. Catecholamines are markedly elevated during bypass.

It is controversial as to whether hyperglycemia increases neurologic complications during CPB. Under conditions of limited cerebral oxygen delivery, anaerobic glucose oxidation becomes the primary method of ATP production, resulting in intracellular lactic acidosis. Hyperglycemia, by providing more glucose for anaerobic oxidation, increases the degree of intracellular acidosis which, in numerous animal studies, correlates with the severity of subsequent injury. Although the deleterious effect of hyperglycemia in the face of both global and focal cerebral ischemia is generally accepted, a recent human study challenges these conclusions. Metz and Keats reported zero neurologic injury in a group of 54 patients undergoing CABG managed with glucose-containing fluids (glucose during bypass—approximately 700 ± 100 mg/dl) versus 1 stroke and 1 case of encephalopathy in 53 patients in whom glucose was avoided during CABG (glucose during bypass—approximately 200 ± 100 mg/dl). The authors contend that glucose does not affect neurologic outcome in the presence of a permanent focal lesion. Although provocative, this study can be faulted for (1) its lack of sensitive monitors of neurologic outcome and (2) its small sample size in relation to the occurrence rate of the event of interest. At the present time, avoidance of hyperglycemia during periods of potential neurologic injury (such as bypass) still appears prudent, although neurologic benefit is by no means proven.

Hindman B: Con: Glucose primary solutions should not be used for cardiopulmonary bypass. J Cardiothorac Vasc Anesth 9:605–606, 1995

Lanier WL: Glucose management during cardiopulmonary bypass: Cardiovascular and neurologic implications. Anesth Analg 72:423–427, 1991

Metz S: Pro: Glucose priming solution should be used for cardiopulmonary bypass. J Cardiothorac Vasc Anesth 9:603–604, 1995

Metz S, Keats AS: Benefits of a glucose-containing priming solution for cardiopulmonary bypass. Anesth Analg 72:428–434, 1991

O'Dwyer C, Prough DS, Johnston WE: Determinants of cerebral perfusion during cardiopulmonary bypass. J Cardiothorac Vasc Anesth 10:54–65, 1996

Stanley TH, Berman L, Green O et al: Plasma catecholamine and cortisol responses to fentanyl-oxygen anesthesia for coronary-artery operations. Anesthesiology 53:250–253, 1980

Wass CT, Lanier WL: Glucose modulation of ischemic brain injury: Review and clinical recommendations. Mayo Clin Proc 71:801–812, 1996

C. II-39. What are the effects of CPB on platelet and coagulation factors?

Platelet dysfunction and thrombocytopenia are found on and after CPB. Platelet dysfunction is the most common cause of a bleeding problem following CPB after heparin is reversed and surgical bleeding is controlled. Transient defects in platelet plug formation and aggregation are seen in all patients put on CPB. Generally, platelet function returns to near normal status 2 to 4 hours following CPB. The defects are exacerbated and prolonged by drugs such as aspirin and persantine, which inhibit platelet function.

Platelet counts fall more with the bubble-type oxygenator than with the membrane-type oxygenator, but rarely below the levels clinically required for hemostasis. Thrombocytopenia is mainly caused by hemodilution, aggregation, adhesion, and the

ADP-release reaction induced by the foreign surfaces and the blood-gas interface. Heparin may potentiate platelet aggregation and adhesions. The level of coagulation factors decreases at the beginning of bypass because of hemodilution; surface absorption by the plastic, glass, and metal; and protein denaturation induced by the blood-gas interface. At the same time, the synthesis of clotting factors by the liver increases so that the concentration of clotting factors returns to normal within a period of hours. Membrane oxygenators cause few changes in clotting factors.

Gravlee GP, Davis RF, Utley JR: Cardiopulmonary Bypass, Principles and Practice, pp 416–430, 450–451. Baltimore, Williams & Wilkins, 1993

C. III. After Cardiopulmonary Bypass

C. III-1. How would you reverse heparin? How much protamine would you use?

It has been recommended that 1.1 to 1.3 mg of protamine sulfate is needed to reverse each 100 units of remaining heparin calculated by ACT dose-response curve or protamine titration test. At the New York Hospital–Cornell Medical Center, we give 1.0 mg of protamine to reverse each 100 units or 1 mg of heparin initially administered. Only the initial dose of heparin is counted. The subsequently added dose of heparin, to keep the ACT level above 480 seconds, is not considered because of its metabolism and elimination. The ACT test is repeated 20 minutes after the administration of protamine. ACT usually returns to its control level. If the ACT is still prolonged, additional protamine is given according to the ACT dose-response curve. However, the ACT is affected by dilution and by hypothermia; dose-response curves utilizing data obtained during hypothermia may be misleading. In addition, severe thrombocytopenia also prolongs the ACT because clot formation using the ACT depends on platelet phospholipid. Furthermore, because heparin rebound is possible, it may be optimal to administer protamine at two times following CPB: once after bypass and again 1 or 2 hours later to prevent heparin rebound.

Other drugs that have been used to neutralize heparin include platelet factor 4 (PF4), polybrene, and toluidine blue. Human or recombinant PF4 has been used in animals and humans to reverse heparin and does not cause systemic arterial hypotension, or pulmonary hypertension, or changes in white blood cell count, platelet count, or complement levels. Polybrene, also known as hexadimethrine bromide, at one time was commonly used, but it was withdrawn from clinical use because of suspected nephrotoxicity and production of pulmonary hypertension. Toluidine blue has also been used for heparin reversal, but it is less effective than protamine and is associated with methemoglobulinemia.

Bull MH, Huse WM, Bull BS: Evaluation of tests used to monitor heparin therapy during extracorporeal circulation. Anesthesiology 43:346–353, 1975

Gravlee GP, Davis RF, Utley JR: Cardiopulmonary Bypass, Principles and Practice, pp 381–388. Baltimore, Williams & Wilkins, 1993

C. III-2. What is the action mechanism of protamine?

Heparin is a strong organic acid (polyanion). Protamine is a strong organic base (polycation). They combine ionically to form a stable salt and lose their own anticoagulant activity.

Gravlee GP, Davis RF, Utley JR: Cardiopulmonary Bypass, Principles and Practice, p 381. Baltimore, Williams & Wilkins, 1993

Hardman JG, Limbird LE, Molinoff PB et al (eds): Goodman and Gilman's The Pharmacological Basis of Therapeutics, 9th ed, p 1346. New York, McGraw-Hill, 1996

C. III-3. What are the complications of too much protamine?

Protamine itself is an anticoagulant. Protamine administered intravenously in the absence of heparin interacts with platelets and with many clotting proteins. Protamine induces transient thrombocytopenia in humans. Platelet aggregation is impaired by the protamine-heparin complex, but protamine alone has no deleterious effects. Protamine may bind to thrombin and inhibit thrombin's ability to convert fibrinogen to fibrin.

However, it has been shown that excess protamine minimally increases the Lee-White whole-blood coagulation time. After 600 mg/70 kg of protamine, the clotting time increased from 6.7 minutes to 8.2 minutes in unheparinized volunteers; the partial thromboplastin time (PTT) was not affected. In addition, the clotting time returned to baseline within 30 minutes. The results were similar in patients undergoing CPB. Therefore, protamine does inhibit coagulation *in vitro* and does minimally prolong clotting time in volunteers and in patients. However, the doses needed to achieve clinical anticoagulant effects are more than double those used routinely and >3 to 4 times the dose shown to result in return of adequate coagulation. Because of protamine's apparent rapid disappearance and because small doses of heparin do exert an important clinical effect, it seems prudent not to withhold additional doses of protamine in moderation whenever a residual heparin effect is suspected. The danger in giving additional doses of protamine for continued bleeding is that the hemostatic defect may not be residual heparin. Thus, the search for and correction of the real hemostatic defect may be delayed or forgotten.

Ellison N, Ominsky AJ, Wollman H: Is protamine a clinically important anticoagulant? Anesthesiology 35:621–629, 1971

Gravlee GP, Davis RF, Utley JR: Cardiopulmonary Bypass, Principles and Practice, pp 381–383. Baltimore, Williams & Wilkins, 1993

Hardman JG, Limbird LE, Molinoff PB et al (eds): Goodman and Gilman's The Pharmacological Basis of Therapeutics, 9th ed, p 1346. New York, Mc Graw-Hill, 1996

C. III-4. Why did the patient develop hypotension after protamine was administered? How do you treat and prevent this condition?

Three different types of circulatory reactions to protamine reversal of heparin have been proposed by Horrow:

Type I: Systemic Hypotension from Rapid Injection—A Predictable Pharmacologic Reaction

Type II: Anaphylactic or Anaphylactoid Reaction
- Antibody-medicated
- Immediate anaphylactoid response without antibody involvement
- Delayed anaphylactoid response (? noncardiac pulmonary edema)

Type III: Catastrophic Pulmonary Vasoconstriction with Systemic Hypotension
However, etiologically there are only two types of reaction: (1) pharmacologic side-ef-

fect reactions and (2) idiosyncratic reactions. Therefore, an alternative classification was proposed by Moorman, Zapl, and Lowenstein as follows:

- Pharmacologic histamine release
- True anaphylaxis (IgE-mediated)
- Anaphylactoid reactions
  - Pulmonary vasoconstriction
  - Noncardiogenic pulmonary edema

Mild to moderate systemic hypotension from pharmacologic side-effects is almost always the reaction seen when protamine is given rapidly or is given to patients who are relatively hypovolemic and vasoconstricted. Since it can be elicited in most patients, it is classified as a pharmacologic side-effect, not an idiosyncratic reaction. This side-effect is possibly mediated by histamine and is characterized by venodilation, reduced cardiac filling pressures, and decreased vascular resistance. Mild cardiac depression by protamine is suggested but probably does not occur. This type of hypotension can be corrected by rapid volume administration from a CPB pump and phenylephrine in 0.1-mg increments. There have been many attempts to modify the hypotensive response (e.g., intraaortic or left atrial administration, protamine pretreatment), with little evidence of predictable success. Only slower rates of intravenous infusion over 5 to 10 minutes and simultaneous maintenance of an adequate blood volume have been shown to decrease the incidence of hypotension.

Anaphylactic or anaphylactoid reaction is uncommon and rarely seen in in-

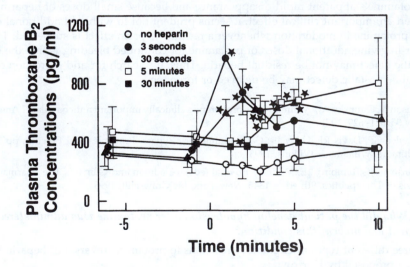

Figure 7-4. Plasma thromboxane B_2 concentrations before and after administration of protamine infused over 3 seconds, 30 seconds, 300 seconds, and 30 minutes. Heparin is injected at time − 5 minutes; protamine infusion is started at 0 minutes. Data points represent mean +/− SE values; n = 6 in each group. *P < 0.05 from unheparinized group. (Reprinted with permission from Morel DR, Costabella PMM, Pittet JF: Adverse cardiopulmonary effects and increased plasma thromboxane concentrations following the neutralization of heparin with protamine in awake sheep are infusion rate-dependent. Anesthesiology 73:415–424, 1990)

fants and children. The reaction varies from mild skin flushing and urticaria to severe vascular collapse. Systemic hypotension is usually accompanied by low pulmonary arterial pressure and low right-sided and left-sided filling pressures. This type of hypotension may be treated and prevented with rapid volume infusion and administration of vasoconstrictors, antihistamines, and steroids. Diabetic patients taking NPH insulin may develop antibodies to protamine and would appear to be at increased risk. However, clinical reactions do not predictably occur in these patients. Suspected cross-sensitivity in cases of fish allergy or autosensitization in men after vasectomy do not seem to put most patients at increased risk.

Catastrophic pulmonary hypertension occurs in about 0.2% to 4.0% of patients.

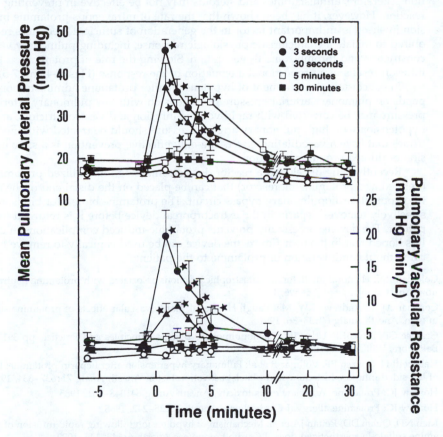

Figure 7-5.   Pulmonary hemodynamics before and after administration of protamine infused over 3 seconds, 30 seconds, 300 seconds, and 30 minutes. Heparin is injected at time −5 minutes; protamine infusion is started at 0 minutes. Data points represent mean +/− SE values; n = 6 in each group. *P < 0.05 from unheparinized group. (Reprinted with permission from Morel DR, Costabella PMM, Pittet JF: Adverse cardiopulmonary effects and increased plasma thromboxane concentrations following the neutralization of heparin with protamine in awake sheep are infusion rate-dependent. Anesthesiology 73:415−424, 1990)

There are several-fold increases in pulmonary artery pressure leading to right ventricular failure, elevated central venous pressure, low flow across the pulmonary circuit, and low left atrial pressure. Elevated plasma levels of C5a anaphylatoxins and thromboxane are responsible for pulmonary vasoconstriction and accompanied bronchoconstriction. Treatment with isoproterenol or amrinone is reasonable; epinephrine in 0.1-mg increments has been successfully used. If severe hypotension persists, the patient should be heparinized again and go back on bypass to maintain circulation. A recent study has shown that left ventricular infusion of protamine provides no protection from pulmonary hypertension and that histamine and platelet-activating factors are not involved in acute pulmonary vasoconstriction. Therefore, antihistamines and steroids may not be effective in preventing this reaction. However, it has been shown that the rate of intravenous protamine infusion in sheep is an important factor in the generation of sufficient mediators required to initiate a characteristic physiologic response, including pulmonary vasoconstriction and thromboxane B_2 generation. Slowing the rate of protamine infusion results in a proportional attenuation of the response (Figs. 7-4 and 7-5).

In conclusion, the treatment of hypotension after protamine administration depends on pulmonary arterial pressure. Hypotension with low pulmonary arterial pressure may be corrected with rapid volume infusion and vasoconstrictors, and hypotension with high pulmonary arterial pressure should be treated with inotropes that have a vasodilating effect. The only effective prevention is a slow infusion of diluted protamine solution.

Recently Yang developed a reactor device containing immobilized protamine (defined as a protamine bioreactor) that can be placed on the distal end of the extracorporeal cardiopulmonary bypass circuit. The protamine bioreactor binds and selectively removes heparin in the extracorporeal device before it is returned to the patient. The device successfully prevents protamine-induced complications in dogs. It is hoped that in the near future, the device can be used clinically to remove heparin without administration of protamine to the patients.

Coleman RN: Humoral mediators of catastrophic reactions associated with protamine neutralization. Anesthesiology 66:595–596, 1987

Conahan TJ III, Andrews RW, MacVaugh H III et al: Cardiovascular effects of protamine sulfate in man. Anesth Analg 60:33–36, 1981

Gravlee GP, Davis RF, Utley JR: Cardiopulmonary Bypass, Principles and Practice, pp 391–402. Baltimore, Williams & Wilkins, 1993

Habazettl H, Conzen PF, Vollmar B et al: Pulmonary hypertension after heparin-protamine: Roles of left-sided infusion, histamine and platelet activation factor. Anesth Analg 71:637–634, 1990

Horrow JC: Protamine: A review of its toxicity. Anesth Analg 64:348–361, 1985

Horrow JC: Protamine allergy. J Cardiothorac Anesth 2:225–242, 1988

Kien ND, Quam DD, Reitan JA et al: Mechanism of hypotension following rapid infusion of protamine sulfate in anesthetized dogs. J Cardiothorac Vasc Anesth 6:143–147, 1992

Morel DR, Costabella PMM, Pittet JF: Adverse cardiopulmonary effects and increased plasma thromboxane concentrations following the neutralization of heparin with protamine in awake sheep are infusion rate-dependent. Anesthesiology 73:415–424, 1990

Morel DR, Zapol WM, Thomas SJ et al: C5a and thromboxane generation associated with pulmonary vaso- and broncho-constriction during protamine reversal of heparin. Anesthesiology 66:597–604, 1987

Rogers K, Milne B, Salerno TA: The hemodynamic effects of intraaortic versus intravenous administration of protamine for reversal of heparin in pigs. J Thorac Cardiovasc Surg 85:851–855, 1983

Yang VC, Port FK, Kim JS et al: The use of immobilized protamine in removing heparin and preventing protamine-induced complications during extracorporeal circulation. Anesthesiology 75: 288–297, 1991

C. III-5. What are the indications for intraaortic balloon pump (IABP)?

IABP is primarily used for pump failure and myocardial ischemia that are not responsive to maximal pharmacologic support. The indications include the following:

Ischemic Heart Disease
- Cardiogenic shock
- Acute myocardial infarction complicated by
  - Mechanical defects—ventricular or septal rupture, acute mitral insufficiency, or ventricular aneurysm
  - Continued ischemic pain and extension of infarction
  - Refractory ventricular arrhythmias
- During cardiac catheterization
- Undergoing noncardiac surgery
- Failed PTCA and awaiting CABG

Cardiac Surgery
- Before CPB and postoperatively
- After CPB—low output syndrome

Pulsatile CPB—rare

Pediatric Congenital Heart Disease—rare

Neurosurgery—temporarily increases total cerebral blood flow in specific circumstances

Barash PG, Cullen BF, Stoelting RK (eds): Clinical Anesthesia, 3rd ed, p 859. Philadelphia, Lippincott-Raven, 1997

C. III-6. What are the principles of IABP?

IABP counterpulsation is designed to increase the myocardial oxygen supply during diastole and to decrease myocardial oxygen demand during systole. The balloon is inflated during diastole to increase the diastolic aortic pressure, resulting in increased coronary blood flow. The balloon should be inflated immediately following the closure of the aortic valve at the dicrotic notch of arterial tracing. The balloon is deflated just prior to the next systole to decrease the intraaortic pressure and afterload, resulting in decreased myocardial oxygen consumption. The cardiac output is increased because of increased coronary perfusion and decreased resistance.

Barash PG, Cullen BF, Stoelting RK (eds): Clinical Anesthesia, 3rd ed, p 859. Philadelphia, Lippincott-Raven, 1997

C. III-7. What are the complications of IABP?

- Ischemia of the leg
- Dissection of the aorta
- Thrombus formation and embolization
- Renal artery occlusion
- Splenic, mesenteric, and spinal cord infarction
- Internal mammary occlusion

- Thrombocytopenia
- Infection
- Gas embolization
- Inability to place the IABP

Barash PG, Cullen BF, Stoelting RK (eds): Clinical Anesthesia, 3rd ed, p 1371. Philadelphia, Lippincott-Raven, 1997

Kaplan J (ed): Cardiac Anesthesia, 3rd ed, pp 1130–1134. Philadelphia, WB Saunders, 1993

C. III-8. Can pulmonary artery wedge pressure (PAWP) represent left ventricular end-diastolic volume (LVEDV) after coronary artery bypass grafting?

It has been demonstrated that in nonsurgical patients, there was a significant correlation between changes in PAWP and LVEDV. However, in patients during the first few hours after CABG there was a poor correlation between changes in PAWP and LVEDV. The poor correlation was not explained by changes in systemic or pulmonary vascular resistance. The altered ventricular pressure-volume relationship may reflect acute changes in ventricular compliance. Although measurement of PAWP remains valuable in clinical management to avoid pulmonary edema, it cannot reliably be used as an index of left ventricular preload while attempting to optimize stroke volume. Transesophageal echocardiography can accurately assess left ventricular end-diastolic volume and cardiac contractility.

Harsen RM, Viquerat CE, Matthay MA et al: Poor correlation between pulmonary arterial wedge pressure and left ventricular end-diastolic volume after coronary artery bypass graft surgery. Anesthesiology 64:764–770, 1986

D. Postoperative Management

D.1. What are the postoperative complications?

Cardiovascular—congestive heart failure, arrhythmias, low output syndrome, myocardial ischemia or infarction due to surgical manipulation, prolonged CPB and aortic cross-clamp (coronary ischemia), use of cardioplegic solution, and occlusion or kinking of grafts

Pulmonary—pump lung or adult respiratory distress syndrome due to the following:
- Decreased blood flow to the lung during total CPB
- Deflated alveoli during CPB, resulting in decreased surfactant and decreased distensibility
- Fluid overloading
- Hyperoxia during CPB
- Left ventricular failure
- Microemboli

Renal
- Polyuria from hemodilution and diuretics
- Oliguria from hypoperfusion

Hemorrhage
- Too much or too little protamine to reverse heparin
- Thrombocytopenia and decreased coagulation factors
- Disseminated intravascular coagulopathy
- Poor surgical hemostasis

Embolism—due to air, destroyed or aggregated formed blood elements, fat, endogenous and exogenous debris

Neurologic—functional changes in behavior, personality, or other brain functions; cerebral embolism

Hyperglycemia—due to increased catecholamine levels

Hypopotassemia—due to hemodilution and diuretics

DiNardo JA, Schwartz MJ (eds): Anesthesia for Cardiac Surgery, pp 313–323. Norwalk, CT, Appleton & Lange, 1990

D.2. Would you reverse the muscle relaxants? Why?

No. We usually keep the patient on the respirator overnight to prevent postoperative respiratory failure. Moreover, atropine and neostigmine may cause severe tachycardia or bradycardia in ischemic cardiac patients.

D.3. When will you wean the patient from the respirator?

Generally, the patient is weaned from the respirator the following morning after surgery. If the operative course is very smooth and if the patient has good ventricular function, the patient may be weaned from the respirator early, usually 2 to 6 hours after surgery.

Early tracheal extubation (fast-track) after CABG surgery has cost benefits and improves resource use when compared with late tracheal extubation. Early tracheal extubation 1 to 6 hours after surgery reduces total cost per CABG surgery by 25% without increasing the rate or costs of complications in patients younger than 75 years.

Cheng DC, Havski J, Peniston C et al: Early tracheal extubation after coronary artery graft surgery reduces costs and improves resource use. Anesthesiology 85:1300–1310, 1996

Kaplan J (ed): Cardiac Anesthesia, 3rd ed, p 1161. Philadelphia, WB Saunders, 1993

D.4. What criteria would you use in deciding when to wean the patient from the respirator?

- Consciousness—awake and alert
- Stable vital signs
- Acceptable arterial blood gases—pH, 7.35 to 7.45; Po_2, over 80 mm Hg with F_IO_2 0.4; Pco_2, 35 to 45 mm Hg
- Acceptable respiratory mechanics
  - Vital capacity >10 to 15 ml/kg
  - Maximal inspiratory force—>20 to 25 cm H_2O
- Hemostasis—<200 ml/h of chest tube drainage
- Stable metabolic state—normal temperature and electrolytes

When the patient can satisfy the above criteria, the patient is put on continuous positive airway pressure (CPAP) of 5 cm H_2O with 50% oxygen. If the patient tolerates the CPAP well for 30 minutes and arterial blood gases are acceptable, the patient is extubated.

Kaplan J (ed): Cardiac Anesthesia, 3rd ed, p 1161. Philadelphia, WB Saunders, 1993

8 Valvular Heart Disease

Gregg S. Hartman
Stephen J. Thomas

A 72-year-old man was admitted with the recent onset of dyspnea on exertion. He was known to have had a heart murmur for many years and had experienced chest pain in the past, but did not see a physician regularly. He had fainted on two occasions in the past year. On physical examination, a loud systolic murmur could be heard at the left sternal border radiating to the neck. His vital signs were: blood pressure, 110/70 mm Hg; heart rate, 88/min with frequent premature beats. The ECG showed sinus rhythm with APCs, LVH with strain. An echocardiogram showed a hypertrophied left ventricle, and Doppler examination demonstrated severe aortic stenosis with a gradient of 64 mm Hg, mild aortic insufficiency, and severe mitral regurgitation. He was scheduled for aortic and mitral valve replacements.

A. Medical Disease and Differential Diagnosis

1. What are the major etiologies of aortic stenosis (AS), aortic insufficiency (AI), mitral stenosis (MS), and mitral regurgitation (MR)?
2. What are the major changes in the loading conditions of the left ventricle (LV) that result from the four different lesions? Why do they occur? What changes result from them?
3. What are pressure-volume (PV) loops? What do the different inflection points represent?
4. What are representative PV loops for the four valvular lesions?
5. Draw the pressure curves for the left ventricle, left atrium, pulmonary artery, and aorta for a normal patient and for patients with each of the four valvular lesions.
6. What are the echocardiographic and cardiac catheterization criteria for the four valvular lesions?

B. Preoperative Evaluation and Preparation

1. What are the presenting signs and symptoms of the four valvular lesions listed above?
2. What is the New York Heart Association classification of heart failure?
3. Discuss the role of premedication for patients with the four different valvular lesions.
4. How would you premedicate this patient with severe AS and MR?

C. Intraoperative Management

1. Outline the hemodynamic management goals for each of the four valvular lesions. What are the anesthetic goals with respect to heart rate and rhythm, preload, afterload, and contractility?

2. What are the hemodynamic goals for this patient with severe AS and MR?
3. How would you monitor this patient with severe AS and MR?
4. Should the patient have a pulmonary artery (PA) catheter placed prior to induction?
5. Is a pulmonary artery catheter with pacing capabilities indicated?
6. What anesthetic technique would you employ? Why?
7. What muscle relaxant would you use for this patient?
8. What special considerations particular to cardiopulmonary bypass (CPB) operations do you have for each of the four lesions? Focus on these concerns with respect to the induction and prebypass, bypass, and postbypass periods.
9. The patient cannot be weaned from bypass following an aortic and mitral valve replacement. What are the possible causes?
10. How would you diagnose right heart failure and pulmonary hypertension? How would you treat it?
11. What role does an intraaortic balloon pump (IABP) have in this setting?
12. How does it work to benefit the failing heart?
13. How would you properly time its cycle?
14. What are the contraindications to the use of an IABP?

D. Postoperative Management

1. In the intensive care unit 4 hours later, the patient became hypotensive with a low cardiac output. How could you distinguish between cardiac tamponade and pump failure? How would the TEE images differ?
2. Would you extubate this patient early in the intensive care unit? Why?
3. What are the advantages and disadvantages of early extubation?

A. Medical Disease and Differential Diagnosis

A.1. What are the major etiologies of aortic stenosis (AS), aortic insufficiency (AI), mitral stenosis (MS), and mitral regurgitation (MR)?

Aortic stenosis occurs as a congenital lesion, but more commonly as an acquired disease. Stenosis may develop on a previously normal valve following rheumatic fever or from progressive calcification. Congenitally bicuspid valves are also prone to calcification with eventual stenosis. Calcification of the leaflets can result in incomplete closure of the valve with associated insufficiency.

Aortic insufficiency is usually an acquired disease. The most common causes include bacterial endocarditis and rheumatic heart disease. Annular dilation may result from diseases such as cystic medial necrosis, collagen disorders, or following aortic dissections with resultant insufficiency. When occurring as a congenital lesion, AI rarely occurs in the absence of other cardiac abnormalities.

Mitral stenosis is almost always caused by rheumatic fever (RF), although only half of patients will have a history of an acute febrile illness. The inflammatory process of RF results in thickening of the leaflets and fusion of the commissures. Other rare causes include congenital stenosis and other systemic diseases including systemic lupus erythematosus and carcinoid. Pathophysiology similar to that seen with valvular MS can occur with obstructing left atrial tumors. MS commonly occurs in conjunction with other valvular heart disease; only 25% of patients present with isolated MS; approximately 40% have combined MS and MR.

Mitral regurgitation can result from defects in either the leaflets, the annular ring, or the supporting chordae and papillary muscles. Primary leaflet dysfunction occurs with rheumatic fever but can also follow bacterial endocarditis, connective tissue disorders, and congenital malformations. Annular dilation can follow ventricular dysfunction. Mitral valve prolapse and/or rupture of papillary muscles results in incomplete leaflet coaptation and MR. Left ventricular ischemia can affect papillary muscle contraction and is the etiology of postischemic or postinfarction MR.

Hartman GS: Management of patients with valvular heart disease. 1994 IARS Review Course Lectures, pp 141–151. Cleveland, Ohio, International Anesthesia Research Society, 1994

Thomas SJ, Kramer JL (eds): Manual of Cardiac Anesthesia, 2nd ed, pp 81–127. New York, Churchill Livingstone, 1993

A.2. What are the major changes in the loading conditions of the left ventricle (LV) that result from the four different lesions? Why do they occur? What changes result from them?

Aortic stenosis represents a chronic systolic pressure load on the left ventricle. This elevation increases wall tension in accordance with LaPlace's law.

$$\text{Wall tension} = (\text{Pressure} \times \text{Radius}) / (2 \times \text{Wall thickness})$$

The ventricle undergoes parallel duplication of muscle fibers in an attempt to compensate for the increase in tension. This results in increased wall thickness or concentric (common center) hypertrophy and some decrease in radius thereby normalizing wall stress. If the mitral valve remains competent, the major pressure overload occurs in the LV and little change in the other cardiac chambers results.

Aortic insufficiency results in the LV diastolic volume overload resulting in eccentric (away from the center) hypertrophy and LV dilation. Compliance, the relationship between volume and pressure, is altered only slightly as both end-systolic and end-diastolic volumes increase. Some concentric hypertrophy occurs as well secondary to the increase in wall stress resulting from an increase in LV radius. The diastolic pressure is lower with AI. Thus the increased volume work required to eject the additional blood, which flowed into the LV during diastole across the incompetent aortic valve, is reduced as the work can be performed against a lower outflow impedance. Stroke volume and ejection fraction therefore may be preserved until late in the disease process. As with aortic stenosis, the presence of a competent mitral valve confines the changes to the LV. However, the LV dilation that follows chronic AI may result in mitral annular dilation or alteration in chordae tendineae geometry with resultant MR. Left atrial enlargement can therefore occur.

Mitral stenosis results in a chronically underfilled left ventricle because of progressive obstruction to left atrial emptying. This chronic underloading condition can result in decreased LV thickness and diminished contractile function (a "disuse atrophy" of sorts). In addition, if the etiology of the MS is rheumatic, myofibril damage may have occurred. While the LV is pressure and volume underloaded, the left atrium is both pressure and volume overloaded. In order to maintain flow across the progressively narrowing mitral orifice, the pressure in the left atrium must be correspondingly increasing. Gorlin's equation for pressure gradient is shown below.

$$\text{Pressure gradient} = [\text{Flow rate}/(K \times \text{Valve area})]^2$$

It would predict that the pressure gradient increases by the square of any increase in flow rate or decrease in valve area. The elevations in LA pressure leads to hypertrophy and eventually dilation, which predisposes to premature atrial contractions and subsequently atrial fibrillation. The loss of atrial contraction further diminishes forward flow across the stenotic mitral valve. The elevations in left atrial pressure limit pulmonary venous flow with consequent pulmonary engorgement. The pulmonary vasculature undergoes reactive changes including intimal fibroelastosis inducing irreversible elevations in pulmonary vascular resistance. Right ventricular failure may develop, as this chamber is poorly equipped to deal with the elevations in afterload (e.g., pulmonary hypertension). Right ventricular dilation combined with increased RV systolic pressures leads to tricuspid regurgitation.

Mitral regurgitation results in volume overload of the left ventricle. The outflow of the left ventricle is divided between the high pressure/low compliance outflow tract of the arterial tree and the low pressure/high compliance outflow route across the incompetent mitral valve into the left atrium. Although the volume work of the LV is increased, the high compliance outflow route permits a large portion of this work to be performed at low pressure; therefore LV wall tension is minimally increased if at all. As with aortic insufficiency, the volume overload results in marked LV dilation and eccentric hypertrophy. In contrast, however, the left atrium is also volume overloaded and undergoes dilation. When the volume overload occurs slowly, the left atrium enlarges and minimal rises in pulmonary pressures result despite large regurgitant volumes. In contrast, the occurrence of acute MR, e.g., an acute myocardial infarction with papillary muscle rupture presents the left atrium with a sudden volume overload. Without the time to dilate, the left atrial pressure rapidly rises limiting pulmonary drainage with resultant pulmonary engorgement.

Braunwald E (ed): Heart Disease: A Textbook of Cardiovascular Medicine, 5th ed, pp 1007–1077. Philadelphia, WB Saunders, 1997

Hartman, GS: Management of patients with valvular heart disease. 1994 IARS Review Course Lectures, pp 141–151. Cleveland, Ohio, International Anesthesia Research Society, 1994

Thomas SJ, Kramer JL (eds): Manual of Cardiac Anesthesia, 2nd ed, pp 81–127. New York, Churchill Livingstone, 1993

A.3. What are pressure-volume(PV) loops? What do the different inflection points represent?

The pressure-volume loop analysis (Figure 8-1) depicts the relationship between left ventricular volume and left ventricular pressure during a single cardiac cycle. Opening and closing of the mitral and aortic valves are represented by the inflection points A, B, C, D, respectively (Fig. 8-1). Moving from points A through D, AB depicts LV filling; BC, isovolumetric contraction; CD, LV ejection; and DA, isovolumetric relaxation. Point A coincides with opening of the mitral valve and represents LV end-systolic volume and early diastolic pressure. Point B is closure of the mitral valve and the end of diastolic pressure (LVEDP) and volume (LVEDV). Point C represents the opening of the aortic valve and coincides with systemic, aortic diastolic pressure. Finally, point D is the closure of the aortic valve and represents LV end-systolic pressure and volume, coinciding with the dicrotic notch in the aortic pressure tracing. LV compliance is the relationship between the change in pressure and change in volume of the chamber and is defined by the slope of the filling phase, or segment

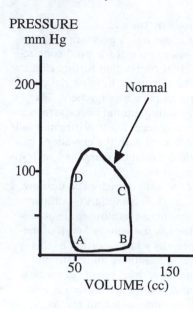

PRESSURE
mm Hg

200—

Normal

100—

D

C

A   B

50   150

VOLUME (cc)

Figure 8-1.   Normal pressure-volume loop and valve positions. *A* = MV opening, *B* = MV closure, *C* = AV opening, *D* = AV closure, *AB* = LV filling, *BC* = isovolumetric contraction, *CD* = ejection, *DA* = isovolumetric relaxation.

AB. Preload is the pressure-volume relationship prior to the onset of contraction (LVEDP). Contractility may be illustrated by the slope of a line called the end-systolic pressure-volume relationship (ESPVR). The ESPVR slope is created by connecting multiple points (D) from mulitple PV loops generated by changing the filling volume to the left ventricle (Fig. 8-2). Increased contractility results in a steeper line, whereas diminished contractility results in a flatter relationship. The PV loop analysis permits illustration of stroke volume (SV) and ejection fraction (EF). Stroke volume is defined as difference in volume from the end of filling to the end of ejection (EDV-ESV), while ejection fraction is the ratio of SV to total volume in the heart at peak filling (SV/EDV). Thus the PV loop analysis permits illustration of the volume-pressure relationships and their changes with each of the four valvular lesions.

Braunwald E (ed): Heart Disease: A Textbook of Cardiovascular Medicine, 5th ed, pp 1007–1077. Philadelphia, WB Saunders, 1997

Thomas SJ, Kramer JL (eds): Manual of Cardiac Anesthesia, 2nd ed, pp 81–127. New York, Churchill Livingstone, 1993

A.4. What are representative PV loops for the four valvular lesions?

The hallmarks of AS illustrated by the pressure-volume loop analysis framework are a high LV systolic pressure and an upward and counterclockwise rotation in the end-diastolic pressure-volume relationship (AB) indicative of decreased chamber compliance (Fig. 8-3). Stroke volume and ejection fraction are well preserved, but the ejection phase of the loop occurs at much higher pressures. This is permitted by an increase in contractility of a counterclockwise rotation of the ESPVR line.

The schematic PV loop for AI depicts the enlarged LV of chronic AI. The minimal change in LVEDP despite the large volume overload is seen by the shift in the

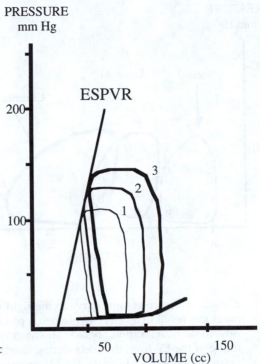

Figure 8-2. Contractility. ESPVR, end-systolic pressure-volume relationships.

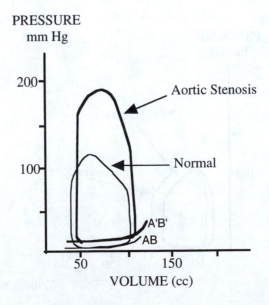

Figure 8-3. Pressure-volume loop of aortic stenosis.

PRESSURE
mm Hg

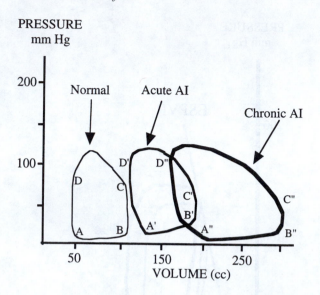

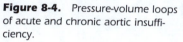

Figure 8-4.   *Pressure-volume loops of acute and chronic aortic insufficiency.*

diastolic pressure-volume curve to the right (A′B′) (Fig. 8-4). Low systemic diastolic pressures result in a brief isovolumetric phase (B′C′) and early complete ejection. The isovolumetric relaxation phase is absent as the incompetent valve permits regurgitant filling of the LV from the aorta during diastole even before opening of the mitral valve. When acute AI occurs, the LV compliance is unchanged. Rapid increases in LVEDP from volume overload along the unshifted LV diastolic PV curve (AB) rapidly lead to increased left atrial pressure and pulmonary congestion.

The PV loop of MS illustrates hypovolemia, the etiology of which cannot be de-

PRESSURE
mm Hg

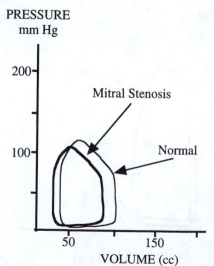

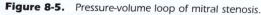

Figure 8-5.   *Pressure-volume loop of mitral stenosis.*

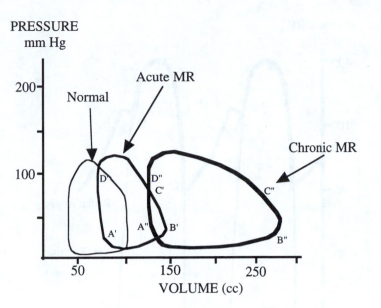

Figure 8-6.   Pressure-volume loop of acute and chronic mitral regurgitation.

termined from the loop alone (Fig. 8-5). Since the predominant impact of MS occurs proximal to the left ventricle, the PV analysis format is less useful.

In MR, the diastolic PV relationship (line AB) is shifted to the right as it is in AI, consistent with a marked increase in compliance (Fig. 8-6). The isovolumetric phase (BC) is nearly absent as the left atrium serves as a low pressure/high compliance route for ejection due to the incompetent mitral valve. Decreases in contractility are depicted by a decrease in the slope of the end-systolic–PV line (line through D). Nevertheless stroke volume and ejection fraction are maintained because of this low pressure left atrial vent.

Hartman GS: Management of patients with valvular heart disease. 1994 IARS Review Course Lectures, pp 141–151. Cleveland, Ohio, International Anesthesia Research Society, 1994

Sagawa K, Maugan L, Suga H, Sunagawa K: Cardiac contraction and the pressure-volume relationship. New York, Oxford University Press, 1988

Thomas SJ, Kramer JL (eds): Manual of Cardiac Anesthesia, 2nd ed, pp 81–127. New York, Churchill Livingstone, 1993

A.5. Draw the pressure curves for the left ventricle, left atrium, pulmonary artery, and aorta for a normal patient and for patients with each of the four valvular lesions.

Normal curves are shown in Figure 8-7. The points A, B, C, D correspond to the same points in the pressure-volume loops.

Aortic Stenosis
The additional systolic pressure work of AS can be seen in the LV pressure tracing (Fig. 8-8). Elevations in LVEDP (point B) can be seen to diminish the perfusion gradient for coronary flow to the left ventricle. The left atrial kick from sinus rhythm is

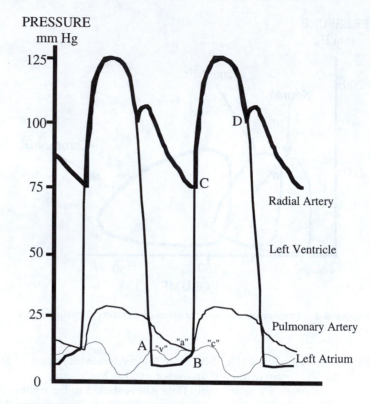

PRESSURE
mm Hg

Figure 8-7. *Pressure curves for the LV, LA, PA and aorta in a normal patient.*

highlighted in the inset. Rising LV diastolic pressures secondary to decreased compliance necessitate elevations in left atrial pressures to permit complete LV volume loading. Atrial systole provides this elevation in LA pressure synchronous with elevations in LVEDP while keeping LA pressures relatively low during the remaining cardiac cycle facilitating pulmonary venous drainage.

Aortic Insufficiency
The rapid upstroke and rapid decline of arterial pressure indicate absence of aortic valve closure and low end-diastolic aortic pressure (Fig. 8-9). Elevations in the LVEDV and LVEDP are typical of AI. The early increase in LVEDP can result in LV pressures exceeding those of the LA during diastole with resultant premature closure of the mitral valve.

Mitral Stenosis
Elevations in pressure are seen in both the LA and PA tracing with MS (Fig. 8-10). The large gradient between LA and LV pressures is highlighted in the inset. Chronic elevations in pulmonary volume leads to pulmonary hypertension.

Mitral Regurgitation
The hallmark of MR is the marked elevations of LA pressure during systole and the occurrence of a giant "v" wave and elevated pulmonary artery pressures (Fig. 8-11).

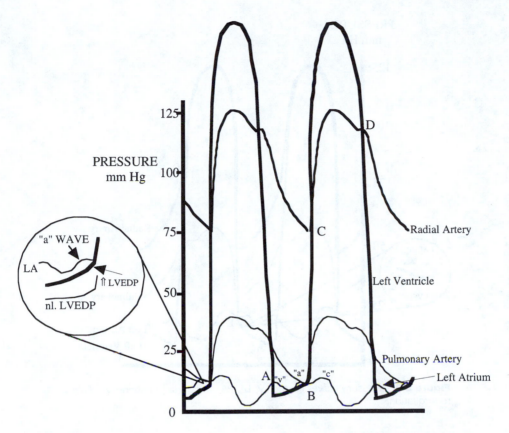

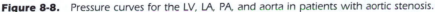

Figure 8-8. Pressure curves for the LV, LA, PA, and aorta in patients with aortic stenosis.

Hartman GS: Management of patients with valvular heart disease. 1994 IARS Review Course Lectures, pp 141–151. Cleveland, Ohio, International Anesthesia Research Society, 1994

A.6. What are the echocardiographic and cardiac catheterization criteria for the four valvular lesions?

The TEE severity scales of the various valvular lesions are summarized in Table 8-1.

Aortic Stenosis
Echocardiographic criteria for AS include two-dimensional (2D) images demonstrating limited aortic valve opening and LV concentric hypertrophy. Doppler examination will reveal a turbulent high velocity jet across the aortic valve. The gradient across the aortic valve measured at cardiac catheterization is different from that measured by echocardiography. The catheterization derived-gradient is the difference of the peak aortic and peak ventricular pressure. In contrast, the gradient from Doppler echocardiography is the maximum instantaneous transvalvular gradient calculated

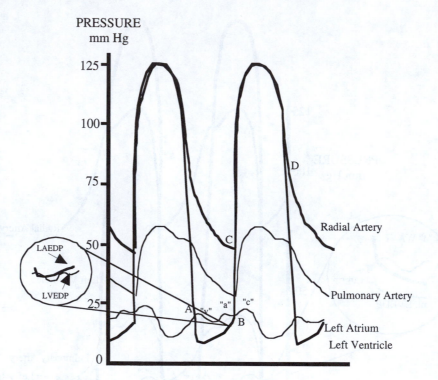

Figure 8-9. Pressure curves for the LV, LA, PA, and aorta in patients with aortic regurgitation.

from the maximal blood velocity. Quantification of this Doppler derived pressure gradient relies on the modified Bernoulli equation:

$$\text{Pressure gradient} = 4 \times v^2$$

where v = velocity (m/sec), pressure (mm Hg)

Since flow is an important determinant of pressure gradients, both these catheterization and Doppler derived values are related to cardiac output and a valve area determined. Severe AS is present when the gradient exceeds 75 mm Hg and/or the valve area is <0.8 cm^2.

Aortic Insufficiency
Catheterization criteria for AI relies on the qualitative estimation of the regurgitation volume and an estimation of LV size. Similar quantification can be made from Doppler color echocardiography-derived data. The most common criteria compare the width of the regurgitant jet at the level of the valve to the width of the LV outflow tract. A ratio of >0.66 represents severe AI.

Mitral Stenosis
The severity of MS can be obtained by the direct measurement of a diastolic gradient between the left atrium and ventricle. However, this requires a transatrial puncture, a procedure largely replaced by echocardiographic techniques. Echocardiographic diag-

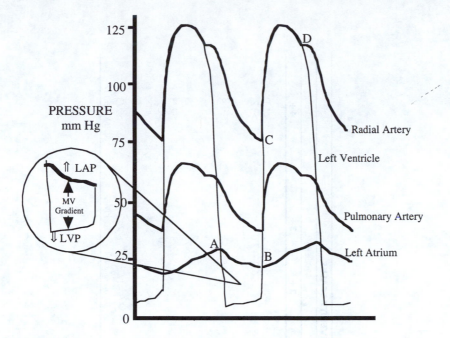

Figure 8-10. Pressure curves for the LV, LA, PA, and aorta in patients with mitral stenosis.

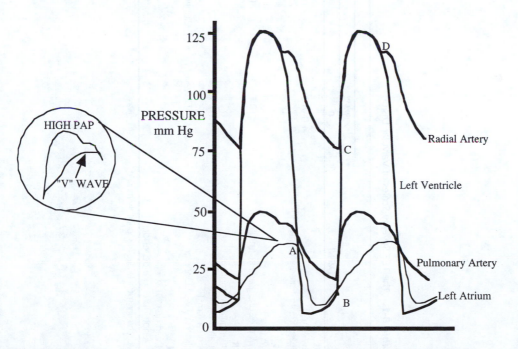

Figure 8-11. Pressure curves for the LV, LA, PA, and aorta in patients with mitral regurgitation.

Table 8-1. The TEE Severity Scales of Valvular Lesions

MEASUREMENT	NORMAL 0	MILD 1+	MODERATE 2+	MODERATE 3+	SEVERE 4+
MS					
MVA (cm^2)	4.0–6.0	1.5–2.5	1.0–1.5		<1.0
Mean pressure gradient (mm Hg)	<2	2.0–6.0	6.0–12.0		>12
AS					
AVA (cm^2)	3.0–5.0	1.2–2.0	0.8–1.1		<0.8
Peak pressure gradient (mm Hg)	<10	16–34	35–75		>75
MR					
Jet length/LA length	0	<1/3	1/3–2/3		>2/3
Jet area/LA area	0	<1/3	1/3–2/3		>2/3
Jet area (cm^2)	0	<3	3.0–6.0		>6
Pulmonary vein Doppler	S wave ≫ D wave	Blunting S wave	S < D	S ≪ D	Systolic reversal of flow
AI					
Jet width/LVOT width	0	<1/4	1/4–1/2	1/2–2/3	>2/3
Jet length (pressure dependent)	0	to middle of AML	to tip of AML	to PM	beyond PM

AML, anterior mitral leaflet; PM, papillary muscle

nosis is based on gradient estimation by Doppler and by measuring the rate of decay in the pressure with the time spent in diastole (pressure half-time). The mitral valve area in cm² equals 220 divided by this pressure half-time. Severe MS is present when the end-diastolic gradient exceeds 12 mm Hg corresponding to a valve area of <1.0 cm².

Mitral Regurgitation
In the presence of MR, ventriculography will demonstrate the reflux of dye from the left ventricle into the left atrium. Severe MR is diagnosed when dye refluxes into the pulmonary veins. Color Doppler echocardiography permits similar quantification. Estimation relies on an estimation of regurgitant jet volume as compared to the left atrium and via analysis of pulmonary venous flow profiles.

In every case, color Doppler echocardiography is often useful in identifying the etiology of the valvular lesion, its extent of involvement within and around the valve, and the associated hemodynamic changes. Thus for many valvular lesions, it may be sufficient for the diagnosis. Catheterization, however, is often performed in order to assess the presence of concomitant coronary artery disease, especially in patients of advanced age.

Braunwald E (ed): Heart Disease: A Textbook of Cardiovascular Medicine, 5th ed, pp 1007–1077. Philadelphia, WB Saunders, 1997

Weyman AE (ed): Principles and Practice of Echocardiography, 2nd ed, pp 391–574. Philadelphia, Lea & Febiger, 1994.

B. Preoperative Evaluation and Preparation

B.1. What are the presenting signs and symptoms of the four valvular lesions listed above?
See Table 8-2.

Aortic Stenosis
The triad of angina, syncope, and congestive heart failure represents the progression of symptoms associated with AS. These symptoms correlate directly with mortality; the 50% survival data for these symptoms are 5, 3, and 2 years from the onset of these symptoms, respectively. Angina results from both increased demand for and a decrease in supply of coronary blood flow. Increased muscle mass from LVH and the high energy requirements to generate increased (high) systolic pressure combine to

Table 8-2. The Signs and Symptoms for the Various Valvular Lesions

LESION	SIGNS AND SYMPTOMS
AS	Angina, syncope, dyspnea/CHF
AI	
Chronic	Fatigability, dyspnea
Acute	Severe pulmonary edema, CHF
MS	Pulmonary congestion, AFib
MR	
Chronic	DOE, PND, AFib
Acute	Severe pulmonary edema, CHF

increase demands for coronary blood flow. In addition, insufficient supply secondary to decreased perfusion gradients and a decrease in coronary vasculature relative to the large amount of myocardium sum to diminish relative myocardial blood supply. Therefore, up to one-third of patients with AS can have angina in the absence of significant coronary artery disease.

Aortic Insufficiency

Patients with AI have variable clinical presentations, primarily depending on the rapidity with which the LV volume overload develops. When the volume increase occurs gradually as in chronic AI, there is usually a long asymptomatic period. The onset of the symptoms of fatigability and dyspnea signals either reduced cardiac output or increased LVEDP indicative of impairment of LV contractile function. When AI occurs acutely, the ventricular compliance is unchanged; increased LV diastolic volumes from regurgitant flow therefore lead to rapid rises in LVEDP and the clinical picture of congestive failure.

Mitral Stenosis

MS is a slowly progressive obstruction to flow across the mitral valve with gradual increase in left atrial pressure and volume. Symptoms of pulmonary congestion result from elevations in left atrial pressures and *not* from poor left ventricular systolic function. Atrial fibrillation develops secondary to atrial dilation.

Mitral Regurgitation

The time course for the development of MR determines the severity of the symptoms. When the volume of regurgitant flow from the left ventricle to the left atrium increases gradually, the left atrium compensates by gradual dilatation. In contrast, the onset of acute MR can lead to rapid increases in left atrial pressures and severe pulmonary congestion and congestive heart failure.

Braunwald E (ed): Heart Disease: A Textbook of Cardiovascular Medicine, 5th ed, pp 1007–1077. Philadelphia, WB Saunders, 1997

Hartman GS: Management of patients with valvular heart disease. 1994 IARS Review Course Lectures, pp 141–151. Cleveland, Ohio, International Anesthesia Research Society, 1994

Thomas SJ, Kramer JL (eds): Manual of Cardiac Anesthesia, 2nd ed, pp 81–127. New York, Churchill Livingstone, 1993

B.2. What is the New York Heart Association classification of heart failure?

The NYHA heart failure classification is based on the amount of symptoms, specifically dyspnea and fatigue. The various classes are listed below.

Class I No symptoms

Class II Symptoms with ordinary activity

Class III Symptoms with less than ordinary activity

Class IV Symptoms at rest

Criteria Committee of the New York Heart Association Inc: Diseases of the Heart and Blood Vessels (Nomenclature and Criteria for Diagnosis), 6th ed. Boston, Little, Brown, 1964

B.3. Discuss the role of premedication for patients with the four different valvular lesions.

The role of premedication is to allay the patient's anxiety of the impending surgical procedure, thereby controlling the sympathetic outflow that may accompany the stress response. However, acute changes in heart rate, venous return, and systemic resistance can have particularly profound effects on patients with valvular heart disease.

Patients with AS benefit from premedication by preventing unnecessary increases in heart rate. Concern, however, must be taken to ensure adequate venous return and preservation of sinus mechanism (see below).

Patients with AI can similarly benefit from premedication, as any increases in afterload that accompany sympathetic stimulation can increase regurgitant volume. Drug doses should be adjusted based on the severity of debilitation and degree of systemic hypoperfusion.

Patients with MS should be premedicated with caution. Elevations in carbon dioxide resulting from narcotic-induced hypoventilation can dramatically elevate pulmonary pressures, further compromising right ventricle output. Conversely venodilation may excessively diminish filling pressures.

Patients with MR can respond similarly to those with MS, particularly when pulmonary hypertension is present. Elevations in systemic pressure from stress can also compromise forward LV output. Proper premedication can be delivered by careful dosage selection and the provision of supplemental oxygen.

Hartman GS: Management of patients with valvular heart disease. 1994 IARS Review Course Lectures, pp 141–151. Cleveland, Ohio, International Anesthesia Research Society, 1994

Thomas SJ, Kramer JL (eds): Manual of Cardiac Anesthesia, 2nd ed, pp 81–127. New York, Churchill Livingstone, 1993

B.4. How would you premedicate this patient with severe AS and MR?

Premedication of this patient with severe AS and MR must be approached with caution. The patient should receive supplemental oxygen. A light premedication could be provided with small doses of benzodiazepines administered intramuscularly (IM). However, I would prefer to titrate in small doses of sedation while the patient was under the closely monitored situation of the operating room. In this setting, incremental doses of midazolam (0.5 mg intravenously [IV]) would be administered. It is important to remember that there may be significant delay in the onset of effect of IV medications secondary to pooling in the pulmonary and left atrial systems. Adequate waiting periods must be observed between each aliquot to avoid overdosage with ensuing respiratory depression, pulmonary hypertension, hypotension, and right heart failure.

C. Intraoperative Management:

C.1. Outline the hemodynamic management goals for each of the four valvular lesions. What are the anesthetic goals with respect to heart rate and rhythm, preload, afterload, and contractility?

Table 8-3 summarizes the hemodynamic goals with respect to heart rate and rhythm, preload, afterload, and contractility.

Table 8-3. The Hemodynamic Goals for the Various Valvular Lesions

LESIONS	HEMODYNAMIC GOALS			
	HR and Rhythm	Preload	Afterload	Contractility
AS	60–70, sinus	Full	Maintain	—
AI	80–90	Maintain	Lower	May need support
MS	60–70	Full	—	—
MR	80–90, sinus if possible	Maintain	Lower	May need support

Aortic Stenosis

Patients with AS need the LV filling obtained through a well-timed atrial contraction. Similarly, LVH renders the ventricle stiff, and adequate preload is required. Reducing vascular tone will do little to relieve the fixed afterload increases from a stenotic valve, but rather it lowers diastolic coronary perfusion gradients and should be avoided. Patients with AS experiencing angina may require the administration of an alpha-agonist like phenylephrine rather than nitroglycerin in order to increase coronary perfusion pressure.

Aortic Insufficiency

The severity of AI is determined by the size of the regurgitant orifice, the pressure gradient between the aorta and LV during diastole, and the time spent in that phase of the cycle. Elevated heart rates decrease the time spent in diastole and decrease heart size. Afterload reduction can decrease the regurgitant driving force, but therapeutic maneuvers to do so may be limited by systemic hypotension.

Mitral Stenosis

Patients with MS can rapidly deteriorate in the setting of rapid heart rates. The decreased filling time necessitates the marked elevation of left atrial pressures, and pulmonary edema can rapidly ensue. Beta-blockade does result in decreased contractility, which, in the setting of decreased cardiac output and blood pressure, could be deleterious. However, the loss in contractility is more than offset by the beneficial effects of the reduction of heart rate. Slower heart rates permit adequate time for transfer of blood from the left atrium to the LV across the stenotic mitral valve (MV) to occur. In addition, the pressure gradient across the MV is also reduced, diminishing pulmonary congestion. Since there is some variability in the individual response, the use of short-acting beta-blockers such as esmolol is prudent, as an adverse response should be evanescent.

Mitral Regurgitation

Patients with MR can rapidly deteriorate with marked increases in systemic blood pressure and afterload. As with other volume overload lesions such as AI, rapid heart rates result in smaller LV volumes. This may lessen any component of MR secondary to annular dilation or chordal malalignment.

C.2. *What are the hemodynamic goals for this patient with severe AS and MR?*

In this patient with combined AS and MR, the situation is more complex than when only a single valvular lesion is present. Careful examination of the hemodynamic goals for each of the two lesions will reveal that therapy beneficial to patients with aortic stenosis may exacerbate the severity of the mitral regurgitation. Early aggressive intervention is the key to these combined lesions. There usually exists less margin for error as minor hemodynamic aberrations can rapidly lead to cardiac collapse. A good rule of thumb is to prioritize the management based on the character of the present symptoms. Patients with AS and MR who present with syncope or angina are best managed for their AS, whereas patients with dyspnea and pulmonary edema are best managed for their congestive symptoms. It is prudent to maintain the patient's own usual hemodynamics and avoid physiologic trespass.

Hartman GS: Management of patients with valvular heart disease. 1994 IARS Review Course Lectures, pp 141–151. Cleveland, Ohio, International Anesthesia Research Society, 1994

Thomas SJ, Kramer JL (eds): Manual of Cardiac Anesthesia, 2nd ed, pp 81–127. New York, Churchill Livingstone, 1993

C.3. How would you monitor this patient with severe AS and MR?

In addition to the standard ASA-recommended monitors, the patient would have a radial-artery and a pulmonary-artery catheter. Following induction of anesthesia and endotracheal intubation, a transesophageal echocardiography (TEE) probe would be inserted to confirm the valvular pathology and to assess ventricular function. Following valve replacement, the TEE would be used to check for adequacy of valvular function and the absence of paravalvular leaks, and to assess postbypass ventricular function.

C.4. Should the patient have a pulmonary artery (PA) catheter placed prior to induction?

Volume status may be particularly difficult to assess in patients with valvular heart disease. Patients with stenotic lesions depend on adequate filling pressures for diastolic filling of the ventricle. Patients with the volume overload lesions of AI and MR can benefit from the careful reductions in pulmonary pressure guided by the simultaneous assessment of cardiac performance. In these capacities, the PA catheter is useful. Patients with current hemodynamic stability, without severe respiratory distress, can be safely anesthetized prior to having the PA catheter placed.

Roizen MF, Berger DL, Gabel RA et al: Practice guidelines for pulmonary artery catheterization: A report by the American Society of Anesthesiologists Task Force on Pulmonary Artery Catheterization. Anesthesiology 78:380–394, 1993.

C.5. Is a pulmonary artery catheter with pacing capabilities indicated?

Patients with AS can become severely compromised with the loss of atrial kick or the presence of slow junctional rhythms. Patients with AI or MR can experience LV dilation in the setting of slow heart rates. In patients with intact conduction systems, rate manipulation can often be achieved pharmacologically. Transesophageal atrial pacing is another option; transthoracic pacing elicits a ventricular response only and does not permit atrial stimulation. Transthoracic pacing is indicated when the ability to rapidly open the pericardium and obtain epicardial pacing is limited. This occurs in the setting of reoperations or with patients having a history of inflammatory pericardial disease.

Risk SC, Brandon D, D'Ambra MN et al: Indications for the use of pacing pulmonary artery catheters in cardiac surgery. J Cardiothorac Vasc Anesth 6:275–279, 1992

C.6. What anesthetic technique would you employ? Why?

For this patient undergoing cardiopulmonary bypass and aortic valve replacement (AVR), general endotracheal anesthesia is the obvious choice. Both narcotics and inhalation anesthetics can be safely administered. When prolonged postoperative ventilation is anticipated, a high-dose narcotic anesthetic has numerous advantages. Recent anesthetic technique for cardiac surgery has focused on the use of techniques permitting earlier extubation, so-called fast-tracking. Anesthetic combinations utilizing smaller total narcotic doses, inhalational anesthetics, and short-acting intravenous sedatives such as propofol are gaining popularity. For uncomplicated valve replacements with good ventricular function, the advantages of early extubation can be safely achieved. In complicated cases with longer bypass periods, poor ventricular function or postbypass bleeding, the hemodynamic stability of a high-dose narcotic technique may be advantageous.

Howie MB, Black HA, Romanelli VA et al: A comparison of isoflurane versus fentanyl as primary anesthetics for mitral surgery. Anesth Analg 83:941–948, 1996

Tuman KJ, McCarthy RJ, Spiess BD, Ivankonich AD: Comparison of anesthetic techniques in patients undergoing heart valve replacement. J Cardiothoracic Anesth 4:159–167, 1990

C.7. What muscle relaxant would you use for this patient?

Muscle relaxants can alter hemodynamics both from the effects of histamine release including vasodilatation and bronchospasm and through effects on rhythm. While slowing of heart rates usually benefits the patient with angina, it may have severe consequences in patients with valvular heart disease. The typical high-dose narcotic anesthesia usually results in bradycardia secondary to the vagotonic actions. Pancuronium-mediated increases in heart rate usually offset these actions and result in a stable heart rate.

Certainly the newly released long-duration relaxants doxacurium and pipercuronium have the potential for minimal effects on hemodynamics. However, as outlined above, the potential side-effect of one agent may be rationally used to counter the adverse effect of another.

Therefore, it is important to choose that combination of agents that will promote hemodynamic stability in a particular patient with their unique hemodynamic presentation. In this patient, I would utilize pancuronium in conjunction with the high-dose narcotic anesthetic.

Fleming N: Con: The choice of muscle relaxants is not important in cardiac surgery. J Cardiothorac Vasc Anesth 9:768–771, 1995

Hudson RJ, Thomson IR: Pro: The choice of muscle relaxants is important in cardiac surgery. J Cardiothor Vasc Anesth 9(6):768–771, 1995

C.8. What special considerations particular to cardiopulmonary bypass (CPB) operations do you have for each of the four lesions? Focus on these concerns with respect to the induction and prebypass, bypass, and postbypass periods.

Aortic Stenosis

Critical to the management of a patient with aortic stenosis is the avoidance of hypotension. Low blood pressure can initiate a cascade of events leading to cardiac arrest. Hypotension decreases the gradient for coronary perfusion with resultant ischemia. Ischemia leads to diminished cardiac output and decreased blood pressure further compromising coronary perfusion. The occurrence of cardiac arrest in a patient with AS is particularly catastrophic because closed chest cardiac massage will provide little gradient for blood flow across a stenosed aortic valve.

Patients with AS are particularly dependent upon their atrial kick for adequate ventricular filling volume and can rapidly become hypotensive and ischemic following the onset of an SVT or atrial fibrillation. These rhythms are not uncommon during atrial cannulation. Therefore it is of particular importance that every preparation for the initiation of cardiopulmonary bypass be made prior to atrial manipulation. Increased muscle mass of left ventricular hypertrophy can be more difficult to adequately protect with cardioplegia. Careful attention to surface cooling, myocardial temperature measurement, and/or the use of retrograde cardioplegia can be helpful. Following aortic valve replacement, hypertension from LV output now unopposed by any valvular lesion can result in stress on suture lines and excessive bleeding. It is important to remember that the compliance of the LV is unchanged by surgery and still critically dependent upon adequate preload and sinus rhythm.

Aortic Insufficiency

Patients undergoing AVR for AI can often present difficult management decisions. The usual treatment measures for hypotension (alpha-agonist) may have deleterious effects by increasing regurgitant volume. The use of combined alpha- and beta-agonists (ephedrine, epinephrine, or infusions of dopamine or dobutamine) may be required. Although it would serve to lessen regurgitant volume, afterload reduction is beneficial in only a subset of patients with AI. Those patients with elevated LVEDP, reduced ejection fractions, diminished cardiac output, and systemic hypertension usually benefit from afterload reduction. In contrast, those patients without the above constellation may experience a decrease in forward cardiac output secondary to diminished preload from reduced venous return. Systemic hypotension usually limits the utility in the acute setting. The presence of AI makes initiation of CPB a critical period. Periods of bradycardia or ventricular fibrillation can lead to rapid volume overload of the LV through the incompetent aortic valve. Pacing, electrical defibrillation and/or cross clamping should be performed to prevent ventricular distention. Myocardial protection is similarly compromised by AI; generation of adequate root pressures is usually not obtainable and delivery of cardioplegia requires aortotomy and cannulation of the coronary ostia. Utilization of retrograde cardioplegia is advantageous. Following AVR, the ventricle no longer has the lower pressure/impedance outflow afforded by the low aortic diastolic pressure. Inotropic support is often required. As with AS, the presence of an aortic suture line necessitates rapid response to hypertension to avoid bleeding and dissection.

Mitral Stenosis

Patients undergoing mitral valve (MV) replacement for MS are particularly challenging. Marked elevations in pulmonary vascular resistance can be present with associated right heart failure. Stasis in the left atrium necessitates the careful echocardiographic examination for the presence of atrial thrombi. Manipulation of the heart prior to cross-clamping should be avoided. Following replacement, the chronically underfilled, underworked LV may be unable to handle the new volume load. Inotropic support is usually required. Afterload reduction and improved systemic perfusion via an intraaortic balloon pump (IABP) may be beneficial.

Mitral Regurgitation

Similarly, patients with MR may have pulmonary hypertension and right heart failure. In contrast to AI, almost all patients with MR can be greatly benefited by afterload reduction, both pharmacologically and/or via an IABP. Diminution of LV systolic pressure via afterload reduction decreases the pressure gradient from the LV to the LA during systole with resultant decreased regurgitant volume.

Prebypass assessment can be misleading. Marked LV systolic dysfunction may be masked by preserved ejection fractions and elevated stroke volumes. It should be remembered that much of the LV volume is ejected into the low pressure/impedance outflow path of the left atrium. This route is no longer available following valve replacement. Following MV replacement, dysfunctional ventricles may be unable to provide adequate forward flow into the systemic circuit with its elevated vascular resistance, which usually necessitates the use of inotropic support.

Patients previously in atrial fibrillation without marked atrial enlargement can often be converted to sinus rhythm following valve replacement. The capacity of maintaining a person in sinus rhythm dramatically decreases when the diameter of the atrium is over 5 cm.

Hartman GS: Management of patients with valvular heart disease. 1994 IARS Review Course Lectures, pp 141–151. Cleveland, Ohio, International Anesthesia Research Society, 1994

Thomas SJ, Kramer JL (eds): Manual of Cardiac Anesthesia, 2nd ed, pp 81–127. New York, Churchill Livingstone, 1993

C.9. The patient cannot be weaned from bypass following an aortic and mitral valve replacement. What are the possible causes?

The adequacy of myocardial preservation should be considered. LVH without or with accompanying coronary artery disease increases myocardial oxygen demands. Prolonged cross-clamp time necessitated by dual valve replacement can lead to inadequate and unhomogeneous myocardial protection. In addition, there may be residual cardioplegia present in the myocardium. Therefore some degree of postbypass LV dysfunction can be anticipated. Inotropic support may be required. It is important to remember that although the obstruction to LV ejection is acutely relieved by replacement of the stenotic valve, LV compliance is largely unchanged. Adequate preload still depends on sinus rhythm and sufficient LV filling pressures (PCWP or LVEDP). Elevations in pulmonary vascular resistance may render estimation of LA pressure via the PA catheter inaccurate. In this setting, placement of an LA catheter is indicated. Transesophageal echocardiography may prove invaluable in identifying surgically correctable etiologies for inability to wean from CPB. Abnormal valve seating may compromise flow into the coronary ostia and return to bypass with valve repositioning and/or coronary artery bypass grafting may be indicated.

Thomas SJ, Kramer JL (eds): Manual of Cardiac Anesthesia, 2nd ed, pp 81–127. New York, Churchill Livingstone, 1993

C.10. How would you diagnose right heart failure and pulmonary hypertension? How would you treat it?

Right heart failure is diagnosed by the elevations in right-sided filling pressures, specifically central venous pressure (CVP). Careful examination is required to rule out tricuspid insufficiency as the etiology of the CVP elevation. A high CVP indicates the inability of the right heart to adequately propel the venous return volume into the pulmonary circulation. Elevation in the pulmonary artery (PA) pressure is indicative of pulmonary hypertension. The combination of high CVP and high PA pressures indicates severe right heart failure. This scenario can be difficult to manage. Attempts to elevate systemic perfusion pressure with alpha-agonists can worsen pulmonary hypertension. Administration of vasodilators to lower PA pressures results in systemic hypotension. In this setting, it is often prudent to return to cardiopulmonary bypass, relieve ventricular distention, and improve myocardial perfusion. During this rest period, adjustments in inotropic therapy, ventilation, and rhythm can be instituted.

Optimization of acid-base status and hemoglobin concentration should also be performed. Separation from bypass can then be reattempted.

Typical inotropic agents effective in this setting are those with high degrees of beta-adrenegic potency. Commonly employed agents include dobutamine, epinephrine, and more recently, the phosphodiesterase-III inhibitors (PDI-III) amrinone and milrinone. It is not uncommon to require the administration of alpha-agonists to counteract the systemic vasodilating effects of prostaglandin E_1 and the PDI-III agents. Selective pulmonary vasodilating action and systemic vasoconstricting effects can often be achieved by administration of pulmonary vasodilating agents such as prostaglandin E_1 via the right-sided access (CVP or PA catheter) and infusion of the alpha-agonists via the left atrial line. Thus, the vasoconstriction of the pulmonary arterial bed can be minimized.

Nitric oxide (NO) is a potent, inhaled pulmonary vasodilator. Its half-life in the systemic circulation is extremely short, permitting its administration with minimal systemic hypotensive effects. In fact, NO can selectively and effectively dilate the pulmonary vasculature. The exact method of delivery and scavenging of waste gases remain as obstacles to its clinical application.

Body SC, Hartigan PM, Shernan SK et al: Nitric oxide: Delivery, measurement, and clinical application. J Cardiothorac Vasc Anesth 9:748–763, 1995

Kieler-Jensen N, Houltz E, Ricksten SE: A comparison of prostacyclin and sodium nitroprusside for the treatment of heart failure after cardiac surgery. J Cardiothorac Vasc Anesth 9:641–646, 1995

C.11. What role does an intraaortic balloon pump (IABP) have in this setting?

An IABP may be useful because unlike any pharmacologic maneuver, it is capable of increasing diastolic pressure critical for coronary perfusion while simultaneously lowering afterload to systolic LV ejection. Myocardial dysfunction secondary to inadequate protection during bypass can be reduced by decreased afterload and augmentation of diastolic pressures through counterpulsation.

C.12. How does it work to benefit the failing heart?

An IABP is a catheter with a large balloon (40 to 60 cc) at its tip. It is positioned in the thoracic aorta distal to the left subclavian artery origin and rests proximal to the takeoff of the renal vessels. It is timed to inflate during diastole to increase diastolic perfusion pressure to the coronary arteries and to deflate just prior to systole to decrease afterload, thereby increasing forward cardiac output. It is the unique modality that can improve coronary perfusion pressures while simultaneously reducing myocardial oxygen demand.

Cheung AT, Savino JS, Weiss SJ: Beat-to-beat augmentation of left ventricular function by intraaortic counterpulsation. Anesthesiology 84:545–554, 1996

C.13. How would you properly time its cycle?

Inflation should occur just following the dicrotic notch and deflation should occur prior to the upstroke in the aortic pressure curve. Augmentation in systolic and mean pressures with a reduction in diastolic pressure should follow its proper function.

C.14. What are the contraindications to the use of an IABP?

The most common contraindications are aortic insufficiency and severe aortic disease, either atheromatous, aneurysmal, or a dissection. Although often listed as absolute contraindications, there are reports of the effective use of IABP in these settings.

Sanfelippo PM, Baker NH, Ewy HG et al: Experience with intraaortic balloon counterpulsation. Ann Thorac Surg 41:36–41, 1986

D. Postoperative Management

D.1. In the intensive care unit 4 hours later, the patient became hypotensive with a low cardiac output. How could you distinguish between cardiac tamponade and pump failure? How would the TEE images differ?

The differentiation between cardiac tamponade and primary pump failure in the immediate postbypass-ICU setting can be difficult. Elevations in filling pressures, systemic hypotension, and low cardiac output are consistent with both diagnoses. The classic teaching of equalization of cardiac pressures seen in a fluid tamponade may not be present because areas of focal compression from clot can markedly reduce filling of only one chamber. Echocardiography can be beneficial in this setting by permitting visualization of chamber volume and function. The transesophageal approach has particular advantage over transthoracic echocardiography in the postoperative setting where the usual transthoracic windows may be obscured by dressings and drainage tubing. Focal compression of the cardiac chambers from a clot or pericardial effusion can readily be distinguished from a volume overloaded, failing heart with poor myocardial contractility. When the diagnosis is not clear, however, surgical reexploration may be indicated.

Bommer WJ, Follette D, Pollock M et al: Tamponade in patients undergoing cardiac surgery: A clinical-echocardiographic diagnosis. Am Heart J 130:1216–1223, 1995

D.2. Would you extubate this patient early in the intensive care unit? Why?

No. This patient has undergone a double valve replacement. In this more complex procedure, coagulopathy and postoperative bleeding, hypothermia from incomplete and nonuniform rewarming, and pulmonary hypertension are not uncommon occurrences in the immediate postoperative period. Sedation, paralysis, and mechanical ventilation can reduce the oxygen requirements during this early phase of recovery, minimize pulmonary hypertension secondary to hypercarbia, and permit reestablishment of core temperatures.

Cheng DCH: Pro: Early extubation after cardiac surgery decreases intensive care unit stay and cost. J Cardiothorac Vasc Anesth 9:460–464, 1995

Guenther CR: Con: Early extubation after cardiac surgery decreases intensive care unit stay and cost. J Cardiothorac Vasc Anesth 9:465–467, 1995

D.3. What are the advantages and disadvantages of early extubation?

The advantages of early extubation are both medical and financial. Early extubation can lessen the adverse sequelae from prolonged endotracheal intubation including epithelial damage, decreased ciliary motility, and diminished mobilization of secretions. Positive-pressure ventilation can have adverse effects on venous return. However, the overwhelming drive toward early extubation is cost. Early extubation can decrease cost by decreasing ICU staff requirements, decreasing the cost of sedatives, lessening the duration of ICU stays, and improving operating room utilization by lessening cancellation of cases secondary to blocked ICU beds.

The potential advantages of early extubation, both financial and physiologic, must be weighed against the potential disadvantages of early extubation. The potential for respiratory compromise leading to hypoxemia, hypercarbia, ischemia, and the potential for infarction and neurologic injury is real. Any savings realized from early extubation can be rapidly lost by one adverse event. Success relies on careful integration of all players in the care of the cardiac surgery patient, from the management of intraoperative anesthetic techniques, to the organization of the ICU and staff, and the provision of postoperative analgesia. Equally important to the success of an early extubation program is appropriate patient selection.

Cheng DCH: Pro: Early extubation after cardiac surgery decreases intensive care unit stay and cost. J Cardiothorac Vasc Anesth 9:460–464, 1995

Guenther CR: Con: Early extubation after cardiac surgery decreases intensive care unit stay and cost. J Cardiothorac Vasc Anesth 9:465–467, 1995

9 Tetralogy of Fallot

Marjorie J. Topkins

A 10-month-old girl was admitted to the hospital for cardiac catheterization. Her history included cyanosis noted at about 6 weeks of age, increasing over the past 7 months and becoming more severe with crying or physical activity. A presumptive diagnosis of Tetralogy of Fallot was made on admission.

A. Medical Disease and Differential Diagnosis

1. What is Tetralogy of Fallot (TOF)?
2. What other conditions might produce cyanosis in the first year of life?
3. Describe the pathophysiology of TOF.
4. What is the natural history of the disease?
5. What are the variables in TOF? How do they affect outcome?
6. What is a "pink tet"?
7. What is a "tet spell"?
8. How do you manage "tet spells"?
9. What techniques or surgical procedures are available for treating this patient?
10. What are some of the reasons for palliative shunting as opposed to definitive correction? When should a definitive correction be considered?
11. What definitive correction is used for TOF? What parts of the tetrad are involved in the repair?

B. Preoperative Evaluation and Preparation

1. What preoperative information or preparation do you want?
2. What premedication do you want given to the patient?
3. Discuss preoperative antibiotics.

C. Intraoperative Management

1. What emergency drugs will you prepare?
2. What monitoring will be needed for a palliative shunt?
3. How will monitoring differ for a definitive correction?
4. How will you anesthetize this patient for a shunt procedure?
5. What is the effect of each of these drugs on pulmonary vascular resistance (PVR): barbiturates, ketamine, narcotics, halothane, isoflurane, and nitrous oxide?
6. How would you manage this patient undergoing definitive correction?
7. How are "tet spells" managed during anesthesia?
8. Discuss fluid replacement in a patient undergoing a palliative shunt and in a patient undergoing a definitive correction.
9. Discuss blood replacement.
10. What is monitored during cardiopulmonary bypass?

11. What is measured after separation from cardiopulmonary bypass? Why?
12. How is heparin reversed?
13. What is a protamine reaction?
14. Discuss inotropic support following definitive correction of TOF.

D. Postoperative Management

1. Discuss postoperative ventilation.
2. What are the requirements for early extubation in a shunt procedure?
3. Discuss postoperative complications in a shunt procedure and in a definitive correction.
4. If this patient were brought to the hospital for an emergency noncardiac procedure, how would you manage the anesthesia?
5. What problems would you anticipate?

A. Medical Disease and Differential Diagnosis

A.1. What is Tetralogy of Fallot (TOF)?

Tetralogy of Fallot describes a complex malformation of the heart having the following components (Fig. 9-1):

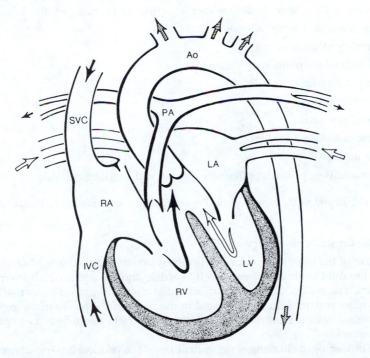

Figure 9-1. Tetralogy of Fallot. (Reprinted with permission from Moller DH, Neal WA, Hoffman WR [eds.]: A Parent's Guide to Heart Disorders, p 44. Minneapolis, University of Minnesota Press, 1988)

Large ventricular septal defect (VSD)

Right ventricular outflow obstruction

Overriding aorta

Right ventricular hypertrophy

The VSD is high, large, and subaortic.

The right ventricular outflow obstruction is usually subvalvular and muscular but may also involve the pulmonary valve, the annulus, the main pulmonary artery, or the right and/or left pulmonary arteries.

The overriding aorta is an essential component of the anomaly.

The right ventricular hypertrophy is compensatory.

Freedom RM, Benson LN, Smallhorn JF (eds): Neonatal Heart Disease, pp 214, 215. London, Springer-Verlag, 1992

Fyler DC (ed): Nadas' Pediatric Cardiology, pp 471–473. Philadelphia, Hanley & Belfus, 1992

A.2. What other conditions might produce cyanosis in the first year of life?

Any condition that results in right-to-left shunting will produce cyanosis. In the first year of life only transposition of the great arteries occurs with a frequency equal to or greater than TOF, but this condition frequently requires intervention in the first few days of life. Other conditions that will produce cyanosis are the following:

Hypoplastic left heart syndrome

Pulmonary stenosis or atresia

Total anomalous pulmonary venous return

Tricuspid atresia

Single ventricle

Truncus arteriosus

Double-outlet right ventricle

Single atrium

In addition, primary pulmonary disease will produce cyanosis.

Fyler DC: Report of the New England Regional Infant Cardiac Program. Pediatrics 65:375–461, 1980

A.3. Describe the pathophysiology of TOF.

Because of the right ventricular outflow obstruction and the large VSD, blood ejected from the right ventricle enters the left ventricle and the aorta, which overrides the septum. The resultant increase in desaturated circulating blood gives rise to the cyanosis most apparent circumorally and in the nail beds. Pressure in the right ventricle is systemic or near systemic. Hypertrophy of the right ventricle is a compensatory mechanism.

The degree of shunting is dependent upon the relationship of pulmonary vascular resistance and systemic vascular resistance. The degree of right ventricular outflow obstruction is relatively fixed but may increase as a result of activity. Systemic vascular resistance is variable.

Garson A, Bricker JT, McNamara DC (eds): The Science and Practice of Pediatric Cardiology, pp 1078–1079. Philadelphia, Lea & Febiger, 1990

A.4. What is the natural history of the disease?

Without treatment, 25% of infants with TOF and pulmonary stenosis die in the first year; 40% will die by the age of 4 years, 70% by 10 years, and 95% by 40 years. The newborn may not exhibit cyanosis until closure of the ductus arteriosus occurs or hypertrophy or spasms of the infundibulum increase. The former decreases flow to the lungs; the latter increases the right ventricular outflow obstruction and therefore the right-to-left shunt. Increasing obstruction and shunting result in compensatory polycythemia. The increased total hemoglobin and increased desaturated hemoglobin result in greater observable cyanosis. If the condition remains uncorrected, the polycythemia increases with age; clubbing of the digits occurs; pulmonary, renal, and cerebral arterial thromboses occur; and cerebral abscesses are a terminal event. Cardiomyopathy secondary to right ventricular hypertrophy, hypoxia, and aortic valve insufficiency with chronic failure are responsible for late deaths. Not until the hematocrit exceeds 65% does hyperviscosity produce problems.

Lake CL (ed): Pediatric Cardiac Anesthesia, 3rd ed, pp 305–306. Stamford, CT, Appleton & Lange, 1998

Moller JH, Neal WA (eds): Fetal, Neonatal and Infant Cardiac Disease, pp 639–640. Norwalk, CT, Appleton & Lange, 1990

A.5. What are the variables in TOF? How do they affect outcome?

The most significant variable is the degree of right ventricular outflow obstruction. This obstruction may involve the infundibulum, the pulmonary valve, the pulmonary annulus, the main pulmonary artery, the right or left pulmonary arteries, or even the distal branches.

The second variable is the nature of the VSD. If the VSD is restrictive and the degree of outflow obstruction is not too severe, the outcome is better. Other variables include the relationship between systemic vascular resistance and pulmonary vascular resistance. As pulmonary vascular resistance increases or systemic vascular resistance decreases, shunting will increase.

Garson A, Bricker JT, McNamara DG (eds): The Science and Practice of Pediatric Cardiology, pp 1070–1074. Philadelphia, Lea & Febiger, 1990

Lake CL (ed): Pediatric Cardiac Anesthesia, 3rd ed, pp 303–305. Stamford, CT, Appleton & Lange, 1998

A.6. What is a "pink tet"?

A "pink tet" is a patient with tetralogy of Fallot, but with a large pulmonary blood flow secondary to naturally occurring large collateral circulation. One major source is a patent ductus arteriosus. Aortopulmonary collateral arteries are another, and finally there can be blood flow from acquired collateral arteries that originate from bronchial arteries, intercostal arteries, and coronary arteries.

More important in the physiology of the "pink tet" or the acyanotic "tet" is the presence of a balanced left-to-right and right-to-left shunt. In this case the obstruction to pulmonary flow is minimal. With time, however, acyanotic TOF becomes cyanotic, usually by 1 to 2 years of age.

Garson A, Bricker JT, McNamara DG (eds): The Science and Practice of Pediatric Cardiology, pp 1071, 1074–1075. Philadelphia, Lea & Febiger, 1990

Park MK: Pediatric Cardiology for Practitioners, 3rd ed, p 120. St. Louis, Mosby, 1996

A.7. What is a "tet spell"?

"Tet spells" occur in 20% to 70% of patients; they are periods of paroxysmal hypoxemia or hypercyanosis. They may be initiated by feeding, crying, or defecating. These activities result in an increase in oxygen demand, a decrease in PaO_2 and pH, an increase in $PaCO_2$, and a decrease in systemic vascular resistance resulting in increased right-to-left shunting. Another suggested mechanism is spasm or increased reactivity of the infundibulum resulting in increased resistance to right ventricular outflow and increased shunting. The incidence of "tet spells" peaks at 2 to 3 to 6 months of age. Other names for "tet spell" include paroxysmal dyspnea, hyperpnea, or hypoxic spell. By 2 to 3 years of age "tet spells" decrease in frequency and severity spontaneously.

Fyler DC (ed): Nadas' Pediatric Cardiology, pp 474–475. Philadelphia, Hanley & Belfus, 1992

Gregory GA (ed): Pediatric Anesthesia, 3rd ed, pp 501–502. New York, Churchill-Livingstone, 1994

Kambam J (ed): Cardiac Anesthesia for Infants and Children, p 219. St Louis, Mosby, 1994

Lake CL (ed): Pediatric Cardiac Anesthesia, 3rd ed, p 305. Stamford, CT, Appleton & Lange, 1998

Park MK (ed): Pediatric Cardiology for Practitioners, 3rd ed, pp 122–123. St. Louis, Mosby, 1996

A.8. How do you manage "tet spells"?

Sodium bicarbonate is given to treat the metabolic acidosis, phenylephrine to increase the systemic vascular resistance, and propranolol is used to decrease the spasm and hypercontractility of the infundibulum. Morphine is useful for its central effect, reducing the hyperpneic response.

Older children are noted to squat during these episodes. The squatting decreases venous return from the legs and increases systemic vascular resistance; both decrease the shunt.

Lake CL (ed): Pediatric Cardiac Anesthesia, 3rd ed, p 305. Stamford, CT, Appleton & Lange, 1998

Park MK (ed): Pediatric Cardiology for Practitioners, 3rd ed, pp 195–196. St. Louis, Mosby, 1996

A.9. What techniques or surgical procedures are available for treating this patient?

Corrective procedures may be palliative or definitive. Palliative procedures include the following:

Balloon dilatation, usually performed during catheterization.

Shunts—creation of systemic to pulmonary artery shunts. These shunts include the classic Blalock-Taussig shunt, subclavian artery to pulmonary artery most commonly on the right, but, if necessary, additionally on the left. The classic shunt is an end-to--

side anastomosis of subclavian artery to pulmonary artery. A modification of the Blalock-Taussig shunt utilizes a tubed Gore-Tex graft between the subclavian artery and the pulmonary artery. Other shunts include the following:

Glenn shunt—superior vena cava to right pulmonary artery

Waterston shunt—ascending aorta to right pulmonary artery

Potts shunt—descending aorta to left pulmonary artery

Central (aortic-pulmonary) shunt—aorta to pulmonary artery with a tube graft

Lake CL (ed): Pediatric Cardiac Anesthesia, 3rd ed, pp 309–310. Stamford, CT, Appleton & Lange, 1998

Moller JH, Neal WA (eds): Fetal, Neonatal and Infant Cardiac Disease, p 653. Norwalk, CT, Appleton & Lange, 1990

A.10. What are some of the reasons for palliative shunting as opposed to definitive correction? When should a definitive correction be considered?

Shunts permit improved blood flow and oxygenation until the infant is larger, stronger, and more capable of withstanding the "open" definitive correction. Similarly, when the pulmonary arteries are small, the increased flow provided by the shunt may enlarge these arteries. When there is atresia of the pulmonary artery, a temporary shunt may permit the infant to grow large enough before a definitive correction such as the Rastelli procedure (right ventricle to distal pulmonary artery) is undertaken.

A successful shunt may become inadequate as the patient grows. A rising hematocrit and increasing symptoms indicate the need for a definitive correction or a second shunt if correction is not feasible. Cardiac catheterization and echocardiography will help to define the possibilities.

Moller JH, Neal WA (eds): Fetal, Neonatal and Infant Cardiac Disease, pp 652, 653, 655. Norwalk, CT, Appleton & Lange, 1990

A.11. What definitive correction is used for TOF? What parts of the tetrad are involved in the repair?

Correction includes dismantling any prior shunt, patch closure of the VSD, excising infundibular bundles of muscle, and, if necessary, patching the outflow tract with pericardium. The patch may include the outflow tract, pulmonary valve annulus, the main pulmonary artery, and even the right or left pulmonary arteries. Nothing is done to the overriding aorta. The patch closure of the VSD effectively places the aorta functionally in the left ventricle. Nothing can be done about the right ventricular hypertrophy. If the correction is adequate, the previous systemic pressure in the right ventricle will be decreased by half and the right ventricular hypertrophy will decrease over time. Definitive correction of TOF requires cardiopulmonary bypass.

In approximately 8% of patients the anterior descending coronary artery will arise from the right coronary artery. The location of this artery will alter the ventriculotomy site and in some cases preclude the conventional repair and outflow tract patch. In this extreme case an external conduit from the right ventricle to the pulmonary artery will be required.

Hensley FA, Martin DE (eds): A Practical Approach to Cardiac Anesthesia, 2nd ed, p 348. Boston, Little, Brown, 1995

Lake CL (ed): Pediatric Cardiac Anesthesia, 3rd ed, p 310. Stamford, CT, Appleton & Lange, 1998

Schwartz SI, Shires GT, Spenser FC (eds): Principles of Surgery, 5th ed, pp 814–817. New York, McGraw-Hill, 1989

B. Preoperative Evaluation and Preparation

B.1. What preoperative information or preparation do you want?

A complete history and physical examination, including laboratory data, is essential. Knowledge of the frequency, severity, duration, and therapy of "tet spells" and the hematocrit is essential. In older children with very high hematocrits, phlebotomy in the operating room with autologous blood to be given at the termination of surgery should be considered. Knowledge of the medication the patient is receiving and its effects is imperative. Knowledge of allergies, especially to medications, is also needed. With older children, the presence of loose deciduous teeth should be evaluated.

The chest x-ray will demonstrate the large hypertrophied right ventricle and the concave pulmonary artery segment, a boot-shaped heart.

The existence of other congenital anomalies is important. The most commonly associated anomalies are patent ductus arteriosus (4%), multiple VSDs (2.4%), complete arteriovenous canal (2.2%), and partial anomalous pulmonary venous return (1%). Atrial septal defect occurs in approximately 9% of patients and persistent left superior vena cava in 8%.

Cardiac catheterization will provide information on peripheral oxygen saturation; knowledge of the pulmonary vascular resistance before and after administration of nitroglycerin, oxygen, or tolazoline will demonstrate whether the resistance is reactive or fixed. The ratio of pulmonary blood flow (Q_p) to systemic blood flow (Q_s) will give some evidence of the degree of shunting and the degree of pulmonary outflow obstruction. The systolic pressure gradient across the pulmonary valve will be useful in evaluating the repair. The pressures in the right ventricle usually equal the pressures in the left ventricle. Angiography will demonstrate the areas of outflow obstruction, other anomalies, the number of VSDs, collateral circulation, and in older patients, the presence of tricuspid regurgitation or aortic regurgitation.

Hensley FA Jr, Martin DE (eds): A Practical Approach to Cardiac Anesthesia, 2nd ed, pp 335–349. Boston, Little, Brown, 1995

Lake CL (ed): Pediatric Cardiac Anesthesia, 3rd ed, pp 307–308. Stamford, CT, Appleton & Lange, 1998

B.2. What premedication do you want given to the patient?

Premedication is generally heavy, with pentobarbital, 5 mg/kg IM, and morphine sulphate, 0.1 mg/kg IM. If an intravenous infusion is present, pentobarbital, 2 to 3 mg/kg, and morphine, 0.05 mg/kg, can be given intravenously. An anticholinergic drug is needed to prevent the bradycardia of anesthestic induction. It can be given prior to induction at 0.01 to 0.015 mg/kg. If the infant is medicated with propranolol, this should be continued up to and including the day of surgery.

Gregory GA (ed): Pediatric Anesthesia, 3rd ed, p 193. New York, Churchill Livingstone, 1994

Hensley FA, Martin DE (eds): A Practical Approach to Cardiac Anesthesia, 2nd ed, p 349. Boston, Little, Brown, 1995

Kambam J (ed): Cardiac Anesthesia for Infants and Children, pp 92–108. St. Louis, Mosby, 1994

Lake CL (ed): Pediatric Cardiac Anesthesia, 3rd ed, pp 307–308. Stamford, CT, Appleton & Lange, 1998

B.3. Discuss preoperative antibiotics.

Antibiotics should be given intravenously (IV) at the time of premedication. If there is no known allergy, cefazolin, 25 mg/kg, can be given intravenously. If it is not given prior to induction, it should be given as soon as an IV route is established. This dose will be repeated after termination of cardiopulmonary bypass.

There is a 10% crossover reaction to cefazolin (cephalosporins) in patients who are allergic to penicillin. If a patient is allergic to cephalosporins or to penicillin, vancomycin can be given. The usual dose is 20 mg/kg IV given very slowly over 1 hour. This dose will be repeated after termination of cardiopulmonary bypass.

Gregory GA (ed): Pediatric Anesthesia, 3rd ed, pp 182–184, 187, 876–877. New York, Churchill Livingstone, 1994

Lake CL (ed): Pediatric Cardiac Anesthesia, 3rd ed, p 308. Stamford, CT, Appleton & Lange, 1998

The New York Hospital Protocol

C. Intraoperative Management

C.1. What emergency drugs will you prepare?

Epinephrine, atropine, sodium bicarbonate, lidocaine, and calcium chloride are the commonly used emergency drugs in the pediatric patient. In TOF phenylephrine and propranolol should be available to treat "tet spells." In addition, infusions for inotropic support after bypass should be prepared or readily available. Dopamine, epinephrine, and isoproterenol are useful in this situation. These patients come to the operating room with a computerized form giving drugs, range of dosage, and standard concentration. Thus all medication is standardized when the patient is transported back to the pediatric intensive care unit. The following concentrations and dosages are used (see also Table 9-1):

Drug	Dose	Route
Epinephrine, 1:10,000 (100 μg/ml)	10 μg/kg	IV, IT
Atropine, 1 mg diluted to 10 ml	10 μg/kg	IV, IM, IT
Sodium bicarbonate, 1 mEq/ml	1 mEq/kg	IV
Lidocaine, 20 mg/ml	1 mg/kg	IV, IT
Calcium chloride, 100 mg/ml	20 mg/kg	IV
Phenylephrine diluted to 0.1 mg/ml (100 μg/ml)	50-μg bolus	IV
Propranolol diluted to 0.1 mg/ml	0.2 mg/kg	IV

IM, intramuscular; IT, intrathecal; IV, intravenous

Table 9.1. Preparation and Dosage of Pediatric Resuscitation Drugs at the New York Hospital

	DOSE–ml/kg [MAX. 50 kgs]		PATIENT DOSE	
IV PUSH RESUSCITATION DRUGS [CONCENTRATION]				
Epinephrine 1:10,000 (100 μg/cc)	0.1 cc	× _____ kgs =	_____ cc (10 μg/kg)	
Atropine (0.1 mg/cc) [min. dose 1.5 cc (0.15 mg); max. dose 10 cc (1 mg)]	0.1 cc	× _____ kgs =	_____ cc (10 μg/kg)	
Sodium bicarbonate (1 mEq/cc)	1.0 cc	× _____ kgs =	_____ cc (1 mEq/kg)	
Calcium chloride 10% (100 mg/cc)	0.2 cc	× _____ kgs =	_____ cc (20 mg/kg)	
Lidocaine (20 mg/cc)	0.05 cc	× _____ kgs =	_____ cc (1 mg/kg)	
Bretylium (50 mg/cc)	0.1 cc	× _____ kgs =	_____ cc (5 mg/kg)	
Naloxone (0.4 mg/cc) [10 × this dose for Rx of intoxication]	0.25 cc	× _____ kgs =	_____ cc (0.1 mg/kg)	
Dextrose 50% (0.5 g/cc)	1 cc	× _____ kgs =	_____ cc (0.5 g/kg)	
25% (0.25 g/cc)	2 cc	× _____ kgs =	_____ cc	
Diazepam (5 mg/cc)	0.04 cc	× _____ kgs =	_____ cc (0.2 mg/kg)	
DRIPS				
Dopamine, dobutamine	6 mg × _____ kgs = _____ mgs in 100 cc D$_5$W:1 cc/h = 1 μg/kg/min			
Epinephrine, norepinephrine, isoproterenol	0.3 mg × _____ kgs = _____ mgs in 100 cc D$_5$W:1 cc/h = 0.05 μg/kg/min			
Nitroprusside, nitroglycerin	3 mg × _____ kgs = _____ mgs in 100 cc D$_5$W:1 cc/h = 0.5 μg/kg/min			
Lidocaine	60 mg × _____ kgs = _____ mgs in 100 cc D$_5$W:1 cc/h = 10 μg/kg/min			

Infusions

Dopamine or dobutamine, 6 mg/kg in 100 ml D$_5$W:
- 1 ml/h = 1 μg/kg/min
- Dose, 2 to 20 μg/kg/min

Epinephrine or norepinephrine, 0.3 mg/kg in 100 ml D$_5$W:
- 1 ml/h = 0.05 μg/kg/min
- Dose, 0.1 to 1.0 μg/kg/min

Isoproterenol, 0.3 mg/kg in 100 ml D$_5$W:
- ml/h = 0.05 μg/kg/min
- Dose, 0.1 to 1.0 μg/kg/min

Lidocaine, 60 mg/kg in 100 ml D$_5$W:
- 1 ml/h = 10 μg/kg/min
- Dose, 20 to 50 μg/kg/min

Nitroprusside or nitroglycerin, 3 mg/kg in 100 ml D$_5$W:
- 1 ml/h = 0.5 μg/kg/min
- Dose, 0.2 to 5.0 μg/kg/min

Gregory GA (ed): Pediatric Anesthesia, 3rd ed, p 841. New York, Churchill Livingstone, 1994
Lake CL (ed): Pediatric Cardiac Anesthesia, 2nd ed, p 217. Norwalk CT, Appleton & Lange, 1993
The New York Hospital Protocol

C.2. What monitoring will be needed for a palliative shunt?

ECG.

Precordial stethoscope.

Pulse oximetry. Care must be taken to avoid placing the pulse oximeter on an extremity that is to be involved in the shunt or that might have been involved in a prior shunt. Occasionally two sites are used, one on an upper extremity and one on a lower extremity.

Blood pressure and pulse. Blood pressure may be taken with the automated blood pressure apparatus until the induction is completed and intubation accomplished. At this point, an intraarterial catheter is inserted (for young infants and children, a 22-gauge intraarterial catheter is used). Again, selection of a site for the arterial line should take into account the planned shunt or prior shunts. The intraarterial catheter will be used for continuous pressure and arterial blood sampling.

End-tidal carbon dioxide for managing ventilation.

Rectal and esophageal temperature.

Urine output.

At least one large-bore peripheral intravenous route is established after induction.

Gregory GA (ed): Pediatric Anesthesia, 3rd ed, pp 465–477, 852–853, 862. New York, Churchill Livingstone, 1994

Kambam J (ed): Cardiac Anesthesia for Infants and Children, pp 92–108. St. Louis, Mosby, 1994

Lake CL (ed): Pediatric Cardiac Anesthesia, 3rd ed, pp 181–210. Stamford, CT, Appleton & Lange, 1998

C.3. How will monitoring differ for a definitive correction?

All of the above will be used for a definitive correction. In addition, a double-lumen catheter is placed in the right internal jugular vein. One lumen is attached to a transducer for central venous pressure; the other lumen is attached to an intravenous line to be used to administer medications and narcotics. This catheter must be short enough to avoid the right atrium and the superior vena caval cannula inserted by the surgeon as part of the right heart drainage system. If prior catheterization or angiography has demonstrated a persistent left superior vena cava (SVC), a left internal jugular catheter may be required to monitor the adequacy of cerebral drainage from this system. This occurs in approximately 2% to 4.3% of patients with congenital heart anomalies. If the left SVC is obstructed by the right SVC cannula, pressure can rise distal to the occlusion. If the persistent left SVC drains directly into the right heart, the operative field (right atrium and/or right ventricle) will be obscured by this venous return not captured by the caval cannulae. The left SVC may have to be ligated or clamped if this occurs.

Goor DA, Lillehei CW: Congenital Malformations of the Heart, pp 400–404. New York, Grune & Stratton, 1975

Lake CL (ed): Pediatric Cardiac Anesthesia, 3rd ed, pp 181–210. Stamford, CT, Appleton & Lange, 1998

C.4. How will you anesthetize this patient for a shunt procedure?

The rationale for induction in a patient with severe cyanosis is to establish anesthesia without increasing the right-to-left shunt. Agents and techniques that decrease systemic vascular resistance (SVR) are to be avoided, and those that increase pulmonary blood flow by decreasing infundibular reactivity or pulmonary vascular resistance (PVR) are to be utilized.

Hypoxia, hypercarbia, acidosis, atelectasis, hypothermia, elevated airway pressures, pulmonary vasoconstriction, light anesthesia, and polycythemia increase pulmonary vascular resistance. Conversely, high inspired oxygen concentration, hypocarbia, alkalosis, anemia, and fentanyl all decrease pulmonary vascular resistance and therefore increase pulmonary blood flow. On the basis of this list, rapid low pressure ventilation with a high percentage of oxygen (F_1O_2) should be employed. In addition, the level of anesthesia should be moderately deep, but not so deep as to depress the myocardium.

Induction can be accomplished with ketamine IM or IV, halothane and oxygen by inhalation, or barbiturate or fentanyl IV. If an intravenous route is present, ketamine 2 mg/kg IV, barbiturate 3 to 5 mg/kg IV, and/or fentanyl 25 µg/kg IV can be used. In the absence of an intravenous route, intramuscular ketamine, 4 mg/kg, is helpful to avoid a crying, thrashing induction, followed by an inhalation agent and oxygen until an intravenous route is established. If the premedication is adequate and the child is sleeping, a careful inhalation induction can be accomplished once the ECG, pulse oximeter, and blood pressure cuff are in place. The child should be disturbed as little as possible.

When an intravenous infusion is prepared, it is essential to eliminate air bubbles trapped in the line. This is absolutely vital for all right-to-left shunts. Even left-to-right shunts may have elements of a bidirectional shunt; care must be taken with any congenital heart lesion associated with a shunt.

Blood should be available, but it is not anticipated that it will be used or necessary.

Intubation is accomplished with an endotracheal tube, which should not leak at 20 cm H_2O when the patient is curarized. Ventilation in our institution is accomplished using the Ohio Ventilator 7000 with a pediatric bellows and lightweight pediatric plastic tubing. Others recommend the Bains system, which has no valves and therefore little resistance.

Anesthetic maintenance can include halothane and oxygen, isoflurane and oxygen, or fentanyl and oxygen with or without small amounts of halothane or isoflurane.

Succinylcholine preceded by atropine, 0.015 to 0.020 mg/kg (0.03 mg/kg is the vagolytic dose in infants), can be used for intubation. The dosage of succinylcholine is 1 mg/kg IV. Similarly, vecuronium can be used without significant evidence of cardiovascular effects or histamine release. For intubation, the dosage is 0.1 mg/kg; for maintenance, 0.05 mg/kg. Pancuronium shows little vagolytic effect in infants but raises the pulse and blood pressure in children. The maintenance dose is 0.10 mg/kg.

Gregory GA (ed): Pediatric Anesthesia, 3rd ed, pp 486–490. New York, Churchill Livingstone, 1994

Hensley FA Jr, Martin DE (eds): A Practical Approach to Cardiac Anesthesia, 2nd ed, p 346. Boston, Little, Brown, 1995

Lake CL (ed): Pediatric Cardiac Anesthesia, 3rd ed, pp 307–308. Stamford, CT, Appleton & Lange, 1998

C.5. What is the effect of each of these drugs on pulmonary vascular resistance (PVR): barbiturates, ketamine, narcotics, halothane, isoflurane, and nitrous oxide?

Barbiturates show no specific beneficial effect on pulmonary vascular resistance. The effect on PVR is the same as the effect on systemic vascular resistance (SVR): both systems are dilated.

Ketamine does not increase PVR if $PaCO_2$ and PaO_2 are maintained in normal range.

Fentanyl and other narcotics have little effect on pulmonary artery pressure (PAP) and PVR. They probably blunt the sympathetically mediated pulmonary hypertensive response.

Halothane and isoflurane: there are conflicting reports on the effects of the volatile anesthetic agents on hypoxic pulmonary vasoconstriction (HPV). Isoflurane and halothane *in vitro* both inhibit HPV. The inhibition of HPV is dose related. However, in intact animal preparations under clinical concentrations of potent inhalation anesthetics, some biologic or physiologic property seems to abolish or greatly decrease the inhibitory effect of inhalation anesthetics on HPV. These volatile agents have little effect on PVR or PAP in the presence of normal $PaCO_2$ and PaO_2 and if there are no concomitant falls in cardiac output, SVR, and myocardial contractility.

Nitrous oxide may increase PVR and probably should be avoided.

Lake CL (ed): Pediatric Cardiac Anesthesia, 3rd ed, pp 131–140. Stamford, CT, Appleton & Lange, 1998

Miller RD (ed): Anesthesia, 4th ed, pp 1678–1681. New York, Churchill Livingstone, 1994

Rogers SN, Benumof JL: Halothane and isoflurane do not decrease PaO_2 during one-lung ventilation in intravenously anesthetized patients. Anesth Analg 64:946–954, 1985

C.6. How would you manage this patient undergoing definitive correction?

Management is essentially the same as for shunt procedure.

The anesthetic agent for induction can be ketamine, 4 mg/kg IM or 2 mg/kg IV. Halothane and oxygen plus a muscle relaxant can be used. If blood pressure decreases, shunting may increase. The pressure will respond to a decrease in anesthetic agent and a peripheral vasoconstrictor such as phenylephrine which is essentially pure alpha in its effect. Maintenance is with fentanyl, 10 to 30 μg/kg, or sufentanil, 2 to 5 μg/kg, plus inhalation agents.

The major difference between shunting procedures and definitive correction is the requirement of cardiopulmonary bypass to accomplish the correction. Monitoring is established as in question C.2. The patient is anticoagulated with heparin, 200 to 300 units/kg. Activated clotting time (ACT) should exceed 400 to 480 seconds before the patient is placed on cardiopulmonary bypass. Heparin is usually given by the surgeon into the right atrium. However, in some cases supplemental heparin is needed and is given by the anesthesiologist into the central line. Some surgeons request that the entire dose be given by the anesthesiologist.

Intravenous narcotics and pancuronium with or without diazepam can be used during bypass. Sodium thiopental can be used in place of diazepam at doses of 2 to 5 mg/kg. The hemodilutional effect of cardiopulmonary bypass will reduce the hematocrit, which should not be allowed to go below 20%. Hypothermia is usually induced to a level of approximately 25° to 28°C. Cardioplegia is given to arrest the heart and for myocardial preservation. Any prior shunt is dissected prior to going on cardiopulmonary bypass and must be clamped after going on bypass before any repair is begun. After correction of the defects, the heart is closed. Careful attention to removing residual air in the heart is the final surgical maneuver, which is accomplished with the patient in steep Trendelenburg position.

In our institution there is no attempt at separation from cardiopulmonary bypass until the rectal temperature is 36°C.

Inotropic support, if necessary, is epinephrine 0.05 to 0.10 µg/kg/min, dopamine 5 to 15 µg/kg/min, and, rarely, isoproterenol 0.05 to 0.1 µg/kg/min.

Gregory GA (ed): Pediatric Anesthesia, 3rd ed, pp 486–490. New York, Churchill Livingstone, 1994

Henley FA Jr, Martin DE (eds): A Practical Approach to Cardiac Anesthesia, 2nd ed, pp 348–350. Boston, Little, Brown, 1995

Kambam J (ed): Cardiac Anesthesia for Infants and Children, pp 223–227. St. Louis, Mosby, 1994

Lake CL (ed): Pediatric Cardiac Anesthesia, 3rd ed. pp 308–309. Stamford, CT, Appleton & Lange, 1998

C.7. How are "tet spells" managed during anesthesia?

"Tet spells" are less common during anesthesia if adequate depths are maintained and systemic blood pressure does not drop excessively. They can be recognized by profound cyanosis, usually of rapid onset heralded by the pulse oximeter, and subsequent bradycardia and hypotension.

Treatment consists of rapid low-pressure ventilation with oxygen, concomitant vasoconstriction with phenylephrine, 5 to 10 µg/kg IV, and propranolol, 0.05 to 0.1 mg/kg, to decrease infundibular reactivity. Treatment with sodium bicarbonate, 1 mEq/kg, should be considered since metabolic acidosis ensues quickly.

Katz J, Steward DJ (eds): Anesthesia and Uncommon Pediatric Diseases, p 108. Philadelphia, WB Saunders, 1987

Lake CL (ed): Pediatric Cardiac Anesthesia, 3rd ed, p 305. Stamford, CT, Appleton & Lange, 1998

C.8. Discuss fluid replacement in a patient undergoing a palliative shunt and in a patient undergoing a definitive correction.

Fluid replacement should be 1 to 1½ maintenance levels of 4 cc/kg/h. If an intravenous route was established the night prior to surgery, there should be no fluid deficit. An elevated hematocrit requires greater-than-maintenance fluid replacement. Blood loss can be replaced milliliter for milliliter using either Ringer's lactate solution or dextrose, 5% in ¼ normal saline. During a definitive corrective procedure, maintenance fluid replacement will be sufficient unless the hematocrit is very high. Adequate hemodilution is usually accomplished during cardiopulmonary bypass.

Patients who are very polycythemic should undergo hemodilution to a hematocrit of 55% to 60% prior to surgery. This improves cardiac output and peripheral perfusion.

Gregory GA (ed): Pediatric Anesthesia, 3rd ed, p 481. New York, Churchill Livingstone, 1994

Henley FA, Martin DE (eds): The Practice of Cardiac Anesthesia, p 402. Boston, Little, Brown, 1990

Katz J, Steward DJ (eds): Anesthesia and Uncommon Pediatric Diseases, p 106. Philadelphia, WB Saunders, 1987

C.9. Discuss blood replacement.

Rarely is blood required for a shunt procedure. However, blood is usually a component of the prime in the oxygenator during definitive correction. This is particularly true in very small patients, where the prime volume constitutes a very large dilutional volume relative to the patient's blood volume.

A fresh warm unit of compatible blood drawn the morning of surgery should be available following reversal of heparin with protamine. This provides the clotting factors and platelets that have been diminished or destroyed during cardiopulmonary bypass.

Gregory GA (ed): Pediatric Anesthesia, 3rd ed, p 491. New York, Churchill Livingstone, 1994

New York Hospital Protocol

C.10. What is monitored during cardiopulmonary bypass?

The perfusion pressure, blood gases, mixed venous oxygen saturation, urine output, temperature, and activated clotting times are measured.

Acceptable perfusion pressures are lower than those in adults. Levels of 30 to 50 mm Hg are satisfactory. Blood flow rates, however, are much higher than those in adults. Neonates require flows of 150 to 175 ml/kg. In older infants and young children flow rates are approximately 100 ml/kg.

A blood gas (arterial) is taken shortly after going on cardiopulmonary bypass and repeated approximately every 20 to 30 minutes thereafter. If necessary, the blood gas will be repeated more often, especially if therapeutic measures have been undertaken. The presence of metabolic or respiratory acidosis requires treatment, the former with sodium bicarbonate, the latter by increasing the sweep through the oxygenator. The hematocrit obtained with the blood gas should be corrected if it falls below 20%.

The mixed venous oxygen saturation is measured continually. A falling mixed venous saturation indicates inadequate perfusion.

A urine output of 1 to 2 ml/kg/h is adequate.

Temperature is usually reduced to 25° to 30°C, which is moderate hypothermia. Greater reductions in temperature are used when flow must be reduced because of surgical requirements.

The activated clotting time (ACT) is measured before anticoagulation for a baseline level and again after heparinization to be sure the ACT is 400 to 480 seconds or greater. Additional heparin is added to the pump volume if the ACT falls below 400 seconds.

Gregory GA (ed): Pediatric Anesthesia, 3rd ed, pp 491–492. New York, Churchill Livingstone, 1994

Hensley FA Jr, Martin DE (eds): A Practical Approach to Cardiac Anesthesia, pp 345–346. Boston, Little, Brown, 1995

Lake CL (ed): Pediatric Cardiac Anesthesia, 3rd ed, pp 308–309. Stamford, CT, Appleton & Lange, 1998

C.11. What is measured after separation from cardiopulmonary bypass? Why?

Pressures in the right ventricle and the left ventricle are measured to determine the adequacy of repair. Pressures in the right ventricle should be below 50% of the left ventricle. Also, pressure in the main pulmonary artery should be measured and compared with the preoperative pressure. Failure to obtain a 50% reduction in right ventricular pressure compared with left ventricular pressure (which before surgery were equal) may require going back on cardiopulmonary bypass for further patching of the outflow tract. If pressures are not high enough in the pulmonary artery, return to bypass for further infundibular muscle resection may be needed. Only if the surgeon is sure that there is nothing more he or she can do surgically will he or she accept less than optimal results.

If multiple ventricular septal defects were present, oxygen saturation taken from the pulmonary artery and the right atrium will help determine the adequacy of the septal repair. A major step up in oxygen saturation in the pulmonary artery compared with the oxygen saturation in the right atrium indicates a significant left-to-right shunt. Small differences can be due to patch leak, which decreases with time.

Waldhausen JA, Orringer MB (eds): Complications in Cardiothoracic Surgery, pp 180–184. St. Louis, Mosby-Year Book, 1991

The New York Hospital Protocol

C.12. How is heparin reversed?

Protamine sulfate is given to reverse the heparin. The dose is dependent on the initial dose given plus additional heparin used for any blood placed in the prime. The initial heparin dose is 200 to 300 units/kg. Each unit of blood added to or used in the prime is prepared with 2500 units of heparin plus calcium chloride. In an adult 1 or 2 units of blood added to the prime would add only 25% to the total heparin given to a 70-kg man. To a 7-kg baby this amount of heparin would constitute a 250% increase. Therefore, though we might overlook the heparin used in blood placed in the prime for adults, we must take this into account when calculating the protamine dose for infants and children. Protamine is given in doses of 1 to 1.3 mg/ 100 units of heparin administered, including the heparin used to convert CPD blood for use in the pump. Protamine is placed in a Soluset and administered slowly to avoid a protamine reaction. The adequacy of reversal of heparin effect is checked 5 to 10 minutes after completion of the protamine infusion by means of the ACT, which should return to control levels. If the ACT remains elevated, additional protamine should be given.

Hensley FA Jr, Martin DE (eds): A Practical Approach to Cardiac Anesthesia, 2nd ed, pp 442–443. Boston, Little, Brown, 1995

Lake CL (ed): Pediatric Cardiac Anesthesia, 3rd ed, pp 228–231. Stamford, CT, Appleton & Lange, 1998

C.13. What is a protamine reaction?

Protamine reactions may include hypotension due to myocardial depression, histamine release, and/or peripheral vasodilatation. The pulmonary effects may include increased pulmonary vasoconstriction and bronchospasm. Elevated pressures in the breathing circuit may be the earliest sign of a protamine reaction. Reactions are relatively rare but can be catastrophic.

Kambam J (ed): Cardiac Anesthesia for Infants and Children, pp 137–139. St. Louis, Mosby, 1994

Lake CL (ed): Pediatric Cardiac Anesthesia, p 224. Norwalk CT, Appleton & Lange, 1993

Ullman DA, Bloom BS, Danker PR et al: Protamine induced hypotension in a two year old child. J Cardiothorac Anesth 2:497–499, 1988

C.14. Discuss inotropic support following definitive correction of TOF.

The following agents can be used for their inotropic effects:

- Epinephrine, 0.05 to 0.1 µg/kg/min
- Dopamine, 5 to 15 µg/kg/min
- Isoproterenol, 0.05 to 0.1 µg/kg/min

Isoproterenol is a beta-sympathomimetic agent that decreases both PVR and SVR but increases cardiac output. Epinephrine stimulates both beta-1 and beta-2 receptors. The beta-1 effects increase contractility and heart rate by accelerating the sinoatrial (SA) node and conductivity.

Epinephrine is useful as a bronchodilator; it also inhibits degranulation of mast cells and release of histamine. For this reason it is valuable in treating protamine reactions.

Dopamine is a naturally occurring catacholamine with both dopaminergic effects and beta-adrenergic effects. At low doses, <5 µg/kg/min, dopaminergic effects are produced with dilatation of the renal, splanchnic, coronary and cerebrovascular beds. Maximal dopaminergic effects are seen at infusion rate of 1 to 2 µg/kg/min. The inotropic effects of dopamine occur at doses of 5 to 10 µg/kg/min and are due to beta adrenergic receptor action. Between 10 and 20 µg/min both beta and alpha effects are present and above 20 µg/kg/min almost pure alpha effects are present. The alpha effects result in vasoconstriction and increased systemic vascular resistance.

Gregory GA (ed): Pediatric Anesthesia, 3rd ed, pp 848–850. New York, Churchill-Livingstone, 1994

Lake CL (ed): Pediatric Cardiac Anesthesia, 3rd ed, p 242. Stamford, CT, Appleton & Lang, 1998

Motayama EK (ed): Smith's Anesthesia for Infants and Children, pp 823–825. St. Louis, CV Mosby, 1990

Stephenson LW, Edmunds LH, Raphaely R et al: Effects of nitroprusside and dopamine on pulmonary arterial vasculature in children after cardiac surgery. Circulation 60:2–104, 1979

Williams DB, Kiernan PD, Schoff HV et al: The hemodynamic response to dopamine and nitroprusside following right atrium pulmonary artery bypass (Fontan procedure). Ann Thorac Surg 34:51–57, 1982

D. Postoperative Management

D.1. Discuss postoperative ventilation.

Pulmonary blood flow is augmented by high F_IO_2, P_{CO_2} between 30 to 35 mm Hg, and alkalosis with a pH of 7.50. Controlled ventilation with the lowest possible pressure is needed to obtain the above requirement. No attempt is made to extubate this patient in the operating room following a definitive correction. Following palliative shunting operations, early extubation may be considered, particularly in the older child. Positive-pressure ventilation may inhibit pulmonary blood flow. If controlled ventilation is required, the above conditions should be met.

Mechanical ventilation is not without possible complications. These include decreased venous return, altered pulmonary and systemic vascular pressures and resistance, and ventricular dysfunction. Pulmonary complications include infection, altered ventilation-perfusion ratios, increased dead space, and parenchymal damage. Airway problems include mucosal damage, pressure necrosis, endotracheal tube obstruction, malposition, or inadvertent extubation. Additionally, muscle relaxants and sedation are required to facilitate mechanical ventilation. Mechanical ventilation should therefore be utilized when necessary but with appreciation of the possible consequences of its use. Earlier extubation is the current trend whenever possible.

Gregory GA (ed): Pediatric Anesthesia, 2nd ed, p 835. New York, Churchill Livingstone, 1989

Heard CC, Lamberti JT, Park SM et al: Extubation after surgical repair of congenital heart disease. Crit Care Med 13:830–832, 1985

Lake CL (ed): Pediatric Cardiac Anesthesia, 3rd ed, pp 582, 593–594. Stamford, CT, Appleton & Lange, 1998

Schuller JL, Bovill JG, Nejveld A et al: Extubation of the trachea after open heart surgery for congenital heart disease. Br J Anaesth 56:1101–1108, 1984

D.2. What are the requirements for early extubation in a shunt procedure?

The patient is awake and ventilating on his or her own, and blood gases are normal. The patient must be normothermic. The patient does not require inotropic support. Other factors may play a part in the decision about extubating in the operating room. At the New York Hospital, the pediatric intensive care unit is too distant from the operating room. Therefore, we transport most patients intubated with oxygen, arterial blood pressure, and ECG and defibrillator. Oxygen saturation can also be monitored during transport.

Hensley FA Jr, Martin DE (eds): A Practical Approach to Cardiac Anesthesia, 2nd ed, pp 347–348. Boston, Little, Brown, 1995

Lake CL (ed): Pediatric Cardiac Anesthesia, 3rd ed, p 582. Stamford, CT, Appleton & Lange, 1998

D.3. Discuss postoperative complications in a shunt procedure and in a definitive correction.

The shunt may be too large, resulting in excessive pulmonary blood flow and pulmonary edema. Conversely, the shunt may be too small, offering little improvement in oxygenation. Kinking of the graft may be a problem, and last, a previously functioning shunt can thrombose. All of these will require shunt revision or a new shunt.

Postoperative complications following definitive correction of TOF may be classified as the following:

- Early proximate—those occurring within the postoperative period
- Early delayed—those occurring within the first year after surgery
- Late—those occurring in the long term after surgery

Early proximate complications include the following:

- Low output states
- Residual right ventricular outflow tract obstruction
- Residual ventricular septal defects
- Pulmonary problems
- Coagulopathies

- Heart block and interventricular conduction defects
- Phrenic nerve injury
- Acute renal failure

Early delayed complications include the following:

- Valvular insufficiency
- Residual VSD
- Infection
- Dysrhythmias

Late complications requiring reoperation include the following:

- Residual VSD
- Residual right ventricular outflow tract obstruction
- Valvular insufficiency
- Right ventricular outflow tract aneurysm

In addition, sudden late death is possible.

Low cardiac output states may be due to injury of an anomalous anterior descending coronary artery, persistent VSD, high right ventricular pressure after repair, large persistent aortopulmonary collaterals, and tamponade. Treatment might include digitalizing the patient; electrical pacing; reduction in SVR, if elevated, with nitroglycerine or nitroprusside; and dopamine for inotropic support. Other drugs that might be useful are dobutamine, epinephrine, or isoproterenol.

Residual right ventricular outflow obstruction and residual VSD should be assessed after cardiopulmonary bypass as described in question C.11. Fresh whole blood is administered after protamine to reduce the possibility of coagulopathy. Heart block and conduction defects and other arrhythmias are rare and are usually related to unusual location of the VSD and consequently the conduction system.

Death following repair is approximately 6% to 8% in patients <2 years of age. Of these deaths in the hospital, 50% are due to acute cardiac failure and 25% due to acute or chronic pulmonary dysfunction. One series reported a mortality of <1% for TOF with pulmonary stenosis but 12% for TOF with pulmonary atresia.

The incidence of reoperation (late complications) has been reported to vary from 1.8% to 13.2%. The average of the five series was 5.4%.

Phrenic nerve injury occurs in approximately 2.9% of patients undergoing repair of TOF. In young children and infants this can be a serious complication because of weak intercostal muscles, horizontal rib cage, and recumbent position.

Fallis JC, Filler RM, Lemoine G (eds): Pediatric Thoracic Surgery, pp 215, 216. New York, Elsevier, 1991

Katz J, Steward DJ (eds): Anesthesia and Uncommon Pediatric Diseases, p 107. Philadelphia, WB Saunders, 1987

Waldhausen JA, Orringer MB (eds): Complications in Cardiothoracic Surgery, pp 180–189. St. Louis, Mosby-Year Book, 1991

D.4. If this patient were brought to the hospital for an emergency noncardiac procedure, how would you manage the anesthesia?

The history and physical examination will be very important. Knowledge of the presence, frequency, and severity of "tet spells" is essential. The mode of treating these spells should be known. The hematocrit, the shunt fraction, and the general condition of the patient must be evaluated. If no prior shunt has been established, "tet spells" are present, and the hematocrit is high, the risk is increased. The presence of a functioning shunt improves the risk.

The general principles of management, from premedication through induction, maintenance, and recovery, parallel the management for cardiac surgery. Anything that favors pulmonary blood flow and increases systemic vascular resistance should be utilized.

Monitoring would depend on the duration and magnitude of the surgery. The following would be monitored:

Blood pressure and pulse. If the planned surgery is short, the noninvasive blood pressure (NIBP) monitor will be sufficient. For longer, more extensive procedures, an intraarterial catheter will permit continuous readings as well as the ability to obtain arterial blood gases and hematocrits.

- A precordial or esophageal stethoscope
- Pulse oximetry
- ECG
- End-tidal carbon dioxide
- A large-bore peripheral intravenous route is established
- Temperature—esophageal or rectal

The agents are the same as for a shunt procedure.

The anesthetic technique could be inhalational or intravenous or a combination of both, as described for a shunting or a definitive repair. Ventilation should be accomplished at the lowest possible peak and mean pressures. Positive end-expiratory pressure (PEEP) should be avoided.

Lake CL (ed): Pediatric Anesthesia, 3rd ed. pp 307–308. Stamford, CT, Appleton & Lange, 1998

D.5. What problems would you anticipate?

Unexpected or excessive blood loss will lower the blood pressure and favor increasing the right-to-left shunt. Fluid depletion or a contracted blood volume will increase the viscosity, decrease perfusion, lower blood pressure, and promote right-to-left shunting. Therefore, blood loss must be measured carefully. Fluid therapy should be 1 to 1½ times maintenance.

Lake CL (ed): Pediatric Cardiac Anesthesia, 3rd ed, pp 307–308. Stamford, CT, Appleton & Lange, 1998

Transposition of the Great Arteries

10

Doreen L. Wray Roth

A six-day-old, full-term, 3.3 kg male infant was scheduled for an arterial switch operation. At birth, he was severely cyanotic and underwent a balloon atrial septostomy during cardiac catheterization with improvement noted in his oxygenation. Prostaglandin E_1 had been administered initially but was discontinued after the septostomy. His arterial oxygen saturation was 70%; BP, 60/35 mm Hg; pulse, 145/min; respirations, 46/min; temperature, 37.0°C.

A. Medical Disease and Differential Diagnosis

1. What is transposition of the great arteries (TGA) and how is it diagnosed?
2. Describe the anatomy and classification of TGA.
3. Describe the pattern of blood flow in TGA. What are the potential sites for mixing?
4. What is meant by congenitally corrected transposition?
5. What is the embryologic development of TGA?
6. What is the most common type of TGA? What anomalies are associated with TGA?
7. What is a balloon atrial septostomy and why is it performed?
8. Why did this patient receive prostaglandin E_1 (PGE_1)? What is the dosage range of PGE_1 and what are its side-effects?
9. With complete TGA, if a ventricular or atrial septal defect coexists, what determines the amount of intercirculatory mixing and shunt direction?
10. What determines the arterial oxygen saturation in TGA?
11. Describe the coronary anatomy in TGA. Why is it important in this patient?
12. What is an arterial switch operation (ASO), how is it performed, and what are the complications associated with it? What is the optimal timing for the procedure and why?
13. What other definitive surgical techniques are there for correction of complete TGA? Explain the advantages and disadvantages of each.

B. Preoperative Evaluation and Preparation

1. What preoperative information would you want to know?
2. Why is it important to know the anatomic communication(s) and the amount of mixing?
3. What is important in the preoperative optimization of this patient?
4. What is pulmonary vascular occlusive disease (PVOD) and why is it important?
5. What premedication would you give?

C. Intraoperative Management

1. How would you prepare the operating room?
2. What monitors would you use? Could transesophageal echocardiography (TEE) be used in this infant?

3. What intraoperative laboratory data would you monitor?
4. What emergency drugs would you have available?
5. How would you anesthetize this infant? Discuss the prebypass hemodynamic management of this patient.
6. In general, how does cardiopulmonary bypass (CPB) for infants differ from that used for adults?
7. How is hypothermia classified and how is it accomplished?
8. What is deep hypothermic circulatory arrest (DHCA) and how long can patients tolerate it? What is Q_{10}?
9. What is low-flow cardiopulmonary bypass and is there an advantage to it over DHCA?
10. What are the physiologic changes and potential complications associated with hypothermia?
11. How is rewarming accomplished?
12. Discuss the major issues in successful weaning from CPB. Why is ventilation pattern important postbypass?
13. What are the potential complications observed immediately postbypass?

D. Postoperative Management

1. Discuss postoperative hemodynamic and ventilatory management. When would you plan to extubate this infant?
2. What are the common complications associated with the ASO that are observed in the early postoperative period?
3. What is JET? How is it treated?

A. Medical Disease and Differential Diagnosis

A.1. What is transposition of the great arteries (TGA) and how is it diagnosed?

TGA is a congenital abnormality of the origin of the great arteries which accounts for approximately 5% to 7% of all congenital heart lesions. TGA refers to the anatomic discordance between the ventricles and the great arteries in that the aorta arises from the right ventricle and the pulmonary artery arises from the left ventricle. This results in a parallel circulation of the systemic and pulmonary circuits which is incompatible with life if no mixing of the circulations occurs. TGA has a high mortality rate without intervention: 30% within the first week of life, 45% within the first month, and 90% within the first year. However, developments in medical and surgical interventions over the last two decades have greatly improved survival in these infants. Such interventions include the use of prostaglandin E_1 to maintain ductal patency, balloon atrial septostomy, and early corrective surgical repair rather than multiple palliative procedures. There is a male preponderance of approximately 3 to 1.

The infant with TGA is usually noticed by attentive nursery personnel who observe cyanosis in an otherwise apparently healthy infant. A high index of suspicion is necessary for an early diagnosis. Infants with TGA who have very little or no intracardiac mixing become critically ill within the first few days after birth. However, if there is some mixing, e.g., via a large ventricular septal defect, then cyanosis may be slight and congestive heart failure symptoms may occur over the first few weeks of life. Chest x-ray findings include the triad of a large egg-shaped heart (classic transposition cardiac silhouette), narrow superior mediastinum with small thymic shadow, and increased pulmonary vascular markings. However, chest x-ray findings may be normal or very near normal in the neonate. The classic x-ray findings are present in only about one-third of the newborn infants with TGA. The electrocardiogram likewise may not be very helpful because the amount of right axis deviation and right ventricular hypertrophy associated with TGA may be considered normal for a neonate.

Echocardiography (two-dimensional and Doppler) is the major diagnostic modality used to delineate the structural anatomy and to assess function. The aorta can be observed to be arising (anteriorly and to the right) from the morphologic right ventricle and the pulmonary artery originating (posteriorly and to the left) from the morphologic left ventricle. The location, size, and direction of shunts can be seen and ventricular pressures may be estimated. The coronary anatomy can also be assessed echocardiographically.

Cardiac catheterization in the neonate affords both diagnostic and therapeutic capabilities. Typical findings include a pulmonary artery oxygen saturation higher than that in the aorta and a pressure difference across the atrial septum (left atrial pressure greater than right atrial pressure). The left ventricular systolic pressure may equal the right ventricular systolic pressure in the newborn with an intact ventricular septum, but it usually decreases to one-half or less of the right ventricular pressure unless there is a degree of left ventricular outflow tract obstruction. The position of the great vessels, the status of the ventricular septum and ductus arteriosus, and the presence of outflow tract obstruction may also be assessed by catheterization. The coronary anatomy is best assessed via catheterization. A balloon atrial septostomy may be performed during catheterization to enhance intercirculatory mixing and improve systemic oxygenation.

Emmanouilides GC, Riemenschneider TA, Allen HD, Gutgesell HP (eds): Moss and Adams' Heart Disease in Infants, Children, and Adolescents, 5th ed, pp 1154–1155. Baltimore, Williams & Wilkins, 1995

Rudolph AM (ed): Rudolph's Pediatrics, 20th ed, pp 1506–1508. Stamford, CT, Appleton & Lange, 1996

Schwartz SI, Shires GT, Spencer FC (eds): Principles of Surgery, 6th ed, pp 824–827. New York, McGraw-Hill, 1994

A.2. Describe the anatomy and classification of TGA.

TGA represents the anatomic discordance between the arteries and ventricles where the aorta originates from the right ventricle and the pulmonary artery arises from the left ventricle. Thus, the right ventricle becomes the systemic ventricle and the left ventricle becomes the pulmonary ventricle. However, the right ventricle is not morphologically designed to function in a high pressure system. In the normally developed heart, the aorta is posterior and to the left, and the pulmonary artery is anterior and to the right. In TGA, this relationship is reversed where the aorta lies anteriorly and the pulmonary artery lies posteriorly. D-TGA refers to the anatomic type where the aorta is situated anterior and to the right (dextro) of the pulmonary artery. With L-TGA, the aorta is anterior and to the left (levo) of the pulmonary artery.

The physiologic classification of TGA results in four anatomic subsets, which

Table 10-1. The Anatomic and Physiologic Classification of Transposition of the Great Arteries

ANATOMY	PBF	MIXING
1. TGA with IVS (atrial septostomy or PDA)	↑(↑)	Small (large)
2. TGA with VSD	↑	Large
3. TGA with VSD and LVOT obstruction	↓	Small
4. TGA with PVOD	↓	Small

have differences in the amount of pulmonary blood flow (PBF) and intercirculatory mixing and is shown in Table 10-1. The four subsets are:

• TGA with intact ventricular septum (IVS)
• TGA with ventricular septal defect (VSD)
• TGA with VSD and left ventricular outflow tract (LVOT) obstruction
• TGA with pulmonary vascular occlusive disease (PVOD).

Emmanouilides GC, Riemenschneider TA, Allen HD, Gutgesell HP (eds): Moss and Adams' Heart Disease in Infants, Children, and Adolescents, 5th ed, pp 1172–1174. Baltimore, Williams & Wilkins, 1995

Lake CL (ed): Pediatric Cardiac Anesthesia, 3rd ed, pp 315–319. Stamford, CT, Appleton & Lange, 1998

A.3. Describe the pattern of blood flow in TGA. What are the potential sites for mixing?

In complete TGA, systemic venous blood is returned to the right atrium, then to the right ventricle, and out via the transposed aorta to the body. Pulmonary venous blood is returned to the left atrium then to the left ventricle and out through the transposed pulmonary artery to the lungs (Figure 10-1). Thus, two separate circula-

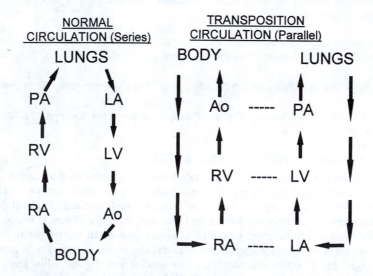

Figure 10-1. Pattern of blood flow in normal (series) and in transposition (parallel) circulations. Dashed lines represent potential sites of intercirculatory mixing.

tions exist in parallel, rather than in series, which is incompatible with life. Some degree of intercirculatory mixing must occur for the oxygenated pulmonary blood to reach the systemic circuit and vice versa for viability. The potential sites for mixing are a patent ductus arteriosus (PDA), atrial septal defect (ASD), patent foramen ovale (PFO), VSD, or bronchopulmonary collaterals.

Emmanouilides GC, Riemenschneider TA, Allen HD, Gutgesell HP (eds): Moss and Adams' Heart Disease in Infants, Children, and Adolescents, 5th ed, pp 1166–1171. Baltimore, Williams & Wilkins, 1995

Rudolph AM (ed): Rudolph's Pediatrics, 20th ed, pp 1506–1507. Stamford, CT, Appleton & Lange, 1996

A.4. What is meant by congenitally corrected transposition?

In corrected transposition, TGA is associated with discordance of the atria and ventricles and the blood flows physiologically. Systemic venous blood returns to the right atrium, then through the tricuspid valve to the left ventricle, and out via the transposed pulmonary artery to the lungs. Pulmonary venous blood returns to the left atrium, then through the mitral valve to the right ventricle, and out to the body via the transposed aorta. The tricuspid and mitral valves remain associated with the appropriate atria. Although blood flow is physiologic, the arteries remain attached to morphologically inappropriate ventricles. Associated abnormalities include VSD (with or without pulmonic stenosis), valvular insufficiency, and conduction abnormalities (AV block). Patients may present with congestive heart failure and cardiomegaly.

Emmanouilides GC, Riemenschneider TA, Allen HD, Gutgesell HP (eds): Moss and Adams' Heart Disease in Infants, Children, and Adolescents, 5th ed, pp 1155–1156. Baltimore, Williams & Wilkins, 1995

Friedberg DZ, Nadas AS: Clinical profile of patients with congenitally corrected transposition of the great arteries. N Engl J Med 282:1053–1059, 1970

Lake CL (ed): Pediatric Cardiac Anesthesia, 3rd ed, p 316. Stamford, CT, Appleton & Lange, 1998

A.5. What is the embryologic development of TGA?

During the first 3 to 4 weeks of gestation, the primitive cardiac tube forms (Fig. 10-2A). It consists of four segments in series: three chambers— sinuatrium (SA), primitive ventricle (V), and bulbus cordis (BC)—and a single main artery, truncus arteriosus (TA). The sinuatrium will divide into the right and left atria (RA and LA), the primitive ventricle will become the left ventricle (LV), and the bulbus cordis will become the right ventricle (RV). The truncus arteriosus will divide into the aorta (Ao) and pulmonary artery (PA).

During the second month of gestation, this simple tube changes to a four-chamber heart with two systems in parallel. Each system has two chambers and a great artery associated with it. The sinuatrium divides into the right and left atria and the truncus arteriosus divides into the aorta and pulmonary artery. Differential growth bends the cardiac tube toward the right (D-loop) with the RV on the right and the LV on the left (Fig. 10-2B). If it bends to the left (L-loop), the RV is situated on the left and the LV on the right. The bulboventricular region of the tube, bulbus cordis, and primitive ventricle (BC and V), folds over on itself, so that the RV and LV lie

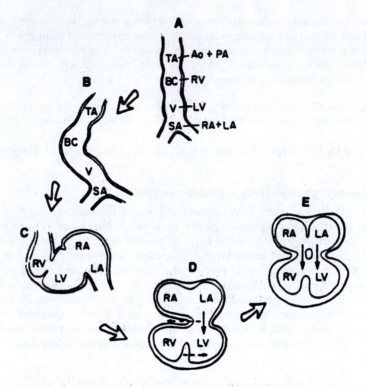

Figure 10-2. Embryologic transition of the straight cardiac tube to the four-chambered heart. (Reprinted with permission from Rudolph AM [ed]: Rudolph's Pediatrics, 20th ed, p 1414. Stamford, CT, Appleton & Lange, 1996)

side by side (Fig. 10-2C). The RA and LA still connect to the LV by the atrioventricular (AV) canal (Fig. 10-2D).

Transition to a normal series pumping system involves alignment of each ventricle with its respective atrioventricular (AV) valve proximally and great artery distally. Proximal alignment is met by migration of the AV canal to the right and migration of the ventricular septum to the left so that the AV canal lies over both ventricles (Fig. 10-2D). The anterior and posterior endocardial cushions meet and divide the AV canal into tricuspid and mitral orifices (Fig. 10-2E). Distal alignment is more complex in that the distal portion of the bulbus cordis is divided into two parts: (1) the subaortic conus, which resorbs as the aorta migrates posteriorly to connect to the LV, and (2) the subpulmonic conus, which increases in length and is connected to the PA. TGA is believed to be an abnormality of conal resorption in that the subpulmonic conus is resorbed instead of the subaortic conus resulting in the aorta arising from the RV and the PA from the LV (D-TGA). TGA thus occurs by the eighth week of gestation.

Anderson RH, Macartney FJ, Shinebourne EA, Tynan M (eds): Paediatric Cardiology, p 83. Edinburgh, Churchill Livingstone, 1987

Emmanouilides GC, Riemenschneider TA, Allen HD, Gutgesell HP (eds): Moss and Adams' Heart Disease in Infants, Children, and Adolescents, 5th ed, pp 1–16. Baltimore, Williams & Wilkins, 1995

Rudolph AM (ed): Rudolph's Pediatrics, 20th ed, pp 1413–1414. Stamford, CT, Appleton & Lange, 1996

A.6. What is the most common type of TGA? What anomalies are associated with TGA?

The most common type of complete TGA is the D-loop where the RV is on the right and the aorta arises anteriorly and to the right of the PA. Systemic venous blood returns to the RA then through the tricuspid valve to the RV and out the aorta to the body and returns to the RA. Pulmonary venous blood returns to the LA then through the mitral valve to the LV and out to the lungs via the PA and back to the LA (Fig. 10-1). Two parallel circuits exist and the affected infant is profoundly cyanotic unless there is some degree of mixing via a PFO, ASD, VSD, PDA, or bronchopulmonary collaterals.

Approximately half of the patients with simple TGA have no coexisting anomaly other than a PFO or a PDA. In the remainder of patients, a coexisting VSD is common (up to 45%). Other associated anomalies include LVOT obstruction, mitral and tricuspid valvular abnormalities, coarctation of the aorta, and interrupted aortic arch.

Fyler DC (ed): Nadas Pediatric Cardiology, pp 557–576. Philadelphia, Hanley & Belfus, 1992

Kirklin JW, Barrett-Boyes BG (eds): Cardiac Surgery, 2nd ed, pp 1383–1467. White Plains, Churchill Livingstone, 1993

A.7. What is a balloon atrial septostomy and why is it performed?

A balloon atrial septostomy is a palliative procedure performed at the time of cardiac catheterization by introducing a balloon-tipped catheter transvenously (femoral or umbilical) into the right atrium and across the foramen ovale into the left atrium, where the balloon is inflated. The catheter with inflated balloon is then rapidly pulled back into the right atrium which ruptures the septum primum valve of the fossa ovalis and effectively enlarges the interatrial communication (creates an ASD) and increases the amount of intercirculatory mixing. It is performed whenever a shunt is needed to improve arteriovenous mixing.

Lake CL (ed): Pediatric Cardiac Anesthesia, 3rd ed, p 322. Stamford, CT, Appleton & Lange, 1998

Rashkind WJ, Miller WW: Creation of an atrial septal defect without thoracotomy: A palliative approach to complete transposition of the great arteries. JAMA 196:991–992, 1966

Rudolph AM (ed): Rudolph's Pediatrics, 20th ed, p 1508. Stamford, CT, Appleton & Lange, 1996

A.8. Why did this patient receive prostaglandin E_1 (PGE_1)? What is the dosage range of PGE_1 and what are its side-effects?

This infant must have been profoundly cyanotic due to insufficient intercirculatory mixing. He probably had TGA with an intact ventricular septum. PGE_1 was initiated to maintain ductal patency and allow some mixing of the circulations. Once the atrial septostomy was performed, sufficient mixing must have been established and the patient stabilized, which allowed for the discontinuation of the PGE_1. The dosage range of PGE_1 infusion to maintain ductal patency is 0.05 to 0.1 μg/kg/min. Important side-effects of PGE_1 include apnea, fever, seizures, arrhythmias, vasodilation, and peripheral edema.

Lake CL (ed): Pediatric Cardiac Anesthesia, 3rd ed, p 319. Stamford, CT, Appleton & Lange, 1998

Lewis A, Freed M, Heymann M et al: Side-effects of therapy with prostaglandin E_1 in infants with critical congenital heart disease. Circulation 64:893–898, 1981

A.9. With complete TGA, if a ventricular or atrial septal defect coexists, what determines the amount of intercirculatory mixing and shunt direction?

The amount of intercirculatory mixing depends on the number, size, and position of the communication sites. One large nonrestrictive communication provides better mixing than two or three restrictive, small communications. In the presence of adequate communication sites, the extent of mixing or improvement in oxygenation is directly related to the total pulmonary blood flow (PBF). For example, patients with subpulmonic stenosis will have reduced intercirculatory mixing due to decreased PBF.

Mixing is a result of anatomic right-to-left and left-to-right shunts that are equal in magnitude. Shunt flow should be bidirectional; however, changes in ventricular compliance, systemic vascular resistance and/or pulmonary vascular resistance will result in changes in shunt direction. Such changes can easily occur intraoperatively, and attempts are made to avoid such changes and maintain adequate mixing.

Emmanouilides GC, Riemenschneider TA, Allen HD, Gutgesell HP (eds): Moss and Adams' Heart Disease in Infants, Children, and Adolescents, 5th ed, pp 1166–1167. Baltimore, Williams & Wilkins, 1995

Lake CL (ed): Pediatric Cardiac Anesthesia, 3rd ed, p 319. Stamford, CT, Appleton & Lange, 1998

A.10. What determines the arterial oxygen saturation in TGA?

Arterial oxygen saturation is determined by the degree of mixing, i.e., the relative volumes and saturations of the recirculated systemic (deoxygenated) blood and the left-to-right shunted (oxygenated) blood reaching the aorta. The greater the amount of shunted blood relative to the amount of recirculated blood, the higher the arterial oxygen saturation will be. The amount of shunt flow, the systemic and pulmonary venous saturations, and cardiac output all may affect the arterial oxygen saturation.

Emmanouilides GC, Riemenschneider TA, Allen HD, Gutgesell HP (eds): Moss and Adams' Heart Disease in Infants, Children, and Adolescents, 5th ed, pp 1166–1167. Baltimore, Williams & Wilkins, 1995

Lake CL (ed): Pediatric Cardiac Anesthesia, 3rd ed, pp 317–318. Stamford, CT, Appleton & Lange, 1998

A.11. Describe the coronary anatomy in TGA. Why is it important in this patient?

There is considerable variability in the coronary anatomy in hearts with TGA. This variability may be related to the embryologic development of this heart defect. As in hearts with normally related great vessels, the coronary arteries in TGA arise from the aortic sinuses (sinuses of Valsalva) that face the pulmonary artery. In normal hearts, the sinuses are located on the anterior portion of the aorta, whereas in TGA, they are located posteriorly. The right coronary artery (RCA) originates from the right sinus and the left main coronary artery (LCA) originates from the left sinus in the majority (60%) of TGA patients. However, considerable variation exists. For example, there may be a single RCA or single LCA with all three major vessels (RCA, left anterior descending, and circumflex) arising from it, the circumflex may arise from the RCA instead of from the LCA, or portions of the coronaries may be intramyocardial (intramural).

The importance of the coronary anatomy in this patient is due to the fact that he is to have an arterial switch operation performed, which involves reimplantation of the coronary arteries, and there are certain variations in coronary anatomy that would preclude or severely limit the successful performance of this corrective procedure (e.g., inverted coronaries, single RCA, intramural LCA). In addition, knowledge of the location of the sinus node artery (usually the first branch of the RCA close to its origin) is important to avoid damaging this vessel during surgery and thus reduce the risk of atrial arrhythmias and heart block.

Emmanouilides GC, Riemenschneider TA, Allen HD, Gutgesell HP (eds): Moss and Adams' Heart Disease in Infants, Children, and Adolescents, 5th ed, pp 1156–1158. Baltimore, Williams & Wilkins, 1995

Lake CL (ed): Pediatric Cardiac Anesthesia, 3rd ed, pp 324–325. Stamford, CT, Appleton & Lange, 1998

A.12. What is an arterial switch operation (ASO), how is it performed, and what are the complications associated with it? What is the optimal timing for the procedure and why?

The arterial switch operation (ASO) is the definitive repair for TGA that anatomically corrects the discordant arterial connections such that the aorta arises from the left ventricle and the pulmonary artery arises from the right ventricle (Fig. 10-3). Jatene was the first to successfully perform and describe the ASO in 1975 and it has gradually become the procedure of choice for TGA in the neonatal period. First, the pulmonary artery and aorta are transected just above their respective valves. The coronaries are excised and mobilized from the ascending aorta with a button of surrounding tissue and then reimplanted into the proximal pulmonary artery (neoaorta). The great

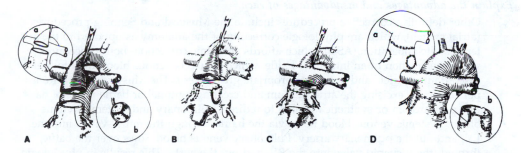

Figure 10-3. The arterial switch procedure. **(A)** First, the pulmonary artery and aorta are transected just above their respective valves. The coronaries are excised and mobilized from the ascending aorta with a button of surrounding tissue and then reimplanted into the proximal pulmonary artery (neoaorta) **(A and B)**. **(C)** The great arteries are then switched: the distal pulmonary artery is brought anterior to the ascending aorta (RV outflow) and the distal aorta is moved posteriorly where it is anastomosed to the proximal pulmonary artery (LV outflow) just above the reimplanted coronary arteries. **(D)** The donor sites of the excised coronary arteries in the proximal aorta are repaired with either pericardium or synthetic material. Finally, anastomosis of the proximal aorta and distal pulmonary artery is completed. (Reprinted with permission from Castaneda AR, Norwood WI, Jonas RI et al: Transposition of the great arteries and intact interventricular septum: Anatomical repair in the neonate. Ann Thorac Surg 38:440, 1984)

arteries are then switched: the distal pulmonary artery is brought anterior to the ascending aorta (RV outflow) and the distal aorta is moved posteriorly where it is anastomosed to the proximal pulmonary artery (LV outflow) just above the reimplanted coronary arteries. The donor sites of the excised coronary arteries in the proximal aorta are repaired with either pericardium or synthetic material, and finally, anastomosis of the proximal aorta and distal pulmonary artery is completed.

Complications associated with the ASO include supravalvular pulmonic stenosis (mild to moderate; 10% to 44% of patients), aortic regurgitation, arrhythmias (PACs and PVCs), and myocardial ischemia related to reimplantation of the coronary arteries.

The success of the ASO depends on the LV (the pulmonary ventricle in TGA) having sufficient mass to be capable of becoming the systemic ventricle. In TGA patients with an intact IVS, there is progressive decrease in LV mass as the physiologic pulmonary hypertension of the neonate regresses within the first few days after birth. In these patients, adequate LV mass exists for only the first 2 to 3 weeks after birth and therefore a primary arterial switch procedure must be performed within the first 2 weeks of life. An ASO may be performed later as a staged procedure after a PA banding (which prepares the LV). However, this is less commonly done.

Emmanouilides GC, Riemenschneider TA, Allen HD, Gutgesell HP (eds): Moss and Adams' Heart Disease in Infants, Children, and Adolescents, 5th ed, pp 1198–1205. Baltimore, Williams & Wilkins, 1995

Jatene AD, Fontes VF, Paulista PP et al: Anatomic correction of transposition of the great vessels. J Thorac Cardiovasc Surg 72:364–370, 1976

Lake CL (ed): Pediatric Cardiac Anesthesia, 3rd ed, pp 323–326. Stamford, CT, Appleton & Lange, 1998

A.13. What other definitive surgical techniques are there for correction of complete TGA? Explain the advantages and disadvantages of each.

Other definitive corrective procedures include the Mustard and Senning procedures (atrial switch), which are physiologic correction of the anatomy as opposed to the arterial switch operation (ASO), which affords anatomic correction. Both procedures involve the creation of an intraatrial baffle, which redirects venous blood flow to the discordant ventricle and out the appropriate great artery. The Mustard procedure is performed by excising the atrial septum and creating a tunnel or baffle made of native pericardium or synthetic material to redirect pulmonary and systemic venous blood. Systemic venous blood flows via the baffle through the mitral valve, into the LV, and out the pulmonary artery. Pulmonary venous blood flows over the baffle, through the tricuspid valve into the RV, and out the aorta. This results in physiologic correction of blood flow; however, the RV remains as the systemic ventricle. The Senning procedure is similar to the Mustard repair in that it results in the same redirection of pulmonary and systemic venous blood flow by creation of an intraatrial baffle. However, in the Senning repair the baffle is constructed of autologous right atrial tissue and interatrial septum instead of pericardium or synthetic material.

The atrial switch procedures (Mustard and Senning) may be complicated by conduction defects and arrhythmias (due to surgical manipulation of conduction tissue), pulmonary venous congestion (due to baffle construction), tricuspid regurgitation, and RV dysfunction (because the RV is not morphologically designed to function as the systemic ventricle). Since the Senning repair involves the use of *in situ* tissues, it may be less restrictive over time than the Mustard repair. The ASO results in anatomic correction and restores the LV as the systemic ventricle. ASO complications include myocardial ischemia, supravalvular pulmonic stenosis, aortic regurgitation, and arrhythmias. Intermediate outcome results of neonatal ASO are very good (early operative survival of 95% or more) and have led to the ASO becoming the procedure of choice in infants with TGA.

Mustard WT: Successful two-stage correction of transposition of the great vessels. Surgery 55:469–472, 1964

Norwood WI, Dobell AR, Freed MD et al: The Congenital Heart Surgeons Society. Intermediate results of the arterial switch repair: a 20-institution study. J Thorac Cardiovasc Surg 96:854–863, 1988

Senning A: Surgical correction of transposition of the great vessels. Surgery 45:966–980, 1959

B. Preoperative Evaluation and Preparation

B.1. What preoperative information would you want to know?

The history and physical examination should include gestational age, birth complications if any, initial treatment and/or interventions, coexisting medical diseases or congenital abnormalities, vital signs, airway, cardiopulmonary examination, peripheral pulses, capillary refill (to assess perfusion), evidence of cyanosis, location of intravenous and arterial catheter sites, and the sites of medication infusions. A summary of the cardiac catheterization data should be available, which defines the anatomy and identifies the locations and size of intercirculatory communications. The chest x-ray and electrocardiogram are also needed. Laboratory data should include complete blood count, electrolytes, BUN, creatinine, glucose, urine analysis, arterial blood gas analysis (acid/base status) and a coagulation profile with prothrombin time and partial thromboplastin time. The infant's blood must be typed and crossmatched and an adequate supply of blood must be available for this infant. Preparations should be made for a donor unit of fresh whole blood to be drawn the morning of surgery.

Kaplan JA (ed): Cardiac Anesthesia, 3rd ed, pp 702–704. Philadelphia, WB Saunders, 1993

Thomas SJ, Kramer JL (eds): Manual of Cardiac Anesthesia, 2nd ed, pp 216–221. New York, Churchill Livingstone, 1993

B.2. Why is it important to know the anatomic communication(s) and the amount of mixing?

The presence of anatomic communications results in the potential for changes in shunt flow direction to occur. It is important to know this information and to understand the pathophysiology of the lesion preoperatively in order to anesthetize the patient safely. Any change in systemic vascular resistance (SVR) relative to pulmonary vascular resistance (PVR) may alter the direction of shunt flow and the amount of mixing. During anesthesia and surgery, there are a multitude of factors that can change the SVR, PVR, and amount of mixing. The anesthesiologist must be prepared to intelligently prevent and appropriately treat such changes should they occur.

Knowledge of the anatomy and anatomic communications allows the anesthesiologist to formulate an individual cardiac physiologic profile of the patient and to outline the optimal hemodynamic goals required to maintain hemodynamic stability intraoperatively. The key hemodynamic factors include PVR, SVR, heart rate, preload, and contractility.

Lake CL (ed): Pediatric Cardiac Anesthesia, 3rd ed, pp 317–320. Stamford, CT, Appleton & Lange, 1998

B.3. What is important in the preoperative optimization of this patient?

The fact that this patient was severely cyanotic at birth and required PGE_1 implies that he was critically ill. It is important that any degree of metabolic acidosis and hemodynamic instability be corrected preoperatively.

Rudolph AM (ed): Rudolph's Pediatrics, 20th ed, p 1508. Stamford, CT, Appleton & Lange, 1996

B.4. What is pulmonary vascular occlusive disease (PVOD) and why is it important?

Pulmonary vascular occlusive disease (PVOD) is a progressive lesion of the pulmonary vascular bed that occurs in infants with congenital heart disease, and patients with TGA are particularly afflicted. In the normal neonate, pulmonary vascular resistance (PVR) progressively decreases in the days and weeks following birth. The normal postnatal pulmonary changes are altered by the development of PVOD. It involves remodeling of the pulmonary vessels with medial and intimal hyperplasia. Contributing factors to the development of PVOD include sustained high pulmonary blood flow and pressures as a result of the congenital heart defect. PVOD results in increases in PVR and pulmonary hypertension, which, in turn, decreases pulmonary blood flow. The decrease in pulmonary blood flow reduces intercirculatory mixing and worsens systemic hypoxemia.

PVOD is important because the resultant pulmonary hypertension limits the corrective surgical options available. Definitive surgical repair must be performed before the development of irreversible PVOD and severe pulmonary hypertension.

Emmanouilides GC, Riemenschneider TA, Allen HD, Gutgesell HP (eds): Moss and Adams' Heart Disease in Infants, Children, and Adolescents, 5th ed, pp 1660–1662. Baltimore, Williams & Wilkins, 1995

B.5. What premedication would you give?

Premedication is unnecessary in an infant this age and could be detrimental if an adverse reaction or overdose occurs.

Lake CL (ed): Pediatric Cardiac Anesthesia, 3rd ed, p 320. Stamford, CT, Appleton & Lange, 1998

C. Intraoperative Management

C.1. How would you prepare the operating room?

The operating room will be warmed to prevent heat loss and stress in the infant during the preinduction period. The anesthetic machine, circuit, and suction apparatus will be checked out. All medications will be prepared, and all intravenous fluid lines and pressure tubing lines will have any air bubbles present meticulously removed (de-aired). A heat–moisture exchanger will be inserted into the airway circuit, and a warming blanket and a blood/fluid warmer will be available. Airway supplies including face masks, an assortment of endotracheal tubes, and laryngoscopic equipment will be prepared. All supplies necessary for intravenous, intraarterial and central line catheter placement will be organized and set up for use. A defibrillator with appropriate sized paddles must be present. Crossmatched blood should be readily available if the need for an emergency transfusion arises.

Lake CL (ed): Pediatric Cardiac Anesthesia, 3rd ed, pp 320–321. Stamford, CT, Appleton & Lange, 1998

C.2. What monitors would you use? Could transesophageal echocardiography (TEE) be used in this infant?

Routine monitors including pulse oximetry, electrocardiography, capnography, and noninvasive blood pressure machine (or arterial line pressure is transduced if already present preoperatively) are used for induction. After induction, an intraarterial catheter is inserted percutaneously for continuous blood pressure monitoring and intermittent blood gas sampling. The radial artery is the usual insertion site, but alternative sites include the femoral, brachial, axillary, superficial temporal, or posterior tibial arteries. A double-lumen central venous pressure (CVP) catheter is inserted via the internal jugular vein or femoral vein for CVP monitoring and drug infusion. A urinary catheter is inserted and attached to a collection reservoir to monitor urine output and to aid in the assessment of intravascular volume and cardiac output (kidney perfusion). Temperature probes, both peripheral and core, are inserted at multiple sites to maximize the accuracy in temperature monitoring during cooling and rewarming. Usual sites for temperature monitoring include rectal, nasopharyngeal, esophageal, and tympanic. Rectal temperature lags behind nasopharyngeal, esophageal, and tympanic during central or core cooling and rewarming. Tympanic and nasopharyngeal most closely reflect brain temperature.

Transesophageal echocardiography (TEE) may be used in an infant this size and affords an excellent assessment of the anatomy, ventricular function, and shunt flow prebypass. Postbypass, TEE is invaluable in the immediate assessment of the surgical repair (i.e., residual shunts, valvular regurgitation), myocardial contractility, and volume status (i.e., preload). New regional wall motion abnormalities due to myocardial ischemia from technical difficulty with reimplantation of the coronary arteries may be observed by TEE.

The usefulness of TEE in neonates has been limited by the availability of an appropriate sized probe. Recent technological developments have resulted in the availability of smaller probes. At our institution, we use a pediatric biplane probe that measures 7.5 mm in diameter, and it may be used in neonates >3 kg in weight.

Muhiudeen IA, Roberson DA, Silverman NH et al: Intraoperative echocardiography for evaluation of congenital heart defects in infants and children. Anesthesiology 76:165–172, 1992

Ritter SB: Transesophageal echocardiography in children: New peephole to the heart. J Am Coll Card 16:447–450, 1990

Stumper OFW, Elzenga NJ, Hess J, Sutherland GR: Transesophageal echocardiography in children with congenital heart disease: An initial experience. J Am Coll Card 16:433–441, 1990

C.3. What intraoperative laboratory data would you monitor?

Intermittent blood sampling will be performed to monitor the following:

- Blood gases (pH, P_{CO_2}, P_{O_2}, oxygen saturation, and bicarbonate)
- Hematocrit

- Glucose
- Electrolytes (sodium and potassium)
- Ionized calcium
- Activated clotting time

Arterial blood gases are monitored to ensure adequate oxygenation and ventilation and to assess the acid/base status. The hematocrit is important to ensure adequate oxygen carrying capacity and to guide transfusion requirements. The glucose concentration should be monitored to avoid unrecognized hypoglycemia (particularly prebypass) or hyperglycemia. The ionized calcium is important because it may decrease significantly during bypass and after rapid transfusion of citrated blood resulting in a decrease in systemic blood pressure and myocardial contractility. Monitoring of the ionized calcium concentration will aid in the differential diagnosis of myocardial dysfunction postbypass and guide appropriate supplementation if necessary. The activated clotting time is monitored to assess the adequacy of anticoagulation before and during bypass and of protamine reversal postbypass.

Kaplan JA (ed): Cardiac Anesthesia, 3rd ed, pp 927–942. Philadelphia, WB Saunders, 1993

Thomas SJ, Kramer JL (eds): Manual of Cardiac Anesthesia, 2nd ed, pp 233–235. New York, Churchill Livingstone, 1993

C.4. What emergency drugs would you have available?

The following drugs will be prepared in advance for emergency bolus administration and diluted appropriately, if necessary, for this patient according to his body weight:

• Atropine sulfate	0.01 mg/kg
• Calcium chloride (or gluconate)	10 mg/kg (30 mg/kg)
• Epinephrine	1 to 10 µg/kg
• Lidocaine	1 mg/kg
• Phenylephrine	1 to 2 µg/kg
• Sodium bicarbonate	0.5 to 1 mEq/kg
• Heparin	200 to 400 units/kg (depends on institutional practice)

An infusion of one of the following vasopressors should be prepared in advance for emergency use:

• Dobutamine	5 to 20 µg/kg/min
• Epinephrine	0.1 µg/kg/min

Kaplan JA (ed): Cardiac Anesthesia, 3rd ed, p 694. New York, Grune & Stratton, 1993

Lake CL (ed): Pediatric Cardiac Anesthesia, 3rd ed, p 109. Stamford, CT, Appleton & Lange, 1998

C.5. How would you anesthetize this infant? Discuss the prebypass hemodynamic management of this patient.

Anesthetic choice must be predicated on the known physiology of the congenital heart lesion. A narcotic-based anesthetic (fentanyl or sufentanil) for induction and maintenance is preferred because of its proven ability to afford hemodynamic stability, not depress the myocardium, and to blunt reactive pulmonary hypertension. In neonates and infants, the cardiac output is more heart-rate dependent due to a lower

Table 10-2. Prebypass Management Goals in the Patient with TGA

- Maintain heart rate, preload, and contractility to maintain adequate CO. ↓ in CO results in a ↓ systemic venous oxygen saturation and thus ↓ in arterial saturation.
- If duct dependent, maintain ductal patency with prostaglandin E_1, 0.05–0.1 μg/kg/min.
- Avoid increased PVR relative to SVR. ↑ PVR results in ↓ PBF and ↓ in intercirculatory mixing. Ventilatory intervention, e.g., hyperventilation with low airway pressures should be used to ↓ PVR. Exception: patients with VSD and symptoms of CHF, do not ↓ PVR because it will further ↑ PBF at the expense of systemic perfusion.
- Avoid decreased SVR relative to PVR. ↓ SVR results in ↑ recirculation of systemic venous blood and ↓ arterial oxygen saturation.

Table 10-3. Factors That Alter Pulmonary Vascular Resistance (PVR) and Blood Flow

INCREASE PVR	DECREASE PVR
Hypoxia	Hyperoxia
Hypercarbia	Hypocarbia
Acidosis	Alkalosis
High mean airway pressure	Prostaglandin E_1/prostacyclin
Sympathetic stimulation	Alpha-Adrenergic antagonists
Alpha-Adrenergic agonists	Vasodilators
Hypervolemia	Anesthetics except ketamine, N_2O
Anesthetic (N_2O)	

ventricular compliance when compared to an adult. The high dose of narcotic may result in bradycardia; thus in order to maintain the heart rate, pancuronium (0.1 mg/ kg for intubation), which is vagolytic, is used to provide muscle relaxation and to offset any slowing of the heart rate. Narcotics alone may not provide adequate amnesia and breakthrough hypertension may be observed that is not responsive to additional narcotics. For these reasons, a benzodiazepine (midazolam, 0.025 to 0.05 mg/kg) or a low dose of inhalational agent may be used as an adjunct. If a benzodiazepine is used, it must be remembered that the combination of it with a narcotic may result in a significant decrease in vascular resistance and, as a result, adversely affect the direction and/or amount of shunt flow in TGA.

The prebypass management goals for the patient with TGA are outlined in Table 10-2. The essence of appropriate management depends on the balance of PVR relative

Table 10-4. Factors That Alter Systemic Vascular Resistance (SVR) and Blood Flow

INCREASE SVR	DECREASE SVR
Sympathetic stimulation	Anesthetics
Alpha-Adrenergic agonists	Vasodilators
Hyperoxia	Alpha-Adrenergic antagonists
Hypercarbia, moderate	Beta-Adrenergic agonists
	Calcium slow channel blocking agents
	Phosphodiesterase III inhibitors
	Hypoxia
	Severe hypercarbia

to SVR, which will directly affect the shunt flow and amount of intercircuitry mixing. An increase in PVR relative to SVR will decrease pulmonary blood flow (PBF), decrease the amount of mixing, and decrease the arterial oxygen saturation. A decrease in SVR relative to PVR results in more recirculation of systemic venous blood and a decrease in arterial saturation. Factors that influence PVR and SVR are listed in Tables 10-3 and 10-4.

Anand KJS, Hickey PR: Halothane-morphine compared with high dose sufentanil for anesthesia and postoperative analgesia in neonatal cardiac surgery. N Engl J Med 326:1–9, 1992

Hickey PR, Hansen DD: Fentanyl- and sufentanil-oxygen-pancuronium anesthesia for cardiac surgery in infants. Anesth Analg 63:117–124, 1984

Kaplan JA (ed): Cardiac Anesthesia, 3rd ed, pp 732–735. Philadelphia, WB Saunders, 1993

Lake CL (ed): Pediatric Cardiac Anesthesia, 3rd ed, pp 320–322. Stamford, CT, Appleton & Lange, 1998

C.6. In general, how does cardiopulmonary bypass (CPB) for infants differ from that used for adults?

The most notable differences are related to the degree of hemodilution and attendant dilution of drugs and clotting factors in the pump prime, higher flow rates, lower perfusion pressures, lower temperatures (in certain cases), more technical difficulty with proper cannula placement, and adequacy of venous drainage. In addition, the necessity to occlude any existing systemic to pulmonary shunts is limited to the pediatric population. The differences in CPB between pediatric and adult patients are outlined in Table 10-5.

Gravlee G, Davis RF, Utley JR (eds): Cardiopulmonary Bypass: Principles and Practice, pp 603–632. Baltimore, Williams & Wilkins, 1993

Lake CL (ed): Pediatric Cardiac Anesthesia, 3rd ed, pp 225–226. Stamford, CT, Appleton & Lange, 1998

C.7. How is hypothermia classified and how is it accomplished?

Hypothermia is used during surgery to decrease metabolism and preserve organ function. Hypothermia is classified as follows:

- Mild hypothermia   > 32°C
- Moderate hypothermia   25°–32°C
- Deep or profound hypothermia   15°–20°C

The choice of which degree of hypothermia will be used during surgery depends on the desired surgical conditions, patient size, the type of operation, and whether

Table 10-5.   The Differences in CPB Between Pediatric and Adult Patients

	ADULT	PEDIATRIC
Perfusion pressure (mm Hg)	50–60	30–40
Flow rates (ml/kg/min, at normothermia)	50–75	100–150
Hemodilution	+	+ + + +
Temperature (°C)	28–32	15–20 (certain cases)
Venous drainage problems	Rare	Common
Aortic cannula obstruction to aortic outflow	Not a problem	Common in small neonates due to Small aortic lumen

the patient can tolerate the desired level of cooling. Moderate hypothermia (25° to 32°C) is utilized in older children and adolescents and in infants undergoing repair of uncomplicated congenital heart defects, e.g., an ASD or VSD. Deep hypothermic cardiopulmonary bypass is primarily utilized for neonates and infants requiring repair of complex congenital heart lesions. Deep hypothermia allows the surgeon to operate under optimal conditions providing a near bloodless field and, in the case of circulatory arrest, a cannula-free field. Hypothermia is accomplished by a combination of surface cooling including ice packs applied around head and cooling blanket, and core cooling utilizing cardiopulmonary bypass. Since cooling is not uniform, multiple temperature sites such as esophageal, rectal, nasopharyngeal, and/or tympanic are monitored simultaneously to assess the temperature correlation and ensure the adequacy of systemic cooling.

Gravlee G, Davis RF, Utley JR (eds): Cardiopulmonary Bypass: Principles and Practice, pp 140–142, 149–150. Baltimore, Williams & Wilkins, 1993

Lake CL (ed): Pediatric Cardiac Anesthesia, 3rd ed, p 232. Stamford, CT, Appleton & Lange, 1998

C.8. What is deep hypothermic circulatory arrest (DHCA) and how long can patients tolerate it? What is Q_{10}?

Deep hypothermic circulatory arrest is utilized during repair of complex congenital heart defects in neonates and infants. It is accomplished by active cooling of the patient on bypass down to a temperature of 15° to 20°C and then turning off the pump so that no blood flow occurs. This allows the surgeon to remove the cannulae (which may have distorted the anatomy) and allows for a more precise repair of the lesion under optimal conditions, i.e., a bloodless and cannula-free field. The maximum duration of a safe circulatory arrest period is approximately 50 to 60 minutes.

All organs are at risk for hypoxic/ischemic injury; however, the brain is the most sensitive. Thus, the determination of a safe duration of circulatory arrest is based on the duration of cerebral protection. Q_{10} is a temperature coefficient that describes the reduction in cerebral metabolism for every 10°C decrease in temperature. It is derived from the ratio of cerebral metabolism ($CMRO_2$) measured at two temperatures, 10°C apart. For every 10°C decrease in temperature, there is an average of 3.6 times reduction in $CMRO_2$. Based on the assumption that 3 to 5 minutes of normothermic arrest does not result in ischemic brain damage, then the Q_{10} data predicts that a safe arrest time at 15°C would be 50 to 90 minutes. However, clinical evidence suggests that the duration of a safe circulatory arrest period is 50 to 60 minutes in neonates, infants, and children. Estimated safe periods of circulatory arrest at various temperatures are listed in Table 10-6.

Table 10-6.   Estimated Safe Duration of Circulatory Arrest at Different Body Temperatures

NASOPHARYNGEAL TEMPERATURE	ESTIMATED SAFE DURATION OF ARREST
37°C	3–5 minutes
32°C	5–9 minutes
30°C	7–12 minutes
25°C	14–24 minutes
20°C	28–46 minutes
15°C	53–89 minutes

In general, cerebral metabolism decreases with hypothermia in an exponential manner: $CMRO_2$ is reduced by 40% to 50% at 30°C, 60% at 25°C, 75% at 20°C, and 85% at 10°C. Infants tolerate hypothermic circulatory arrest better than older children and adults.

Gravlee G, Davis RF, Utley JR (eds): Cardiopulmonary Bypass: Principles and Practice, pp 606, 608–609. Baltimore, Williams & Wilkins, 1993

Greeley WJ, Kern FH, Ungerleider RM et al: The effect of hypothermic cardiopulmonary bypass and total circulatory arrest on cerebral metabolism in neonates, infants and children. J Thorac Cardiovasc Surg 101:783–794, 1991

Lake CL (ed): Pediatric Cardiac Anesthesia, 3rd ed, pp 233–235. Stamford, CT, Appleton & Lange, 1998

C.9. What is low-flow cardiopulmonary bypass and is there an advantage to it over DHCA?

Low-flow cardiopulmonary bypass is an alternative to DHCA in the management of cardiopulmonary bypass for repair of complex congenital cardiac defects. Low-flow cardiopulmonary bypass is conducted at a temperature of 15° to 18°C and using flows of 30 to 35 cc/kg/min or 1 to 1.2 liters/min/m². The hypothermia reduces cerebral metabolism and the metabolism of all vital organs to allow such low flows to be tolerated. The low flow rate provides a near bloodless field and near optimal operating conditions. However, the cannulae remain in place and may distort the anatomy, making repair of the defect less precise.

The theoretical advantage of low-flow cardiopulmonary bypass over DHCA is that by maintaining a small amount of blood flow during deep hypothermia, this will afford better protection than no flow at all. Indeed, early studies on neurologic outcome of infants randomized to either low-flow or DHCA for repair of TGA have shown that there is better neurologic outcome with low-flow cardiopulmonary bypass. Specifically, in the early postoperative period, the low-flow bypass infants had a lower incidence of seizures and neurologic morbidity than those randomized to DHCA. Additionally, it has been shown that low-flow bypass is associated with a lower risk of delayed motor development and neurologic abnormalities at 1 year of age when compared to infants managed with DHCA.

Bellinger DC, Jonas RA, Rappaport LA et al: Developmental and neurologic status of children after heart surgery with hypothermic circulatory arrest or low-flow cardiopulmonary bypass. N Engl J Med 332:549–555, 1995

Gravlee G, Davis RF, Utley JR (eds): Cardiopulmonary Bypass: Principles and Practice, pp 605, 609–610. Baltimore, Williams & Wilkins, 1993

Newburger JW, Jonas RA, Wernovsky G et al: A comparison of the perioperative neurologic effects of hypothermic circulatory arrest versus low-flow cardiopulmonary bypass in infant heart surgery. N Engl J Med 329:1057–1064, 1993

C.10. What are the physiologic changes and potential complications associated with hypothermia?

The goal of hypothermia is to afford organ protection by reducing cellular metabolism and thereby preserving high-energy phosphate (ATP) stores. Hypothermia decreases metabolism as long as shivering is prevented. Shivering can increase whole-body metabolic demand by severalfold. It can be prevented by the use of muscle re- laxants and sedatives. Hypothermia induces the following physiologic changes:

- *Oxygen delivery and acid/base status*
  Oxygen-hemoglobin dissociation curve is shifted to left, which reduces the release of oxygen from hemoglobin. There is an increase in the solubility of oxygen, carbon dioxide, and anesthetic gases in the blood. If perfusion, and therefore cooling, is not uniform then metabolic acidosis may occur.
- *Hematologic*
  Increase in blood viscosity (offset by the hemodilution of bypass), prolongation of prothrombin time and bleeding time, decrease in fibrinogen activity.
- *Cardiovascular*
  Initial cooling results in vasoconstriction and an increase in SVR. Heart rate progressively slows as cooling continues. Electrocardiographic changes include prolongation of the PR, QRS, and QT intervals. Nonspecific ST and T-wave changes may be observed. The J wave is a characteristic EKG change associated with hypothermia (at about 30°C) and consists of a small positive wave on the downstroke of the R wave. Cardiac output decreases as the heart rate slows; stroke volume is not significantly changed above a temperature of 25°C.
- *Hepatic and renal*
  Hepatic function decreases as hypothermia ensues and drug metabolism is significantly reduced. Glucose and citrate are not metabolized. As temperature and cardiac output fall, renal blood flow decreases. This is in part due to the release of renin, angiotensin, and antidiuretic hormone. Tubule reabsorption decreases due to cold-induced inhibition of transport mechanisms. Urinary output may be maintained down to 20°C; however below this, urine production stops.
- *Endocrine*
  Epinephrine, adrenal cortical steroids, and ACTH levels increase with hypothermia, indicating that it induces a stress response.

Potential complications include tissue ischemia and irreversible damage to peripheral tissues such as the nose, fingers, toes, external genitalia, and ears.

Gravlee G, Davis RF, Utley JR (eds): Cardiopulmonary Bypass: Principles and Practice, pp 140–149. Baltimore, Williams & Wilkins, 1993

C.11. How is rewarming accomplished?

Rewarming is accomplished via cardiopulmonary bypass using a heat exchanger. The rewarming process is performed slowly by maintaining a temperature gradient of approximately 8° to 10°C between the arterial perfusate and the venous blood temperature. Larger temperature gradients may increase the risk of gas bubbles coming out of solution. As the patient is rewarmed, flows are increased accordingly, and any metabolic acidosis that may occur during this time is treated with sodium bicarbonate. Once the tympanic (or nasopharyngeal) and rectal temperatures reach 36°C, the patient is weaned from CPB.

C.12. Discuss the major issues in successful weaning from CPB. Why is ventilation pattern important postbypass?

The major considerations in successful weaning from CPB following repair of TGA are the heart rate and rhythm, preload, afterload, and contractility. The hemodynamic goals in weaning from CPB and post-CPB management are listed below:

- Maintain heart rate at age-appropriate rate. Sinus rhythm is preferred. Cardiac output is more rate-dependent post-CPB due to reduced ventricular compliance. Pacing may be required.
- Systemic ventricular dysfunction (RV for atrial switch, LV for arterial switch) may occur post-CPB due to myocardial ischemia from ASO, inadequate ventricular mass, poor myocardial protection during cross-clamping, or a combination of these factors. If left ventricular myocardial contractility is reduced, inotropic support with afterload reduction may be required. This can be achieved with a combination of dobutamine and nitroprusside infusions or alternatively with an amrinone bolus and infusion.
- Adequate ventilation is imperative. Lung compliance may be severely reduced post-CPB and requires adequate inspiratory pressures for lung inflation. A long expiratory time is recommended to allow exhalation of CO_2 (i.e., I:E ratio of 1:3) and to avoid stacking of the lungs. Hyperventilation may be necessary to reduce PVR and enhance pulmonary blood flow and oxygenation.
- Monitoring for ischemia is crucial, especially if following the ASO procedure. If ischemia occurs, it should be managed aggressively by maintaining adequate coronary perfusion pressure and treatment with nitroglycerin. If it is due to an anatomic problem with the reimplanted coronaries, then surgical intervention is indicated.
- Systemic and pulmonary hypertension is avoided to minimize bleeding and reduce the tension on suture lines.

Kaplan JA (ed): Cardiac Anesthesia, 3rd ed, pp 732–735. Philadelphia, WB Saunders, 1993

Lake CL (ed): Pediatric Cardiac Anesthesia, 3rd ed, pp 327–328. Stamford, CT, Appleton & Lange, 1998

C.13. What are the potential complications observed immediately postbypass?

The ASO procedure is associated with the potential for myocardial ischemia related to reimplantation of the coronary arteries (kinking of the vessels, air, etc.), arrhythmias, bleeding, and ventricular dysfunction. The atrial switch procedure (Senning or Mustard) is associated with a higher incidence of arrhythmias and heart block than the ASO. Since the atrial switch procedure does not involve reimplantation of the coronary arteries, there is a lower incidence of myocardial ischemia associated with it than the ASO.

Lake CL (ed): Pediatric Cardiac Anesthesia, 3rd ed, pp 327–328. Stamford, CT, Appleton & Lange, 1998

D. Postoperative Management

D.1. Discuss postoperative hemodynamic and ventilatory management. When would you plan to extubate this infant?

In the immediate postoperative period, the infant should have controlled mechanical ventilation with adequate airway pressures and tidal volumes to avoid atelectasis and shunt. If elevated PVR is an issue, then mild hyperventilation may be indicated to reduce PVR. The infant who has had an ASO procedure should remain intubated and sedated until he is hemodynamically stable and the adequacy of the repair has been ascertained. There should be no evidence of myocardial ischemia, and any arrhythmias should be controlled. There should be no evidence of continued bleeding and/or coagulopathy. It has been shown that a high-dose sufentanil anesthetic with postoperative opioid infusion for 24 hours in ASO patients reduces the stress response and conveys a better outcome than infants managed with a lighter anesthetic, i.e., halothane and morphine intraoperatively with intermittent doses of morphine and diazepam postoperatively. The infants who remained intubated on an opioid infusion postoperatively had a lower mortality and a lower incidence of complications such as sepsis, disseminated intravascular coagulation, and metabolic acidosis.

Anand KJS, Hickey PR: Halothane-morphine compared with high dose sufentanil for anesthesia and postoperative analgesia in neonatal cardiac surgery. N Engl J Med 326:1–9, 1992

D.2. What are the common complications associated with the ASO that are observed in the early postoperative period?

- Myocardial ischemia due to air or anatomic problems with reimplanted coronary arteries
- LV dysfunction due to ischemia, poor protection during cross-clamp, and/or inadequate muscle mass to support the systemic circulation
- Bleeding at suture lines or coagulopathy
- Arrhythmias, most commonly are asymptomatic atrial and ventricular premature beats

Lake CL (ed): Pediatric Cardiac Anesthesia, 3rd ed, pp 328–329. Stamford, CT, Appleton & Lange, 1998

D.3. What is JET? How is it treated?

JET is junctional ectopic tachycardia, which is an uncommon tachycardia that is observed in the early postoperative period following cardiopulmonary bypass in infants and toddlers with congenital heart disease. There is also a rarer congenital form of JET. The classic ECG findings include a tachycardia with a normal QRS at a rate of 180 to 240 bpm with atrioventricular dissociation. The etiology remains unknown but it is believed to be due to enhanced automaticity of tissues in or near the AV node as a result of surgical trauma.

The arrhythmia is usually transient in nature and is unusually resistant to most antiarrhythmic therapy. The hemodynamic instability associated with JET warrants aggressive intervention to slow the rate and, if possible, restore sinus rhythm. Procainamide and propafenone have been used effectively but, due to their negative inotropic effects, may not be appropriate agents if the patient is hemodynamically unstable. Due to the lack of response and risks of other therapies, induced hypothermia has become the treatment of choice in treating postoperative JET. Cooling to a temperature of 31° to 34°C has been shown to decrease the heart rate to below 180 bpm, but may result in peripheral vasoconstriction, metabolic acidosis, and agitation. Postoperative JET is usually transient, and slowing of the heart rate to allow return to normal sinus rhythm usually occurs within 24 to 72 hours regardless of the intervention used. Refractory or prolonged JET in the postoperative period conveys a poor prognosis.

Emmanouilides GC, Riemenschneider TA, Allen HD, Gutgesell HP (eds): Moss and Adams' Heart Disease in Infants, Children, and Adolescents, 5th ed, pp 1585–1587. Baltimore, Williams & Wilkins, 1995

11 Pacemaker

Fun-Sun F. Yao

A 76-year-old man was scheduled for insertion of a permanent transvenous pacemaker. He had had an anterior myocardial infarction 8 months earlier. His blood pressure was 120/80 mm Hg; heart rate, 40/min. He was taking propranolol, digoxin, furosemide, and isosorbide dinitrate.

A. Medical Disease and Differential Diagnosis

1. What is the possible ECG rhythm when the heart rate is 40/min?
2. What is the problem of complete atrioventricular (AV) block?
3. What are the common causes of heart block?
4. What are the indications for permanent pacemakers?
5. What is sick sinus syndrome?
6. How would you diagnose first-, second-, and third-degree AV block, right bundle branch block with, left anterior fascicular hemiblock, and left posterior fascicular hemiblock?
7. Is it necessary to insert a temporary pacemaker before general anesthesia for an asymptomatic patient with bifascicular block?
8. How many types of pacemakers are there? How do they work?
9. What are the three-letter and five-letter identification codes for pacemaker classification?
10. What is activity-mode or rate-responsive pacing? What are the precautions during anesthesia?
11. What are the differences between unipolar and bipolar electrode systems?
12. How would you know if it is atrial, ventricular, or AV sequential pacing?
13. What are the advantages and disadvantages of atrial pacing?
14. What are the indications and contraindications for AV sequential pacemakers?
15. In a permanent pacemaker battery, what are the usual values for pulse amplitude, pulse width, pulse rate, and sensing threshold?
16. What is the hysteresis rate?
17. How do you set the external pacemaker to test the pacing threshold, sensing R wave, and diaphragmatic pacing?
18. What are the acceptable values of pacing threshold, sensing R wave, and resistance?
19. What is "slew rate"?
20. What are the factors affecting pacing threshold?
21. What are the usual life spans of pacemakers?
22. How do you know if the implanted demand pacemaker is working?

B. Preoperative Evaluation and Preparation

1. What kind of workup would you like the patient to have?
2. What premedication would you give for local anesthesia?

C. Intraoperative Management

1. Would you give general or local anesthesia for insertion of a transvenous pacemaker? Why?
2. If it is an epicardial electrode, would you give local or general anesthesia?
3. Can regional anesthesia be used for pacemaker insertion?
4. How would you monitor the patient?
5. What drugs and equipment would you like to have on hand in the operating room?
6. How do you sedate the patient?
7. After the endocardial pacemaker was inserted, the ECG pattern suddenly changed from left bundle branch block to right bundle branch block. What is the possible diagnosis?

D. Postoperative Management

1. What are the complications of transvenous implantation of pacemakers?
2. What are the causes of pacemaker failure?
3. What is pacemaker syndrome?
4. What kinds of environmental electromagnetic interference may affect the function of a demand pacemaker?
5. Two months later, the patient came back for transurethral resection of the prostate because of prostatic hypertrophy. How would you prevent interference to the pacemaker from the electrocautery?
6. How do you detect inhibition of pacemaker function?
7. Are there any possible complications in applying a magnet over a demand pacemaker when electrocautery is used during surgery?
8. Would you use nitrous oxide anesthesia if a patient just had a permanent pacemaker implanted the day before surgery?
9. Is magnetic resonance imaging (MRI) contraindicated in patients with pacemakers?
10. What precautions should be taken when a patient with a pacemaker is undergoing extracorporeal shock wave lithotripsy (ESWL)?

A. Medical Disease and Differential Diagnosis

A.1. What is the possible ECG rhythm when the heart rate is 40/min?

Bradycardia may come from any part of the conduction system, including sinus bradycardia, nodal bradycardia, second-degree or third-degree AV block, atrial fibrillation with slow ventricular rate, and idioventricular rhythm.

Braunwald E (ed): Heart Disease, a Textbook of Cardiovascular Medicine, 5th ed, pp 642–643. Philadelphia, WB Saunders, 1997

A.2. What is the problem of complete atrioventricular (AV) block?

Complete heart block is the failure of the electrical activity from the atrium to progress through the AV node into the His-Purkinje system. When an impulse is not initiated immediately in the bundle of His, arrest occurs for a brief period and Stokes-Adams syndrome occurs, which causes light-headedness, dizziness, or loss of consciousness, sometimes accompanied by convulsions. During bradycardia, cardiac output is maintained by an increasing stroke volume. When the stroke volume is maximally increased, any further decrease in the heart rate will compromise cardiac output and cause circulatory failure.

Braunwald E (ed): Heart Disease, a Textbook of Cardiovascular Medicine, 5th ed, pp 691–692. Philadelphia, WB Saunders, 1997

Kusumoto FM, Goldschlager N: Cardiac pacing. N Engl J Med 334:89–98, 1996

A.3. What are the common causes of heart block?

Organic Disease
- Disease affecting primary conduction tissue
  - Lenegre's disease—sclerodegenerative process of the terminal portions of His bundles
  - Lev's disease—fibrous encroachment of the proximal His conduction pathway
- Disease affecting cardiac tissue
  - Coronary artery disease with ischemia or infarction
  - Cardiomyopathy
  - Myocarditis
- Surgically produced
- Congenital block

Functional Disturbances
- Increased vagal tone
- Drug therapy with quinidine, digitalis, procainamide, propranolol, verapamil, or potassium

Braunwald E (ed): Heart Disease, a Textbook of Cardiovascular Medicine, 5th ed, pp 687–692. Philadelphia, WB Saunders, 1997

Wynands JE: Anesthesia for patients with heart block and artificial cardiac pacemakers. Anesth Analg 55:626–631, 1976

A.4. What are the indications for permanent pacemakers?

Artificial pacing is indicated for treatment of persistent bradycardia of any origin if it compromises hemodynamics or predisposes to ventricular irritability manifested by premature beats or ventricular tachycardia. The two major indications for permanent pacing are failure of impulse formation and failure of cardiac conduction. Clinically, sick sinus syndrome and complete heart block are the most common indications for pacemakers. The following types of arrhythmias are common indications for pacemakers:

- Sinoatrial (SA) node—sick sinus syndrome, bradytachyarrhythmia, sinus bradycardia, hypersensitive carotid sinus syndrome, or vasovagal syncope
- AV node—second-degree or third-degree AV block
- Trifascicular block or bifascicular block with prolonged infranodal conduction
  - Right bundle branch block and left anterior hemiblock with hemodynamic symptoms
  - Right bundle branch block and left posterior hemiblock with hemodynamic symptoms
  - Alternating left bundle branch block and right bundle branch block
  - Left bundle branch block and first-degree AV block

- Hemodynamically disabling tachyarrhythmias with resistance to or intolerance of drug therapy or DC cardioversion
- Syncope without an ECG diagnosis
- Cardiomyopathy—severely symptomatic patients with hypertrophic obstructive cardiomyopathy

Braunwald E (ed): Heart Disease, a Textbook of Cardiovascular Medicine, 5th ed, pp 707–709. Philadelphia, WB Saunders, 1997

Kusumoto FM, Goldschlager N: Cardiac pacing. N Engl J Med 334:89–98, 1996

A.5. What is sick sinus syndrome?

Sick sinus syndrome describes an array of clinical disorders of sinus node function characterized by intrinsic inadequacy of the sinus node to perform its pacemaking function because of automatic dysfunction or failure of sinus node impulse to activate the rest of the atrium. Continuous tape recording for 24 hours by Holter monitor is necessary to make a diagnosis. The bradytachycardia syndrome is a common form of sick sinus syndrome. It is one of the most common indications for pacemakers and is characterized by the following:

- Unexpected persistent severe sinus bradycardia
- Episodes of sinus arrest or exit block
- Paroxysmal or chronic atrial fibrillation or atrial flutter
- Alteration of paroxyms of rapid regular or irregular atrial tachyarrhythmias and periods of slow atrial and ventricular rates (bradycardia-tachycardia syndrome)
- Slow return to sinus rhythm following cardioversion
- Lack of increase in sinus rate above 90/min following intravenous administration of 1.5 to 2.0 mg atropine.

Braunwald E (ed): Heart Disease, a Textbook of Cardiovascular Medicine, 5th ed, pp 648–649. Philadelphia, WB Saunders, 1997

Ferrer MI: The sick sinus syndrome. Circulation 47:635–641, 1973

A.6. How would you diagnose first-, second-, and third-degree AV block, right bundle branch block with left anterior fascicular hemiblock, and left posterior fascicular hemiblock?

First-degree AV block is characterized by a PR interval of >0.20 seconds. Second-degree AV block is subdivided into two types. Mobitz type I, or Wenckebach block, is characterized by a progressively lengthening PR interval, which occurs until an impulse is not conducted and a beat is dropped. Mobitz type II block is characterized by a sudden dropping of the QRS complex, with no progressive lengthening of the PR interval occurring. Third-degree AV block, also called complete heart block, occurs when all electrical activity from the atrium fails to progress into the Purkinje system. The atrial and ventricular contractions have no relationship with each other. The QRS complex is normal in complete AV nodal block. The QRS complex with complete infranodal block is frequently wide, and the ventricular rate is slow, averaging 40/min. Right bundle branch block with left anterior superior hemiblock is indicated when ECG shows right bundle branch block and left axis deviation. Complete right bundle branch block with right axis deviation is indicative of right bundle branch block and left postero-inferior hemiblock.

Braunwald E (ed): Heart Disease, a Textbook of Cardiovascular Medicine, 5th ed, pp 121–123, 688–692. Philadelphia, WB Saunders, 1997

Wynands JE: Anesthesia for patients with heart block and artificial cardiac pacemakers. Anesth Analg 55:626–631, 1976

A.7. Is it necessary to insert a temporary pacemaker before general anesthesia for an asymptomatic patient with bifascicular block?

Only a small minority of patients with bifascicular block may develop transient or established complete heart block and require implantation of a permanent pacemaker. The risk of progress to complete heart block in asymptomatic patients is very small, and such patients do not require a permanent pacemaker; it is not necessary to insert a temporary pacemaker before general anesthesia. However, it is advisable to have an external pacemaker available in the operating room.

Berg GR, Kotler MN: The significance of bilateral bundle branch block in the preoperative patient. Chest 59:62–67, 1971

Bloomfield P, Bowler GMR: Anaesthetic management of the patient with a permanent pacemaker. Anaesthesia 44:42–46, 1989

Braunwald E (ed): Heart Disease, a Textbook of Cardiovascular Medicine, 5th ed, pp 708–709. Philadelphia, WB Saunders, 1997

Kusumoto FM, Goldschlager N: Cardiac pacing. N Engl J Med 334:89–98, 1996

A.8. How many types of pacemakers are there? How do they work?

There are four types of pacers—asynchronous, single-chamber synchronous, double-chamber AV sequential, and programmable.

- Asynchronous or fixed-rate (AOO, VOO, DOO) pacemakers discharge at a preset rate that is independent of the inherent heart rate. They can be atrial, ventricular, or dual-chamber. Competition and ventricular fibrillation are the potential complications when normal heart rate reappears.
- Single-chamber synchronous or demand (AAI, AAT, VVI, VVT) pacemakers discharge at a preset rate only when the spontaneous heart rate drops below the preset rate. There are three types of synchronous pacers—ventricular-inhibited, ventricular-triggered, and atrial-triggered. The ventricular-inhibited pacer is the most popular type and is suppressed by normal electrical activity of the QRS complex. The ventricular-triggered pacers sense the QRS complex and then discharge into the absolute refractory period; therefore, they do not trigger another contraction. Atrial synchronous (triggered) pacers function through a double electrode system. When the P wave is sensed, the ventricle is stimulated to contract. When the P wave is not sensed, the ventricle is paced at the preset rate.
- Dual-chamber AV sequential pacing usually uses two electrodes, one in the atrial appendage and one in the right ventricular apex. The atrium is stimulated to contract first; then, after an adjustable PR interval, the ventricle is stimulated to contract. The atrial sequential ventricular-inhibited pacer is a combination of atrial, ventricular, sequential, and demand pacing. It may be totally dormant, may stimulate only the atrium, or may stimulate both atria and ventricles with a preset sequence. In AV synchronous (VAT, VDD) pacemakers, sensed atrial activity triggers a ventricular pacing stimulus. In AV sequential (DVI) pacemakers, sensing occurs

within the ventricle and pacing occurs sequentially within the atrium and ventricle. AV universal (DDD) pacemakers are essentially three pacemakers in one: VDD pacing during sinus rhythm with abnormal AV conduction; AAI pacing during sinus bradycardia with normal AV conduction; and DVI pacing during sinus bradycardia with abnormal AV conduction.

- Programmable pacemakers have been widely used since 1980. Pacing rate, pulse duration, voltage output, and R-wave sensitivity are the most common programmable functions. Refractory periods, PR intervals, mode of pacing, hysteresis, and atrial tracking rate can be programmed in modern pacemakers. Continuous and pulsed magnetic fields and radiofrequency wave are common methods of programming.

Braunwald E (ed): Heart Disease, a Textbook of Cardiovascular Medicine, 5th ed, pp 711–722. Philadelphia, WB Saunders, 1997

Eckenbrecht PD: Pacemaker and implantable cardioverter defibrillators. ASA Refresher Courses in Anesthesiology 23:55–67, 1995

Kusumoto FM, Goldschlager N: Cardiac pacing. N Engl J Med 334:89–98, 1996

Zaidan JR: Pacemakers. Anesthesiology 60:319–334, 1984

A.9. What are the three-letter and five-letter identification codes for pacemaker classification?

With the growing complexity of mode of pacing, location, and function of cardiac electrodes, difficulties with terminology became apparent. In the 1970s, the Inter-Society Commission for Heart Disease Resources (ICHD) suggested a classification code, which is now widely accepted. The original nomenclature involved a three-letter identification code, as shown in the first three columns of Table 11-1. In 1980, this code was extended to five letters; the last two letters can be deleted when not applicable. In 1987, the North American Society of Pacing and Electrophysiology (NASPE) adopted a new five-letter code to describe the operation of implantable pacemakers and defibrillators (Table 11-1). For example, a VOO pacemaker is a ventricular asynchronous type without sensing capability; a VVI pacemaker paces the ventricle and senses intrinsic R waves to inhibit artificial pacing.

Bernstein AD, Camm AJ, Flecher RD et al: The NASPE/BPEG generic pacemaker code for antibradyarrhythmias and adaptive-rate pacing and antitachyarrhythmias devices. Pace 10:794, 1987

Table 11-1. The NASPE/BPEG Generic (NBG) Pacemaker Identification Code

LETTER I	LETTER II	LETTER III	LETTER IV	LETTER V
Chamber(s) Paced	Chamber(s) Sensed	Mode of Response	Programmability, Rate Modulation	Antitachyarrhythmia Function(s)
0 = None	0 = None	0 = None	0 = None	0 = None
A = Atrium	A = Atrium	T = Triggered	P = Single programmable	P = Pacing
V = Ventricle	V = Ventricle	I = Inhibited	M = Multi-programmable	S = Shock
D = Dual (A + V)	D = Dual (A + V)	D = Dual (T + I)	C = Communicating	D = Dual (P + S)
			R = Rate modulation	

NASPE, North American Society of Pacing and Electrophysiology; BPEG, British Pacing and Electrophysiology Group; NBG, North American and British Generic.

Braunwald E (ed): Heart Disease, a Textbook of Cardiovascular Medicine, 5th ed, p 706. Philadelphia, WB Saunders, 1997

Eckenbrecht PD: Pacemaker and implantable cardioverter defibrillators. ASA Refresher Courses in Anesthesiology 23:55–67, 1995

Parsonnet V, Furman S, Smyth NPD: Implantable cardiac pacemakers: Status report and resource guideline. Report of the Inter-Society Commission for Heart Disease Resources. Am J Cardiol 34:487, 1974

Parsonnet V, Furman S, Smyth NPD: A revised code for pacemaker identification. Pace 4:440, 1981

A.10. What is activity-mode or rate-responsive pacing? What are the precautions during anesthesia?

In recent years, a new generation of pacemakers (AAIR, VVIR, DDIR and DDDR) has been developed to adjust the pacing rate according to the patient's level of activity, in order to obtain a more physiologic response to exercise. Various activity-detecting systems have been developed to create a reliable rate-responsive pacemaker; they include muscle movement, respiratory rate, minute ventilation, central venous temperature, QT interval, myocardial contractility (dp/dt), oxygen saturation and pH in mixed venous blood, and ventricular depolarization gradient. Currently, the sensors of motion or minute ventilation are used most widely in the United States.

It has been reported that pacemakers with a rate-responsive function based on calculation of ventilatory minute volume such as METAMV 1202 (Telectronics) may induce tachycardia in patients who undergo hyperventilation during general anesthesia. If hyperventilation is desired (e.g., in neurosurgery), it is suggested that the pacemaker be reprogrammed to exclude the rate-responsive function. If the programming device is not available, a magnet may be placed over the pacemaker site to convert it to fixed-rate pacing.

Braunwald E (ed): Heart Disease, a Textbook of Cardiovascular Medicine, 5th ed, pp 723–725. Philadelphia, WB Saunders, 1997

Eckenbrecht PD: Pacemaker and implantable cardioverter defibrillators. ASA Refresher Courses in Anesthesiology 23:55–67, 1995

Kusumoto FM, Goldschlager N: Cardiac pacing. N Engl J Med 334:89–98, 1996

Madsen GM, Andersen C: Pacemaker-induced tachycardia during general anaesthesia: A case report. Br J Anaesth 63:360–361, 1989

A.11. What are the differences between unipolar and bipolar electrode systems?

A unipolar lead has only one electrode—the cathode, or active lead. Current flows from the cathode, stimulates the heart, and must return to the anode on the casing of the pulse generator to complete the circuit. A bipolar lead has two poles on the lead a short distance from each other at the distal end, and both electrodes lie within the heart. Usually, the tip electrode is the cathode, while behind it is the ring anode. Generally, bipolar leads are preferred because of greater signal-to-noise ratio, less sensitivity to extraneous interference (especially skeletal myopotentials), less frequent crosstalk (atrial stimulus sensed by ventricular lead in a dual-chamber system), and avoidance of muscle stimulation occasionally seen at the anodal site of unipolar pulse generators. With modern pacemakers, there is little difference between unipolar and bipolar lead systems. The major difference between the two systems is the superiority of the unipolar system with sensing. Because of the larger distance between electrodes, the unipolar system has a larger area for sensing. Because of its enhanced sensing capability, the unipolar system is more sensitive to extracardiac electromagnetic interference than the bipolar system. However, the fibrillation threshold is lower for the bipolar compared with the unipolar cathodal stimulation. Therefore, bipolar pacing is more likely to cause ventricular fibrillation than unipolar pacing.

Braunwald E (ed): Heart Disease, a Textbook of Cardiovascular Medicine, 5th ed, p 771. Philadelphia, WB Saunders, 1997

A.12. *How would you know if it is atrial, ventricular, or AV sequential pacing?*

In atrial pacing, an electrical spike appears before the P wave and the QRS complex is usually normal. In ventricular pacing, the electrical spike is followed immediately by a widened QRS complex. In AV sequential pacing, there are two spikes, one before the P wave and another preceding the QRS complex.

Braunwald E (ed): Heart Disease, a Textbook of Cardiovascular Medicine, 5th ed, pp 712–715. Philadelphia, WB Saunders, 1997

A.13. *What are the advantages and disadvantages of atrial pacing?*

Atrial pacing increases cardiac output 26% over the cardiac output during ventricular pacing, because atrial contraction contributes 15% to 25% of the preload to the ventricle. It has been shown that coronary blood flow increases and coronary resistance decreases during atrial pacing. Atrial pacing is useless if atrioventricular block is present.

Yoshida S et al: Coronary hemodynamics during successive elevation of heart rate by pacing in subjects with angina pectoris. Circulation 44:1062, 1971

A.14. *What are the indications and contraindications for AV sequential pacemakers?*

AV sequential pacing increases cardiac output 34% over the cardiac output during ventricular pacing. This is achieved by the atrial systolic boost (atrial kick) to ventricular filling. When ventricular pacing cannot maintain adequate cardiac output and atrial pacing is not justified, as in complete AV block, AV sequential pacing is indicated. Because of the success of atrial endocardial leads, thin polyurethane insulation, miniature electronic circuits, and programmability, the indications for dual-chamber pacing are broadened. It can be used for the sick sinus syndrome and all degrees of heart block. DDD pacemaker is the ultimate form of physiologic pacing. Programmable features include the mode of pacing, the AV delay, the maximum atrial rate that the ventricle will follow (atrial tracking), and the minimum atrial rate for sensing at which atrial pacing commences. The major advantage of such pacing is the ability to increase the cardiac output by 200% to 300% under extreme stress. However, the major deficiency of DDD pacing is the dependence on the atrium as the physiologic sensor. Like VDD pacing, DDD pacing is contraindicated in patients with persistent or recurrent atrial fibrillation or flutter or significant atrial tachyarrhythmias, because it can cause pacemaker-mediated reentry tachyarrhythmia in the presence of retrograde conduction.

Braunwald E (ed): Heart Disease, a Textbook of Cardiovascular Medicine, 5th ed, pp 714–720. Philadelphia, WB Saunders, 1997

Eckenbrecht PD: Pacemaker and implantable cardioverter defibrillators. ASA Refresher Courses in Anesthesiology 23:55–67, 1995

Hatzler G et al: Hemodynamic benefits of AV sequential pacing after cardiac surgery. Am J Cardiol 40:323, 1977

A.15. *In a permanent pacemaker battery, what are the usual values for pulse amplitude, pulse width, pulse rate, and sensing threshold?*

The specifications of pacemakers differ slightly from one model to the next. The pulse amplitude or the output of stimulation usually is 4.8 to 5.0 volts or 9.6 to 10 milliamps. The pulse width or the duration of stimulation is usually preset at 0.5 to 0.8 msec. The pulse rate or the frequency of stimulation is usually set at 70/min. The sensing threshold or sensitivity is approximately 2.0 to 3.5 millivolts. The specifications may be programmed to suit special needs of the individual patient in a programmable pacemaker. The sensing threshold is the minimal electrical output from the heart to suppress the demand pacemaker.

Braunwald E (ed): Heart Disease, a Textbook of Cardiovascular Medicine, 5th ed, pp 710–711. Philadelphia, WB Saunders, 1997

A.16. *What is the hysteresis rate?*

Some types of pacemakers have a built-in hysteresis rate below the demand pacing rate. In pacing, hysteresis refers to an escape interval, which is different from an automatic interval. The escape interval is the period from the sensed patient's own beat to the next paced beat; the automatic interval is the period between two paced beats. Hysteresis is particularly useful for patients with sick sinus syndrome. If the hysteresis rate is 60/min and the pacing rate is 70/min the pacemaker will discharge at 70/min when the spontaneous cardiac rate falls below 60/min. However, hysteresis appears to have no advantage over a simple decrease in the pacing rate, and its advantages are more theoretical than real during single-chamber pacing.

Braunwald E (ed): Heart Disease, a Textbook of Cardiovascular Medicine, 5th ed, p 712. Philadelphia, WB Saunders, 1997

Eckenbrecht PD: Pacemaker and implantable cardioverter defibrillators. ASA Refresher Courses in Anesthesiology 23:55–67, 1995

A.17. *How do you set the external pacemaker to test the pacing threshold, sensing R wave, and diaphragmatic pacing?*

Any kind of electrical stimulation should have the following three components: strength (pulse amplitude), duration (pulse width), and frequency (pulse interval or rate). The pulse rate should be set approximately 10% higher than the patient's intrinsic heart rate in order to overdrive the heart. If the patient is in complete heart block, the rate is set to a physiologic level, 70 to 80/min. The pulse width depends on the factory preset value of the pacemaker generator to be implanted. It should be set at either the same number or slightly lower than the factory preset value in order to ensure that the implanted generator will work.

The pulse width of new generators is usually preset at 0.5 to 0.6 msec. The energy output of each impulse depends on the product of pulse amplitude and pulse width. If we test the pacing threshold with pulse width higher than that of the generator to be implanted, the generator may not work because of low energy output. The pulse amplitude is set at 10 milliamps or 5 volts, which is the output of the internal pacemaker to be implanted. Decrease the output until the ventricle is no longer paced, then increase the output until pacing begins. The pacing threshold is the minimal output necessary to pace the ventricle. It may be represented by voltage or current. Resistance may be obtained from Ohm's law, dividing voltage by current. In the Medtronic 5300 Pacing System Analyzer, the R wave may be tested by turning the control function to R wave and pushing the R-wave test button. The number of millivolts in the QRS complex, sensed by the pacemaker, passing from the ventricle through the electrode, is essential for the demand type of pacemaker. The most likely parameter to be inadequate, thus requiring lead repositioning, is R-wave size and this should be measured first. The R wave should also be measured prior to pacing because, on occasion, pacemaker dependence occurs immediately, making it very difficult to reestablish a satisfactory spontaneous rhythm after measuring pacing thresholds. Low pacing threshold, low resistance, and a high sensing R wave indicate a satisfactory position of the pacing electrode. Diaphragmatic pacing may be detected by increasing the pacing output to 5 to 10 volts or 10 milliamps and watching diaphragm movements and hiccups while the patient is asked to breathe deeply.

Braunwald E (ed): Heart Disease, a Textbook of Cardiovascular Medicine, 5th ed, pp 710–711. Philadelphia, WB Saunders, 1997

Kaplan JA (ed): Cardiac Anesthesia, 3rd ed, p 900. Philadelphia, WB Saunders, 1993

A.18. What are the acceptable values of pacing threshold, sensing R wave, and resistance?

Since the implant generators have a maximal initial output of 5 volts or 10 milliamps, the pacing threshold cannot exceed the above values. The acceptable values are 0.3 to 2.0 milliamps or 0.3 to 1.0 volts in acute or initial implants and up to 2.0 to 3.5 milliamps or 2.0 to 3.5 volts in chronic implants. There is an initial sharp rise in the pacing threshold during the first 2 weeks of up to ten times the acute level because of tissue reaction around the tip of the electrode. Then it falls to two to three times the acute level from the scar formation. In the chronic state, it remains essentially at the same level in 80% of patients; only 20% of patients exhibit a late rise in threshold. The sensing R wave should be at least 5 to 6 millivolts amplitude to inhibit or trigger a demand pacemaker, because the preset sensitivity is approximately 2.0 to 4.0 millivolts. Resistance should be between 250 and 1000 ohms. In atrial lead implantation, the acceptable sensing P-wave values are at least 1.5 to 2.0 millivolts, and pacing threshold is 0.6 to 2.0 volts or 1.0 to 3.0 milliamps.

Braunwald E (ed): Heart Disease, a Textbook of Cardiovascular Medicine, 5th ed, pp 710–711. Philadelphia, WB Saunders, 1997

A.19. What is "slew rate"?

Slew rate is the maximum rate of voltage change (dv/dt) in the sensed ventricular electrocardiogram and represents the steepness of the slope over a 2-millivolts voltage excursion. The slew rate can be measured by the pacing system analyzer or directly from an intracardiac electrogram. Adequate R-wave slew rates are of the order of 1 to 4 volts/sec and the minimum usually required to inhibit a pulse generator is 0.5 volts/sec.

Hurst JW (ed): The Heart, 7th ed, p 2102. New York, McGraw-Hill, 1990

A.20. What are the factors affecting pacing threshold?

Myocardial Factors
- Increased threshold—moderate hypoxia, hypercarbia, increased intracellular potassium, hypernatremia, sleep, postprandial state, propranolol, verapamil, quinidine, procainamide
- Decreased threshold—extreme hypoxia, hyperkalemia, exercise, ischemia, catecholamines

Electrode Factors
- Current density—the larger the electrode surface, the lower the pacing threshold
- Impulse duration—the longer the impulse, the lower the pacing threshold

Ream AK, Fogdall RP (eds): Acute Cardiovascular Management: Anesthesia and Intensive Care, pp 207–208. Philadelphia, JB Lippincott, 1982

A.21. What are the usual life spans of pacemakers?

The mercury-zinc pacemakers have a life span of 2 to 3 years, whereas the lithium-powered pacemakers can last 5 to 10 years for dual-chamber pacing and 7 to 12 years for single-chamber pacing.

Braunwald E (ed): Heart Disease, a Textbook of Cardiovascular Medicine, 5th ed, p 705. Philadelphia, WB Saunders, 1997

A.22. How do you know if the implanted demand pacemaker is working?

Slow the intrinsic heart rate to a rate below that of the pacemaker by carotid massage or a Valsalva maneuver. Carotid massage to slow the heart rate should be used cautiously because it could result in an arteriosclerotic plaque embolizing to the cerebral circulation. If the rate does not slow down enough for the pacemaker to take over the ventricle, a magnet can be applied over the pacemaker to convert it to the fixed-rate mode, and captured beats can be observed by watching the ECG and palpating the pulse. A 10% reduction in the magnet or automatic rate indicates a weakened battery supply.

Eckenbrecht PD: Pacemaker and implantable cardioverter defibrillators. ASA Refresher Courses in Anesthesiology 23:55–67, 1995

Zaidan JR: Pacemakers. Anesthesiology 60:319–334, 1984

B. Preoperative Evaluation and Preparation

B.1. What kind of workup would you like the patient to have?

Preoperative evaluation should include the routine systemic workup, paying particular attention to cardiovascular disorders. The systemic routine includes complete blood count, urinalysis, coagulation screening with prothrombin time and partial thromboplastin time, serum electrolytes, BUN, blood sugar, chest x-ray film, and ECG. Special attention should be paid to the history, symptoms, and signs of myocardial infarction, congestive heart failure, and arrhythmia. Serum electrolytes, especially potassium level, must be in the normal range. Blood pressure and consciousness level are checked to ensure adequate perfusion before implantation of the pacemaker.

Eckenbrecht PD: Pacemaker and implantable cardioverter defibrillators. ASA Refresher Courses in Anesthesiology 23:55–67, 1995

Simon AB: Perioperative management of the pacemaker patient. Anesthesiology 46:127–131, 1977

B.2. What premedication would you give for local anesthesia?

We prefer light sedation with pentobarbital, 1.5 mg/kg, intramuscularly. Because most patients with pacemakers are elderly and have cardiac disease, heavy sedation should be avoided to prevent cardiopulmonary depression.

C. Intraoperative Management

C.1. Would you give general or local anesthesia for insertion of a transvenous pacemaker? Why?

We prefer local anesthesia because patients who have heart block with symptoms and are given general anesthesia may develop cardiac standstill, ventricular tachycardia, or ventricular fibrillation. During local anesthesia, we can request that patients cough to check for the possibility of electrode dislodge or breathe deeply to test diaphragmatic pacing.

Braunwald E (ed): Heart Disease, a Textbook of Cardiovascular Medicine, 5th ed, p 709. Philadelphia, WB Saunders, 1997

Thomas SJ (ed): Manual of Cardiac Anesthesia, 2nd ed, p 385. New York, Churchill Livingstone, 1993

C.2. If it is an epicardial electrode, would you give local or general anesthesia?

Although local anesthesia with sedation has been used successfully for transthoracic implantation of epicardial electrodes, general anesthesia is commonly administered at our institution. If a complete block or severe bradycardia is present before the induction of general anesthesia, it is necessary to insert a transvenous temporary pacemaker under local anesthesia. When the patient is in sinus rhythm at the time of induction, a temporary pacer probably is not indicated. If a complete block suddenly develops after induction, isoproterenol may be given. An external transcutaneous pacemaker (PHYSIOCONTROL QUIK-PACE) should be available in emergency situations, especially during anesthesia.

Kaplan JA (ed): Cardiac Anesthesia, 3rd ed, p 990. Philadelphia, WB Saunders, 1993

C.3. Can regional anesthesia be used for pacemaker insertion?

Raza et al reported that the combination of an interscalene cervical plexus block and blocks of the second, third, and fourth intercostal nerves provided safe and effective anesthesia for pacemaker insertion. This technique provided complete surgical anesthesia without the need for large doses of either local anesthetics or narcotic analgesics.

Raza SM, Vasiveddy AR, Candido KD et al: A complete regional anesthesia technique for cardiac pacemaker insertion. J Cardiothorac Vasc Anesth 5:54–56, 1991

C.4. How would you monitor the patient?

The patient should have a blood pressure cuff, ECG with simultaneous V_5 and II leads display, precordial stethoscope, and pulse monitor for hemodynamic status. A pulse oximeter is especially helpful to detect hypoxia caused by excessive use of sedatives and narcotics.

C.5. What drugs and equipment would you like to have on hand in the operating room?

A complete array of drugs and equipment must be ready for cardiopulmonary resuscitation. The minimal requirements include a finger on the pulse, ECG monitor, a DC defibrillator, and the usual drugs for resuscitation. Atropine and isoproterenol are used to treat bradycardia. Lidocaine or a DC defibrillator is necessary to treat ventricular arrhythmia during the insertion of endocardial electrodes. A transcutaneous external pacemaker is very convenient in cases of extreme bradycardia or cardiac standstill.

Wynands JE: Anesthesia for patients with heart block and artificial cardiac pacemakers. Anesth Analg 55:626–631, 1976

C.6. How do you sedate the patient?

We usually titrate small doses of short-acting sedatives, such as thiopental sodium in 25-mg increments, midazolam in 0.5-mg increments, or diazepam in 1- to 2-mg increments. Fentanyl in 0.025-mg increments is used to supplement the local anesthesia. Oxygen is given by mask to prevent hypoxia from sedation. Hypoventilation is avoided by reminding the patient to take deep breaths intermittently. A precordial stethoscope is applied over the right chest to monitor respiration. A pulse oximeter is used to monitor arterial oxygen saturation.

C.7. After the endocardial pacemaker was inserted, the ECG pattern suddenly changed from left bundle branch block to right bundle branch block. What is the possible diagnosis?

The endocardial electrode has perforated the interventricular septum and paces the left ventricle. When the electrode is in the right ventricle, the ECG pattern is usually that of left bundle branch block.

Chung EK: Artificial Cardiac Pacing, p 338. Baltimore, Williams & Wilkins, 1978

D. Postoperative Management

D.1. What are the complications of transvenous implantation of pacemakers?

The complications are displacement of electrode, inability to pace or sense, skin erosion, infection, myocardial perforation, ventricular fibrillation, diaphragm stimulation, endocarditis, cardiac tamponade, skeletal muscle stimulation, pacemaker malfunction, pacemaker syndrome, and psychological distress and reliance.

Braunwald E (ed): Heart Disease, a Textbook of Cardiovascular Medicine, 5th ed, pp 726–729. Philadelphia, WB Saunders, 1997

D.2. What are the causes of pacemaker failure?

Failure of pacing may be due to battery failure, disruption of electrodes, or failure of capture at a myocardial level.

- Battery failure—exhausted battery, leak in seal, suppression, runaway pacemaker
- Disruption of electrode—broken wire, short circuit, insulation break
- Failure of capture—increasing threshold, myocardial perforation, malposition of pacing leads

Braunwald E (ed): Heart Disease, a Textbook of Cardiovascular Medicine, 5th ed, p 727. Philadelphia, WB Saunders, 1997

D.3. What is pacemaker syndrome?

Pacemaker syndrome is a clinical constellation of signs and symptoms produced by adverse hemodynamic and electrophysiologic responses to VVI pacing because of inappropriate timing of atrial and ventricular contractions. During VVI pacing, pacemaker syndrome most commonly occurs in patients with normal or near-normal LV function and retrograde ventriculoatrial (VA) conduction. A retrograde P wave or VA conduction follows each ventricular complex. In some patients this retrograde atrial contraction may have a negative effect on cardiac output. Loss of AV synchrony can decrease cardiac output by 20% to 30% at rest, but hemodynamic compromise in pacemaker syndrome is more complex because retrograde VA conduction causes a negative atrial kick with more profound hemodynamic disadvantages than simple loss of AV synchrony. Atrial contraction against closed mitral and tricuspid valves causes systemic and pulmonary venous regurgitation and congestion (cannon "a" waves).

Pacemaker syndrome includes hypotension, syncope, vertigo, light-headedness, fatigue, exercise intolerance, malaise, weakness, lethargy, dyspnea, induction of congestive heart failure, cough, awareness of beat-to-beat variations of cardiac response from spontaneous to paced beats, neck pulsations or pressure sensation in the chest, neck or head, headache and chest pain.

Pacemaker syndrome can be eliminated by restoring AV synchrony either with atrial pacing alone (if AV conduction is normal) or with dual-chamber pacing with an appropriate AV delay. Occasionally, restoration of AV synchrony can be accomplished by decreasing the VVI pacing rate (or using hysteresis) to minimize competition with sinus rhythm.

Braunwald E (ed): Heart Disease, a Textbook of Cardiovascular Medicine, 5th ed, pp 722–723. Philadelphia, WB Saunders, 1997

Miller M, Fox S, Jenkins R et al: Pacemaker syndrome: A noninvasive means to its diagnosis and treatment. Pace 4:503, 1981

D.4. What kinds of environmental electromagnetic interference may affect the function of a demand pacemaker?

- Microwave oven—The patient with the old type of pacemaker should not approach within 3 feet of an operating microwave oven. However, a modern pacemaker system can easily reject the interference.
- Diathermy—contraindicated.
- Electrocautery—Do not use within 15 cm of the implanted pulse generator.
- Electric razor—Do not use on the skin area over the implant site.
- Amateur radio transmitting equipment—Linear power amplifiers are contraindicated.
- Power transmission lines—High-voltage electric fields produced by 765 KV power lines should be avoided.
- Arc welding—contraindicated.
- Telephone transformer—contraindicated.
- Radiofrequency catheter ablation of arrhythmias potentially can produce similar disturbances of pacemaker behavior caused by electrocautery and can produce upper rate pacing in a minute ventilation-driven DDDR pacemaker.
- MRI—generally contraindicated
- Radiation therapy—This can damage pacemaker electronics and can cause unpredictable transient or permanent malfunction including runaway behavior. The effect is cumulative and similar whether the dose is given at one time or spread over several treatments. Given a sufficiently high cumulative absorbed dose, all pulse generators will fall catastrophically. Appropriate shielding of the pulse generator during radiation therapy is mandatory. Barring reset and other responses related to sensing electromagnetic interference, malfunction requires pacemaker replacement because long-term reliability becomes questionable.

Braunwald E (ed): Heart Disease, a Textbook of Cardiovascular Medicine, 5th ed, pp 728–729. Philadelphia, WB Saunders, 1997

D.5. Two months later, the patient came back for transurethral resection of the prostate because of prostatic hypertrophy. How would you prevent interference to the pacemaker from the electrocautery?

Electrocautery used in the presence of a demand pacemaker may cause inhibition, reversion into fixed-rate pacing, power-up sequence, and, rarely, myocardial burns and ventricular fibrillation. The following precautions should be taken:

- The grounding plate of the cautery should be placed as close to the operative site as possible and as far from the pacemaker as possible.
- The cautery should not be used within 15 cm of the pacemaker not only because it may interfere with the battery circuitry, but also because if the cautery should come in contact with a break in the insulation of the electrode, it may cauterize the myocardium at the tip of the electrode, rendering it insensitive to pacing impulses.
- The use of cautery should be limited to 1-second bursts every 10 seconds to prevent repetitive asystolic periods.
- If the pacemaker is inhibited by the cautery, a high-powered magnet can be safely applied over the demand nonprogrammable pacemaker to convert it to fixed-rate mode. Programmable pacemakers can undergo random reprogramming to almost

any conceivable mode of function while the electrocautery is being used. This risk is increased when a magnet is applied because the magnet activates a radio receiver that accepts radiofrequency signals emitted from the electrocautery.
- The use of bipolar electrocautery forceps reduces electromagnetic interference.
- Transcutaneous pacemaker and isoproterenol should be available for unexpected sudden cessation of pacing.

Bloomfield P, Bowler GMR: Anaesthetic management of the patient with a permanent pacemaker. Anaesthesia 44:42–46, 1989

Eckenbrecht PD: Pacemaker and implantable cardioverter defibrillators. ASA Refresher Courses in Anesthesiology 23:55–67, 1995

Simon AB: Perioperative management of the pacemaker patient. Anesthesiology 46:127–131, 1977

Wynands JE: Anesthesia for patients with heart block and artificial cardiac pacemakers. Anesth Analg 55:626–631, 1976

D.6. How do you detect inhibition of pacemaker function?

During electrocautery, the ECG is frequently useless because of interference. The best monitor available to determine if inhibition is taking place is a hand on the pulse. The precordial or esophageal stethoscope, pulse monitor, or blood pressure is also acceptable.

Eckenbrecht PD: Pacemaker and implantable cardioverter defibrillators. ASA Refresher Courses in Anesthesiology 23:55–67, 1995

Zaidan JR: Pacemakers. Anesthesiology 60:319–334, 1984

D.7. Are there any possible complications in applying a magnet over a demand pacemaker when electrocautery is used during surgery?

Most modern demand pacemakers automatically revert to the fixed-rate pacing mode in the presence of electromagnetic interference. However, reversion may not occur with intermittent or rapidly changing fields of electromagnetic interference, as with the rapid turning on and off of the electrocautery. A magnet may be placed to convert a demand pacemaker to the asynchronous mode. However, in certain programmable pacemakers, such as the Medtronic Xyrel-VP, magnets may activate the rate-changing circuit that allows electromagnetic waves emitted from the electrocautery to reprogram and change the pacing rate. Varying pacing rates from 30/min to 100/min have been reported. Therefore, we recommend that a specific pacemaker programmer should be available to program the demand pacer to a fixed-rate mode and remove the magnet from the precordial area.

Eckenbrecht PD: Pacemaker and implantable cardioverter defibrillators. ASA Refresher Courses in Anesthesiology 23:55–67, 1995

Komino KB, Smith TC: Electrocautery-induced reprogramming of a pacemaker using a precordial magnet. Anesth Analg 62:609–612, 1983

D.8. Would you use nitrous oxide anesthesia if a patient just had a permanent pacemaker implanted the day before surgery?

It has been reported that nitrous oxide could cause pacemaker malfunction by increasing gas in the prepectoral pacemaker pocket. Despite air evacuation with antibiotic solution before closure of the prepectoral pocket, a small amount of air remains entrapped in the pocket. In general, this small amount of air should have no clinical significance. However, nitrous oxide is 35 times more soluble in blood than nitrogen. When nitrous oxide is used for anesthesia, the amount of nitrous oxide diffused from blood to the air pocket is much more than the amount of nitrogen diffused from the air pocket to blood. Therefore, this causes an expansion of the gas in the pocket, which leads to loss of anodal contact and pacing system malfunction. It is advisable not to use nitrous oxide in a patient with a newly implanted pacemaker.

Lamas GA, Rebecca GS, Braunwald NS et al: Pacemaker malfunction after nitrous oxide anesthesia. Am J Cardiol 56:995, 1985

D.9. Is magnetic resonance imaging (MRI) contraindicated in patients with pacemakers?

MRI is generally contraindicated in patients with pacemakers. MRI can cause rapid pacing, inhibition, resetting of DDD pacemakers, and transient reed switch malfunction with asynchronous pacing. Serious malfunction with no output or rapid pacing may occur because pulsed energy from MRI can enter the lead by capacitive coupling and cause rapid ventricular pacing. When an MRI is considered absolutely essential, it is reasonable to program the pacemaker to its lowest voltage and pulse width or to OOO mode, provided the patient has an adequate underlying rhythm.

Braunwald E (ed): Heart Disease, a Textbook of Cardiovascular Medicine, 5th ed, p 729. Philadelphia, WB Saunders, 1997

D.10. What precautions should be taken when a patient with a pacemaker is undergoing extracorporeal shock wave lithotripsy (ESWL)?

ESWL is no longer contraindicated for patients with pacemakers. The only exception to this general statement is the abdominally placed pacemaker generators that are used for epicardial pacing. Because these generators are in the blast path of the shock wave, such patients should not be treated with ESWL. However, most transvenous pacemaker generators are placed in a pectoral location which is at a safe distance from the blast path.

While most pacemakers are not affected by ESWL, sometimes it may cause pacemaker malfunctions which include:

- Switching to magnet mode
- Reaching upper rate limit
- Pacing irregularity
- Oversensing of asynchronous shocks
- Damage to rate-sensing piezoelectric crystal
- Intermittent inhibition of ventricular output in dual-chamber pacemaker
- Electromagnetic interference

Therefore, special precautions should be taken preoperatively. The type of pacemaker, indications for its placement, degree of patient dependence, and pacemaker programmability must be determined prior to lithotripsy. A dedicated pacemaker programmer should be available in the lithotripsy suite should pacemaker malfunction be caused by the shock waves. In addition, an alternative means of pacing, such as transcutaneous pacing, should also be available in case the pacemaker becomes permanently damaged. Low-energy shock waves (<16 kilovolts) should be used initially; then the energy level is gradually increased while pacemaker function is monitored carefully.

Dual-chamber demand pacemakers are especially sensitive to shock waves. They may need to be programmed to a ventricular pacing mode or switched from demand to fixed-rate pacing so that lithotripsy can be conducted safely.

Malhotra V (ed): Anesthesia for Renal and Genito-Urologic Surgery, pp 126–128. New York, McGraw-Hill, 1996

12 Thoracic Aortic Aneurysm

Fun-Sun F. Yao

A 76-year-old man suffered for 2 days from severe chest pain radiating to his back. He was scheduled for repair of a dissecting descending thoracic aneurysm. Past history revealed hypertension and three episodes of myocardial infarction. The last heart attack took place 5 months ago. He was taking propranolol, nitroglycerin, and diltiazem.

A. Medical Disease and Differential Diagnosis

1. Discuss the differential diagnosis of chest pain.
2. How would you classify dissecting aneurysm?
3. What is Crawford classification of thoracoabdominal aneurysms?
4. What is the treatment for aortic dissection? What are the indications for surgery?
5. What is the statistical incidence of perioperative myocardial reinfarction for this patient?

B. Preoperative Evaluation and Preparation

1. Would you discontinue propranolol, nitroglycerin, and diltiazem?
2. How would you premedicate this patient?

C. Intraoperative Management

1. How would you monitor this patient?
2. Where would you put the arterial line for monitoring?
3. How could you differentiate the true and false lumens of the aorta by transesophageal echocardiography (TEE)?
4. How would you induce anesthesia?
5. How would you maintain anesthesia?
6. Would you do one-lung anesthesia for resection of a descending thoracic aneurysm? Why?
7. How would you achieve one-lung anesthesia? Would you use a left-sided or right-sided double-lumen tube (DLT)? How would you know if the tube is in the proper position?
8. What are the cardiovascular effects of cross-clamping the descending thoracic aorta?
9. What are the metabolic effects of cross-clamping the descending thoracic aorta?
10. How do you control hypertension when the aorta is cross-clamped?
11. Why is distal aortic perfusion recommended when the thoracic aorta is cross-clamped? How can it be done?
12. What levels of blood pressure would you maintain when the aorta is cross-clamped?

276

13. Describe the blood supply of the spinal cord.
14. How do you detect spinal cord ischemia?
15. What are the effects of anesthetics on somatosensory evoked potentials in humans?
16. How would you protect the spinal cord when the descending aorta is cross-clamped?
17. What are determinants of postoperative renal failure after descending thoracic aneurysm repair? How would you protect the kidneys during surgery?
18. What are hemodynamic and metabolic effects of aortic unclamping? How would you prevent and treat them?

D. Postoperative Management

1. What are the postoperative complications from resection of an aortic aneurysm?

A. Medical Disease and Differential Diagnosis

A.1. Discuss the differential diagnosis of chest pain.

Chest pain is one of the most frequent complaints for which patients seek medical attention. Careful history taking, complete physical examination, chest x-ray film, and ECG are essential for accurate diagnosis. The differential diagnosis includes the following: angina pectoris, myocardial infarction, pericarditis, pleurisy, pneumothorax, pulmonary tumors, pulmonary emboli, mediastinal emphysema, mediastinitis, mediastinal tumors, acute dissection of the aorta, expanding aortic aneurysm, subacromial bursitis, arthritis of the shoulder and spine, esophagitis, abdominal disorders, and emotional disorders.

The abrupt onset of excruciating pain, which almost immediately reaches its peak intensity, is very characteristic of an aortic dissection. The pain is localized to the center of the chest, and often radiates into the back. A myocardial infarction, by contrast, may gradually develop pain of increasing severity over several minutes. Electrocardiographic changes are diagnostic.

The diagnostic findings of aortic aneurysm include a widened mediastinum or a left pleural effusion from extravasation. CT scanning or transesophageal echocardiography to demonstrate the double lumen created by the dissection is the most definitive diagnostic procedure.

Fauci AS, Braunwald E, Isselbacher KJ et al (eds): Harrison's Principles of Internal Medicine, 14th ed, pp 60–63. New York, McGraw-Hill, 1998

Schwartz SI (ed): Principles of Surgery, 6th ed, pp 916–917. New York, McGraw-Hill, 1994

A.2. How would you classify dissecting aneurysm?

The term "dissecting aneurysm" is a misnomer, because the condition is not an aneurysm but an "aortic dissection," a dissection of the aortic wall. An aneurysm develops when elastica of the aorta is weakened so that the pressure of blood causes dilation of the wall. Aortic dissections result from cystic medial necrosis with mucoid and cystic degeneration of the elastic fibers in the medial of the aorta. Currently, there are two classifications for aortic dissections. Aortic dissection is classified by De-

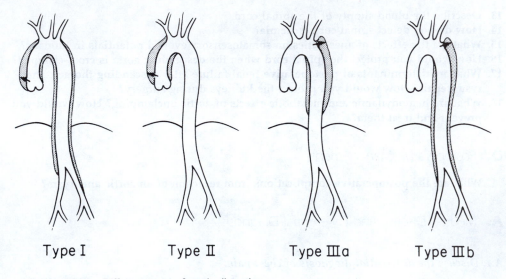

Type I   Type II   Type IIIa   Type IIIb

Figure 12-1. Different types of aortic dissection.

Bakey and associates according to the site of origin and the extent of distal dissection, as shown in Figure 12-1.

- Type I dissection begins in the ascending aorta near the aortic valve and extends throughout the aorta down to the common iliac arteries. Unfortunately, this is a common type of aortic dissection.
- Type II dissection is limited to the ascending aorta. This is commonly seen in Marfan's syndrome. This is the rarest form of dissection.
- Type IIIa dissection begins distal to the left subclavian artery and ends in the descending thoracic aorta. Its localized nature makes it accessible to surgical excision if needed.
- Type IIIb dissection begins distal to the left subclavian artery and extends into the abdominal aorta. Type IIIb dissections rarely require surgical intervention.

Based on clinical course and surgical significance, Daily at Stanford reclassified dissections into two types:

- Type A dissection originates in the ascending aorta and includes DeBakey's type I and type II dissections.
- Type B dissection originates only in the descending aorta and is equivalent to DeBakey's type III dissection. These may dissect retrograde into the aortic arch or ascending aorta.

Crawford ES: The diagnosis and management of aortic dissection. JAMA 264:2537–2541, 1990

Daily PO, Trueblood H, Stinson E et al: Management of acute aortic dissections. Ann Thorac Surg 10:237–247, 1990

DeBakey ME, Cooley DA, Crawford ES et al: Aneurysms of the thoracic aorta. J Thorac Surg 36:393–420, 1958

O'Connor CJ, Rothenberg DM: Anesthetic considerations for descending thoracic aortic surgery: Part I. J Cardiothorac Vasc Anesth 9:581–588, 1995

O'Connor CJ, Rothenberg DM: Anesthetic considerations for descending thoracic aortic surgery: Part II. J Cardiothorac Vasc Anesth 9:734–749, 1995

Schwartz SI (ed): Principles of Surgery, 6th ed, pp 915–916. New York, McGraw-Hill, 1994

A.3. What is Crawford classification of thoracoabdominal aneurysms?

Thoracoabdominal aneurysm is classified by Crawford into four types:

- Type I extends from the proximal descending thoracic aorta (DTA) to the upper abdominal aorta but terminates before the renal arteries.
- Type II extends below the renal arteries.
- Type III begins in the distal half of the DTA and extends for a variable length into the abdomen.
- Type IV involves most of the abdominal aorta.

O'Connor CJ, Rothenberg DM: Anesthetic considerations for descending thoracic aortic surgery: Part I. J Cardiothorac Vasc Anesth 9:581–588, 1995

Svensson LG, Crawford ES: Aortic dissection and aortic aneurysm surgery: Clinical observations, experimental investigations, and statistical analyses, Part II. Curr Probl Surg December: 922–1011, 1992

A.4. What is the treatment for aortic dissection? What are the indications for surgery?

The above classification schemes have therapeutic implications because patients with acute distal dissections (type B or type III) are initially treated medically, whereas proximal dissections (type A, type I, or type II) are immediately repaired.

Medical treatment should be started as soon as the diagnosis is suspected, preferably in the emergency room, because it may stop the dissection process and prevent complications such as aortic valve insufficiency, myocardial infarction, or rupture. Immediate drug therapy includes controlling hypertension with sodium nitroprusside and decreasing forceful contractility of the left ventricle with a beta-blocking agent, such as propranolol. Long-acting drugs such as methyldopa and hydralazine may be used. Immediate and 5-year survival is improved in type B dissection with medical therapy versus surgical intervention. A patent false lumen is predictive of the need for surgical intervention in the future.

Dissections of the ascending aorta are promptly operated upon, generally as an emergency. With dissections of the ascending thoracic aorta, surgical treatment corrects associated aortic regurgitation, coronary ischemia, cardiac tamponade, and cerebral malperfusion. Surgery for type B dissections is indicated for occlusion of limb circulation, renal or visceral ischemia, or chronic dissection with an aneurysm >6 cm in diameter or frank rupture. Surgical treatments include complete resection and prosthetic replacement of the involved aorta. If the ascending aorta is to be repaired, cardiopulmonary bypass should be used. For aneurysms of the aortic arch, total circulatory arrest with profound hypothermia, retrograde cerebral perfusion, or antegrade perfusion of arch vessels is used to provide cerebral perfusion during arch replacement. For repair of a descending thoracic aneurysm, the aorta is clamped distal to the left subclavian or left common carotid artery, using partial bypass or a shunt to unload the left ventricle and to perfuse the lower parts of the body. The mortality of emergency operations is presently 22% with ascending dissections and 14% with descending dissections.

Hillenberg A, Rainier W, Sadler T: Aneurysm of the descending thoracic aorta: Replacement with the use of a shunt or bypass. J Thorac Cardiovasc Surg 81:818, 1981

Schwartz SI (ed): Principles of Surgery, 6th ed, pp 923–924. New York, McGraw-Hill, 1994

A.5. What is the statistical incidence of perioperative myocardial reinfarction for this patient?

The incidence of perioperative reinfarction depends on the time interval between the previous myocardial infarction and surgery. Because this patient had an infarction 5 months ago, the reinfarction rate is between 2.3% and 16%. Other factors increasing the risk of perioperative reinfarction are discussed in Chapter 7, question A.4. The incidence of reinfarction for this patient is increased because of the following factors: age over 70 years, myocardial infarction in previous 6 months, preoperative hypertension, aortic surgery, long duration of surgery (>3 hours), and intraoperative hypertension and hypotension.

Goldman L, Caldera DL, Nussbaum SR et al: Multifactorial index of cardiac risk in noncardiac surgical procedures. N Engl J Med 297:845–850, 1977

Mangano DT: Perioperative cardiac morbidity. Anesthesiology 72:153–184, 1990

Rao TLK, Jacobs KH, El-Etr AA: Reinfarction following anesthesia in patients with myocardial infarction. Anesthesiology 59:499–505, 1983

B. Preoperative Evaluation and Preparation

B.1. Would you discontinue propranolol, nitroglycerin, and diltiazem?

No. All the antihypertensive drugs and medications for angina pectoris and hypertension should be continued until the time of surgery to prevent rebound hypertension, which may cause rupture of the aortic aneurysm or dissection and precipitate a myocardial infarction.

Barash PG, Cullen BF, Stoelting RK (eds): Clinical Anesthesia 3rd ed, pp 1139–1140. Philadelphia, Lippincott-Raven, 1997

Prichard BWC et al: The syndrome associated with the withdrawal of beta-adrenergic receptor blocking drugs. Br J Clin Pharm 13:337, 1982

B.2. How would you premedicate this patient?

Morphine sulfate, 4 mg, may be given intramuscularly if the patient still has chest pain. Diazepam, 5 mg, may be taken orally to relieve anxiety. In elderly patients, narcotics and sedatives should be administered cautiously because severe respiratory depression and hypotension may occur.

C. Intraoperative Management

C.1. How would you monitor this patient?

Invasive hemodynamic monitoring is required.

- ECG—simultaneous leads V_5 and II for myocardial ischemia and arrhythmias
- Arterial line for blood pressure and blood gases
- Swan-Ganz catheter for PCWP, PAP, and cardiac output measurement

- Foley catheter for urine output
- Temperature
- Oxygen analyzer for inspired gas mixture
- Pulse oximeter for continuous arterial oxygen saturation
- End-tidal CO_2 monitor
- Laboratory studies—arterial blood gases, electrolytes, hematocrit, coagulation study
- Transesophageal two-dimensional echocardiography for confirmation of the aortic dissection, identification of the true and false lumens, locating the site of intimal tears, and monitoring ventricular function, myocardial ischemia, volume status, and valvular function.
- Somatosensory evoked potentials for spinal cord function, if available
- Esophageal stethoscope
- CSF pressure—CSF drainage keeping the ICP <10 mm Hg for extensive operations on the thoracoabdominal aorta.

C.2. *Where would you put the arterial line for monitoring?*

The arterial line should be placed in the right radial or brachial artery and the femoral or dorsalis pedis artery when descending thoracic aneurysms are resected using extracorporeal circulation. Left radial catheterization is not useful because the left subclavian artery may be clamped during aortic resection. Both radial and femoral arterial lines monitor systemic pressure above and below the aortic clamp. Without a pressure monitor below the clamp, hypertension above the clamp may be treated too vigorously and cause hypoperfusion of the lower half of the body. However, monitoring arterial blood pressure during ascending aorta repair, unlike descending aorta repair, is performed from the left radial or brachial artery because the innominate artery may be cross-clamped during surgery.

O'Connor CJ, Rothenberg DM: Anesthetic considerations for descending thoracic aortic surgery: Part I. J Cardiothorac Vasc Anesth 9:581–588, 1995

C.3. *How could you differentiate the true and false lumens of the aorta by transesophageal echocardiography (TEE)?*

Color Doppler and pulsed Doppler modes can show systolic forward flow with high velocities in the true lumen and slow flow or flow reversal in the false lumen. Two-dimensional TEE often demonstrates spontaneous echo density in the false lumen. In addition, the true lumen tends to expand during systole and collapse during diastole. The entry tears in the intimal flap may be located with color Doppler by illustrating systolic flow from the true lumen to the false lumen. Absent flow in the false lumen indicates no communication or a more distal communication between the two lumens or that the false lumen is filled with thrombus.

Erbel R: Role of transesophageal echocardiography in dissection of the aorta and evaluation of degenerative aortic disease. Cardiol Clin 11:461–472, 1993

Neustein SM, Lansman SL, Quintana CS et al: Transesophageal Doppler echocardiographic monitoring for malperfusion during aortic dissection repair. Ann Thorac Surg 56:358–361, 1993

O'Connor CJ, Rothenberg DM: Anesthetic considerations for descending thoracic aortic surgery: Part I. J Cardiothorac Vasc Anesth 9:581–588, 1995

Simon P, Owen AN, Havel M et al: Transesophageal echocardiography in the emergency surgical management of patients with aortic dissection. J Thorac Cardiovasc Surg 103:1113–1118, 1992

C.4. How would you induce anesthesia?

A smooth induction is essential to prevent hypotension, tachycardia, and hypertension, which may precipitate myocardial ischemia and rupture of the aortic aneurysm. We prefer to induce anesthesia with fentanyl, 5 to 10 μg/kg, and the hypnotic dose of thiopental sodium, 1 to 2 mg/kg. The patient is ventilated with 100% oxygen by mask. After administration of succinylcholine, 1 mg/kg, and lidocaine, 1 mg/kg intravenously, the patient is intubated with a double-lumen tube. Intravenous lidocaine is used to block a hypertensive response to laryngoscopy and intubation. Nitroprusside or nitroglycerin drip should be prepared to control hypertension whenever necessary. Another acceptable induction technique is performed by slowly administering a hypnotic dose of midazolam or etomidate followed by an intubating dose of a nondepolarizing muscle relaxant after demonstrating a patent airway. This will attenuate the risk of chest wall rigidity following administration of high dose narcotics. Fentanyl-induced chest wall rigidity may cause hypercarbia and hypoxemia resulting in sympathetic mediated tachycardia and hypertension. Once mask ventilation and oxygenation is established, fentanyl may then be titrated to blunt the cardiovascular effects of subsequent endotracheal intubation. Esmolol or propranolol should be readily available to control tachycardia induced by tracheal intubation.

Cork RC, Weiss JL, Hameroff SR et al: Fentanyl preloading for rapid-sequence induction of anesthesia. Anesth Analg 63:60–64, 1984

Martin DE, Rosenberg H, Aukburg SJ et al: Low-dose fentanyl blunts circulatory responses to tracheal intubation. Anesth Analg 61:680–684, 1982

O'Connor CJ, Rothenberg DM: Anesthetic considerations for descending thoracic aortic surgery: Part I. J Cardiothorac Vasc Anesth 9:581–588, 1995

C.5. How would you maintain anesthesia?

A smooth anesthetic course is essential for the patient with ischemic heart disease undergoing aortic aneurysm repair. Moderate-dose fentanyl and low concentrations of inhalation anesthetics, such as isoflurane or halothane, are titrated to achieve this. Enflurane has been shown to increase cerebrospinal fluid (CSF) production and decrease CSF removal in dogs and theoretically should be avoided to minimize the risk of spinal cord ischemia from excessive CSF pressure. Nitrous oxide is avoided during one-lung anesthesia because high concentrations of oxygen are needed to prevent hypoxemia. It is easier to control hypertension with inhalation anesthetics, especially in patients with a history of hypertension. However, high concentrations of inhalation anesthetics should be avoided because they are potent cardiac depressants and may cause hypoxemia from inhibition of hypoxic pulmonary vasoconstriction. Moreover, isoflurane at concentrations of >1% probably may induce coronary steal and myocardial ischemia in patients with coronary artery disease and steal-prone anatomy. However, isoflurane can be safely administered to patients with coronary artery disease as long as hypotension and tachycardia are avoided.

Artru AA: Relationship between cerebral blood volume and CSF pressure during anesthesia with halothane or enflurane in dogs. Anesthesiology 58:533–539, 1983

Carlsson AJ, Bindslev L, Hedenstierna G: Hypoxia-induced pulmonary vasoconstriction in the human lung: The effect of isoflurane anesthesia. Anesthesiology 66:312–316, 1987

Cheng DCH, Moyers JR, Knutson RM et al: Dose-response relationship of isoflurane and halothane versus coronary perfusion pressures. Anesthesiology 76:113–122, 1992

Domino KB, Boronec L, Alexander CM et al: Influence of isoflurane on hypoxic pulmonary vasoconstriction in dogs. Anesthesiology 64:423–429, 1986

Merin RG, Buffington CW: Is isoflurane hazardous for the patient with coronary artery disease? ASA Refresher Courses in Anesthesiology 17:193–200, 1989

O'Connor CJ, Rothenberg DM: Anesthetic considerations for descending thoracic aortic surgery: Part I. J Cardiothorac Vasc Anesth 9:581–588, 1995

Pulley DD, Kirvassilis GV, Ketermenos N et al: Regional and global myocardial circulatory and metabolic effects of isoflurane and halothane in patients with steal-prone coronary anatomy. Anesthesiology 75:756–766, 1991

C.6. Would you do one-lung anesthesia for resection of a descending thoracic aneurysm? Why?

The indications for one-lung anesthesia are listed in the answer to question C.10. in Chapter 2, Bronchoscopy and Thoracotomy. One-lung anesthesia is especially advantageous for resection of a descending aortic aneurysm. First, surgical exposure is considerably enhanced by collapse of the left lung. Second, the nondependent left lung is protected from the trauma of surgical retraction. Third, initial surgical dissection and manipulation can cause bleeding into the bronchi of the left lung, especially when the patient is heparinized, because the aneurysm is often adherent to the adjacent lung tissue. A double-lumen endotracheal tube can separate the involved from the uninvolved lung, providing one functional lung both intraoperatively and postoperatively.

O'Connor CJ, Rothenberg DM: Anesthetic considerations for descending thoracic aortic surgery: Part I. J Cardiothorac Vasc Anesth 9:581–588, 1995

C.7. How would you achieve one-lung anesthesia? Would you use a left-sided or right-sided double-lumen tube (DLT)? How would you know if the tube is in the proper position?

A double-lumen endobronchial tube, such as a Robertshaw tube, may be used to achieve one-lung anesthesia. The left-sided DLT is preferred because the right-sided DLT may occlude the right upper bronchus. However, a left-sided DLT may be impossible to insert in some patients because very large descending aneurysms may distort the trachea or left mainstem bronchus. Moreover, repetitive blind attempts at DLT placement risk potential rupture of the aneurysm. Patients with aortic aneurysm may also have a distorted left mainstem bronchus. A right endobronchial tube may be used, but proper alignment with the right upper lobe bronchus should be confirmed with a fiberoptic bronchoscope.

The position of the double-lumen endobronchial tube may be checked by listening to the breath sounds of each lung while clamping each lumen of the endobronchial tube. If the breath sounds are unclear, as in patients with emphysema, a fiberoptic bronchoscope should be used to make sure that the tracheal opening is 1 to 2 cm above the carina and that the left endobronchial cuff is just below the tracheal carina and not blocking the opening of the left upper lobe bronchus.

O' Connor CJ, Rothenberg DM: Anesthetic considerations for descending thoracic aortic surgery: Part I. J Cardiothorac Vasc Anesth 9:581–588, 1995

C.8. What are the cardiovascular effects of cross-clamping the descending thoracic aorta?
Cross-clamping of the descending thoracic aorta causes marked proximal aortic hypertension, elevations in intracranial, central venous, pulmonary artery, pulmonary wedge, and left-ventricular end-diastolic pressures. It also markedly decreases distal aortic and spinal cord perfusion pressures as well as renal blood flow. Aortic cross-clamping also causes myocardial systolic and diastolic dysfunction and may produce myocardial ischemia by alterations in coronary blood flow and increased myocardial oxygen consumption.

The most consistent and dramatic response is severe proximal arterial hypertension. The main hemodynamic effects induced by aortic cross-clamping result from an increase in impedance to aortic flow and an increase in systemic vascular resistance and afterload, blood volume redistribution caused by collapse and constriction of venous vasculature distal to aortic clamp, and a subsequent increase in preload. Preload may not increase if the aorta is clamped distal to celiac artery; in that case blood volume from distal venous vasculature may be redistributed into splanchnic vasculature without associated increase in preload. Increases in afterload and preload demand an increase in contractility, which results in an autoregulatory increase in coronary blood flow. If an increase in coronary blood flow and myocardial contractility does not occur, as in patients with severe coronary artery disease, decompensation follows. Aortic cross-clamping is associated with the formation and release of many humoral mediators such as renin, angiotensin, catecholamines, oxygen free radicals, prostaglandins, complement activation system, endotoxins, cytokines, and myocardial-depressant factors. These mediators represent a double-edged sword. They may reduce or aggravate the harmful effects of aortic cross-clamp and unclamping. Injury to the lungs, kidneys, spinal cord and abdominal viscera is caused mainly by ischemia and reperfusion of organs distal to aortic cross-clamping (local effects) or to a release of mediators from ischemic and reperfused tissue (distal effects).

Barash PG, Cullen BF, Stoelting RK (eds): Clinical Anesthesia 3rd ed, pp 889–892. Philadelphia, Lippincott-Raven, 1997

Gelman S: The pathophysiology of aortic cross-clamping and unclamping. Anesthesiology 82:1026–1060, 1995

O'Connor CJ, Rothenberg DM: Anesthetic considerations for descending thoracic aortic surgery: Part II. J Cardiothorac Vasc Anesth 9:734–749, 1995

C.9. What are the metabolic effects of cross-clamping the descending thoracic aorta?
Cross-clamping of the descending thoracic aorta causes anaerobic metabolism and lac-

tic acid production in tissues below the cross-clamp. High aortic cross-clamping also reduces hepatic blood flow, resulting in decreased hepatic clearance of lactate, and further contributes to metabolic acidosis.

Gelman S: The pathophysiology of aortic cross-clamping and unclamping. Anesthesiology 82:1026–1060, 1995

O'Connor CJ, Rothenberg DM: Anesthetic considerations for descending thoracic aortic surgery: Part II. J Cardiothorac Vasc Anesth 9:734–749, 1995

O'Rourke K, Beattie C, Walman AT et al: Acidosis during high cross-clamp surgery. Anesthesiology 63:A266, 1985

C.10. How do you control hypertension when the aorta is cross-clamped?

The control of proximal hypertension must begin before the aortic cross-clamp is fully applied and, therefore, vasodilators are titrated to reduce the preclamp systolic blood pressure to approximately 90 mm Hg. Hypertension may be controlled by partial bypass, shunt, vasodilation, and anesthesia. If partial bypass is employed, proximal blood pressure can be lowered by increasing venous return to the pump with subsequent decrease in venous return to the heart. Shunting blood from the proximal aorta, left atrium, or left ventricle to the distal aorta or femoral artery may decrease systemic vascular resistance and lower blood pressure, but shunt flow cannot be controlled. A vasodilator, such as trimethaphan, nitroprusside or nitroglycerin, may be added to inhalational anesthetics to decrease systemic vascular resistance. However, if shunt or bypass is not used, only the upper part of the body proximal to the aortic clamp can be vasodilated to accommodate total cardiac output. Therefore, vasodilator therapy is not very effective. In addition, regional blood flow studies have shown that nitroprusside may decrease renal and spinal cord blood flow in a dose-related fashion. In addition, nitroprusside can also increase cerebral blood flow and intracranial and intraspinal pressures, further compromising spinal cord perfusion. Thus, sodium nitroprusside should be used with caution during aortic cross-clamping. Inhalation anesthetics, such as halothane or isoflurane, may be used in combination with trimethaphan, nitroprusside, and nitroglycerin to lower blood pressure by their cardiac depression and vasodilator effects. In addition, judicious titration of short-acting beta-blocker such as esmolol or labetalol can control heart rate and lower the dose requirement for nitroprusside. Recently, trimethaphan has been compared with nitroprusside to control proximal aortic hypertension during aortic cross-clamping in a canine model. Simpson et al demonstrated that distal aortic pressure was higher, CSF pressure was lower, spinal cord perfusion pressure was higher, and the neurologic outcome was better in the trimethaphan group.

O'Connor CJ, Rothenberg DM: Anesthetic considerations for descending thoracic aortic surgery: Part II. J Cardiothorac Vasc Anesth 9:734–749, 1995

Simpson JI, Zide TR, Newman SB et al: Trimethaphan versus sodium nitroprusside for the control of proximal hypertension during thoracic aortic cross-clamping: the effects on spinal cord ischemia. Anesth Analg 82:68–74, 1996

C.11. Why is distal aortic perfusion recommended when the thoracic aorta is cross-clamped? How can it be done?

Distal aortic perfusion is recommended to attenuate proximal hypertension and to increase tissue perfusion below the aortic cross-clamp. Distal aortic perfusion protects the cerebral circulation from the resultant hypertension. It also protects the left ventricle from increased afterload and provides blood flow to the lower body to prevent spinal cord and renal ischemia. In addition, it prevents the metabolic acidosis and dramatic hypotension characteristic of the declamping syndrome. Mortality associated with repair of DTA aneurysm or thoracoabdominal aneurysm is approximately 10%. Neurologic injury from spinal cord ischemia ranges from 3% to 15% depending on the extent of the aneurysm. Renal failure can be present up to 10% of the time. The risk of spinal cord injury increases dramatically when cross-clamp times exceed 30 minutes. Although there have been no randomized prospective trials demonstrating a benefit to distal perfusion, distal perfusion methods are recommended for complex reconstructions.

There are three common methods to perfuse the distal aorta: partial left heart bypass, femoral venoarterial bypass, and a heparin-bonded (Gott) shunt.

In partial left heart (atriofemoral) bypass, the left atrium and femoral artery are cannulated after heparinization. A portion of the left atrial blood is diverted into a receiving reservoir or directly into a roller or centrifugal pump and returned to the femoral artery. Although reservoir systems require full heparinization, centrifugal pumps require either minimal or no heparin to maintain an activated clotting time (ACT) of 150 to 200 seconds.

In femoral venoarterial bypass, femoral venous blood is drained to the pump oxygenator and then returned by a roller pump to the femoral artery to provide blood circulation below the aortic cross-clamp. Systemic heparinization is mandatory.

In the shunt technique, a metal cannula or one end of the shunt is placed into the left ventricular apex or proximal aorta and the other end into the distal aorta or femoral artery. The heparin-coated Gott shunt eliminates the need for systemic anticoagulation.

Barash PG, Cullen BF, Stoelting RK (eds): Clinical Anesthesia 3rd ed, p 854. Philadelphia, Lippincott-Raven, 1997

Najafi H: Descending aortic aneurysmectomy without adjuncts to avoid ischemia: 1993 update. Ann Thorac Surg 55:1042–1045, 1993

O'Connor CJ, Rothenberg DM: Anesthetic considerations for descending thoracic aortic surgery: Part II. J Cardiothorac Vasc Anesth 9:734–749, 1995

Svensson LG, Crawford ES, Hess KR et al: Experience with 1509 patients undergoing thoracoabdominal aortic operations. J Vasc Surg 17:357–370, 1993

C.12. *What levels of blood pressure would you maintain when the aorta is cross-clamped?*
When the aorta is cross-clamped, the flow through the extracorporeal circuit should be regulated to provide 25 to 40 ml/kg/min to the body below the clamp at pressures of 40 to 60 mm Hg. The systolic pressure above the clamp is maintained at 100 to 150 mm Hg or 20 mm Hg above the pre-cross-clamp value. It is very important to maintain blood pressure above the clamp to perfuse the heart and brain. Frequently, in order to maintain blood pressure and flow below the clamp, to perfuse the spinal cord and kidney, venous return to the heart is so decreased that blood pressure above the clamp becomes very low, resulting in hypoperfusion to the heart and brain. Volume should be added to increase venous return.

Livesay JL, Cooley DA, Ventemiglia RA et al: Surgical experience in descending thoracic aneurysmectomy with and without adjuncts to avoid ischemia. Ann Thorac Surg 39:37–46, 1985

O'Connor CJ, Rothenberg DM: Anesthetic considerations for descending thoracic aortic surgery: Part II. J Cardiothorac Vasc Anesth 9:734–749, 1995

C.13. *Describe the blood supply of the spinal cord.*

The spinal cord has a system of longitudinal arteries and a system of transverse arteries as shown in Figure 12-2. Anatomic studies have shown that the most important longitudinal arteries are a single anterior spinal artery supplying 75% of the cord and a pair of posterior spinal arteries supplying 25% of the cord. Although in humans the anterior spinal artery is a continuous vessel, modern anatomy has emphasized the importance of the reinforcing transverse arteries rather than the meager longitudinal vessels. The territory supplied by the anterior spinal artery is divided into three functionally distinct levels: cervicodorsal, intermediate or midthoracic, and thoracolumbar

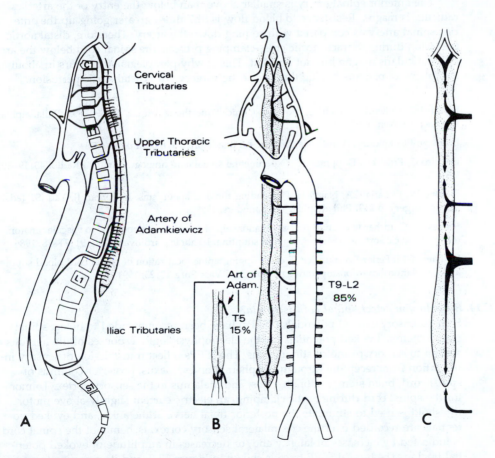

Figure 12-2. Diagram to show components of the anterior spinal artery. **(A)** Lateral view. **(B)** Anteroposterior view showing origins of artery of Adamkiewicz. **(C)** Schematic representation of direction and volume of flow from nutrient vessels supplying the anterior spinal artery. Size of arrows is proportional to flow contribution. (Reprinted with permission from Bromage PR: Epidural Anesthesia, pp 50–54. Philadelphia, WB Saunders, 1978)

(see Fig. 12-2). The cervicodorsal region receives its blood supply from the vertebral, subclavian, thyrocervical, and costocervical arteries. The midthoracic region is supplied by a meager left or right intercostal artery arising between the fourth and the ninth thoracic vertebrae. The thoracolumbar region of the anterior spinal artery receives its blood supply mainly from one of the intercostal arteries called the arteria radicularis magna or the artery of Adamkiewicz. It provides one-fourth to one-third of the blood supply to the spinal cord. It originates from the aorta between T8 and T12 in 75% of cases, between L1 and L2 in 10% of cases, and at T5 in 15% of cases. When the thoracic aorta is cross-clamped, the blood supply to the spinal cord may be seriously compromised, with resultant paraplegia. However, reimplantation of intercostal arteries during surgery has been shown to reduce the incidence of neurologic injury.

The anterior spinal artery is smaller above than below the entry of the arteria radicularis magna. Resistance to blood flow is 51.7 times greater going up the anterior spinal artery as compared with coming down the artery. Therefore, distal aortic perfusion during thoracic aortic cross-clamping protects the spinal cord below the arteria radicularis magna but not above it. This is why paraplegia still occurs in about 2% to 15% of patients having thoracic aortic surgery with distal aortic perfusion.

Barash PG, Cullen BF, Stoelting RK (eds): Clinical Anesthesia 3rd ed, pp 892–893. Philadelphia, Lippincott-Raven, 1997

Bromage PR: Epidural Anesthesia, pp 50–54. Philadelphia, WB Saunders, 1978

DiChiro G, Fried LC, Doppman JL: Experimental spinal cord angiography. Br J Radiol 43:19–30, 1970

Piccone W, DeLaria GA, Najafi H: Descending thoracic aneurysms. In Bergan JJ, Yao JST (eds): Aortic Surgery, p 249. Philadelphia, WB Saunders, 1989

Svensson LG, Richards E, Coull A et al: Relationship of spinal cord blood flow to vascular anatomy during thoracic aortic cross-clamping and shunting. J Thorac Cardiovasc Surg 91:71–78, 1986

Williams GM, Perler BA, Burdick JF et al: Angiographic localization of spinal cord blood supply and its relationship to postoperative paraplegia. J Vasc Surg 13:23, 1991

C.14. *How do you detect spinal cord ischemia?*

Somatosensory evoked potentials (SSEPs) have been recommended to detect spinal cord ischemia. Evoked potentials are the electrophysiologic responses of the nervous system to sensory or motor stimulations. The SSEPs reflect transmission of sensory information from receptors through peripheral nerves, plexus, posterior columns of spinal cord, brain stem, midbrain, pons, and thalamus to the sensory cortex. To monitor the spinal cord during aortic clamping, an electric current slightly above motor threshold is used to stimulate the posterior tibial nerve at the ankle, and evoked potentials are recorded over the contralateral sensory cortex. Ischemia of the spinal cord is indicated by increases in latency and/or decreases in amplitude of evoked potential tracing. The typical SSEP trace is shown in Figure 12-3, and its response to aortic cross-clamping is shown in Figure 12-4. The latency increases as early as 4 minutes following aortic cross-clamping, with progress to cessation of spinal cord conduction within 7 minutes of cross-clamping. Return of spinal cord conduction occurs 47 minutes following distal aortic reperfusion, with return to normal spinal cord conduction

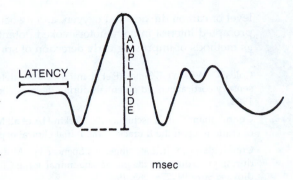

Figure 12-3. Typical somatosensory evoked potential trace. (Reprinted with permission from Cunningham JN Jr, Laschinger JC, Merkin HA et al: Measurement of spinal cord ischemia during operations upon the thoracic aorta: Initial clinical experience. Ann Surg 196:285–296, 1982)

within 24 hours after operation. It has been shown that the loss of SSEP signals for longer than 14 to 30 minutes was associated with postoperative neurologic deficit.

Intraoperative monitoring of the physiologic integrity of the spinal cord should permit the early detection of spinal cord ischemia, the judicious and timely institution of corrective measures, including bypass or shunting, and the preservation of important intercostal arteries in appropriate circumstances. However, postoperative paraplegia has been reported despite normal intraoperative somatosensory evoked potentials. This suggests that SSEP monitoring may fail to reflect cord dysfunction on two counts: (1) if the insult does not involve the dorsal columns, or (2) if it does involve the dorsal columns but is not of sufficient magnitude to affect the SSEP. High incidence of false-positive, and occasional false-negative SSEPs, as well as technical difficulties associated with SSEP monitoring (e.g., effects of anesthetics, temperature,

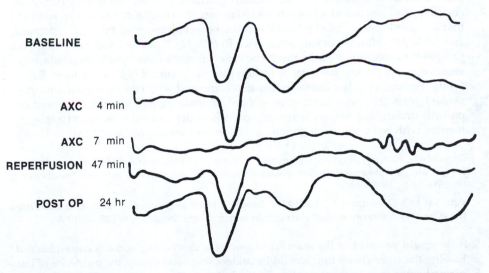

Figure 12-4. Somatosensory evoked potential response to aortic cross-clamping (AXC). (Reprinted with permission from Cunningham JN Jr, Laschinger JC, Merkin HA et al: Measurement of spinal cord ischemia during operations upon the thoracic aorta: Initial clinical experience. Ann Surg 196:285–296, 1982)

level of carbon dioxide and oxygen, and associated peripheral neuropathies) have prompted interest in both motor-evoked potentials and spinal cord-evoked potentials as methods of improving early detection of spinal cord ischemia.

Coles JC, Wilson GJ, Sima AF et al: Intraoperative detection of spinal cord ischemia using somatosensory cortical evoked potentials during thoracic aortic occlusion. Ann Thorac Surg 34:299–306, 1982

Cunningham JN Jr, Laschinger JC, Merkin HA et al: Measurement of spinal cord ischemia during operations upon the thoracic aorta: Initial clinical experience. Ann Surg 196:285–296, 1982

Cunningham JN Jr, Laschinger JC, Spencer FC: Monitoring of somatosensory evoked potentials during procedures on the thoracoabdominal aorta: Clinical observations and results. J Thorac Cardiovasc Surg 94: 275–285, 1987

Ginsbury HH, Shetter AG, Raudzens PA et al: Postoperative paraplegia with preserved intraoperative somatosensory evoked potentials. J Neurosurg 63:296–300, 1985

Grundy BL: Intraoperative monitoring of sensory-evoked potentials. Anesthesiology 58:72–87, 1983

O'Connor CJ, Rothenberg DM: Anesthetic considerations for descending thoracic aortic surgery: Part II. J Cardiothorac Vasc Anesth 9:734–749, 1995

Takaki O, Okumura F: Application and limitation of somatosensory evoked potential monitoring during thoracic aortic aneurysm surgery: A case report. Anesthesiology 63:700–703, 1985

C.15. *What are the effects of anesthetics on somatosensory evoked potentials in humans?*
Halothane, enflurane, and isoflurane all produce dose-related reductions in the amplitude and increases in the latency of the cortical component of the SSEP. These changes are most pronounced with enflurane and least with halothane. At 1.5 minimum alveolar concentration (MAC) of each volatile agent, cortical latency decreased and amplitude increased when nitrous oxide was discontinued. The results suggest that in neurologically intact patients, end-tidal concentrations of 1.0 MAC halothane and 0.5 MAC enflurane or isoflurane (each in 60% N_2O) can be compatible with effective SSEP monitoring. Volatile anesthetic concentrations consistent with satisfactory somatosensory evoked potential recording may be greater if N_2O is not used. Recently, Bernard et al has demonstrated that compared with cortical somatosensory-evoked potentials, neurogenic motor-evoked potential signals are well preserved in patients undergoing surgery to correct scoliosis under general anesthesia supplemented with isoflurane or desflurane in concentrations as great as 1 MAC.

Bernard JM, Pereon Y, Tayet G, Guiheneuc P: Effects of isoflurane and desflurane on neurogenic motor- and somatosensory-evoked potential monitoring for scoliosis surgery. Anesthesiology 85:1013–1019, 1996

Peterson DO, Drummond JC, Todd MM: Effects of halothane, enflurane, isoflurane and nitrous oxide on somatosensory evoked potentials in humans. Anesthesiology 65:35–40, 1986

C.16. *How would you protect the spinal cord when the descending aorta is cross-clamped?*
Ideally, the cross-clamp time should be under 30 minutes, since the incidence of paraplegia begins to increase above this limit. However, the cross-clamp time depends on the complexity of the surgical repair, which is out of our control. Nevertheless, various methods have been used to prevent paraplegia during aortic cross-clamping. These include the following:

- Maintaining perfusion pressures of the proximal and distal aorta
- Reimplantation of intercostal and lumbar arteries
- Hypothermia (systemic, regional, intrathecal)
- Cerebrospinal fluid (CSF) drainage
- Avoiding hyperglycemia
- Open distal anastomosis
- Pharmacologic measures

Maintenance of Proximal and Distal Perfusion Pressures
Systemic (proximal) blood pressure is increased to 15% to 20% above baseline to aid in collateral perfusion to the spinal cord. Distal aortic perfusion can be accomplished by partial left heart bypass, femoral venoarterial bypass, or shunts, as described in question C.11. Perfusion pressure of 40 to 60 mm Hg or above 60 mm Hg has been recommended to protect the spinal cord. However, as described in question C.13., because the resistance of the anterior spinal artery above the arteria radicularis magna is very high, distal aortic perfusion protects the spinal cord only below the arteria radicularis magna but not above it.

Reimplantation of Intercostal and Lumbar Arteries
This has been associated with a lower incidence of spinal cord ischemia. Identification of the artery of Adamkiewicz has been performed preoperatively by selective intercostal angiography. However, the procedure itself carries a small risk of paraplegia. Arteries identified intraoperatively as critical to spinal cord perfusion are reimplanted or preserved.

Hypothermia
Mild hypothermia of 33° to 34°C will decrease the metabolic rate and may protect the spinal cord from ischemic injury. Surface cooling with cooling blankets and infusion of cool intravenous fluids may achieve mild hypothermia. However, precise control of temperature is difficult, and at temperatures below 32°C, the heart may become more irritable and prone to ventricular arrhythmia. Therefore, hypothermia should be used cautiously.

Profound hypothermia (15° to 19°C) with circulatory arrest has been safely used for selected patients who require extensive aortic resections and who are at substantial risk for the development of spinal cord injury.

Regional spinal cord hypothermia with epidural cooling has been reported to have satisfactory neurologic outcome. An epidural catheter was placed at T11–12, and a subarachnoid thermistor catheter was placed at L3–4. Approximately 30 minutes before aortic cross-clamping, iced (4°C) saline solution (80 to 1700 ml) was infused into the epidural catheter until CSF temperature decreased to 25°C. The infusion was then adjusted to maintain this temperature until the aorta was unclamped. The subarachnoid catheter was also used to measure CSF pressure and provide for CSF drainage.

Cerebrospinal Fluid Drainage
Aortic cross-clamping increases CSF pressure 3 to 5 mm Hg. CSF drainage decreases the intraspinal pressure and thus increases the perfusion pressure of the spinal cord. The CSF pressure is maintained at or below 10 mm Hg. CSF drainage has been shown to reduce the incidence of paraplegia in the dog. However, a recent clinical study by Crawford et al did not show CSF drainage to be beneficial in preventing

paraplegia. Additional concerns of CSF drainage relate to the risks of cerebral herniation and the risks of epidural hematoma.

Avoidance of Hyperglycemia

There is consistent evidence of glucose-induced enhancement of injury in studies of global cerebral ischemia, and the majority of studies in focal cerebral ischemia also suggest that glucose worsens outcome. The proposed mechanism by which glucose exacerbates postischemic neurologic injury is as follows. The anaerobic metabolism of glucose during ischemia results in an intracellular lactic acidosis. This acidosis facilitates a cascade of secondary processes that cause permanent neurologic injury. Therefore, glucose-containing solutions should be avoided during this surgery. If the glucose level rises above 220 mg/dl, exogenous insulin is given to normalize the blood glucose.

Open Distal Anastomosis

Using rapid autotransfusion, some surgeons repair the descending thoracic aneurysms by using an open technique in which a single cross-clamp is placed proximal to the aneurysm to exsanguinate the lower body. A lower incidence of spinal cord injury and renal insufficiency using this technique may result from the free drainage of the intercostal and lumbar arteries during aortic occlusion, which decreases CSF and central venous pressures and increases spinal cord perfusion pressure.

Pharmacologic Measures

These include the use of various drugs, such as steroids, oxygen radical scavengers, mannitol, barbiturates, magnesium, antagonists of N-methyl-D-asparate (NMDA) receptor, intrathecal papaverine and magnesium, and calcium channel blockers. Recently, Fluosol-DA, an artificial blood substitute, has been shown to improve the neurologic outcome in dogs with spinal cord ischemia produced by aortic cross-clamping. However, large-scale clinical studies have not been able to demonstrate that any of these methods are superior to simple cross-clamping and proximal blood pressure control. In addition, no single technique has proven consistently safe and effective in preventing spinal cord injury.

Barash PG, Cullen BF, Stoelting RK (eds): Clinical Anesthesia 3rd ed, pp 894–895. Philadelphia, Lippincott-Raven, 1997

Crawford ES, Svensson LG, Hess KR et al: A prospective randomized study of cerebrospinal fluid drainage to prevent paraplegia after high-risk surgery on the thoracoabdominal aorta. J Vasc Surg 13:36–46, 1990

Davison JK, Cambria RP, Vierra DJ et al: Epidural cooling for regional spinal cord hypothermia during thoracoabdominal aneurysm repair. J Vasc Surg 20:304–310, 1994

DelRossi AJ, Cernaianu AC, Cilley JH et al: Preventive effect of Fluosol-DA for paraplegia encountered after surgical treatment of the thoracic aorta. J Thorac Cardiovasc Surg 99:665–669, 1990

Hollier LH, Money SR, Naslund TG et al: Risk of spinal cord dysfunction in patients undergoing thoracoabdominal aortic replacement. Am J Surg 164:210–214, 1992

Kouchoukos NT, Wareing TH, Izumoto H et al: Elective hypothermia cardiopulmonary bypass and circulatory arrest for spinal cord protection during operations on the thoracoabdominal aorta. J Thorac Cardiovasc Surg 99:659–664, 1990

Lanier WL: Glucose management during cardiopulmonary bypass: Cardiovascular and neurologic implications. Anesth Analg 72:423–427, 1991

Mauney MC, Blackbourne LH, Langenburg SE et al: Prevention of spinal cord injury after repair of the thoracic or thoracoabdominal aorta. Ann Thorac Surg 59:245–252, 1995

O'Connor CJ, Rothenberg DM: Anesthetic considerations for descending thoracic aortic surgery: Part II. J Cardiothorac Vasc Anesth 9:734–749, 1995

Shenaq SA, Svensson LG: Paraplegia following aortic surgery. J Cardiothorac Vasc Anesth 7:81–94, 1993

C.17. What are determinants of postoperative renal failure after descending thoracic aneurysm repair? How would you protect the kidneys during surgery?

The duration of aortic cross-clamp time (in excess of 30 minutes) appears to be the major determinant associated with postoperative renal failure. Advanced age, preoperative renal dysfunction, and failure to use atriofemoral bypass have been identified as additional predictors of acute renal failure. However, intraoperative urine output has been shown to be a poor predictor of postoperative renal failure.

Renal function may be protected by the following measures:

- Maintenance of intravascular volume and cardiac function to perfuse the kidney
- Minimization of aortic cross-clamp time
- Avoidance of distal hypotension during aortic clamping
- Atriofemoral bypass for distal perfusion
- Cold perfusion of renal arteries
- Systemic hypothermia
- Low dose dopamine (<4 μg/kg/min) to increase renal blood flow and glomerular filtration rate
- Mannitol for osmotic diuresis, renovasodilation, shifting blood flow to the renal cortex, and scavenging oxygen free radicals
- Furosemide for natriuretic effect and renovasodilation by stimulating prostaglandin E_1.

Although it is common practice for anesthesiologists to give one or all of these last three agents before aortic cross-clamping as prophylaxis against renal failure, little data exist to demonstrate any outcome differences with this approach.

- Experimental agents: calcium-channel blockers, fenoldopam (a DA_2-specific agonist), prostaglandin E_1, oxygen free radical scavengers (superoxide dismutase).

Barash PG, Cullen BF, Stoelting RK (eds): Clinical Anesthesia 3rd ed, pp 894–895. Philadelphia, Lippincott-Raven, 1997

Bush HG Jr, Huse JB, Johnson WC et al: Prevention of renal insufficiency after abdominal aortic aneurysm resection by optimal volume loading. Arch Surg 116:1517–1524, 1981

O'Connor CJ, Rothenberg DM: Anesthetic considerations for descending thoracic aortic surgery: Part II. J Cardiothorac Vasc Anesth 9:734–749, 1995

C.18. What are hemodynamic and metabolic effects of aortic unclamping? How would you prevent and treat them?

If distal aortic perfusion is not provided by shunting procedures, release of the aortic cross-clamp can cause severe hypotension and metabolic acidosis that has been termed declamping shock. The typical changes include marked decreases in blood pressure and systemic vascular resistance, and increases in pulmonary artery pressures, end-tidal CO_2, arterial P_{CO_2}, and serum lactate levels with severe metabolic acidosis. Although initially the pulmonary wedge pressure and central venous pressure decrease, cardiac output and stroke volume increase because of substantial decrease in afterload upon release of aortic clamp. The pulmonary hypertension is produced by lactic acidosis and hypercarbia. Severe arterial hypotension is primarily caused by peripheral vasodilation; other mechanisms include redistribution of blood from the upper body to the lower body, reactive hyperemia in previously unperfused vascular beds, sequestration of blood in venous capacitance vessels, the systemic effects of ischemic metabolites released from unperfused tissues, myocardial depression, hypovolemia, and increases in intestinal permeability probably due to translocation of endotoxin and bacteria into portal circulation.

Preventing the adverse effects of aortic unclamping may be achieved by:

- Aggressive expansion of intravascular volume before release of the aortic clamp
- Discontinuation of anesthetics, vasodilators, and beta-blockers well in advance of aortic declamping
- Increasing minute ventilation
- Slow release of the aortic clamp over 2 to 4 minutes
- Sodium bicarbonate drip during cross-clamping, 3 mEq/kg/h without distal perfusion and 1 mEq/kg/h with distal perfusion.

If severe hypotension or significant bleeding occurs, the aorta can be reclamped. Volume loading is the key to correct hypotension. A sample of arterial blood should be analyzed shortly after unclamping, and metabolic acidosis should be corrected with sodium bicarbonate, if necessary. If blood pressure is unstable or stays below 80 mm Hg within 3 to 5 minutes, small doses of phenylephrine by 0.1-mg increments may be given to raise blood pressure temporarily before additional volume loading is accomplished. Intraoperative TEE allows real-time evaluation of ventricular function and may aid in selection of appropriate inotropic agents to help with the cross-clamping and declamping periods.

Gelman S: The pathophysiology of aortic cross-clamping and unclamping. Anesthesiology 82:1026–1060, 1995

O'Connor CJ, Rothenberg DM: Anesthetic considerations for descending thoracic aortic surgery: Part II. J Cardiothorac Vasc Anesth 9:734–749, 1995

Silverstein PR, Caldera DL, Cullen DJ et al: Avoiding the hemodynamic consequences of aortic cross-clamping and unclamping. Anesthesiology 50:462–466, 1979

D. Postoperative Management

D.1. What are the postoperative complications from resection of an aortic aneurysm?
Myocardial infarction, arrhythmias, hemorrhage, and renal or respiratory failure may occur after resection of a thoracic aneurysm. Hypothermia and hypertension are frequent problems after aneurysmectomy, while the most serious complication is paraplegia. The incidence of paraplegia is 0.9% to 40%. In some instances spinal cord injury is unexplained, probably resulting from ligating an intercostal artery from which an important source of circulation to the spinal cord originated. The important fac-

tors causing paraplegia include long duration of aortic clamping, resection of long aortic segments, clamping or interruption of flow to radicular branches, hypotension, arteriosclerosis of cord vessels, compression of intercostal arteries by the dissecting aneurysm, and subclavian steal. Postoperative respiratory failure may result from the pulmonary contusion and occasionally from injury to the left phrenic or left recurrent nerves during surgical dissection.

Barash PG, Cullen BF, Stoelting RK (eds): Clinical Anesthesia 3rd ed, pp 894–895. Philadelphia, Lippincott-Raven, 1997

Gelman S: The pathophysiology of aortic cross-clamping and unclamping. Anesthesiology 82:1026–1060, 1995

O'Connor CJ, Rothenberg DM: Anesthetic considerations for descending thoracic aortic surgery: Part II. J Cardiothorac Vasc Anesth 9:734–749, 1995

13 Abdominal Aortic Aneurysm Resection and Postoperative Pain Management

Lori A. Rubin
Howard L. Rosner

The patient was a 55-year-old woman with a 6.0-cm infrarenal aortic aneurysm discovered on routine physical examination and confirmed with abdominal computed tomography (CT) scan. She was a two-pack-per-day smoker and complained of dyspnea on exertion. Her electrocardiogram showed Q waves in leads II, III, and aV_F. Chest x-ray displayed mild hyperinflation of the lung fields, and her hematocrit was 46%.

A. Medical Disease and Differential Diagnosis

1. What are the major causes of morbidity and mortality in the patient with an abdominal aortic aneurysm (AAA)?
2. What other diseases are commonly found in patients with aortic aneurysms?
3. What is the incidence of morbidity and mortality in these patients if they undergo elective surgical repair? What is the natural history of the disease without surgical repair?
4. What is the risk of perioperative myocardial infarction in patients with ischemic heart disease? Are there any means by which we can reduce the risk of further ischemic events in these patients?
5. Does the morbidity and mortality of elective repair of an aortic aneurysm differ significantly from that of an emergency repair?

B. Preoperative Evaluation and Preparation

1. Which preoperative laboratory tests would you require for this patient?
2. Was this patient's preoperative ECG significant? Would you wish to pursue further preoperative cardiac workup? What tests would you request, and what would they tell you?
3. Is it necessary to evaluate this patient's pulmonary status?
4. Preoperative arterial blood gases showed pH, 7.38; PCO_2, 45 mm Hg; PO_2, 68 mm Hg on room air. What was the significance of this result?
5. How would you measure creatinine clearance in this patient and why is it an important value in this case?
6. Describe the blood flow to the spinal cord. What is its relevance to surgery of the abdominal aorta?
7. What are the various surgical approaches to the abdominal aorta? How does the choice of surgical technique affect the anesthetic management?
8. How would you premedicate this patient?

C. Intraoperative Management

1. Would you use an arterial line? What are the complications of an arterial line placement?
2. What various monitors are available for myocardial ischemia? Is a pulmonary artery catheter helpful in determining the occurrence of ischemia?
3. What additional monitors would you employ?
4. How would you anesthetize this patient? Discuss the various anesthetic techniques which can be employed for this surgery.
5. This patient is to be heparinized intraoperatively and anticoagulation is to be continued postoperatively. Is this a contraindication to the preoperative placement of either an epidural or intraspinal catheter?
6. What are your plans for fluid and blood replacement during surgery?
7. What are the hemodynamic changes of aortic cross-clamp placement? What efforts can be made to minimize these changes both prior to and during cross-clamping? If the patient develops ST-segment depressions with a rising pulmonary capillary wedge pressure (PCWP) during cross-clamp, what maneuvers should be taken?
8. As this case involves an infrarenal aneurysm, is renal blood flow affected with the placement of the cross-clamp? Are there any treatment maneuvers that can be taken to minimize these changes?
9. What are the hemodynamic consequences of aortic cross-clamp removal? What can be done to minimize the effects of removing the aortic cross-clamp? If the systemic blood pressure remains depressed after removal of the cross-clamp, what is the differential diagnosis? How would you define and correct the problem?

D. Postoperative Management

1. What are the parameters used to extubate this patient?
2. What are the anticipated changes in postoperative pulmonary function in these patients? How does the surgical technique affect postoperative pulmonary function? Are there any postoperative maneuvers that can maximize respiratory parameters?
3. How would you control postoperative pain? What are the alternatives in the management of this patient's postoperative pain? Is there a role for nonnarcotic medications or alternative pain management techniques for this patient?

A. Medical Disease and Differential Diagnosis

A.1. What are the major causes of morbidity and mortality in the patient with an abdominal aortic aneurysm (AAA)?

Myocardial infarction is the single most common cause of early morbidity in AAA resection patients, accounting for approximately 55% of perioperative deaths. Of all patients who suffer a perioperative myocardial infarction, 70% will not survive. Other postoperative complications include renal insufficiency, pulmonary infections and insufficiency, colon ischemia, hepatic failure, and paraplegia resulting from spinal cord ischemia. However, these events account for <1% of the total number of deaths from this operation. Risk factors affecting postoperative mortality are the presence of coronary artery disease, serum creatinine of >2.0 mg/dl, age over 60, and aneurysmal rupture. Postoperative complications also increase with increasing transfusion requirements, and are more likely with emergency surgery on the abdominal aorta.

Barash PG, Cullen BF, Stoelting RK (eds): Clinical Anesthesia, 3rd ed, pp 888–900. Philadelphia, Lippincott-Raven, 1997

Dieke JT, Cali RF, Hertzer NR, Beven EG: Complications of abdominal aortic reconstruction: An analysis of perioperative risk factors in 557 patients. Ann Surg 197:49–56, 1983

A2. What other diseases are commonly found in patients with aortic aneurysms?

The major pathologic cause of aneurysmal disease is atherosclerosis. In addition to peripheral vascular disease, this population has a high incidence of coronary artery disease (50% to 70%), cerebrovascular and renal disease. Commonly, these patients also suffer from hypertension, diabetes mellitus, and pulmonary disease. Patients with diffuse aortoiliac disease are more likely to be smokers and have hypertension, diabetes, and/or hypercholesterolemia, which contributes to their vascular disease. The above risk factors, combined with advanced age (>60), are often exacerbated by the extreme physiologic changes during aneurysmal surgery.

DeBakey ME: Changing concepts in vascular surgery. J Cardiovasc Surg 27:367–409, 1986

Roizen MF (ed): Anesthesia for Vascular Surgery, pp 12–22. New York, Churchill Livingstone, 1990

A.3. What is the incidence of morbidity and mortality in these patients if they undergo elective surgical repair? What is the natural history of the disease without surgical repair?

Morbidity in this patient group is most commonly due to cardiovascular, pulmonary, and renal complications. Perioperative mortality for elective abdominal aortic aneurysm repair is 2% to 5%. The major cause of mortality in the nonsurgically treated patient is rupture of the aneurysm. In one study, resection of the aneurysm doubled life expectancy. The incidence of rupture within 5 years of diagnosis of an abdominal aortic aneurysm is 80%. The incidence of rupture increases with aneurysmal size: 25% for lesions of 4 to 7 cm in diameter, 45% for lesions 7 to 10 cm, and 60% for lesions larger than 10 cm. Mortality rates for ruptured aneurysms are higher, 25% to 75%. After 10 years, graft patency is worse for patients with disease in more distal vessels, as is survival rate, being 28% in patients with isolated aortoiliac disease and increasing to 41% in patients with femoral popliteal or tibial disease.

Roizen MF (ed): Anesthesia for Vascular Surgery, pp 12–13, 253. New York, Churchill Livingstone, 1990

A.4. What is the risk of perioperative myocardial infarction in patients with ischemic heart disease? Are there any means by which we can reduce the risk of further ischemic events in these patients?

The occurrence of a recent myocardial infarction is one of the most important independent predictors of perioperative morbidity and mortality. The statistical rate of reinfarction is related to the length of time since the initial myocardial infarction. In a group of patients studied prospectively for perioperative reinfarction by Rao et al, there was a 5% to 8% incidence if the prior infarction was <3 months old, 2% to 3% if it was 4 to 6 months old, and <2% if the infarction occurred >6 months earlier.

Patients were monitored with pulmonary artery catheters and arterial lines, and were aggressively treated and monitored in an intensive care unit setting for 3 to 4 days postoperatively.

Prior studies indicated that reinfarction rates in patients 0 to 6 months postinfarction were significantly greater than those in Rao's study. If there was no previous infarction, the rate of perioperative infarction was 0.1% to 0.7%. In most studies, the mortality following a perioperative myocardial infarction approaches 50%. Fleisher and Barash suggest that risk after a myocardial infarction may be best linked to the ongoing risk of ischemia. Patients who have survived a non-Q wave infarction are potentially at greatest risk of further ischemia. These patients should be evaluated by symptom-limited exercise testing and/or cardiac catheterization.

In a prospective randomized study by Stone et al, it was shown that a small oral dose of a beta-blocking agent preoperatively reduces the risk of intraoperative ischemic events. The most helpful means of decreasing the risk of a perioperative cardiac event is to optimize the patient's current cardiovascular status. Treating congestive heart failure, if present, and controlling hypertension (although not definitively shown to improve outcome) are important preoperative maneuvers.

Fleisher LA, Barash PG: Preoperative cardiac evaluation for noncardiac surgery. A functional approach. Anesth Analg 74:586–598, 1992

Mangano DT: Perioperative cardiac morbidity. Anesthesiology 72:153–184, 1990

Prys-Roberts C, Meloche R, Foëx P: Studies of anesthesia in relation to hypertension. I. Cardiovascular responses of treated and untreated patients. Br J Anaesth 43:122–137, 1971

Rao TL, Jacobs KH, El-Etr AA: Reinfarction following anesthesia in patients with myocardial infarction. Anesthesiology 59:499–505, 1983

Steen PA, Tinker JH, Tarhan S: Myocardial reinfarction after anesthesia and surgery. JAMA 239:2566–2570, 1978

Stone JG, Foëx P, Sear JW et al: Myocardial ischemia in untreated hypertensive patients: Effect of a single small oral dose of a beta-adrenergic blocking agent. Anesthesiology 68:495–500, 1988

A5. Does the morbidity and mortality of elective repair of an aortic aneurysm differ significantly from that of an emergency repair?

Overall mortality for a ruptured aortic aneurysm is 75%. One study showed an overall survival rate of 19.8% as compared with an elective surgical survival rate of 95%. The worst prognosis occurred in patients with a systolic blood pressure of <80 mm Hg on admission; a prior history of hypertension, angina, or previous myocardial infarction; and an operating time of >4 hours. Retroperitoneal rupture was more likely to be associated with survival. Elective surgical intervention is indicated if the aneurysm changes rapidly or if its diameter is >6 cm.

Ingoldby CJ, Wuyanto R, Mitchell JE: Impact of vascular surgery on community mortality from ruptured aortic aneurysms. Br J Surg 73:551–553, 1986

Lambert ME, Baguley P, Charlesworth D: Ruptured abdominal aortic aneurysms. J Cardiovasc Surg 27:256, 1986

B. Preoperative Evaluation and Preparation

B.1. Which preoperative laboratory tests would you require for this patient?

The patient should have the following laboratory tests as part of her preoperative evaluation: complete blood count, serum electrolytes (sodium, potassium), blood urea nitrogen, creatinine, coagulation profile (platelet count, prothrombin time, partial thromboplastin time), arterial blood gas, urinalysis, chest x-ray, bedside spirometry, and electrocardiogram.

Vandam LD (ed): To Make the Patient Ready for Anesthesia; Medical Care of the Surgical Patient, 2nd ed, pp 44–45, 68, 155. Menlo Park, CA, Addison-Wesley, 1984

B.2. Was this patient's preoperative ECG significant? Would you wish to pursue further preoperative cardiac workup? What tests would you request, and what would they tell you?

The patient's preoperative ECG was consistent with a prior inferior wall myocardial infarction. Patients having a history of a prior myocardial infarction or a history of angina in conjunction with an abnormal ECG have a fivefold increase in postoperative mortality when compared with those with no clinical evidence of coronary artery disease (CAD). If this patient's dyspnea on exertion is a symptom of congestive heart failure, this would further increase her perioperative morbidity. This increased risk may be altered by measurement and maintenance of normal hemodynamics with a pulmonary artery catheter. In selected patients with severe or unstable cardiac ischemia, prior myocardial revascularization may be indicated. When coronary angiography was performed on patients undergoing elective peripheral vascular surgery it

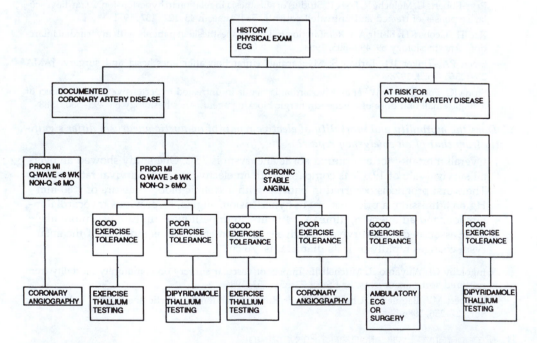

Figure 13-1. Proposed algorithm for patients undergoing surgical procedures associated with a high risk of perioperative myocardial ischemia (i.e., abdominal aortic aneurysm resection). In these patients, further cardiovascular evaluation to delineate the extent of coronary artery disease is warrantd if the information obtained influences clinical care (see text).

was revealed that more than half of the 1000 patients had significant coronary artery disease (> 50% stenosis), and 33% had severe stenosis (> 70%). Of the asymptomatic patients with no history or ECG evidence of ischemic heart disease, 15% had severe CAD and 22% of these seemingly normal patients had impaired left ventricular function.

A comparison of this patient's current ECG with a prior ECG may aid in assessing the timing of the previous infarction if the history is not helpful. The patient's history or ECG may not be accurate predictors of risk in this patient population. A functional approach is advocated by Fleisher and Barash. The aortic aneurysm patients are those whose surgery is likely to increase their perioperative ischemia. They recommend that patients with documented coronary artery disease or a history of diabetes who are having aortic aneurysm surgery undergo further testing. The proposed algorithm for patients undergoing surgical procedures associated with a high risk of perioperative myocardial ischemia is shown in Figure 13-1.

Many vascular surgery patients are unable to undergo exercise stress testing due to limitations presented by their cardiac, pulmonary, or peripheral vascular disease. A dipyridamole-thallium stress test or a dobutamine stress test are pharmacologic tests to assess myocardial ischemic potential. Dipyridamole causes vasodilation of normal coronary arteries. This results in a steal of blood flow from the area beyond a coronary stenosis. Blood flow redistributes as the drug dissipates. Boucher found that redistribution is predictive of a 20-fold increase in postoperative ischemic events in patients undergoing peripheral vascular surgery. Those without redistribution had no perioperative cardiac events.

Boucher CA, Brewster DC, Darling RC et al: Determination of cardiac risk by dipyridamole-thallium imaging before peripheral vascular surgery. N Engl J Med 312:389–394, 1985

Fleisher LA, Barash PG: Preoperative cardiac evaluation for noncardiac surgery: A functional approach. Anesth Analg 74:586–598, 1992

Goldman L: Cardiac risk in non-cardiac surgery: An update. Anesth Analg 80:810–820, 1995

Hertzer NR, Bevan EG, Young JR et al: Coronary artery disease in peripheral vascular patients: A classification of 1,000 coronary angiograms and results of surgical management. Ann Surg 199:223–233, 1984

Sirrek CC, Watson DD, Smith WH et al: Dipyridamole thallium-201 imaging versus dobutamine echocardiography for the evaluation of coronary artery disease in patients unable to exercise. Am J Cardiol 72:1257–1262, 1993

Whittemore AD, Clowes AW, Hechtman HB, Mannick JA: Aortic aneurysm repair: Reduced operative mortality associated with maintenance of optimal cardiac performance. Ann Surg 192:414–421, 1980

B3. Is it necessary to evaluate this patient's pulmonary status?

Yes. This patient was a two-pack-per-day smoker with dyspnea on exertion and the anticipated surgery required an upper abdominal incision. These factors affect her baseline pulmonary function and presage postoperative ventilatory problems. A vital capacity (VC) <50% of predicted, or <2 liters total, is an indicator of increased risk because a VC at least three times tidal volume is necessary for an effective cough. FEV_1 <2 liters, maximum breathing capacity (MBC) <50% of predicted, and maximum mid-expiratory flow rate (MMEFR) <50% of predicted are also values associated with increased risk.

An assessment of pulmonary function should include an arterial blood gas analysis and spirometry. Arterial blood gas measurement evaluates the patient's ability to oxygenate and ventilate. Preoperative spirometry evaluates baseline forced vital capacity (FVC) and forced expiratory volume in 1 second (FEV_1). MMEFR is an effort-independent value and a sensitive index of small airway obstruction. Peak expiratory flow rate (PEFR) is related to the FEV_1 and MMEFR, although it is often less reproducible.

These tests should be performed before and after bronchodilator therapy to assess reversibility of airway obstruction. A 15% improvement is considered a positive response. Discontinuation of smoking for 48 hours preoperatively increases oxygen tissue availability and, if stopped 4 to 6 weeks prior to surgery, may decrease postoperative complications.

Gass GD, Olsen GN: Clinical significance of PFT: Preoperative pulmonary testing to predict postoperative morbidity and mortality. Chest 89:127, 1986

Tisi GM: Preoperative identification and evaluation of the patient with lung disease. Med Clin North Am: 71:399–412, 1987

B.4. Preoperative arterial blood gases showed pH, 7.38; P_{CO_2}, 45 mm Hg; P_{O_2}, 68 mm Hg on room air. What was the significance of this result?

The normal value for PaO_2 in young adults ranges from 85 to 100 mm Hg with an average of about 95 mm Hg. This value falls steadily with aging to an average P_{O_2} of 80 mm Hg at age 60. A method of estimating the expected PaO_2 is 100 − (age in years/3). The normal $PaCO_2$ is 37 to 43 mm Hg and is unaffected by aging. For every 10-mm Hg increase in $PaCO_2$, pH decreases by 0.05. For every 10-mm Hg decrease in $PaCO_2$, pH increases by 0.1.

The main causes of hypoxemia in arterial blood are hypoventilation, diffusion impairment, shunting, and ventilation/perfusion ($\dot{V}/\dot{Q}$) mismatch. The major causes of hypercarbia or carbon dioxide retention are hypoventilation and ventilation/perfusion mismatch. Not all $\dot{V}/\dot{Q}$ mismatches cause increases in arterial CO_2 because the chemoreceptors can recognize increasing CO_2 tension and cause an increase in ventilation. This, however, will not lead to a normalization of the hypoxemia caused by ventilation/perfusion imbalances.

The assessment of this patient's blood gas analysis reveals moderate hypoxemia with a high normal carbon dioxide tension. The pH is consistent with the CO_2. The most likely reason for this patient's blood gas abnormalities is $\dot{V}/\dot{Q}$ mismatches secondary to the multiyear history of smoking. It is also likely that she has developed some obstructive lung disease with resultant $\dot{V}/\dot{Q}$ mismatches.

Nunn JF: Nunn's Applied Respiratory Physiology, 4th ed, pp 156–197. London, Butterworth-Heinemann, 1993

West JB: Respiratory Physiology, 5th ed, pp 51–69. Baltimore, Williams & Wilkins, 1995

B5. How would you measure creatinine clearance in this patient and why is it an important value in this case?

Preoperative renal dysfunction indicates potential postoperative impairment. Despite maximal medical management, including hemodialysis, acute renal failure after aortic reconstruction carries a mortality of >30% postoperatively. Maintenance of intravascular volume and adequate blood pressure is the best means of avoiding postoperative renal failure. This complication is more likely in patients requiring a suprarenal cross-clamp.

Pretreatment with mannitol may lessen postischemic increases in creatinine. Additionally, furosemide, vasodilating prostaglandins, and dopamine may attenuate the reduction of renal cortical blood flow and increase glomerular filtration pressure, thereby increasing glomerular filtration rate (GFR).

Operative mortality is 19% when aortic reconstruction is performed on patients with a creatinine >2 mg/dl, but 4.6% if the levels are lower. Therefore, should the creatinine be >2 mg/dl, reversible factors, such as renal stenosis, should be investigated. The most direct measurement of GFR is the measurement of creatinine clearance. Although blood urea nitrogen (BUN) and serum creatinine are related to renal function, they are altered by such nonrenal factors as protein metabolism, diet, liver dysfunction, or skeletal muscle mass. A 24-hour collection of urine is measured, and the following equation is used to calculate GFR: GFR = U × V/P, where U = urine concentration of creatinine (mg/dl), V = volume of urine measured (ml/min), P = plasma concentration of creatinine (mg/dl). A 2-hour sample collected through a Foley catheter correlates well with the 24-hour sample.

Diehl JT, Cali RF, Hertzer NR, Bevan EG: Complications of abdominal aortic reconstruction: An analysis of perioperative risk factors in 557 patients. Ann Surg 197:49–56, 1983

Miller DC, Myer BD: Pathophysiology and prevention of acute renal failure associated with thoracoabdominal or abdominal aortic surgery. J Vasc Surg 5:518–523, 1987

Ostri P, Mouritsen L, Jorgensen B, Frimodt-Moller C: Renal function following aneurysmectomy of the abdominal aorta. J Cardiovasc Surg 27:714–718, 1986

Sladen RN, Endo E, Harrison T: Two hour versus 24 hour creatinine clearance in critically ill patients. Anesthesiology 67:1013, 1987

B.6. Describe the blood flow to the spinal cord. What is its relevance to surgery of the abdominal aorta?

The spinal cord receives blood through radicular arteries which arise from three main sources: upper, branches of the subclavian artery; middle, branches off a few intercostal and lumbar arteries from T3 to L4; and lower, branches of the internal iliac artery. Of these sources, the least significant is the lower supply. These radicular arteries give rise to spinal branches that enter the spinal canal through the intervertebral foramen and divide into three parts: the anterior and posterior arteries of the vertebral canal, which supply the vertebral column, and the neuromedullary artery, which supplies the spinal cord and meninges through the anterior and posterior radicular arteries. The largest artery of the spinal cord is the anterior radicular artery in the vicinity of the thoracolumbar junction. It is the main blood supply to the lumbar enlargement of the cord and is known as the *Artery of Adamkiewicz*. This artery usually arises from one of the lowermost intercostal arteries, usually on the left side, and rarely from the upper two lumbar arteries.

Spinal cord ischemia can develop during aortic cross-clamping as a result of one of two mechanisms: decreased blood flow through critical intercostal arteries (important in infrarenal cross-clamping) and hypotension in the aorta distal to the cross-clamp, leading to a "steal" phenomenon through the collateral circulation to the distal aorta (important in thoracic cross-clamping).

Barash PG, Cullen BF, Stoelting RK (eds): Clinical Anesthesia, 3rd ed, pp 889–893. Philadelphia, Lippincott-Raven, 1997

Richenbacher J, Landolt AM, Theiler K: Applied Anatomy of the Back, pp 268–280. Berlin, Springer-Verlag, 1985

B.7. What are the various surgical approaches to the abdominal aorta? How does the choice of surgical technique affect the anesthetic management?

The classic approach to the abdominal aorta is through a vertical anterior midline incision with a transperitoneal approach to the retroperitoneal space. This gives access to all major arteries in the abdomen and pelvis. A transverse abdominal incision (supraumbilical) is also adequate for a transperitoneal approach. Although the entry is slower, there is less pain and pulmonary impairment postoperatively. The transperitoneal approach, with the necessary exposure of the abdominal organs, causes major heat and fluid loss and prolonged postoperative ileus.

The retroperitoneal approach is performed through a left flank incision with the patient in the right lateral decubitus position. In some studies, this approach has been shown to have less respiratory and wound complications, less postoperative ileus, less blood loss, lower fluid requirements, and earlier discharge from the hospital. Monitor and line placement must take the lateral position into consideration.

Rob C: Extraperitoneal approach to the abdominal aorta. Surgery 53:87–89, 1963

Sicard GA, Freeman MB, VanderWoude JC, Anderson CB: Comparison between the transabdominal and retroperitoneal approach for reconstruction of the infrarenal abdominal aorta. J Vasc Surg 5:19–27, 1987

Williams GM, Ricotta J, Zimmer M, Burdick J: The extended retroperitoneal approach for treatment of extensive atherosclerosis of the aorta and renal vessels. Surgery 88:846–855, 1980

B.8. How would you premedicate this patient?

The most common problem patients face in presentation to the operating room is anxiety. For this reason we would suggest a low-dose anxiolytic as sufficient premedication for the vast majority of patients. The remainder of preoperative medications can be given intravenously after arrival in the operating room. A small dose of a benzodiazepine, e.g., diazepam, 10 mg, or lorazepam, 0.05 to 4 mg orally, should be sufficient for premedication. Additionally, psychological preparation for surgery is an important preoperative task for the anesthesiologist.

Additional specific pharmacologic regimens should be tailored to individual patient needs. Various medications and combinations have been used, including narcotics, anticholinergics, barbiturates, and benzodiazepines. No single agent or combination has been demonstrated to be greatly superior to others. Certainly respiratory depressants should be avoided in patients who are at risk to develop hypoventilation (e.g., after carotid repair or chronic CO_2 retention).

Barash PG, Cullen BF, Stoelting RK (eds): Clinical Anesthesia, 3rd ed, p 897. Philadelphia, Lippincott-Raven, 1997

Kaplan JA (ed): Vascular Anesthesia, pp 187–204. New York, Churchill Livingstone, 1991

C. Intraoperative Management

C.1. Would you use an arterial line? What are the complications of an arterial line placement?

Arterial pressure monitoring is exceedingly important in this case, from induction of anesthesia through emergence. For patients without coronary or cerebral artery disease, the arterial line can be placed after induction. However, since this patient has coronary artery disease, an arterial line is important for blood pressure management during induction and should be placed prior to institution of anesthesia.

Vascular insufficiency and infection are the two major complications of arterial line placement. Catheter size and duration of cannulation are implicated in vascular occlusion. The etiologies of most vascular injuries are embolic. Radial artery cannulation is a low-risk, high-benefit method used to closely monitor blood pressure in this patient with labile blood pressure, who also requires frequent sampling of arterial blood gases and hematocrits.

Bedford RF: Radial arterial function following percutaneous cannulation with 18 and 20 gauge catheters. Anesthesiology 47:37–39, 1977

Bedford RF, Wollman H: Complications of radial artery cannulation: An objective prospective study in man. Anesthesiology 38:228–236, 1973

Slogoff S, Keats AS, Arkind C: On the safety of radial artery cannulation. Anesthesiology 59:42–47, 1983

C2. What various monitors are available for myocardial ischemia? Is a pulmonary artery catheter helpful in determining the occurrence of ischemia?

Monitoring of the patient undergoing aortic reconstruction surgery should be aimed at preserving myocardial, pulmonary, and renal function as well as maintaining intravascular volume. Therefore, it is mandatory, particularly in the patient with known coronary artery disease, to monitor for myocardial ischemia. Monitoring of the V_5 lead as well as lead II of the ECG for ST-segment changes is the most common intraoperative assessment of myocardial ischemia. Lead V_5 or lead V_4 (sensitivities of 75% and 61%, respectively) are useful in detecting intraoperative myocardial ischemia. Simultaneous viewing of both V_5 and V_4 leads have a sensitivity of 90%, while simultaneous viewing of leads II and V_5 yields a sensitivity of 80%. However, in some studies, this alone was insufficient to recognize from 40% to 75% of intraoperative ischemic events as detected by regional wall motion abnormalities (RWMA) seen with a transesophageal two-dimensional echocardiogram (TEE).

Monitoring the pulmonary artery pressure tracing for the appearance of V waves and increasing pulmonary capillary wedge pressure (PCWP) with decreasing cardiac output are other relatively insensitive means of detecting intraoperative myocardial ischemia. As with the ECG, wall motion abnormality changes associated with early ischemia as detected by transesophageal echocardiography are found far earlier than the appearance of V waves or changes in PCWP.

A microcomputer-based ECG reader (ST-segment trend monitor) has also been advocated as a monitor of myocardial ischemia. These systems can pick up more subtle changes in ST segments than by simple observation. The most sensitive means for monitoring patients to determine the development of myocardial ischemia at its earliest presentation is, in fact, wall-motion dyskinesis demonstrated by two-dimensional transesophageal echocardiography. As yet, no improvement in outcome has been demonstrated by the use of these monitors.

Barash PG, Cullen BF, Stoelting RK (eds): Clinical Anesthesia, 3rd ed, p 877. Philadelphia, Lippincott-Raven, 1997

Kalman PG et al: Cardiac dysfunction during abdominal aortic operation: The limitations of pulmonary wedge pressures. J Vasc Surg 3:773–781, 1986

Kotrly KJ et al: Intraoperative detection of myocardial ischemia with an ST segment trend monitoring system. Anesth Analg 63:343–345, 1984

Mangano DT: Perioperative cardiac morbidity. Anesthesiology 72:153–184, 1990

C.3. What additional monitors would you employ?

A monitor of central venous pressures is recommended to determine volume status in these patients. The choice of monitor, central venous pressure (CVP) or pulmonary artery (PA) catheter, can be based on the level of aortic cross-clamping and the severity of the patient's underlying cardiac disease. The CVP is informative only if it is very low or very high. Since the right side of the heart is usually a compliant system, large changes in intravascular volume can occur without significant changes in the CVP. The PCWP, as obtained by a PA catheter, is far more accurate in determining intravascular volume status. Additionally, the PA catheter allows for the simple measurement of cardiac output, which is exceedingly helpful during aortic cross-clamp in the patient with left ventricular dysfunction. In this situation particularly, CVP is not an accurate reflection of left-sided pressures reflected by the PCWP. This is also true of the patient with severe pulmonary disease.

Another useful measure of intravascular volume status as well as renal blood flow is the collection of urine through a Foley catheter. Urine output will diminish with decreasing glomerular filtration caused by decreased renal blood flow.

Somatosensory evoked potentials (SSEPs) during aortic reconstruction surgery monitor spinal cord function. It has been demonstrated for thoracic aortic surgery that SSEPs remain stable if the distal aortic pressure is maintained above 60 mm Hg. At lower pressures SSEPs disappear gradually. In one study, paraplegia resulted in 5 of 6 patients whose SSEPs remained absent for >30 minutes. Patients should be monitored for SSEP changes if they are at higher risk of spinal cord ischemia. SSEPs are changed or lost with aortic cross-clamp most commonly in those patients who are already at increased risk for neurologic complications. Higher (especially thoracic) or prolonged cross-clamp placement also places the patient at increased risk for development of spinal cord ischemia. With a conduction block in place, as in epidural or spinal anesthesia, SSEPs will be ablated.

These patients can undergo tremendous heat and insensible fluid loss as a result of the enormous surface area of the bowel exposed to room air. Therefore, body temperature should be monitored and aggressively maintained. Forced hot air thermal blankets are contraindicated on the lower extremities when an aortic cross-clamp is applied, but may be used on the upper body along with fluid warmers to maintain temperature.

Ansley DM, Ramsay JG, Whalley DG et al: The relationship between central venous pressure and pulmonary capillary wedge pressure during aortic surgery. Can J Anaesth 34:594–600, 1987

Barash PG, Cullen BF, Stoelting RK (eds): Clinical Anesthesia, 3rd ed, pp 894–895. Philadelphia, Lippincott-Raven, 1997

Bush H Jr, Hydo LU, Fischer E et al: Hypothermia during elective abdominal aortic aneurysm repair: The high price of avoidable morbidity. J Vasc Surg 21:392–402, 1995

Nuwer MR: Evoked Potential Monitoring in the Operating Room, pp 93–95. New York, Raven Press, 1986

Practice Guidelines for PA Catheterization. A Report by the ASA Task Force on PA Catheterization. Anesthesiology 78:380–394, 1993

Teplick R: Measuring central vascular pressures: A surprisingly complex problem. Anesthesiology 67:289–291, 1987

C.4. How would you anesthetize this patient? Discuss the various anesthetic techniques which can be employed for this surgery.

Balanced anesthesia with narcotics, relaxants, and volatile agents is a good technique for the anesthetic management of this patient. Loading intravenous narcotic such as fentanyl 5 to 10 μg/kg prior to induction of anesthesia promotes cardiovascular stability during induction.

All anesthetic techniques have been used and advocated for abdominal aortic surgery. Pure general anesthesia, combined general and regional techniques, and pure regional anesthesia have all been described. Outcome studies seem to indicate no particular difference with respect to technique or agents used. Benefits and problems can be argued from any side and a case made for each technique and agent selected. Tailoring the anesthetic to the individual patient is the single most important approach. In some, an inhalational technique may be indicated. In others, an opiate or mixed technique would better serve the patient's medical problems. The most important goals in the anesthetic management of patients undergoing aortic reconstruction include protection of myocardial and renal function. As long as these goals are met, the actual technique is probably less important. Some studies indicate that for patients with ischemic heart disease isoflurane may not be an ideal drug. It is clear that in patients with ischemic heart disease, a slow heart rate is exceedingly beneficial. An anesthetic technique should be constructed with this goal in mind. Combined regional (epidural) and general anesthesia techniques usually involve an additional fluid requirement of up to 2 liters per case. This can be offset by the concomitant use of an alpha-agonist for vasoconstriction. The placement of an epidural catheter may also be of benefit in the postoperative management of the patient.

Dodds TM, Burns AK, DeRoo DB et al: Effects of anesthetic technique on myocardial wall motion abnormalities during abdominal aortic surgery. J Cardiothoracic Vasc Anesth 11:129–136, 1997

Kaplan JA (ed): Vascular Anesthesia, pp 309–332. New York, Churchill Livingstone, 1991

Liu S, Carpenter RL, Neal JM: Epidural anesthesia and analgesia: Their role in postoperative outcome. Anesthesiology 82:1474–1506, 1995

Raggi R, Dardik H, Mauro A: Continuous epidural anesthesia and postoperative narcotics in vascular surgery. Am J Surg 154:192–197, 1987

Yeager M, Glass DD, Neff RK, Brinck-Johnsen T: Epidural anesthesia and analgesia in high-risk surgical patients. Anesthesiology 66:729–736, 1987

*C5. This patient is to be heparinized intraoperatively and anticoagulation is to be contin-
ued postoperatively. Is this a contraindication to the preoperative placement of either an
epidural or intraspinal catheter?*

There is concern that placement of an epidural catheter in a patient to be anticoagulated increases the risk of an epidural hematoma and a subsequent neurologic deficit.
Indeed, for those cases where there is significant risk of spinal cord ischemia, the diagnostic confusion of epidural hematoma versus cord ischemia may preclude the
placement of an epidural catheter. However, an epidural catheter can be placed with
a relative degree of confidence in patients who are not anticoagulated at the time of
the puncture but who will be anticoagulated later, with careful maintenance of the
partial thromboplastin time (PTT) at 1.5 to 2 times the control value. Removal of the
catheter should occur either when the PTT is normalized or when it is well controlled if heparinization is to be continued postoperatively.

Rao TLK, El-Etr AA: Anticoagulation following placement of epidural and subarachnoid catheters:
An evaluation of neurologic sequelae. Anesthesiology 55:618–620, 1981

Vandermeulen EP, Van Aken H, Vermylen J: Anticoagulants and spinal-epidural anesthesia. Anesth
Analg 79:1165–1177, 1994

C.6. What are your plans for fluid and blood replacement during surgery?

Fluid replacement should be aimed at maintaining the patient's intravascular filling
pressures. The use of a pulmonary artery catheter simplifies this matter greatly. In
the majority of patients, crystalloid fluid should be isotonic. All preoperative fluid
deficits must be accounted for early in the procedure (e.g., half the deficit in the first
hour, half the remainder in the second hour, etc.); one must also watch the hourly
fluid requirement for the weight of the patient (which takes into account the urine
output and the usual insensible loss from skin and lungs) and the insensible loss
from the large abdominal incision. Additional third-space loss from surgical trauma
ranges from 3 to 5 ml/kg/h for small incisions to 8 to 10 ml/kg/h for large incisions
as in abdominal aortic aneurysm repair. Blood loss should be replaced milliliter for
milliliter with blood or colloid, or in a 3:1 ratio with crystalloid. The concurrent use
of an autotransfuser (e.g., Cell Saver) decreases the need for homologous blood transfusions. Transfusions have been shown to cause a clinically significant depression of
immune function. Clinical studies have shown a beneficial effect of blood transfusion
on transfusion graft survival, but an adverse effect on cancer recurrence and postoperative infection. With the hemodynamic changes associated with aortic cross-clamping, it is vital to maintain adequate intravascular volume in order to ensure adequate
renal perfusion and normotension after removal of the cross-clamp.

Barash PG, Cullen BF, Stoelting RK (eds): Clinical Anesthesia, 3rd ed, pp 897–898. Philadelphia,
Lippincott-Raven, 1997

Keane RM, Munster AM, Birmingham W et al: Suppression of lymphocyte function after aortic
reconstruction: Use of non-immunosuppressive anesthesia. Arch Surg 117:1133–1135, 1982

Landers DF, Hill GE, Wong KC, Fox IJ: Blood transfusion-induced immunomodulation. Anesth
Analg 82:187–204, 1996

C.7. What are the hemodynamic changes of aortic cross-clamp placement? What efforts can be made to minimize these changes both prior to and during cross-clamping? If the patient develops ST-segment depressions with a rising pulmonary capillary wedge pressure (PCWP) during cross-clamp, what maneuvers should be taken?

The systemic hemodynamic response to aortic cross-clamping is shown in Figure 13-2. Arterial hypertension is the most dramatic and consistent result of the application of an aortic cross-clamp. This is easily envisioned as a result of a sudden increase in afterload resulting in increased left ventricular end-systolic wall stress and systemic arterial pressure. Usually these changes are accompanied by decreased cardiac output. Some of these changes may also be due to redistribution of blood volume from the venous vasculature to the upper part of the body. All of the previously stated factors are more profound in the case of a supraceliac or thoracic cross-clamp placement. Variations in blood volume status or splanchnic vascular tone are affected by the depth of anesthesia, type of anesthesia, and the extent of fluid load, all of which affect the pattern of blood volume redistribution.

A sudden increase in afterload can lead to left ventricular failure, particularly in the patient with a noncompliant left ventricle. Ideally, the patient should have lower filling pressures for the half hour prior to cross-clamp placement. This helps to minimize these responses to cross-clamp placement. The PA catheter is helpful in accurately assessing and maintaining the preclamp values for the left side of the heart. A

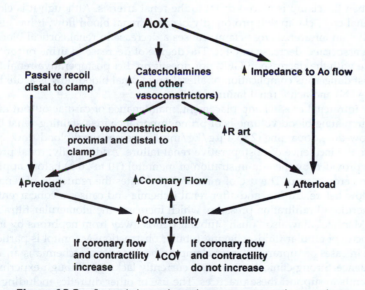

Figure 13-2. Systemic hemodynamic response to aortic cross-clamping. Preload does not necessarily increase. If during infrarenal aortic cross-clamping blood volume shifts into the splanchnic vasculature, preload does not increase (Fig. 13-1). AoX, aortic cross-clamping; Ao, aortic; R art, arterial resistance; ↑ and ↓, increase and decrease, respectively. *Different patterns are possible. (Reprinted with permission from Gelman S: The patholophysiology of aortic cross-clamping and unclamping. Anesthesiology 82:1026–1060, 1995)

potent agent and/or a vasodilator such as nitroprusside is used to return afterload to near normal. This also helps increase the cardiac output and decrease stress on the left ventricle. Should this be insufficient to reverse the left ventricular failure, the addition of an inotrope such as dopamine may be necessary.

The increase in afterload may also result in myocardial ischemia. Ischemia, reflected as ST-segment depressions or RWMA from TEE, can be managed with intravenous nitroglycerin, a potent dilator of the capacitance vessels. This drug is used to decrease left ventricular end-diastolic volume (LVEDV) and end-diastolic pressure (LVEDP). By decreasing LVEDP, one also decreases the transluminal pressure in the coronary vasculature. Blood flow to the myocardium is thereby increased. When LVEDV is decreased, heart work and myocardial oxygen consumption are also decreased.

Barash PG, Cullen BF, Stoelting RK (eds): Clinical Anesthesia, 3rd ed, pp 889–892. Philadelphia, Lippincott-Raven, 1997

Gelman S: The pathophysiology of aortic cross-clamping and unclamping. Anesthesiology 82:1026–1060, 1995

C8. As this case involves an infrarenal aneurysm, is renal blood flow affected with the placement of the cross-clamp? Are there any treatment maneuvers that can be taken to minimize these changes?

Decreased renal function is observed in many patients after aortic cross-clamping, even when the clamp is placed distal to the renal arteries. Although it is clear that a suprarenal cross-clamp will profoundly decrease renal blood flow, it has also been noted that an infrarenal cross-clamp causes a decrease in renal cortical blood flow with an associated decrease in GFR. The degree of decrease in urine output does not correlate with the decrease in GFR, nor does it predict postoperative renal failure. The most dangerous complication of alteration in renal blood flow is acute tubular necrosis (ATN) and acute renal failure (ARF).

For infrarenal cross-clamp placement, maintenance of cardiac output and adequate circulating blood volume is of prime importance in sustaining renal blood flow. Low-dose dopamine (2 to 4 µg/kg/min) increases renal blood flow and may decrease the incidence of postoperative renal failure. Additionally, renal protection may be provided by the administration of mannitol (10 to 20 g) before application of the aortic cross-clamp. The use of mannitol attenuates the reduction of renal cortical blood flow before, during, and after renal ischemia and causes a concurrent increase in glomerular ultrafiltration pressure, which increases the glomerular filtration rate (GFR). Mannitol may also "flush" tubular debris away from nephrons by increasing the velocity of tubular fluid, relieving tubular obstruction. Mannitol is particularly important in cases of suprarenal cross-clamping because renal ischemia is an inevitable consequence. Strong clinical evidence is currently lacking, although experimental evidence tends to support these practices. The use of other diuretics including furosemide and/or ethacrynic acid has never been proven to prevent renal failure.

Alpert RA, Roizen MF, Hamilton WK et al: Intraoperative urinary output does not predict postoperative renal function in patients undergoing abdominal aortic revascularization. Surgery 95:707–710, 1984

Barash PG, Cullen BF, Stoelting RK (eds): Clinical Anesthesia, 3rd ed, p 895. Philadelphia, Lippincott-Raven, 1997

Gamulin Z et al: Effects of infrarenal aortic cross-clamping on renal hemodynamics in humans. Anesthesiology 61:394–399, 1984

Miller DC, Myers BD: Pathophysiology and prevention of acute renal failure associated with thoracoabdominal or abdominal aortic surgery. J Vasc Surg 5:518–523, 1987

Paul MD, Mazer CD, Byrick RJ et al: Influence of mannitol and dopamine on renal function during elective infrarenal aortic clamping in man. Am J Nephrol 6:427–434, 1986

C.9. What are the hemodynamic consequences of aortic cross-clamp removal? What can be done to minimize the effects of removing the aortic cross-clamp? If the systemic blood pressure remains depressed after removal of the cross-clamp, what is the differential diagnosis? How would you define and correct the problem?

The hemodynamic response to aortic unclamping is shown in Figure 13-3. During cross-clamping, blood flow to the lower extremities is halted. Metabolism switches from aerobic to anaerobic as ischemia develops. This results in maximal vasodilation and lactic acid production. When the cross-clamp is released, systemic vascular resistance and arterial blood pressure decrease dramatically. Reactive hyperemia is a consequence of unclamping. This may be the result of arterial relaxation (myogenic mechanism), an accumulation of vasodilating substances below the occlusion, or anoxic relaxation of smooth muscles. Peripheral vasodilation can result in relative volume depletion and hypotension. Vasodilation may become systemic as the lactic acid is washed out of the extremities into the central circulation. This condition is sometimes known as "declamping shock."

In order to minimize the hypotensive response, volume loading for the 30 minutes prior to cross-clamp release is suggested to raise filling pressures to slightly above normal. Vasodilators such as nitroprusside and/or nitroglycerin during this

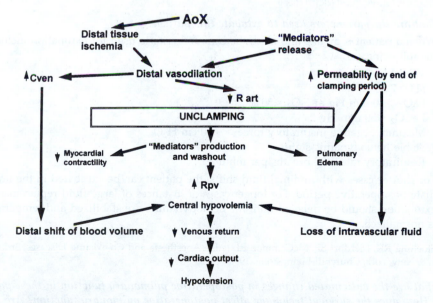

Figure 13-3.   Systemic hemodynamic response to aortic unclamping. AoX, aortic cross-clamping; Cven, venous capacitance; R art, arterial resistance; Rpv, pulmonary vascular resistance; ↑ and ↓, increase and decrease, respectively. (Reprinted with permission from Gelman S: The pathophysiology of aortic cross-clamping and unclamping. Anesthesiology 82:1026–1060, 1995)

pre-unclamping period allow additional volume loading with maintenance of filling pressures. In addition, gradual release of the clamp allows time for adjustments in volume, pressors, and sodium bicarbonate replacement.

Sometimes, even in the face of adequate volume loading, the blood pressure remains low following cross-clamp removal. The more cephalad the cross-clamp placement, the greater the incidence of this problem. In this situation it is advisable to ask the surgeon to reapply the aortic cross-clamp in various degrees depending on the severity of the hypotension. This allows more time for correction of blood volume or acidosis.

Other causes of sustained hypotension in the face of adequate management include a continued site of hemorrhage and myocardial ischemia and/or failure. Measurement of filling pressures would help in this differentiation. Ischemia or failure would have elevated filling pressures with hypotension, whereas hemorrhage would naturally have low filling pressures.

Eklof B, Neglen P, Thomson D: Temporary incomplete ischemia of the legs induced by aortic clamping in man: Effects on central hemodynamics and skeletal muscle metabolism by adrenergic block. Ann Surg 193:89–98, 1981

Gelman S: The pathophysiology of aortic cross-clamping and unclamping. Anesthesiology 82:1026–1060, 1995

Reiz S, Peter T, Rais O: Hemodynamic and cardiometabolic effects of infrarenal aortic and common iliac artery declamping in man: An approach to optimal volume loading. Acta Anesth Scand 23:579–586, 1979

D. Postoperative Management

D.1. What are the parameters used to extubate this patient?

When a patient is awake and alert, the common criteria used for extubation include the following:

- VC >15 ml/kg
- pH >7.30
- PaO_2 >60 mm Hg at F_IO_2 <50%
- $PaCO_2$ <50 mm Hg
- Maximal negative inspiratory force >-20 cm H_2O
- Stable hemodynamic status
- Respiratory rate <30 breaths per minute

For shorter cases with minimal fluid shifts, the patient can be extubated in the immediate postoperative period. For longer cases or instances of large fluid replacement, extubation should be delayed until the hemodynamics are stabilized and temperature is normalized.

Stoelting RK, Dierdorf SF, McCammon RL (eds): Anesthesia and Co-existing Diseases, 3rd ed, p 178. New York, Churchill Livingstone, 1993

D.2. What are the anticipated changes in postoperative pulmonary function in these patients? How does the surgical technique affect postoperative pulmonary function? Are there any postoperative maneuvers that can maximize respiratory parameters?

The transabdominal approach to the aorta involves an upper abdominal incision. Total lung capacity (TLC) and its subdivisions decrease after upper abdominal surgery. Vital capacity (VC) decreases 25% to 50% and returns to normal in 1 to 2 weeks, and residual volume (RV) increases 13%. Functional residual capacity (FRC) declines 20% and is most marked on the fourth postoperative day. Expiratory reserve volume (ERV) declines 20% after lower abdominal surgery, and up to 60% after upper abdominal and thoracic incisions. Tidal volume decreases 20% on the first postoperative day and gradually returns to normal. The retroperitoneal approach to the aorta involves a flank incision, which leads to far less respiratory compromise. Ambulation and control of postoperative pain diminish splinting and help maximize respiratory parameters.

Barash PG, Cullen BF, Stoelting RK (eds): Clinical Anesthesia, 3rd ed, pp 1287–1294. Philadelphia, Lippincott-Raven, 1997

D.3. How would you control postoperative pain? What are the alternatives in the management of this patient's postoperative pain? Is there a role for nonnarcotic medications or alternative pain management techniques for this patient?

The goal of effective postoperative pain relief is to produce a high quality of pain control with the fewest number of side-effects and complications. Neuraxial analgesia in the immediate postoperative period is the preferred method of pain management in this high-risk patient population. The ideal opiate and its concentration and combination with local anesthetic has yet to be defined. Table 13-1 lists different suggested protocols.

It remains controversial whether epidural opioids when used alone are superior to the intravenous administration of opioids. Epidural opioids have the advantage of producing analgesia without motor or sympathetic blockade. The most commonly used opioids are morphine and fentanyl. Spinal cord concentrations of an opiate after epidural administration are the balance between vascular and meningeal permeability. Fentanyl (more lipophilic) is preferentially absorbed by the vasculature rather than the meninges, accounting for its systemic effect. When fentanyl is administered via a thoracic epidural infusion similar pain relief is achieved at a lower dose of narcotic than with an intravenous infusion. Lipid-soluble opioids should be administered near the dermatomal region of the incision. Epidural morphine can be administered by bolus dosing or a continuous infusion. Respiratory depression is less and the quality of analgesia is better with a continuous infusion.

The combination of epidural opioids and local anesthetics provides synergistic analgesia, especially with patient movement. The advantage of the combination is enhanced pain relief with a reduced dose of both drugs, decreasing the number of side-effects of both. Further relief is not achieved by the addition of NSAIDs. They are better administered in combination with systemic narcotics. Epidural adrenergic agonists are another class of antinociceptive agents. Their use continues to be explored.

The final link between the quality of postoperative analgesia and outcome remains ill-defined. The confounding issues include the location of the epidural catheter, the composite of the opioid/local anesthetic mixture, and the timing of the administration of the epidural mixture (intraoperatively or postoperatively).

Studies suggest that intraoperative and/or postoperative epidural anesthesia is associated with reduced postoperative cardiac morbidity and mortality in high-risk populations. In addition, there appears to be a reduction in the incidence of postoper-

Table 13-1. Epidural Opioid/Bupivacaine Combinations Administered by Continuous Infusion[a]

DRUG COMBINATIONS	SOLUTION[b]	BOLUS DOSE OF BUPIVACAINE	BASAL INFUSION[c]	BREAKTHROUGH DOSES	INCREMENTS IN BREAKTHROUGH[d]
Morphine Bupivacaine[e]	0.01% 0.05%–0.1%	0.5%–0.25%	6–8 ml/h	1–2 ml every 10–15 min	1 ml of the solution
Hydromorphone Bupivacaine[f]	0.0025%–0.005% 0.05%–0.1%	0.5%–0.25%	6–8 ml/h	1–3 ml every 10–15 min	1 ml of the solution
Fentanyl Bupivacaine[g]	0.001% 0.05%–0.1%	0.5%–0.25%	0.1–0.15 ml/kg/h	1–1.5 ml every 10–15 min	1 ml of the solution
Sufentanil Bupivacaine[h]	0.0001% 0.05%–0.1%	0.5%–0.25%	0.1–0.2 ml/kg/h	1–1.5 ml every 10–15 min	1 ml of the solution

[a] Catheter insertion site is the dermatome corresponding to the middle of the surgical incision. Administer a bolus dose of 0.5% bupivacaine or 2% lidocaine to establish surgical anesthesia, or 0.25% bupivacaine to induce postoperative analgesia in 5-ml aliquots.
[b] Due to infectious control, a total volume of 150 ml is recommended.
[c] Initial basal infusion rates will depend on the age, general condition, and weight of the patient.
[d] If analgesia is inadequate after 1 h, increase the breakthrough dose by the recommended amount. If analgesia is inadequate after one additional hour, decrease the lockout interval by 5 min.
[e] Prepare this solution by mixing 75–150 mg of bupivacaine with 15 mg of preservative-free morphine in a total volume of 150 ml of perservative-free normal saline.
[f] Prepare this solution by mixing 75–150 mg of bupivacaine with 3.75–7.5 mg of hydromorphone in a total volume of 150 ml of perservative-free normal saline.
[g] Prepare this solution by mixing 75–150 mg of bupivacaine with 1500 μg of fentanyl in a total volume of 150 ml of perservative-free normal saline.
[h] Prepare this solution by mixing 75–150 mg of bupivacaine with 150–300 μg of sufentanil in a total volume of 150 ml of perservative-free normal saline.
(Reprinted with permission from deLeon-Cosa Sola OA, Lema MJ: Postoperative epidural opioid analgesia. What are the choices? Anesth Analg 83:867–875, 1996.)

ative graft occlusion, thromboembolic complications and pulmonary complications, and an earlier recovery from postoperative ileus.

Complications of the epidural route of analgesia include dural puncture, epidural hematoma, and epidural abscess. The risk of epidural hematoma is small in patients receiving appropriate doses of anticoagulation postoperatively, but is prohibitively high in patients receiving thrombolytic treatment. The risk of complications are similar whether the catheter is placed at the thoracic or lumbar level. Other complications include pruritus, nausea, urinary retention, and delayed respiratory depression. The latter is <1% when epidural morphine is used, similar to the oral and parenteral route. Difficulty ambulating and orthostatic hypotension are minimized when catheters are placed in the thoracic region and the bupivacaine concentration is <0.08%.

Alternatively, a systemic narcotic analgesic can be used. Rapid onset of serum levels is of prime importance in the administration of systemic narcotics. This can be accomplished through parenteral bolus techniques such as intramuscular, subcutaneous, or intravenous injections. One of the most successful means of administering systemic narcotics during the postoperative period is by patient-controlled analgesia (PCA), which uses modified infusion pumps that are able to administer infusions of narcotics, small preprogrammed bolus doses on patient demand, and larger bolus doses by prescription. This allows patients to titrate their narcotic doses to need while avoiding the toxic side-effects which result from high peak serum levels.

Nonnarcotic medications, particularly nonsteroidal anti-inflammatory drugs (NSAIDs) such as ketorolac (15 to 30 mg IV or IM every 6 hours) or indomethacin (50 to 100 mg suppository PR twice daily), can be a helpful adjunct to systemic narcotic analgesics in a total pain management program. Prostaglandins, locally released in response to tissue injury, interact with nociceptors (sensory nerve endings) to start the pain cascade. By inhibiting prostaglandin synthesis, the peripheral input in the pain cascade is diminished. NSAIDs should be avoided in the anticoagulated patient, the patient with ulcer disease, or those with impaired renal function.

Transcutaneous electrical nerve stimulation (TENS) can diminish incisional pain through a counterirritant mechanism. Electrodes placed on either side of the incision can, in some cases, diminish the narcotic requirement.

Bell SD, Seltzer JL: Postoperative pain management. In Kaplan JA (ed): Vascular Anesthesia, pp 565–586. New York, Churchill-Livingstone, 1991

deLeon-Casa Sola OA, Lema MJ: Postoperative epidural opioid analgesia: What are the choices? Anesth Analg 83:867–875, 1996

Eisenach JC, DeKock M, Klimscha W: α-Adrenergic agonists for regional anesthesia: A:clinical review of clonidine (1984–1995). Anesthesiology 85:655–674, 1996

Gold MS, Rockman CB, Riles TS: Comparison of lumbar and thoracic epidural narcotics for postoperative analgesia in patients undergoing abdominal aortic aneurysm repair. J Cardiothoracic Vasc Anesth 11:137–140, 1997

Kavanagh BP, Katz J, Sandler AN: Pain control after thoracic surgery: A review of current techniques. Anesthesiology 81:737–759, 1994

Liu S, Carpenter RL, Neal JM: Epidural anesthesia and analgesia: Their role in postoperative outcome. Anesthesiology 82:1474–1506, 1995

Simon LS, Mills JA: Non-steroidal anti-inflammatory drugs. N Engl J Med 302:1179–1185, 1237–1243, 1980

Yeager M, Glass DD, Neff RK, Brinck-Johnsen T: Epidural anesthesia and analgesia in high-risk surgical patients. Anesthesiology 66:729–736, 1987

14 Hypertension

Fun-Sun F. Yao

A 70-year-old man with cholelithiasis was scheduled for a cholecystectomy. His blood pressure (BP) was 230/120 mm Hg; pulse 60/min. Hematocrit was 38%; serum sodium, 140 mEq/liter; serum potassium, 2.7 mEq/liter. His medications included propranolol and hydrochlorothiazide.

A. Medical Disease and Differential Diagnosis

1. Define hypertension and classify its severity.
2. What is the prevalence of hypertension?
3. What is the general classification of hypertension? Enumerate the causes of each type of hypertension.
4. What is the pathophysiology of essential hypertension?
5. Are hypertensive patients at an increased risk for perioperative cardiac morbidity?
6. Are hypertensive patients at increased risk for perioperative cerebral and renal complications? Why?
7. Would you employ a controlled hypotensive technique for hypertensive patients? How much would you safely lower the blood pressure?
8. What is the mechanism of action of antihypertensive drugs?
9. Does the choice of antihypertensive therapy influence hemodynamic responses to induction, laryngoscopy, and intubation?
10. Does chronic angiotensin-converting enzyme inhibition influence anesthetic induction?

B. Preoperative Evaluation and Preparation

1. How would you evaluate this patient preoperatively?
2. Would you postpone the surgery? Why? What blood pressure would you like the patient to achieve before surgery?
3. Should all or any of the chronic medications be discontinued prior to the operation?
4. Should hypokalemia be treated prior to anesthesia? Why?
5. Should hypomagnesemia be treated prior to anesthesia? Why?
6. Does an asymptomatic carotid bruit increase the risk in these patients?
7. The surgery was postponed for 2 weeks. The patient has been on propranolol, captopril, hydrochlorothiazide and KCl. His blood pressure was 160/95 mm Hg and potassium 4.0 mEq/liter. How would you premedicate this patient?
8. If the patient is an untreated hypertensive patient with blood pressure 170/100 mm Hg, would you pretreat the patient preoperatively with an antihypertensive agent?

C. Intraoperative Management

1. How would you monitor this patient?
2. What are the anesthetic goals for hypertensive patients?

3. How would you induce anesthesia for the hypertensive patient?
4. How does tracheal intubation produce hypertension?
5. What happens to the left ventricular ejection fraction during and immediately following intubation?
6. What other measures can prevent hypertension and tachycardia at the time of intubation?
7. After induction and intubation, the blood pressure went down to 70/40 mm Hg. What would you do?
8. What is your choice of agents for maintenance of anesthesia? Why?
9. How would you manage fluid therapy for hypertensive patients?
10. During the surgery, blood pressure went up to 220/120 mm Hg. How would you treat the hypertension?
11. What could you do to prevent hypertension during extubation and emergence?
12. Would you consider regional anesthesia for this patient?

D. Postoperative Management

1. The patient developed hypertension BP 210/110 mm Hg in the postanesthesia care unit. What would you do?

A. Medical Disease and Differential Diagnosis

A.1. Define hypertension and classify its severity.

True systemic hypertension can be diagnosed when there is an increase in arterial pressure above accepted normal pressure for age, sex, and race. The accepted upper limits of normal blood pressure are as follows:

Adult	140/90 mm Hg
Adolescent	100/75 mm Hg
Early childhood	85/55 mm Hg
Infant	70/45 mm Hg

The accepted upper limit of normal pressure in the adult was chosen as 140/90 rather than 160/95 mm Hg (World Health Organization criteria) because systolic blood pressure levels above 140 mm Hg and diastolic levels above 90 mm Hg are associated with increased risk for eventual cardiovascular disease.

The classification of severity of hypertension is shown in Table 14-1.

Table 14-1.   Severity of Hypertension in Adults

SEVERITY	RANGE (mm Hg)	
	Systole	Diastole
Normal	<140	<90
Hypertension		
Mild	140–159	90–99
Moderate	160–179	100–109
Severe	180–209	110–119
Very Severe	>210	>120

Braunwald E: Heart Disease, 5th ed, pp 807–810. Philadelphia, WB Saunders, 1997

Braunwald E, Isselbacher KJ, Fauci AS et al: Harrison's Principles of Internal Medicine, 14th ed, pp 202–203. New York, McGraw-Hill, 1998

The 1988 report of the Joint National Committee on detection, evaluation and treatment of high blood pressure. Arch Intern Med 148:1023, 1989

A.2. What is the prevalence of hypertension?

The prevalence of hypertension depends on both the racial composition of the population and the criteria used to define hypertension. In a white suburban population like that in the Framingham Study, nearly one-fifth have blood pressure >160/95 mm Hg, while almost one-half have blood pressures >140/90 mm Hg. A higher prevalence has been found in the nonwhite population. The frequency increases with the age of the population. The number of hypertensive persons in the United States in 1983 was estimated to be 57.7 million—more than double the estimate made in 1960 to 1962.

Braunwald E: Heart Disease, 5th ed, pp 811–812. Philadelphia, WB Saunders, 1997

Braunwald E, Isselbacher KJ, Fauci AS et al: Harrison's Principles of Internal Medicine, 14th ed, pp 1380. New York, McGraw-Hill, 1998

A.3. What is the general classification of hypertension? Enumerate the causes of each type of hypertension.

The classification is outlined in Table 14-2.

Systolic and Diastolic Hypertension

- Essential hypertension
  Unknown etiology
- Renal
  Acute and chronic glomerulonephritis, chronic pyelonephritis, polycystic kidney, hydronephrosis, renovascular stenosis, renin-producing tumors, primary sodium retention
- Endocrine
  Adrenal: Cushing's syndrome, primary aldosteronism, congenital adrenal hyperplasia, pheochromocytoma, acromegaly, hypothyroidism, carcinoid, oral contraceptives, corticosteroids

Table 14-2.   Classification of Hypertension

SYSTOLIC AND DIASTOLIC HYPERTENSION
• Essential
• Renal
• Endocrine
• Neurogenic
• Miscellaneous
SYSTOLIC HYPERTENSION WITH WIDE PULSE PRESSURE
• Increased cardiac output
• Rigidity of aorta

- Neurogenic
    Psychogenic, increased intracranial pressure, spinal cord section, familial dysau-
    tonomia, lead poisoning, Guillain-Barré syndrome, sleep apnea
- Miscellaneous
    Coactation of aorta, increased intravascular volume, pregnancy-induced hyper-
    tension, polyarteritis nodosa, acute porphyria, hypercalcemia

Systolic Hypertension with Wide Pulse Pressure
- Arteriosclerosis, rigidity of aorta
- Increased cardiac output
    Arteriovenous fistula, thyrotoxicosis, patent ductus arteriosus, Beriberi heart,
    fever, aortic valvular insufficiency

Braunwald E: Heart Disease, 5th ed, p 811. Philadelphia, WB Saunders, 1997

Braunwald E, Isselbacher KJ, Fauci AS et al: Harrison's Principles of Internal Medicine, 14th ed,
p 1380. New York, McGraw-Hill, 1998

A.4. What is the pathophysiology of essential hypertension?

The underlying mechanism of essential hypertension is unknown. A variety of abnormalities including heredity, fetal undernutrition, abnormal sympathetic nervous system (SNS) activity, cell membrane defects, renal retention of excess salt, microcirculatory alterations, vascular hypertrophy, and altered renin-angiotensin system
regulation are implicated. However, characteristic hemodynamic changes are present
as follows:

- Increased systemic vascular resistance (SVR) with normal cardiac output
- Markedly increased sympathetic response to stress such as endotracheal intubation
- A greater increase in blood pressure with vasoconstriction and a greater decrease
  in blood pressure with vasodilation due to the increased thickening of arterial wall
  and high ratio of wall thickness to internal diameter

The higher the level of blood pressure, the more likely that various cardiovascular
diseases will develop prematurely through acceleration of atherosclerosis. If untreated, about 50% of hypertensive patients die of coronary heart disease or congestive heart failure, about 33% of stroke, and 10% to 15% of renal failure.

Braunwald E: Heart Disease, 5th ed, pp 816–820. Philadelphia, WB Saunders, 1997

Domino KB: Perioperative hypertension. ASA Annual Refresher Course Lectures, no. 115, 1996

Braunwald E, Isselbacher KJ, Fauci AS et al: Harrison's Principles of Internal Medicine, 14th ed,
pp 1380–1382. New York, McGraw-Hill, 1998

A.5. Are hypertensive patients at an increased risk for perioperative cardiac morbidity?

Hypertensive patients are at increased risk for coronary artery disease, silent myocardial ischemia, congestive heart failure, and stroke. However, whether preoperative
hypertension is predictive of perioperative major cardiac morbidity remains controversial. Some investigators have shown that patients with untreated, poorly controlled, or labile preoperative hypertension are at increased risk for perioperative
blood pressure lability, dysrhythmias, myocardial ischemia, and transient neurologic
complications. Some suggested that preoperative hypertension predicted perioperative myocardial infarction. However, Goldman et al demonstrated that mild-to-
moderate hypertension did not increase the risk of major morbid events. Rather,

preoperative hypertension may predict several intermediates of outcome, such as blood pressure lability and myocardial ischemia. The controversy may be due to the wide variability in the hypertensive population. Hypertension may affect perioperative morbidity through the extent of end-organ damage and not the manifestation of the disease itself. Left ventricular hypertrophy, which signifies long-standing poorly controlled hypertension, can increase the risk of myocardial ischemia from imbalances of myocardial oxygen supply and demand regardless of the presence or absence of coronary artery disease.

Allman KG, Muir A, Howell SJ et al: Resistant hypertension and preoperative silent myocardial ischaemia in surgical patients. Br J Anaesth 73:574–578, 1994

Foëx P, Prys-Roberts C: Anaesthesia and the hypertensive patient. Br J Anaesth 46:575, 1974

Goldman L: Cardiac risk in noncardiac surgery: An update. Anesth Analg 80:810–820, 1995

Goldman L, Caldera DL: Risks of general anesthesia and elective operation in the hypertensive patient. Anesthesiology 50:285–292, 1979

Mangano DT: Perioperative cardiac morbidity. Anesthesiology 72:153–184, 1990

Hollenberg M, Mangano DT, Browner WS et al: Predictors of postoperative myocardial ischemia in patient undergoing noncardiac surgery. JAMA 268:205–209, 1992

A.6. Are hypertensive patients at increased risk for perioperative cerebral and renal complications? Why?

Hypertensive patients are at increased risk for perioperative cerebrovascular accidents and acute renal failure. Most anesthetic agents produce a dose-related depression of myocardial contractility with a fall in cardiac output and a decreased blood flow to brain and kidneys. Since autoregulation may be impaired in these patients, there is a greater susceptibility of the brain and kidney to sudden changes in pressure. In hypertensive patients, autoregulation of cerebral blood flow is reset to a higher range than normal, and although it protects the brain against sudden increases in pressure, it makes it more vulnerable to hypotension. Thus, when blood pressure is lowered acutely, hypertensive patients will show signs of cerebral ischemia at a higher level of blood pressure than normotensive patients.

Finnerty FA, Witkin L, Fazekas JF: Cerebral hemodynamics during cerebral ischemia induced by acute hypotension. J Clin Invest 34:1227, 1955

Goldman L, Caldera DL: Risks of general anesthesia and elective operation in the hypertensive patient. Anesthesiology 50:285, 1979

Matthews DM, Miller ED: Mechanism and treatment of perioperative hypertension. ASA Refresher Courses in Anesthesiology 18:237–250, 1990

Strangaard S, Olsen J, Skinhof E et al: Autoregulation of brain circulation in severe arterial hypertension. Br Med J 1:507, 1973

A.7. Would you employ a controlled hypotensive technique for hypertensive patients? How much would you safely lower the blood pressure?

Uncontrolled or untreated severe hypertension is a contraindication to controlled hypotension. However, controlled hypotension may be used with caution in treated hypertensive patients. Since cerebral autoregulation is shifted to the right with chronic hypertension, the lower limit of controlled hypotension should be higher for hypertensive patients. However, with long-term treatment, the autoregulation curve shifts leftward to approach that in normals. Strangaard found that the lower limit of autoregulation was 113 mm Hg in severe untreated or uncontrolled hypertensives; 96 mm Hg in formerly severe, now-treated hypertensives; and 73 mm Hg in normotensive patients. The lowest level of mean blood pressure tolerated without symptoms of hypoperfusion was 65 mm Hg in severe hypertensives, 53 mm Hg in treated hypertensives, and 43 mm Hg in normal patients. However, while the autoregulation may shift towards normal with treatment, in many patients the autoregulation did not shift towards normal even after 12 months of treatment. Since we can not measure our patients' autoregulation, a useful clinical guide is that a 25% decrease in mean arterial pressure (MAP) reaches the lower limit of autoregulation and a 55% decrease in MAP reaches symptomatic cerebral hypoperfusion. Another suggested rule is that the systolic pressure of controlled hypotension should not be lower than the diastolic pressure of the patient's usual pressure.

Domino KB: Perioperative hypertension. ASA Annual Refresher Course Lectures, no. 115, 1996

Lindop MJ: Complications and morbidity of controlled hypotension. Br J Anaesth 47:799, 1975

Strangaard S: Autoregulation of cerebral blood flow in hypertension patients. Circulation 53:720–727, 1976

A.8. What is the mechanism of action of antihypertensive drugs?

Antihypertensive drugs are categorized by their mechanism of action as follows:

Diuretics
They include thiazides (e.g., hydrochlorothiazide), loop diuretics (e.g., furosemide, ethacrynic acid), and potassium-sparing agents (e.g., spironolactone, triamterene). All diuretics initially lower the BP by increasing urinary sodium excretion and by reducing plasma volume, extracellular fluid volume, and cardiac output. Within 6 to 8 weeks the cardiac output returned to normal. The lowered BP is related to a fall in peripheral resistance. Diuretics may cause hypokalemia, hypomagnesemia, hyperuricemia, hypercalcemia, and hyperglycemia.

Antiadrenergic Agents
- Centrally acting drugs—clonidine, methyldopa, guanfacine, and guanabenz.
  These drugs and their metabolites are primarily alpha-2 receptor agonists. Stimulation of alpha-2 receptors in the vasomotor centers of the brain reduces sympathetic outflow.
- Peripherally acting drugs—reserpine, guanethidine, guanadrel, and bethanidine.
  These drugs inhibit the release of norepinephrine from peripheral adrenergic neurons, each in a different manner.
  - Alpha-receptor blockers
    - Alpha-1 and alpha-2 receptors— phenoxybenzamine (Dibenzyline), phentolamine (Regitine)
    - Alpha-1 receptor—prazosin (Minipress), doxazosin (Cardura)
      By blocking alpha-mediated vasoconstriction, these drugs induce a fall in peripheral resistance with both arteriolar and venous dilation.
  - Beta-receptor blockers—atenolol (Tenormin), metoprolol (Lopressor), nadol (Corgard), pindolol (Visken), propranolol (Inderal), esmolol (Brevibloc).
    These drugs lower the blood pressure by decreasing heart rate, contractility, cardiac output, and renin levels.

Table 14-3. Cardiovascular Effects of Calcium Channel Blockers

	VERAPAMIL	DILTIAZEM	NIFEDIPINE	NICARDIPINE
Heart rate	↓	↓	↑−	↑−
Nodal conduction	↓↓	↓	↓−	−−
Myocardial depression	↑↑	↑	−−	−−
Vasodilation	↑	↑	↑↑	↑↑

Note: ↑, increase; ↓, decrease; −, no change.

- Alpha- and beta-receptor blockers—labetalol (Trandate)

Direct Vasodilators

They include hydralazine, diazoxide, minoxidil, nitroprusside, and nitroglycerin. These drugs directly relax the smooth muscle of resistance and capacitance vessels to different degrees.

Calcium Channel Blockers

The cardiovascular effects of calcium antagonists are listed in Table 14-3. These drugs decrease blood pressure mainly by peripheral vasodilation. Renin and aldosterone secretion may be reduced as well.

Angiotensin-Converting Enzyme (ACE) Inhibitors

They include captopril, enalapril, lisinopril, quinapril, and ramipril. The renin-angiotensin system may be inhibited in four ways as shown in Figure 14-1. These drugs inhibit the conversion of the inactive decapeptide angiotensin I to the active octapeptide angiotensin II. Lower levels of angiotensin II may decrease blood pressure by reducing angiotensin II-induced vasoconstriction, and by decreasing aldosterone synthesis. ACE inhibitors also retard the degradation of a potent vasodilator (bradykinin), alter prostaglandin production (most notably with captopril), and can modify the activity of the adrenergic nervous system.

Barash PG, Cullen BF, Stoelting RK (eds): Clinical Anesthesia, 3rd ed, pp 299–301. Philadelphia, Lippincott-Raven, 1997

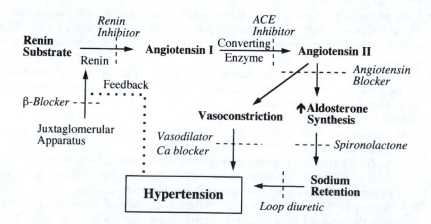

Figure 14-1. The renin-angiotensin system and the mechanism of action of antihypertensive drugs.

Braunwald E: Heart Disease, 5th ed, pp 846–856. Philadelphia, WB Saunders, 1997

Braunwald E, Isselbacher KJ, Fauci AS et al: Harrison's Principles of Internal Medicine, 14th ed, pp 1386–1390. New York, McGraw-Hill, 1998

A.9. Does the choice of antihypertensive therapy influence hemodynamic responses to induction, laryngoscopy, and intubation?

The pressor responses to induction, laryngoscopy, and intubation differ little whether patients with mild to moderate hypertension receive a beta-blocker, a calcium channel blocker, an ACE inhibitor, or a diuretic. Even changes of a similar magnitude are also observed in untreated hypertensive patients.

Sear JW, Jewkes C, Teller JC, Foëx P: Does the choice of antihypertensive therapy influence haemodynamic responses to induction, laryngoscopy and intubation? Br J Anaesth 73:303–308, 1994

A.10. Does chronic angiotensin-converting enzyme inhibition influence anesthetic induction?

Coriat et al reported that in hypertensive patients chronically treated with ACE inhibitors, therapy until the day of surgery is a major factor influencing blood pressure responsiveness to anesthetic induction for vascular surgery. If enalapril, a long-acting ACE inhibitor, treatment is continued, a very low plasma-converting enzyme activity will be observed and an exaggerated hypotensive response may occur at induction. If captopril, a short-acting ACE inhibitor, treatment is continued, the magnitude of the decrease in blood pressure in response to induction, although lower than with enalapril, is enhanced compared with that noted in patients in whom captopril had been stopped. All of the hypotensive episodes in patients who received ACE inhibitors until the day of surgery were easily corrected by ephedrine infusion. The temporary withdrawal of these two ACE inhibitors attenuated the hypotensive response to induction but did not lead to an abnormal blood pressure response to induction and intubation. However, recently Ryckwaert et al reported that ACE inhibitor treatment in patients with infarction-induced myocardial dysfunction does not increase the incidence of severe hypotension after induction of anesthesia.

Coriat P, Richter C, Douraki T et al: Influence of chronic angiotensin-converting enzyme inhibition on anesthetic induction. Anesthesiology 81:299–307, 1994

Ryckwaert F, Colson P: Hemodynamic effects of anesthesia in patients with ischemic heart failure chronically treated with angiotensin-converting enzyme inhibitors. Anesth Analg 84:945–949, 1997

B. Preoperative Evaluation and Preparation

B.1. How would you evaluate this patient preoperatively?

In addition to the routine systemic preoperative physical and history, special attention should be paid to the following: etiology and severity of hypertension, current therapy, and the end-organ damage by chronic hypertension.

The underlying cause of hypertension should be clear. Surgical mortality is relatively high in patients with renovascular hypertension. Moreover, failure to diagnose a pheochromocytoma preoperatively may prove fatal, because anesthetic agents are well known to precipitate a crisis in such patients. Meanwhile, the severity of hypertension alters anesthetic risk.

Antihypertensive drugs have different anesthetic implications. Diuretics frequently cause chronic hypokalemia and hypomagnesemia, which may increase the risk of arrhythmia. Therefore, serum electrolytes should be checked preoperatively.

The presence of target-organ damage in the brain, heart, and kidney signifies long-standing poorly controlled hypertension.

For cardiac evaluation, ECG and chest x-ray film serve as minimal test. The echocardiogram will be helpful. Left ventricular hypertrophy (LVH) can increase the risk of perioperative myocardial ischemia from imbalances of myocardial oxygen supply and demand regardless of the presence or absence of coronary artery disease. Some authorities believe that hypertensive patients without evidence of LVH or other risk factors are at a lower perioperative cardiac risk and do not require further evaluation for most operations. Patients with severe hypertension are also at increased risk for congestive heart failure and pulmonary edema.

For renal evaluation, urinalysis, serum creatinine, and blood urea nitrogen should be measured to define the presence and extent of renal parenchymal disease. If chronic renal failure exists, hyperkalemia and elevated plasma volume should be considered.

For cerebrovascular evaluation, a history of cerebrovascular accidents (CVA) and transient ischemia attacks (TIA), and the presence of hypertensive retinopathy should be looked for.

Barash PG, Cullen BF, Stoelting RK (eds): Clinical Anesthesia, 3rd ed, p 447. Philadelphia, Lippincott-Raven, 1997

Domino KB: Perioperative hypertension. ASA Annual Refresher Course Lectures, No. 115, 1996

Fleisher LA, Barash PH: Preoperative cardiac evaluation for noncardiac surgery. Anesth Analg 74:586–598, 1992

Tubau JF, Szlachcic J, Meyer L et al: Left ventricular hypertrophy increases the risk of postoperative myocardial ischemia (abstract). Circulation 82:111–163, 1990

Yurenev AP, Dequattro V, Devereux RB: Hypertensive heart disease: Relationship of silent ischemia to coronary artery disease and left ventricular hypertrophy. Am Heart J 120:928–933, 1990

B.2. Would you postpone the surgery? Why? What blood pressure would you like the patient to achieve before surgery?

Yes. I would postpone the elective surgery because the blood pressure was 230/120 mm Hg. In general, elective surgery should be delayed for patients with severe hypertension (diastolic BP >115 mm Hg) or with severe isolated systolic hypertension (systolic BP >200 mm Hg) until the blood pressure is below 180/110 mm Hg. If time permits, the blood pressure should be lowered over several weeks to 140/90 mm Hg. Acute control within several hours is inadvisable prior to elective surgery.

In moderate hypertensive patients with severe end-organ involvement, preoperative BP should be normalized as much as possible. While in asymptomatic patients with mild to moderate hypertension (diastolic BP <110 mm Hg), elective surgery may proceed without increased cardiovascular risks.

Domino KB: Perioperative hypertension. ASA Annual Refresher Course Lectures, No.115, 1996

Fleisher LA, Barash PH: Preoperative cardiac evaluation for noncardiac surgery. Anesth Analg 74:586–598, 1992

B.3. Should all or any of the chronic medications be discontinued prior to the operation?

Current opinion generally favors continuation of antihypertensive medications, especially beta-blockers, up to the time of surgery. There is concern that acute withdrawal of these medications may precipitate ischemic myocardial events. Since beta-blockade does not impair the hemodynamic response to hemorrhage and does not adversely affect responses to hypoxia, the medications should be continued. The withdrawal syndrome is characterized by an enhanced sensitivity to sympathetic stimulation and has been attributed to various factors, including sympathetic overactivity and increased triiodothyronine levels, but most probably it is a result of increased beta-receptor density.

The safety of beta-blockers and their benefits (prevention of hypertensive responses, dysrhythmias, and myocardial ischemia) have been long established. Similarly, treatment with calcium channel blockers, ACE inhibitors, and diuretics can be maintained. Indeed, the responses to induction of anesthesia, laryngoscopy, and intubation differ little whether patients receive a beta-blocker, a calcium channel blocker, an ACE inhibitor, or a diuretic. However, Coriat reported that maintenance of ACE inhibitor therapy until the day of surgery might increase the probability of hypotension at induction and the hypotensive episodes were easily corrected by ephedrine infusion.

Barash PG, Cullen BF, Stoelting RK (eds): Clinical Anesthesia, 3rd ed, pp 1139–1140. Philadelphia, Lippincott-Raven, 1997

Coriat P, Richters C, Douraki T et al: Influence of chronic angiotensin-converting enzyme inhibition on anesthetic induction. Anesthesiology 81:299–307, 1994

Mangano DT (ed): Preoperative cardiac assessment, pp 141–163. Philadelphia, JB Lippincott, 1990

Prichard BWC et al: The syndrome associated with the withdrawal of beta-adrenergic receptor blocking drugs. Br J Clin Pharm 13:337, 1982

Sear JW, Jewkes C, Tellez JC, Foëx P: Does the choice of antihypertensive therapy influence haemodynamic responses to induction, laryngoscopy and intubation? Br J Anaesth 73:303–308, 1994

B.4. Should hypokalemia be treated prior to anesthesia? Why?

Hypokalemia is a frequent finding in hypertensive patients treated with the diuretic thiazides. It is important to maintain normal electrolyte balance in patients with heart or coronary artery disease. A low value of potassium (3.0 to 3.5 mEq/liter) in these patients may cause arrhythmias, increase sensitivity to digitalis, and depress neuromuscular function. In patients without risk of cardiac complications of surgery and anesthesia, this modest reduction (3.0 to 3.5 mEq/liter) should not prompt postponement of surgery or immediate potassium replacement. Patients with more severe potassium depletion (2.9 mEq/liter or lower) should be treated. For those patients, at least 1 week prior to surgery supplemental potassium should be given if renal function is not impaired. In surgical emergencies, potassium may be given at a rate not to exceed 0.5 mEq/kg of body weight per hour. Administration should be stopped during surgery and restarted postoperatively, depending on serial potassium determinations. It should be noted that Vitez et al concluded that chronic hypokalemia per se is not associated with a higher incidence of intraoperative arrhythmia.

Barash PG, Cullen BF, Stoelting RK (eds): Clinical Anesthesia, 3rd ed, pp 176–178. Philadelphia, Lippincott-Raven, 1997

McGovern B: Editorial: Hypokalemia and cardiac arrhythmias. Anesthesiology 63:127, 1985

Schwartz SI, Shires GT, Spencer FC (eds): Principles of Surgery, 6th ed, pp 71–72. New York, McGraw-Hill, 1994

Vitez TS, Soper LE, Wong KC et al: Chronic hypokalemia and intraoperative dysrhythmias. Anesthesiology 63:130–133, 1985

B.5. Should hypomagnesemia be treated prior to anesthesia? Why?

The normal level of magnesium is between 1.5 and 2.5 mEq/liter. Magnesium ion is essential for the proper function of most enzyme systems. Depletion is characterized by neuromuscular and central nervous system hyperexcitability. These signs are similar to those of calcium deficiency. Replacement should be done only in cases of severe depletion. Magnesium should not be given to the oliguric patient and should be given very carefully to patients with renal insufficiency. Small intravenous doses should be used, with careful observation for toxicity (lethargy, weakness, and loss of deep tendon reflexes).

Barash PG, Cullen BF, Stoelting RK (eds): Clinical Anesthesia, 3rd ed, pp 183–184. Philadelphia, Lippincott-Raven, 1997

Schwartz SI, Shires GT, Spencer FC (eds): Principles of Surgery, 6th ed, pp 73–74. New York, McGraw-Hill, 1994

B.6. Does an asymptomatic carotid bruit increase the risk in these patients?

Yes. The incidence of stroke is increased in such patients, although the stroke may not be thrombotic or related to the carotid artery in which the bruit was heard. Bruits are general predictors of vascular disease and may be predictors of perioperative strokes.

Wolf P, Kannel WB, Sorlie P et al: Asymptomatic carotid bruit and the risk of stroke: The Framingham Study. JAMA 245:1442, 1981

Yatsu FM, Hart RG: Asymptomatic carotid bruit and stenosis: A reappraisal. Curr Concepts Cerebrovascular Disease 17:21, 1982

B.7. The surgery was postponed for 2 weeks. The patient has been on propranolol, captopril, hydrochlorothiazide, and KCl. His blood pressure was 160/95 mm Hg and potassium 4.0 mEq/liter. How would you premedicate this patient?

Since most hypertensive patients still have elevated blood pressures in spite of treatment, the anesthesiologist should determine the anxiety level of the patient. With this knowledge, the premedication with diazepam, lorazepam, or midazolam can be regulated to have the patient arrive in the operating room sedated. This will help to prevent a starting blood pressure well above the optimal level. Glycopyrrolate is the preferred anticholinergic because it produces less tachycardia than atropine. All the antihypertensive medications are continued up to the day of surgery with the possible exception of ACE inhibitors, which may be discontinued the evening before surgery. Coriat reported that the incidence of induction-induced hypotension was significantly less when enalapril or captopril has been discontinued. If ACE inhibitors are maintained until the day of surgery, phenylephrine or ephedrine should be ready to treat the possible induction-induced hypotension.

Coriat P, Richters C, Douraki T et al: Influence of chronic angiotensin-converting enzyme inhibition on anesthetic induction. Anesthesiology 81:299–307, 1994

B.8. If the patient is an untreated hypertensive patient with blood pressure 170/100 mm Hg, would you pretreat the patient preoperatively with an antihypertensive agent?

Yes. The preoperative administration of clonidine, beta-blockers, or ACE inhibitors has been advocated to reduce the intraoperative hemodynamic lability and myocardial ischemia in hypertensive patients. Clonidine, a central alpha-2 agonist, decreases sympathetic outflow and reduces plasma catecholamines, aldosterone levels and renin activity. A single dose of clonidine, 5 μg/kg orally, 2 hours prior to surgery significantly decreases anesthetic requirements and hemodynamic lability in patients with mild to moderate hypertension. However, preoperative clonidine did not decrease blood pressure lability during aortic operation.

A single small oral dose of a beta-adrenergic blocking agent such as labetalol, atenolol, or oxyprenolol given preoperatively to untreated, asymptomatic, mildly hypertensive patients effectively attenuated tachycardia with tracheal intubation and emergence. The incidence of myocardial ischemia was reduced from 28% in the control group to 2% in the beta-blocker groups. An oral-dose ACE inhibitor such as enalapril given preoperatively also attenuates the hemodynamic responses to intubation and surgical stimulation.

Engelman E et al: Effects of clonidine on anesthetic drug requirements and hemodynamic response during aortic surgery. Anesthesiology 71:178–187, 1989

Ghignone M et al: Anesthesia and hypertension: The effect of clonidine on perioperative hemodynamics and isoflurane requirements. Anesthesiology 67:3–10, 1987

Stone JG et al: Myocardial ischemia in untreated hypertensive patients: Effect of a single small oral dose of a beta-adrenergic blocking agent. Anesthesiology 68:495–500, 1988

Yeates AP: Anaesthesia and angiotensin-converting enzyme inhibitors. Anaesthesia 43:935–939, 1988

C. Intraoperative Management

C.1. How would you monitor this patient?

- ECG—Simultaneous leads V_5 and II, multiple lead ST analysis, if possible, are essential because hypertensive patients are at increased risk for myocardial ischemia regardless of the presence or absence of coronary disease.
- Blood pressure—A continuous monitoring of blood pressure is essential because of lability of blood pressure in these patients. Direct intraarterial measurement of blood pressure permits beat to beat observation. However, noninvasive automatic sphygmomanometric techniques are usually sufficient.
- Swan-Ganz catheter—Only for those hypertensive patients with a history of congestive heart failure or a recent myocardial infarction, a Swan-Ganz catheter may be extremely helpful in managing fluid replacement and monitoring ventricular function.
- Pulse oximeter—This should be used to monitor peripheral blood flow and oxygenation.
- End-tidal CO_2 analyzer—This monitor will help maintain normocarbia.
- Temperature

C.2. What are the anesthetic goals for hypertensive patients?

The anesthetic goal is to minimize wide lability of blood pressure in response to anesthetic and surgical stimuli to prevent:

- Myocardial ischemia from either hypertension or, less commonly, hypotension
- Cerebral hypoperfusion from hypotension
- Cerebral hemorrhage and hypertensive encephalopathy due to hypertension
- Renal failure from renal hypoperfusion

Careful control of the hemodynamic responses to noxious stimuli such as endotracheal intubation, surgical incision and manipulation, and emergence from anesthesia is essential in the hypertensive patient.

Thomas S (ed): Manual of Cardiac Anesthesia, p 226. New York, Churchill Livingstone, 1984

C.3. How would you induce anesthesia for the hypertensive patient?

Before induction of anesthesia, I would like to hydrate the patient with at least 200 ml of lactated Ringer's solution. While the patient is being preoxygenated, fentanyl, 7 to 8 μg/kg, is given slowly to achieve drowsiness. Then, either thiopental in 50-mg increments or midazolam in 1-mg increments is titrated to produce unconsciousness, followed by succinylcholine, 1-mg/kg, to facilitate tracheal intubation.

All anesthetic agents are acceptable with the possible exception of ketamine, which may produce significant hypertension and tachycardia. However, deeper anesthesia with potent inhalation agents to attenuate tachycardia and hypertension is not recommended because of higher incidence of hypotension due to both vasodilation and cardiac depression.

Martin DE, Rosenberg H, Aukburg SJ et al: Low-dose fentanyl blunts circulatory responses to tracheal intubation. Anesth Analg 61:680, 1982

C.4. How does tracheal intubation produce hypertension?

Translaryngeal intubation of the trachea stimulates laryngeal and tracheal receptors, resulting in marked increase in the elaboration of sympathomimetic amines. This sympathetic stimulation results in tachycardia and a rise in blood pressure. In normotensive patients, this rise is approximately 20 to 25 mm Hg; it is much greater in hypertensive patients. This increase in blood pressure results from vasoconstriction, owing to unopposed alpha stimulation in hypertensive patients taking beta-blocking drugs.

Prys-Roberts C, Greene LT, Meloche R et al: Studies of anaesthesia in relation to hypertension. II: Haemodynamic consequences of induction and endotracheal intubation. Br J Anaesth 43:531, 1971

C.5. What happens to the left ventricular ejection fraction during and immediately following intubation?

During and immediately following intubation associated with tachycardia and hypertension, there is a decrease in the left ventricular ejection fraction. This is particularly marked in patients with coronary artery disease.

Giles RW, Berger JH, Barash PG et al: Continuous monitoring of left ventricular performance with the computerized nuclear probe during laryngoscopy and intubation before coronary artery bypass surgery. Am J Cardiol 50:735, 1982

C.6. What other measures can prevent hypertension and tachycardia at the time of intubation?

The rise in blood pressure and heart rate occurs about 14 seconds after the start of laryngoscopy and becomes maximal after 30 to 45 seconds of direct laryngoscopy. If possible, laryngoscopy time should be 15 seconds or less to minimize blood pressure elevation. Simultaneous administration of fentanyl 7 to 8 μg/kg with the induction dose of thiopental can blunt the cardiovascular response to tracheal intubation. Other measures are described as follows:

- Lidocaine 1.5 mg/kg is given 2 minutes prior to intubation
- Sodium nitroprusside 1 to 2 μg/kg has been recommended
- Esmolol, up to 2 mg/kg, appears to be especially effective in providing consistent and reliable protection against hypertension and tachycardia with intubation. It is easy to titrate and does not exacerbate postintubation hypotension because of its short duration of action.
- Labetalol 0.15 to 0.45 mg/kg is comparable to esmolol 1.5 to 4.5 mg/kg in attenuating hemodynamic effects. However, the half-lives of intravenous esmolol and labetalol are 9 minutes and 5 hours, respectively.
- Diltiazem, 0.1 or 0.2 mg/kg, given 2 minutes before extubation was of value in attenuating the cardiovascular responses occurring in association with tracheal extubation and emergence of anesthesia. This alleviative effect of diltiazem was equal or superior to that of intravenous lidocaine, 1 mg/kg.
- Verapamil, 0.1 mg/kg, given 2 minutes before tracheal extubation is a more effective prophylactic for attenuating the cardiovascular responses associated with extubation than is diltiazem, 0.2 mg/kg.

It is important to remember that all the above mentioned dosages are used with a single agent only. If a combination of different agents or anesthetics is used, dosages should be decreased accordingly. Otherwise, severe hypotension may ensue.

Barash PG, Cullen BF, Stoelting RK (eds): Clinical Anesthesia, 3rd ed, pp 587, 855. Philadelphia, Lippincott-Raven, 1997

Cucchiara RF et al: Evaluation of esmolol in controlling increases in heart rate and blood pressure during endotracheal intubation in patients undergoing carotid endarterectomy. Anesthesiology 65:528–531, 1986

Gold MI et al: Use of esmolol during anesthesia to treat tachycardia and hypertension. Anesth Analg 68:101–104, 1989

Helfman SM et al: Which drug prevents tachycardia and hypertension associated with tracheal intubation: Lidocaine, fentanyl, or esmolol? Anesth Analg 72:482–486, 1991

Kapnoudhis P, Vaghadia H, Jenkins LC et al: Esmolol versus fentanyl for preventing haemodynamic response to intubation in cardiovascular disease. Can J Anaesth 37:S145, 1990

Martin DE, Rosenberg H, Aukburg SJ et al: Low-dose fentanyl blunts circulatory responses to tracheal intubation. Anesth Analg 61:680, 1982

Mikawa K, Nishina K, Maekawa N et al: Attenuation of cardiovascular responses to tracheal extubation: Verapamil versus diltiazem. Anesth Analg 82:1205–1210, 1996

Nishina K et al: Attenuation of cardiovascular responses to tracheal extubation with diltiazem. Anesth Analg 80:1217–1222, 1995

Stoelting RK: Attenuation of blood pressure response to laryngoscopy and tracheal intubation with sodium nitroprusside. Anesth Analg 58:116, 1979

Stoelting RK: Blood pressure and heart rate changes during short-duration laryngoscopy for tracheal intubation: Influence of viscous or intravenous lidocaine. Anesth Analg 57:197, 1978

C.7. After induction and intubation, the blood pressure went down to 70/40 mm Hg. What would you do?

Hypotension after induction of anesthesia is usually due to combination of vasodilation, hypovolemia, and cardiac depression. Vasodilation can be caused by inducing agents such as thiopental, diazepam, or midazolam; moderate to high doses of narcotics; and potent inhalation agents. Hypertensive patients are in relative hypovolemia due to chronic vasoconstriction and/or diuretic therapy. Preoperative bowel preparation and nothing by mouth further contribute to hypovolemia. Barbiturates, benzodiazepines, and inhalation agents can cause a mild to moderate degree of cardiac depression.

Hypotension after induction of anesthesia usually can be easily corrected by volume replacement and simultaneous titration of vasopressors such as ephedrine 5 to 10 mg or phenylephrine in 0.1-mg increments.

Coriat P, Richters C, Douraki T et al: Influence of chronic angiotensin-converting enzyme inhibition on anesthetic induction. Anesthesiology 81:299–307, 1994

C.8. What is your choice of agents for maintenance of anesthesia? Why?

I would use nitrous oxide and low to moderate doses of fentanyl and isoflurane for maintenance of anesthesia. No particular anesthetic technique or specific drug combinations have been demonstrated to be superior to others in hypertensive patients. Potent inhalation anesthetics or narcotics should be titrated to the desired level of central nervous system depression while the blood pressure is monitored continuously.

Narcotics and nitrous oxide provide an anesthetic with less overall lability of blood pressure, but commonly intraoperative hypertension is difficult to control by moderate doses of narcotics. High doses of narcotics are not suitable for early extubation.

Potent inhalation agents provide greater control of hypertension but seem to produce less stability. Isoflurane possesses the advantage of more peripheral vasodilation and less cardiac depression. Enflurane may be least useful in patients receiving beta-blockers because of the potential for greater cardiac depression than is observed with halothane or isoflurane. The combination of nitrous oxide and low to moderate doses of narcotics and potent inhalation agents may provide the most stable intraoperative course.

Kaplan JA (ed): Cardiac Anesthesia, 3rd ed, pp 167–168. Philadelphia, WB Saunders, 1993

C.9. How would you manage fluid therapy for hypertensive patients?

Patients with essential hypertension are usually hypovolemic because of vasoconstriction and diuretic therapy. Hydration of the hypertensive patient should be started prior to induction of anesthesia to minimize the roller-coasters often seen with hypertension. However, overhydration should be avoided because it may contribute to postoperative hypertension when the vasodilating effects of anesthetics are gone. Therefore, careful estimation of fluid intake and output is essential. Foley catheter and central venous pressure monitor are indicated for major surgery with extensive fluid exchange.

Domino KB: Perioperative hypertension. ASA Annual Refresher Course Lectures, No. 115, 1996

C.10. During the surgery, blood pressure went up to 220/120 mm Hg. How would you treat the hypertension?

Intraoperative control of hypertension is outlined in Table 14-4. Severe hypertension that occurs during a surgical procedure is most frequently due to inadequate anesthesia. Inadequate blockade of sensory input from the surgical procedure stimulates the elaboration of sympathomimetic amines, resulting in hypertension and tachycardia. If a potent inhalation anesthetic is being used, the level of anesthesia should be deepened by increasing the inspired concentration of the anesthetic. A narcotic may not control the rise in blood pressure, and it may be necessary to switch to a potent inhalation anesthetic.

Droperidol, 2.5-mg increments up to 10 mg, may be titrated to control hypertension since it not only deepens anesthesia but also dilates peripheral vessels from its alpha-blocking effect.

Hydralazine, 5-mg increments, may be titrated to decrease blood pressure safely with little chance of excessive reduction. The onset of action is in 10 to 15 minutes with 1 to 2 hours duration.

Phentolamine, 5-mg increments, may be titrated to control hypertension, especially for patients with pheochromocytoma.

Labetalol, 5- to 10-mg increments, is very useful in controlling hypertension and tachycardia.

Rarely, continuous infusion of *trimethaphan*, a ganglionic blocker, or *nitroprusside*, 1 to 2 μg/kg/min, a direct arteriolar vasodilator, is needed to control hypertension during anesthesia. It is necessary to monitor blood pressure by an intraarterial catheter.

Table 14-4. Inraoperative Control of Hypertension

Anesthetics
    Narcotics, inhalation agents, butorphanol, lidocaine
Antihypertensives
    Adrenergic Blockers
        Alpha-blocker: Phentolamine
        Beta-blocker: Propranolol, Metoprolol
        Alpha- and beta-blocker: Labetalol
    Calcium Channel Blockers
        Diltiazem, nicardipine, verapamil
    ACE Inhibitors
        Enalapril
    Direct Vasodilators
        Hydralazine, nitroglycerin, nitroprusside

Lake CL: Cardiovascular Anesthesia, p 138. New York, Springer-Verlag, 1985

Matthews DM, Miller ED: Mechanism and treatment of perioperative hypertension. ASA Refresher Courses in Anesthesiology 18:237–250, 1990

C.11. What could you do to prevent hypertension during extubation and emergence?

Intraoperative hypertension can be controlled either by adequate anesthesia with moderate to high doses of narcotics or inhalation agents, or by antihypertensive agents listed in question A.8. It is logical to use anesthetic agents to prevent hypertension during induction and intubation and to use antihypertensive agents during extubation and emergence, since the patient has to be awakened at the end of surgery. The alternative measures listed in question C.7 may be applied to prevent hypertension. I prefer to give lower doses of preventive medications such as 1 mg/kg of lidocaine or esmolol, or 0.1 mg/kg of labetalol, diltiazem, or verapamil 2 minutes before extubation. If blood pressure goes over desired levels after extubation, additional doses may be titrated to control blood pressure.

Mikawa K, Nishina K, Maekawa N et al: Attenuation of cardiovascular responses to tracheal extubation: Verapamil versus diltiazem. Anesth Analg 82:1205–1210, 1996

Nishina K et al: Attenuation of cardiovascular responses to tracheal extubation with diltiazem. Anesth Analg 80:1217–1222, 1995

C.12. Would you consider regional anesthesia for this patient?

Certainly, regional anesthesia can avoid marked increases in sympathetic tone and hemodynamic changes that occur with intubation and extubation. Spinal or epidural anesthesia may be used for lower abdominal surgery. For cholecystectomy, higher levels of regional anesthesia are needed and may compromise respiratory function. Meanwhile, prolonged surgery can cause anxiety and irritability that may induce hypertension and tachycardia.

D. Postoperative Management

D.1. The patient developed hypertension BP 210/110 mm Hg in the postanesthesia care unit. What would you do?

The management of postoperative hypertension depends on the etiology of the hypertension, the clinical scenario, and the level of hypertension. First, the cause of hypertension should be determined and treated accordingly. Hypertension per se should also be treated by an antihypertensive agent. The causes of postoperative hypertension include pain, emergence excitement, hypoxemia, hypercarbia, reaction to endotracheal tube, full bladder, hypothermia, relative hypervolemia from intraoperative administration of excess fluid and chronic medication and withdrawal. The most common cause of postoperative hypertension is incisional pain. As the patient awakens, pain triggers an outpouring of catecholamines. The extreme lability of blood pressure in many hypertensive patients makes this rapid increase critical to control. Depending on the cause of hypertension, intravenous analgesics and antihypertensives or diuretics should be titrated to control hypertension. If both tachycardia and hypertension occurred postoperatively, calcium channel blockers such as verapamil, diltiazem or nicardipine, and beta-blocking agents such as propranolol, esmolol, labetalol or metoprolol are preferred agents.

Barash PG, Cullen BF, Stoelting RK (eds): Clinical Anesthesia, 3rd ed, pp 301–302, 1285. Philadelphia, Lippincott-Raven, 1997

Davis RF: Acute postoperative hypertension. ASA Refresher Courses in Anesthesiology 17:59–70, 1989

Gal TJ, Cooperman LH: Hypertension in the immediate postoperative period. Br J Anesth 47:70, 1975

15 Postoperative Hemorrhage with Cardiac Tamponade

Onofrio Patafio

A 54-year-old man underwent an uneventful triple coronary artery bypass surgery. Six hours postoperatively the combined drainage from both the mediastinal and pleural tubes was 1400 ml. His heart rate was 130/min; systemic blood pressure, 85/60 mm Hg; pulmonary artery pressure, 40/23; pulmonary artery wedge pressure, 22 mm Hg; central venous pressure, 21 mm Hg; and cardiac output, 2.4 liters/min. He was responsive to verbal commands.

A. Medical Disease and Differential Diagnosis

1. What is the differential diagnosis of postoperative hypotension?
2. What is cardiac tamponade?
3. How common is cardiac tamponade in cardiac surgery?
4. Enumerate the common etiologies of cardiac tamponade.
5. When does delayed cardiac tamponade develop?
6. What is the difference between acute and chronic cardiac tamponade?
7. What is regional cardiac tamponade?
8. What is pulsus paradoxus? Can positive ventilation affect the severity of cardiac tamponade?
9. How is excessive postoperative bleeding defined in cardiac surgery patients?
10. What is in the differential diagnosis of post–cardiopulmonary–bypass (CPB) bleeding?
11. How are platelets affected by cardiopulmonary bypass? What do platelet alpha-granules contain?
12. How does desmopressin aid hemostasis? What is aprotinin? What is iloprost?
13. What is the major arachidonic acid metabolite in platelets? How does aspirin inhibit platelet function?
14. What is fibrinolysis?
15. How does heparin prevent clot formation?
16. What is the mechanism of heparin antagonism by protamine?
17. What is "heparin rebound"?
18. Can heparin cause thrombocytopenia? Can protamine sulfate cause thrombocytopenia?
19. What do the following measure: prothrombin time, activated partial thromboplastin time, thrombin time, activated clotting time, bleeding time?
20. What is a thromboelastograph? What is the Sonoclot?
21. What are the electrocardiographic abnormalities associated with cardiac tamponade?
22. What roentgenography and echocardiogram findings are noted in cardiac tamponade?

B. Preoperative Evaluation and Preparation

1. How would you evaluate this patient's coagulation status?
2. What do fresh-frozen plasma and cryoprecipitate contain?

3. What are the indications for transfusing fresh-frozen plasma (FFP), platelet concentrate, and cryoprecipitate?
4. What are the complications associated with blood component transfusions?
5. What is the statistical incidence of exposure to HIV through blood transfusion?
6. Does the patient's temperature affect coagulation? Why are patients often cold after cardiopulmonary bypass?
7. In what situation might epsilon-aminocaproic acid improve hemostasis?
8. How would you assess the hemodynamic status of this patient?
9. How would you treat hypotension due to cardiac tamponade?
10. How would you prepare the patient for surgery?
11. What premedication would you prescribe for this patient?

C. Intraoperative Management

1. How would you monitor this patient during transport from the intensive care unit to the operating room? What emergency drugs would you bring with you?
2. What effect on contractility and systemic blood pressure in this patient would be expected from ketamine, thiopental, fentanyl, propofol, and diazepam?
3. How would you induce anesthesia in this patient? After anesthesia was induced, the systemic blood pressure fell to 55/30 mm Hg. What were likely causes of hypotension in this situation? How would you treat this hypotension?
4. Why does stroke volume change when the sternum is opened?
5. How would you manage hypertension following relief of the tamponade?
6. What complications may arise from this procedure?

D. Postoperative Management

1. How would you manage hypertension in the intensive care unit?

A. Medical Disease and Differential Diagnosis

A.1. What is the differential diagnosis of postoperative hypotension?

Hypotension can be due to reductions in preload, contractility, systemic vascular resistance, and heart rate. Blood pressure (BP) is a function of both cardiac output (CO) and systemic vascular resistance (SVR). This relationship may be represented as

$$BP = CO \times SVR. \qquad CO = HR \times SV, \text{ where } SV = \text{stroke volume}$$

therefore,

$$BP = HR \times SVR \times SV$$

The differential diagnosis of hypotension includes:
- Decreased preload—hypovolemia, cardiac tamponade
- Decreased contractility—myocardial ischemia, myocardial depression secondary to drugs, myocardial stunning
- Decreased afterload—drugs (nitroprusside, nitroglycerin). Allergic or anaphylactic reactions, excessive warming, septicemia.
- Heart rate and rhythm—nonsinus rhythms, bradycardia

A.2. What is cardiac tamponade?

Cardiac tamponade is characterized by a reduction in stroke volume and blood pressure due to increased intrapericardial pressure. When fluid accumulates in the pericardial sac, intrapericardial pressure increases and restricts atrial and ventricular filling. In the postoperative cardiac surgical patient, tamponade is usually limited to a region of the heart.

Fowler NO, Gabel M, Buncher CR: Cardiac tamponade: A comparison of right heart versus left heart compression. JACC 12:187, 1988

Kaplan JA (ed): Cardiac Anesthesia, 3rd ed, p 847. Philadelphia, WB Saunders, 1993

A.3. How common is cardiac tamponade in cardiac surgery?

The incidence of cardiac tamponade following cardiac surgery ranges from 1% to 5%, whereas pericardial effusions after cardiac surgery is quite common. Weitzman et al found by echocardiographic study that 103 of 122 consecutive patients had pericardial effusions. Effusions reach their maximum size on about the 10th postoperative day, generally regressing spontaneously after that time. Despite the common event of pericardial effusion from cardiac surgery, tamponade develops in only about 1% of patients with pericardial fluid.

D'Cruz IA, Overton DH, Pai GH: Pericardial complications of cardiac surgery: Emphasis on the diagnostic role of echocardiography. J Card Surg 7:257–268, 1992

Kirklin JK, Barratt-Boyes BG (eds): Cardiac Surgery, 2nd ed, p 1685. New York, Churchill Livingstone, 1993

Nelson RM, Jeson CB, Smoot WM: Pericardial tamponade following open heart surgery. J Thorac Cardiovascular Surg 58:510–516, 1969

Weitzman LB, Tinker WC, Kronzon I et al: The incidence and natural history of pericardial effusions after cardiac surgery: An echocardiographic study. Circulation 69:506, 1984

A.4. Enumerate the common etiologies of cardiac tamponade.

Malignant diseases, idiopathic pericarditis, uremia, acute cardiac infarction (receiving heparin), diagnostic procedures with cardiac perforation, tuberculosis, radiation, myxedema, dissecting aortic aneurysm, postpericardium syndrome, systemic lupus erythematous.

Braunwald E (ed): Heart disease: A Textbook of Cardiovascular Medicine, 5th ed, p 1489. Philadelphia, WB Saunders, 1997

Kirklin JW, Barratt-Boyes BG (eds): Cardiac Surgery, 2nd ed, pp 1694–1695. New York, Churchill Livingstone, 1993

A5. When does delayed cardiac tamponade develop?

Delayed cardiac tamponade may develop several days to several weeks after the patient leaves the operating room. Delayed tamponade is uncommon. There is an increased incidence of delayed cardiac tamponade among patients being treated with anticoagulants.

Kirklin JK, Barratt-Boyes BG (eds): Cardiac Surgery, 2nd ed, pp 1694–1695. New York, Churchill Livingstone, 1993

A6. What is the difference between acute and chronic cardiac tamponade?

Acute cardiac tamponade must always be considered when low cardiac output is presented early postoperatively. Undrained intrapericardial bleeding may cause acute cardiac tamponade. Acute pericardial tamponade can also occur as a result of masked myocardial edema and chamber dilation inside the closed chest.

Patients in whom cardiac tamponade develops slowly differ from those with acute pericardial tamponade in that they usually appear acutely ill, but not *in extremis*, and the major complaint is dyspnea. Patients with chronic tamponade may have additional symptoms of weight loss, anorexia, and profound weakness.

Braunwald E (ed): Heart Disease: A Textbook of Cardiovascular Medicine, 5th ed, p 1489. Philadelphia, WB Saunders, 1997

A.7. What is regional cardiac tamponade?

Regional cardiac tamponade occurs less often. It is often misdiagnosed since classic features of tamponade are frequently absent. Single-chamber tamponade may be facilitated by an unclosed pericardium after surgery. This allows blood and blood clots to distribute unevenly around the heart compressing individual chambers. Postoperative right atrial hematomas often become localized to the anterior and lateral walls, whereas left atrial clots are more commonly found behind the left atrium where they become encysted in the posterior space in the oblique sinus.

Hutchins GM: Isolated right atrial tamponade caused by hematoma complicating coronary artery bypass graft surgery (letter). Arch Pathol Lab Med 104:612–614, 1980

Kochar GS, Jocab LE, Holter MN: Right atrial impression in postoperative patients: Detection by transesophageal cardiography. J Am Coll Cardiol 16:511–516, 1990

A.8. What is pulsus paradoxus? Can positive ventilation affect the severity of cardiac tamponade?

Normally there is an inspiratory fall of <10 mm Hg in the arterial systolic pressure and an accompanying inspiratory fall in the venous pressure. However, a paradoxical pulse differs from the normal situation in two aspects: (1) the inspiratory fall of the arterial pressure exceeds 10 mm Hg and (2) the inspiratory venous pressure remains steady or increases (Kussmaul sign). Pulsus paradoxus occurs only when intrapericardial pressure exceeds the diastolic filling pressures of both ventricles. Two factors are involved in the physiology of pulsus paradoxus: (1) intrathoracic pressure change during ventilation and (2) the anatomic interrelationship between the ventricles. Venous return increases slightly during spontaneous inspiration increasing right ventricular size. Because cardiac size is restricted by the tamponading fluid, the right ventricle can enlarge only at the expense of left ventricular size. Left ventricular preload, stroke volume, and systemic pressure thus decrease during inspiration. Positive pressure ventilation may worsen cardiac tamponade by further restricting venous return to the heart.

Braunwald E, Isselbacher KJ, Petersdorf RG et al (eds): Harrison's Principles of Internal Medicine, 13th ed, p 948. New York, McGraw-Hill, 1994

McGregor M: Pulsus paradoxus. N Engl J Med 301:480, 1979

A.9. How is excessive postoperative bleeding defined in cardiac surgery patients?

Excessive postoperative bleeding is variable but is generally considered to be present if 500 ml is lost in 1 hour, 100 to 200 ml/h is lost in over 2 to 4 hours, or a total of 1500 ml has been lost in the first 12 hours postoperatively. Other evidence of bleeding includes the presence of a widened cardiac silhouette on a postoperative chest radiograph or the presence of acute cardiac tamponade.

Kirklin JW, Barrett-Boyes BG (eds): Cardiac Surgery, 2nd ed, p 224. New York, Churchill Livingstone, 1993

A.10. What is in the differential diagnosis of post–cardiopulmonary–bypass (CPB) bleeding?

Inadequate surgical hemostasis is the most common cause of post-CPB bleeding. Platelet function is altered as a result of multiple factors and may be a cause of transient excessive bleeding. Another contributing factor for bleeding postoperatively is the state of health of the patient prior to surgery. Many of these patients are malnourished with decreased absorption of vitamin K via the gastrointestinal tract. Many of these patients are given coumadin or fribinolytic therapy prior to surgery causing inadequate concentrations of circulating coagulation factors. Primary fibrinolysis, caused by activation of endogenous plasminogen activators, is a rare cause of postoperative bleeding. Unneutralized heparin and excessive protamine are uncommon causes of bleeding.

Woodman RC, Harker LA: Bleeding complications associated with cardiopulmonary bypass. Blood 76:1680, 1990

A.11. How are platelets affected by cardiopulmonary bypass? What do platelet alpha-granules contain?

The platelet count is reduced during and following cardiopulmonary bypass as a result of hemodilution. Generally the platelet count remains above $100,000/\mu l$, which should not contribute to a bleeding diathesis. However, platelet function is also adversely affected by cardiopulmonary bypass. Platelets appear to be activated by contact with artificial surfaces. An early step in platelet activation is secretion of the contents of several types of granules. During cardiopulmonary bypass alpha-granules, containing peptides such as fibrinogen, thrombospondin, factors V and VIII, and beta-thromboglobulin, are reduced in both number and content. Probably of greater importance is the loss of several membrane glycoproteins (Ib, IIa–IIIb). These glycoproteins are involved in platelet-cellular interactions and lead to platelet aggregation on blood vessel walls, the first step in thrombosis formation.

Harker L, Malpass TW, Branson HE: Mechanism of abnormal bleeding in patients undergoing cardiopulmonary bypass: Acquired transient platelet dysfunction associated with selective α-granule release. Blood 56:824, 1980

A.12. How does desmopressin aid hemostasis? What is aprotinin? What is iloprost?

Desmopressin (1-deamino-8-D-arginine vasopressin, DDAVP) increases von Willebrand's factor and factor VIII activity in plasma. Von Willebrand's factor, which binds to platelets, is found in subendothelial tissue and is in part responsible for platelet adhesion to damaged blood vessels. DDAVP was initially shown to significantly decrease postoperative bleeding. More recent studies have failed to support this conclusion.

Aprotinin, a nonspecific serine protease inhibitor, decreases bleeding if administered prior to cardiopulmonary bypass. The mechanism of action is unclear at present.

Iloprost is a synthetic analogue of prostacyclin, PGI_2, a potent inhibitor of platelet activation. Iloprost has been used to protect platelets from the activating influences of the cardiopulmonary bypass circuit.

Cosgrove DM III, Heric B, Lytle BW et al: Aprotinin therapy for reoperative myocardial revascularization: A placebo-controlled study. Ann Thorac Surg 54:1031–1038, 1992

George JN, Pickett EB, Saucerman S et al: Platelet surface glycoproteins: Studies on resting and activated platelets and platelet membrane microparticles in normal subjects, and observations in patients during adult respiratory distress syndrome and cardiac surgery. J Clin Invest 78:340, 1986

Hackman T, Gascoyne CD, Naiman SC et al: A trial of desmopressin to reduce blood loss in uncomplicated cardiac surgery. N Engl J Med 321:1437, 1989

Salzman EW, Weinstein MJ, Weintraub RM et al: Treatment with desmopressin acetate to reduce blood loss after cardiac surgery. N Engl J Med 314:1402, 1986

A.13. What is the major arachidonic acid metabolite in platelets? How does aspirin inhibit platelet function?

The major component of platelet membrane phospholipids is arachidonic acid. Arachidonic acid cascade is activated by a disturbance of the cell membrane, which in turn activates phospholipase A_2. The cascade proceeds through the cyclooxygenase pathway, initiating prostaglandin synthesis. Thromboxane A_2, a potent platelet aggregant, is the major arachidonic acid metabolite formed in platelets. The release of thromboxane A_2 may occur to a great extent in the lungs.

Aspirin binds irreversibly to platelets and inhibits cyclooxygenase and platelet aggregation. Preoperative aspirin use has been associated with increased postoperative bleeding.

Colman RW, Hirsh J, Marder VJ, Salzman EW (eds): Hemostasis and Thrombosis: Basic Principles and Clinical Practice, 2nd ed, p 676. Philadelphia, JB Lippincott, 1987

Michelson EL, Morganroth J, Torosian M et al: Relation of preoperative use of aspirin to increased mediastinal blood loss after coronary artery bypass surgery. J Thorac Cardiovasc Surg 78:694, 1978

A.14. What is fibrinolysis?

Fibrinolysis is fibrin breakdown in thrombi. Plasmin, derived from plasminogen, is the enzyme involved in this process. Physiologic fibrinolysis involves clot remodeling and removal during the healing process. Pathologic fibrinolysis occurs when fibrin in a thrombus is broken down prior to healing. Though elevated concentrations of plasminogen activators are found during cardiopulmonary bypass, their half-lives are very short after bypass. Fibrinolysis is therefore a rare cause of postoperative bleeding in cardiac surgery patients.

Colman RW, Hirsh J, Marder VJ, Salzman EW (eds): Hemostasis and Thrombosis: Basic Principles and Clinical Practice, 2nd ed, p 358. Philadelphia, JB Lippincott, 1987

Stibbe J, Kluft C, Brommer EJP et al: Enhanced fibrinolytic activity during cardiopulmonary bypass in open heart surgery in man was caused by extrinsic (tissue-type) plasminogen activator. Eur J Clin Invest 14:375, 1984

A.15. How does heparin prevent clot formation?

Thrombin, the final product of the coagulation factor cascade, is inhibited by a naturally occurring inhibitor termed antithrombin III. Heparin binds reversibly to antithrombin III, accelerating the thrombin-antithrombin III interaction approximately 100-fold. Thrombin bound to antithrombin III is unable to bind to fibrinogen, thus inhibiting clot formation at a very early stage. The heparin-antithrombin III complex also inhibits the activated factors of the "intrinsic" coagulation pathway.

Colman RW, Hirsh J, Marder VJ, Salzman EW (eds): Hemostasis and Thrombosis: Basic Principles and Clinical Practice, 2nd ed, p 1373. Philadelphia, JB Lippincott, 1987

A.16. What is the mechanism of heparin antagonism by protamine?

Heparin is strongly negatively charged and binds ionically to protamine, a highly positively charged molecule. Heparin bound to protamine is incapable of binding to antithrombin III. Protamine has minimal intrinsic anticoagulant effects.

Ellison N, Ominsky AJ, Wollman H: Is protamine a clinically important anticoagulant? Anesthesiology 35:621, 1971

A.17. What is "heparin rebound"?

Heparin rebound is an abnormal coagulation assay, usually the activated clotting time (ACT), after initial correction by protamine infusion. This phenomenon was reported after *in vitro* protamine titration techniques were used. Presumably heparin is sequestered in tissues and released slowly into the circulation, where it performs its anticoagulant function again. Studies in which 1 mg of protamine is given per 100 units of heparin (total dose) found no evidence of heparin rebound. It is unlikely that heparin rebound is a common cause of bleeding in the postoperative cardiac surgical patient.

Woodman RC, Harker LA: Bleeding complications associated with cardiopulmonary bypass. Blood 76:1680, 1990

A.18. Can heparin cause thrombocytopenia? Can protamine sulfate cause thrombocytopenia?

Heparin can cause thrombocytopenia. Heparin from beef lung induces thrombocytopenia significantly more often than heparin derived from porcine intestinal mucosa. The plasma of some patients with heparin-induced thrombocytopenia contains a factor, probably an immunoglobulin, that is capable of inducing platelet aggregation and platelet immunoinjury in the presence of heparin. Thus, heparin appears to induce platelet activation and aggregation that involve the platelet fibrinogen receptor. In some patients, thromboxane A_2 synthesis seems to be involved, though aspirin does not seem to alter the clinical course of these patients. *In vitro* studies have demonstrated that antiplatelet antibodies may lead to endothelial cell damage and establish a prothrombotic environment. Thrombotic events are very common in heparin-induced thrombocytopenia compared with thrombocytopenias of other etiologies.

Cardiac surgery in the patient with heparin-induced thrombocytopenia should be postponed until the platelet count returns to normal. This may occur over a very variable length of time. In addition, a single dose of heparin may induce thrombocytopenia again. Heparin preparations commonly used clinically are a mixture of large and small molecules. Heparins of lower molecular weights have been found to have fewer effects on platelets and have been used in patients with heparin-induced thrombocytopenia. Prostacyclin, PGI_2, is a potent inhibitor of platelet activation. A synthetic analogue of prostacyclin, iloprost, has been used successfully to prevent further reduction of the platelet count when heparin is used during cardiac surgery.

Following intravenous injection of protamine sulfate, platelet levels were reduced within 5 minutes by about one-third in patients recovering from surgery on cardiopulmonary bypass and by about one half in normal subjects. The effect was transient, lasting <1 hour. On the basis of body surface scanning following transfusion of platelets labeled with indium[III], it was concluded that protamine induces temporary sequestration of platelets in the liver.

Ellison N, Jobes DR (eds): Effective Hemostasis in Cardiac Surgery, p 123. Philadelphia, WB Saunders, 1988

Hieyns A, du P et al: Kinetics and in vivo redistribution of [III]Indium-labelled human platelets after intravenous protamine sulfate. Thromb Haemost 44:65, 1980

A.19. What do the following measure: prothrombin time, activated partial thromboplastin time, thrombin time, activated clotting time, bleeding time?

- Prothrombin time measures the activity of the "extrinsic" pathway: factors I (fibrinogen), II (prothrombin), V, VII, and X (Fig. 15-1). Deficiencies of factors V, VII, and X (50% of normal) significantly prolong the prothrombin time. Much lower concen-

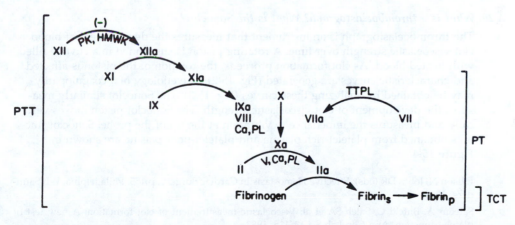

Figure 15-1. The coagulation cascade, illustrating the coagulation factors required for various screening tests. PTT, partial thromboplastin time; PT, prothrombin time; TCT, thrombin clotting time; PK, prekallikrein; HMWK, high-molecular-weight kininogen; PL, phospholipid by platelets; TTPL, tissue thromboplastin. (Reprinted with permission from Coleman RW, Hirsch J, Marder VJ et al [eds]: Hemostasis and Thrombosis: Basic Principles and Clinical Practice, 2nd ed, p 1052. Philadelphia, JB Lippincott, 1987)

trations of fibrinogen and prothrombin are required to prolong the prothrombin time. Activities of 3 of the 4 vitamin K-dependent factors (II, VII, IX, and X) are measured by the prothrombin time. Normal values are <12 seconds.
- Activated partial thromboplastin time (aPTT) measures the activity of the "intrinsic" pathway: factors XII, XI, IX, VIII, V, X, prothrombin, and fibrinogen (Fig. 15-1). The aPTT is prolonged by concentrations of <20% to 30% of these factors. Normal values are 25 to 40 seconds.
- Thrombin time measures the conversion of fibrinogen to fibrin by thrombin, the final step in the coagulation cascade (Fig. 15-1). The thrombin time is decreased in the presence of low concentrations of fibrinogen and thrombin. Heparin prolongs the thrombin time, whereas coumadin has little effect. Normal values are <10 seconds.
- Activated clotting time measures the general function of the coagulation system. It is used primarily to measure the adequacy of heparinization during cardiopulmonary bypass and protamine reversal of heparin following cardiopulmonary bypass. Prolonged activated clotting times may be due to heparin, low levels of coagulation factors, or thrombocytopenia. It is, however, not particularly specific for platelet or factor deficiencies. Normal values are 110 to 140 seconds.
- Bleeding time measures platelet activity, including both platelet number and aggregation. The bleeding time becomes prolonged with platelet counts <50,000/ml and in the presence of inhibitors of platelet aggregation such as aspirin. Normal values are <5 minutes.

Colman RW, Hirsh J, Marder VJ, Salzman EW (eds): Hemostasis and Thrombosis: Basic Principles and Clinical Practice, 2nd ed, p 1048. Philadelphia, JB Lippincott, 1987

Ellison N, Jobes DR (eds): Effective Hemostasis in Cardiac Surgery, p 155. Philadelphia, WB Saunders, 1988

A.20. What is a thromboelastograph? What is the Sonoclot?

The thromboelastograph is an instrument that measures the development of blood clot viscoelastic strength over time. A rotating piston is suspended in a cuvette filled with heated blood. As clot formation proceeds, the rotation of the piston is affected and characteristic curves are generated (Fig. 15-2). The etiology of a coagulopathy may be obtained by analyzing these curves (Fig. 15-3). The Sonoclot similarly measures the development of clot viscoelastic strength. The Sonoclot piston moves vertically and measures the impedance to vibration at the tip of the probe. Sonoclot tracings obtained from platelet-rich plasma and platelet-poor plasma are shown in Figure 15-4.

Ellison N, Jobes DR (eds): Effective Hemostasis in Cardiac Surgery, p 155. Philadelphia, WB Saunders, 1988

Saleem A, Blifeld C, Saleh SA et al: Viscoelastic measurement of clot formation: A new test of platelet function. Ann Clin Lab Sci 13:115, 1983

A.21. What are the electrocardiographic abnormalities associated with cardiac tamponade?

Electrical alternans is a specific indicator of pericardial tamponade and reflects swinging of the heart within the pericardial space. Echocardiographic findings suggest,

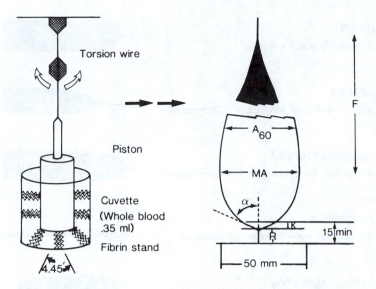

Figure 15-2. Production of normal thromboelastogram and measured parameters. R, reaction time, 7–14 min; K value, 3–7 min; α, clot formation rate, 40° to 60°; MA, maximum amplitude, 40–60 mm, A60/MA, amplitude 60 min after MA; whole blood clot lysis index, > 0.85; F, whole blood clot lysis time, > 300 min. (Reprinted with permission from Tumen KJ, spiess BD, McCathy RJ et al: Effects of progressive blood loss on coagulation as measured by thromboelastography. Anesth Analg 66:856–863, 1987)

however, that electrical alternans may be related to a beat-to-beat alternans of right and left ventricular filling.

Thus the appearance of electrical alternans in a patient with known pericardial effusion is very suggestive of cardiac tamponade. Electrical alternans is usually limited to the QRS complex and T waves.

Braunwald E (ed): Heart Disease: A Textbook of Cardiovascular Medicine, 5th ed, pp 1490–1492. Philadelphia, WB Saunders, 1997

A.22. What roentgenography and echocardiogram findings are noted in cardiac tamponade?

The heart may appear normal in size in an acute process developed or may appear enlarged if an effusion accumulates slowly to >25 ml. Patients who are status post–coronary bypass surgery can show wider cardiac silhouette within hours after surgery. Thus if cardiac tamponade is suspected, several chest films can help make the diagnosis with other clinical evidence. Other roentgenography features include obscuring of the pulmonary vessels at the hilum, aglobular or water bottle configuration of the heart, clear lungs, and separation of epicardial and pericardial pads.

Echocardiogram is an other extremely useful diagnostic tool in documenting the presence and magnitude of a pericardial effusion. Echocardiogram will increase the

NORMAL
R/K/MA/ANGLE = Normal

HEPARIN
R/K = Prolonged, MA/Angle = Decreased

THROMBOCYTOPENIA
R=Normal, K = Prolonged, MA= Decreased

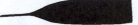

FIBRINOLYSIS
R = Normal, MA = Continuous decrease

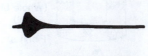

HYPERCOAGULATION
R/K = Decreased, MA/Angle = Increased

NO PLATELET FUNCTION
R = Prolonged, MA/Angle = Decreased

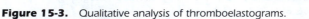

Figure 15-3. Qualitative analysis of thromboelastograms.

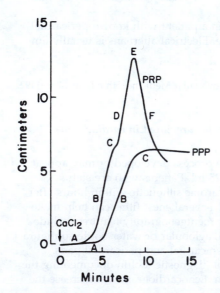

Figure 15-4. Sonoclot tracings of platelet-rich plasma (PRP) and platelet-poor plasma (PPP). *(A)* lag period; *(B)* primary wave; *(C)* shoulder; *(D)* secondary wave; *(E)* peak; *(F)* downward wave. (Reprinted with permission from Saleem A, Blifeld C, Saleh SA et al: Viscoelastic measurement of clot formation: A new test of platelet function. Ann Clin Lab Sci 13:115, 1983)

likelihood of diagnosing cardiac tamponade correctly and preventing inappropriate pericardiocentesis or pericardiotomy. The absence of a pericardial effusion virtually excludes the diagnosis of cardiac tamponade.

The application of M-mode and two-dimensional echocardiogram, the presence of a reduction in the E to F slope and excursion of the anterior mitral valve leaflet, and early systolic notching of the anterior right ventricular wall provide important features that a pericardial effusion is associated with cardiac tamponade.

Braunwald E (ed): Heart Disease: A Textbook of Cardiovascular Medicine, 5th ed, p 1490. Philadelphia, WB Saunders, 1997

Kaplan JA (ed): Cardiac Anesthesia, 2nd ed, p 811. Philadelphia, WB Saunders, 1993

B. Preoperative Evaluation and Preparation

B.1. How would you evaluate this patient's coagulation status?

The activated clotting time (ACT) should be measured because this is the most readily available test. If this is prolonged, additional protamine may be indicated. If the ACT is not corrected by protamine, then a platelet count, prothrombin time (PT), and an activated partial thromboplastin time (aPTT) will allow a relatively rapid screen of the coagulation system. Though most patients exhibit abnormalities in concentrations of coagulation factors because of dilution during cardiopulmonary bypass, PT and aPTT tests are rarely markedly prolonged, and platelet count is rarely markedly decreased.

Ellison N, Jobes DR (eds): Effective Hemostasis in Cardiac Surgery, p 195. Philadelphia, WB Saunders, 1988

B.2. What do fresh-frozen plasma and cryoprecipitate contain?

Fresh-frozen plasma contains the labile (factors V and VIII) as well as the stable coagulation factors (factors II, VII, IX, X, XI). In addition, fresh-frozen plasma contains other plasma proteins and lipids normally found in human plasma. Cryoprecipitate forms when fresh-frozen plasma is thawed at 4°C. Cryoprecipitate contains factor VIII, von Willebrand's factor, and fibrinogen.

Ellison N, Jobes DR (eds): Effective Hemostasis in Cardiac Surgery, p 69. Philadelphia, WB Saunders, 1988

B.3. What are the indications for transfusing fresh-frozen plasma (FFP), platelet concentrate, and cryoprecipitate?

Blood usually coagulates appropriately when coagulation factor concentrations are at least 20% to 30% of normal and when fibrinogen levels are >75 mg/dl. Although laboratory values such as prothrombin time (PT) and partial thromboplastin time (PTT) may be abnormal, American Society of Anesthesiologist Task Force on Blood Component Therapy believes, however, that there are few clinical circumstances in the perioperative setting resulting in coagulopathies that require replacement of coagulation factors with FFP. Although massive blood replacement can produce prolongation of PT and/or PTT, the Task Force believes that a true dilution coagulopathy does not ordinarily occur until >100% of the patient's blood volume has been replaced. The

Task Force believes that FFP can be beneficial in patients with minor vascular bleeding with PT/PTT values >1.5 times the laboratory's normal value. FFP should be administrated in doses calculated to achieve a minimum of 30% of plasma factor concentration. This can be done with the administration of 10 to 15 ml/kg of FFP.

Fresh-Frozen Plasma is Indicated in the Following:

- Replacement of factor deficiencies
- Reversal of coumadin effect
- Massive blood transfusions
- Treatment of antithrombin III deficiency in patients who must be anticoagulated with heparin.

In 1994 the College of American Pathologists recommended platelet transfusions after cardiopulmonary bypass in patients with normal coagulation values and platelet count below 100,000/μl when major unexplained bleeding occurs. Transfusion of one platelet concentrate will increase the platelet count by approximately 5 to 10 × 10^3/μl in the average adult. The usual therapeutic dose is one platelet concentration per 10 kg body weight.

Platelet Concentrate is Indicated in the Following:

- Active bleeding associated with thrombocytopenia
- Massive blood transfusions

The American Society of Anesthesiologists Task Force on Blood Component Therapy recommends the administration of cryoprecipitate for

- Prophylaxis in nonbleeding perioperative or peripartum patients with congenital fibrinogen deficiencies or von Willenbrand's disease unresponsive to DDAVP (whenever possible, these decisions should be made in consultation with the patient's hematologist
- Bleeding patients with von Willenbrand's disease, and
- Correction of microvascular bleeding in massively transfused patients with fibrinogen concentrations <80 to 100 mg/dl.

One unit of cryoprecipitate per 10 kg body weight raises plasma fibrinogen concentration approximately 50 mg/dl in the absence of continued consumption or massive bleeding.

Bleeding following cardiac surgery without demonstrable abnormalities of coagulation is not considered to be an indication for transfusion of fresh-frozen plasma, platelets, or cryoprecipitate.

American Society of Anesthesiologists: Guidelines for blood component therapy. A report by the American Society of Anesthesiologists' Task Force on Blood Component Therapy. Anesthesiology 84:732–747, 1996

British Committee for Standards in Haematology: Guidelines for the use of fresh frozen plasma. Transfus Med 2:57–63, 1992

Fresh frozen plasma: Indications and risks. NIH Consensus Development Conference Statement 5(5):1, 1985

Goodnough RL, Rutman RL, Silberstein LE: Guidelines for transfusion support in patients undergoing coronary artery bypass grafting. Ann Thorac Surg 50:675–683, 1990

Murray DJ, Pennell BJ, Weinstein SL, Olson JD: Packed red cells in acute blood loss: Dilutional coagulopathy as a course of surgical bleeding. Anesth Analg 80:336–342, 1995

Platelet transfusion therapy. NIH Consensus Development Conference Statement 6(7):1, 1986

B.4. What are the complications associated with blood component transfusions?

Complications associated with all types of blood component transfusions include transmission of infectious agents (e.g., hepatitis, human immunodeficiency virus [HIV] infection), hemolytic and nonhemolytic transfusion reactions, immunosuppression, anaphylactic or anaphylactoid reactions, and alloimmunization to platelet-specific antigens and the Rh-antigen (due to erythrocyte contamination). Platelets in particular may contain proliferating bacteria because they are stored at room temperature. Graft-versus-host disease may occur in immunodeficient patients receiving platelet transfusion.

Fresh frozen plasma: Indications and risks. NIH Consensus Development Conference Statement 5(5):1, 1985

Lacritz EM, Sullen GA, Aberle-Grasse J et al: Estimated risk of transmission of the human immunodeficiency virus by screened blood in the United States. N Engl J Med 333:1721–1725, 1995

Platelet transfusion therapy. NIH Consensus Development Conference Statement 6(7):1, 1986

Sazama K: Reports of 355 transfusion-associated deaths: 1976 through 1985. Transfusion 30:583–590, 1990

B.5. What is the statistical incidence of exposure to HIV through blood transfusion?

The current risk of HIV infection in the United States is 1:450,000 to 1:660,000 per transfused unit of blood. However, with the implementation of donor screening tests for HIV-1 antigen, there is an expectation of preventing up to 25% of the window period cases (the period between viral infection and its detection by tests for the presence of antibodies). Perhaps the immunoviral agent most transmitted by blood transfusion is cytomegalovirus.

Lacritz EM, Sullen GA, Aberle-Grasse J et al: Estimated risk of transmission of the human immunodeficiency virus by screened blood in the United States. N Engl J Med 333:1721–1725, 1995

B.6. Does the patient's temperature affect coagulation? Why are patients often cold after cardiopulmonary bypass?

Platelet aggregation decreases as temperature decreases and is virtually abolished at 33°C *in vitro*. The specific defect induced by hypothermia is unknown. Even though patients are warmed to nasal pharyngeal temperatures of 37°C, they still have a large caloric deficit equal to about one third of the total caloric loss during cardiopulmonary bypass. In addition, temperature loss due to evaporation, radiation, conduction, and convection continues.

Thrombocytopenia, usually transient, sometimes very severe, occurs both in animals and in humans, during induced hypothermia, and it has been implicated as a cause of the hemorrhagic diathesis that sometimes follows restoration of normal body temperature following surgical hypothermia. The reduction in platelet levels is much less severe in patients given heparin (as those in cardiopulmonary bypass surgery) than in those who receive no anticoagulant.

Davis FM, Parinelazhagan KN, Harris EA: Thermal balance during cardiopulmonary bypass with hypothermia in man. Br J Anaesth 49:1127, 1977

Ellison N, Jobes DR (eds): Effective Hemostasis in Cardiac Surgery, p 100. Philadelphia, WB Saunders, 1988

Grant RA, Peerschke EI, Zucker MB: Altered surface properties of human blood platelets associated with the loss of aggregability. J Cell Biol 83:64, 1979

B.7. In what situation might epsilon-aminocaproic acid improve hemostasis?

Epsilon-aminocaproic acid (EACA) inhibits plasminogen activation by binding to plasminogen. It inhibits primary fibrinolysis, which is caused by excessive plasminogen activation by endogenous plasminogen activators (e.g., urokinase, tissue-type plasminogen activator) occasionally seen in urinary tract bleeding and subarachnoid hemorrhage from an intracranial aneurysm. Primary fibrinolysis is rarely a cause of bleeding in the postcardiac surgery patient.

Colman RW, Hirsh J, Marder VJ, Salzman EW (eds): Hemostasis and Thrombosis: Basic Principles and Clinical Practice, 2nd ed, p 1026. Philadelphia, JB Lippincott, 1987

B.8. How would you assess the hemodynamic status of this patient?

Hypotension and low cardiac output in the presence of elevated right and left heart filling pressures and significant postoperative bleeding are probably due to acute cardiac tamponade. However, any increase in intrathoracic pressure may present with this hemodynamic scenario. In addition, severe biventricular heart failure may also present in a similar manner. Although it is important to consider these alternative diagnoses, tamponade is the most likely and must be treated with some urgency since surgical reexploration of the mediastinum will cure the hemodynamic problem as well as terminate surgical bleeding.

B.9. How would you treat hypotension due to cardiac tamponade?

Mechanical restriction of cardiac filling is the etiology of the hypotension associated with cardiac tamponade. Therefore, the definitive treatment of tamponade is removal of the fluid (or clot) compressing the heart, by either pericardiocentesis, subxiphoid pericardial window, or sternotomy. In this patient, temporizing measures must be taken until return to the operating room is feasible. Since volume status is difficult to analyze in this patient, fluids should be administered in an attempt to maximize ventricular filling. Tissue perfusion may be maintained by maximizing contractility with inotropes. Adequate systemic perfusion pressure is provided by the careful use of vasoconstrictors. Finally, although stroke volume is limited, cardiac output may be increased by judiciously increasing heart rate. If all else fails, the chest must be opened in the intensive care unit in order to relieve the tamponade.

Thomas SJ (ed): Manual of Cardiac Anesthesia, 2nd ed, pp 135–136. New York, Churchill Livingstone, 1993

B.10. How would you prepare the patient for surgery?

Patients who arrive at the operating room with the diagnosis of cardiac tamponade usually have hemodynamic alterations. The net effect of the increased pressure around the heart causes impairment of diastolic filling of the right and left ventricles. This results in a subsequent reduction in stroke volume. Initiation of general anesthesia and positive pressure ventilation can lead to severe hypotension and possible cardiac arrest. Thus inotropic support in the form of continuous infusions and bolus doses should be prepared. Since these patients are bleeding, it is critical to maintain the intravascular volume. The patient should be typed and crossmatched for at least 4 to 6 units of packed red blood cells. However, if the patient has not been typed and crossmatched, balanced salt solution may be used. Fluid volume replacement with balanced salt solution will provide enough circulatory volume to maintain the cardiac output.

B.11. What premedication would you prescribe for this patient?

Since these patients are usually hypotensive and are dependent on activation of the sympathetic nervous system, it is not recommended to premedicate these patients. The potential adverse effects of either narcotics or barbiturates can place the patient in a dangerous situation and should be avoided.

C. Intraoperative Management

C.1. How would you monitor this patient during transport from the intensive care unit to the operating room? What emergency drugs would you bring with you?

Systemic blood pressure and an electrocardiogram must be monitored. Emergency drugs should include a vasoconstrictor such as:

- Phenylephrine: pure alpha agonist vasoconstrictor. Dose: bolus, 100 to 500 µg; infusion, 10 µg/min
- Norepinephrine: direct-acting alpha- and beta-agonist. Dose: 1 to 8 µg/min
- Metaraminol: direct alpha- and beta-agonist with indirect action by causing release of norepinephrine. Dose: 0.5 µg/kg/min.

Inotropes such as:

- Epinephrine: endogenous catecholamine with alpha and beta effects. Dose: 45 to 150 µg/kg may be used to induce a diastolic pressure of 30 mm Hg or more for up to 5 minutes if there is no blood pressure or the patient is arrested.
- Calcium chloride is essential to the process of excitation-contraction coupling. The transient increase in intracellular calcium concentration activates actin-myosin coupling through interaction regulatory proteins. Dose: 2 to 4 mg/kg.

In addition, lidocaine and atropine may occasionally prove useful during transport of an unstable patient.

C.2. What effect on contractility and systemic blood pressure in this patient would be expected from ketamine, thiopental, fentanyl, propofol, and diazepam?

Ketamine has a rapid onset of action with a peak plasma concentration reached in <1 minute after intravenous administration. Ketamine has a relatively short duration of action. Patients remain unconscious for 10 to 15 minutes after intravenous induction dose, but analgesia (somatic greater than visceral) will persist into the postoperative period. Ketamine increases blood pressure, heart rate, cardiac output, and myocardial oxygen demand because of direct central sympathetic stimulation and inhibition of norepinephrine uptake into postganglionic sympathetic nerve endings. Ketamine intrinsically depresses myocardial contractility. Therefore, in patients without hemodynamic compromise this effect is offset by central sympathetic stimulation leading to increased contractility and blood pressure. However, in this patient, in whom sympathetic tone was likely to be quite high, depression of myocardial contractility and blood pressure might occur as the intrinsic effects of ketamine were manifested.

Thiopental is a mild to moderate myocardial contractility depressant and a mild vasodilator. Small doses (1 to 2 mg/kg) would be unlikely to affect this patient adversely. Higher doses might lead to myocardial depression and further hypotension.

Fentanyl has little direct effect on myocardial contractility. Fentanyl might attenuate sympathetic tone, thereby causing hypotension, particularly if large doses are used.

Propofol is a potent vasodilator and might cause severe hypotension in this patient when used in large doses. It appears to have little effect on myocardial contractility.

Diazepam might cause mild to moderate vasodilation, particularly when used in combination with narcotics. Myocardial contractility might be mildly depressed.

Barash PG, Cullen BF, Stoelting RK (eds): Clinical Anesthesia, 3rd ed, pp 316–320, 341–342. Philadelphia, Lippincott-Raven, 1997

Kaplan JA (ed): Cardiac Anesthesia, 3rd ed, pp 513–525. Philadelphia, WB Saunders, 1993

Tweed WA, Minuck M, Mymin D: Circulatory responses to ketamine anesthesia. Anesthesiology 37:612, 1972

C.3. How would you induce anesthesia in this patient? After anesthesia was induced, the systemic blood pressure fell to 55/30 mm Hg. What were likely causes of hypotension in this situation? How would you treat this hypotension?

Any induction sequence may be safely used provided the hemodynamic parameters discussed above are maintained. Vasoactive drugs should be readily available and used quickly to maintain these parameters. Hypotension following induction was likely due to a combination of vasodilation and depression of myocardial contractility. Also with the decrease in preload secondary to positive pressure ventilation there will be a drop in cardiac output and stroke volume. Hand ventilation with a slight decrease in minute ventilation may be necessary until surgical correction is applied. Administration of a vasoconstrictor and an inotrope might be necessary to correct the hypotension. These would be merely temporizing measures; surgical relief of tamponade would be the definitive treatment of this problem.

Thomas SJ (ed): Manual of Cardiac Anesthesia, 2nd ed, p 135. New York, Churchill Livingstone, 1993

C.4. Why does stroke volume change when the sternum is opened?

As discussed, the primary problem in cardiac tamponade is limited filling of the ventricles due to elevated intrapericardial pressure. When the pressure is relieved by sternotomy, the ventricles can fill normally and therefore eject a normal stroke volume.

Thomas SJ (ed): Manual of Cardiac Anesthesia, 2nd ed, pp 135–136. New York, Churchill Livingstone, 1993

C.5. How would you manage hypertension following relief of the tamponade?

Hypertension following relief of tamponade may be due to increased left ventricular stroke volume, hypervolemia, the effects of exogenously administered inotropes and vasoconstrictors, and inadequate anesthesia. The first consideration should be the depth of anesthesia. Vasodilators may then be necessary. Sodium nitroprusside infusion decreases blood pressure via relaxation of vessel wall smooth muscle. The maximum recommended dose is 8.0 $\mu g/kg/min$ over 1 to 3 hours or 500 $\mu g/kg/h$. The usual perioperative rate is 0.5 to 20 $\mu g/kg/min$.

C.6. What complications may arise from this procedure?

The complications include exsanguinating hemorrhage, disruption of aortocoronary or internal mammary artery grafts with subsequent ischemia, disruption of valve prostheses, particularly in the mitral position if the heart is raised out of the pericardial cavity, and rhythm disturbances when the heart is manipulated.

Reoperation for bleeding has not been a risk factor for sternal infection. However, imperfect aseptic technique in the operating room is the basic cause of infected median sternotomy wounds. Also the prolonged operative time is a risk factor for the development of mediastinal wound infections. Those patients who return to the operating room for acute or delayed cardiac tamponade following either coronary or vascular surgery have an increased incidence of breaking sterile technique. The prolonged operation time and the simple fact that they have undrained retrosternal hematoma is an increased risk of infection.

Demmy TL, Park SB, Liebler F et al: Recent experience with major sternal wound complications. Ann Thorac Surg 49:458, 1990

Wilson APR, Livesey SA, Treasure T et al: Factors predisposing to wound infection in cardiac surgery: A prospective study of 517 patients. Eur J Cardiothoracic Surg 1:158, 1987

D. Postoperative Management

D.1 How would you manage hypertension in the intensive care unit?

The patient following relief of acute postoperative tamponade is no different from any other post–cardiopulmonary bypass patient. Ischemia, depressed contractility, and rhythm disturbances may appear and would be treated. Because these patients are not deeply anesthetized, a common problem in the intensive care unit is hypertension. Treatment may include sedatives, analgesics, vasodilators, beta-adrenergic antagonists, and calcium entry blockers.

Thomas SJ (ed): Manual of Cardiac Anesthesia, 2nd ed, p 469. New York, Churchill Livingstone, 1993

16 Patent Ductus Arteriosus and Prematurity

Fun-Sun F. Yao
Robert E. Kelly

A 10-day-old male infant weighing 950 g was scheduled for ligation of patent ductus arteriosus (PDA). He was born at 29 weeks gestation and was intubated immediately after delivery because of respiratory distress. His condition improved over the following 4 days. However, on the 5th day of his life the respiratory distress worsened and a murmur was heard over his chest. Medical treatment for patent ductus arteriosus was attempted unsuccessfully. His blood pressure was 60/40 mm Hg; heart rate, 150 beats/min. The laboratory data were as follows: WBC, 17,000/mm^3; hemoglobin, 11 g/dl; hematocrit, 34%; urine specific gravity 1.005; protein 1+; sugar 1+; serum calcium, 6.0 mg/dl; blood glucose, 60 mg/dl; arterial blood gases: pH 7.30; PaCO$_2$, 45 mm Hg; PaO$_2$, 60 mm Hg on F$_I$O$_2$ 50%, inspiratory pressure, 30/4 cm H$_2$O; and ventilation rate, 25/min.

A. Medical Disease and Differential Diagnosis

1. How would you classify prematurity? What are the common problems associated with prematurity?
2. What are the survival rates of preterm infants?
3. What are the incidence and survival rates of respiratory distress syndrome (RDS)? Discuss its pathophysiology.
4. What is bronchopulmonary dysplasia? How would you treat it?
5. What are the possible causes of apneic spells?
6. Discuss the incidence and pathophysiology of patent ductus arteriosus (PDA) in preterm infants.
7. How would you make a diagnosis of PDA? Describe its treatment.
8. Would you give digitalis to treat congestive heart failure in preterm infants? Why?
9. How does indomethacin close the ductus?
10. What is retinopathy of prematurity (retrolental fibroplasia)? Discuss its etiology, pathophysiology, prognosis, and prevention.
11. Define neutral and critical temperatures. What are these values in the preterm neonate, in the term neonate, and in the adult? Discuss temperature regulation in the neonate.

B. Preoperative Evaluation and Preparation

1. How would you evaluate this patient preoperatively?
2. What are the normal values of arterial blood gases and *p*H in preterm and term pediatric patients?
3. Interpret the arterial blood gases: *p*H, 7.30; P$_{CO_2}$, 45 mm Hg; P$_{O_2}$, 60 mm Hg; HCO$_3$$^-$,

20 mEq/liter on 60% oxygen; and 5 cm H_2O of positive end-expiratory pressure (PEEP). How would you improve them?

4. What are the normal values of arterial blood pressure, heart rate, and respiratory rate for preterm infants?
5. What are the normal values of WBC, RBC, hemoglobin, glucose, electrolytes, calcium, BUN, and creatinine for preterm infants?
6. Would you transfuse blood to this patient preoperatively?
7. How would you interpret the urinalysis: specific gravity 1.005, sugar 1+, protein 1+?
8. Would you correct a serum calcium of 6.0 mg/dl? What other information would you like to have? Which contains more calcium, 10 cc of 10% calcium chloride or 10 cc of 10% calcium gluconate? Could you hyperventilate this child safely?
9. How would you premedicate this patient?

C. Intraoperative Management

1. What monitors would you use for this child during surgery?
2. How does the oxygen analyzer work?
3. What is the Doppler effect? How does the Doppler transducer measure blood pressure?
4. What is the mechanism of pulse oximetry? Why is it important to monitor arterial oxygen saturation? What levels of arterial oxygen saturation would you like to keep during surgery?
5. How would you maintain the patient's body temperature?
6. How do the anesthetic requirements of the preterm infant differ from those of the adult?
7. What size endotracheal tube would you have used if the patient had not been intubated?
8. How would you have induced anesthesia if the patient had not been intubated?
9. How would you maintain anesthesia?
10. How would you ventilate the patient? What tidal volume, respiratory rates, and F_1O_2 would you set for the infant?
11. Discuss blood and fluid therapy in this preterm infant.
12. During dissection of the ductus arteriosus, the arterial oxygen saturation dropped from 92% to 80% and the heart rate decreased from 140 beats/min to 80 beats/min. What were the causes? How would you correct this situation?

D. Postoperative Management

1. Would you reverse the muscle relaxants and extubate the patient at the end of surgery?
2. How can one minimize the risk of transporting the patient to the neonatal intensive care unit after surgery?
3. The patient's condition deteriorated postoperatively in the intensive care unit. Physical examination revealed persistent cardiac murmur. What was the possible diagnosis?

Table 16-1. Classification of Prematurity

	BORDERLINE PREMATURITY	MODERATE PREMATURITY	EXTREME PREMATURITY
Gestational age (wk)	37 to 38	31 to 36	24 to 30
Percentage live births	16%	6% to 7%	<1%
Weight (gs)	2500 to 3200	1500 to 2500	500 to 1500
Associated problems	Poor suck	Poor suck	Poor suck
	RDS	RDS	RDS
	Temperature regulation	Temperature regulation	Temperature regulation
		Sepsis	Sepsis
		Intracranial hemorrhage	Intracranial hemorrhage
			Necrotizing enterocolitis
			Congestive heart failure
			Birth asphyxia
Level of care	Careful observation in newborn nursery	Neonatal ICU	Neonatal ICU

A. Medical Disease and Differential Diagnosis

A.1. How would you classify prematurity? What are the common problems associated with prematurity?

Preterm infants can be classified into three groups, as shown in Table 16-1. Infants of borderline prematurity usually require no special care, but, because of their susceptibility to respiratory distress syndrome (RDS), they should be observed closely for 24 to 48 hours in the newborn nursery. Further, those with a poor suck reflex may require gavage feedings. Infants classified as moderately premature require intense neonatal care, and neonatal mortality correlates inversely with gestational age. Neonates of extreme prematurity constitute only 1% of all preterm infants; however, mortality in this group is extremely high, accounting for >70% of all neonatal deaths. Furthermore, morbidity in surviving infants is substantial, often secondary to irreversible neurologic or respiratory insult.

Avery GB (ed): Neonatology. Philadelphia, JB Lippincott, 1981

Behrman RE, Kliegman RM, Arvin AM (eds): Nelson Textbook of Pediatrics, 15th ed, p 454. Philadelphia, WB Saunders, 1996

Gregory GA (ed): Pediatric Anesthesia, 3rd ed, p 351–352. New York, Churchill Livingstone, 1994

Usher RH, Allen AC, McLean RH: Risk of respiratory distress syndrome related to gestational age, route of delivery and maternal diabetes. Am J Obstet Gynecol 111:826, 1971

A.2. What are the survival rates of preterm infants?

The survival rates of preterm infants depend mainly on their maturity or birth weights. Because of the advancement in neonatal care, survival rates have increased twofold in the last two decades. Recently, the survival rates for infants with birth weights 500 to 750 g, 750 to 1000 g, 1000 to 1250 g, 1250 to 1500 g and 1500 to 2000 g have been approximately 20% to 70%, 75%, 85%, 92%, and 97% respectively.

Behrman RE, Kliegman RM, Arvin AM (eds): Nelson Textbook of Pediatrics, 15th ed, p 452–454. Philadelphia, WB Saunders, 1996

Gregory GA (ed): Pediatric Anesthesia, 3rd ed, p 352. New York, Churchill Livingstone, 1994

A.3. What are the incidence and survival rates of respiratory distress syndrome (RDS)? Discuss its pathophysiology.

Respiratory distress syndrome, formerly called hyaline membrane disease, is common in preterm infants. Respiratory distress syndrome (RDS) is a life-threatening condition associated with 50% to 75% of all deaths of premature infants. It occurs three times more often in those born by cesarean section than in those born vaginally. The incidence of RDS depends on the birth weight. It happens in 30% to 55% of preterm infants weighing 1000 to 1500 g, 20% to 40% of those weighing 1501 to 2000 g, and 0.3% to 0.4% of those weighing >2000 g.

The survival rate has increased dramatically over the past 50 years. Survival depends on the infant's size. Ninety percent of those weighing 900 to 1000 g survive, whereas about 70% of those weighing 500 to 700 g survive. Recently, an increase in survival and a decrease in serious complications have been associated with administration of surfactant into the lungs at birth. This may pose a problem for the anesthesiologist if these patients require surgery. Ventilation with high positive pressures and large volumes increases the likelihood of pulmonary gas leaks and lung injury.

Physical examination of the infant with RDS will likely reveal cyanosis, tachypnea, intercostal retractions, and bilateral rales that fail to clear with suctioning. An arterial blood gas sample will demonstrate hypoxemia, metabolic acidosis, and respiratory alkalosis; a chest radiograph will show diffuse, hazy ("ground glass") infiltrates.

RDS is thought to be caused by a deficiency of the alveolar phospholipid surfactant. The surfactant is produced by the type II alveolar cells and is necessary for the maintenance of alveolar stability. Surfactant production is usually inadequate prior to 35 weeks of gestational age. In its absence, alveolar collapse occurs, with consequent right-to-left shunting, arterial hypoxemia, and metabolic acidosis.

Coates AL, Desmond K, Willis D et al: Oxygen therapy and long-term pulmonary outcome of respiratory distress syndrome in newborns. Am J Dis Child 136:892, 1982

Gregory GA (ed): Pediatric Anesthesia, 3rd ed, p 352. New York, Churchill Livingstone, 1994

Stoelting RK, Dierdorf SF (eds): Anesthesia and Coexisting Disease, 3rd ed, pp 587–588. New York, Churchill Livingstone, 1993

A.4. What is bronchopulmonary dysplasia? How would you treat it?

Bronchopulmonary dysplasia is a chronic lung disease found in many small preterm infants as a result of mechanical ventilation, oxygen toxicity, infection, or a combination of these factors. It usually progresses through 4 stages:

Stage I
At 2 to 3 days of age, the chest x-ray shows classic respiratory distress syndrome. There are atelectasis, hyaline membrane, hyperemia, lymphatic dilation, metaplasia, and necrosis of bronchiolar mucosa.

Stage II
At 4 to 10 days of age, the chest x-ray shows obscure cardiac borders and nearly complete opacification of lung fields. The pathology reveals necrosis and repair of epithelium, persisting hyaline membrane, emphysematous coalescence of alveoli, and thickening of alveolar and capillary membranes.

Stage III

At 10 to 20 days of age, the chest film shows small rounded areas of sponge-like radiolucency. There are few hyaline membranes, regeneration of clear cells, bronchiolar metaplasia, mucous secretion, emphysematous alveoli, and focal thickening of basement membrane.

Stage IV

After 30 days of age, the radiolucent areas seen in stage III enlarge and alternate with thin strands of radiodensity. The pathology reveals emphysematous alveoli and marked hypertrophy of epithelium.

Bronchopulmonary dysplasia causes maldistribution of ventilation and perfusion, resulting in hypoxemia and hypercarbia. The treatment includes mechanical ventilation with positive end-expiratory pressure and large doses of furosemide (Lasix), 5 to 10 mg/kg every 6 hours, to decrease pulmonary edema and improve gas exchange. Furosemide therapy induces metabolic alkalosis; therefore, an adequate amount of potassium and chloride should be supplemented.

Gregory GA (ed): Pediatric Anesthesia, 3rd ed, pp 354–355. New York, Churchill Livingstone, 1994

Northway WH Jr, Rosan R, Porter D: Pulmonary disease following respiratory therapy of hyaline membrane disease: Bronchopulmonary dysplasia. N Engl J Med 276:357, 1967

A.5. What are the possible causes of apneic spells?

Apneic spells are common in preterm infants, especially after the first week of life. The causes are multiple and include the following:

- Hypothermia and hyperthermia
- Hypoglycemia and hyperglycemia
- Hypocalcemia and hypercalcemia
- Hypovolemia and hypervolemia
- Anemia
- Decreased functional residual capacity
- Patent ductus arteriosus
- Constipation
- Hypothyroidism
- Poorly developed control of respiration
- Excessive handling

Repeated apnea increases the likelihood of central nervous system damage because of repeated episodes of hypoxemia. Infants who have apneic spells do not breathe during anesthesia; therefore, they should be ventilated throughout anesthesia, including during its induction.

Gregory GA (ed): Pediatric Anesthesia, 3rd ed, pp 354–355. New York, Churchill Livingstone, 1994

Rigatto H, Brady JP: Periodic breathing and apnea in preterm infants. I. Evidence of hypoventilation possibly due to central respiratory depression. Pediatrics 50:202, 1972

Rigatto H, Brady JP: Periodic breathing and apnea in preterm infants. II. Hypoxia as a primary event. Pediatrics 50:219, 1972

A.6. Discuss the incidence and pathophysiology of patent ductus arteriosus (PDA) in preterm infants.

Forty-two percent of infants weighing <1000 g and 20.2% of infants under 1750 g have hemodynamically significant PDA. In term infants, the ductus arteriosus closes soon after birth in response to the increased arterial oxygen tension. However, in preterm infants, it has a thinner, poorly contractile muscular layer with diminished responsiveness to the increasing oxygen levels after birth. In addition, preterm infants often suffer from hypoxemia because of respiratory distress syndrome, so that there are both a reduced stimulus to and a reduced response to physiologic closure. However, on the third to fifth day of life, some resolution of the RDS usually occurs, with a concurrent decrease in pulmonary resistance. This allows blood shunting from the systemic to the pulmonary circulation by way of the patent ductus arteriosus, resulting in pulmonary vascular overload and ultimately left heart failure. The pulmonary congestion worsens respiratory failure, resulting in further hypoxemia and CO_2 retention.

Emmanouilides GC, Riemenschneider TA, Allen HD, Gutgesell HP (eds): Moss and Adams' Heart Disease in Infants, Children and Adolescents, Including the Fetus and Young Adult, 5th ed, pp 746–761. Baltimore, Williams & Wilkins, 1995

Lake CL (ed): Pediatric Cardiac Anesthesia, 3rd ed, pp 453–454. Stamford, CT, Appleton & Lange, 1998

Siassi B, Blanco C, Cabal LA et al: Incidence and clinical features of patent ductus arteriosus in low birth weight infants: A perspective analysis of 150 consecutively born infants. Pediatrics 57:347, 1976

A.7. How would you make a diagnosis of PDA? Describe its treatment.

The diagnosis of PDA in preterm infants may be suspected when there is sudden increase in respiratory failure, tachycardia, tachypnea, and a widened pulse pressure. The typical continuous or machinery murmur of PDA is usually not present in this population, but a systolic murmur, sometimes extending into diastole, and a hyperdynamic precordium are nearly always present. The diagnosis is confirmed by echocardiography that demonstrates left atrial enlargement. Two-dimensional echocardiography can identify the aortic end of the ductus. Continuous-wave Doppler can detect abnormal flow in the pulmonary artery. Color Doppler can visualize the jet of abnormal flow.

The initial treatment of PDA is medical. It includes fluid restriction and administration of diuretics and indomethacin. Indomethacin, 0.1 to 0.2 mg/kg, three doses for every 12 hours, usually closes the ductus within 24 hours. If the ductus fails to close with medical treatment, surgical ligation is indicated.

Gregory GA (ed): Pediatric Anesthesia, 3rd ed, pp 355–356. New York, Churchill Livingstone, 1994

Lake CL (ed): Pediatric Cardiac Anesthesia, 3rd ed, pp 455–456. Stamford, CT, Appleton & Lange, 1998

A.8. Would you give digitalis to treat congestive heart failure in preterm infants? Why?

Digitalis should not be given to small preterm infants because it does not effectively improve stroke volume or ventricular emptying. However, it does decrease the heart rate, resulting in detrimental decrease in cardiac output.

Berman W Jr, Dubynsky O, Whitman V et al: Digoxin therapy in low birth weight infants with patent ductus arteriosus. J Pediatr 93:652, 1978

Emmanouilides GC, Riemenschneider TA, Allen HD, Gutgesell HP (eds): Moss and Adams' Heart Disease in Infants, Children and Adolescents, Including the Fetus and Young Adult, 5th ed, pp 746–761. Baltimore, Williams & Wilkins, 1995

Gregory GA (ed): Pediatric Anesthesia, 3rd ed, p 355. New York, Churchill Livingstone, 1994

A.9. How does indomethacin close the ductus?

The ductus arteriosus functionally closes shortly after birth in term infants when the vascular smooth muscle contracts. The muscular contraction of the ductus is initiated by the increased oxygen content and is influenced by other factors, such as release of vasoactive substances, the relative resistances in the aorta and pulmonary artery, and the differences in sensitivity of the vessel to oxygen. The ductus arteriosus produces several prostaglandins, including PGI_2 and PGE_2; both prostaglandins relax the smooth muscle of the ductus and keep the ductus patent. Meanwhile, the ductus of preterm infants is far more sensitive to the vasodilating effects of prostaglandins than is the ductus of term infants. Indomethacin is one of the most potent inhibitors of the prostaglandin-forming cyclooxygenase. Therefore, indomethacin decreases the synthesis of prostaglandins, resulting in closure of the ductus.

Clyman RI: Ontogeny of the ductus arteriosus response to prostaglandins and inhibitors of their synthesis. Semin Perinatol 4:115, 1980

Emmanouilides GC, Riemenschneider TA, Allen HD, Gutgesell HP (eds): Moss and Adams' Heart Disease in Infants, Children and Adolescents, Including the Fetus and Young Adult, 5th ed, p 747. Baltimore, Williams & Wilkins, 1995

Gregory GA (ed): Pediatric Anesthesia, 3rd ed, p 355. New York, Churchill Livingstone, 1994

Hardman JG, Limbird LE (eds): Goodman and Gilman's The Pharmacological Bases of Therapeutics, 9th ed, p 634. New York, McGraw-Hill, 1996

A.10. What is retinopathy of prematurity (retrolental fibroplasia)? Discuss its etiology, pathophysiology, prognosis, and prevention.

Retinopathy of prematurity (ROP) is seen in 3% to 43% of preterm infants, depending on the patient's gestational age. ROP begins with retinal vascular obliteration, which is followed by increased vascularity, hemorrhage, cicatrization, and finally retinal detachment. ROP refers to all stages of the disease and its sequelae. Retrolental fibroplasia (RLF), the term previously used for this disease, described only the cicatricial stages.

The factors that cause ROP and determine its outcome are not fully known, but prematurity, the degree of retinal immaturity at birth, and hyperoxia are major factors. Other contributing factors include respiratory distress, apnea, bradycardia, heart disease, infection, hypoxia, hypercarbia, acidosis, anemia, and the need for transfusion. Generally, the lower the birth weight and the sicker the infant, the greater the risk for ROP.

The retinal vasculature in the developing fetus spreads outward from the optic disc, reaching the nasal side of the retinal periphery by 36 weeks gestational age and the temporal side at 40 weeks. Classically, it was postulated that hyperoxia constricts the retinal arterioles, resulting in swelling and degeneration of the endothelium. This causes paradoxical retinal ischemia in spite of systemic hyperoxia. When normoxic conditions are restored, vascularization resumes in an aberrant manner, leading to retinal detachment and blindness.

Eighty-five percent of ROP cases undergo spontaneous recovery. Mild ROP regresses in 2 to 3 months, and moderate ROP in 6 months. The most severe ROP usually results in blindness or limited vision.

It is unclear what level of PaO_2 causes ROP, but a PaO_2 of 150 mm Hg for as short a time as 1 to 2 hours can do so. Furthermore, the retinal vessels of these neonates certainly constrict maximally with a PaO_2 of 100 mm Hg. In addition, it is also possible that ROP might develop at lower PaO_2 levels because infants of this age are normally exposed to a much lower PaO_2 (30 to 40 mm Hg) *in utero* than the levels found during the neonatal period. Therefore, in order to reduce the possibility of ROP, it is wise to maintain the PaO_2 levels between 50 and 70 mm Hg or the SaO_2 between 87% and 92% for infants <44 to 50 weeks gestation. However, prevention of ROP ultimately depends on the prevention of premature birth and its attendant problems. Oxygen alone is neither sufficient nor necessary to produce ROP, and no safe level of oxygen has yet been determined. Each infant must be treated with whatsoever is necessary to sustain life and neurologic function. Some investigations have suggested the use of vitamin E for its antioxidant effects in infants at risk for ROP. However, its efficacy has not been proven.

Behrman RE, Kliegman RM, Arvin AM (eds): Nelson Textbook of Pediatrics, 15th ed, pp 1790–1792. Philadelphia, WB Saunders, 1996

Betts EK, Downes JJ, Schaffer DB et al: Retrolental fibroplasia and oxygen administration during general anesthesia. Anesthesiology 47:518, 1977

Gregory GA (ed): Pediatric Anesthesia, 3rd ed, pp 358–359. New York, Churchill Livingstone, 1994

Lucey JF, Dongman B: A reexamination of the role of oxygen in retrolental fibroplasia. Pediatrics 73:82, 1984

Stark DJ, Manning LM, Lenton L: Retrolental fibroplasia today. Med J Aust 1:275, 1981

A.11. *Define neutral and critical temperatures. What are these values in the preterm neonate, in the term neonate, and in the adult? Discuss temperature regulation in the neonate.*

Neutral temperature is the ambient temperature that results in minimal oxygen consumption. Critical temperature is the ambient temperature below which an unclothed, unanesthetized individual cannot maintain a normal core temperature (see Table 16-2).

Normally, body heat is lost by conduction, convection, radiation, and evaporation. The neonate is particularly susceptible to heat loss owing to a large surface:volume ratio, lack of insulating fat, and naturally flaccid and open posture. When stressed by a cold environment, vasoconstriction occurs, but the neonate is unable to shiver. Further cold stress stimulates norepinephrine release, promoting the exothermic metabolism of brown fat deposits in an attempt to maintain core temperature. Continued cold stress often results in episodes of bradycardia, apnea, hypoglycemia, and metabolic acidosis.

Table 16-2. Neutral and Critical Temperature

	NEUTRAL TEMPERATURE °C	CRITICAL TEMPERATURE °C
Preterm neonate	34	28
Term neonate	32	23
Adults	28	1

Table 16-3. Normal Values of Arterial Blood Gases and *p*H in Pediatric Patients

AGE	PRETERM	TERM	1 MONTH	1 YEAR
*p*H	7.37 ± 0.03	7.40 ± 0.02	7.41 ± 0.04	7.39 ± 0.02
PaO$_2$ (torr)	60 ± 8	70 ± 11	95 ± 8	93 ± 10
PaCO$_2$ (torr)	37 ± 6	39 ± 7	40 ± 6	41 ± 7

When the infant's temperature reaches 36.6°C, dilation of peripheral vessels occurs. The term neonate will perspire at 37.2°C in an attempt to maintain a normal core temperature, whereas those infants born before 37 weeks gestation are unable to sweat.

Gregory GA (ed): Pediatric Anesthesia, 3rd ed, pp 353–354. New York, Churchill Livingstone, 1994

Silverman WA, Sinclair JC: Temperature regulation in the newborn infant. N Engl J Med 279:146, 1966

Stoelting RK, Dierdorf SF (eds): Anesthesia and Coexisting Disease, 3rd ed, p 584. New York, Churchill Livingstone, 1993

B. Preoperative Evaluation and Preparation

B.1. How would you evaluate this patient preoperatively?

The preoperative evaluation of preterm infants should be based on a clear understanding of the pathophysiology of prematurity. The preoperative evaluation of this patient should begin with a careful review of the medical record, followed by a systemic physical examination and laboratory evaluation. Specifically:

- History—birth trauma, asphyxia, maternal drug history, respiratory, cardiovascular, and fluid status
- Physical examination—evaluation of the airway, cardiopulmonary system, fluid status (skin texture, turgor, mucous membranes, and fontanelles), abdominal examination
- Laboratory data—white blood count; hemoglobin and hematocrit; serum electrolytes; serum coagulation profile, including PT, PTT, and platelet count; serum calcium and serum protein; arterial blood gases; urinalysis and urine-specific gravity; chest and abdominal radiographs

B.2. What are the normal values of arterial blood gases and pH in preterm and term pediatric patients?

The normal blood gas and *p*H values for pediatric patients are shown in Table 16-3. The normal *p*H and Pco$_2$ values for pediatric patients are similar to those for adults, whereas the normal PaO$_2$ values are lower in pediatric patients than in adult patients.

Behrman RE, Kliegman RM, Arvin AM (eds): Nelson Textbook of Pediatrics, 15th ed, pp 2051–2038. Philadelphia, WB Saunders, 1996

Gregory GA (ed): Pediatric Anesthesia, 3rd ed, p 361. New York, Churchill Livingstone, 1994

Orzalesi MM, Mendicini M, Bucci G et al: Arterial oxygen studies in premature newborns with and without mild respiratory disorders. Arch Dis Child 42:174, 1967

Table 16-4.   Normal Blood Pressure of Infants Between 1000 g and 4000 g

BIRTH WEIGHT	1000 g	2000 g	3000 g	4000 g
Systolic BP (torr)	50 ± 10	55 ± 10	60 ± 10	70 ± 10
Diastolic BP (torr)	25 ± 10	30 ± 10	35 ± 10	40 ± 10
Mean BP (torr)	35 ± 10	40 ± 10	45 ± 10	50 ± 10

B.3. Interpret the arterial blood gases: pH, 7.30; P_{CO_2}, 45 mm Hg; P_{O_2}, 60 mm Hg; HCO_3^-, 20 mEq/liter on 60% oxygen; and 5 cm H_2O of positive end-expiratory pressure (PEEP). How would you improve them?

The blood gases show mild respiratory and metabolic acidosis. The P_{O_2} of 60 mm Hg is within normal range of preterm infants, although it is lower than normal values for adult patients. In order to prevent retinopathy of prematurity, it is wise to keep P_{O_2} between 50 and 70 mm Hg. P_{CO_2} of 45 mm Hg indicates hypoventilation, which can be corrected by increasing respiratory rate or tidal volume. In order to avoid the pulmonary oxygen toxicity, F_IO_2 should be lowered to <40% by increasing levels of PEEP. Mild acidosis may be corrected by hypervention and by improving fluid balance and circulation.

B.4. What are the normal values of arterial blood pressure, heart rate, and respiratory rate for preterm infants?

The blood pressure is related to the size of infants, as shown in Table 16-4. The heavier the birth weight, the higher the blood pressure. The normal heart rate is 120 to 160 beats/min. The respiratory rate is normally between 30 and 60 breaths/min. However, it can increase to 100 to 150 breaths/min depending on how severely the lung compliance is decreased.

Gregory GA (ed): Pediatric Anesthesia, 3rd ed, p 362. New York, Churchill Livingstone, 1994

B.5. What are the normal values of WBC, RBC, hemoglobin, glucose, electrolytes, calcium, BUN, and creatinine for preterm infants?

The WBC count usually ranges from 9000 to 30,000/mm^3 at birth and decreases to 5000 to 20,000/mm^3 during the fifth week of life.

The normal RBC and hemoglobin are $5.1 \pm 1.0 \times 10^6$/mm^3 and 19.5 ± 5.0 g/dl, respectively, at birth and decrease to $4.5 \pm 0.7 \times 10^6$/mm^3 and 12.2 ± 2.3 g/dl at 3 months of age. At birth, most of the hemoglobin is fetal hemoglobin, which has a greater affinity for oxygen. Thus the oxygen saturation (and content) of blood for a given PaO_2 is higher. By 7 months of age, all hemoglobin is of the adult type.

The normal blood glucose level is between 45 and 90 mg/dl. A glucose level below 40 mg/dl is common in preterm infants. It should be corrected with a bolus of 10% to 20% glucose (2 to 5 g/kg) given over 5 minutes, followed by a continuous infusion of glucose. Severe hypoglycemia (<10 mg/dl) may cause brain damage.

The serum calcium concentration of preterm infants is normally lower than that of term infants because preterm infants have decreased serum proteins. Normal calcium level is over 8.0 mg/dl.

The normal values of sodium, potassium, and chloride are 135 to 145, 3.0 to 5.0, and 105 to 115 mEq/liter, respectively.

The creatinine levels of term infants at birth are 0.6 to 1.2 mg/dl, but within 1 month fall to levels of 0.1 to 0.2 mg/dl. Preterm infants have relatively high serum creatinine levels compared with term infants. They are 0.8 to 1.8 mg/dl at birth and fall to 0.2 to 0.8 mg/dl in 1 month.

The normal BUN level is 10 to 20 mg/dl in term infants, whereas it is 16 to 28 mg/dl in preterm infants.

Behrman RE, Kliegman RM, Arvin AM (eds): Nelson Textbook of Pediatrics, 15th ed, pp 2035–2056. Philadelphia, WB Saunders, 1996

Gregory GA (ed): Pediatric Anesthesia, 3rd ed, pp 356–364. New York, Churchill Livingstone, 1994

B.6. Would you transfuse blood to this patient preoperatively?

The patient had a hemoglobin of 11 g/dl; I would not transfuse this patient. To ensure oxygen-carrying capacity, most clinicians agree that a hemoglobin of 10 g/dl is the lowest acceptable level if cardiorespiratory disease exists. If infants are well, a hemoglobin level of above 7.0 g/dl is usually tolerable. Blood transfusion is best avoided in order to prevent the transmission of hepatitis and AIDS.

Gregory GA (ed): Pediatric Anesthesia, 3rd ed, pp 357, 364. New York, Churchill Livingstone, 1994

B.7. How would you interpret the urinalysis: specific gravity 1.005, sugar 1+, protein 1+?

In infants weighing 1000 to 3300 g, the normal urine-specific gravity is 1.005 to 1.010. A urine specific gravity of >1.020 suggests dehydration.

Glucosuria 1+ normally presents in 13% of preterm infants who are <34 weeks gestational age because the preterm infant has a decreased renal tubular reabsorption for glucose. After 34 weeks of gestational age, glucosuria is usually associated with hyperglycemia.

Albumin is normally filtered by the glomerulus and is completely reabsorbed. However, because of tubular immaturity, 16% to 21% of preterm infants have proteinuria.

Grant BS Jr: Developmental patterns of renal functional maturation compared in the human neonate. J Pediatr 92:705, 1978

Jones MD, Gersham EL, Battaglia FC: Urinary flow rates and urea excretion rates in newborn infants. Biol Neonate 21:321, 1972

Rhodes PG, Hammel CL, Berman LB: Urinary constituents of the newborn infant. J Pediatr 60:18, 1962

B.8. Would you correct a serum calcium of 6.0 mg/dl? What other information would you like to have? Which contains more calcium, 10 cc of 10% calcium chloride or 10 cc of 10% calcium gluconate? Could you hyperventilate this child safely?

Normally, the serum calcium is maintained at 8.0 mg/dl; however, in the preterm infant a level of 7.0 mg/dl is acceptable. This child's serum calcium is 6.0 mg/dl. Therefore, supplementation with 100 to 200 mg/kg of calcium gluconate is appropriate.

When evaluating the serum calcium levels, it is important to know the serum protein concentration; neonatal hypocalcemia is usually due to hypoproteinemia. It is also important to determine the ionized calcium concentration (usually 45% of the total calcium concentration), since this is the calcium immediately available at the cellular level. The chloride molecule is approximately one-third the weight of the gluconate molecule. For this reason, approximately three times more calcium is given when an equivalent volume of calcium chloride is administered instead of 10% calcium gluconate. Respiratory alkalosis following hyperventilation will reduce serum ionized calcium levels and for this reason should be avoided in this infant.

Gregory GA (ed): Pediatric Anesthesia, 3rd ed, p 364. New York, Churchill Livingstone, 1994

Stoelting RK, Dierdorf SF (eds): Anesthesia and Coexisting Disease, 3rd ed, pp 329–331. New York, Churchill Livingstone, 1993

B.9. How would you premedicate this patient?

Children under 1 year of age do not need sedation. However, atropine, 0.01 to 0.02 mg/kg, may be given to attenuate the vagal response to a host of different stimuli.

Lake CL (ed): Pediatric Cardiac Anesthesia, 3rd ed, p 455. Stamford, CT, Appleton & Lange, 1998

C. Intraoperative Management

C.1. What monitors would you use for this child during surgery?

Proper monitoring of this child for safe administration of anesthesia includes the following:

- Respiratory—precordial or esophageal stethoscope, end-tidal CO_2, inspiratory oxygen monitor, pulse oximeter, arterial blood gases, inspiratory pressure gauge
- Cardiovascular—precordial or esophageal stethoscope, electrocardiogram, blood pressure cuff and Doppler transducer, urinary bag
- Thermoregulatory—esophageal or axillary temperature probe with servoloop overhead heater, thermal blanket

If the patient has an umbilical artery catheter in place, it is useful for the measurement of blood pressure and arterial blood gases. However, it is probably unnecessary to establish an arterial line for the surgery alone because invasive monitoring in this age group is not without risk.

C.2. How does the oxygen analyzer work?

Oxygen analysis can be done by either parametric or ampometric analysis. Parametric analysis is based on the fact that oxygen is a dipole molecule. When a gas containing oxygen is passed through a magnetic field, the gas is deflected in proportion to the concentration of oxygen. Sensors can detect this deflection and give a readout of oxygen concentration. Ampometric analysis can be done with 1 of 2 devices: the galvanic cell analyzer and the polarographic cell analyzer. In the galvanic or fuel cell analyzer, oxygen diffuses through a membrane of the sensor into an electrolyte solution from which the oxygen absorbs electrons and forms hydroxide ions. The hydroxide ions then diffuse to a lead anode where oxidation to lead oxide and water occurs with the resultant liberation of free electrons. An electron flow (current) is thereby generated between the anode and the cathode, which is proportional to the oxygen level at the sensor. This current is directly displayed by a meter that indicates oxygen percentage. These devices are relatively inexpensive to purchase but carry a high operating cost because the sensor is eventually exhausted and must be replaced.

The polarographic cell, or Clark electrode, uses a battery to induce a negative potential of 0.75 volts between the anode and the cathode. As oxygen diffuses across a membrane and into the electrolyte solution separating the anode and cathode, the polarizing voltage at the cathode causes electrons to combine with oxygen molecules, reducing them to hydroxide ions. The hydroxide ions then move to the anode, causing electron flow (current) that is proportional to the initial oxygen concentration. This flow is read by a meter that translates to oxygen percentages. These monitors are initially more expensive than galvanic cell monitors, but they are less expensive to maintain, requiring only inexpensive electrolyte solution and battery replacement.

Saidman LJ, Smith NT (eds): Monitoring in Anesthesia, 3rd ed, p 384. Boston, Butterworth-Heinemann, 1993

C.3. What is the Doppler effect? How does the Doppler transducer measure blood pressure?

In 1841 Christian Doppler noted the change in observed frequency from a constant frequency sound generator when the source moved with respect to the observer. Ballot confirmed this "Doppler effect" in 1845 with the simple example of the frequency increase in a train's steam whistle as the train approached an observer. In the 1960s Ware described a practical ultrasonic system for transducing arterial wall motion to obtain blood pressure. The ultrasonic system consists of an occlusive cuff and a dual-crystal ultrasonic transducer placed over the artery distal to the occlusion. One crystal transmits the ultrasonic signal while the other receives the signal reflected from the artery. While the artery is occluded by the cuff, there is no arterial wall movement and the crystal receives a signal with an unchanged frequency. When the cuff pressure falls below systolic pressure, arterial wall motion occurs, causing a Doppler frequency shift, indicating systolic blood pressure. When the cuff pressure falls to diastolic pressure, the artery is open throughout the cycle: rhythmic arterial opening and closing does not occur and there is a loss of Doppler frequency shift. Thus, one can easily and accurately obtain systolic and diastolic blood pressure.

Saidman LJ, Smith NT (eds): Monitoring in Anesthesia, 3rd ed, p 121. Boston, Butterworth-Heinemann, 1993

C.4. What is the mechanism of pulse oximetry? Why is it important to monitor arterial oxygen saturation? What levels of arterial oxygen saturation would you like to keep during surgery?

The mechanism of pulse oximetry is described in Chapter 2, question C.20.

Safe anesthesia practice requires the monitoring of arterial oxygen saturation in all patients to prevent hypoxia. However, in infants of <44 to 50 weeks gestation, it is also vital to guard against hyperoxia, which may cause retinopathy of prematurity.

The arterial oxygen saturation should be kept between 86% and 92% (some say 85% to 95%).

Lake CL (ed): Pediatric Cardiac Anesthesia, 3rd ed, pp 455–456. Stamford, CT, Appleton & Lange, 1998

Purohit DM, Ellison RC, Fierler S et al: Risks of retrolental fibroplasia: Experience with 3025 premature infants. Pediatrics 76:339, 1985

Wasunna A, Whitlaw AGL: Pulse oximetry in preterm infants. Arch Dis Child 62:957, 1987

C.5. How would you maintain the patient's body temperature?

Hypothermia greatly increases the metabolic rate and oxygen consumption of preterm infants. The preterm infant is particularly susceptible to heat loss because of a large surface-to-volume ratio, lack of insulating fat, and a naturally flaccid and open posture. In addition, the preterm infant often has impaired thermal regulatory ability; therefore, all precautions must be taken to ensure normothermia. The patient may be transported to the operating room in a battery-operated transport incubator if available. Otherwise, the infant should be covered with Saran Wrap and a warm blanket, and a cap should be put on his or her head to prevent heat loss. The operating room should be warmed to 35° to 37°C and a servo-controlled infrared heater placed over the operating table. A water-circulating heating blanket should be put under the table sheet and kept at 37° to 38°C. All extremities should be wrapped in sheet wadding. All intravenous fluids and inspired gases should be warmed to help maintain the patient's body temperature.

Gregory GA (ed): Pediatric Anesthesia, 3rd ed, p 368. New York, Churchill Livingstone, 1994

C.6. How do the anesthetic requirements of the preterm infant differ from those of the adult?

Achieving proper anesthetic depth in the preterm infant presents a unique challenge to the anesthesiologist. Whereas anesthetic requirements (as determined by MAC) are decreased in the preterm infant as compared with the adult, cardiovascular sensitivity is greatly pronounced because of greater myocardial depression and a reduced peripheral response to catecholamines. Further, the baroreceptor reflex, often poorly developed in the preterm infant, is totally ablated by even light levels of inhalation anesthesia. Thus, the preterm infant is extremely susceptible to anesthetic overdose, which produces cardiovascular depression leading to hypotension or cardiovascular collapse.

Unfortunately, an inadequate depth of anesthesia is also uniquely hazardous in the neonate. Because there is a lack of cerebral autoregulation, any systemic hypertension from inadequate depth of anesthesia may be transmitted directly to the cerebral circulation, resulting in intraventricular hemorrhage.

For these reasons, it is essential to carefully tailor anesthetic depth to surgical conditions, since the therapeutic margin between underdose and overdose is extremely narrow.

Gregory GA: The baroresponses of preterm infants during halothane anesthesia. Can Anaesth Soc J 29:105, 1982

Lou HC, Lassen PH, Fris-Hansen B: Impaired autoregulation of cerebral blood flow in the distressed newborn infant. J Pediatr 94:118, 1979

C.7. What size endotracheal tube would you have used if the patient had not been intubated?

The larynx of a full-term neonate usually accommodates a 3.0-mm or 3.5-mm endotracheal tube, whereas infants weighing <3500 g tolerate a 3.0-mm tube. In infants weighing <1500 g, a 2.5-mm (ID) tube is usually recommended. The endotracheal tube should be large enough to allow easy ventilation but small enough to permit leaking of gas between the tube and trachea when the lung is ventilated with 15 to 20 cm H_2O pressure. However, a higher leak pressure of 25 to 35 cm H_2O may be aimed for when high peak inspiratory pressures may be required during anesthesia, e.g., during a thoracotomy or an upper laparotomy, or if the patient has decreased pulmonary compliance.

Gregory GA (ed): Pediatric Anesthesia, 3rd ed, pp 215–228. New York, Churchill Livingstone, 1994

C.8. How would you have induced anesthesia if the patient had not been intubated?

Preterm infants do need anesthesia for surgery. The patient should be preoxygenated with 100% oxygen, and ventilation should be controlled; otherwise, the preterm infant develops apnea and bradycardia. Anesthesia is induced with fentanyl, 5 µg/kg, and thiopental sodium, 1 mg/kg intravenously. When the lid reflexes are lost, the infant is intubated without muscle relaxants. As the endotracheal tube is being inserted, an assistant should place a finger in the suprasternal notch to feel the tip of the tube. When it hits his or her finger, the tube is fixed and taped in place. Of course, breath sounds should be checked bilaterally to ensure that the tube is properly positioned.

Alternatively, anesthesia may be induced with an inhalation anesthetic such as halothane. However, halothane often causes hypotension and bradycardia in preterm infants because of its cardiovascular depression.

High doses of fentanyl, 30 to 50 µg/kg, have been used for induction. However, hypotension often occurs because of vasodilation, and the infant has to be resuscitated with a relatively large amount of Ringer's lactate, 10 ml/kg. Therefore, we recommend the use of fentanyl 10 to 30 µg/kg alone or fentanyl 5 µg/kg with thiopental 1 mg/kg for induction.

Robinson SR, Gregory GA: Fentanyl-air oxygen anesthesia for ligation of patent ductus arteriosus in preterm infants. Anesth Analg 60:504, 1981

C.9. How would you maintain anesthesia?

Because preterm infants are extremely sensitive to cardiovascular depression from inhalation anesthetics, we prefer to use fentanyl with or without nitrous oxide for maintenance of anesthesia. Increments of fentanyl, 5 µg/kg, are titrated to maintain hemodynamic stability. A bolus injection of high-dose fentanyl, 30 to 50 µg/kg, often causes hypotension since the infant is usually dehydrated as a result of fluid restriction and diuretic therapy for congestive heart failure from patent ductus arteriosus. Ketamine may be used alone or as a supplement to fentanyl-air-oxygen anesthesia.

Pancuronium, 0.1 mg/kg, is an attractive choice for muscle relaxation because it causes mild tachycardia and the infant's blood pressure is dependent on heart rate.

Lake CL (ed): Pediatric Cardiac Anesthesia, 3rd ed, p 456. Stamford, CT, Appleton & Lange, 1998

Robinson SR, Gregory GA: Fentanyl-air-oxygen anesthesia for ligation of patent ductus arteriosus in preterm infants. Anesth Analg 60:504, 1981

C.10. How would you ventilate the patient? What tidal volume, respiratory rates, and F_1O_2 would you set for the infant?

Controlled ventilation should be employed because preterm infants do not breathe well under anesthesia. The patient may be ventilated by hand with a Jackson-Reese device. The technique allows instantaneous compensation for changes in pulmonary compliance and resistance, especially during thoracotomy. It also permits the use of PEEP. If extra hands are not available, a mechanical ventilation, preferably with a pediatric bellows, may be used to ventilate the infant.

During spontaneous respiration, normal tidal volume is 7 ml/kg for all ages. However, the ventilator tidal volumes calculated on the basis of body weight for adult patients, such as 10 ml/kg, are not applicable for pediatric patients, especially small infants. A large amount of ventilator-delivered tidal volume is lost through the large compression volume of the anesthesia breathing circuit and the leak around the uncuffed endotracheal tube. For example, if the compression volume of the anesthesia ventilator is 4.5 ml/cm H_2O (a value typical for adult ventilators) and the ventilator is set to deliver a 100-ml tidal volume to a patient at 20 cm H_2O peak inspiratory pressure, 90 ml is lost to compression volume: only 10 ml is delivered to the patient. In addition, if pulmonary and chest wall compliances change during anesthesia and surgery, the delivered tidal volume to the patient will also be changed. Therefore, it is wise to set tidal volume whatever necessary to achieve the desired inspiratory pressures, such as those used in the neonatal intensive care unit prior to surgery. Usually the peak inspiratory pressures are set between 15 and 25 cm H_2O, depending on the patient's respiratory condition, to ensure adequate chest expansion.

The respiratory rates and inspiratory pressures are adjusted as needed to maintain the $PaCO_2$ between 35 and 40 mm Hg or the end-tidal CO_2 between 30 and 35 mm Hg. The F_1O_2 is adjusted to keep the PaO_2 between 50 and 70 mm Hg or the arterial oxygen saturation between 87% and 92% (practically 90% to 95%).

Gregory GA (ed): Pediatric Anesthesia, 3rd ed, p 366. New York, Churchill Livingstone, 1994

Robins L, Crooker D, Smith RM: Tidal volume losses of volume limited ventilators. Anesth Analg 46:428, 1967

C.11. Discuss blood and fluid therapy in this preterm infant.

Fluid therapy should be aimed at correcting the preoperative deficit, providing maintenance fluid, and replacing intraoperative evaporative, third-space, and blood loss.

Intraoperative blood loss must be carefully estimated by weighing the sponges and using small calibrated suction bottles in plain view of the anesthesiologist. The preterm infant's blood volume is only 80 to 95 ml (85 to 100 ml/kg); therefore, even a 10-ml blood loss can be critical. Despite these precautions, estimation of blood loss is inevitably inaccurate because of the unmeasured loss in the drapes and tissues. For this reason, it is recommended that 125% to 150% of measured blood loss be replaced. Each milliliter of estimated blood loss is replaced with 3 ml of Ringer's lactate or 1 ml of 5% albumin in saline. If the hematocrit is low (<30%) to begin with, blood losses are replaced with packed red blood cells.

Maintenance fluids consisting of 5% dextrose in one-fourth strength normal saline are given at 4 ml/kg/h, whereas evaporative and third-space losses are replaced with Ringer's lactate at 8 to 12 ml/kg/h for abdominal or thoracic procedures. The adequacy of blood and fluid therapy may be ensured by stable blood pressure, normal central venous pressure (over 3 cm H_2O), and an adequate urine output of >0.75 ml/kg/h and specific gravity of <1.010. In addition, the infant's fontanelle should be above the inner table of the skull if there is no volume depletion.

Dierdorf SF, Krishna G: Anesthetic management of neonatal surgical emergencies. Anesth Analg 60:204–214, 1981

Gregory GA (ed): Pediatric Anesthesia, 3rd ed, pp 366–368. New York, Churchill Livingstone, 1994

C.12. *During dissection of the ductus arteriosus, the arterial oxygen saturation dropped from 92% to 80% and the heart rate decreased from 140 beats/min to 80 beats/min. What were the causes? How would you correct this situation?*

Pediatric patients, especially preterm infants, develop hypoxemia quickly after hypoventilation because they have high metabolism (increased oxygen demand) and low functional residual capacity (decreased oxygen reserve). During dissection of the ductus arteriosus, the ipsilateral lung is retracted and compressed by the surgeon. Therefore, the pulmonary resistance increases and pulmonary compliance decreases. Consequently, the delivered tidal volume to the patient decreases and the gas leak around the endotracheal tube increases if the inspiratory pressures remain unchanged. Decreasing tidal volume causes hypoventilation, resulting in hypoxemia and CO_2 retention. In addition, compressing the lung tissue increases intrapulmonary shunt, which causes further hypoxemia. In pediatric patients, bradycardia is most commonly caused by hypoxemia. During dissection of the ductus arteriosus, surgical manipulation of the vagus nerve and lung tissue may initiate vagal reflex, with resultant bradycardia.

The infant should be manually ventilated with 100% oxygen to correct hypoxemia and bradycardia. If bradycardia persists, atropine, 0.01 to 0.02 mg/kg, should be given. The surgical manipulation should be stopped and the collapsed lung reexpanded. Blood loss or hypovolemia should also be corrected.

When the hemodynamic status and oxygenation are stabilized, the F_1O_2 and respiratory pressures should be adjusted to ensure adequate ventilation and oxygenation.

D. Postoperative Management

D.1. *Would you reverse the muscle relaxants and extubate the patient at the end of surgery?*

No. Postoperative ventilatory support would be necessary for this preterm infant with respiratory distress syndrome; therefore, reversal of muscle relaxation and extubation are not indicated.

D.2. *How can one minimize the risk of transporting the patient to the neonatal intensive care unit after surgery?*

The anesthesiologist's responsibilities do not end with the successful completion of the operative procedure. Removal of the surgical drapes must be done with caution to prevent inadvertent extubation or removal of the arterial or venous cannula. Transportation of the infant to the neonatal intensive care unit is an extremely hazardous transition and requires watchful vigilance. Arrangements must be made in advance so that elevators are waiting and the nursery is ready to accept the patient. The anesthesiologist must accompany the child until satisfied that care has been appropriately transferred to the neonatal nursery staff.

The same monitors that were employed for surgery must be used in transport, including ECG and monitors for arterial blood pressure and oxygen saturation. Ventilation should be maintained by hand with a Jackson-Reese device or by a battery-operated transport ventilator, and the child should not be transported with 100% oxygen unless it was used for the operative procedure. A precordial stethoscope is especially helpful to monitor the adequacy of respiration and heart sounds. Finally, every effort to ensure thermal stability must be made, including the use of a heated isolette (if possible), Saran Wrap, warm blankets, and a cap on the infant's head.

D.3. The patient's condition deteriorated postoperatively in the intensive care unit. Physical examination revealed persistent cardiac murmur. What was the possible diagnosis?

It has been reported that a large ductus arteriosus arising from the aortic arch proximal to the subclavian artery creates the illusion of the arch, leading to surgical closure of the distal left pulmonary artery instead of ductus arteriosus (Fig. 16-1). The ductus arteriosus was not ligated; therefore, the ductus murmur persisted. Inadvertent ligation of the distal left pulmonary artery resulted in pulmonary ischemia distal to the ligation. Meanwhile, the right lung was further flooded with the shunted

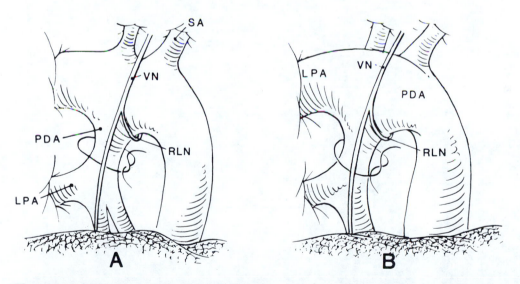

Figure 16-1. **(A)** Anatomically atypical patent ductus arteriosus arising proximal to the left subclavian artery. **(B)** Large patent ductus arteriosus sweeping into the descending aorta and appearing to be the arch. The ductus overlies the arch and hides it from view. A large distal left pulmonary artery is misinterpreted as the patent ductus (encircled by ligature). PDA, patent ductus arteriosus; LPA, left pulmonary artery; SA, subclavian artery; VN, vagus nerve; RLN, recurrent laryngeal nerve. (Reprinted with permission from Pontius RG, Danielson GK, Noonan JA et al: Illusions leading to surgical closure to the distal left pulmonary artery instead of the ductus arteriosus. J Thorac Cardiovasc Surg 82:103-107, 1981)

blood through the unligated PDA. The resultant ventilation/perfusion maldistribution ($\dot{V}/\dot{Q}$ abnormalities) caused further hypoxemia and CO_2 retention in this infant. The patient should be brought to the operating room for repair of the left pulmonary artery and ligation of the ductus arteriosus.

To prevent this complication, an esophageal stethoscope should be placed to monitor the change or disappearance of the murmur upon temporary occlusion of the suspected ductus.

Pontius RG, Danielson GK, Noonan JA et al: Illusions leading to surgical closure to the distal left pulmonary artery instead of the ductus arteriosus. J Thorac Cardiovasc Surg 82:103–107, 1981

Heart Transplantation and Subsequent Noncardiac Surgery

17

Davy C.H. Cheng

A 56-year-old man with end-stage ischemic heart disease and recurrent congestive heart failure was scheduled for heart transplantation. He had a long-standing history of coronary artery disease with multiple myocardial infarctions and had two coronary revascularization surgeries 11 and 8 years prior to this admission. His condition continued to deteriorate in the last 6 months with clinical signs of low output failure, loss of appetite, cachexia, and a significant decrease in exercise capacity. His medications included digoxin, furosemide, nitroglycerin, cilazapril, warfarin, potassium chloride, and fluoxetine. An electrocardiogram (ECG) showed a sinus rhythm with frequent premature ventricular contractions (PVC) and a left bundle branch block. A nuclear ventriculogram showed a left ventricular ejection fraction of 9% that fell to 5% with exercise. Pulmonary arterial pressure (PAP) was 40/22 mm Hg and pulmonary capillary wedge pressure (PCWP) was 19 mm Hg.

A. Medical Disease and Differential Diagnosis

1. What are the common diagnoses for adult heart transplant?
2. What are the criteria for recipient selection?
3. What are the criteria for donor heart selection?
4. What is the current survival rate for heart transplantation?
5. What are the risk factors associated with post-transplant mortality?
6. What is the sequence of surgical anastomoses in heart transplantation?

B. Preoperative Evaluation and Preparation

1. How would you assess this patient preoperatively?
2. What is particularly important for the patient who has had previous cardiac surgery?
3. How would you premedicate this patient? Why?

C. Intraoperative Management

1. What anesthetic equipment and monitors would you set up? Why?
2. How would you conduct the anesthesia induction?
3. How would you manage the patient safely onto cardiopulmonary bypass (CPB)?
4. How would you manage this patient during CPB?

D. Postoperative Management

1. What are the early postoperative complications?
2. What are the mechanisms of right ventricular failure following heart transplantation?
3. How would you treat right ventricular failure following heart transplantation?

4. How does inhaled nitric oxide (NO) work as a selective pulmonary vasodilator?
5. What is the pathophysiology of denervated heart?
6. What are the common cardiac dysrhythmias following heart transplant?
7. What are the causes of post-transplant bleeding?
8. How would you treat post-transplant bleeding?
9. What are the causes of early graft failure?
10. How would you manage this patient in the intensive care unit?

E. Subsequent Noncardiac Surgery

The patient had a successful heart transplant. However, 5 months after heart transplant, he developed urinary retention and was scheduled for a transurethral resection of the prostate.
1. How would you monitor this patient?
2. What type of anesthetic is best for the heart transplanted patient?
3. Which anesthetic technique would you give this patient?
4. Do you need to use a muscarinic antagonist with anticholinesterase to reverse the muscle relaxant in heart transplanted patients?
5. What are the anesthetic implications for heart transplanted patients?
6. What is the significant implication of the denervated heart?
7. What is the significant implication of allograft rejection?
8. What is the significant implication of infection?
9. What is the significant implication of drug interaction?
10. What is the significant implication of allograft coronary artery disease (CAD)?
11. What is the significant implication of post-transplant hypertension?
12. What is the significant implication of renal dysfunction?

A. Medical Disease and Differential Diagnosis

A.1. What are the common diagnoses for adult heart transplant?

Heart transplantation is now considered to be a viable treatment option for selected patients with end-stage heart disease. At present, >3000 heart transplants are done annually worldwide. The indications or diagnoses for adult heart transplant as reported to the Registry of the International Society for Heart and Lung Transplantation are shown in Figure 17-1. Ischemic coronary artery disease (47.2%) and cardiomyopathy (43.5%) represent the most frequent causes for transplantation.

A.2. What are the criteria for recipient selection?

The criteria include all of the following:

- End-stage heart disease with a life expectancy of <6 to 12 months
- Physiologic age <60 years
- Absence of:
  - Active systemic or pulmonary infection
  - Irreversible pulmonary hypertension: pulmonary vascular resistance (PVR) >5 wood units, or transpulmonary pressure gradient >15 mm Hg (1 wood unit = 80 dyne·sec·cm^{-5})
  - Renal or hepatic dysfunction

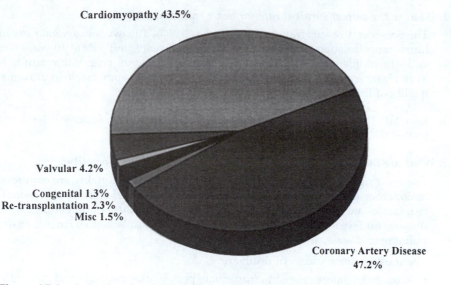

Figure 17-1. *Indications for adult heart transplantation. (Reprinted with permission from Hosenpud JD, Novick RJ, Breen TJ et al: The Registry of the International Society for Heart and Lung Transplantation: Eleventh Official Report—1994. J Heart Lung Transplant 13:561–570, 1994)*

- Severe chronic obstructive pulmonary disease, peripheral vascular disease, stroke, or active peptic ulcer
- Incurable malignancy
- Compliance, psychological stability, supportive social environment

Jhaveri R, Tardiff B, Stanley TE III: Anesthesia for heart and heart-lung transplantation. Anesthesiol Clin North Am 12:729–747, 1994

A.3. What are the criteria for donor heart selection?

The limiting factor in heart transplantation is the shortage of donor organs. It has been documented that 20% to 40% of patients on transplant lists will die while waiting for an allograft. Some specific criteria are important to the cardiac donor. The donor should not have sustained prolonged cardiac arrest, severe chest trauma, intracardiac injections, septicemia, or excessive inotropic support. In all cases, a careful clinical examination of the potential donor heart is definitive to rule out coronary artery atherosclerosis and contractile dysfunction at harvest.

Blood ABO compatibility is important as mismatch may result in hyperacute rejection. The donor body weight should be within 20% of that of the recipient. In fact, it is often desirable for the donor to be larger than the recipient if the latter has an elevated PVR. The donor heart ischemic time, defined as the time from aortal cross-clamp at harvest to cross-clamp removal following transplant, is under 4 to 6 hours and is considered to be an acceptable limit.

Jhaveri R, Tardiff B, Stanley TE III: Anesthesia for heart and heart-lung transplantation. Anesthesiol Clin North Am 12:729–747, 1994

A.4. What is the current survival rate for heart transplantation?

The postoperative survival rate at 30 days is 91.5%. The overall survival rates in heart transplantation are 80% at 1 year, 75% at 3 years, and 50% at 10 years worldwide. In addition, heart transplant survivors have a >90% chance to return to New York Heart Association Class I functional capacity with appreciable improvement in quality of life.

Kaye MP: The Registry of the International Society for Heart Transplantation: Tenth official report—1993. J Heart Lung Transplant 12:541–548, 1993

A.5. What are the risk factors associated with post-transplant mortality?

The most significant preoperative risk factors for 30-day mortality are requirement of amiodarone therapy, being on life support, and hypertension; for 1-year mortality the risk factors are retransplantation, insulin-dependent diabetes, and peripheral vascular disease; for 5-year mortality the risk factors are retransplantation, chronic obstructive pulmonary disease, and ventricular assist device.

The most common causes of death are:

- Acute heart failure related to inadequate preservation methods and other intraoperative problems resulting in graft failure
- Severe pulmonary hypertension with secondary right ventricular failure
- Less commonly, early allograft rejection

Bourge RC, Naftel DC, Costanzo-Nordin MR et al: Pre-transplantation risk factors for death after heart transplantation: A multi-institutional study. J Heart Lung Transplant 12:549–562, 1993

Kaye MP: The Registry of the International Society for Heart Transplantation: Tenth official report—1993. J Heart Lung Transplant 12:541–548, 1993

A.6. What is the sequence of surgical anastomoses in heart transplantation?

The heart is excised transecting the great vessels and leaving cuffs of both left and right atria to minimize the number of anastomoses that need to be performed. The donor heart is prepared by creating a left atrial and right atrial cuff. The sinoatrial node is preserved. Following atrial anastomoses, the aortal anastomosis is often performed before the pulmonary artery to allow for earlier removal of the aortal crossclamp.

Gallagher RC, Kormos RL: Heart transplantation. In: Makowka L (ed): Handbook of Transplantation Management, p 254. Austin, RG Landes Co, 1991

B. Preoperative Evaluation and Preparation

B.1. How would you assess this patient preoperatively?

Because of time constraints associated with the coordination of donor and recipient matching and organ procurement, anesthesia is usually informed of the impending transplant only a few hours before operation. Preoperatively, the anesthesiologist should review the recipient's pertinent anesthetic history, concomitant diseases, current cardiac status including medications and level of mechanical support, and in particular, the hemodynamic parameters and reversibility of elevated PVR. Because of the emergency basis of these procedures, it should be taken into consideration that these patients probably have a full stomach.

Recipients with preoperative significant transpulmonary pressure gradient (>15 mm Hg) and high PVR (>5 wood units), and not responsive to vasodilator challenge, have a poor chance of survival following cardiac transplantation. Typically two types of patients present for heart transplantation. The first type of patient is relatively compensated requiring possible intravenous inotropic support or may even be ambulatory in a nonhospital setting, whereas the second type is moribund and decompensated requiring mechanical ventilation or mechanical circulatory support. The relative distribution of patients in the second group is subject to institutional differences, varying from 2% to 22% incidence.

Costard-Jackle A, Hill I, Schroeder JS et al: The influence of preoperative patient characteristics on early and late survival following cardiac transplantation. Circulation 84:329–337, 1991

Hensley FA Jr, Martin DE, Larach DR et al: Anesthetic management for cardiac transplantation in North America—1986 survey. J Cardiothorac Anesth 1:429–437, 1987

B.2. What is particularly important for the patient who has had previous cardiac surgery?

Recipients who have undergone prior cardiac surgery need to be identified to increase the surgical time to achieve cardiopulmonary bypass (CPB) because of adhesion and bleeding. Coordination with the surgical team is imperative so that anesthesia induction time and donor heart ischemic time can be minimized.

B.3. How would you premedicate this patient? Why?

Patients should be transported to the operating room with oxygen supplementation. Premedication, if any, should be limited to H_2-receptor antagonists, rather than narcotic or sedative drugs. With minimal cardiac reserve, sedation may blunt the patient's respiratory and sympathomimetic drive, leading to hypoxemia, hypercapnia, and even hypotension. Infection prophylaxis includes preoperative cephazolin (1 g) intravenous (IV), postoperative trimethoprim and sulfamethoxazole, acyclovir, and immunogamma globulin therapy. Immunosuppression protocol includes preoperative methylprednisolone (0.25 mg/kg every 6 hours) and postoperative prednisone, azathioprine, rabbit antithymocyte serum, and cyclosporine therapy.

Jhaveri R, Tardiff B, Stanley TE III: Anesthesia for heart and heart-lung transplantation. Anesthesiol Clin North Am 12:729–747, 1994

C. Intraoperative Management

C.1. What anesthetic equipment and monitors would you set up? Why?

Anesthetic equipment includes a ventilator with air mixture capability, airway and intubation set-up, fluid and blood warmer, extracorporeal bypass machine with membrane oxygenator, nitric oxide (NO) delivery, and a monitoring system (Pulmonox II electrochemical analyzer) if the patient has severe pulmonary hypertension.

The patient is taken to the operating room breathing supplemental oxygen. Monitors include a 5-lead ECG, digital pulse oximeter, blood pressure cuff, capnography, temperature probe, and peripheral nerve stimulator. All invasive lines are placed with meticulous attention to aseptic technique and titrated sedation. A No. 14 gauge IV line and a No. 20 gauge radial arterial catheter for continuous blood pressure monitoring are inserted. We routinely inserted a pulmonary arterial (PA) catheter via the right internal jugular vein for preinduction, post-CPB, and postoperative measurement of pulmonary arterial pressure, pulmonary vascular resistance, and cardiac output. The PA catheter is withdrawn back to about 20-cm position in a 80-cm sterile sleeve before cardiectomy. In some centers, transesophageal echocardiography is routinely used to monitor ventricular filling and contractility.

C.2. How would you conduct the anesthesia induction?

It is important to time both anesthesia induction and surgery carefully to achieve CPB at the time of donor heart arrival to minimize ischemia time, particularly for a resternotomy patient. We routinely perform a modified rapid-sequence induction, as the recipient is not always properly fasted for transplantation surgery. The patient is anesthetized with fentanyl (10 to 15 µg/kg), midazolam (1 to 2 mg), and muscular paralysis is achieved with pancuronium (0.15 mg/kg) while maintaining cricoid pressure. Succinylcholine is not usually used because of concern of bradycardia during induction, as blood pressure in a heart transplant recipient is heart rate dependent.

We routinely infuse an antifibrinolytic agent, tranexamic acid (100 mg/kg), over 20 minutes prior to sternotomy to prevent excess blood loss post-CPB. A variety of regimens have been used successfully for induction and maintenance of anesthesia including fentanyl, sufentanil, etomidate, ketamine, and midazolam. Drug dosage should be titrated and adjusted for a prolonged circulation time and reduced volume of distribution associated with low cardiac output state. Direct laryngoscopy is performed and the trachea is intubated. A nasogastric or orogastric tube, oral pharyngeal temperature probe, and urinary catheter are inserted carefully to avoid trauma, nasal bleeding, and bacteremia.

Jhaveri R, Tardiff B, Stanley TE III: Anesthesia for heart and heart-lung transplantation. Anesthesiol Clin North Am 12:729–747, 1994

C.3. How would you manage the patient safely onto cardiopulmonary bypass (CPB)?

The primary objective postinduction is to maintain the patient safely onto CPB. The overall performance of the failing native heart is determined by impaired contractility, preload dependence, and afterload sensitivity. Because the recipient's diseased heart will no longer be needed after the transplant, the major concern is to augment an adequate perfusion pressure within the autoregulatory range for both the brain and kidney. Hypotension can be treated by an inotrope, vasoconstrictor, and fluid. Anesthesia is maintained with supplemental fentanyl (up to 20 µg/kg), midazolam (0.1 mg/kg), and isoflurane. Controlled ventilation is accomplished with oxygen or oxygen and air mixtures. Nitrous oxide is avoided because of the blunting of hypoxic pulmonary vasoconstrictive reflex, and the possibility of causing pulmonary hypertension by increasing pulmonary vascular resistance. Heparin (400 U/kg) is administrated and activated clotting time (ACT) is checked prior to aortal, inferior, and superior vena cavae cannulation.

Clark NJ, Martin RD: Anesthetic considerations for patients undergoing cardiac transplantation. J Cardiothorac Anesth 2:519–542, 1988

Schulte-Sasse U, Hess W, Tarnow J: Pulmonary vascular responses to nitrous oxide in patients with normal and high pulmonary vascular resistance. Anesthesiology 57:9–13, 1982

C.4. How would you manage this patient during CPB?

The anesthetic management of CPB in these patients does not differ from that in nontransplant patients, except that rewarming is usually prolonged because of the profound cooling of the donor heart and the prolonged ischemic time. Early in the perfusion, mixed venous oxygen desaturation and metabolic acidosis must be corrected. The fluid balance, hematocrit, and electrolyte composition of the blood must be closely monitored. During CPB, anesthesia maintenance has been achieved by narcotic supplementation, an inhalational agent and/or benzodiazepine. We routinely use propofol (2 to 6 mg/kg/h and lower to 2 mg/kg/h on rewarming) or supplement with isoflurane. If spontaneous defibrillation has not occurred when core temperature is 35° to 36°C, electrical defibrillation is undertaken. Once cardiac rhythm has been established and anastomosis of the pulmonary artery is completed, the patient is placed in a head-down position for air evacuation from the left side of the heart. Once the heart is in place and the aorta unclamped, isoproterenol infusion (1 to 5 µg/min) is begun to improve contractility and to increase heart rate to about 90 to 110 beats/min.

D. Postoperative Management

D.1. What are the early postoperative complications?

The early postoperative complications include:

- Right ventricular failure/Pulmonary hypertension
- Denervated heart
- Bleeding
- Early graft failure

D.2. What are the mechanisms of right ventricular failure following heart transplantation?

Right ventricular failure is a major cause of early mortality (0 to 2 days) in heart transplantation. This results from persistent or abruptly elevated pulmonary vascular resistance after CPB, which places a significant afterload on the newly implanted heart with stunned myocardium.

The stunned myocardium has just undergone an extended period of global ischemia. It must work against a significant right ventricular afterload because of increased PVR in patients with refractory cardiomyopathy, particularly if the donor heart is relatively smaller in size. This results in a heart with depressed contractility, relatively fixed stroke volume, and increased right ventricular afterload. Cardiac output is therefore dependent on improving the above parameters and on heart rate.

Bhatia SJ, Kirshenbaum JM, Shemin RJ et al: Time course of resolution of pulmonary hypertension and right ventricular remodeling after orthotopic cardiac transplantation. Circulation 76:819–826, 1987

D.3. How would you treat right ventricular failure following heart transplantation?

Phosphodiesterase inhibitors such as amrinone or milrinone, which have systemic and pulmonary vasodilatory effects in addition to positive inotropy, are particularly useful. Prostacyclin (PGI_2), prostaglandin E_1, isoproterenol (1 to 5 µg/min), and nitrates have also been successfully used to treat transient increases in pulmonary vascular resistance. Recently, inhaled NO appears to hold promise in the management of patients with elevated PVR and right ventricular failure. It is the only selective pulmonary vasodilator that should be used in cases of severe pulmonary hypertension and right ventricular failure associated with systemic hypotension.

We routinely begin with isoproterenol infusion (1 to 5 µg/min) or dopamine infusion (2 to 5 µg/kg/min) to improve contractility and to increase heart rate to about 90 to 110 beats/min prior to weaning from CPB. With life-threatening right ventricular failure, PGE_1 (200 ng/kg/min) or PGI_2 (16 ng/kg/min) infusion has been shown to effectively unload the right ventricle, although simultaneous norepinephrine infusion via a left atrial catheter is required to support systemic blood pressure. Under this circumstance, we use inhaled NO (10 to 40 ppm) for selective treatment of severe pulmonary hypertension and right ventricle failure associated with systemic hypotension.

Kieler-Jensen N, Lundin S, Ricksten SE: Vasodilator therapy after heart transplantation: Effects of inhaled nitric oxide and intravenous prostacyclin, prostaglandin E_1, and sodium nitroprusside. J Heart Lung Transplant 14:436–443, 1995

D.4. How does inhaled nitric oxide (NO) work as a selective pulmonary vasodilator?

The advantage of inhaled NO as a pulmonary vasodilator lies mainly in the fact that its smooth muscle relaxant effect is limited to the airway and the pulmonary vasculature; it has little effect on the systemic circulation because of its rapid inactivation by hemoglobin and it does not induce systemic hypotension, unlike IV vasodilators such as nitroprusside, nitroglycerin, prostaglandins, and calcium channel blockers. Inhaled NO (10 to 15 ppm) resulted in significant decreases in PAP, PVR, and central venous pressure (CVP), and increases in mean arterial pressure (MAP), cardiac output (CO), and arterial oxygenation (PaO_2). In addition, transesophageal echocardiography documented alteration of the ventricular septal shift with a significant reduction in right ventricular chamber and tricuspid valvular annulus size.

Girard C, Durand PG, Vedrinne C et al: Inhaled nitric oxide for right ventricular failure after heart transplantation. J Cardiothorac Vasc Anesth 7:481–485, 1993

Konstadt S: Nitric oxide: Has it progressed from molecule of the year to wonder drug of the decade? J Cardiothorac Vasc Anesth 9:625–626, 1995

D.5. What is the pathophysiology of a denervated heart?

Following cardiac transplantation, the cardiac plexus is interrupted and the heart is denervated. The recipient atrium remains innervated but hemodynamically unimportant, while the donor atrium is denervated and responsible for the electrophysiologic responses of the transplanted heart. The ECG often contains two P waves. The denervated heart retains its intrinsic control mechanisms, which include a normal Frank-Starling effect and intact alpha- and beta-adrenoreceptor responses to circulating catecholamines. This denervated heart lacks the ability to respond acutely to hypovolemia or hypotension with reflex tachycardia, but it responds to stress primarily by an increase in stroke volume. This reflects dependence of the sinus node on direct stimulation by endogenously released catecholamines and the absence of control via neural mechanisms. This is why heart transplanted patients are said to be preload dependent.

Cheng DCH, Ong DD: Anaesthesia for non-cardiac surgery in heart transplanted patients. Can J Anaesth 40:981–986, 1993

D.6. What are the common cardiac dysrhythmias following heart transplant?

Cardiac dysrhythmias can occur because of lack of vagal tone or denervated heart. The sinus node may have an increased refractory period and atrial conduction may be prolonged. Thus, first-degree atrioventricular block is common. It has been reported that 18% to 27% of orthotopic heart transplant patients develop prolonged (>24 hours) bradyarrhythmias within 5 days of transplantation. These bradyarrhythmias are also attributable to ischemic time at harvest; they may be symptomatic and require permanent cardiac pacing. In contrast, the presence of right bundle branch block is benign and without hemodynamic significance. Arrhythmia occurrences are potentially associated with prolonged donor heart ischemic time, elevated pulmonary arterial pressure, and a lower ejection fraction.

Miyamoto Y, Curtiss EI, Kormos RL et al: Bradyarrhythmia after heart transplantation: Incidence, time course, and outcome. Circulation 82:313–317, 1990

D.7. What are the causes of post-transplant bleeding?

Perioperative bleeding is a significant (6%) cause of mortality following heart transplantation. The causes of post-transplant bleeding are anastomosis leaks, bronchial artery injury, and coagulopathy. Immediately prior to weaning from bypass, with the heart filled, the posterior anastomosis is carefully checked again by the surgeon for water tightness because leaks in this area are more difficult and riskier to repair later. Patients with pulmonary hypertension develop enlarged bronchial vessels that are particularly liable to bleed if meticulous hemostasis has not been achieved. Coagulopathy can occur when CPB time is prolonged.

Bourge RC, Naftel DC, Costanzo-Nordin MR et al: Pre-transplantation risk factors for death after heart transplantation: A multi-institutional study. J Heart Lung Transplant 12:549–562, 1993

D.8. How would you treat post-transplant bleeding?

We routinely infuse an antifibrinolytic agent, tranexamic acid (100 mg/kg), over 20 minutes prior to sternotomy to prevent excess blood loss after CPB. A conventional dose of protamine is used to neutralize heparin following CPB, and it is verified by returning the ACT to baseline level. Desmopressin (16 to 20 µg or an additional dose of tranexamic acid (50 mg/kg) may be administered if excessive bleeding persists. Use of blood products such as fresh-frozen plasma, platelets, or cryoprecipitate should be guided by the laboratory coagulation profile and surgical bleeding must be ruled out. Packed red blood cells are administered to achieve a hemoglobin over 8 g/dl. Some centers use aprotinin with the standard regimen of 2×10^6 KIU bolus plus 2×10^6 KIU in CPB prime, plus 5×10^5 KIU/h during CPB. However, meta-analysis by Fremes et al. does not show any difference in the reduction of blood loss between patients pretreated either with aprotinin or a synthetic antifibrinolytic.

Fremes SE, Wong BI, Lee E et al: Meta-analysis of prophylactic drug treatment in the prevention of postoperative bleeding. Ann Thorac Surg 58:1580–1588, 1994

Karski JM, Teasdale SJ, Norman PH et al: Prevention of bleeding after cardiopulmonary bypass with high-dose tranexamic acid. Double-blind, randomized clinical trial. J Thorac Cardiovasc Surg 110:835–842, 1995

D.9. What are the causes of early graft failure?

Early graft failure is one of the most common causes (22%) of death following heart transplantation. The peak hazard for early graft failure occurs in the operating room, and it includes deaths attributed to unknown causes, pulmonary hypertension, right ventricular failure, and hyperacute rejection.

Bourge RC, Naftel DC, Costanzo-Nordin MR et al: Pre-transplantation risk factors for death after heart transplantation: A multi-institutional study. J Heart Lung Transplant 12:549–562, 1993

D.10. How would you manage this patient in the intensive care unit?

The three most common causes of death are infection, early graft failure, and acute rejection. Therefore, early management goals include prevention of infection and rejection, treatment of bleeding and dysrhythmias, and cardiovascular support. We routinely aim to wean the patient from the ventilator and extubate within 24 hours. To facilitate oxygenation and weaning, fluid balance and body weight are strictly supervised. The average duration of ventilation in our transplant population has been 1.0 day (range 0 to 5 days), and the average stay in the intensive care unit has been 3.7 days (range 1 to 11 days).

E. Subsequent Noncardiac Surgery

The patient had a successful heart transplant. However, 5 months after heart transplant, he developed urinary retention and was scheduled for a transurethral resection of the prostate.

E.1. How would you monitor this patient?

This patient should have monitoring requirements similar to nontransplant patients undergoing similar procedures. Those patients in our series who required invasive monitoring did so in keeping with a particular procedure (e.g., arterial line for thoracotomy and open lung biopsy, central venous pressure monitor for small bowel resection, or because the patient was unstable preoperatively). Smooth and safe anesthesia is contingent on careful preoperative assessment, which may reduce the need for invasive monitoring with all its attendant risks. Adequate preload must be ascertained preoperatively and intravascular volume status maintained intraoperatively because these patients are "preload dependent." I would monitor this patient with an ECG, pulse oximeter, automatic blood pressure cuff, and a CVP line.

Cheng DCH, Ong DD: Anaesthesia for non-cardiac surgery in heart transplanted patients. Can J Anaesth 40:981–986, 1993

E.2. What type of anesthetic is best for the heart transplanted patient?

In a series of 86 heart transplanted recipients, 18 returned for 32 noncardiac surgical procedures. Eighteen procedures received neuroleptic anesthesia, 12 received general anesthesia with a combination of N_2O/O_2/narcotic/relaxant and low doses of volatile agents, and 2 received spinal anesthesia. The patients had normal requirements of intravenous and inhalational agents, muscle relaxants, and local anesthetics. There was no prolonged action of any anesthetic agents. This indicates that general, neuroleptic, or spinal anesthesia does not affect postoperative outcome in heart transplanted recipients undergoing subsequent noncardiac surgery.

Cheng DCH, Ong DD: Anaesthesia for non-cardiac surgery in heart transplanted patients. Can J Anaesth 40:981–986, 1993

E.3. Which anesthetic technique would you give this patient?

Perioperative blood loss in patients undergoing transurethral resection of the prostate is not affected by either spinal or general anesthesia. I would give this patient spinal anesthesia with 75 mg hyperbaric lidocaine after 1 liter of crystalloid priming.

Smyth R, Cheng D, Asokumar B, Chung F: Coagulopathies in patients after transurethral resection of the prostate: Spinal versus general anesthesia. Anesth Analg 81:680–685, 1995

E.4. Do you need to use a muscarinic antagonist with anticholinesterase to reverse the muscle relaxant in heart transplanted patients?

Although it does not compromise the hemodynamic parameters, neostigmine recently has been shown to produce a dose-response decrease in heart rate in heart transplanted patients. In remote transplanted patients (>6 months), a muscarinic antagonist should be administered simultaneously with anticholinesterases to block the cardiac and muscarinic side-effects, as slow development of cardiac reinnervation may be possible.

Backman SB, Fox GS, Stein RD et al: Neostigmine decreases heart rate in heart transplant patients. Can J Anaesth 43:373–378, 1996

Wilson RF, Christensen BV, Olivari MT et al: Evidence for structural sympathetic reinnervation after orthotopic cardiac transplantation in humans. Circulation 83:1210–1221, 1991

E.5. What are the anesthetic implications for heart transplanted patients?

The anesthetic implications for heart transplanted patients include:

- Denervated heart
- Allograft rejection
- Infection
- Drug interaction
- Allograft coronary artery disease
- Hypertension
- Renal dysfunction

Cheng DCH, Ong DD: Anaesthesia for non-cardiac surgery in heart transplanted patients. Can J Anaesth 40:981–986, 1993

E.6. What is the significant implication of the denervated heart?

The denervated heart retains its intrinsic control mechanisms, which include a normal Frank-Starling effect, normal impulse formation and conductivity, and intact alpha- and beta-adrenoreceptors responding normally to circulating catecholamines without evidence of denervation hypersensitivity to exogenous and endogenous catecholamines. However, the normal respiratory variations or response to carotid sinus massage and Valsalva's maneuver are absent. At rest the heart rate reflects the intrinsic rate of depolarization at the donor sinoatrial node in the absence of any vagal tone, and is faster than normal at about 90 to 100 beats/min. Thus, increasing preload is useful before anesthetic maneuvers such as rapid thiopental induction or high spinal anesthesia. The heart rate shows minimal response to drugs such as muscle relaxants (pancuronium, gallamine), anticholinergics (atropine, glycopyrrolate, scopolamine), anticholinesterases (neostigmine, edrophonium, pyridostigmine, physostigmine), digoxin, nifedipine, phenylephrine, or nitroprusside, but will respond to isoproterenol, ephedrine, dopamine, and glucagon.

Cardiac dysrhythmias can occur in heart transplanted patients. First-degree atrioventricular (AV) block is common. Dual AV nodal pathways are frequently observed, but re-entry dysrhythmias are rare. Bradyarrhythmic therapy in these patients should be a direct α-adrenergic stimulating agent (epinephrine, isoproterenol). Glucagon is also useful as a positive chronotrope and inotrope. Verapamil, procainamide, and quinidine are useful for supraventricular tachyarrhythmia of atrial flutter and fibrillation. Lidocaine should be used cautiously in treating ventricular dysrhythmias because of its negative inotropic action.

Stein KL, Darby JM, Grenvik A: Intensive care of the cardiac transplant recipient. J Cardiothorac Anesth 2:543–553, 1988

E.7. What is the significant implication of allograft rejection?

Most rejection episodes occur within the first 3 months of transplantation with a peak at about 4 to 6 weeks. Usually, these episodes resolve with modification of the immunosuppression regimen by augmentation of steroid therapy; however, refractory rejection remains an important cause of early mortality after transplantation.

Bourge RC, Naftel DC, Costanzo-Nordin MR et al: Pre-transplantation risk factors for death after heart transplantation: A multi-institutional study. J Heart Lung Transplant 12:549–562, 1993

E.8. What is the significant implication of infection?

Immunosuppressive drugs are continued indefinitely in heart transplanted patients and infection remains a major cause of death. It is most prevalent in the first several weeks after transplantation when immunosuppressive therapy is most intense. Early postoperative bacterial infections (e.g., mediastinitis) and opportunistic infections (e.g., cytomegalovirus, *Pneumocystis carinii*, toxoplasma, and legionella) are the most common. The leading cause of infection is direct contact with contaminated material. Thus, invasive monitoring techniques and all forms of instrumentation should be kept to the minimum consistent with safe anesthesia. Attention to aseptic technique should be paramount. Intubation via the orotracheal route is preferable to the nasotracheal route because the latter is associated with infection by diphtheroids and staphylococcal commensals from the nasopharynx and skin.

Shaw IH, Kirk AJB, Conacher ID: Anaesthesia for patients with transplanted hearts and lungs undergoing non-cardiac surgery. Br J Anaesth 67:772–778, 1991

E.9. What is the significant implication of drug interaction?

Chronic steroid treatment can result in an abnormal stress response, so patients should receive perioperative steroid coverage. Azathioprine has been reported to antagonize the competitive neuromuscular blocking drug by its phosphodiesterase inhibiting properties; therefore larger doses of relaxants may be required. In experimental animals, cyclosporine infusions have been shown to potentiate the neuromuscular blocking effects of atracurium and vecuronium, and single doses of cyclosporine may result in increased duration of action of both barbiturates and narcotics.

Cirella VN, Pantuck CB, Lee YJ, et al: Effects of cyclosporine on anesthetic action. Anesth Analg 66:703–706, 1987

E.10. What is the significant implication of allograft coronary artery disease (CAD)?

The denervated heart is vulnerable to an accelerated process of coronary atherosclerosis. Angiographic evidence of allograft CAD is present in 10% to 20% of patients 1 year after transplantation and in up to 50% by 5 years. Even in angiographically normal coronary arteries, coronary luminal narrowing can develop insidiously. The cause of allograft CAD is likely multifactorial. Some CAD is transplanted with the donor heart. Other factors include immunologic or vital injury to vascular endothelium with a resultant proliferative response, ischemic injury at time of transplantation, and other risk factors such as smoking, hypertension, hyperlipidemia, and diabetes. The lack of afferent innervation renders episodes of myocardial ischemia silent in these patients. Therefore, diagnostic ECG is essential in the perioperative period.

Miller LW: Long-term complications of cardiac transplantation. Prog Cardiovasc Dis 33:229–282, 1991

E.11. What is the significant implication of post-transplant hypertension?

Nearly 75% of post-transplant recipients develop mild to moderate hypertension as a result of cyclosporine therapy. Current therapy may consist of a calcium channel blocker such as diltiazem. However, diltiazem will interfere with the metabolism of cyclosporine and increase cyclosporine blood levels; therefore dosage adjustments may be required. Nifedipine may be less tolerated by these patients because of its prominent vasodilator effect. When necessary, an angiotensin-converting enzyme inhibitor can be added. Because cardiac responsiveness during exercise is dependent on circulating catecholamines, alpha-blockers are best avoided after heart transplantation.

Rudas L, Pflugfelder PW, Kostuk WJ: Comparison of hemodynamic responses during dynamic exercise in the upright and supine postures after orthotopic cardiac transplantation. J Am Coll Cardiol 16:1367–1373, 1990

E.12. What is the significant implication of renal dysfunction?

Because of the nephrotoxic effects of cyclosporine, serum creatinine concentrations gradually increase after cardiac transplantation, but generally plateau around 170 to 180 mmol.L^{-1}. Simultaneous administration of nephrotoxic drugs (e.g., nonsteroidal anti-inflammatory drugs or trimethoprim-sulfamethoxazole) or agents that elevate cy-closporine blood concentrations (e.g., erythromycin or diltiazem) must be monitored closely to avoid acute deterioration of renal function. Anesthetic drugs that are excreted mainly by renal clearance should be avoided.

Miller LW: Long-term complications of cardiac transplantation. Prog Cardiovasc Dis 33:229–282, 1991

Ischemic Heart Disease and Noncardiac Surgery

18

Fun-Sun F. Yao

A 72-year-old man was scheduled for right hemicolectomy because of colon cancer. Past history revealed a myocardial infarction (MI) 5 months ago. He has been on atenolol, diltiazem, and occasional sublingual nitroglycerin.

A. Medical Disease and Differential Diagnosis

1. What are the preoperative predictors for perioperative cardiac morbidity (PCM)?
2. What is the incidence of perioperative reinfarction for noncardiac surgery at 0 to 3 months, 4 to 6 months, and >6 months after myocardial infarction?
3. Would you recommend that the surgery be postponed for a certain period of time? If so, why?
4. What is the Canadian Cardiovascular Society (CCS) classification of angina pectoris?
5. What is the New York Heart Association (NYHA) classification of heart failure?
6. What is the specific activity scale of cardiac function?
7. What are the determinants of myocardial oxygen demand? How are they measured clinically?
8. What factors determine myocardial oxygen supply?
9. What is the mechanism of myocardial ischemia?
10. Describe antianginal drugs and their mechanism of action.
11. How many types of calcium channels are there? How are calcium channel blockers classified?

B. Preoperative Evaluation and Preparation

1. How would you evaluate the patient's cardiac condition? What laboratory tests would you like to have done?
2. Would you recommend further cardiac testing or coronary revascularization prior to surgery?
3. How would you classify the cardiac risk according to the type of surgery?
4. Are patients with a Q-wave infarction at greater risk of reinfarction than those with a non-Q wave infarction?
5. Is preoperative myocardial ischemia detected by Holter monitor related to postoperative myocardial ischemia and infarction?
6. Would you discontinue any medications for angina before surgery?
7. How would you premedicate this patient?

C. Intraoperative Management

1. What are the intraoperative predictors for perioperative cardiac morbidity (PCM)?
2. How would you monitor the patient?

385

3. How would you monitor electrocardiography (ECG)? Why V_5? If you do not have precordial leads in your ECG machine, how can you monitor ischemia of the left ventricle?
4. Would you use a pulmonary artery catheter (PAC)?
5. Would you monitor transesophageal echocardiography (TEE)?
6. Is regional anesthesia better than general anesthesia for patients with cardiac disease?
7. How would you induce anesthesia?
8. What is the best choice of anesthetic agents for maintenance of anesthesia? Why?
9. What agents would you use for maintenance of anesthesia?
10. What muscle relaxant would you choose?
11. In the middle of surgery significant depression of ST segment was noticed. How would you treat it?
12. Would you give prophylactic intravenous nitroglycerin to prevent myocardial ischemia?
13. When would you extubate this patient? What could you do to prevent hypertension and tachycardia during extubation and emergence?

D. Postoperative Management

1. What are the postoperative predictors of perioperative cardiac morbidity?
2. How would you control postoperative pain?
3. Is postoperative anemia associated with adverse cardiac outcome?
4. Is postoperative hypothermia associated with postoperative myocardial ischemia?
5. How would you make a diagnosis of perioperative myocardial infarction?

A. Medical Disease and Differential Diagnosis

A.1. What are the preoperative predictors for perioperative cardiac morbidity (PCM)?

Goldman and associates found nine factors to have statistically significant independent correlations with cardiac outcome. They are as follows:

- Age >70 years
- Myocardial infarction in previous 6 months
- S_3 gallop or jugular vein distention
- Important valvular aortic stenosis
- Rhythm other than sinus or premature atrial contractions on preoperative ECG
- Premature ventricular contractions >5/min at any time before surgery
- Poor general medical status—PaO_2 <60 mm Hg, or $PaCO_2$ >50 mm Hg, potassium <3.0 mEq/liter, or HCO_3^- <20 mEq/liter, blood urea nitrogen (BUN) >50 mg/dl or creatinine > 3.0 mg/dl, abnormal serum glutamic-oxaloacetic transaminase (SGOT) or signs of chronic liver disease
- Intraperitoneal, intrathoracic, or aortic operation
- Emergency operation

Mangano extensively reviewed articles of perioperative cardiac morbidity (PCM) and found the following conclusions.

Preoperative Predictors
Preoperative historical predictors include age, previous myocardial infarction, angina,

congestive heart failure (CHF), hypertension, diabetes mellitus, dysrhythmias, peripheral vascular disease, cholesterol, cigarette smoking, previous coronary artery bypass graft (CABG) surgery, previous angioplasty, cardiovascular therapy, and risk indices. Most predictors had as many studies supporting as refuting their prognostic value. Only a recent (within 6 months) MI and current congestive heart failure are consistently proven preoperative predictors of PCM. The efficacy and cost-effectiveness of specialized preoperative cardiac testing, such as exercise stress testing or dipyridamole thallium imaging, remain controversial.

Recently, the Perioperative Ischemia Research Group led by Hollenberg and Mangano identified five major preoperative predictors of postoperative myocardial ischemia:

- Left ventricular hypertrophy by ECG
- History of hypertension
- Diabetes mellitus
- Definite coronary artery disease (CAD)
- Digoxin use

The risk of postoperative myocardial ischemia increased progressively with the number of predictors present: in 22% of patients with no predictors, in 31% with one predictor, in 46% with two predictors, in 70% with three predictors, and in 77% with four predictors.

Forrest JB, Cahalan MK, Rehder K et al: Multicenter study of anesthesia. II. Results. Anesthesiology 72:262–268, 1990

Forrest JB, Rehder K, Cahalan MK et al: Multicenter study of general anesthesia. III. Predictors of severe perioperative adverse outcomes. Anesthesiology 76:3–15, 1992

Goldman L, Calders DL, Nussbaum SR et al: Multifactorial index of cardiac risk in noncardiac surgical procedures. N Engl J Med 297:845–850, 1977

Hollenberg, M, Mangano DT, Browner WS et al: Predictors of postoperative myocardial ischemia in patients undergoing non-cardiac surgery. JAMA 268:205–209, 1992

Mangano DT: Perioperative cardiac morbidity. Anesthesiology 72:153–184, 1990

Mangano DT, Browner WS, Hollenberg M et al: Association of perioperative myocardial ischemia with cardiac morbidity and mortality in men undergoing noncardiac surgery. N Engl J Med 323:1781–1788, 1990

Mangano DT, Siliciano D, Hollenberg M et al: Postoperative myocardial ischemia: Therapeutic trials using intensive analgesia following surgery. Anesthesiology 76:342–353, 1992

A.2. What is the incidence of perioperative reinfarction for noncardiac surgery at 0 to 3 months, 4 to 6 months, and >6 months after myocardial infarction?

The incidence of perioperative reinfarction depends on the time interval between myocardial infarction and operation. Topkins and Artusio in 1964 reported a 55% incidence of reinfarction in male patients >50 years of age, undergoing surgery within 6 months of an MI. Between 6 months and 2 years, the reinfarction rate was 22% to 25%. After 3 years, the incidence decreased to 1%. The more recent reports are shown in Table 18-1. All reports showed a significant decline in reinfarction rate after 6 months of an MI. In 1983, Rao and associates claimed the reinfarction rate to be 5.8% and 2.3% in patients who developed infarction 3 and 6 months before surgery.

Table 18-1. The Incidence and Mortality of Perioperative Reinfarction for Noncardiac Surgery

	TIME INTERVAL			MORTALITY OF REINFARCTION
	0–3 mo	4–6 mo	>6 mo	
Tarhan and Moffitt (1972)	37%	16%	5%	66%
Steen and Tarhan (1978)	27%	11%	4.1%	69%
Rao, Jacobs, and El-Etr (1983)	5.8%	2.3%	1.5%	36%
Shah, Kleinman, Sami et al (1990)	4.3%	0%	5.7%	23%

Close hemodynamic monitoring for up to 72 to 96 hours following operation, including systemic and pulmonary arterial pressures and chest lead V_5 ECG, with immediate and appropriate therapy to control various hemodynamic aberrations, has contributed to the lower reinfarction rate. In 1990, Rao's group reevaluated the reinfarction rate and reported similar results as in 1983. The mortality rate of reinfarction was about 70% in all reports except Rao's, in which it was 36% and 23%.

Rao TLK, Jacobs KH, El-Etr AA: Reinfarction following anesthesia in patients with myocardial infarction. Anesthesiology 59:499–505, 1983

Shah KB, Kleinman BS, Sami H, et al: Reevaluation of perioperative myocardial infarction in patients with prior myocardial infarction undergoing noncardiac operations. Anesth Analg 71:231–235, 1990

Steen P, Tinker JH, Tarhan S: Myocardial reinfarction after anesthesia and surgery. JAMA 239:2566, 1978

Tarhan S, Moffitt EA: Myocardial infarction after general anesthesia. JAMA 220:1451, 1972

Topkins MJ, Artusio JF: Myocardial infarction and surgery: A five year study. Anesth Analg 43:716, 1964

A.3. Would you recommend that the surgery be postponed for a certain period of time? If so, why?

As mentioned in question A.2., all reports showed a significant decrease in reinfarction rate after 6 months of a myocardial infarction. Therefore, it is generally recommended to delay surgery 6 months after an MI. However, Teplick and Lowenstein recently questioned the validity of this practice. The recommendation to delay is based on only four studies, each of which contains design flaws. The most important of these is selection bias. Thus, those patients who survived longer are likely to constitute groups with progressively lower risk from their coronary artery disease. Most studies are also retrospective and lack a concurrent control group. Interestingly, in the Shah study (Table 18-1), the mortality was numerically lower in the first 6 months after MI than later. The bottom line is that the optimal duration for delaying surgery remains in doubt, and that to arbitrarily delay surgery either 3 or 6 months has inadequate statistical validity. Only well-defined studies with sufficient power have the potential for determining the truth.

Lowenstein E: Review of recent information on myocardial ischemia. ASA Annual Refresher Course No. 234, 1996

Teplick R, Lowenstein E: There is no proven benefit of delaying surgery for three to six months following a myocardial infarction. Anesthesiology 83:A122, 1995

A.4. What is the Canadian Cardiovascular Society (CCS) classification of angina pectoris?

The Canadian Cardiovascular Society classification is currently being used to describe the amount of effort required to produce angina pectoris.

- Class I: Ordinary physical activity, such as walking and climbing stairs, does not cause angina. Angina with strenuous or rapid or prolonged exertion at work or recreation.
- Class II: Slight limitations of ordinary activity. Walking or climbing stairs rapidly, walking uphill, walking or stair climbing after meals, in cold, in wind, under emotional stress, or only during the few hours after awakening. Walking more than two blocks on the level and climbing more than one flight of ordinary stairs at a normal pace and in normal conditions.
- Class III: Marked limitation of ordinary physical activity. Walking one to two blocks on the level and climbing one flight of stairs in normal conditions and at normal pace.
- Class IV: Inability to carry on any physical activity without discomfort; anginal syndrome may be present at rest.

Braunwald E (ed): Heart Disease, A Textbook of Cardiovascular Medicine, 5th ed, pp 12–13. Philadelphia, WB Saunders, 1997

Campeau L: Grading of angina pectoris. Circulation 54:522, 1975

A.5. What is the New York Heart Association (NYHA) classification of heart failure?

The NYHA classification of heart failure is determined by the number of symptoms including dyspnea and fatigue.

- Class I: No symptoms
- Class II: Symptoms with ordinary activity
- Class III: Symptoms with less than ordinary activity
- Class IV: Symptoms at rest

Braunwald E (ed): Heart Disease, A Textbook of Cardiovascular Medicine, 5th ed, pp 12–13. Philadelphia, WB Saunders, 1997

The Criteria Committee of the New York Heart Association: Nomenclature and Criteria for Diagnosis, 9th ed. Boston, Little, Brown, 1994

A.6. What is the specific activity scale of cardiac function?

- Class I: Can carry at least 24 lb up eight steps, carry objects that are at least 80 lb, shovel snow, spade soil, jog or walk 5 mph, ski, or play basketball, football, squash, or handball.
- Class II: Can carry anything up a flight of eight steps without stopping, have sexual intercourse without stopping, garden, rake, weed, roller skate, dance, or walk at a 4-mph rate on level ground.
- Class III: Can shower without stopping, strip and make bed, mop floors, hang washed clothes, clean windows, walk 2.5 mph, bowl, play golf (walk and carry clubs), push power lawn mower, or dress without stopping because of symptoms.
- Class IV: Can do none of the above or has symptoms at rest.

Goldman L: Cardiac risk in noncardiac surgery: An update. Anesth Analg 80:810–820, 1995

A.7. What are the determinants of myocardial oxygen demand? How are they measured clinically?

The three major determinants are myocardial wall tension, which is determined by left ventricular preload and afterload, contractility, and heart rate. See also Chapter 7, question B.7.

A.8. What factors determine myocardial oxygen supply?

The factors include aortic diastolic pressure, left ventricular end-diastolic pressure, coronary artery patency, coronary vascular tone, arterial oxygen saturation and tension, and hemoglobin concentration. See also Chapter 7, question B.9.

A.9. What is the mechanism of myocardial ischemia?

Myocardial ischemia occurs whenever myocardial oxygen supply cannot match myocardial oxygen demand. Intraoperative ischemia can be precipitated by increases in myocardial oxygen demand caused by tachycardia, hypertension, anemia, stress, sympathomimetic drugs, or discontinuation of beta-blockers. However, as many as 50% or more of the ischemic episodes may be unrelated to the indices of oxygen demand, suggesting decreased oxygen supply as the primary cause. Potential causes of decreased supply include external factors such as hypotension, tachycardia, increased filling pressures, anemia, or hypoxemia. In addition, internal factors such as acute coronary artery thrombosis and spasm also may play a role, although no data are available for determining their importance in the perioperative setting. Finally, the relationship of intraoperative ECG, TEE, or cardiokymographic changes to outcome has not been investigated in patients undergoing noncardiac surgery.

Mangano DT: Perioperative cardiac morbidity. Anesthesiology 72:153–184, 1990

A.10. Describe antianginal drugs and their mechanism of action.

The major antianginal drugs are nitrovasodilators, calcium channel blockers, beta-adrenergic antagonists, and, especially in unstable angina, antiplatelet agents. All approved agents function by improving the balance of myocardial oxygen supply and demand: increasing supply by dilating the coronary vasculature or decreasing demand by reducing cardiac work. The effects of antianginal agents on myocardial oxygen supply and demand are shown in Figure 18-1. See also Chapter 14, question A.8.

Nitrovasodilators (Nitroglycerin, Isosorbide Dinitrate)
- Decreased left ventricle (LV) preload (low dose)
  - Systemic venous dilation
  - Pulmonary arterial bed dilation
  - Pulmonary vein dilation
  - Decreased LV filling pressure
  - Decrease in LV diastolic compressive forces
  - Decreased LV diastolic chamber size
- Decreased LV afterload (high dose)
  - Decreased systolic pressure
  - Decreased systemic vascular resistance
  - Decreased aortic impedance

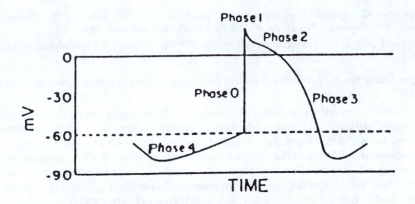

Figure 18-1. Action potential of a cell of the cardiac conducting system demonstrating automaticity. (Reprinted with permission from Bigger JT, Braunwald E [eds]: Heart Disease: Mechanism and Diagnosis of Arrhythmias, p 136. Philadelphia, WB Saunders, 1980)

- Coronary circulation
  - Coronary artery and arteriolar dilation (high dose)
  - Spasm reversal or prevention
  - Stenosis dilation
  - Increased collateral flow
  - Improvement of regional subendocardial ischemia

Beta-Adrenergic Antagonists (Propranolol, Esmolol, Atenolol)
- Reductions in myocardial oxygen consumption
- Improvements in coronary blood flow
  - Prolonged diastolic perfusion period
  - Improved collateral flow
  - Increased flow to ischemic areas
- Overall improvement in supply:demand ratio
- Stabilization of cellular membranes
- Improved oxygen dissociation from hemoglobin
- Inhibition of platelet aggregation
- Reduced mortality after myocardial infarction

Calcium Channel Blockers (Verapamil, Diltiazem, Nifedipine, Nicardipine)
Calcium channel blockers reduce myocardial oxygen demand by depression of myocardial contractility and dilation of coronary and collateral vessels, which improve blood flow. However, the most important effects may be the prevention of sympathetically mediated and ergonovine-induced coronary vasoconstriction.

Antiplatelet and Antithrombotic Agents (Aspirin, Dipyridamole, Ticlopidine)
Aspirin inhibits platelet aggregation by blocking the production of thromboxane A_2 by covalently acetylating a serine residue near the active site of cyclooxygenase, the enzyme that produces the cyclic endoperoxide precursor of thromboxane A_2. Low doses of aspirin appear to reduce the incidence of MI in chronic stable angina.

Hardman JG, Limbird LE, Molinoff PB et al (eds): Goodman and Gilman's The Pharmacological Basis of Therapeutics, 9th ed, pp 88–116. New York, McGraw-Hill, 1996

Kaplan J (ed): Cardiac Anesthesia, 3rd ed, pp 759–776, 1353–1354. Philadelphia, WB Saunders, 1993

A.11. How many types of calcium channels are there? How are calcium channel blockers classified?

Calcium enters cellular membranes through voltage-dependent channels or receptor-operated channels. The voltage-dependent channels depend on a transmembrane potential for activation (opening). Receptor-operated channels are either linked to a voltage-dependent channel after receptor stimulation or directly allow calcium passage through cell or organelle membranes independent of transmembrane potentials.

Three types of voltage-dependent channels exist: the T (transient), L (long-lasting), and N (neuronal) channels. The T and L channels are located in cardiac and smooth muscle tissue, whereas the N channels are located only in neural tissues. The T channel is activated at low voltages (-50 mV) in cardiac tissue; it plays a major role in cardiac depolarization (phase 0) as shown in Figure 18-1, and is not blocked by calcium antagonists. The L channels are the classic slow channels; they are activated at higher voltages (-30 mV) and are responsible for phase 2 of the cardiac action potential. These channels are blocked by calcium antagonists. N channels are also resistant to blockade by the calcium channel blocking agents.

Calcium channel blockers interact with the L-type calcium channel and are composed of drugs from five classes: (1) the 1,4-dihydropyridine (DHP) derivatives, represented by nifedipine, nicardipine, nimodipine, and nitrendipine; (2) the phenylalkylamines, represented by verapamil; (3) the benzodiazepines, represented by diltiazem; (4) the diarylaminopropylamine ester, represented by bepridil; and (5) the diphenylpiperazine. The L-type calcium channel has specific receptors that bind to each of the different chemical classes of calcium channel blockers. The binding to calcium blocker receptors by DHP derivatives (nifedipine) is voltage dependent. Calcium channels transform from a closed resting form that potentially open, to an activated open form, to an inactive conformation that cannot open, and finally back to the closed resting form. Nifedipine binds preferentially to the inactive receptor that has just recently undergone activation and cannot open. Nifedipine essentially acts as a plug to block the channel. Verapamil binds to the L-type channel preferentially when it is active or open. The greater the period of activation of the channel, the more effective is the blockade (use dependent). Any repetitive activity, such as cardiac pacemaker activity, is sensitive to use-dependent agents.

Hardman JG, Limbird LE, Molinoff PB et al (eds): Goodman and Gilman's The Pharmacological Basis of Therapeutics, 9th ed, pp 767–769. New York, McGraw-Hill, 1996

Kaplan J (ed): Cardiac Anesthesia, 3rd ed, p 108. Philadelphia, WB Saunders, 1993

B. Preoperative Evaluation and Preparation

B.1. How would you evaluate the patient's cardiac condition? What laboratory tests would you like to have done?

The initial history, physical examination, and ECG assessment should focus on identification of potentially serious cardiac disorders, including coronary artery disease (e.g., prior myocardial infarction, angina pectoris), congestive heart failure, and electrical instability (e.g., symptomatic arrhythmias).

In addition to identifying preexisting manifested heart disease, it is essential to define disease severity, stability, and prior treatment. Other factors that help determine cardiac risk include functional capacity, age, comorbid conditions (e.g., diabetes mellitus, peripheral vascular disease, renal dysfunction, chronic pulmonary disease), and type of surgery (vascular procedures and prolonged, complicated thoracic, abdominal, and head and neck procedures considered higher risk). See also question A.1.

Executive summary of the ACC/AHA task force report: guidelines for perioperative cardiovascular evaluation for noncardiac surgery. Anesth Analg 82:854–860, 1996

Fleisher LA, Barash PG: Preoperative cardiac evaluation for noncardiac surgery: A functional approach. Anesth Analg 74:586–598, 1992

Goldman L: Cardiac risk in noncardiac surgery: An update. Anesth Analg 80:810–820, 1995

Mangano DT, Goldman L: Preoperative assessment of patients with known or suspected coronary disease. N Engl J Med 333: 1750–1756, 1995

B.2. Would you recommend further cardiac testing or coronary revascularization prior to surgery?

Successful perioperative evaluation and treatment of cardiac patients undergoing noncardiac surgery requires careful teamwork and communication between patient, primary care physician, anesthesiologist, and surgeon. In general, indications for further cardiac testing and treatments are the same as those in the nonoperative setting, but their timing is dependent on such factors as the urgency of noncardiac surgery, the patient's risk factors, and specific surgical considerations. Coronary revascularization before noncardiac surgery to enable the patient to get through the noncardiac procedure is appropriate only for a small subset of patients at very high risk. Preoperative testing should be limited to circumstances in which the results will affect patient treatment and outcomes. A conservative approach to use of expensive tests and treatments is recommended.

The patient suffered from a myocardial infarction 5 months ago and was scheduled for an intermediate-risk procedure, hemicolectomy. It is recommended that further testing should be considered for all patients with a previous MI whose planned surgery raises the risk of perioperative ischemia. I would recommend a noninvasive stress test such as exercise ECG. Fleisher and Barash proposed a functional approach (Fig. 18-2). Further cardiac testing depends on the type of surgery and the functional status of the patient. If the exercise ECG is negative, the patient is cleared for surgery. When it is positive, then exercise thallium imaging or dipyridamole thallium imaging (if unable to exercise) is performed. If the ischemic area is small, surgery is allowed. If the ischemic area is moderate to large, the patient is recommended for coronary revascularization after cardiac catheterization prior to the planned surgery (Fig. 18-2 and Fig. 18-3).

Another approach combines clinical and thallium data to optimize preoperative assessment of cardiac risk. Using the clinical historical variables of presence of (1) a Q wave on ECG, (2) age >70 years, (3) angina pectoris, (4) ventricular ectopic activity requiring therapy, and (5) diabetes mellitus requiring therapy, Eagle et al. have been able to identify patients who are at high-risk for a postoperative ischemic event (three or more variables) and patients at low-risk (no variables). An intermediate

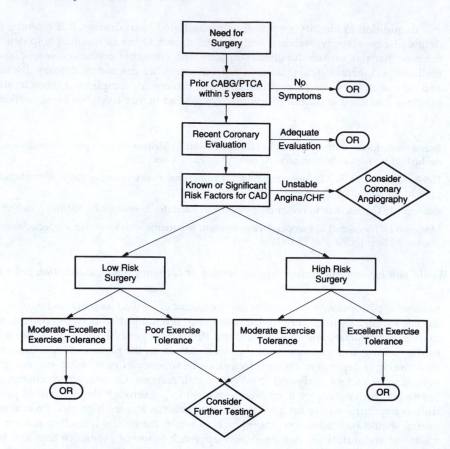

Figure 18-2. Proposed algorithm for the preoperative cardiac evaluation of the patient undergoing noncardiac surgery. The risk of the surgery and functional capacity of the patient are important in determining the need for noninvasive and invasive testing. (Reprinted with permission from Fleisher LA, Barash PG: Preoperative cardiac evaluation for noncardiac surgery: A functional approach. Anesth Analg 74:586–598, 1992)

group in which a patient has one or two clinical variables can be stratified into high- and low-risk groups by thallium scintigraphy.

The third approach proposed by Goldman is as follows:

- Assess functional capacity by history.
- If the history is reliable and the patient is Class I or early Class II (can carry two grocery bags up a flight of stairs), surgery is low risk.
- If history is unreliable, do an exercise tolerance test.
- If history is unreliable or unhelpful and the patient is unable to exercise, do dipyridamole thallium scintigraphy, ambulatory ischemia monitoring, or stress echocardiography.

See also Chapter 13, question B.2.

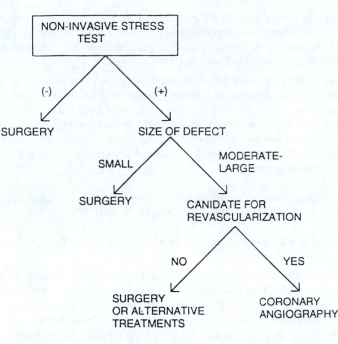

Figure 18-3. Algorithm for the use of information obtained from noninvasive stress testing (exercise and dipyridamole-thallium testing). The size of the defect on thallium imaging should be used to determine which patients may benefit from further evaluation and coronary revascularization. (Reprinted with permission from Fleisher LA, Barash PG: Preoperative cardiac evaluation for noncardiac surgery: A functional approach. Anesth Analg 74:586–598, 1992)

Eagle KA, Coley CM, Newell JB et al: Combining clinical and thallium data optimizes preoperative assessment of cardiac risk before major vascular surgery. Ann Intern Med 110:859, 1989

Executive summary of the ACC/AHA task force report: guidelines for perioperative cardiovascular evaluation for noncardiac surgery. Anesth Analg 82:854–860, 1996

Fleisher LA: Perioperative management of the cardiac patient undergoing noncardiac surgery. ASA Refresher Course in Anesthesiology 24:71–84, 1996

Fleisher LA, Barash PG: Preoperative cardiac evaluation for noncardiac surgery: A functional approach. Anesth Analg 74:586–598, 1992

Goldman L: Cardiac risk in noncardiac surgery: An update. Anesth Analg 80:810–820, 1995

Lowenstein E: Review of recent information on myocardial ischemia. ASA Annual Refresher Course No. 234, 1996.

Mangano DT, Goldman L: Preoperative assessment of patients with known or suspected coronary disease. N Engl J Med 333: 1750–1756, 1995

B.3. How would you classify the cardiac risk according to the type of surgery?

Surgery-specific cardiac risk of noncardiac surgery is related to two important factors: the type of surgery itself and the degree of hemodynamic stress associated with surgery-specific procedures. The duration and intensity of coronary and myocardial stressors can be helpful in estimating the likelihood of perioperative cardiac events, particularly for emergency surgery. Surgery-specific risk for noncardiac surgery can be stratified as high, intermediate, and low.

- High-risk surgery includes major emergency surgery, particularly in the elderly; aortic and other major vascular surgery; peripheral vascular surgery; and anticipated prolonged procedures associated with large fluid shifts and/or blood loss.
- Intermediate-risk procedures include carotid endarterectomy, head and neck surgery, intraperitoneal and intrathoracic, orthopedic, and prostate surgery.
- Low-risk procedures include endoscopic and superficial procedures, cataract surgery, and breast surgery.

Executive summary of the ACC/AHA task force report: guidelines for perioperative cardiovascular evaluation for noncardiac surgery. Anesth Analg 82:854–860, 1996

B.4. Are patients with a Q-wave infarction at greater risk of reinfarction than those with a non-Q wave infarction?

Recent studies indicate that individuals who survive a non-Q wave infarction are at greater risk of reinfarction than those who survive a Q-wave infarction. Patients who have not had a transmural wall infarction probably have border zones of that infarction that remain at high-risk for subsequent damage. These border zones might not be present with a clear-cut transmural Q-wave infarction. In contradistinction, patients with complicated Q-wave infarctions frequently do not survive the immediate postinfarction period, but they have a lower rate of reinfarction than non-Q wave MI after this period. Theoretically, patients who have had a solitary coronary artery lesion and sustained a transmural infarction may be considered at a significantly lower risk for reinfarction as the area that was at risk of ischemia is already necrotic. Although their risk of reinfarction may be low, an increased risk of dysrrhythmias is present because of the necrotic myocardium. It is important to remember (1) that the distinction between the Q and non-Q wave MI is an electrocardiographic classification and it does not necessarily correlate with the pathologic findings of transmural and subendocardial infarctions and (2) that overlap exists, especially with thrombolytic therapy.

Fleisher LA, Barash PG: Preoperative cardiac evaluation for noncardiac surgery: A functional approach. Anesth Analg 74:586–598, 1992

B.5. Is preoperative myocardial ischemia detected by Holter monitor related to postoperative myocardial ischemia and infarction?

It is controversial. A group at Harvard and a group at Yale have related preoperative silent ischemia by Holter monitoring to an increased risk in both vascular and nonvascular surgical patients. Nevertheless, a group from the West Coast does not agree with this, and they believe that only postoperative ischemia is related to postoperative MI. The resolution of this question has obvious important implications. If it were as simple as expanding Holter monitoring to preoperative patients, one would think that would be most worthwhile. If not, it would be an enormous waste of effort and resources.

Fleisher LA, Rosenbaum SH, Nelson AH et al: The predictive value of preoperative silent ischemia for postoperative ischemic cardiac events in vascular and nonvascular surgery patients. Am Heart J 122:980, 1991

Lowenstein E: Review of recent information on myocardial ischemia. ASA Annual Refresher Course No. 234, 1996

Raby KE, Goldman L, Creager MA, et al: Correlation between perioperative ischemia and major cardiac events after peripheral vascular surgery. N Engl J Med 321:1296, 1989

B.6. Would you discontinue any medications for angina before surgery?

No. All antianginal medications, especially beta-blockers, should be continued up to the time of surgery. Sudden withdrawal of antianginal drugs may produce rebound tachycardia and hypertension, which may precipitate acute myocardial ischemia or infarction.

Barash PG, Cullen BF, Stoelting RK (eds): Clinical Anesthesia, 3rd ed, pp 454–457. Philadelphia, Lippincott-Raven, 1997

Mangano DT (ed): Preoperative Cardiac Assessment, pp 141–163. Philadelphia, JB Lippincott, 1990

B.7. How would you premedicate this patient?

The patient with ischemic heart disease should be sedated before surgery to avoid anxiety-induced tachycardia and hypertension, which may cause adverse myocardial ischemic events. Appropriate doses of diazepam, lorazepam, or midazolam may be given with the antianginal medications.

C. Intraoperative Management

C.1. What are the intraoperative predictors for perioperative cardiac morbidity (PCM)?

Intraoperative Predictors
Among the classic intraoperative predictors, emergency surgery, major vascular surgery, and prolonged (>3 hours) thoracic or upper abdominal surgery appear to be independent predictors of PCM, whereas choice of anesthesia does not. Among the dynamic predictors, both hypotension and tachycardia predict PCM. Hypertension remains a controversial predictor. Myocardial ischemia is a suggestive predictor. Left ventricular end-diastolic pressure is a sensitive measure of ischemia, but preliminary studies suggest that pulmonary capillary wedge pressure (PCWP) may be too insensitive.

Mangano DT: Perioperative cardiac morbidity. Anesthesiology 72:153–184, 1990

C.2. How would you monitor the patient?

The patient would be monitored as follows:

- ECG—simultaneous leads V_5 and II, multiple-lead ST-segment analysis if available
- Blood pressure—noninvasive automatic Doppler sphygmomanometric technique
- Swan-Ganz catheter—PCWP, pulmonary artery diastolic pressure (PADP), hemodynamic study only for patients with ventricular dysfunction

- Central venous pressure (CVP) line—if the patient has good left ventricular function
- Urine output
- Temperature—esophageal
- Oxygen analyzer for inspired gas mixture
- End-tidal CO_2 analyzer
- Pulse oximeter for arterial oxygenation

C.3. How would you monitor electrocardiography (ECG)? Why V_5? If you do not have precordial leads in your ECG machine, how can you monitor ischemia of the left ventricle?

ST segment changes in ECG are most commonly used to detect intraoperative myocardial ischemia. Multiple-lead ECG monitoring provides the best clinically available method of detecting perioperative ischemia. Based primarily on results obtained from exercise treadmill testing, combined ECG leads II and V_5, which can detect 96% of ischemic events, are suggested optimal leads for detecting intraoperative myocardial ischemia. However, London et al. recently found that the standard combination of leads II and V_5 was only 80% sensitive, whereas combining leads V_4 and V_5 increased sensitivity to 90% in patients with known or suspected coronary artery disease undergoing noncardiac surgery with general anesthesia. The sensitivity increased to 96% by combining leads II, V_4, and V_5.

If only one lead can be displayed, V_5 should be used because lead V_5 has the greatest sensitivity, 75% intraoperatively and 89% during exercise treadmill testing.

A modified V_5 or CM_5 may be used. Place the right arm (RA) electrode on the middle part of the manubrium, the left leg (LL) electrode on the V_5 position, and the left arm electrode on any area of the body for ground, and monitor lead II. Recent claims suggest that the CB_5 lead is simple to apply and provides tracings equivalent to the V_5 when monitoring for ischemia, while allowing easier recognition of P waves. Lead CB_5 is a bipolar lead consisting of a negative (RA) electrode over the center of the right scapula and a positive (LL) electrode over the V_5 position monitoring lead II. The CB_5 lead is useful for thoracic surgery.

However, certain prerequisites must be met to use the ECG effectively.

- The diagnostic mode allows detection of ST segment changes, which are filtered out by the monitoring mode.
- The number of ECG leads and their location affect detection of ischemic events.
- Immediate availability of a hardcopy of the ECG leads for more detailed analysis. Studies have reported that even trained observers recognize only 15% to 40% of ECG ischemic events displayed on oscilloscope.
- The introduction of ST segment trending helps as an early warning detection system, but it should not replace examination of the ECG printout.
- The quantitative increase in PCWP and the characteristic changes in its waveform have been suggested as an ischemia monitor.

Barash PG: Monitoring myocardial ischemia: A sequential clinical approach. ASA Annual Refresher Course Lecture No. 112, 1996

Blackburn H, Katigbak R: What ECG leads to take after exercise. Am Heart J 67:184–185, 1964

London MJ, Hollenberg M, Wong MG et al: Intraoperative myocardial ischemia: Localization by continuous 12-lead electrocardiography. Anesthesiology 69:232–241, 1988

C.4. Would you use a pulmonary artery catheter (PAC)?

A number of studies report that PAC is an insensitive monitor for myocardial ischemia and should not be inserted with this as a primary indication. (See also Chapter 7, questions CI-6. and CI-8.)

Although few studies have reported on comparison of patient outcomes after treatment with or without PAC, the following three variables are particularly important in assessing benefit versus risk of PAC use: disease severity, magnitude of anticipated surgery, and practice setting. The extent of expected fluid shifts is a primary concern. Patients most likely to benefit from perioperative use of a PAC appear to be those with a recent MI complicated by CHF, those with significant CAD who are undergoing procedures associated with significant hemodynamic stress, and those with systolic or diastolic left ventricular dysfunction, cardiomyopathy, and valvular disease undergoing high-risk operations.

Barash PG: Monitoring myocardial ischemia: A sequential clinical approach. ASA Annual Refresher Course Lecture No. 112, 1996

Executive summary of the ACC/AHA task force report: Guidelines for perioperative cardiovascular evaluation for noncardiac surgery. Anesth Analg 82:854–860, 1996

C.5. Would you monitor transesophageal echocardiography (TEE)?

Transesophageal echocardiography is a highly sensitive ischemia monitor, which is based on the development of new regional wall motion abnormalities (RWMA), decreased systolic wall thickening, and ventricular dilation to recognize ischemic events. Usually a cross-sectional view of the left ventricle is imaged because this view displays the myocardial perfusion territories of the three coronary arteries. The incremental value of adding TEE to ECG monitoring is small. In CABG patients postbypass RWMA were related to adverse clinical outcome. In contrast, no association was found with ECG-detected ischemia or prebypass RMWA and perioperative cardiac morbidity. In addition to cost, significant limitations exist to the use of this technique. The ability to detect RWMA is decreased in an operating room setting. Preintubation events are missed. The image plane can miss vents in other areas of the myocardium. The type of analysis technique (fixed versus floating) will affect interpretation of RWMA. See also Chapter 7, question CI-10.

Barash PG: Monitoring myocardial ischemia: a sequential clinical approach. ASA Annual Refresher Course Lecture No. 112, 1996

Executive summary of the ACC/AHA task force report: Guidelines for perioperative cardiovascular evaluation for noncardiac surgery. Anesth Analg 82:854–860, 1996

C.6. Is regional anesthesia better than general anesthesia for patients with cardiac disease?

A number of studies in patients with cardiac disease have compared the effects of regional versus general anesthesia on the incidence of perioperative infarction, dysrhythmias, and CHF. Most studies have suggested no difference in infarction rate during general and regional (spinal, epidural, nerve block, local) anesthesia. However, regional anesthesia may benefit patients with prior MI undergoing transurethral prostatectomy; the reinfarction rate for spinal anesthesia has been reported to be

<1%, versus 2% to 8% for general anesthesia. Yaeger et al. reported that only 1 of 28 (3.6%) patients receiving epidural anesthesia (and light levels of general anesthesia) and postoperative epidural analgesia developed CHF versus 10 of 25 (40%) patients given general anesthesia and postoperative parenteral narcotic analgesia. The potential advantages of regional anesthesia in patients undergoing vascular surgery including modifying the cardiovascular and metabolic stress response to surgery are diminished postoperative respiratory depression and decreased postoperative hypercoagulability when compared with general anesthesia. However, a recent larger study (423 patients) by Bode et al. has concluded that the choice of anesthetic techniques does not significantly influence cardiac morbidity and overall mortality in patients undergoing peripheral vascular surgery. Thus, regional anesthesia may offer an advantage over general anesthesia for certain types of surgery (prostate resection) or for specific patients (history of CHF). Otherwise, no one technique demonstrates a consistent advantage. Therefore, the choice of anesthesia is best left to the discretion of the anesthesia care team, which will consider the need for postoperative ventilation; cardiovascular effects, including myocardial depression; sympathetic blockade; and dermatomal level of the procedure.

Bode RH Jr, Lewis KP, Zarich SW et al: Cardiac outcome after peripheral vascular surgery: Comparison of general and regional anesthesia. Anesthesiology 84:3–13, 1996

Go AS, Browner WS: Cardiac outcomes after regional or general anesthesia, do we have the answer? Anesthesiology 84:1–2, 1996

Mangano DT: Perioperative cardiac morbidity. Anesthesiology 72:153–184, 1990

Yaeger M, Glass DD, Neft RK, Brinck-Johnsen T: Epidural anesthesia and analgesia in high-risk surgical patients. Anesthesiology 66:729–736, 1987

C.7. How would you induce anesthesia?

A smooth induction is essential to prevent hypotension, hypertension, and tachycardia, which can precipitate myocardial ischemia. Different induction techniques can be employed to achieve this goal. While the patient is being preoxygenated, fentanyl (7 to 8 μg/kg) is given slowly to achieve drowsiness. Then, thiopental in 50-mg increments or midazolam in 1-mg increments is titrated to produce unconsciousness, followed by succinylcholine (1 mg/kg) or an intermediate nondepolarizing relaxant to facilitate tracheal intubation. All anesthetic agents are acceptable with the exception of ketamine, which can produce significant hypertension and tachycardia. High-dose fentanyl technique is not recommended because we like to extubate the patient early. See also Chapter 14, question C.6 for other measures used to prevent hypertension and tachycardia at the time of intubation.

Martin DE, Rosenberg H, Aukburg SJ et al: Low-dose fentanyl blunts circulatory responses to tracheal intubation. Anesth Analg 61:680, 1982

C.8. What is the best choice of anesthetic agents for maintenance of anesthesia? Why?

No one best myocardial protective agent or technique currently exists. Inhalational versus narcotic anesthesia in patients with cardiac disease is still debated, although the cardiovascular effects of both techniques and the physiologic differences between them are well documented. Their differences imply that one anesthetic can perform better than another in selected risk groups. However, most outcome studies have not demonstrated a difference between anesthetics in the patient with cardiac disease. Ten of 11 outcome studies of >3000 noncardiac surgical patients with CAD have concluded that anesthetic type does not affect outcome. Only one study (Rao et al.) has suggested a difference: narcotic–nitrous oxide–relaxant anesthesia was found to be associated with a significantly (P <0.005) higher incidence of myocardial reinfarction: 7.0% versus 0.5% to 1.5% for other general anesthetics, and 2.7% for regional anesthesia. However, 5 of these 11 studies were retrospective, resulting in incomplete and nonstandardized data collection. Of the six prospective studies, only two thoroughly measured cardiac outcomes and none used a random anesthetic assignment. More rigorous methods may (or may not) demonstrate differences between the inhalation and intravenous narcotic techniques. Rao et al.'s unique findings have been challenged by two large-scale outcome studies of patients undergoing CABG surgery, which report that anesthetic choice does not affect outcome.

Mangano DT: Perioperative cardiac morbidity. Anesthesiology 72:153–184, 1990

Rao TK, Jacobs KH, El-Etr AA: Reinfarction following anesthesia in patients with myocardial infarction. Anesthesiology 59:499–505, 1983

Slogoff S, Keats AS: Randomized trial of primary anesthetic agents on outcome of coronary bypass operations. Anesthesiology 70:179–188, 1989

Tuman KJ, McCarthy RJ, Spiess BD et al: Does choice of anesthetic agent significantly affect outcome after coronary artery surgery? Anesthesiology 70:189–198, 1989

C.9. What agents would you use for maintenance of anesthesia?

Because I like to extubate the patient at the end of surgery, I would use nitrous oxide and a combination of low-dose isoflurane and fentanyl for maintenance of anesthesia. High-dose narcotics should be avoided if postoperative ventilation is not planned. Isoflurane has been shown to cause coronary steal and myocardial ischemia. However, recent animal and clinical studies conclude that isoflurane in clinical concentrations can be used safely in patients with coronary heart disease provided that hypotension and tachycardia are avoided. See also Chapter 7, question CI-15.

C.10. What muscle relaxant would you choose?

The hemodynamic goals are to avoid hypotension, tachycardia, and hypertension. Intermediate acting neuromuscular blocking agents such as vecuronium, cisatracurium, and rocuronium can be used safely because they do not produce significant cardiovascular changes. A peripheral nerve stimulator should be used to monitor the degree of blockade.

Fleming N: Con: The choice of muscle relaxants is not important in cardiac surgery. J Cardiothorac Vasc Anesth 9:772–774, 1995

Hudson RJ, Thomson IR: Pro: The choice of muscle relaxants is important in cardiac surgery. J Cardiothorac Vasc Anesth 9:768–771, 1995

C.11. In the middle of surgery significant depression of ST segment was noticed. How would you treat it?

ST segment depression indicates myocardial ischemia, either from increased myocardial oxygen demand or from decreased oxygen supply. Treatment includes the following:

- Increase O_2 supply—correct hypotension, hypoxemia, and severe anemia
- Decrease O_2 demand—correct hypertension and tachycardia by deepening the level of anesthesia or by using vasodilator, beta-blockers, and calcium channel blockers.
- With no obvious changes in hemodynamics (silent intraoperative ischemia), nitroglycerin drips, sublingual nifedipine, or intravenous nicardipine may be used to relieve suspected coronary spasm.

Mangano DT: Perioperative cardiac morbidity. Anesthesiology 72:153–184, 1990

C.12. Would you give prophylactic intravenous nitroglycerin to prevent myocardial ischemia?

Insufficient data exist about the effects of prophylactic intraoperative intravenous nitroglycerin in patients at high-risk. Nitroglycerin should be used only when the hemodynamic effects of other agents in use are considered. See also Chapter 7, question CI-19.

Executive summary of the ACC/AHA task force report: Guidelines for perioperative cardiovascular evaluation for noncardiac surgery. Anesth Analg 82:854–860, 1996

C.13. When would you extubate this patient? What could you do to prevent hypertension and tachycardia during extubation and emergence?

At the end of surgery I would extubate the patient when the patient is awake, breathing adequately, and neuromuscular blockade is fully reversed. To prevent tachycardia and hypertension associated with extubation and emergence, I would give the patient low doses of preventive medication such as 1 mg/kg of lidocaine or esmolol, or 0.1 mg/kg of labetalol, diltiazem, or verapamil 2 minutes before extubation. See also Chapter 14, questions C.7. and C.11.

Helfman SM, Gold MI, De Lisser EA et al: Which drug prevents tachycardia and hypertension associated with tracheal intubation: Lidocaine, fentanyl, or esmolol? Anesth Analg 72:482–486, 1991

Mikawa K, Nishina K, Maekawa N et al: Attenuation of cardiovascular responses to tracheal extubation: Verapamil versus diltiazem. Anesth Analg 82:1205–1210, 1996

Nishina K, Mikawa K, Maekawa N et al: Attenuation of cardiovascular responses to tracheal extubation with diltiazem. Anesth Analg 80:1217–1222, 1995

Stoelting RK: Blood pressure and heart rate changes during short-duration laryngoscopy for tracheal intubation: Influence of viscous or intravenous lidocaine. Anesth Analg 57:197–198, 1978

D. Postoperative Management

D.1. What are the postoperative predictors of perioperative cardiac morbidity?

The postoperative period appears to present the highest risk for cardiac morbidity for the noncardiac surgical patient. Depending on surveillance duration, the postoperative period may have the highest incidence of ischemic events with the most important clinical and prognostic implications. Most of these events are silent (without angina). Studies involving large numbers of patients suggest that postoperative ischemia is the most important marker of immediate and long-term adverse cardiovascular events. Traditionally ischemia monitoring has been of short duration following operation (24 to 72 hours), but new data suggest that period should be increased to 7 days. Heart rate commonly increases postoperatively by 25% to 50% over intraoperative values, and tachycardia occurs in 10% to 25% of patients. Postoperative myocardial ischemia occurs in 27% to 41% of high-risk patients, and >70% of episodes are silent. It is associated with a 2.8 times increase in the odds of all PCM. Moreover, postoperative unintentional hypothermia and anemia are associated with increased incidence of myocardial ischemia.

Mangano DT, Browner WS, Hollenberg M et al: Association for perioperative myocardial ischemia with cardiac morbidity in men undergoing noncardiac surgery. N Engl J Med 323:178–188, 1990

Mangano DT, Browner WS, Hollenberger M et al: Long-term cardiac prognosis following noncardiac surgery. JAMA 268:233–239, 1992

D.2. How would you control postoperative pain?

The postoperative period can be stressful because of the onset of pain during emergence from anesthesia, fluid shifts, temperature changes, and alteration of respiratory function. Marked changes occur in plasma catecholamine concentration, hemodynamics, ventricular function, and coagulation following noncardiac surgery, particularly in patients with preexisting cardiac disease. These stresses place the patient at increased risk for development of adverse cardiac outcome. Therefore, effective pain management is essential to prevent adverse outcome. Patient-controlled intravenous and/or epidural analgesia is a popular method for reducing postoperative pain. Several studies suggest that effective pain management leads to a reduction in postoperative catecholamine surges and hypercoagulability. See also Chapter 13, question D.3.

Executive summary of the ACC/AHA task force report: guidelines for perioperative cardiovascular evaluation for noncardiac surgery. Anesth Analg 82:854–860, 1996

Mangano DT: Perioperative cardiac morbidity. Anesthesiology 72:153–184, 1990

D.3. Is postoperative anemia associated with adverse cardiac outcome?

The acceptance of acute anemia during and after cardiac surgery in an attempt to conserve blood and prevent the transmission of bloodborne diseases has led to aggressive application of this principle to noncardiac surgery. Thus, high-risk patients undergoing major surgical procedures are being exposed to unprecedented levels of acute anemia. Logically, and based on fluid physics, this should result in decreased oxygen delivery and regional myocardial oxygen imbalance in those areas supplied by a critically stenotic coronary artery.

Two groups have now documented adverse clinical consequences of postoperative, iatrogenic acute anemia. Nelson et al. have identified a hematocrit of 28% as being the threshold associated with increased incidence of morbid cardiac events in postoperative vascular surgical patients. A second study documented that a hematocrit on postoperative day 2 of <29% was associated with a high degree of ischemia on the first two postoperative days (55% versus 16%; P <0.01). This appears to be evidence that myocardial revascularization enables patients undergoing effective revascularization to tolerate lower hematocrits than patients whose coronary stenoses have not been bypassed. Therefore, when confronted with high-risk patients or those who demonstrate myocardial ischemia, we are more likely to transfuse packed cells to raise the hematocrit to 30%.

Christopherson R, Frank S, Norris E et al: Low postoperative hematocrit is associated with cardiac ischemia in high-risk patients. Anesthesiology 75:A99, 1991

Nelson AH, Fleisher LA, Rosenbaum SH: Relationship between postoperative anemia and cardiac morbidity in high-risk vascular patients in the intensive care unit. Crit Care Med 21:860, 1993

D.4. Is postoperative hypothermia associated with postoperative myocardial ischemia?

Frank et al. studied 100 patients undergoing lower extremity vascular surgery. They found that unintentional hypothermia (sublingual temperature <35°C on arrival to postoperative intensive care unit) is associated with a significantly higher incidence of myocardial ischemia (36% versus 13%), angina (18% versus 15%) and PaO_2 <80 mm Hg (52% versus 30%) during the early postoperative period. Therefore, aggressive warming and heat conservation are mandatory during and after surgery. It is recommended to continue forced-air warming for the first several hours after surgery in hypothermic patients.

Frank SM, Beattie C, Christopherson R et al: Unintentional hypothermia is associated with postoperative myocardial ischemia: The Perioperative Ischemia Randomized Anesthesia Trial Study Group. Anesthesiology 78:468–476, 1993

D.5. How would you make a diagnosis of perioperative myocardial infarction?

Few studies have examined the optimal method for diagnosing a perioperative MI. Clinical symptoms, postoperative ECG changes, and elevation of the MB fraction of creatine kinase (CK) have been most extensively studied. Newer myocardial-specific enzyme elevations such as troponin-L, troponin-T, or CK-MB isoforms may also have value. In patients with known or suspected CAD undergoing high-risk procedures, ECG obtained at baseline, immediately after surgery, and the first 2 days after surgery appear to be cost-effective. Use of cardiac enzymes is best reserved for patients at high risk and those with clinical, ECG, or hemodynamic evidence of cardiovascular dysfunction.

Barash PG: Monitoring myocardial ischemia: A sequential clinical approach. ASA Annual Refresher Course Lecture No. 112, 1996

Executive summary of the ACC/AHA task force report: Guidelines for perioperative cardiovascular evaluation for noncardiac surgery. Anesth Analg 82:854–860, 1996

The Gastrointestinal System   III

Intestinal Obstruction

19

Joseph Tjan

A 62-year-old woman was admitted to the emergency room with complaints of a 2-day history of diffuse crampy abdominal pain associated with several episodes of emesis and a mild fever. Blood pressure (BP), 85/60 mm Hg; pulse, 115 beats/min; hematocrit, 45%.

A. Medical Disease and Differential Diagnosis

1. What is the differential diagnosis of the acute abdomen?
2. What are the causes of intestinal obstruction of the small bowel? Of the large bowel?
3. Differentiate between simple and strangulated bowel obstruction.
4. Is it important to differentiate whether the bowel obstruction is located in the small bowel or large bowel? Why?
5. What are the signs and symptoms of intestinal obstruction?
6. What are the causes and effects of bowel distention?
7. Describe the fluid shifts during small bowel intestinal obstruction.
8. Discuss the systemic derangements that occur with intestinal obstruction.
9. Can there be actual losses of red cell mass?
10. What is an ileus? Discuss its causes and treatment.
11. What are the systemic effects from the absorption of bacteria and bacterial products?

B. Preoperative Evaluation and Preparation

1. Is it important to decompress the abdomen prior to surgical intervention? Why?
2. Describe the respiratory implications.
3. What are the implications of the tense abdominal wall?
4. Outline the methods of abdominal decompression.
5. Discuss the goals of fluid management.
6. What would you use as a guide to fluid volume replacement?
7. Would you premedicate this patient?

C. Intraoperative Management

1. What dangers are present during induction? How are they planned for?
2. Does the administration of antacids and/or H_2-blockers prior to the induction of anesthesia have a significant value in patients with small bowel obstruction?
3. In what position would you intubate this patient? Would you use Sellick's maneuver?
4. Is succinylcholine the best muscle relaxant to use for the rapid-sequence induction?
5. Would you remove or leave the nasogastric tube in place before inducing anesthesia?
6. Would you use nitrous oxide (N_2O) in this patient?

D. Postoperative Management

1. What are the principles of postoperative care in this patient?
2. Are there any postoperative respiratory problems not associated with aspiration? When would you extubate this patient?
3. If the patient did aspirate gastric contents, what are the possible sequelae of this event? What is the treatment?
4. What is gram-negative sepsis? Describe the clinical picture and treatment.

A. Medical Disease and Differential Diagnosis

A.1. What is the differential diagnosis of the acute abdomen?

Intestinal obstruction accounts for approximately 15% to 20% of hospitalized patients with an acute abdomen. Abdominal pain can be divided into three categories: visceral, somatic, and referred. Visceral pain is transmitted through the autonomic nervous system via C fibers located intramurally in hollow viscera and in the capsule of abdominal organs. Visceral pain is dull, crampy, or aching in nature, and the factors that produce it include stretching and distention, which result in increased wall tension, inflammation, ischemia, torsion, compression, and certain chemicals. Transmission of somatic pain occurs via A-delta fibers of spinal nerves to produce pain that is characteristically sharp, severe, and persistent. Somatic pain is caused by irritation of the parietal peritoneum, and it arises as a response to acute changes in pH or temperature, as seen with bacterial or chemical inflammation. Referred pain is that which is felt in a region of the body different from the point of its origin due to the sharing of common pathways for afferent neurons arising from different sites. A proper history and physical examination with early diagnosis is of utmost importance in the management of the patient with an acute abdomen. In a recent review of >1100 patients with abdominal pain who presented to the emergency room, the most common diagnosis overall was nonspecific abdominal pain. Appendicitis, intestinal obstruction, urologic disorders, and gallstones were the most common surgical causes in order of decreasing frequency. In 47% of the patients, surgical intervention was required. The gastrointestinal and intraperitoneal causes of abdominal pain are listed in Table 19-1. Many extraperitoneal causes of abdominal pain are found, and these include pulmonary, cardiac, neurologic, metabolic, toxic, infectious, vascular, and hematologic conditions.

Schwartz SI, Shirer GT, Spencer FC et al (eds): Principles of Surgery, 6th ed, pp 1016–1019, 1028–1031. New York, McGraw-Hill, 1994

A.2. What are the causes of intestinal obstruction of the small bowel? Of the large bowel?

Intestinal obstruction can be of extraluminal (adhesions), intraluminal (gallstones), or intramural (Crohn's disease) origin. The term "mechanical bowel obstruction" denotes an actual physical barrier that interferes with the normal progression of intestinal contents. The most common cause of small bowel obstruction is postoperative adhesions, followed by incarcerated hernias and malignant tumors, respectively. Alternatively, neoplasms account for most cases of large bowel obstruction. Other causes of large bowel obstruction include diverticulitis and volvulus.

Table 19-1.　Gastrointestinal and Intraperitoneal Causes of Abdominal Pain

I. Inflammation/Infection	II. Mechanical (obstruction, acute distention)
A. Peritoneum	A. Hollow intestinal organs
1. Chemical and nonbacterial peritonitis—perforated peptic ulcer, gallbladder, ruptured ovarian cyst, mittelschmerz	1. Intestinal obstruction—adhesions, hernia, tumor, volvulus, intussusception
	2. Biliary obstruction—calculi, tumor, choledochal cyst, hematobilia
2. Bacterial peritonitis	B. Solid viscera
a. Primary peritonitis—pneumococcal, streptococcal, tuberculous	1. Acute splenomegaly
b. Perforated hollow viscus—stomach, intestine, biliary tract	2. Acute hepatomegaly—cardiac failure, Budd-Chiari syndrome
B. Hollow intestinal organs	C. Mesentery
1. Appendicitis	1. Omental torsion
2. Cholecystitis	D. Pelvic organs
3. Peptic ulceration	1. Ovarian cyst
4. Gastroenteritis	2. Torsion or degeneration of fibroid
5. Regional enteritis	3. Ectopic pregnancy
6. Meckel's diverticulitis	III. Vascular
7. Colitis—ulcerative, bacterial, amebic	A. Intraperitoneal bleeding
8. Diverticulitis	1. Ruptured liver
C. Solid viscera	2. Ruptured spleen
1. Pancreatitis	3. Ruptured mesentery
2. Hepatitis	4. Ruptured ectopic pregnancy
3. Hepatic abscess	5. Ruptured aortic, splenic, or hepatic aneurysm
4. Splenic abscess	B. Ischemia
D. Mesentery	1. Mesenteric thrombosis
1. Lymphadenitis	2. Hepatic infarction—toxemia, purpura
E. Pelvic organs	3. Splenic infarction
1. Pelvic inflammatory disease	4. Omental ischemia
2. Tuboovarian abscess	IV. Miscellaneous
3. Endometritis	A. Endometriosis

(Reprinted with permission from Schwartz SI, Shirer GT, Spencer FC, et al [eds]: Principles of Surgery, 6th ed, p 1016. New York, McGraw-Hill, 1994)

Rogers MC, Covino BG, Tinker JH et al (eds): Principles and Practice of Anesthesiology, pp 1978–1979. St. Louis, Mosby-Year Book, 1993

Schwartz SI, Shirer GT, Spencer FC et al (eds): Principles of Surgery, 6th ed, pp 1028–1031. New York, McGraw-Hill, 1994

A.3. Differentiate between simple and strangulated bowel obstruction.

Simple obstruction occurs when the lumen is obstructed and the blood supply remains normal. Occlusion of the blood supply to the obstructed bowel results in a strangulated obstruction. Toxic fluid is discharged into the bowel lumen, bowel wall, and peritoneal cavity when venous outflow obstruction occurs. It is important to recognize strangulation preoperatively because the implications are more serious and the mortality rate is high at between 20% to 40%. However, the overall mortality rate for intestinal obstruction is <10%. A closed-loop obstruction is present when both limbs of the loop are obstructed. This leads rapidly to strangulation, occasionally even before clinical evidence of intestinal obstruction exists.

Rogers MC, Covino BG, Tinker JH et al (eds): Principles and Practice of Anesthesiology, pp 1978–1979. St. Louis, Mosby-Year Book, 1993

Schwartz SI, Shirer GT, Spencer FC et al (eds): Principles of Surgery, 6th ed, pp 1028–1031. New York, McGraw-Hill, 1994

A.4. Is it important to differentiate whether the bowel obstruction is located in the small bowel or large bowel? Why?

Yes. Simple mechanical obstruction of the small bowel results in altered bowel motility, bowel distention with progressive accumulation of fluid and gas, and systemic derangements. Strangulation ensues if the obstruction is not relieved promptly, which leads to bowel necrosis and the leakage of blood, fluid, and toxic substances into the bowel and peritoneal cavity. About 60% to 80% of intestinal obstruction occurs in the small bowel.

Although the signs and symptoms may be similar, large bowel obstruction is usually more insidious than small bowel obstruction. Except for a volvulus, large bowel obstruction has less of a propensity to strangulate. The colon is essentially a storage organ with little secretory and absorptive functions. Therefore, systemic derangements are less severe with large bowel obstruction. The most important complication is progressive distention and rupture of the colon, especially in the presence of a competent ileocecal valve. The cecum is the usual site of rupture.

Rogers MC, Covino BG, Tinker JH et al (eds): Principles and Practice of Anesthesiology, pp 1978–1979. St. Louis, Mosby-Year Book, 1993

Schwartz SI, Shirer GT, Spencer FC et al (eds): Principles of Surgery, 6th ed, pp 1028–1031. New York, McGraw-Hill, 1994

A.5. What are the signs and symptoms of intestinal obstruction?

The four cardinal signs and symptoms of intestinal obstruction are crampy abdominal pain, vomiting, obstipation, and abdominal distention. The colicky pain is often diffuse, and it alternates with quiescent periods. The duration of the quiescent period depends on the site of intestinal obstruction. With a high obstruction, the duration is approximately 4 to 5 minutes, and 15 to 20 minutes with lower ileal obstruction. Steady severe abdominal pain usually indicates strangulation.

Vomiting commonly occurs immediately after the onset of bowel obstruction, followed by a variable quiescent period before recurrence. Vomiting becomes more frequent and bilious the higher the level of obstruction, and with the exception of a volvulus, it is uncommon in colonic obstruction. Abdominal distention, a late finding, may be absent in high small bowel obstruction that is associated with frequent bouts of emesis. Other signs of intestinal obstruction include localized tenderness, fever, tachycardia, and leukocytosis. A white blood cell count of 15,000 to 25,000/mm^3 is strongly suggestive of strangulation but this is not a sensitive test because 40% of patients with strangulation have normal white blood cell counts. With the development of dehydration serum chemistries will change, hemoconcentration occurs, and urine output diminishes and becomes concentrated.

The most important diagnostic procedure is radiographic study of the abdomen in the supine and upright positions with upright and lateral chest radiographs. In intestinal obstruction, gas-fluid levels are seen on the radiographs. Although normal within the stomach and colon, intestinal gas is usually minimal and infrequent in the small bowel. Therefore, gas-fluid levels are indicative of obstruction, but they may

Table 19-2.   Radiologic Signs in Intestinal Obstruction

SIGN	SIMPLE MECHANICAL OBSTRUCTION	ADYNAMIC ILEUS
Gas in intestine	Large bow-shaped loops in ladder pattern	Copious gas diffusely through intestine
Gas in colon	Less than normal	Increased, scattered through colon
Fluid levels in intestine	Definite	Often very large throughout
Tumor	None	None
Peritoneal exudate	None	Present with peritonitis; otherwise absent
Diaphragm	Somewhat elevated; free motion	Elevated; diminished motion

(Reprinted with permission from Schwartz SI, Shirer GT, Spencer FC, et al [eds]: Principles of Surgery, 6th ed, p 1030. New York, McGraw-Hill, 1994)

also be seen in gastroenteritis, severe constipation, sprue, and severe aerophagia. The radiologic findings and those features that differentiate simple mechanical obstruction from an ileus are summarized in Table 19-2.

Katz J, Benumof JL, Kadis LB (eds): Anesthesia and Uncommon Diseases, 3rd ed, pp 439–446, 474. Philadelphia, WB Saunders, 1990

Rogers MC, Covino BG, Tinker JH et al (eds): Principles and Practice of Anesthesiology, pp 1978–1984. St. Louis, Mosby-Year Book, 1993

Schwartz SI, Shirer GT, Spencer FC et al (eds): Principles of Surgery, 6th ed, pp 1028–1031. New York, McGraw-Hill, 1994

A.6. What are the causes and effects of bowel distention?

Intestinal obstruction results in the sequestration of fluid and gas within the lumen. Accumulation of fluid accounts for most cases of the bowel distention. As intraluminal pressure increases, the secretory function of the bowel increases progressively. Prostaglandin release seems to mediate this hypersecretion of fluid. In addition, reabsorption is impaired once intraluminal pressure exceeds 20 cm H_2O. The basic composition of the intestinal gas is that of swallowed air. As bowel distention continues, progressive interference with the mesenteric blood supply occurs, resulting in a strangulated obstruction with its associated morbidity and mortality.

Rogers MC, Covino BG, Tinker JH et al (eds): Principles and Practice of Anesthesiology, pp 1978–1984. St. Louis, Mosby-Year Book, 1993

Schwartz SI, Shirer GT, Spencer FC et al (eds): Principles of Surgery, 6th ed, pp 1028–1031. New York, McGraw-Hill, 1994

A.7. Describe the fluid shifts during small bowel intestinal obstruction.

Normally, approximately 7 to 9 liters of fluid are secreted daily into the upper gastrointestinal tract. The secretions include saliva (500–2000 ml), gastric juice (1000–2000 ml), bile (300–600 ml), pancreatic juice (300–800 ml), and succus entericus (2000–4000 ml) (Table 19-3). Due to small intestinal reabsorption only 400 ml of fluid passes the ileocecal valve.

In small bowel obstruction, several mechanisms contribute to fluid and electrolyte loss. The most important is the accumulation of fluid in the bowel lumen be-

Table 19-3. Volume and Composition of Gastrointestinal Fluids

SOURCE	24-HR VOL	Na (mEq/L)	K (mEq/L)	Cl (mEq/L)	HCO₃ (mEq/L)
Saliva	500–2000	2–10	20–30	8–18	30
Stomach	1000–2000	60–100	10–20	100–130	0
Pancreas	300–800	135–145	5–10	70–90	95–120
Bile	300–600	135–145	5–10	90–130	30–40
Jejunum	2000–4000	120–140	5–10	90–140	30–40
Ileum	1000–2000	80–150	2–8	45–140	30
Colon	–	60	30	40	—

(Reprinted with permission from Miller RD [ed]: Anesthesia, 4th ed, p 1610. New York, Churchill Livingstone, 1994)

cause the obstructed bowel becomes overly secretory instead of absorptive. Sequestration of fluid within the bowel wall accounts for its edematous appearance. This in turn results in free peritoneal fluid because of transudation of fluid across the serosal surface of the bowel. Fluid accumulation above the obstruction can be remarkable. In early small bowel obstruction, 1500 ml of fluid accumulates in the bowel. Once intestinal obstruction is well established and vomiting occurs, 3000 ml of fluid may be present. When the patient exhibits hypotension and tachycardia, indicating circulatory instability, as much as 6000 ml of fluid is in the gut. Lastly, vomiting or nasogastric suctioning further increases fluid losses.

Katz J, Benumof JL, Kadis LB (eds): Anesthesia and Uncommon Diseases, 3rd ed, pp 437–443, 481–482. Philadelphia, WB Saunders, 1990

Miller RD (ed): Anesthesia, 4th ed, pp 1610–1613. New York, Churchill Livingstone, 1994

Rogers MC, Covino BG, Tinker JH et al (eds): Principles and Practice of Anesthesiology, pp 1978–1984. St. Louis, Mosby-Year Book, 1993

Schwartz SI, Shirer GT, Spencer FC et al (eds): Principles of Surgery, 6th ed, pp 1028–1031. New York, McGraw-Hill, 1994

A.8. Discuss the systemic derangements that occur with intestinal obstruction.

The systemic derangements that occur can be categorized as hemodynamic changes, electrolyte abnormalities, and disturbances in acid-base balance.

Hemodynamically, if fluid and electrolyte losses are not corrected, central venous pressure falls. Hypotension and tachycardia follow as the vascular volume decreases in relation to the size of the vascular bed. The shock state develops as the body calls forth sympathomimetic amines to increase cardiac output and decrease the size of the vascular bed.

Small bowel obstruction results in the loss of vast quantities of isotonic extracellular fluid. The extent of extracellular fluid loss can be monitored by serial hematocrit determinations. A rise in the hematocrit is proportionate to the amount of fluid loss. For example, if the hematocrit has risen to 55%, approximately 40% of plasma and extracellular fluid volume has been lost.

As the obstruction continues, a gradual decrease is seen in the plasma sodium and chloride concentrations. Hyponatremia will aggravate hypovolemic hypotension, and confusion and somnolence will ensue. Hypokalemia will be manifested in delayed ventricular conduction, ST-T segment changes, and ventricular arrhythmias.

With respect to acid-base balance, the most common occurrence is metabolic acidosis due to the effects of dehydration, starvation, ketosis, and loss of alkaline secretions. Metabolic alkalosis, which is rare, is the result of marked loss of acidic gastric fluid. Monitoring includes serial determinations of sodium, potassium, chloride, and CO_2.

Katz J, Benumof JL, Kadis LB (eds): Anesthesia and Uncommon Diseases, 3rd ed, pp 437–443, 474. Philadelphia, WB Saunders, 1990

Miller RD (ed): Anesthesia, 4th ed, pp 1612–1613. New York, Churchill Livingstone, 1994

Rogers MC, Covino BG, Tinker JH et al (eds): Principles and Practice of Anesthesiology, pp 1978–1984. St. Louis, Mosby-Year Book, 1993

Schwartz SI, Shirer GT, Spencer FC, et al (eds): Principles of Surgery, 6th ed, pp 1028–1031. New York, McGraw-Hill, 1994

A.9. Can there be actual losses of red cell mass?

Yes. In long-standing intestinal obstruction, especially when it is associated with strangulation, increased permeability of the bowel wall occurs with loss of red cells into the bowel and peritoneal cavity. Whole blood or packed cells may be needed to restore circulating red blood cells.

Schwartz SI, Shirer GT, Spencer FC et al (eds): Principles of Surgery, 6th ed, pp 1028–1031. New York, McGraw-Hill, 1994

A.10. What is an ileus? Discuss its causes and treatment.

An ileus is a functional failure of normal aboral intestinal transit. Except for the discomfort of abdominal distention, it is usually not painful. The pathogenesis of ileus is poorly understood, but stimulation of the inhibitory adrenergic neurons may play an important role. Classification of ileus is as follows:

- Adynamic or inhibition ileus—diminished or absent motility from neuromuscular inhibition
- Spastic ileus—contracted bowel musculature with resultant uncoordinated motility
- Ileus of vascular occlusion—disordered motility secondary to ischemia

Adynamic ileus is the most common form because it is present following every intra-abdominal operation. Postoperative ileus affects different parts of the gastrointestinal tract differently. Small bowel function recovers within 24 hours, whereas gastric motility may take 24 to 48 hours to return. The colon is the most severely affected organ, where ileus can persist for as long as 3 to 5 days.

If postoperative ileus is prolonged, other contributing causes should be sought, which include:

- Metabolic—hypokalemia, hyponatremia, hypomagnesemia
- Drugs—narcotics, antacids, anticoagulants, phenothiazines, ganglionic blockers
- Other—intraperitoneal inflammation (e.g., acute appendicitis or acute pancreatitis), sepsis, hematoma, wound infection, ureteral colic, spine or rib fractures, basal pneumonia

Spastic ileus, which is rare, occurs with heavy metal poisoning, porphyria, and uremia.

Management of ileus involves treatment of the underlying cause, nasogastric decompression, intravenous hydration, correction of metabolic abnormalities, and nutritional support if needed. No specific drug therapy has been shown to be effective.

Rogers MC, Covino BG, Tinker JH et al (eds): Principles and Practice of Anesthesiology, pp 1978–1979. St. Louis, Mosby-Year Book, 1993

Schwartz SI, Shirer GT, Spencer FC et al (eds): Principles of Surgery, 6th ed, p 1031. New York, McGraw-Hill, 1994

A.11. What are the systemic effects from the absorption of bacteria and bacterial products?

The normal mucosa is impermeable to bacteria and toxins produced by bacterial degradation, but permeability is affected when the blood supply is impaired in a strangulated segment of bowel. Thus, transperitoneal absorption of toxins can result in septic shock.

Schwartz SI, Shirer GT, Spencer FC et al (eds): Principles of Surgery, 6th ed, pp 1028–1031. New York, McGraw-Hill, 1994

B. Preoperative Evaluation and Preparation

B.1. Is it important to decompress the abdomen prior to surgical intervention? Why?

Yes. Because of the respiratory and circulatory complications that ensue.

Katz J, Benumof JL, Kadis LB (eds): Anesthesia and Uncommon Diseases, 3rd ed, pp 443–444. Philadelphia, WB Saunders, 1990

Schwartz SI, Shirer GT, Spencer FC et al (eds): Principles of Surgery, 6th ed, pp 1028–1031. New York, McGraw-Hill, 1994

B.2. Describe the respiratory implications.

The distended bowel produces pressure on the diaphragm, limiting its downward movement and resulting in inadequate ventilation. The decrease in tidal volume and the reduction in functional residual capacity result in a low PaO_2 and an elevated $PaCO_2$. It is especially true if the stomach is also distended. An additional reason for gastric decompression is to remove fluid and air from the stomach to lessen the likelihood of aspiration of gastric contents into the tracheobronchial tree during anesthesia induction. A long-standing obstruction and its associated respiratory compromise will result in a gasping, dusky, cyanotic, semicomatose patient.

Katz J, Benumof JL, Kadis LB (eds): Anesthesia and Uncommon Diseases, 3rd ed, pp 443–444. Philadelphia, WB Saunders, 1990

Schwartz SI, Shirer GT, Spencer FC et al (eds): Principles of Surgery, 6th ed, pp 1028–1031. New York, McGraw-Hill, 1994

B.3. What are the implications of the tense abdominal wall?

The first implication is related to the higher incidence of reverse peristalsis. Second, the stretched abdominal wall requires deeper anesthesia and more muscle relaxant to provide adequate operating conditions. These implications can increase morbidity. The distended abdomen significantly affects venous return by two mechanisms. First, abdominal distention decreases negative intrathoracic pressure and thereby decreases venous return. The second is caused by direct vena caval compression from intraperitoneal tension. In long-standing intestinal obstruction, a large volume of intraperitoneal fluid may be present in the abdominal cavity. At the time of surgical incision, care must be taken to prevent the fluid from escaping rapidly from the abdomen to minimize severe hypotension. As fluid is slowly released from the abdominal cavity, the blood pressure should be checked frequently and the rate of fluid release adjusted to minimize a fall in blood pressure.

Katz J, Benumof JL, Kadis LB (eds): Anesthesia and Uncommon Diseases, 3rd ed, pp 451–452, 486–487. Philadelphia, WB Saunders, 1990

Schwartz SI, Shirer GT, Spencer FC et al (eds): Principles of Surgery, 6th ed, pp 1028–1031. New York, McGraw-Hill, 1994

B.4. Outline the methods of abdominal decompression.

Two types of tubes are available for abdominal decompression: short tubes placed in the stomach and long tubes placed in the small intestine. To reduce the likelihood of regurgitation of gastric contents, it is important that the stomach be empty prior to anesthesia induction. This is best done by the sump tube, which is more efficient than the simple Levin tube. The sump tube is composed of a double lumen, one for aspiration and the other to allow air into the stomach. The Miller-Abbott tube is a long intestinal tube that is initially passed into the stomach; an incorporated balloon containing mercury at its tip aids in its passage through the pylorus into the small bowel.

Although gastric and intestinal tubes are used to relieve abdominal distention, they do not function solely as definitive therapy for bowel obstruction except in postoperative ileus, partial small bowel obstruction, and intestinal obstruction caused by inflammation that is expected to subside with conservative therapy. For all other bowel obstructions, the mainstay of therapy is surgical intervention.

Schwartz SI, Shirer GT, Spencer FC et al (eds): Principles of Surgery, 6th ed, pp 1028–1031. New York, McGraw-Hill, 1994

B.5. Discuss the goals of fluid management.

Estimating the degree of fluid deficit in intestinal obstruction is extremely difficult and often underestimated. Significant sequestration of fluid is found within the bowel lumen, bowel wall, and transudation into the peritoneal cavity. Poor preoperative nutrition and protein loss into the bowel can lead to hypoalbuminemia and further fluid losses. The primary goal of fluid management is the initial restoration of intravascular volume to a state of normovolemia. This will lead to the optimization of oxygen delivery to the tissues and organs. The second goal is the correction of any existing electrolyte disturbances, including acid-base derangements. Because the fluid lost to an obstructed segment of bowel is similar to plasma in composition, a balanced salt solution such as lactated Ringer's solution is appropriate to use for fluid resuscitation.

Katz J, Benumof JL, Kadis LB (eds): Anesthesia and Uncommon Diseases, 3rd ed, pp 437–443, 481–482. Philadelphia, WB Saunders, 1990

Miller RD (ed): Anesthesia, 4th ed, pp 1610–1613. New York, Churchill Livingstone, 1994

Schwartz SI, Shirer GT, Spencer FC et al (eds): Principles of Surgery, 6th ed, pp 1028–1031. New York, McGraw-Hill, 1994

B.6. What would you use as a guide to fluid volume replacement?

Fluid losses can be calculated knowing that the body turns over 17 to 18 liters of fluid a day, made up of intestinal secretions, urine excreted by the kidneys, fluid loss through the feces, and insensible losses from the lungs and skin. As mentioned, tremendous fluid loss occurs into the gut, which may amount to 4500 to 9000 ml of functional fluid loss, including loss owing to vomiting and nasogastric suctioning. With significant bowel wall edema and leakage of fluid into the peritoneal cavity due to peritonitis, an additional 7 liters of fluid may be sequestered in the peritoneal space. Measurement of central venous pressure, hourly urine output, arterial blood pressure, heart rate, and skin turgor can be used to guide fluid replacement. Additionally, ongoing modifications are made in the management of fluid and electrolytes to achieve the desired physiologic goals.

Katz J, Benumof JL, Kadis LB (eds): Anesthesia and Uncommon Diseases, 3rd ed, pp 439–442, 481–482. Philadelphia, WB Saunders, 1990

Miller RD (ed): Anesthesia, 4th ed, pp 1610–1613. New York, Churchill Livingstone, 1994

Schwartz SI, Shirer GT, Spencer FC et al (eds): Principles of Surgery, 6th ed, pp 1028–1031. New York, McGraw-Hill, 1994

B.7. Would you premedicate this patient?

Because these individuals may have a diminished respiratory reserve owing to the distended abdomen, any premedication that depresses respiratory drive will diminish the ability of the patient to ventilate. This will exaggerate any preexisting hypoxia and hypercarbia. Despite the fact that the patient may be in considerable pain from the abdominal distention, narcotic analgesics should be avoided. Anticholinergic drug use has some value in protecting the heart from potent vagal stimulation associated with the use of vagomimetic drugs and endotracheal intubation. In those patients with preexisting tachycardia or hyperthermia, atropine or glycopyrrolate is omitted. Some physicians have advocated the use of antacids to increase the pH of gastric contents prior to anesthesia induction, but this may actually stimulate vomiting in the bowel-obstructed patient. Antacids themselves, especially particulate antacids, can produce serious pulmonary insufficiency if aspirated. In general, oral premedication should not be given to patients with intestinal obstruction.

Barash PG, Cullen BF, Stoelting RK (eds): Clinical Anesthesia 3rd ed, pp 984–985, 1293–1295. Philadelphia, JB Lippincott, 1997

Katz J, Benumof JL, Kadis LB (eds): Anesthesia and Uncommon Diseases, 3rd ed, pp 443–444, 448–456. Philadelphia, WB Saunders, 1990

Longnecker DE, Murphy FL (eds): Introduction to Anesthesia, 9th ed, pp 27–35. Philadelphia, WB Saunders, 1997

Rogers MC, Covino BG, Tinker JH et al (eds): Principles and Practice of Anesthesiology, pp 1978–1984. St. Louis, Mosby-Year Book, 1993

C. Intraoperative Management

C.1. What dangers are present during induction? How are they planned for?

Regurgitation of stomach contents and subsequent aspiration into the tracheobronchial tree is the principal danger during induction of anesthesia for the patient with intestinal obstruction.

Mortality associated with aspiration of gastric contents ranges widely from 3% to 70%. Abdominal surgery in particular has been associated with up to 75% of the perioperative mortality due to aspiration pneumonitis. The incidence of aspiration for all anesthetics is almost 5 per 10,000. Anesthesia should proceed with a rapid-sequence and cricoid pressure induction or an awake intubation, especially if a difficult intubation is anticipated.

If the awake intubation route is chosen, the patient's lips, tongue, and upper oral pharynx should be sprayed with a topical anesthetic. When this is accomplished, additional spray further down into the pharynx can be done, but care must be taken to avoid the laryngeal mechanism. Do not anesthetize the larynx because the defense mechanism for laryngeal closure will be lost in the event that regurgitation or vomiting should occur. Therefore, a superior laryngeal nerve block or a transtracheal injection is not warranted in these patients. Sedation should be limited or avoided altogether. A rapid-sequence induction allows the completion of tracheal intubation with a cuffed endotracheal tube in the shortest possible time from the onset of loss of consciousness. The sequence consists of denitrogenation with 100% oxygen for approximately 2 to 3 minutes, precurarization with 3 mg of d-tubocurarine to prevent vigorous fasciculations produced by succinylcholine, which may increase intragastric pressure; administration of thiopental sodium; application of cricoid pressure; rapid paralysis with succinylcholine; and endotracheal intubation with immediate cuff inflation. Cricoid pressure should not be released until the cuff is inflated and correct placement of the endotracheal tube has been verified by measures including auscultation and capnometry. Should the patient remain hemodynamically unstable following fluid and electrolyte resuscitation, ketamine or etomidate is preferable for anesthesia induction.

Katz J, Benumof JL, Kadis LB (eds): Anesthesia and Uncommon Diseases, 3rd ed, pp 446–451, 476–481. Philadelphia, WB Saunders, 1990

Miller RD (ed): Anesthesia, 4th ed, pp 1437–1464. New York, Churchill Livingstone, 1994

Rogers MC, Covino BG, Tinker JH et al (eds): Principles and Practice of Anesthesiology, pp 1978–1984. St. Louis, Mosby-Year Book, 1993

C.2. Does the administration of antacids and/or H_2-blockers prior to the induction of anesthesia have a significant value in patients with small bowel obstruction?

The volume and pH of gastric contents and the presence or absence of particulate matter appear to be the three most important factors determining the degree of pulmonary injury following aspiration. The classic term "at risk" is thought to imply a gastric volume >25 ml with a pH <2.5. About 40% of emergency surgical patients have a gastric pH <2.5. The more critical factor involved in determining the degree of lung injury appears to be the pH of gastric contents. Thus, outcomes are better with aspirations of large volumes of nonacidic material compared with that of small volumes of acidic material. Normally, clear, nonparticulate antacids (0.3 M sodium citrate) are effective in raising gastric pH and, likewise, H_2-blocking agents are effective in reducing gastric volume and acidity. However, because of the large volumes of fluid sequestered in the bowel, antacids and/or H_2-blockers have little or no value in high mechanical intestinal obstruction. When time permits to prepare the patient, these agents may be of some value in partial small bowel obstruction to reduce both gastric volume and acidity.

Katz J, Benumof JL, Kadis LB (eds): Anesthesia and Uncommon Diseases, 3rd ed, pp 446–451, 476–481. Philadelphia, WB Saunders, 1990

Miller RD (ed): Anesthesia, 4th ed, pp 1437–1464. New York, Churchill Livingstone, 1994

Rogers MC, Covino BG, Tinker JH et al (eds): Principles and Practice of Anesthesiology, pp 1978–1984. St. Louis, Mosby-Year Book, 1993

C.3. In what position would you intubate this patient? Would you use Sellick's maneuver?

Because gravity aids in keeping gastrointestinal contents within the stomach, the sitting or semisitting position decreases the incidence of regurgitation itself and thereby lessens the risk of pulmonary aspiration. Some clinicians advise that the patient be intubated in the supine position for fear that if the patient did vomit and was in the sitting or semisitting position, there would be a greater tendency to aspirate. However, we believe the head-up position is preferable. Should massive reverse peristalsis and regurgitation occur, vigorous suctioning and the head-down position are the best methods of preventing soilage of the tracheobronchial tree. The head-down position must be at least 10 degrees to prevent aspiration into the lungs. Sellick's maneuver will aid in preventing refluxed material from reaching the pharynx by compression of the cricoid cartilage against the esophagus. When properly done, cricoid pressure provides a barrier for at least 100 cm H_2O of esophageal pressure. Although some clinicians caution against using Sellick's maneuver in the vomiting patient for fear of rupture of the esophagus, this is mostly a theoretical concern. In fact, Sellick recently recommended that cricoid pressure should not be released in these situations.

Barash PG, Cullen BF, Stoelting RK (eds): Clinical Anesthesia, 3rd ed, pp 984–985, 1293–1295. Philadelphia, JB Lippincott, 1997

Katz J, Benumof JL, Kadis LB (eds): Anesthesia and Uncommon Diseases, 3rd ed, pp 446–447. Philadelphia, WB Saunders, 1990

Miller RD (ed): Anesthesia, 4th ed, pp 1455–1456. New York, Churchill Livingstone, 1994

Rogers MC, Covino BG, Tinker JH et al (eds): Principles and Practice of Anesthesiology, pp 1981–1983. St. Louis, Mosby-Year Book, 1993

C.4. Is succinylcholine the best muscle relaxant to use for the rapid-sequence induction?

Yes. Succinylcholine is still the best muscle relaxant for use in the rapid-sequence induction technique despite the known complications associated with its use. Recently, however, several studies have appeared advocating large doses of nondepolarizing muscle relaxants for rapid-sequence anesthesia induction. Schwartz and Mehta and their associates, in separate studies, described the priming principle. For the technique, they recommend a small dose of a nondepolarizing muscle relaxant, followed 3 to 6 minutes later by a second intubating dose. These authors claim that patients

Table 19-4.   Rapid Tracheal Intubation[a] with Succinylcholine or Various Nondepolarizing Relaxants (Dosages in mg/kg)[b,c]

DRUG	PRIMING DOSE[c]	INTUBATING DOSE[d]	CLINICAL DURATION[e]	FULL RECOVERY[f]
Succinylcholine	None	1.0	5–10	12–15
Succinylcholine	Nondepolarizer pretreatment	1.5	5–10	12–15
Rocuronium	None	0.6–1.0	30–60	60–120
Mivacurium	0.02	0.25	15–20	25–35
Atracurium	0.05	0.7–0.8	45–60	60–90
Vecuronium	0.01	0.15–0.2	60–75	90–120
Vecuronium	None	0.3–0.4	90–150	120–180
Cisatracurium	0.01	0.2–0.25	55–75	75–100
Cisatracurium	None	0.4	75–100	100–120

[a] Intubation within 60 to 90 seconds following injection of the intubating dose of the relaxant.
[b] The administration of adequate dosage of intravenous anesthetic is assumed.
[c] This dose is given as preoxygenation is begun.
[d] This dose is given 2 to 4 minutes following the priming dose. For atracurium and mivacurium, slower injection (30 seconds) is recommended to minimize circulatory effects.
[e] Minutes from injection of the intubating dose to recovery of twitch to 25 percent of control.
[f] Minutes from injection of the intubating dose to recovery of twitch to 95 percent of control.
(Reprinted with permission from Miller RD [ed]: Anesthesia, 4th ed, p 431. New York, Churchill Livingstone, 1994)

can be intubated significantly earlier, by about 30 to 60 seconds, than if they are given a single intubating dose of a nondepolarizing muscle relaxant. With use of the priming principle, tracheal intubation can be achieved approximately 90 seconds following the second intubating dose of muscle relaxant. However, some argue that 90 seconds is not fast enough for a rapid-sequence induction technique and, furthermore, the intubating conditions at 90 seconds may not be as ideal as that achieved at 60 seconds following succinylcholine administration. Also keep in mind that large doses of nondepolarizing muscle relaxants result in a longer duration of neuromuscular blockade. See Table 19-4 for the priming dose and intubating dose of various muscle relaxants.

Katz J, Benumof JL, Kadis LB (eds): Anesthesia and Uncommon Diseases, 3rd ed, pp 450–451. Philadelphia, WB Saunders, 1990

Mehta MP, Choi W, Gergis SD et al: Rapid-sequence endotracheal intubation with nondepolarizing muscle relaxants. Anesthesiology 62: 392, 1985

Miller RD (ed): Anesthesia, 4th ed, pp 430–437. New York, Churchill Livingstone, 1994

Schwarz S, Ilias W, Lackner F et al: Rapid tracheal intubation with vecuronium: The priming principle. Anesthesiology 62: 288, 1985

C.5. Would you remove or leave the nasogastric tube in place before inducing anesthesia?

Evidence indicates that many patients who aspirate have lower esophageal sphincter dysfunction. If a nasogastric tube (simple Levin or sump) or a nasointestinal tube (Miller-Abbott) is in place prior to anesthesia induction, it should be promptly removed. The tube will render the lower esophageal sphincter incompetent, making it possible for passive reflux of gastric contents to occur during induction. Furthermore, tube presence may hinder laryngoscopy and tracheal intubation.

Barash PG, Cullen BF, Stoelting RK (eds): Clinical Anesthesia 3rd ed, pp 984–985, 1293–1295. Philadelphia, JB Lippincott, 1997

C.6. Would you use nitrous oxide (N₂O) in this patient?

Nitrous oxide should be avoided because its administration is associated with an undesirable increase in intraluminal gas volume and pressure which can lead to detrimental consequences. The blood:gas partition coefficient of N_2O is 34 times that of nitrogen. Therefore, N_2O in the blood can enter gas-filled cavities 34 times more rapidly than nitrogen can leave those cavities to enter the blood. When this happens during abdominal surgery, bowel distention will occur. The amount of distention depends on the amount of gas already within the bowel and the duration of N_2O administration. Normally, the bowel contains about 100 ml of gas, which is mostly swallowed air, and N_2O use results in a slow increase in bowel distention and intraluminal pressure. However, with bowel obstruction, the volume of gas within the bowel is greatly increased. Under these conditions, the increased intraluminal pressure associated with N_2O administration may lead to bowel ischemia and necrosis. More commonly, it will cause difficulties with abdominal closure at the conclusion of surgery. Thus, anesthesia should be maintained with oxygen and a volatile agent and increments of opioids and muscle relaxants as needed.

Barash PG, Cullen BF, Stoelting RK (eds): Clinical Anesthesia 3rd ed, pp 984–985. Philadelphia, JB Lippincott, 1997

Katz J, Benumof JL, Kadis LB (eds): Anesthesia and Uncommon Diseases, 3rd ed, pp 486–487. Philadelphia, WB Saunders, 1990

Rogers MC, Covino BG, Tinker JH et al (eds): Principles and Practice of Anesthesiology, p 1983. St. Louis, Mosby-Year Book, 1993

D. Postoperative Management

D.1. What are the principles of postoperative care in this patient?

The principles of postoperative management are the same as those in the preoperative care of the patient, namely fluids and electrolytes, antibiotics, and gastrointestinal decompression. In the immediate postoperative period, significant ongoing fluid loss is seen, mostly secondary to third spacing. However, this fluid loss gradually diminishes over time; usually by about the third postoperative day it reverses in direction as fluid is transferred back into the vascular compartment. The significant autoinfusion that ensues must therefore be accounted for in the computations of the daily fluid requirements of the patient. Otherwise, congestive heart failure may follow, especially because patients with intestinal obstruction are often elderly with limited reserves in several organ systems. As electrolyte loss continues postoperatively, serial determinations of serum sodium and potassium levels may be necessary. Hyponatremia and hypokalemia are factors that contribute to prolonged postoperative ileus. Because return of normal intestinal motility is usually prolonged after surgical relief of bowel obstruction, abdominal decompression often needs to be continued for 5 or 6 days postoperatively, whereas bowel function returns on about the third postoperative day after a routine abdominal operation. Finally, postoperative management may also include frequent monitoring of hemodynamic parameters, hemoglobin concentration, and urine output.

Miller RD (ed): Anesthesia, 4th ed, pp 1612–1613. New York, Churchill Livingstone, 1994

Schwartz SI, Shirer GT, Spencer FC et al (eds): Principles of Surgery, 6th ed, pp 1028–1031. New York, McGraw-Hill, 1994

D.2. Are there any postoperative respiratory problems not associated with aspiration? When would you extubate this patient?

Yes. The postoperative respiratory problems are those related to hypoventilation. Although the intestinal obstruction has been relieved, significant abdominal distention may remain, which will inhibit diaphragmatic motion, and the patient may develop hypoxia and hypercarbia. In addition, abdominal pain and the residual effects of inhaled anesthetics, intravenous anesthetics, and neuromuscular blockers can contribute to respiratory inadequacy. The 15% to 20% reduction in functional residual capacity (FRC) associated with general anesthesia continues into the postoperative period, and following upper abdominal surgery vital capacity remains abnormal for more than a week. In summary, several pulmonary changes occur, including reductions in the following parameters: tidal volume, vital capacity, functional residual capacity, residual volume, and forced expiratory volume in 1 second (FEV_1). For these reasons, the endotracheal tube may be left in place to decrease anatomic dead space and make it possible to ventilate the patient during the immediate postanesthesia period. Leaving the endotracheal tube in place is also desirable for those patients with previous respiratory disease or in the morbidly obese individual. In both of these situations, the respiratory support will decrease residual atelectasis in the basilar portions of the lung. This will decrease any pulmonary shunt and lessen the need for a high inspired oxygen concentration (F_iO_2). As the patient gradually regains full consciousness, and respiratory adequacy (as shown by measuring inspiratory force and vital capacity), ventilation returns to normal and the patient can be safely extubated.

Katz J, Benumof JL, Kadis LB (eds): Anesthesia and Uncommon Diseases, 3rd ed, pp 443–444, 454–455. Philadelphia, WB Saunders, 1990

Rogers MC, Covino BG, Tinker JH et al (eds): Principles and Practice of Anesthesiology, pp 1981–1984. St. Louis, Mosby-Year Book, 1993

D.3. If the patient did aspirate gastric contents, what are the possible sequelae of this event? What is the treatment?

Aspiration of gastric contents produces a chemical pneumonitis characterized initially by hypoxemia, bronchospasm, and atelectasis. Additionally, the patient may exhibit signs of tachypnea, tachycardia, coughing, cyanosis, and shock. Arterial hypoxemia is the earliest and most reliable sign of aspiration. Even saline, when aspirated, causes significant hypoxemia.

Destruction of pneumocytes, lung parenchyma, and pulmonary microvasculature ensues, resulting in decreased surfactant activity, interstitial and alveolar edema, alveolar hemorrhage, and pulmonary hypertension, which is mainly caused by hypoxic pulmonary vasoconstriction. The clinical picture may resemble that of the adult respiratory distress syndrome. Radiographic findings are variable and may not appear for several hours. In at least 10% of cases, the radiographic films are normal. Positive findings usually consist of diffuse infiltrates bilaterally located in either the perihilar or basal regions.

Once vomiting or regurgitation occurs, immediate lateral head positioning, vigorous suctioning, and the head-down position should be instituted. To avoid disseminating the aspirated material further distally, the trachea is suctioned prior to beginning positive pressure ventilation. Bronchoscopy is indicated only for those patients who have aspirated solid material resulting in significant airway obstruction. Use of saline or bicarbonate solution is of little value and may actually be more detrimental than beneficial. Management includes keeping the patient intubated and well ventilated, following arterial blood gases, and obtaining serial chest radiographs. Depending on the arterial blood gases, it will be necessary to regulate the inspired oxygen concentration and the amount of ventilation to maintain PaO_2 and $PaCO_2$ within normal limits. If the F_IO_2 has to be maintained above 60%, positive end-expiratory pressure (PEEP) may be necessary to recruit additional alveoli and improve oxygenation. The best PEEP will have the least effect on venous return and at the same time allow F_IO_2 to be reduced to a safe level (40% or lower), thus decreasing the likelihood of oxygen toxicity. It is important to realize that although a patient may look well and have a clear chest without rhonchi or wheezes in the immediate postanesthetic period following aspiration, respiratory distress can still develop. It may take as long as 6 to 12 hours before the syndrome becomes manifest. The patient should be observed closely over 24 to 48 hours for the development of aspiration pneumonitis. Corticosteroid therapy remains controversial and the routine use of prophylactic antibiotics is not recommended because it may alter the normal flora of the respiratory tract and promote colonization by resistant organisms. However, antibiotics should be administered to those patients who show clinical signs of a secondary bacterial pulmonary infection with positive Gram stain and cultures, or to those patients known to have aspirated gross fecal material, as with lower intestinal obstruction.

Barash PG, Cullen BF, Stoelting RK (eds): Clinical Anesthesia, 3rd ed, pp 984–985, 1293–1295. Philadelphia, JB Lippincott, 1997

Katz J, Benumof JL, Kadis LB (eds): Anesthesia and Uncommon Diseases, 3rd ed, pp 446–447, 476–481. Philadelphia, WB Saunders, 1990

Miller RD (ed): Anesthesia, 4th ed, pp 1437–1464. New York, Churchill Livingstone, 1994

D.4. What is gram-negative sepsis? Describe the clinical picture and treatment.

Gram-negative sepsis frequently leads to a shock state caused by endotoxins from the cell walls of gram-negative bacteria circulating in the blood. The earliest signs of a gram-negative infection include an elevated temperature above 101°F, the development of shaking chills, mild hyperventilation, respiratory alkalosis, and an altered sensorium. The hemodynamic abnormalities of gram-negative sepsis are not clearly understood, but they seem to follow two distinct hemodynamic patterns, depending on the patient's volume status.

The first is a hyperdynamic circulatory pattern associated with early septic shock that occurs in patients who are normovolemic prior to the onset of sepsis. These patients present with hypotension, high cardiac output, normal or increased blood volume, normal or high central venous pressure, decreased peripheral resistance, warm and dry extremities, hyperventilation, and respiratory alkalosis. However, in a patient who is hypovolemic prior to the onset of sepsis as with a strangulated obstruction of the small bowel, a hypodynamic pattern is seen characterized by hypotension, low cardiac output, high peripheral resistance, low central venous pressure, and cold, clammy extremities. Both types of patterns will have a better outcome with early treatment, but if therapy is delayed or unsuccessful, cardiac and circulatory failure ensues associated with a low, fixed cardiac output and a resistant metabolic acidosis.

Definitive therapy of gram-negative sepsis includes the administration of appropriate antibiotics and early surgical debridement or drainage of the source of infection when indicated. Supportive measures are provided by fluid replacement and vasoactive drugs. Corticosteroid administration as part of the treatment regimen for sepsis is still a controversial issue. Direct arterial blood pressure monitoring and insertion of a Swan-Ganz catheter may be necessary for proper management.

Schwartz SI, Shirer GT, Spencer FC et al (eds): Principles of Surgery, 6th ed, pp 140–143. New York, McGraw-Hill, 1994

Wyngaarden JB, Smith LH Jr (eds): Cecil Textbook of Medicine, 19th ed, pp 1584–1588. Philadelphia, WB Saunders, 1992

20 Pyloric Stenosis

Vinod Malhotra

A 3-week-old first-born male infant had projectile vomiting, which contained the ingested formula but no bile. His body weight was 2.5 kg. Serum electrolytes: K, 2.2 mEq/liter; Cl, 86 mEq/liter. Blood pH 7.68.

A. Medical Disease and Differential Diagnosis

1. What is the diagnosis in this patient?
2. What is the differential diagnosis of pyloric stenosis?
3. What are the metabolic problems in this newborn, secondary to his disease?
4. What are the adverse effects of metabolic alkalosis?
5. How would you treat this infant?
6. How would you determine fluid replacement in a newborn and what fluids would you use?
7. How would you correct metabolic alkalosis in this patient?

B. Preoperative Evaluation and Preparation

1. How would you evaluate this patient preoperatively?
2. How would you prepare this patient rapidly for emergency surgery? Is surgical intervention an acute emergency in this case?
3. How would you prepare this patient for anesthesia?

C. Intraoperative Management

1. What anesthetic techniques or agents would you use?
2. What induction-intubation sequence would you use?
3. What are the anatomic characteristics of the airway in the newborn and how do they differ from those in the adult?
4. How do you determine the size of the endotracheal tube in pediatric patients?
5. What anesthesia system would you use and why?
6. What are the advantages and disadvantages of commonly employed non-rebreathing systems?
7. How would you monitor this patient intraoperatively?
8. How does the pulse oximeter function?
9. What factors affect the measurement of oxygen saturation by the pulse oximeter?

D. Postoperative Management

1. What are the complications that can occur in the postanesthesia recovery period?
2. How would you treat postextubation "croup" in this infant?

A. Medical Disease and Differential Diagnosis

A.1. What is the diagnosis in this patient?

The most likely diagnosis in this patient is pyloric stenosis. The factors that favor the diagnosis are as follows:

- Age—3 weeks (average age at onset; range 5 days to 5 months)
- Male child (male:female ratio = 4:1)
- Projectile vomiting (characteristic)
- Contents—ingested formula, no bile

The resultant biochemical abnormality in this patient is a hypokalemic, hypochloremic alkalosis.

Nelson WE, Behrman RE, Kleigman RM et al (eds): Nelson Textbook of Pediatrics, 15th ed, pp 1060–1062. Philadelphia, WB Saunders, 1996

A.2. What is the differential diagnosis of pyloric stenosis?

Pyloric stenosis is distinguished from other congenital anomalies that cause obstruction of the alimentary tract in the newborn. These other anomalies include chalasia of the esophagus, hiatus hernia, duodenal atresia, jejunal atresia, ileal atresia, pancreatic annulus, malrotation of the gut, intra-abdominal hernias, extra-abdominal hernias, and Meckel's diverticulum. Pathognomonic features of pyloric stenosis include absence of bile-staining of the vomitus and visible gastric peristaltic waves on abdominal examination along with a palpable pyloric mass. The diagnosis is commonly made clinically. Occasionally, an upper gastrointestinal (GI) series with barium or abdominal ultrasound may be necessary.

Hall SC: Pediatric Surgical Emergencies. American Society of Anesthesiologists. Annual Refresher Course Lectures 116:1–7, 1996

Maher M, Hehir DJ, Horgan A: Infantile hypertrophic pyloric stenosis: Long-term audit from a general surgical unit. Ir J Med Sci 165:115–117, 1996

Nelson WE, Behrman RE, Kleigman RM et al (eds): Nelson Textbook of Pediatrics, 15th ed, pp 1060–1062. Philadelphia, WB Saunders, 1996

A.3. What are the metabolic problems in this newborn, secondary to his disease?

Metabolic changes occur secondary to protracted vomiting, and they comprise the characteristic hypokalemic, hypochloremic alkalosis, as evident in this patient. Hyponatremia, although present, may not be manifested in serum value determinations owing to severe dehydration. Compensatory respiratory acidosis is a frequent finding; it results from hypoventilation that may be marked and associated with periods of apnea. In severe dehydration leading to circulatory shock, the lack of adequate perfusion, coupled with impaired renal and hepatic function, may produce an entirely different picture of metabolic acidosis with hyperventilation, resulting in respiratory alkalosis. Therefore, depending on the severity and duration of the vomiting and the type of fluid replenishment, one can encounter wide variations in findings on arterial blood gas and electrolyte determinations. However, the most frequent findings are hypokalemia, hyponatremia, hypochloremia, and primary metabolic alkalosis with secondary respiratory acidosis. These findings are summarized in Table 20-1.

Table 20-1. Metabolic Findings in the Newborn Secondary to Pyloric Stenosis

SEVERITY OF DEHYDRATION	ARTERIAL BLOOD GASES				SERUM ELECTROLYTES			
	*p*H	P_{CO_2}	CO_2	P_{O_2}	Na	K	Cl	HCO_3
Mild	↑	↑	↑	↔	↓ (↔)	↓	↓↓	↑
Moderate	↑↑	↑↑	↑↑	↔	↓	↓↓	↓↓↓	↑↑
Severe circulatory shock	↓↓	↓	↓↓	↓	↓	↓↓	↓↓↓	↓↓

(↔), no change; ↑/↓, slight change; ↑↑/↓↓, moderate change; ↑↑↑/↓↓↓, marked change.

Andropoulos DB, Heard MB, Johnson KL: Postanesthetic apnea in full term infants after pyloromyotomy. Anesthesiology 80:216–219, 1994

Hall SC: Pediatric Surgical Emergencies. American Society of Anesthesiologists. Annual Refresher Course Lectures 116:1–7, 1996

Nelson WE, Behrman RE, Kleigman RM et al (eds): Nelson Textbook of Pediatrics, 15th ed, pp 1060–1062. Philadelphia, WB Saunders, 1996

A.4. What are the adverse effects of metabolic alkalosis?

- An increase in *p*H results in the shifting of the oxygen dissociation curve to the left, thereby binding more oxygen to the hemoglobin and unloading less oxygen at the tissue level. This phenomenon assumes even more importance in newborns because at 3 weeks they still have up to 70% fetal hemoglobin with an already low value of P_{50} (i.e., 20 to 22 mm Hg).
- Respiratory compensation is affected by hypoventilation with resultant increased potential for atelectasis, as well as periods of apnea.
- Decrease in ionized calcium.
- Increased potential for seizures.

Barash PG, Cullen BF, Stoelting RK (eds): Clinical Anesthesia, 3rd ed, pp 157–158. Philadelphia, Lippincott-Raven, 1997

A.5. How would you treat this infant?

Medical management of the infant with pyloric stenosis is of acute urgency and should be undertaken early and vigorously. The principles of management can be grouped under the following three categories: supportive therapy, to stabilize the patient; diagnostic tests, to confirm the diagnosis and to monitor therapy; and surgery as the corrective therapy.

Supportive Therapy
- Circulatory support
- Correction of electrolyte derangement
- Prevention of aspiration

Fluids
The infant with pyloric stenosis is hypovolemic and dehydrated secondary to repeated vomiting. Dehydration severity can vary from mild hypovolemia to circulatory shock. The following parameters are good indicators of dehydration severity:

- Physical appearance—skin turgor, parched mucous membranes, sunken fontanelles, sunken eyeballs
- Blood pressure—decreased

- Pulse—increased
- Urine output—decreased
- Weight (birth and present) and weight loss

Quantitative assessment of these parameters gives a fair estimate of the amount of total body fluid depletion.

A wide-bore intravenous cannula should be placed and an infusion started immediately to correct the deficits and provide maintenance fluids.

Electrolytes

The patient is alkalotic, hypokalemic, hypochloremic, and hyponatremic and must be provided with the necessary ions to replenish the deficit. Albumin or Ringer's lactate might be used to treat the shock first. Next, the deficit should be corrected; 0.45% to 0.9% saline is adequate for this purpose. Potassium (usually 40 mEq/L) must be added to this to correct hypokalemia and aid in the correction of alkalosis. However, potassium infusion should be withheld until satisfactory renal function is established. Maintenance fluid should be added to this regimen, and for this purpose 5% dextrose in 0.225% saline is usually adequate.

Prevention of Aspiration

A nasogastric tube should be inserted to thoroughly empty the stomach, and the upper airway reflexes should be preserved.

Diagnostic Tests

- To assess the severity of the fluid and electrolyte derangement and to monitor therapy, the following should be evaluated: complete blood count, serum electrolytes, blood gases, blood urea nitrogen (BUN), urinalysis, and electrocardiogram (ECG) (for marked hypokalemia).
- To confirm the diagnosis—barium swallow, ultrasound imaging.

Surgery

Pyloromyotomy is the only definitive treatment for these infants. It should be carried out early, but only after the patient has been stabilized satisfactorily.

Barash PG, Cullen BF, Stoelting RK (eds): Clinical Anesthesia, 3rd ed, pp 1110–1111. Philadelphia, Lippincott-Raven, 1997

Hall SC: Pediatric Surgical Emergencies. American Society of Anesthesiologists. Annual Refresher Course Lectures 116:1–7, 1996

Nelson WE, Behrman RE, Kleigman RM et al (eds): Nelson Textbook of Pediatrics, 15th ed, pp 1060–1062. Philadelphia, WB Saunders, 1996

A.6. How would you determine fluid replacement in a newborn and what fluids would you use?

The general principles of fluid therapy are based on fluid maintenance, correction of deficits, and replacement of losses.

Maintenance Fluids

In the newborn maintenance fluids are as follows:

- First 48 hours of life—75 ml/kg/d or 3 ml/kg/h
- 2 days to 1 month—150 ml/kg/d or 5 ml/kg/h
- 1 month onward (up to 10 kg)—100 ml/kg/d or 4 ml/kg/h

Table 20-2. Estimation of the Degree of Dehydration in a Newborn

	MILD	**MODERATE**	**SEVERE**
Percent fluid loss	5	10	15–20
Skin turgor	Poor	Very poor	Parched
Mucous membrane and tongue	Dry	Dry	Parched
Other		Sunken fontanelle	Sunken eyes
Urine	Concentrated oliguria	Oliguria with maximal concentration	Oliguria to anuria
Pulse	Normal	Tachycardia	Marked tachycardia
Blood pressure	Normal	Hypotension	Marked hypotension to shock

The maintenance fluids take into account the fluid losses occurring normally through the kidney, bowel, skin, and lungs. At birth, the kidney is still undergoing maturation and what may be called "a glomerulotubular imbalance" exists. What this implies is that some mature glomeruli may be connected to immature tubules and vice versa. Hence, the kidney is functionally limited at birth but undergoes rapid maturation during the first week of life.

Electrolytes

The newborn is an obligate sodium loser as well as a poor tolerator of excessive sodium overload. The maintenance electrolytes are as follows:

- Sodium—3 to 5 mEq/kg/d
- Potassium—2 to 3 mEq/kg/d
- Chloride—1 to 3 mEq/kg/d

Correction of Deficits

Deficits take into account the previous unreplaced losses owing to a period of no intake by mouth and dehydration secondary to increased losses (e.g., from vomiting, diarrhea, and increased body temperature). The amount of deficit can be assessed by physical examination (see Table 20-2), body weight loss, and hematocrit.

Replacement of Losses

Replacing losses covers ongoing abnormal losses not covered by maintenance fluids, and intraoperatively it covers evaporative losses from the operating site, third spacing, and losses from the lungs if dry gases are used in non-rebreathing circuits (see Table 20-3).

Berry FA: Fluid and electrolyte therapy in pediatrics. ASA Refresher Course Lecture No. 132, American Society of Anesthesiologists, 1996

Miller RD (ed): Anesthesia, 4th ed, pp 2112–2113. New York, Churchill Livingstone, 1994

Table 20-3. Fluid Requirement to Replace Intraoperative Fluid Losses (Except Blood Loss) in the Newborn

	FLUID REPLACEMENT (ml/kg/h)
Minor surgery (e.g., hemiorrhaphy)	1–3
Moderate surgery (e.g., pyloromyotomy)	3–5
Major surgery (e.g., intestinal)	5–7
Respiratory water loss owing to dry gases	2

A.7. How would you correct metabolic alkalosis in this patient?

To correct the metabolic alkalosis in this patient the underlying electrolyte derangements must be corrected; namely, hyponatremia, hypokalemia, and hypochloremia. We correct the deficits by using calculated volumes of 5% dextrose in normal saline or Ringer's lactate solution, which helps to restore sodium and chloride mainly. Dextrose, 5%, with one-fourth strength normal saline, may be used to provide maintenance fluids. Once renal function is established, potassium supplements are added to the infusion. Depending on the deficit, this therapy can require anywhere from 12 to 72 hours. In severely alkalotic patients, HCl and NH_4Cl have been used to correct the derangement. However, we have rarely found it necessary.

Barash PG, Cullen BF, Stoelting RK (eds): Clinical Anesthesia, 3rd ed, pp 1120–1121. Philadelphia, Lippincott-Raven, 1997

Berry FA: Fluid and electrolyte therapy in pediatrics. ASA Refresher Course Lecture No. 132, pp 1–6, 1996

Motoyama EK, Davis PJ (eds): Smith's Anesthesia for Infants and Children, 5th ed, pp 592–593. St. Louis, CV Mosby, 1990

B. Preoperative Evaluation and Preparation

B.1. How would you evaluate this patient preoperatively?

The following information is necessary in evaluating this patient.

History
- Onset of illness, frequency and amount of vomiting, last feeding, diarrhea, urine output, activity of the newborn (active or lethargic), birth weight

Physical Examination
- Present body weight (to determine weight loss), temperature, signs of dehydration (skin turgor, mucous membranes, fontanelles, eyeballs, blood pressure, pulse, color, and volume of urine), muscle tone, level of consciousness

Laboratory Findings
- Complete blood count, electrolytes—BUN and blood sugar, urinalysis, arterial blood gases

Based on the data available, we can determine the fluid and electrolyte status of the patient and correct these accordingly to stabilize for surgery and anesthesia.

B.2. How would you prepare this patient rapidly for emergency surgery? Is surgical intervention an acute emergency in this case?

Surgical intervention is never an acute emergency in hypertrophic pyloric stenosis. Therefore, no newborn should be subjected to the additional hazards of anesthesia and surgery until stabilized medically. Medical intervention is of acute urgency to stabilize the patient.

Hall SC: Pediatric Surgical Emergencies. American Society of Anesthesiologists. Annual Refresher Course Lectures 116:1–7, 1996

Nelson WE, Behrman RE, Kleigman RM et al (eds): Nelson Textbook of Pediatrics, 15th ed, pp 1060–1062. Philadelphia, WB Saunders, 1996

B.3. How would you prepare this patient for anesthesia?

Fluid and electrolyte replacement must be accomplished satisfactorily and this may take anywhere from 12 to 72 hours depending on the patient's status.

The next step is to empty the stomach through a wide-lumen nasogastric tube and lavage out any barium left over after the x-ray studies. We find that we can use a tube with a wider lumen and ensure better emptying if we pass the tube orally. Premedication is usually atropine (0.01 to 0.02 mg/kg) intramuscularly. Light or no sedation is ordered to prevent loss of airway reflexes and aspiration.

Barash PG, Cullen BF, Stoelting RK (eds): Clinical Anesthesia, 3rd ed, pp 1110–1111. Philadelphia, Lippincott-Raven, 1997

Hall SC: Pediatric Surgical Emergencies. American Society of Anesthesiologists. Annual Refresher Course Lectures 116:1–7, 1996

Motoyama EK, Davis PJ (eds): Smith's Anesthesia for Infants and Children, 5th ed, pp 592–593. St. Louis, CV Mosby, 1990

C. Intraoperative Management

C.1. What anesthetic techniques or agents would you use?

We have found that using inhalation anesthesia, such as halothane, with the trachea intubated, is satisfactory. Halothane provides a rapid, smooth, and easy induction in these patients. However, with the recent introduction of sevoflurane in clinical practice, it has become the preferred anesthetic because of its more rapid induction and emergence when compared with halothane. Intubation of the trachea is performed and cricoid pressure is used to minimize the risk of aspiration. Muscle relaxants are rarely if ever necessary for this procedure, and the patient is extubated after regaining consciousness and airway reflex at the end of surgery in the operating room. Some commonly choose an intravenous rapid-sequence technique using thiopental, propofol, or ketamine for induction and succinylcholine or cisatracurium to facilitate intubation.

Barash PG, Cullen BF, Stoelting RK (eds): Clinical Anesthesia, 3rd ed, pp 1110–1111. Philadelphia, Lippincott-Raven, 1997

Dubois MC, Troje C, Martin C: Anesthesia in the management of pyloric stenosis. Evaluation of propofol-halogenated anesthetics. Ann Fr Anesth Reanim 12:566–570, 1993

Hall SC: Pediatric Surgical Emergencies. American Society of Anesthesiologists. Annual Refresher Course Lectures 116:1–7, 1996

MacDonald NJ, Fitzpatrick GJ, Moore KP et al: Anesthesia for congenital hypertrophic pyloric stenosis: A review of 350 patients. Br J Anaesth 59:672–677, 1987

C.2. What induction-intubation sequence would you use?

The patient is induced with a mixture of 50% O_2 and 50% N_2O and sevoflurane or halothane, with spontaneous ventilation and gentle assist as respiration is depressed. The trachea is intubated without muscle relaxant use once the proper depth of anesthesia is obtained. More recently, however, the intravenous technique of anesthesia with rapid-sequence induction-intubation has gained popularity, and it has been recommended as the technique of choice by some authorities. Both techniques have proved to be safe. The safety of induction depends on ensuring, as far as possible, that the stomach is emptied by prior aspiration through a large-bore orogastric tube. Awake intubation may be accomplished in skillful hands for a lethargic neonate or a very sick infant. However, the stabilized baby is usually fit and healthy, and we feel that awake intubation in the active infant is more traumatic than beneficial.

Barash PG, Cullen BF, Stoelting RK (eds): Clinical Anesthesia, 3rd ed, pp 1110–1111. Philadelphia, Lippincott-Raven, 1997

Hall SC: Pediatric Surgical Emergencies. American Society of Anesthesiologists. Annual Refresher Course Lectures 116:1–7, 1996

MacDonald NJ, Fitzpatrick GJ, Morre KP et al: Anesthesia for congenital hypertrophic pyloric stenosis: A review of 350 patients. Br J Anaesth 59:672–677, 1987

C.3. What are the anatomic characteristics of the airway in the newborn and how do they differ from those in the adult?

The special characteristics of the upper airway in the newborn are as follows:

- Nasopharynx—narrow nasal passages, obligate nasal breather
- Oropharynx—large tongue, long and pendulous epiglottis
- Larynx—the distinctive features are shown in Table 20-4

It is apparent, therefore, that the newborn who has low respiratory reserves can develop airway obstruction easily. The infant may present problems during intubation and tolerate airway trauma poorly.

Barash PG, Cullen BF, Stoelting RK (eds): Clinical Anesthesia, 3rd ed, p 575. Philadelphia, Lippincott-Raven, 1997

De Soto H: The child with a difficult airway: Recognition and management. ASA. Annual Refresher Course Lecture No. 236, 1–7, 1996

C.4. How do you determine the size of the endotracheal tube in pediatric patients?

The two parameters of endotracheal tube sizes are the tube length and diameter, depending on the age of the child, as shown in Table 20-5. However, these are approximate sizes and one must have one size bigger and one size smaller tube available when selecting any size tube. A simple way to remember these numbers is to know the sizes at newborn, 6 months, and 1 year of age. Between 2 and 12 years the following guides may be used:

Table 20-4. Comparative Anatomy of the Larynx and Trachea in the Newborn and the Adult

ANATOMIC FEATURES	NEWBORN	ADULT
Size	4 cm	10–13 cm
Shape	Funnel	Cylindrical
Position of glottis	C_{3-4}	C_6
Narrowest point	1 cm below vocal cords	At vocal cords
Vocal cords	Slanting anteriorly	Transverse or slight slanting posteriorly
Mucous membrane	Loose (swells easily)	More firmly bound

Table 20-5.   Estimated Tube Sizes for the Pediatric Patient

AGE	LENGTH (cm)	INTERNAL DIAMETER (mm)	FRENCH SIZES
Newborn	10	3.0	14
6 mo	12	3.5	16
1 y	14	4.0	18
2 y	15	4.5	20
4 y	16	5.0	22
6 y	17	5.5	24
8 y	18	6.0	26
10 y	19	6.5	28
12 y	20	7.0	30

$$\text{Tube length (cm) (ages 2–12 yrs)} = 14 + \frac{\text{age}}{2}$$

$$\text{Tube internal diameter (mm)} = 4 + \frac{\text{age}}{4}$$

$$\text{French size (French)} = 18 + \text{age}$$

$$\text{External circumference (French)} = I\,D\ (mm) \times 4 + 2$$

(French size means external circumference in millimeters, which equals π times external diameter; $\pi = 3.1416$.)

Barash PG, Cullen BF, Stoelting RK (eds): Clinical Anesthesia, 3rd ed, p 575. Philadelphia, Lippincott-Raven, 1997

Miller RD (ed): Anesthesia, 4th ed, pp 2112–2113. New York, Churchill Livingstone, 1994

C.5. What anesthesia system would you use and why?

We employ the circle system with a light circuit. The circle system is more advantageous because it maintains heat and humidification better and offers the freedom of choosing varying fresh gas flows. The controversy about the increased resistance in the adult circuit system is discounted by the fact that the respiration is assisted or controlled intraoperatively.

Barash PG, Cullen BF, Stoelting RK (eds): Clinical Anesthesia, 3rd ed, pp 1120–1121. Philadelphia, Lippincott-Raven, 1997

Miller RD (ed): Anesthesia, 4th ed, pp 2112–2113. New York, Churchill Livingstone, 1994

C.6. What are the advantages and disadvantages of commonly employed non-rebreathing systems?

Commonly used non-rebreathing systems include Bain Breathing circuit (Mapleson D system) and the Jackson-Rees modification of Ayre's T-piece. They offer the following:

Advantages
- Minimal dead space
- No valves, low resistance
- Lightweight

- Reservoir bag to assist ventilation
- Good appreciation of patient's respiratory exchange

Disadvantages
- High flows of fresh gas required
- Low flows may allow rebreathing of gases without CO_2 absorption
- Loss of heat and humidity owing to high flow of cold, dry gases (Bain's circuit allows some heating of inspired gases by surrounding fresh gas flow tubing with expired gas tubing)
- Scavenging problems of waste gases

Barash PG, Cullen BF, Stoelting RK (eds): Clinical Anesthesia, 3rd ed, pp 1120–1121. Philadelphia, Lippincott-Raven, 1997

Miller RD (ed): Anesthesia, 4th ed, pp 203–207. New York, Churchill Livingstone, 1994

C.7. How would you monitor this patient intraoperatively?

Monitoring should include blood pressure, ECG, rectal temperature, precordial stethoscope, pulse oximeter, and an end-tidal CO_2 monitor.

C.8. How does the pulse oximeter function?

The commonly used pulse oximeter (Nellcor pulse oximeter Model 100) combines the scientific principles of spectrophotometric oximetry and plethysmography. Light of two wavelengths, 660 nm (red) and 925 nm (infrared), is emitted by a pair of light-emitting diodes (LED) and is passed through the tissue being measured to a photodetector. Because the saturated hemoglobin absorbs more blue light than unsaturated hemoglobin, the absorption of the light for each color is an indication of the ratio of oxygen-saturated blood to unsaturated blood. The pulsating vascular bed, by expanding and relaxing, creates a change in the light-path length that modifies the amount of light detected. The microprocessor-controlled circuitry in the unit senses the pulsatile waveform, which is solely produced by the arterial blood, thus allowing measurement of pulse rate and arterial saturation. The oximeter is reliably accurate in 50% to 100% saturation range.

Nellcor Pulse Oximeter Model N-100, Instruction Manual. Hayward, CA, Nellcor Inc, 1984

Tremper KK, Barker SJ: Pulse oximetry. Anesthesiology 70:98–108, 1989

Yelderman M, New W Jr: Evaluation of pulse oximetry. Anesthesiology 59:349–352, 1983

C.9. What factors affect the measurement of oxygen saturation by the pulse oximeter?

Dysfunctional hemoglobin, as with carboxyhemoglobin and methoxyhemoglobin, can affect the accuracy of the oximeter. Intravascular dyes such as cardiogreen can also interfere with the accuracy of the instrument. Skin color, tissue thickness, venous blood, light intensity, and ambient light do not affect the accuracy of the instrument because they do not pulse.

Nellcor Pulse Oximeter Model N100, Instruction Manual. Hayward, CA, Nellcor Inc, 1984

Tremper KK, Barker SJ: Pulse oximetry. Anesthesiology 70:98–108, 1989

D. Postoperative Management

D.1. What are the complications that can occur in the postanesthesia recovery period?

The patient should be carefully observed for signs of respiratory depression and periods of apnea secondary to a combination of metabolic alkalosis, general anesthesia, and decreased body temperature. Hypoventilation predisposes to atelectasis. Patients should be awake and responsive to avoid aspiration. Severe hypoglycemia resulting from depletion of liver glycogen stores has been reported 2 to 3 hours after surgery. Postextubation "croup" is a potentially dangerous complication in this age group.

Andropoulos DB, Heard MB, Johnson KL: Postanesthetic apnea in full term infants after pyloromyotomy. Anesthesiology 80:216–219, 1994

Barash PG, Cullen BF, Stoelting RK (eds): Clinical Anesthesia, 3rd ed, pp 1110–1111. Philadelphia, Lippincott-Raven, 1997

Hall SC: Pediatric Surgical Emergencies. American Society of Anesthesiologists. Annual Refresher Course Lectures 116:1–7, 1996

D.2. How would you treat postextubation "croup" in this infant?

Treatment of the potentially catastrophic postextubation laryngeal edema should be immediate, vigorous, and carried out under direct observation of the anesthesiologist. It consists of the following:

- Increasing inspired-oxygen concentration (50% to 60%)
- Humidification of inspired gases
- Adequate hydration using parenteral fluids
- Light sedation to calm the patient and allow for cooperation in therapy
- Avoidance of any significant respiratory depression
- Epinephrine through hand-held nebulizer and mask, 50 mg/kg/min of active isomer
  - Racemic epinephrine (2.25%) diluted in 5-ml saline solution
  - Dose—0.05 ml/kg delivered in 10 minutes
  - Aqueous epinephrine (0.1%) diluted in 5-ml saline solution
  - Dose—0.1% 0.5 ml/kg delivered in 10 minutes

Treatment should be given over 10 minutes and may be repeated every 30 minutes, as necessary.

Rebound phenomenon may be expected about 2 hours after cessation of this therapy.

- Steroids—dexamethasone, 0.5 to 1 mg/kg intravenously
- Reintubation—if signs of deterioration or hypoxia appear
- Tracheostomy, if necessary—rarely, subglottic edema may be so rapid and so severe that tracheostomy is the only choice

The age group most likely to manifest this complication is from 1 to 4 years. At most risk is an infant <1 year of age, mainly because of the size of the airway. Fortunately, an infant this age is most amenable to early and vigorous intervention and should always be treated as an emergency requiring the continued presence of and evaluation by a physician who is adept at securing an airway for the child.

Barash PG, Cullen BF, Stoelting RK (eds): Clinical Anesthesia, 3rd ed, p 1122. Philadelphia, Lippincott-Raven, 1997

Berry FA: Management of the pediatric patient with croup or epiglottitis. ASA Annual Refresher Course Lecture No. 261, 1990

Ledwith CA, Shea LM, Mauro RD: Safety and efficacy of nebulized racemic epinephrine in conjunction with oral dexamethasone and mist in the outpatient treatment of croup. Ann Emerg Med 25: 331–337, 1995

Nutman J, Brooks LJ, Deakins KM: Racemic versus L-epinephrine aerosol in the treatment of post-extubation laryngeal edema: Results from a prospective randomized, double-blind study. Crit Care Med 22:1591–1594, 1994

The Nervous System

IV

Brain Tumor and Craniotomy **21**

Alan Van Poznak

The patient was a 67-year-old man in mild congestive heart failure. He had 1 month of increasing lethargy, headache, aphasia, and right-sided weakness. Moderate bilateral papilledema was present. Because he was restless and uncooperative, he required sedation and anesthesia for accomplishing arteriograms, computed tomography (CT) scans, and magnetic resonance imaging (MRI) studies. When completed, these studies showed a left convexity meningioma, which invades the superior sagittal sinus.

A. Medical Disease and Differential Diagnosis

1. What are the determinants of intracranial pressure (ICP) under normal healthy conditions?
2. By what mechanisms may the presence of a brain tumor change the intracranial pressure?
3. What are the determinants of cerebral blood flow under normal healthy conditions?
4. How may intracranial diseases modify cerebral blood flow? Discuss cerebral steal syndromes.
5. What are the special dangers of posterior cranial fossa pathology?

B. Preoperative Evaluation and Preparation

1. What are some problems that can be associated with neuroradiologic anesthesia?
2. What are some reactions that can occur from the use of radiopaque iodine-containing contrast agents?
3. What are the special anesthetic considerations for cerebral angiography?
4. What are the special anesthetic considerations for computed tomography?
5. What are the special problems of anesthesia for magnetic resonance imaging?
6. How would you prepare the patient for surgery? Discuss medical management, fluids, and drugs.
7. What premedication would you choose?

C. Intraoperative Management

1. How would you conduct the anesthesia induction?
2. What special dangers are there during induction?
3. What are the significant monitors to use during surgery?
4. Discuss air embolism—its cause, symptoms, recognition, avoidance, and treatment.
5. What are the special problems associated with large meningiomas?
6. What are the two special requirements of anesthesia for brain tumor removal?
7. Enumerate four techniques with which one can make room for the surgeon to work in the head.
8. How does hyperventilation increase the room within the head?

9. How much hyperventilation is desirable?
10. If a little hyperventilation is good, will a lot be better?
11. What is the claimed danger of extreme hyperventilation?
12. What do you think about this?
13. Vigorously hyperventilated patients take longer to awaken. What else besides hypoxia could cause this?
14. Should all brain tumor patients be hyperventilated?
15. Why are hypertonic solutions used?
16. Why do hypertonic solutions have a preferential effect on the brain?
17. What percentage of total cardiac output is the cerebral blood flow?
18. What hypertonic solution is currently in use?
19. What is the dose?
20. Can excessive mannitol draw so much water from the heart cells that irreversible cardiac arrest ensues?
21. Give four reasons why intraoperative fluid restriction is desirable.
22. How can one increase the chances of successful spinal fluid drainage?
23. What four factors should be sequentially considered for the safe induction of hypotension during craniotomy?
24. Why is it important to follow the above sequence?
25. If the use of antihypertensive drugs is indicated, which would you choose? Why? Discuss the effects of antihypertensives on intracranial pressure.
26. What are the effects of anesthetic agents on intracranial pressure?

D. Postoperative Management

1. Discuss the more common early postoperative problems following craniotomy.
2. How does anesthesia management for carotid endarterectomy differ significantly from craniotomy management?
3. Discuss special problems that may be seen after posterior cranial fossa procedures.

A. Medical Disease and Differential Diagnosis

A.1. What are the determinants of intracranial pressure under normal healthy conditions?

The intracranial pressure (ICP) is ultimately determined by the volume relationships between the intracranial contents and the enclosure around them. Intracranial contents are largely fluid and therefore almost incompressible. The cranial enclosure is largely a rigid bony box in the adult, although it does have areas of lesser rigidity, such as various foramina and membranes. In the infant with open fontanelles and open skull sutures, the enclosure is far more compliant. The accumulation of blood, cerebrospinal fluid, tumor tissue, or other substances within the adult cranium will at first cause only a slight pressure rise. However, when the system compliance has been exceeded, the accumulation of only a little more fluid or tumor will result in a sharp rise in pressure. These relationships between the cranium and its contents are known as the "Monro-Kellie hypothesis," which in its original form regarded the cranium as a rigid bony box. The principal determinants of the intracranial pressure under normal healthy conditions are the cerebral and spinal cord blood flow and cerebrospinal fluid mechanisms.

Cutler RWP, Page LK, Galicich J et al: Formation and absorption of cerebrospinal fluid in man. Brain 91:707, 1968

Davison H: Physiology of the Cerebrospinal Fluid. London, J&A Churchill, 1967

Marmarou A, Shulman K, LaMorgese J: Compartmental analysis of compliance and outflow resistance of the cerebrospinal fluid system. J Neurosurg 43:523–524, 1975

Marmarou A, Shulman K, Rosende RM: A nonlinear analysis of the cerebrospinal fluid system and intracranial pressure dynamics. J Neurosurg 48:332–344, 1978

A.2. By what mechanisms may the presence of a brain tumor change the intracranial pressure?

A brain tumor may initially be so small as to have no effect on ICP. This is because there may be a compensatory reduction in the volume of cerebrospinal fluid. With continued enlargement of the tumor, the ability of other structures to compensate will be exceeded and ICP will begin to rise. This rise is caused in part by the bulk of the tumor, but is also caused by the increase in cerebral blood flow in the areas surrounding the tumor and by cerebral edema in adjacent normal brain. If venous thrombosis results, an abrupt rise can occur in intracranial pressure. If local tissue pressure exceeds perfusion pressure of the arterioles supplying the area, hypoxic injury of local tissue may ensue, with endothelial injury and increased transudation across the capillary membrane.

Crutchfield JS, Narayan RK, Robertson CS et al: Evaluation of a fiberoptic intracranial pressure monitor. J Neurosurg 72:482, 1990

Langfitt TW: Increased intracranial pressure. Clin Neurosurg 16:436, 1968

Lundberg N: Continuous recording and control of ventricular fluid pressure in neurosurgical practice. Acta Psychiatr Neurol Scand 36(Suppl 1):149, 1960

Marmarou A, Anderson RL, Ward JD et al: NINDS traumatic coma data bank: Intracranial pressure monitoring methodology. J Neurosurg 75:S21, 1991

Shapiro HM, Wyte SR, Harris AB et al: Acute intra-operative intra-cranial hypertension in neurosurgical patients: Mechanical and pharmacologic factors. Anesthesiology 37:399, 1972

A.3. What are the determinants of cerebral blood flow under normal healthy conditions?

Under normal healthy conditions, cerebral blood flow is determined by $PaCO_2$, perfusion pressure, brain extracellular fluid pH, and nerve cell activity. The cerebral blood flow tends to be held constant by the process of autoregulation within limits of about 50 to 150 mm Hg mean arterial blood pressure. Outside of these limits, cerebral blood flow tends to become more pressure-dependent as autoregulation becomes less effective.

Lassen NA: Cerebral blood flow and oxygen consumption in man. Physiol Rev 39:183, 1959

Sato M, Pawlik G, Heiss WB: Comparative studies of regional CNS blood flow autoregulation and responses to CO_2 in the cat. Stroke 15:91, 1984

Siesjo BK: Cerebral circulation and metabolism. J Neurosurg 60:883, 1984

A.4. How may intracranial diseases modify cerebral blood flow? Discuss cerebral steal syndromes.

Intracranial disease may modify cerebral blood flow by producing brain tissue regions with vasodilatation and high cerebral blood flow. This phenomenon is called "luxury perfusion." It may allow shunt of blood from diseased areas into normal areas of brain with intact autoregulation, producing what is known as "cerebral steal." The phenomenon of "inverse steal" may be seen when hyperventilation produces vasoconstriction in normal, but not in damaged, brain tissue thus causing more blood to flow into the brain tumor or other damaged tissue. Also see Chapter 22 (Carotid Endarterectomy), questions A.13, A.14 and A.15.

Haggendal E, Lofgren J, Nilsson NJ et al: Effects of varied cerebrospinal fluid pressure on cerebral blood flow in dogs. Acta Physiol Scand 79:262, 1970

Matsuda M, Yondea S, Handa H et al: Cerebral hemodynamic changes during plateau waves in brain tumor patients. J Neurosurg 50:483, 1979

Miller JD, Stanek AE, Langfitt TW: A comparison of autoregulation to changes in intracranial pressure and arterial pressure in the same preparation. Eur Neurol 6:34, 1974

Risberg J, Lundberg N, Ingvar DH: Regional cerebral blood volume during acute transient rises of the intracranial pressure (plateau waves). J Neurosurg 31:303, 1969

A.5. What are the special dangers of posterior cranial fossa pathology?

The special dangers of posterior fossa pathology include compression of the lower cranial nerves in the brain stem with resultant difficulty in maintaining an open airway free of secretions. In addition, compression of respiratory and vasomotor centers in the medulla can produce severe compromise of cardiorespiratory function.

Drummond JC, Todd MM: Acute sinus arrhythmia during surgery in the fourth ventricle: An indicator of brain-stem irritation. Anesthesiology 60:232, 1984

Frost EAM (ed): Clinical Anesthesia in Neurosurgery, 2nd ed, p 221. Boston, Butterworth-Heinemann, 1991

Rosenwasser RH, Kleiner LI, Krzeminski JP et al: Intracranial pressure monitoring in the posterior fossa: A preliminary report. J Neurosurg 71:503, 1989

B. Preoperative Evaluation and Preparation

B.1. What are some problems that can be associated with neuroradiologic anesthesia?

Radiologic suites present several additional hazards for the patient and the anesthesiologist. They may be located at a considerable distance from the operating rooms, and specialized equipment and skilled assistance may be difficult to obtain in case of emergency. Illumination and ventilation are often suboptimal; rarely is there provision for scavenging of expired gases and anesthetic agents. Radiologic personnel are often unfamiliar with working with anesthetized patients and anesthesiologists. Anesthesiologists may mistakenly assume that physiologic trespass will be minimal. Patients may be placed in positions that compromise respiration and circulation. Radiologic contrast agents can produce sudden severe reactions.

Barnwell SL: Interventional neuroradiology. West J Med 158:162, 1993

B.2. What are some reactions that can occur from the use of radiopaque iodine-containing contrast agents?

Radiopaque iodine-containing media may be injected into veins, arteries, or cerebrospinal fluid spaces, and they can produce allergic or toxic reactions, ranging from mild skin reactions to anaphylaxis. The fatality rate is about 0.01%, and the total incidence of nonfatal reactions is about 2.3%. With a history of previous reaction to iodine-containing compounds, the probability of a reaction is about tripled. Such patients should receive steroid prophylaxis at 24, 12, and 2 hours before the study and intravenous diphenhydramine immediately before the study. If the study is prolonged and much contrast agent is given, significant osmotic diuresis can occur. Nonionic contrast agents produce a lower osmotic load but they are much more expensive, currently limiting their use to only those patients who specifically need them.

Junck L, Marshall WH: Neurotoxicity of radiological contrast agents. Ann Neurol 13:469, 1983

Lasser EC, Berry CC, Talner LB et al: Pretreatment with corticosteroids to alleviate reactions to intravenous contrast material. N Engl J Med 317:845, 1987

Numaguchi Y, Fleming MS, Hasao K et al: Blood brain barrier disruption due to cerebral arteriography: CT findings. J Comput Assist Tomogr 8:936, 1984

B.3. What are the special anesthetic considerations for cerebral angiography?

In addition to the reactions from contrast agents mentioned, sudden changes may occur in pulse, blood pressure, or respiration when intravascular injections are made into cerebral vessels. Some of these may be of a reflex nature due to baroreceptor discharge. Most cerebral angiograms in adults can be done using only local anesthesia. In uncooperative adults and in children, various degrees of sedation or general anesthesia may be required.

Manipulation of vascular structures can produce spasm, thrombosis, hemorrhage, or edema; these will produce neurologic changes that must be differentiated from any effects caused by the anesthesia being administered.

Dallas SH, Moxon CP: Controlled ventilation for cerebral angiography. Br J Anaesth 41:597, 1979

Field JR, Robertson JT, DeSaussurer L: Complications of cerebral angiography in 2000 consecutive cases. J Neurosurg 19:775, 1962

B.4. What are the special anesthetic considerations for computed tomography?

Most computed tomography is done without any anesthesia. It is painless and noninvasive, but it is necessary for the patient to remain motionless. For this reason, uncooperative adults and children may require sedation or general anesthesia. The patient's head is not easily accessible. Airway patency may be precarious and management consequently difficult. If general anesthesia is chosen, little room is available for the anesthesia machine, and long breathing tubes may be needed. Kinking of the endotracheal tube is an ever-present hazard, especially when the patient is moved in and out of the scanning machinery.

Aidinis SJ, Zimmerman RA, Shapiro HM et al: Anesthesia for brain computer tomography. Anesthesiology 44:420, 1976

B.5. What are the special problems of anesthesia for magnetic resonance imaging?

The physical constraints of magnetic resonance imaging are similar to those for computed tomography, but in addition a very strong magnet is used whose pull on ferromagnetic materials can draw them with dangerous speed and force into the machine and the patient contained within it. For this reason, it is necessary either to use ferromagnetic materials only at a safe distance or with secure anchoring if they must be brought close to the machine. The radiofrequency waves emitted by the machine can cause the malfunction of anesthesia monitoring equipment; conversely, anesthesia monitoring equipment may emit signals that degrade the quality of the image produced by the machine. Close cooperation between anesthesiologists and radiologists is needed to develop safe and effective systems for patients while satisfying the requirements of both specialties. Also see Chapter 56 (Magnetic Resonance Imaging).

Dunn V, Coffman CE, McGowan JE: Mechanical ventilation during magnetic resonance imaging. Magn Reson Imaging 3:169, 1985

Geiger RS, Cascorbi HF: Anesthesia in an NMR scanner. Anesth Analg 63:622, 1985

Patteson SK, Chesney JT: Anesthetic management for magnetic resonance imaging: Problems and solutions. Anesth Analg 74:121–128, 1992

Roth JL, Nugent M, Gray JE et al: Patient monitoring during magnetic resonance imaging. Anesthesiology 62:80, 1985

Vengerven M, Van Hemelrijck J, Wouters P et al: Light anaesthesia with propofol for paediatric MRI. Anaesthesia 47:706, 1992

B.6. How would you prepare the patient for surgery? Discuss medical management, fluids, and drugs.

Preparation for surgery would include control of the congestive heart failure with whatever means were appropriate, including digitalization, diuretics, antihypertensives, and antiarrhythmic drugs as needed for the particular situation.

B.7. What premedication would you choose?

Choice of premedication should be limited to whatever dose of sedative is required to control anxiety, if present. Because the patient is not in pain, narcotics are not needed; their respiratory depressant effect may dangerously elevate the intracranial pressure. Atropine or glycopyrrolate may be given as a premedicant intramuscularly or intravenously just prior to anesthetic induction.

C. Intraoperative Management

C.1. How would you conduct the anesthesia induction?

Regardless of the method chosen, the anesthesiologist should avoid hypoxia or hypercarbia. Hyperventilation prior to intubation and use of potent inhalation anesthetics is desirable. A thiopental–muscle relaxant sequence would be a thoroughly acceptable technique.

Shapiro HM: Intracranial hypertension: Therapeutic and anesthetic considerations. Anesthesiology 43:445, 1975

C.2. What special dangers are there during induction?

The special dangers of induction are hypoxia, hypercarbia, coughing, and wide swings in blood pressure.

Bedford RJ, Morris L, Jane JA: Intracranial hypertension during surgery for supratentorial tumor: Correlation with preoperative computed tomography scans. Anesth Analg 61:430, 1982

Greenfield JC, Rembert JC, Tindall GT: Transient changes in cerebral vascular resistance during the Valsalva maneuver in man. Stroke 15:76, 1984

Hammil JF, Bedford RF, Weaver DC et al: Lidocaine before endotracheal intubation: Intravenous or laryngotracheal. Anesthesiology 55:578, 1981

Martin DE, Rosenberg H, Aukburg SJ et al: Low-dose fentanyl blunts circulatory responses to tracheal intubation. Anesth Analg 61:680, 1982

Moss E, Powell D, Gibson NM et al: Effects of tracheal intubation on intracranial pressure following induction of anesthesia with thiopental. Br J Anaesth 50:353, 1978

Shapiro W, Wasserman AJ, Patterson JL: Human cerebrovascular response to combined hypoxia and hypercapnia. Circ Res 19:903, 1966

Yukioka H, Yoshimoto N, Nishimura K et al: Intravenous lidocaine as a suppressant of coughing during tracheal intubation. Anesth Analg 64:1189, 1985

C.3. What are the significant monitors to use during surgery?

Significant monitors include blood pressure, electrocardiogram (ECG), end-tidal CO_2, precordial Doppler, temperature, O_2, and pulse oximeter monitors.

C.4. Discuss air embolism—its cause, symptoms, recognition, avoidance, and treatment.

Air embolism can occur when atmospheric air enters an open vein in the operative area. Dangerous conditions develop if the amount of air is sufficient to interfere with the ability of the right ventricle to pump blood to the lungs. Air in the pulmonary capillaries can cause reflex pulmonary vasoconstriction, further decreasing the already compromised pulmonary function. Precordial Doppler monitoring is the most efficient way of recognizing a small amount of air in the heart. Avoidance of air embolism is most easily done by proper positioning of the patient so that a small positive pressure is present in the veins of the operative site. If blood is coming out, air cannot be going in. Expansion of intravascular volume and controlled ventilation with positive end-expiratory pressure also help to maintain a continuous positive pressure in the veins of the operative site. The best treatment of this condition is not as good as prevention, but it includes such measures as large-bore right atrial catheters, Swan-Ganz catheters, and the rapid employment of steep head-down tilt to force the foamy blood from the right atrium. Paradoxic passage of air through a patent foramen ovale into the left atrium and systemic circulation is another rare complication of air embolism.

Nitrous oxide (N_2O) use is controversial. Opponents claim that its use will expand air bubbles and worsen problems in the event of venous air embolism. Proponents claim that this enlargement of bubbles will favor earlier Doppler detection of small air emboli. In a recent study, Losasso et al. concluded that administration of N_2O did not improve the sensitivity of transesophageal echocardiography or precordial Doppler, but it did improve sensitivity of end-tidal CO_2 and pulmonary artery pressure monitoring in the detection of venous air embolism.

Albin MS, Carroll RG, Maroon JC: Clinical considerations concerning detection of venous air embolism. Neurosurgery 3:390, 1978

Brechner VL, Bethune WM, Soldo NJ: Pathological physiology of air embolism. Anesthesiology 28:240, 1967

Buckland RW, Manners IM: Venous air embolism during neurosurgery: A comparison of various methods of detection in man. Anaesthesia 31:633, 1976

Losasso TJ, Black S, Muzzi DA et al: Detection and hemodynamic consequences of venous air embolism. Does nitrous oxide make a difference? Anesthesiology 77:148–152, 1992

Losasso TJ, Muzzi DA, Dietz NM et al: Fifty percent nitrous oxide does not increase the risk of venous air embolism in neurosurgical patients operated upon in the sitting position. Anesthesiology 77:21, 1992

Michenfelder JD, Miller RH, Gronert GA: Evaluation of an ultrasonic device (Doppler) for the diagnosis of venous air embolism. Anesthesiology 36:164, 1972

Voorhies RM, Fraser RAR, Van Poznak A: Prevention of air embolism with positive end-expiratory pressure. Neurosurgery 12:503–506, 1983

C.5. What are the special problems associated with large meningiomas?

Meningiomas arise from dural cells; they may invade or compress the venous sinuses that are formed by dural duplications. The special hazards are venous thrombosis, bleeding, and air embolism, as mentioned.

Iwabuchi T, Sobata E, Suzuki M et al: Dural sinus pressure related to neurosurgical position. Neurosurgery 12:203, 1983

C.6. What are the two special requirements of anesthesia for brain tumor removal?
- Make room for the surgeon to work in the head
- Control excessive bleeding

C.7. Enumerate four techniques with which one can make room for the surgeon to work in the head.
- Hyperventilation
- Hypertonic intravenous fluids
- Spinal fluid removal
- Controlled hypotension

Artru A: Partial preservation of cerebral vascular responsiveness to hypocapnia during isoflurane induced hypotension. Anesth Analg 65:660, 1986

Bozza Marrubini ML, Rossanda M, Tretola L: The role of artificial hyperventilation in control of brain tension during neurosurgical operations. Br J Anaesth 36:415, 1961

Cottrell JE, Robustelli A, Post K et al: Furosemide and mannitol induced changes in intracranial pressure and serum osmolality and electrolytes. Anesthesiology 47:28, 1977

Hayes GJ, Slocum HC: The achievements of optimal brain relaxation by hyperventilation techniques of anesthesia. J Neurosurg 19:65, 1962

Hooshang H, Dove J, Houff S et al: Effects of diuretics and steroids on CSF pressure. Arch Neurol 21:499, 1969

Javid M, Anderson J: The effect of urea on cerebrospinal fluid pressure in monkeys before and after bilateral nephrectomy. J Lab Clin Med 53:484, 1959

Ravussin P, Abou-Madi M, Archer D et al: Changes in CSF pressure after mannitol in patients with and without elevated CSF pressure. J Neurosurg 69:869, 1988

Rosenberg GA, Saland L, Kyner WT: Pathophysiology of periventricular tissue changes with raised CSF pressure in cats. J Neurosurg 59:606, 1983

Sivarajan M, Amory DW, McKenzie SM: Regional blood flows during induced hypotension produced by nitroprusside or trimethaphan in the rhesus monkey. Anesth Analg 64:759, 1985

Tinker JH, Michenfelder JD: Sodium nitroprusside: Pharmacology, toxicology and therapeutics. Anesthesiology 45:340, 1976

C.8. How does hyperventilation increase the room within the head?

Reduction of P_{CO_2} decreases vascular engorgement and brain bulk. Cerebral blood flow changes 2% to 4% for each 1 mm Hg change in $PaCO_2$ within the range of 25 to 80 mm Hg.

Bozza Marrubini ML, Rossanda M, Tretola L: The role of artificial hyperventilation in control of brain tension during neurosurgical operations. Br J Anaesth 36:415, 1961

Hayes GJ, Slocum HC: The achievement of optimal brain relaxation by hyperventilation techniques of anesthesia. J Neurosurg 19:65, 1962

Shapiro HM: Intracranial hypertension. Anesthesiology 43:445, 1975

Shuptrine JR, Auffant RA, Gal TJ: Cerebral and cardiopulmonary responses to high frequency jet ventilation and conventional mechanical ventilation in a model of brain and lung injury. Anesth Analg 63:1065, 1984

C.9. How much hyperventilation is desirable?

To an end-expiratory CO_2 of approximately 4%, corresponding to a P_{CO_2} of approximately 30 mm Hg.

Rossanda M, Collice M, Porta M et al: Intracranial hypertension in head injury: Clinical significance and relation to respiration. In Lundberg M, Penten U, Brock M: Intracranial Pressure II, p 475. New York, Springer-Verlag, 1975

C.10. If a little hyperventilation is good, will a lot be better?

Not necessarily. A reasonable limit is found to the reduction of brain bulk that can be produced by hyperventilation. In addition, some have pointed out a theoretical danger of extreme hyperventilation.

Artru AA, Katz RA, Colley PS: Autoregulation of cerebral blood flow during normocapnia and hypocapnia in dogs. Anesthesiology 70:288, 1989

Cold GE: Does acute hyperventilation provoke cerebral oligaemia in comatose patients after acute head injury? Acta Neurochir 96:100, 1989

James HE, Langfitt TW, Kumar VS et al: Treatment of intracranial hypertension: Analysis of 105 consecutive recordings of intracranial pressure. Acta Neurochir 36:189, 1977

C.11. What is the claimed danger of extreme hyperventilation?

Hypoxia caused by extreme cerebral vasoconstriction.

Bruce DA: Effects of hyperventilation on cerebral blood flow and metabolism. Clin Perinatol 11:673, 1984

Grote J, Zimmer K, Schubert R: Effects of severe arterial hypocapnia on regional blood flow regulation, tissue PO_2 and metabolism in the brain cortex of cats. Eur J Physiol 391:195, 1981

Hansen NB, Nowicki PT, Miller RR et al: Alterations in cerebral blood flow and oxygen consumption during prolonged hypocarbia. Pediatr Res 20:147, 1986

Michenfelder JD, Theye RA: The effects of profound hypocapnia and dilutional anemia on canine cerebral metabolism and blood flow. Anesthesiology 31:449, 1969

C.12. What do you think about this?

It is something to argue about. Harp and Wollman have presented a review of the conflicting claims.

Harp JR, Wollman H: Cerebral metabolic effects of hyperventilation and deliberate hypotension. Br J Anaesth 43:256, 1973

C.13. Vigorously hyperventilated patients take longer to awaken. What else besides hypoxia could cause this?

Hyperventilation lowers P_{CO_2} and raises pH, causing a fall in ionized calcium that is needed for proper synaptic function. The time required for restoration of ionized calcium to optimal levels could explain the prolonged awakening time.

Christensen MS, Brodersen P, Olesen J et al: Cerebral apoplexy (stroke) treated with or without prolonged artificial hyperventilation: Cerebrospinal fluid acid-base balance and intracranial pressure. Stroke 4:620, 1973

C.14. Should all brain tumor patients be hyperventilated?

No. Sometimes the neurosurgeon will prefer spontaneous respiration if working near the medulla. All factors should be considered.

C.15. Why are hypertonic solutions used?

Hypertonic solutions are used to draw water from the cells by their osmotic effect.

Albright AL, Latchaw RE, Robinson AG: Osmotic and oncotic therapy in experimental cerebral edema. J Neurosurg 60:481, 1984

Wise DL, Chater N: Effects of mannitol on cerebrospinal fluid pressure. The actions of hypertonic mannitol solutions and of urea compared. Arch Neurol 4:200, 1961

C.16. Why do hypertonic solutions have a preferential effect on the brain?

Hypertonic solutions have a preferential effect because the brain receives a relatively large percentage of the cardiac output.

C.17. What percentage of total cardiac output is the cerebral blood flow?

Approximately 15% of total cardic output is found in the cerebral blood flow.

Cottrell JE, Smith DS: Anesthesia and Neurosurgery, 3rd ed, pp. 17–57. St. Louis, CV Mosby, 1994

Hansen TD, Warner DS, Todd MM et al: The role of cerebral metabolism in determining the local cerebral blood flow effects of volatile anesthetics: evidence for persistent flow-metabolism coupling. J Cereb Blood Flow Metab 9:323, 1989

C.18. *What hypertonic solution is currently in use?*

Mannitol, 20%.

C.19. *What is the dose?*

From 0.6 to 1.5 g/kg body weight.

Miller JD, Leech P: Effects of mannitol and steroid therapy on intracranial volume-pressure relationship in patients. J Neurosurg 42:274–281, 1975

C.20. *Can excessive mannitol draw so much water from the heart cells that irreversible cardiac arrest ensues?*

Yes.

C.21. *Give four reasons why intraoperative fluid restriction is desirable.*

- A given dose of mannitol will exert a greater osmotic effect if put into a smaller circulating blood volume.
- If circulating volume has been expanded with isotonic fluids, the addition of mannitol to patients with marginally compensated circulation may increase circulatory failure. Pulmonary edema can occur before the kidneys can remove the excess water from the circulation.
- Restriction of intraoperative intravenous fluids facilitates the management of induced hypotension.
- The probability of postoperative cerebral edema, a major neurosurgical concern, is lessened by intraoperative fluid restriction. Edema cannot occur without water.

Durward QL, Del Maestro RF, Amacher AL et al: The influence of systemic arterial pressure and intracranial pressure on the development of cerebral vasogenic edema. J Neurosurg 59:803, 1983

Fishman RA: Brain edema. N Engl J Med 293:706, 1975

Greenwood J: Mechanisms of blood-brain barrier breakdown. Neuroradiology 33:95, 1990

Ohnishi T, Sher PB, Posner JB et al: Capillary permeability factor secreted by malignant brain tumor. Role in peritumoral brain edema and possible mechanism for antiedema effect of glucocorticoids. J Neurosurg 72:245, 1990

Reulen HJ, Graham R, Spatz M et al: Role of pressure gradients and bulk flow in dynamics of vasogenic brain edema. J Neurosurg 46:24, 1977

C.22. *How can one increase the chances of successful spinal fluid drainage?*

Proper positioning of the patient for lumbar puncture—hip and shoulders vertical on the table, large-bore needles entered horizontally in the midline—increases the chances of successful spinal fluid drainage. Let fluid drip into a sterile syringe barrel. Do not exert strong negative pressure with a syringe. You may draw tissue against the bevel of the needle and jam the system.

C.23. *What four factors should be sequentially considered for the safe induction of hypotension during craniotomy?*

- Depth of anesthesia
- Tilt of operating table

- Relative blood volume of patient
- Use of drugs

Adams RW, Gronert GA, Sundt TM et al: Halothane, hypocapnia and cerebral spinal fluid pressure in neurosurgery. Anesthesiology 37:510, 1972

Artru AA, Hornbein TF: Prolonged hypocapnia does not alter the rate of CSF production in dogs during halothane anesthesia or sedation with nitrous oxide. Anesthesiology 67:66, 1987

Crosby G, Todd MM: On neuroanesthesia, intracranial pressure and a dead horse. J Neurosurg Anesth 2:143, 1990

Drummond JC, Todd MM: The response of the feline cerebral circulation to $PaCO_2$ during anesthesia with isoflurane and halothane during sedation with nitrous oxide. Anesthesiology 62:268, 1985

Todd MM, Warner DS, Sokoll MD et al: A prospective comparative trial of three anesthetics for elective supratentorial craniotomy: Propofol/fentanyl, isoflurane/nitrous oxide and fentanyl/nitrous oxide. Anesthesiology 78:1005, 1993

Van Poznak A, Jenkins MT, Artusio JF Jr: Anesthesia for surgery of the pituitary gland. Clinical Anesthesia, Vol 3, pp 118–125. Philadelphia, FA Davis, 1963

C.24. Why is it important to follow the above sequence?

The depth of anesthesia and tilt of the table may be sufficient to establish reduction of both arterial and venous pressures in the brain. In such cases, drugs are rarely needed, and then only in small amounts, thus minimizing the likelihood of toxic reactions. Should excessive hypotension occur, usually it can be easily reversed by lessening the doses of inhalation agent and lessening the tilt of the table. Conversely, if the anesthetic depth and table tilt are minimal, then more hypotensive drug will be required and a greater probability of toxic accumulation exists. Should excessive hypotension occur, further lessening of anesthetic depth may invite coughing on the endotracheal tube, which can be disastrous if the dura has been opened. If the table is brought level or head down, profuse venous bleeding may occur.

Madsen JB, Gold GE, Hansen ES et al: The effect of isoflurane on cerebral blood flow and metabolism in humans during craniotomy for small supratentorial cerebral tumors. Anesthesiology 66:332, 1987

Van Poznak A, Jenkins MT, Artusio JF Jr: Anesthesia for surgery of the pituitary gland. Clinical Anesthesia, Vol 3, pp 118–125. Philadelphia, FA Davis, 1963

C.25. If the use of antihypertensive drugs is indicated, which would you choose? Why? Discuss the effects of antihypertensive drugs on intracranial pressure.

The currently popular antihypertensive drugs for intraoperative use are sodium nitroprusside and trimethaphan. Sodium nitroprusside has the advantage of rapid onset of action and recovery but it has the disadvantages of increasing ICP and producing cyanide toxicity if used in excessive amounts. Trimethaphan is a little slower in its onset and recovery time. It produces widespread ganglionic blockade with resultant pupillary dilatation, and it may impair renal blood flow in excessive doses. My personal choice is to use sufficiently deep inhalation anesthesia with isoflurane, so that little, if any, hypotension-inducing drug is needed. In this way, toxicity of injected drug is avoided.

Ghani GA, Sung F, Weinstein MS et al: Effects of intravenous nitroglycerin on the intracranial pressure and volume response. J Neurosurg 58:562, 1983

Marsh ML, Aidinis SJ, Naughton KVH et al: The technique of nitroprusside administration modifies the intracranial pressure response. Anesthesiology 51:538, 1979

C.26. What are the effects of anesthetic agents on intracranial pressure?

All potent inhalation anesthetic agents increase cerebral blood flow. This will cause an increase in ICP. If a mass lesion is present, dangerously sharp increase may occur in intracranial pressure when a potent inhalation anesthetic, such as halothane, is added to the inspired mixture. Much of this pressure rise can be prevented by hyperventilation of the patient to reduce the P_{CO_2} prior to adding halothane to the inspired mixture.

Enflurane and isoflurane, although qualitatively similar to halothane in their effects on intracerebral blood flow, do not seem to produce as much of a rise in ICP in either normal or diseased states. Some authors have felt that extreme hyperventilation is not necessary before adding enflurane or isoflurane to the inspired mixture and that it is sufficient to ventilate the patient to a $PaCO_2$ of about 30 mm Hg. Nitrous oxide has also been reported to increase cerebral blood flow, but not nearly as much as the potent volatile inhalation anesthetics.

Two newer inhalation agents are currently undergoing trial. Desflurane has the advantage of low water solubility, allowing rapid changes in anesthetic depth and prompt emergence when desired. Sevoflurane is less irritating to the respiratory tract, but it is partly decomposed by soda lime and also is metabolized to produce compounds that may have implications for possible toxicity. At present it has had extensive trial in Japan but not yet in the United States.

Barbiturates and benzodiazepines such as diazepam and midazolam decrease cerebral blood flow and may also produce a selective cerebral vasoconstriction, according to some authors. This effect, along with a reduction in cerebral metabolic rate O_2, has made barbiturates, such as thiopental, desirable not only for neurosurgical anesthesia, but also for attempts at minimizing brain damage after cerebral trauma or hypoxic insult. Although in laboratory studies on animals barbiturates have shown a protective effect when given prior to global cerebral ischemic insult, clinical studies have been less clear-cut in demonstrating a protective or therapeutic effect if the barbiturate has been given after the ischemic or hypoxic event has occurred.

Propofol, a substituted phenol, although chemically different from them, has many pharmacologic similarities to the barbiturates. In addition, it has a distinctly shorter duration of action with minimal residual effect even after prolonged infusion. For these reasons, it has become a popular intravenous agent both for induction and maintenance of anesthesia, and for various degrees of sedation in intensive care units.

Narcotics such as morphine or fentanyl and its derivatives (e.g., alfentanil and sufentanil) reduce neuronal activity and blood pressure, but they also decrease ventilatory drive. In the spontaneously ventilating patient, the $PaCO_2$ will rise, thereby causing an increase in both cerebral blood flow and ICP. For this reason, narcotics should be used cautiously if at all in spontaneously ventilating patients with brain tumors or other intracranial lesions. If respiration is assisted or controlled to hold the $PaCO_2$ to an acceptably low level, narcotic analgesics can be safely used.

Ketamine increases both cerebral blood flow and ICP. Despite these effects, ketamine is a useful drug in small doses during neuroradiologic diagnostic procedures, especially in children.

Succinylcholine and other depolarizing neuromuscular blocking drugs may transiently increase intracranial pressure during the period of fasciculation, but not afterward, provided that respiration is adequately controlled. Pancuronium and *d*-tubocurarine likewise have no effects on intracranial pressure in the presence of adequately controlled respiration. Other nondepolarizing relaxants such as vecuronium, atracurium, doxacurium, and pipecuronium are probably similar.

Intravenous lidocaine (1.5 mg/kg) reduces the bucking response to endotracheal intubation, and it can lessen the rise of ICP, which may occur at this time. The dose may be repeated as needed, provided that cardiac toxicity does not develop.

Bristow A, Shalev D, Rice B et al: Low-dose synthetic narcotic infusions for cerebral relaxation during craniotomies. Anesth Analg 66:413, 1987

Drummond JC, Todd MM, Scheller MS et al: A comparison of the direct cerebral vasodilating potencies of halothane and isoflurane in the New Zealand white rabbit. Anesthesiology 62:462, 1986

Frizzell RT, Meyer YJ, Borchers DJ et al: The effects of etomidate on cerebral metabolism and blood flow in a canine model for hypoperfusion. J Neurosurg 74:263, 1991

Hoffman WE, Miletich DJ, Albrecht RF: The effects of midazolam on cerebral blood flow and oxygen consumption and its interaction with nitrous oxide. Anesth Analg 65:729, 1986

Jung R, Shah N, Reinsel R et al: Cerebral fluid pressure in patients with brain tumors: Impact of fentanyl versus alfentanil during nitrous oxide-oxygen anesthesia. Anesth Analg 71:419, 1990

Kotani J, Sugioka S, Momota Y et al: Effect of sevoflurane on intracranial pressure, saggital sinus pressure, and the intracranial volume-pressure relation in cats. J Neurosurg Anesthesiol 4:194, 1992

Lebowitz PW, Ramsey FM, Savarese JJ et al: Combination of pancuronium and metocurine: Neuromuscular and hemodynamic advantages over pancuronium alone. Anesth Analg 60:8, 1981

Milde LN, Milde JH, Gallagher WJ: Effects of sufentanil on cerebral circulation and metabolism in dogs. Anesth Analg 70:138, 1990

Minton MD, Grosslight K, Stirt JA et al: Increases in intracranial pressure from succinylcholine: Prevention by prior nondepolarizing block. Anesthesiology 65:165, 1986

Muzzi DA, Losasso TJ, Dietz NM et al: The effect of desflurane and isoflurane on cerebrospinal fluid pressure in humans with supratentorial mass lesions. Anesthesiology 74:504, 1992

Pinaud M, Lelausque JN, Chetanneau A et al: Effects of propofol on cerebral hemodynamics and metabolism in patients with brain trauma. Anesthesiology 73:404, 1990

Ravussin P, Guinard JP, Ralley F et al: Effect of propofol on cerebrospinal fluid pressure and cerebral perfusion pressure in patients undergoing craniotomy. Anaesthesia 43:37, 1988

Scheller MS, Nakakimura K, Fleisher JE, et al: Cerebral effects of sevoflurane in the dog: Comparison with isoflurane and enflurane. Br J Anaesth 65:388, 1990

Shapiro HM, Galindo A, Wyte SR et al: Rapid intra-operative reduction of intracranial pressure with thiopentone. Br J Anaesth 45:1057, 1973

Shapiro HM, Wyte SR, Harris AB: Ketamine anesthesia in patients with intracranial pathology. Br J Anaesth 44:1200, 1972

Stirt JA, Maggio W, Haworth C et al: Vecuronium: Effect on intracranial pressure and hemodynamics in neuro-surgical patients. Anesthesiology 67:570, 1987

Van Hemelrijck J, Van Aken H, Merckx L et al: Anesthesia for craniotomy: Total intravenous anesthesia with propofol and alfentanil compared to anesthesia with thiopental sodium, isoflurane, fentanyl, and nitrous oxide. J Clin Anesth 3:131, 1991

Yano M, Nishiyami H, Yokota H et al: Effect of lidocaine on ICP response to endotracheal suctioning. Anesthesiology 64:651, 1986

D. Postoperative Management

D.1. Discuss the more common early postoperative problems following craniotomy.

The principal postoperative problems following craniotomy relate partly to mechanical manipulations by the surgeon and chemical manipulations by the anesthesiologist. To allow early assessment of neurologic function, one should choose anesthetic drugs that are rapidly excreted or metabolized, or that can be readily reversed. Temperature should be near normal. Intravenous fluids should be restricted to lessen the probability of cerebral edema, which can be a major early postoperative complication. Intracranial pressure monitoring has been advocated by some authors.

James HE, Bruno LA, Schut L: Intracranial subarachnoid pressure monitoring in children. Surg Neurol 3:313, 1975

Johnston IH, Jennett B: The place of continuous intracranial pressure monitoring in neurosurgical practice. Acta Neurochir (Wien) 29:53, 1973

Thompson WM, Ell SR: Neurogenic pulmonary edema: A review of the literature and a perspective. Invest Radiol 26:499, 1991

D.2. How does anesthesia management for carotid endarterectomy differ significantly from craniotomy management?

Carotid endarterectomy anesthesia management is significantly different in that it is desirable to optimize cerebral blood flow rather than reduce it, as is usually done in anesthesia management for craniotomy.

Cucchiara RF, Benefiel DJ, Matteo RS et al: Evaluation of esmolol in controlling increases in heart rate and blood pressure during endotracheal intubation in patients undergoing carotid endarterectomy. Anesthesiology 65:528, 1986

Drummond JC, Oh Y-S, Cole DJ, et al: Phenylephrine-induced hypertension decreased the area of ischemia following middle cerebral artery occlusion. Stroke 20:1538, 1989

Piatt JH, Schiff SJ: High-dose barbiturates therapy in neurosurgery and intensive care. Neurosurgery 15:427, 1984

Shapiro HM: Brain resuscitation: The chicken should come before the egg. Anesthesiology 60:85, 1984

Wade JG: Carotid endarterectomy: The anesthetic challenge. ASA Refresher Courses in Anesthesiology 6:145–152, 1978

D.3. Discuss special problems that may be seen after posterior cranial fossa procedures.

Following posterior fossa craniotomies, special problems may arise from brain stem edema or hematoma, which may compress respiratory centers or lower cranial nerve nuclei causing difficulty in swallowing or holding the airway open for managing secretions, such as saliva or mucus. Macroglossia is a rare but serious complication. Midcervical quadriplegia may also be seen.

Cottrell JE, Turndorf H: Anesthesia and Neurosurgery, 2nd ed, pp 145–146. St. Louis, CV Mosby, 1986

Ellis SC, Bryan-Brown CW, Hyderally H: Massive swelling of the head and neck. Anesthesiology 42:102, 1975

McAllister RG: Macroglossia—a positional complication. Anesthesiology 40:199, 1974

Teeple E, Maroon J, Rueger R: Hemimacroglossia and unilateral ischemic necrosis of the tongue in a long-duration neurosurgical procedure. Anesthesiology 64:845, 1986

Wilder BL: Hypothesis: The etiology of midcervical quadriplegia after operation with the patient in the sitting position. Neurosurgery 11:530, 1982

Carotid Endarterectomy

22

Cynthia A. Lien
Alan Van Poznak

A 65-year-old man suffered from two episodes of amaurosis fugax during the previous 3 weeks. His medical history revealed angina on exertion. His medications included sublingual nitroglycerin as required and diuretic/hypertensive (Dyazide) 25 mg daily. His blood pressure was 190/100 mm Hg and his pulse was 70 beats/min and regular. He was scheduled for a right carotid endarterectomy.

A. Medical Disease and Differential Diagnosis

1. What is amaurosis fugax?
2. What is the prevalence of carotid artery disease?
3. What is the natural course of carotid artery disease?
4. What are the indications for surgical intervention in the management of carotid atherosclerotic disease?
5. Discuss the anatomy of the cerebral blood flow (CBF), including the carotid artery and the circle of Willis.
6. Discuss cerebral perfusion in the presence of carotid artery disease.
7. Discuss the different surgical approaches to carotid endarterectomy.
8. What is normal cerebral blood flow?
9. What is critically low cerebral blood flow as measured by the electroencephalogram (EEG)?
10. What is cerebral autoregulation?
11. How does P_{CO_2} affect autoregulation?
12. What are the principal determinants of cerebral blood flow?
13. What is meant by the term "luxury perfusion?"
14. What is meant by the term "intracerebral steal?"
15. What is the "inverse steal" or "Robin Hood" syndrome?

B. Preoperative Evaluation and Preparation

1. What would you be looking for in your preoperative evaluation?
2. Was this patient's blood pressure too high for elective surgery?
3. What laboratory data would be required preoperatively?
4. Would you premedicate this patient?

C. Intraoperative Management

1. How would you monitor this patient?
2. Would you monitor this patient with an intra-arterial catheter and a pulmonary artery catheter?

3. How would you know that the patient's cerebral perfusion is adequate during surgery?
4. Discuss the differences and relative advantages and disadvantages of both the unprocessed and the processed EEG.
5. How would you measure cerebral blood flow intraoperatively? What are the relative advantages and disadvantages of each technique? How much cerebral blood flow is considered adequate?
6. Does internal carotid stump pressure accurately reflect cerebral perfusion?
7. Do jugular venous oxygen saturation and transconjunctival oxygen tension correlate with cerebral perfusion?
8. Discuss somatosensory evoked potentials (SSEPs) as a monitor of cerebral blood flow during carotid endarterectomy.
9. Describe the role of the transcranial Doppler as a monitor of cerebral perfusion during carotid endarterectomy.
10. What type of anesthesia would you choose for this patient? Why?
11. How would you induce and maintain general anesthesia in this patient?
12. How would you proceed if the patient were to receive regional anesthesia?
13. Discuss the effects of anesthetics on cerebral blood flow.
14. Discuss the protective effects of anesthetic agents on cerebral function.
15. How would you manage this patient's ventilation under general anesthesia?
16. How would you manage this patient's blood pressure intraoperatively?
17. Discuss reperfusion injury following carotid endarterectomy.
18. What intravenous fluids would you give this patient intraoperatively?

D. Postoperative Management

1. The patient did not "wake up" from general anesthesia. Why?
2. Postoperatively the patient's blood pressure was 170/96 mm Hg. Would you treat this? If so, why and how?
3. What immediate postoperative complications might you expect?

A. Medical Disease and Differential Diagnosis

A.1. What is amaurosis fugax?

Amaurosis fugax is transient monocular blindness that is caused by cerebral ischemia; it is an indication of an evolving arterial thrombus in the internal carotid artery. This artery is the main blood supply to the optic nerve and retina via the ophthalmic artery. Approximately 25% of cases of symptomatic carotid occlusion are antedated by a transient ischemic attack (TIA) that takes the form of amaurosis fugax. The symptoms of amaurosis fugax, which have been described as a shade descending over one eye, often last <10 minutes, and are ipsilateral to the evolving and symptomatic vascular disease.

Bennett JC, Plum F (eds): Cecil Textbook of Medicine, 20th ed, p 2064. Philadelphia, WB Saunders, 1996

A.2. What is the prevalence of carotid artery disease?

Carotid artery disease is a manifestation of generalized arteriosclerosis. A review of data contained in the medical records of Mayo Medical Center showed the incidence of TIAs to be 31 per 100,000 people in Rochester, Minnesota. The incidence rate increases with age (1 per 100,000 in people <45 years to 293 per 100,000 in people 75 years and older). Similar rates have been reported in the former USSR. Stroke is the third most common cause of death in the United States.

Meyer FB (ed): Sundt's Occlusive Cerebrovascular Disease, 2nd ed, p 60. Philadelphia, WB Saunders, 1994

A.3. What is the natural course of carotid artery disease?

In atherosclerotic carotid artery disease plaques develop at branches of the carotid artery. The severity of the process parallels that in other major vessels. Thrombosis is most likely to occur where the plaque narrows the lumen to the greatest degree. The most common sites of thrombosis in the cerebral circulation are the internal carotid artery at the level of the carotid sinus, the vertebral and basilar arteries at the region of their junction, the main bifurcation of the middle cerebral artery, the posterior communicating artery as it courses around the cerebral peduncle, and the anterior communicating artery as it curves upward over the corpus callosum. Rarely a cerebral vessel is affected beyond its first major branch. Embolism can occur from any plaque-covered region. Thromboembolic stroke accounts for the greatest percentage of cerebral vascular accidents.

Sixty percent of thrombotic strokes are preceded by one or more TIAs. This is in direct contrast to embolic and hemorrhagic strokes, which are rarely preceded by transient ischemic attacks. Most frequently one or two TIAs will occur before the final stroke, and each will be <10 minutes. In >25% of cases, a complete stroke will follow a TIA within 1 month. In approximately 30% of cases, TIAs do not precede a stroke.

In a patient population in Rochester, Minnesota, the 50% survival time after the first TIA was 7 to 8 years. The highest mortality rate was in the first 2 years following a TIA. However, 2 years following a TIA, the mortality rate stabilized at one and one-half times that of the general population.

Fields WS, Maslenikov V, Meyer JS et al: Joint study of extracranial arterial occlusion. V. Progress report of prognosis following surgery or nonsurgical treatment for cerebral ischemic attacks and cervical carotid artery lesions. JAMA 211:1993, 1970

Matsumoto N, Whisnant JP, Kurland LT et al: Natural history of stroke in Rochester Minnesota, 1955 through 1969: An extension of a previous study, 1945 through 1954. Stroke 4:20, 1973

Meyer FB (ed): Sundt's Occlusive Cerebrovascular Disease, 2nd ed, p 60. Philadelphia, WB Saunders, 1994

A.4. What are the indications for surgical intervention in the management of carotid atherosclerotic disease?

The indications for surgical management of carotid artery disease are continuing to evolve. Until recently approximately 100,000 carotid endarterectomies were performed per year, with 40% of procedures performed for the treatment of asymptomatic disease. The standard criteria for surgical intervention have come into question. Although the role for surgical management in preventing stroke in symptomatic carotid disease is widely accepted, its usefulness in treating asymptomatic patients is a matter of debate. Because carotid endarterectomy itself carries with it a significant morbidity and mortality of 1% to 20%, the risk:benefit relationship needs to be studied. Accepted indications for surgery currently include the following:

- Transient ischemic attacks
- Reversible ischemic neurologic deficits with >70% stenosis of the vessel wall or an ulcerated plaque, with or without stenosis
- TIAs lasting longer than 1 hour with angiographic evidence of stenosis
- An unstable neurologic status that persists despite anticoagulation

Most recently in a multicenter study of 1662 patients with asymptomatic carotid stenosis of 60% or more, as determined by Doppler examination, patients receiving carotid endarterectomy in addition to medical therapy were found to have a 53% reduction in aggregate risk for stroke or death when compared with patients receiving only medical therapy. Patients included in this study were between the ages of 40 and 79, and they were in general good health.

Some authors feel that still larger outcome studies are required before carotid endarterectomy could be recommended for asymptomatic carotid artery disease.

Barnett HJM, Meldrum HE, Eliasziw M: The dilemma of surgical treatment for patients with asymptomatic carotid disease. Ann Intern Med 123:723–725, 1995

Bogousslavsky J, Despland PA, Regli F: Asymptomatic tight stenosis of the internal carotid artery: Long-term prognosis. Neurology 36:861–863, 1986

The CASANOVA Study Group: Carotid surgery versus medical therapy in asymptomatic carotid stenosis. Stroke 22:1229–1235, 1991

Colgan MP, Kingston W, Shanik DG: Asymptomatic carotid stenosis: Is prophylactic endarterectomy justifiable? Br J Surg 72:313–314, 1985

Executive Committee for the Asymptomatic Carotid Atherosclerosis Study: Endarterectomy for asymptomatic carotid artery stenosis. JAMA 273:1421–1428, 1995

Hobson RW, Weiss DG, Fields WS et al: Efficacy of carotid endartectomy for asymptomatic carotid stenosis. The Veterans Affairs Cooperative Study Group. N Engl J Med 328:221–227, 1993

Mayo Asymptomatic Carotid Endarterectomy Study Group: Results of a randomized controlled trial of carotid endarterectomy of asymptomatic carotid stenosis. Mayo Clin Proc 67:513–518, 1992

Schwartz SI, Shires GT, Spencer FC (eds): Principles of Surgery, 6th ed, p 1846. New York, McGraw-Hill, 1994

Thompson JE: Don't throw out the baby with the bath water. A perspective on carotid endarterectomy. J Vasc Surg 4:543–545, 1986

Young WL: Carotid endarterectomy: Preventing neurologic complications. Anesthesiology Report 1:401–420, 1989

A.5. Discuss the anatomy of the cerebral blood flow (CBF), including the carotid artery and the circle of Willis.

The common carotid arteries originate in the thorax. The right common carotid artery originates at the bifurcation of the brachiocephalic trunk, and the left originates from the aortic arch. In the neck, the common carotid arteries travel within the carotid sheath. At the level of the thyroid cartilage each common carotid artery bifurcates into internal and external carotid arteries.

The external carotid artery supplies structures that are external to the skull. Its

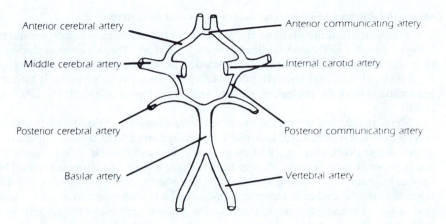

Figure 22-1. Arterial circle of Willis.

branches include the superior thyroid, lingual, facial, ascending pharyngeal, occipital, and posterior auricular arteries.

The internal carotid artery passes through the neck without branching to enter the middle cranial fossa via the carotid canal of the temporal bone, adjacent to the sphenoid bone. It supplies the hypophysis cerebri, the orbit, and the major portion of the supratentorial region of the brain.

Cerebral arteries are derived from the internal carotid and vertebral arteries. The anastomosis they form at the base of the brain is known as the "circle of Willis." The circle is formed anteriorly by the two anterior cerebral arteries; it is connected by the anterior communicating artery and posteriorly by the two posterior cerebral arteries at the junction of which the basilar artery ends. The posterior cerebral arteries are connected to the internal carotid arteries by the two posterior communicating arteries (Fig. 22-1). The lateral surface of each cerebral hemisphere is supplied primarily by the middle cerebral artery. The medial and inferior surfaces of the cerebral hemisphere are supplied by the anterior cerebral and posterior cerebral arteries.

Moore KL: Clinically Oriented Anatomy, pp 1129–1133. Baltimore, Williams & Wilkins, 1980

A.6. Discuss cerebral perfusion in the presence of carotid artery disease.

It can be assumed that autoregulation has been lost in areas of threatened ischemia. Vascular regions subjected to chronic hypoperfusion and relative ischemia are maximally vasodilated and unresponsive to factors that induce vasoconstriction in normally reactive vascular beds. Therefore, in patients with carotid artery disease, blood flow through ischemic regions is passive and dependent on systemic blood pressure. For this reason, hypotension is best avoided in the period prior to restoration of unobstructed cerebral blood flow.

Ehrenfeld WK, Hamilton FN, Larson CP et al: Effect of CO_2 and systemic hypertension on downstream cerebral arterial pressure during carotid endarterectomy. Surgery 67:87, 1970

Fourcade HE, Larson CP, Ehrenfeld WK et al: The effects of CO_2 and systemic hypertension on cerebral perfusion pressure during carotid endarterectomy. Anesthesiology 33:383, 1970

A.7. Discuss the different surgical approaches to carotid endarterectomy.

Carotid endarterectomy involves the removal of atheromatous plaque from the vessel lumen through a fairly standardized surgical procedure. This involves occluding the common, external, and internal carotid arteries, isolating the diseased segment, opening the vessel wall, and removing the plaque. The vessel is then closed. If the remaining intima is too thin, the vessel is closed with a vein graft or a synthetic (Dacron) patch.

Shunt use during the period of carotid cross-clamping varies depending on whether evidence of cerebral ischemia becomes apparent with cross-clamping of the carotid artery. Variations in shunt usage coexist because there is little evidence that one is superior to the others. Placement of a shunt allows hemispheric cerebral blood flow to be maintained during a carotid endarterectomy and may be especially advantageous when the endarterectomy is expected to be complex and to require a long period of time. On the other hand, placement of a shunt may make the surgery technically more difficult; it does not guarantee adequate cerebral blood flow and may cause plaque or air embolization.

Sundt TM, Houser OW, Sharbrough FW et al: Carotid endarterectomy: Results, complications and monitoring techniques. Adv Neurol 16:97–119, 1977

Thompson JE, Talkington CM: Carotid endarterectomy. Ann Surg 184:1–15, 1978

Wylie EJ, Stoney RJ, Ehrenfield WK (eds): Manual of Vascular Surgery. Vol. I. Comprehensive Manuals of Surgical Specialities Series, pp 49–84. New York, Springer-Verlag, 1980

A.8. What is normal cerebral blood flow?

Normal cerebral blood flow is approximately 50 ml/100 g/min for the entire brain. However, blood flow is about four times higher in gray matter than it is in white matter, the flows being respectively 80 and 20 ml/100 g/min.

Kety SS, Schmidt CF: The nitrous oxide method for the quantitative determination of cerebral blood flow in man: Theory, procedure and normal values. J Clin Invest 27:476, 1948

Lassen NA, Munch O: The cerebral blood flow in man determined by the use of radioactive krypton. Acta Physiol Scand 33:30, 1955

A.9. What is critically low cerebral flow as measured by the electroencephalogram (EEG)?

The cerebral blood flow at which ischemia becomes apparent on the EEG is approximately 20 ml/100 g/min.

Assuming a normal temperature and hematocrit, 100 ml of blood contains approximately 20 ml of oxygen. A normal global cerebral blood flow of 50 ml/100 g/min delivers oxygen to the brain at a rate of 10 ml/100 g/min. This is in excess of the high metabolic requirements of the brain for oxygen (3 to 5 ml/100 g/min), which affords a relative margin of safety. Once CBF is decreased to 17 to 18 ml/100 g/min, evidence of ischemia can be detected on the electroencephalogram. Electroencephalographic changes can be delayed for up to 150 seconds following the onset of ischemia. It is impossible to define the specific changes that represent irreversible ischemia. In the setting of an isoelectric EEG, oxygen delivery to the brain may be adequate to keep the neurons alive but insufficient energy for them to function.

The development of cerebral infarction depends on both the degree and duration of ischemia. Jones et al. showed, in an animal model of reversible ischemia, that with cerebral blood flow of 18 to 23 ml/100 g/min animals would recover from impaired neurologic function when blood flow was returned to normal levels, regardless of the duration of the ischemic period. Infarction development at lower flows depends on both the degree of regional cerebral blood flow (rCBF) reduction and the duration of ischemia. Neurons that are nonfunctional but that will recover fully with restoration of adequate flow are said to be in an ischemic penumbra. Neuronal destruction occurs with CBF <10 ml/100 g/min.

Boysen G, Engell HC, Pitolese GR et al: On the critical level of cerebral blood flow in man with particular reference to carotid surgery. Circulation 49:1023, 1974

Jones TH, Morawetz RB, Crowell RM et al: Threshold of focal cerebral ischemia in awake monkeys. J Neurosurg 54:773, 1981

Levy WJ: Intraoperative EEG patterns: Implications for EEG monitoring. Anesthesiology 60:430, 1984

Trojaborg W, Boysen G: Relation between EEG, regional cerebral blood flow and internal carotid artery pressure during carotid endarterectomy. Electroencephalogr Clin Neurophysiol 34:61, 1973

A.10. What is cerebral autoregulation?

Cerebral autoregulation is the tendency of the tissue to maintain normal blood flow despite variations in blood pressure. In normotensive individuals, cerebral blood flow is constant between mean arterial pressures of 50 and 150 mm Hg. What this means is that cerebrovascular resistance increases, through vasoconstriction, as mean arterial pressure increases from 50 to 150 mm Hg. At pressures >150 mm Hg, the cerebral vasculature is maximally vasoconstricted and cerebral blood flow increases with increasing pressure. At pressures <50 mm Hg, cerebral vessels are maximally vasodilated, so that as mean arterial pressure falls cerebral blood flow decreases. In hypertensive patients autoregulation still exists. The upper and lower limits of the autoregulatory curve, however, have been shifted to the right, to higher pressures. What this means is that a mean arterial pressure of 60 mm Hg, which would be well tolerated in a normotensive individual, may actually be below the lower limit of autoregulation in the hypertensive individual, resulting in cerebral hypoperfusion. Conversely, hypertensive patients tolerate marked increases in mean arterial pressure much better than their normotensive counterparts. With chronic antihypertensive medication the limits of autoregulation are shifted toward normal.

Haggendal E, Lofgren J, Nilsson NJ et al: Effects of varied cerebrospinal fluid pressure on cerebral blood flow in dogs. Acta Physiol Scand 79:262, 1970

Symon L, Pasztor E, Dorsch NWC et al: Physiological responses of local areas of the cerebral circulation in experimental primates determined by the method of hydrogen clearance. Stroke 4:632, 1973

A.11. How does P_{CO_2} affect autoregulation?

Cerebral blood flow increases about 4% for each mm Hg increase in arterial P_{CO_2} for partial pressures of arterial carbon dioxide between 20 and 80 mm Hg.

Skinhoj E, Paulson OB: Carbon dioxide and cerebral circulatory control: Evidence of a nonfocal site of action of carbon dioxide on the cerebral circulation. Arch Neurol 20:249, 1969

A.12. *What are the principal determinants of cerebral blood flow?*

The principal determinants of cerebral blood flow are nerve cell activity, cerebral perfusion pressure, $PaCO_2$, the brain extracellular fluid pH, Po_2, and neurogenic influences.

Cottrell JE, Turndorf H: Anesthesia and Neurosurgery, 3rd ed, pp 17–48. St. Louis, CV Mosby, 1994

A.13. *What is meant by the term "luxury perfusion?"*

Luxury perfusion is blood flow that is in excess of metabolic need (increased cerebral blood flow to cerebral metabolic rate O_2 ratio). It is most frequently observed in tissues surrounding tumors or areas of infarction. It has also been observed in tissues that have been manipulated during surgery.

Paulson OB: Cerebral apoplexy (stroke): Pathogenesis, pathophysiology and therapy as illustrated by regional blood flow measurements in the brain. Stroke 2:327–360, 1971

A.14. *What is meant by the term "intracerebral steal?"*

Intracerebral steal is a paradoxic response to carbon dioxide in which hypercapnea decreases the blood flow in an ischemic area. It can be the consequence of the vasodilatory effect of carbon dioxide on the normally perfused arterioles at the periphery of an ischemic lesion. Because chronically ischemic vascular beds are maximally vasodilated, they cannot dilate further in response to hypercapnea.

Paulson OB: Cerebral apoplexy (stroke): Pathogenesis, pathophysiology and therapy as illustrated by regional blood flow measurements in the brain. Stroke 2:327–360, 1971

A.15. *What is the "inverse steal" or "Robin Hood" syndrome?*

Inverse steal is the paradoxic effect of hypocapnea producing increased blood flow to ischemic regions of the brain. Vasoconstriction occurs in adjacent, normal arterioles, thereby causing a local increase in perfusion pressure and augmenting collateral flow to the ischemic, unreactive, maximally vasodilated area of the brain.

Betz E: Cerebral blood flow: Its measurement and regulation. Physiol Rev 52:595–630, 1972

B. Preoperative Evaluation and Preparation

B.1. *What would you be looking for in your preoperative evaluation?*

It can be assumed that once the anesthesiologist is asked to evaluate a patient for surgery, the presence of a carotid lesion amenable to surgical treatment has already been documented through Doppler, angiographic, or oculoplethysmographic studies. The anesthesiologist should be prepared to look for other manifestations of generalized arteriosclerosis, such as coronary artery disease, hypertension, and renal disease. Medical conditions associated with arteriosclerosis, such as obesity, diabetes, and pulmonary disease secondary to cigarette smoking, should be sought. The patient's neurologic status and airway also should be evaluated.

Because 30% to 50% of patients undergoing carotid endarterectomy have coronary artery disease, evidence of heart disease should be sought in the patient's history. Patients should be specifically asked whether they have angina, or have ever had a myocardial infarction or congestive heart failure. An indication of daily activity level should be obtained. A patient unable to ambulate for distances because of claudication may never develop angina or left ventricular failure, and further, more invasive evaluation of the patient's cardiac function may be required. Evidence of cardiac disease should also be sought on physical examination. This would include heart rate and rhythm, and presence of jugular venous distention, basilar rales on auscultation of the chest, cardiac enlargement as determined by lateral displacement of the point of maximal impulse, and a cardiac gallop.

The anesthesiologist should determine whether or not the patient has hypertension. Hypertension is present in 55% to 80% of patients with carotid artery disease, and its presence would alter intraoperative blood pressure management. Blood pressure should be measured in both arms with the patient in both the supine and the upright positions. A range of acceptable blood pressures, where the patient is free of symptoms of both cardiac and cerebral ischemia, should be determined. This is done, in part, by reviewing the patient's chart and making note of the highest and the lowest blood pressures that were measured. Knowing this range allows the anesthesiologist to determine the range of blood pressures that will be tolerated without treatment in the operating room. In these patients, raising the blood pressure excessively to improve cerebral perfusion may exacerbate myocardial ischemia, and lowering the blood pressure to reduce the work of the heart may compromise cerebral perfusion, exacerbating cerebral ischemia.

Other disorders associated with vascular disease, such as obesity, diabetes, and cigarette smoking with its sequelae, should be determined. Evidence of other end-organ effects of vascular disease, such as renal disease, should also be sought.

The patient's neurologic status needs to be evaluated preoperatively by the anesthesiologist. Although it would be preferable to medically optimize the patient with uncontrolled hypertension or untreated metabolic disease or, if possible, delay surgery in the patient with a myocardial infarction <6 months old, the presence of crescendo TIAs may not allow that option.

Finally, the patient's airway needs to be assessed preoperatively for ease of ventilation and intubation. A patient in whom it is difficult to establish ventilation may become hypercarbic during induction, and the increase in $PaCO_2$ may have adverse effects on CBF. As part of this evaluation, the range of motion of the patient's neck tolerated without evidence of cerebral ischemia needs to be determined so that extreme extension and lateral rotation of the neck during ventilation, intubation, and finally patient positioning can be avoided. Such extreme extension and rotation of the neck may occlude the patient's vertebral artery and contribute to postoperative deficits.

Asiddao CB, Donegan JH, Whitesell RC et al: Factors associated with perioperative complications during carotid endarterectomy. Anesth Analg 61:631, 1982

Coriat P, Baron JF, Natali J et al: Incidence of myocardial ischemia during carotid endarterectomy. Int Angiol 5:203, 1986

Donegan JH: Anesthesia for patients with cerebrovascular disease. ASA Refresher Courses in Anesthesiology 10:63, 1982

Sherman DG, Hart RG, Easton JD: Abrupt change in head position and cerebral infarction. Stroke 12:2–6, 1981

Sundt TM, Sandok BA, Whisment JP: Carotid endarterectomy: Complications and preoperative assessment of risk. Mayo Clin Proc 50:301, 1975.

B.2. Was this patient's blood pressure too high for elective surgery?

Although hypertension is present in most patients presenting for carotid endarterectomy, its rapid correction is not recommended because this may exacerbate cerebral ischemia. If this patient had evidence of myocardial ischemia at this blood pressure and was stable from a neurologic standpoint, blood pressure could be gradually decreased with antihypertensive medications. Normal myocardial and cerebral function needs to be preserved. These goals are not necessarily at odds with each other. To decrease myocardial oxygen consumption, one would want to decrease heart rate, blood pressure, and myocardial contractility. Myocardial work can, in this patient population, be decreased by decreasing heart rate, while cerebral perfusion pressure is maintained with an adequate mean arterial pressure. If a patient presents with an unstable neurologic status, it may be necessary to control blood pressure once the obstruction to cerebral blood flow has been relieved.

A single blood pressure measurement is of little use to the anesthesiologist in the preoperative assessment of the patient. It is the range of the blood pressures normally tolerated by the patient that will guide perioperative blood pressure management. For example, if a patient's blood pressure is measured at 80/50 mm Hg preoperatively and at this blood pressure he or she does not develop any new neurologic deficits, and, if at 170/100 he or she does not develop any signs of myocardial ischemia, the clinician will be inclined to treat blood pressures only beyond these two extremes.

Because this patient has a history of hypertension, one can expect that under anesthesia wide swings will occur in his blood pressure. The anesthesiologist must be prepared for these fluctuations by having both vasopressors and vasodilators readily available. Variations in blood pressure should be minimized because these have been shown to be related to increased cardiac and neurologic morbidity.

Hamilton WP: Do let the blood pressure drop and do use myocardial depressants! Anesthesiology 45:273–274, 1976

Roizen MF (ed): Anesthesia for Vascular Surgery, pp 125–128. New York, Churchill Livingstone, 1990

Smith JS, Roizen MF, Calahan MK et al: Does anesthetic technique make a difference? Augmentation of systolic blood pressure during carotid endarterectomy: Effects of phenylephrine versus light anesthesia and of isoflurane versus halothane on the incidence of myocardial ischemia. Anesthesiology 69:846–853, 1988

B.3. What laboratory data would be required preoperatively?

Laboratory tests should be ordered to determine the patient's baseline cardiac, respiratory, and metabolic status.

Hemoglobin and hematocrit should be obtained preoperatively because values may be abnormal in patients with respiratory disease and because a significant blood loss can occur intraoperatively.

An electrocardiogram should be examined preoperatively to look for arrhythmias, evidence of ischemia, previous infarction, or left ventricular hypertrophy. Where appropriate, this should be compared with earlier studies to determine whether interval changes have occurred.

A chest x-ray should be examined to look for cardiomegaly, evidence of chronic obstructive pulmonary disease (COPD), or pneumonia. If the patient has a history of COPD, a preoperative arterial blood gas should be obtained to identify the patient's baseline $PaCO_2$. In patients who are chronically hypercarbic, rapid adjustment to normocarbia intraoperatively will be interpreted by the body as relative hypocarbia. Cerebral blood flow will be reduced accordingly. Management of intraoperative ventilation should be aimed at maintaining the patient's normal arterial carbon dioxide level.

Finally, a urine analysis and data on blood urea nitrogen and creatinine should be obtained to determine the patient's baseline renal status.

Further preoperative evaluation would be based on the presence of concurrent disease.

Roizen MF (ed): Anesthesia for Vascular Surgery, p 125. New York, Churchill Livingstone, 1990

B.4. Would you premedicate this patient?

Some disagreement exists as to whether patients should be premedicated prior to a carotid endarterectomy. Ideally the patient should be calm and awake. Preoperative anxiety should be alleviated in these patients because anxiety can lead to perioperative hypertension, which has been associated with adverse neurologic outcome. Increases in heart rate and blood pressure observed in the anxious patient lead to increased myocardial oxygen consumption and, potentially, ischemia, ventricular dysfunction, and arrhythmias.

Overmedication can lead to ventilatory suppression, with resultant hypercarbia and alterations in cerebral blood flow that can exacerbate cerebral ischemia. Oversedation can also interfere with the immediate postoperative neurologic assessment of the patient because it may cause delayed awakening from anesthesia. One of the anesthetic goals for carotid endarterectomy is to have a patient who promptly awakens from anesthesia and is able to cooperate with a basic neurologic evaluation. A patient who is too sedated at the end of surgery is problematic.

To achieve these goals, a thorough and reassuring preoperative visit alone may provide sufficient anxiolysis. The anesthesiologist should explain the preoperative procedure and what can be expected in the postoperative period, answering any questions that the patient has. If a pharmacologic premedication is required, a benzodiazepine (e.g., diazepam 5 mg orally, 1 hour preoperatively) will provide anxiolysis and minimal respiratory depression.

Bailey PL, Andriano KP, Goldman M et al: Variability of the respiratory response to diazepam. Anesthesiology 64:460, 1986

Freeman LJ, Nixon PGF, Sallabank P et al: Psychological stress and silent myocardial ischemia. Am Heart J 114:477, 1987

Leigh JM, Walker J, Janaganathan P: Effect of preoperative anaesthetic visit on anxiety. BMJ 2:987, 1977

C. Intraoperative Management

C.1. How would you monitor this patient?

Patients who are about to undergo carotid endarterectomy are monitored with the routine monitors of cardiovascular, pulmonary, and metabolic function, which include leads II and V_5 of the electrocardiogram; noninvasive blood pressure monitor; end-tidal capnometry; esophageal temperature; and pulse oximetry. In addition, invasive blood pressure monitors and a monitor of cerebral perfusion should be used.

C.2. Would you monitor this patient with an intra-arterial catheter and a pulmonary artery catheter?

An intra-arterial catheter should be used to monitor the patient's blood pressure. It would permit immediate identification of blood pressure changes and allow for repetitive sampling of arterial blood gases.

Whether a pulmonary artery catheter is required to monitor the patient's cardiac function would be dictated solely by the patient's preoperative cardiac status. Carotid endarterectomy is not an operation in which large fluid shifts are anticipated. A pulmonary artery catheter is not required in the patient with normal left ventricular function.

C.3. How would you know that the patient's cerebral perfusion is adequate during surgery?

In the awake patient undergoing carotid endarterectomy under local anesthesia, repeated neurologic examinations can be done to assess the adequacy of cerebral perfusion. If the patient receives general anesthesia, cerebral perfusion or function should be monitored. No currently available clinical monitor is as sensitive and specific for cerebral dysfunction as repeated neurologic examinations, and no one monitor is used routinely in all operating rooms. A number of monitors have been used to look at cerebral perfusion or function. These include the EEG, somatosensory evoked potentials (SSEP), regional cerebral blood flow, internal carotid stump pressure, jugular venous oxygen saturation, transconjunctival oxygen tension, and transcranial Doppler.

Evans WE, Hayes JP, Waltke EA et al: Optimal cerebral monitoring during carotid endarterectomy: Neurologic response under local anesthesia. J Vasc Surg 2:775, 1985

Grundy BL, Sanderson AC, Webster MW et al: Hemiparesis following carotid endarterectomy: Comparison of monitoring methods. Anesthesiology 55:462, 1981

Rosenthal D, Stanton PE Jr, Lamis PA: Carotid endarterectomy: The unreliability of intraoperative monitoring having had stroke or reversible ischemic neurological deficit. Arch Surg 116:1569, 1981

C.4. Discuss the differences and relative advantages and disadvantages of the unprocessed electroencephalogram and the processed electroencephalogram.

The EEG is neither a measure of cerebral blood flow nor a way to determine whether irreversible neuronal damage has occurred. Rather, it is an indicator that areas of the brain may be at risk for infarction. Electroencephalographic changes that occur with hypothermia, hypocarbia, hypoxemia, and deep anesthesia mimic electroencephalographic signs of ischemia. In patients who have had a cerebral vascular accident (CVA), the EEG does not predict cerebral ischemia.

A number of problems associated with monitoring the 16-lead EEG intraoperatively have detracted from its popularity. These include difficulty in obtaining a meaningful recording in the electrically noisy environment of the operating room, the bulk of the equipment required, and the need for specially trained personnel for interpretation. The 16-channel electroencephalogram is, however, a sensitive indicator of ischemia.

The processed EEG has eliminated many of the problems associated with the 16-channel EEG. The equipment is generally compact and the data display allows for ease of interpretation. The most commonly used processed electroencephalogram is the power spectrum analysis. For this analysis the EEG is studied in short time intervals of 2 to 16 minutes, called epochs. Each epoch then is subjected to a fast Fourier transform analysis during which the complex waveform of the unprocessed EEG is broken down into its component sine waves of varying amplitudes and frequencies. The power spectrum is calculated by squaring the amplitude of the individual frequency components. The power spectrum can then be displayed in a number of graphic forms, two of which are the compressed spectral array and the density modulated spectral array. Data are displayed in these two forms as relative power versus frequency (Fig. 22-2).

It must be remembered that the processed EEG is only as good as the original from which it was obtained. Therefore, meticulous recording techniques are required even when monitoring a processed EEG. During carotid endarterectomy generally two or four EEG channels are monitored.

Harris EJ, Brown WH, Pavy RN et al: Continuous electroencephalographic monitoring during carotid artery endarterectomy. Surgery 83:306, 1978

Kearse LA, Lopez-Bresnahan M, McPeck K et al: Preoperative cerebrovascular symptoms and electroencephalographic abnormalities do not predict cerebral ischemia during carotid endarterectomy. Stroke 26:1210, 1995

Levy W, Shapiro HM, Maruchak G et al: Automated EEG processing for intraoperative monitoring. Anesthesiology 53:223, 1980

Rampil IJ, Holzer JA, Quest DO et al: Prognostic value of computerized EEG analysis during carotid endarterectomy. Anesth Analg 62:186, 1983

Sundt TM, Sharbrough FW, Piepgras DG et al: Correlation of cerebral blood flow and electroencephalographic changes during carotid endarterectomy. Mayo Clin Proc 56:533, 1981

C.5. How would you measure cerebral blood flow intraoperatively? What are the relative advantages and disadvantages of each technique? How much cerebral blood flow is considered adequate?

Measurement of regional cerebral blood flow is the single best method for detecting focal cerebral ischemia during general anesthesia. A number of different ways are used to measure cerebral blood flow. These include the Kety-Schmidt method, later modifications on this, the intracarotid injection method, and the inhalation and intravenous techniques.

The Kety-Schmidt method, as originally described, involved 10 to 15 minutes of inhalation of 15% nitrous oxide. During this period of time equilibration would occur

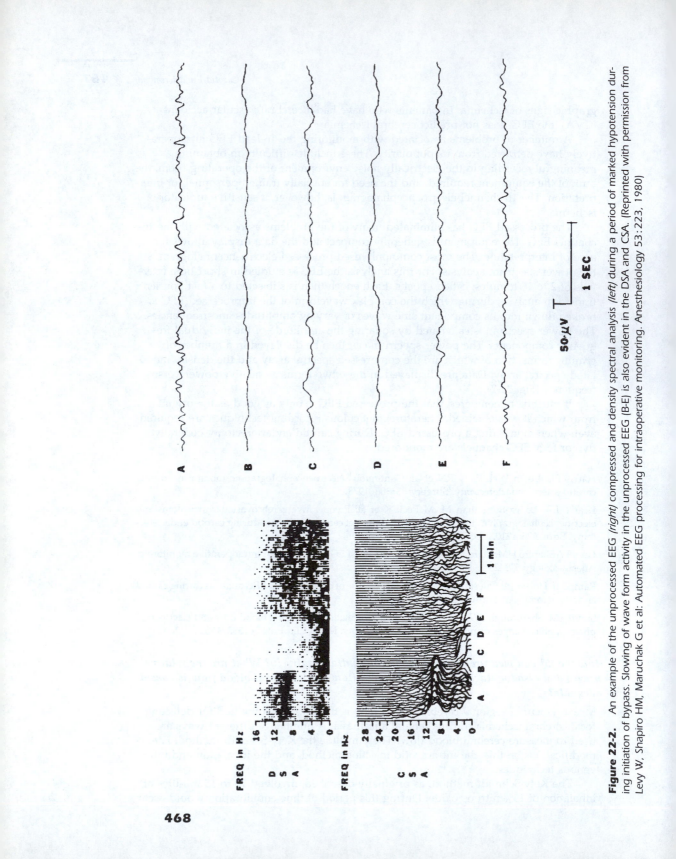

Figure 22-2. An example of the unprocessed EEG *(right)* compressed and density spectral analysis *(left)* during a period of marked hypotension during initiation of bypass. Slowing of wave form activity in the unprocessed EEG (B-E) is also evident in the DSA and CSA. (Reprinted with permission from Levy W, Shapiro HM, Maruchak G et al: Automated EEG processing for intraoperative monitoring. Anesthesiology 53:223, 1980)

between arterial, venous, and tissue concentrations of nitrous oxide. Blood samples would intermittently be taken from a peripheral artery and the jugular bulb to determine tracer concentration. The amount of tracer taken up by the brain in a certain period of time is equivalent to the amount delivered to the brain in the arterial blood supply minus that recovered in the cerebral venous blood in the same period of time. If it is assumed that brain concentrations of the tracer are proportional to the tracer concentrations in the cerebral venous blood, global cerebral blood flow can be determined with knowledge of the blood brain partition coefficient for the tracer used.

Later modifications of this technique employ the radioactive tracers ^{85}krypton or ^{133}xenon. Cerebral blood flow, as measured using the Kety-Schmidt method, may overestimate CBF in the case of low perfusion states in which brain and venous blood may not equilibrate. One cannot measure rCBF using this technique because jugular venous blood is a mixed venous sample with varying amounts of contamination from the contralateral hemisphere.

The intracarotid injection method of cerebral blood flow determination was described by Lassen and Ingvar in 1961. The technique involves injecting a radioactive tracer, ^{85}krypton or ^{133}xenon, as a bolus into the cerebral arterial supply and following the cerebral washout with external scintillation counting. Use of external scintillation counters makes it possible to determine rCBF, and the sensitivity of the technique can be increased by increasing the number of detectors. The tracer is injected directly into either an internal carotid or a vertebral artery, minimizing the number of counts obtained from the extracranial circulatory distribution. This method assumes that the tracer mixes completely with brain. Because the tracer is almost completely exhaled on passage through the lungs, it has essentially no recirculation. A typical tracer washout curve in normal brain is the summation of two exponential curves. Two separate flows, fast (gray matter) and slow (white matter), can be calculated using compartmental analysis.

The most noninvasive techniques to determine cerebral blood flow are the inhalation and the intravenous techniques. The inhalation method involves a 1-minute period of inhalation of ^{133}xenon followed by a 10-minute period of washout with external detection. The washout of tracer from the brain is similar to that obtained with intra-arterial injection except that, because of mixing in the heart and the lungs, the input of tracer is not instantaneous. Because the slow component of CBF is contaminated by extracranial clearance of the tracer, the noninvasive methods are suited primarily for determination of gray matter flow. The inhalation and intravenous methods may be less reliable in the presence of pulmonary disease because the end-tidal concentration of tracer may not adequately reflect arterial concentration. With these techniques, extracranial contamination can result in an underestimation of CBF results, and, under extremely low flow states, they may not give reliable quantitative information.

One thing to bear in mind with all tracer washout techniques is that, in general, they only provide flow information about cortical cerebral blood flow and not about deeper structures. Furthermore, with any of these techniques, CBF is a calculated number, and it will vary depending on the specific technique used to measure it. Average global cerebral blood flow is 50 ml/100 g/min, gray matter flow is 80 ml/100 g/min, and white matter flow is 20 ml/100 g/min. A measured flow intraoperatively of >24 ml/100 g/min is considered to be sufficient and that of <18 ml/100 g/min is inadequate. The specific flow differences compatible with ischemia depend on the anesthetic agents used. The expense and expertise required to collect and interpret CBF data have limited its use to only a few centers.

Bell BA: A history of the study of the cerebral circulation and the measurement of cerebral blood flow. Neurosurgery 14:238, 1984

Kety SS, Schmidt CF: The nitrous oxide method for the quantitative determination of cerebral blood flow in man: Theory, procedure and normal values. J Clin Invest 27:476, 1948

Lassen NA, Hoedt-Rasmussen K, Sorensen SC et al: Regional cerebral blood flow in man determined by krypton 85. Neurology 13:719, 1963

Messick JM, Casement B, Sharbrough FW et al: Correlation of regional cerebral blood flow (rCBF) with EEG changes during isoflurane anesthesia for carotid endarterectomy: Critical rCBF. Anesthesiology 66:344, 1987

Obrist WD, Thompson HK, Wand HS et al: Regional cerebral blood flow estimated by [133]xenon inhalation. Stroke 6:245, 1975

Paulson OB, Cronqvist S, Risberg J et al: Regional cerebral blood flow: A comparison of 8 detector and 16 detector instrumentation. J Nucl Med 10:164, 1968

C.6. Does internal carotid stump pressure accurately reflect cerebral perfusion?

The internal carotid stump pressure, the pressure in the portion of the internal carotid artery cephalad to the carotid cross-clamp, has been used to determine whether CBF during cross-clamping was adequate to avoid neuronal damage. The stump pressure presumably reflects pressure transmitted through collateral vessels. However, because maintaining stump pressures of from 25 to 70 mm Hg have been touted as necessary to avoid neurologic injury, the stump pressure does not appear to reliably represent the adequacy of collateral cerebral blood flow. It does not correlate consistently with changes in the electroencephalogram, rCBF, or changes in the neurologic status of the awake patient. Anesthetic agents can alter carotid stump pressure without changing regional CBF.

Inadequate stump pressures have been demonstrated when measured rCBF was adequate. Therefore, if shunting during carotid endarterectomy were to be done only on the basis of stump pressures, some patients would unnecessarily receive shunts.

Harada RN, Comerota AJ, Good GM et al: Stump pressure, electroencephalographic changes, and the contralateral carotid artery: Another look at selective shunting. Am J Surg 170:148, 1995

Hays RJ, Levinson SA, Wylie EJ: Intraoperative measurement of carotid back pressure as a guide to operative management for carotid endarterectomy. Surgery 72:953, 1972

Kelly JJ, Callow AD, O'Donnell TF et al: Failure of carotid stump pressure: Its incidence as a predictor for a temporary shunt during carotid endarterectomy. Arch Surg 114:1361, 1979

McKay RD, Sundt TM, Michenfelder JD et al: Internal carotid artery stump pressure and cerebral blood flow during carotid endarterectomy: Modification by halothane, enflurane and Innovar. Anesthesiology 45:390, 1976

Sublett JW, Seidenberg AB, Hobson RW: Internal carotid artery stump pressures during regional anesthesia. Anesthesiology 41:505, 1974

C.7. Do jugular venous oxygen saturation and transconjunctival oxygen tension correlate with cerebral perfusion?

Noninvasive measurement of transconjunctival oxygen tension has been used as a monitor of cerebral perfusion during carotid endarterectomy. However, no correlation appears to exist between this and changes in rCBF during cross-clamping.

Jugular venous oxygen saturation is an accurate monitor of global, rather than regional, cerebral blood flow and oxygen consumption. It is not capable of reflecting focal cerebral perfusion because of interhemispheric mixing of venous blood. As long as arterial oxygen content remains stable, a decrease in jugular venous oxygen saturation reflects a decrease in cerebral blood flow or an increase in cerebral metabolic oxygen requirements not associated with an increase in cerebral blood flow. Because changes in rCBF can occur without changes in jugular venous oxygen saturation, this monitor is not adequate for use in the clinical setting.

Gibson BE, McMichan JC, Cucchiara RF: Lack of correlation between transconjunctival O_2 and cerebral blood flow during carotid artery occlusion. Anesthesiology 64:277, 1986

Kram HB, Shoemaker WC, Bratanow N et al: Noninvasive conjunctival oxygen monitoring during carotid endarterectomy. Arch Surg 121:914, 1986

Larson CP Jr, Ehrenfeld WK, Wade JG et al: Jugular venous oxygen saturation as an index of adequacy of cerebral oxygenation. Surgery 62:31, 1967

C.8. Discuss somatosensory evoked potentials (SSEPs) as a monitor of cerebral blood flow during carotid endarterectomy.

Somatosensory evoked potentials are a specialized form of electrophysiologic monitoring that reflects the presence of intact sensory pathways from a stimulated peripheral nerve to the cortex where electrical activity is being monitored. Evidence exists that distortion of certain waveforms is associated with ischemia. These SSEP changes, however, are not consistently associated with changes in the electroencephalogram. Questions have been raised regarding whether SSEPs can overpredict the presence of ischemia and the need for shunting. Further work in this area is certainly warranted because, if SSEPs are a useful indicator of ischemia, they may be used when ischemia cannot be detected on an EEG tracing, such as during barbiturate anesthesia. During barbiturate anesthesia the isoelectric EEG can only indicate that neurons are not functioning and, therefore, maximally protected. It cannot indicate whether these same neurons are ischemic. The SSEP tracing would remain intact with barbiturate anesthesia and, therefore, would potentially be more useful as a clinical monitor.

Lam AM, Teturswamy G: Monitoring of evoked responses during carotid endarterectomy and extracranial-intracranial anastomosis. Int Anesth Clin 22:107, 1984

Moorthy SS, Markand ON, Dilley RS et al: Somatosensory-evoked responses during carotid endarterectomy. Anesth Analg 61:879, 1982

C.9. Describe the role of the transcranial Doppler as a monitor of cerebral perfusion during carotid endarterectomy.

By allowing for continuous assessment of the velocity of the blood flow in the ipsilateral middle cerebral artery, the transcranial Doppler may be useful throughout carotid endarterectomy. It can aid in determining the need for a shunt by detecting a decrease in the middle cerebral artery velocity with placement of the carotid cross-clamp. It allows for continuous assessment of shunt function. It can be used to assess the adequacy of pharmacologically induced intraoperative hypertensive therapy. Finally, the transcranial Doppler allows for the detection of air embolization or particulate matter.

A good correlation has been shown between intraoperative electroencephalography and transcranial Doppler. Although patients who have unchanged electroencephalograms have a middle cerebral artery velocity of 24.1 cm/sec during cross-clamping, those with a middle cerebral artery velocity of 14.7 cm/sec develop EEG changes. The ratio of the mean velocity while the cross-clamp is in place compared with the mean velocity prior to placement of the clamp may also be used to predict alteration in neurologic function. A ratio below 0.4 detects 97% of patients with EEG flattening.

Jansen C, Vriens EM, Eikelboom BC et al: Carotid endartectomy with transcranial Doppler and electroencephalographic monitoring: A prospective study in 130 operations. Stroke 24:665–669, 1993

Jorgensen LG, Schroeder TV: Transcranial Doppler for detection of cerebral ischaemia during carotid endarterectomy. Eur J Vasc Surg 6:142–147, 1992

Schneider PA, Rossman ME, Torem S et al: Transcranial Doppler in the management of extracranial cerebrovascular disease: Implications in diagnosis and monitoring. J Vasc Surg 7:223–231, 1988

C.10. *What type of anesthesia would you choose for this patient? Why?*

Patients undergoing carotid endarterectomy may have either regional or general anesthesia. Each type of anesthesia has its own advantages and disadvantages, which must be considered when choosing the optimal anesthetic for a patient. Benefits of general anesthesia include a still patient and a quiet operative field, early control of the airway and ventilation, and the ability to "protect" the brain should ischemia, which cannot be eliminated, develop. A disadvantage of general anesthesia is the inability to perform repeated neurologic evaluations during surgery. Therefore, patients receiving general anesthesia should have their cerebral blood flow or function monitored as previously discussed.

The primary advantage of a regional anesthetic is that the patient remains awake so that repeated neurologic evaluations are possible. Some authors believe that regional anesthesia allows for greater stability of blood pressure, decreased requirement for vasoactive support of blood pressure, and decreased incidence of perioperative myocardial infarction. Although anecdotal reports may support these claims, further studies are required. Potential complications associated with regional anesthesia include:

- Total spinal anesthesia
- Seizures
- Alteration of mental status
- Loss of patient cooperation associated with cerebral hypoperfusion, inadequate ventilation, cardiac arrest
- Loss of the cerebral protective effects of general anesthesia

Patient outcome appears to be unrelated to the type of anesthesia administered.

Allen BT, Anderson CB, Rubin BG et al: The influence of anesthetic technique on perioperative complications after carotid endarterectomy. J Vasc Surg 19:834, 1994

Corson JD, Chang BB, Shah DM et al: The influence of anesthetic choice on carotid endarterectomy outcome. Arch Surg 122:807, 1987

Gelb AW: Anesthetic considerations for carotid endarterectomy. Int Anesth Clin 22:153, 1984

Ombrellaro MP, Freeman MB, Stevens SL et al: Effect of anesthetic technique on cardiac morbidity following carotid artery surgery. Am J Surg 171:387, 1996

Peitzman AB, Webster MW, Loubeau J et al: Carotid endarterectomy under regional (conductive) anesthesia. Ann Surg 196:59, 1982

Yared I, Martinis AJ, Mack RM: Carotid endarterectomy under local anesthesia: A retrospective study. Am Surg 45:709, 1979

C.11. How would you induce and maintain general anesthesia in this patient?

Following preoxygenation, all anesthetics should be titrated in slowly with special attention being paid to their effect on the patient's blood pressure. Control of the airway should be taken as soon as the patient is no longer able to adequately breathe spontaneously.

While breathing oxygen, the patient is first given either a precurarizing dose or a priming dose of nondepolarizing muscle relaxant. Small doses of fentanyl are then given intravenously. The patient is reminded to breathe to maintain normocapnea. Narcotics are given until the patient is comfortably sedated. This is usually accomplished with a dose of 3 µg/kg of fentanyl. The patient is also given 1 mg/kg of lidocaine intravenously at least 2 minutes prior to laryngoscopy and intubation to blunt the hyperdynamic response to airway manipulation. A 2 to 3 mg/kg dose of thiopental is then given, and controlled ventilation is instituted with 100% oxygen to avoid hypoxia and hypercarbia. A muscle relaxant is then given to facilitate endotracheal intubation. Succinylcholine should be avoided in hemiparetic patients because of the possibility of a hyperkalemic response to its administration. Nondepolarizing muscle relaxants with significant hemodynamic effects such as sympathomimetic activity, vagolysis, or histamine release should be avoided. Either cisatracurium or vecuronium is suitable for administration to these patients. Once the patient is relaxed, an expeditious laryngoscopy and intubation are performed. The time spent intubating the patient is minimized to decrease the hemodynamic response to airway manipulation.

During the induction and intubation sequence, the patient's blood pressure is kept in a normal range by the use of vasopressors such as phenylephrine and vasodilators such as nitroglycerin or sodium nitroprusside as indicated.

Anesthesia can be maintained with a combination of nitrous oxide, volatile anesthetics, and narcotics. Any anesthetic regimen is suitable if it provides hemodynamic stability, does not exacerbate cerebral ischemia, and allows for a prompt emergence from anesthesia at the conclusion of surgery.

Narcotics can be used judiciously as part of the anesthetic. Their addition to an isoflurane anesthetic will decrease heart rate, maintain blood pressure, and, when properly dosed, allow for a prompt, smooth emergence from general anesthesia. Their use should not be avoided because of anecdotal reports of adverse neurologic outcome after focal ischemia in rodents.

Maintenance of a light anesthesia appears to have several advantages over deep anesthesia. It allows ischemic patterns on the EEG to be recognized easily. It also facilitates maintenance of the patient's blood pressure. It has been shown that light anesthesia, compared with deep anesthesia and phenylephrine for maintenance of blood pressure, results in a lower incidence of perioperative myocardial infarction.

Coriat P, Baron JF, Natali J et al: Incidence of myocardial ischemia during carotid endarterectomy. Int Angiol 5:203, 1986

Hosobuchi Y, Baskin DS, Woo SK: Reversal of induced ischemic neurologic deficit in gerbils by the opiate antagonist naloxone. Science 215:69, 1982

Prough DS, Scuderi PE, Stullken E et al: Myocardial infarction following regional anaesthesia for carotid endarterectomy. Can Anaesth Soc J 31:192, 1984

Roizen MF (ed): Anesthesia for Vascular Surgery, p 107. New York, Churchill Livingstone, 1990

Smith JS, Roizen MF, Cahalan MK et al: Does anesthetic technique make a difference? Augmentation of systolic blood pressure during carotid endarterectomy: Effects of phenylephrine versus light anesthesia and of isoflurane versus halothane on the incidence of myocardial ischemia. Anesthesiology 69:846, 1988

C.12. How would you proceed if the patient were to receive regional anesthesia?

Patient consent and cooperation are mandatory for a regional anesthetic for carotid endarterectomy to proceed successfully. For a patient to be adequately anesthetized, a sensory blockade is required in the C2 to C4 dermatomes. This can be accomplished with deep and superficial cervical plexus blocks. In doing the blocks, care must be taken not to excessively palpate the neck, because part of the plaque can dislodge and embolize.

Superficial cervical plexus blocks are performed by superficially infiltrating along the middle third of the posterior border of the sternocleidomastoid muscle with local anesthesia. Deep cervical plexus blocks are performed with three injections along a line drawn from Chassaignac's tubercle to the mastoid process. The C4 nerve root is located at the intersection of that line with one drawn horizontally from the lower border of the mandible. C2 and C3 are located by dividing the distance between the mastoid process and the horizontal line into thirds. Alternatively, a single injection of local anesthetic can be made on the line between the mastoid process and Chassaignac's tubercle at the level of C4 with the needle directed medially and slightly caudad. Cervical plexus blocks entail all of the risks of other regional anesthetics, namely, total spinal anesthesia, seizures, and cardiac arrest.

Patients receiving regional anesthesia must be both cooperative and not oversedated with intravenous medications. If they are unable to cooperate and become obtunded, the primary advantage of regional anesthesia (which is continuous neurologic evaluation) is lost. Intravenous sedation therefore must be given judiciously, if at all, to these patients.

Bosilejevac JE, Farha SJ: Carotid endarterectomy: Results using regional anesthesia. Am J Surg 46:403, 1980

Cousins MJ, Bridenbaugh PO (eds): Neural Blockade in Clinical Anesthesia and Management of Pain, pp 550–555. Philadelphia, JB Lippincott, 1988

Peitzman AB, Webster MW, Loubeau J et al: Carotid endarterectomy under regional (conductive) anesthesia. Ann Surg 196:59, 1982

Rich NM, Hobson RW: Carotid endarterectomy under regional anesthesia. Am J Surg 41:253, 1975

Yared I, Martinis AJ, Mack RM: Carotid endarterectomy under local anesthesia: A retrospective study. Am J Surg 45:709, 1979

C.13. Discuss the effects of anesthetics on cerebral blood flow.

It is important to remember that all general anesthetics affect cerebral blood flow and cerebral metabolic oxygen consumption. This can be used to the anesthesiologist's advantage when the decrease in oxygen consumption is greater than the decrease in CBF.

In general, volatile anesthetics are vasodilators and intravenous anesthetics are vasoconstrictors. Ketamine is one of the exceptions to this generalization. It has been suggested that only the blood flow in normally perfused areas of the brain is affected by anesthetic agents. If this is the case, volatile anesthetics would cause a steal phenomenon, where the blood vessels in normal brain dilate and steal blood flow away from ischemic areas of the brain that are both already maximally vasodilated and unresponsive to the vasodilating effects of the anesthetics.

Barash PG, Cullen BF, Stoelting RK (eds): Clinical Anesthesia, 3rd ed, pp 702–705. Philadelphia, Lippincott-Raven, 1997

C.14. Discuss the protective effects of anesthetic agents on cerebral function.

Although it has not been proved that general anesthetics afford brain protection, the risk of cerebral ischemia should be lessened by agents that cause the greatest decrease in cerebral metabolic oxygen consumption. Which particular anesthetic is optimal for these patients is an area of debate. Obviously, avoiding or eliminating ischemia is essential to protecting against it.

Messick et al. looked at the effects of volatile anesthetics on critical regional cerebral blood flow, that is, the regional cerebral blood flow at which EEG evidence of cerebral ischemia became apparent. They found that critical regional cerebral blood flow in patients receiving isoflurane was <10 ml/100 g/min and in patients receiving halothane was 18 to 20 ml/100 g/min. This decrease in critical CBF suggests that isoflurane may offer some protective effect and may be the best of the volatile anesthetics for use in this operation. Because of its adverse effects on hemodynamics, however, it probably should not be used at high concentrations as the sole anesthetic. A significant portion of patients with carotid artery disease also have coronary artery disease, and they may not tolerate the hypotension and tachycardia associated with the use of high-dose isoflurane. By using this anesthetic in low concentrations in combination with other anesthetic agents, one can maintain better hemodynamic stability while providing for an increased tolerance of cerebral hypoperfusion. Isoflurane, however, may not offer protection during the regional cerebral ischemia which would be expected during carotid endarterectomy.

Thiopental affords cerebral protection against focal cerebral or incomplete global ischemia. It is a cerebral vasoconstrictor, as are most other intravenous anesthetics. It will also transiently decrease cerebral metabolism to 40% to 50% of baseline. The combined effect is that cerebral metabolic oxygen consumption is decreased more than oxygen delivery. The reduction in oxygen demand is the result of inhibition of functioning neurons, which can be seen as a quiet or isoelectric electroencephalogram. When dosing barbiturates for cerebral protection, the EEG should be monitored and repeated doses given to achieve and then maintain a burst suppression pattern on the EEG. Once the EEG is isoelectric, indicating lack of neuronal function, further doses of thiopental do not provide additional protection. It is generally not recommended that thiopental be used for cerebral protection during carotid endarterectomy. As mentioned previously, avoidance of ischemia is preferable to its treatment. If thiopental is used, the EEG, because of its isoelectricity, becomes useless as a monitor of cerebral ischemia. This is especially problematic if selective shunting is to be done. Furthermore, the doses of thiopental required to suppress the EEG may cause hypotension.

Barbiturate use to minimize the possibility of cerebral ischemia has been advocated for the patient undergoing carotid bypass procedures where temporary occlusion of the recipient vessel is required. Whether treatment of patients with a 3 to 5 mg/kg dose of thiopental affects their outcome in terms of neurologic deficit is not known. It has, however, been shown to be efficacious in animal models.

Hicks RG, Kerr DR, Horton DA: Thiopentone cerebral protection under EEG control during carotid endarterectomy. Anaesth Intens Care 14:22, 1988

Messick JM Jr, Casement B, Sharbrough FW et al: Correlation of regional cerebral blood flow (rCBF) with EEG changes during isoflurane anesthesia for carotid endarterectomy: Critical rCBF. Anesthesiology 66:344, 1987

Michenfelder JD, Milde JD: Cerebral protection by anaesthetics during ischaemia. Resuscitation 4:219, 1975

Michenfelder JD, Sundt TM, Fode N et al: Isoflurane when compared to enflurane and halothane decreases the frequency of cerebral ischemia during carotid endarterectomy. Anesthesiology 67:336, 1987

Michenfelder JD, Theye RA: Cerebral protection by thiopental during hypoxia. Anesthesiology 39:510, 1973

Moffat JA, McDougall MJ, Brunet D et al: Thiopental bolus during carotid endarterectomy—rational drug therapy? Can Anaesth Soc J 30:615, 1983

Nehls DG, Todd MM, Spetzler RF et al: A comparison of the cerebral protective effects of isoflurane and barbiturates during temporary focal ischemia in primates. Anesthesiology 66:453, 1987

Nussmeier NA, Arlund C, Slogoff S: Neuropsychiatric complications after cardiopulmonary bypass: Cerebral protection by a barbiturate. Anesthesiology 64:165, 1986

Roizen MF (ed): Anesthesia for Vascular Surgery, p 132. New York, Churchill Livingstone, 1990

Shapiro HM: Barbiturates in brain ischaemia. Br J Anaesth 57:82, 1985

C.15. *How would you manage this patient's ventilation under general anesthesia?*

Because carbon dioxide is a potent cerebral vasodilator, it was initially recommended that patients undergoing carotid endarterectomy be hypoventilated intraoperatively to achieve hypercarbia. It is now well accepted that hypercapnea should be avoided in patients with carotid artery disease. Carbon dioxide causes vasodilation in normally reactive, nonischemic, vascular beds. In patients with carotid artery disease this means that blood flow is diverted away from the already maximally dilated vessels in the territory of the occluded carotid and toward normal areas of the brain. This decrease in rCBF in ischemic areas of the brain with increased CBF in normal areas of the brain is known as "intracerebral steal."

Other authors have recommended extreme hypocapnea during carotid endarterectomy, reasoning that this would result in an inverse steal or Robin Hood phenomenon. Hypocapnea would cause constriction of cerebral vessels in normally perfused areas of the brain, diverting blood flow into the maximally vasodilated, unreactive, hypoperfused regions of the brain. Clinical trials have been unable to demonstrate any real benefit from hypocapnea, and animal studies have shown that it may, in fact, exacerbate ischemia. This most likely happens, not because of intense vasoconstriction, but because of a leftward shift of the oxyhemoglobin dissociation curve so that hemoglobin is less able to give its oxygen to tissues.

The general recommendation for patients with cerebrovascular disease is that normocarbia or mild hypocarbia be maintained. After repair of their carotid stenosis, some patients will have a marked hyperemia with cerebral blood flows of 100 ml/ 100 g/min. In these patients decreasing both blood pressure and arterial carbon dioxide tension to decrease their CBF is indicated. Without a decrease in CBF, these patients are at risk for a postoperative intracerebral hemorrhage.

Baker WH, Rodman JA, Barnes RW et al: An evaluation of hypocarbia and hypercarbia during carotid endarterectomy. Stroke 7:451, 1976

Boysen G, Ladegaard-Pederson HJ, Hendrikson H et al: The effects of $PaCO_2$ on regional cerebral blood flow and internal carotid arterial pressure during carotid clamping. Anesthesiology 35:286, 1971

Christensen M, Paulson O, Olesen J et al: Cerebral apoplexy (stroke) treated with or without prolonged artificial hyperventilation. I. Cerebral circulation, clinical course, and cause of death. Stroke 4:568, 1973

Roizen MF (ed): Anesthesia for Vascular Surgery, pp 128–129. New York, Churchill Livingstone, 1990

C.16. How would you manage this patient's blood pressure intraoperatively?

A number of factors figure into the management of blood pressure in patients during carotid endarterectomy. In the patient with carotid artery disease, a loss of autoregulation occurs in ischemic areas of the brain. In the area of the brain distal to the vascular stenosis, which is chronically hypoperfused, vessels are maximally vasodilated and unresponsive to vasomotor stimuli. Perfusion in these ischemic areas is pressure dependent.

Because of the adjustment of the autoregulatory limits in hypertensive patients and because of a lack of autoregulation in ischemic areas of the brain, hypotension should be avoided. The patient's blood pressure should be maintained in its high normal range or up to 15% to 25% above this when the carotid cross-clamp is in place. Both maintenance and increases in blood pressure can be accomplished with light anesthesia and, when necessary, infusion of the alpha-agonist phenylephrine. Phenylephrine has no direct effect on the cerebral vasculature, so cerebral perfusion is increased by an increase in the perfusion pressure. Phenylephrine increases blood pressure, cerebral perfusion pressure, stump pressure, and regional cerebral blood flow. Phenylephrine also increases myocardial oxygen consumption. Because it increases afterload, care must be taken when it is used in patients with coronary artery disease because it can exacerbate ischemia and failure. In patients with coronary artery disease, blood pressure should probably not be increased above baseline unless evidence of cerebral ischemia develops.

Extreme increases in blood pressure can, and should, be managed with easily titratable intravenous vasodilators such as sodium nitroprusside or nitroglycerin.

After the bifurcation of the carotid artery is exposed, the surgeon often infiltrates the carotid sinus with lidocaine to eliminate the unpredictable hemodynamic response to manipulation of the carotid artery.

Once the stenosis has been relieved and the carotid cross-clamp removed, the patient's blood pressure should be maintained in its low normal range. This lowering of blood pressure offers several advantages. It decreases myocardial oxygen consumption by decreasing the work of the heart, it decreases the amount of stress on the suture line in the carotid artery, and finally, it minimizes the possibility of reperfusion hemorrhage.

Aaslid R, Lindegaard KF, Sorteberg W et al: Cerebral autoregulation dynamics in humans. Stroke 20:45, 1989

Boysen G, Engell HC, Henrickson H: The effect of induced hypertension on internal carotid artery pressure and regional cerebral blood flow during temporary carotid clamping for endarterectomy. Neurology 17:891, 1986

Halsey JH, McDowell HA, Gelman S et al: Blood flow velocity in the middle cerebral artery and regional cerebral flow during carotid endarterectomy. Stroke 20:53, 1989

Smith JS, Roizen MF, Cahalan MK et al: Does anesthetic technique make a difference? Augmentation of systolic blood pressure during carotid endarterectomy: Effects of phenylephrine versus light anesthesia and of isoflurane versus halothane on the incidence of myocardial ischemia. Anesthesiology 69:846, 1988

C.17. Discuss reperfusion injury following carotid endarterectomy.

Reperfusion injury involves cerebral hemorrhage or edema. Although rare, it is an often fatal complication of carotid endarterectomy. Patients with a previous stroke are most likely to suffer reperfusion hemorrhage, but it can occur in otherwise normal brain tissue. Poorly controlled blood pressure contributes to this complication. One proposed mechanism for this injury is that once flow is returned to normal, vascular beds in previously chronically hypoperfused areas of the brain are unable to respond properly by vasoconstricting to maintain normal flow with increased perfusion. Because hypoperfusion distal to the carotid stenosis has been long-standing, these vessels have lost their ability to autoregulate. Once the carotid stenosis is eliminated, the perfusion pressure distal to the former site of the stenosis is markedly increased. Because of a lack of autoregulation in this area, cerebral blood flow increases with increasing perfusion. The patients at highest risk for reperfusion injury have the greatest degree of stenosis and the greatest pressure drop across the carotid lesion. Again, maintaining good blood pressure control with antihypertensives once the carotid obstruction is eliminated decreases the incidence of reperfusion injury.

Breen JC, Caplan LR, DeWitt LD et al: Brain edema after carotid surgery. Neurology 46:175, 1996

Piepgras D, Morgan M, Sundt T et al: Intracerebral hemorrhage after carotid endarterectomy. J Neurosurg 68:532, 1988

Schroeder T, Sillisen H, Sorensen O et al: Cerebral hyperperfusion following carotid endarterectomy. J Neurosurg 66:824, 1987

Solomon R, Loftus C, Quest DQ et al: Incidence and etiology of intracerebral hemorrhage following carotid endarterectomy. J Neurosurg 64:29, 1986

C.18. What intravenous fluids would you give this patient intraoperatively?

Which specific crystalloid is chosen for use during carotid endarterectomy probably does not matter as long as it does not contain dextrose. Because moderate hyperglycemia has been shown to worsen neurologic outcome after ischemia, care must be taken to avoid increasing the patient's glucose with exogenously administered sugar. Intravenous fluids such as Normosol R, lactated Ringer's, or normal saline would be appropriate choices for patients undergoing carotid endarterectomy.

These patients should not be vigorously hydrated intraoperatively. It is best to limit their intraoperative fluids to 10 to 15 ml/kg of crystalloid, with additional colloid and blood replacement being given as needed. Intraoperative overhydration may lead to some of the frequently observed postoperative hypertension and, in patients with myocardial disease, may exacerbate congestive heart failure.

Farias LA, Willis M, Gregory GA: Effects of fructose-1,6-diphosphate, glucose and saline on cardiac resuscitation. Anesthesiology 65:595, 1986

Pulsinelli WA, Levy DE, Sigsbee B et al: Increased damage after ischemic stroke in patients with hyperglycemia with or without established diabetes mellitus. Am J Med 74:540, 1983

Pulsinelli WA, Waldman S, Rawlingson D et al: Moderate hyperglycemia augments ischemic brain damage: A neuropathologic study in the rat. Neurology 33:222, 1983

D. Postoperative Management

D.1. The patient did not "wake up" from general anesthesia. Why?

Once other causes of slow emergence from general anesthesia (e.g., hyperglycemia or hypoglycemia, hypothermia, anesthetic overdose, hypercarbia, and hypoxemia) have been ruled out, the possibility of an adverse intraoperative event having occurred needs to be considered. Patency of the carotid artery on which the surgery was done needs to be evaluated. This can be done by means of Doppler studies while the patient is still in the operating room. If no blood flow is seen in the carotid artery, the incision can be immediately re-explored. If Doppler studies are normal, the possibility of a cerebral infarction from prolonged hypoperfusion or from emboli associated with shunt placement needs to be considered. The patient should remain intubated while further studies, including a computed tomography scan and cerebral angiography, are done as expeditiously as possible. The incidence of new perioperative neurologic deficits is 3% in centers where the operation is done commonly.

Graber JN, Vollman RW, Johnson WC et al: Stroke after carotid endarterectomy: Risk as predicted by preoperative computerized tomography. Am J Surg 147:492, 1984

Sundt TM, Houser OW, Sharbrough FW et al: Carotid endarterectomy: Results, complications and monitoring techniques. Adv Neurol 16:97, 1977

D.2. Postoperatively the patient's blood pressure was 170/96 mm Hg. Would you treat this? If so, why and how?

This patient's blood pressure needs to be carefully controlled because postoperative hypertension is associated with bleeding at the operative site, myocardial ischemia, arrhythmias, and intracerebral hemorrhage.

Hypertension is observed more commonly than hypotension after carotid endarterectomy. Causes of hypertension include hypoxemia, hypercarbia, pain, and a full bladder. Obviously, if any or all of these causes are present, they need to be dealt with promptly and appropriately. Another common cause of postoperative hypertension and tachycardia has been attributed to blunting of the carotid baroreceptor mechanism secondary to carotid sinus dysfunction caused by surgical trauma. If this is the cause of hypertension, therapy with antihypertensive agents needs to be started.

The patient's blood pressure should be maintained in his low normal range postoperatively. Elevated blood pressure can be treated with 5-mg increments of hydralazine or infusions of sodium nitroprusside or nitroglycerin. If the patient is not bradycardic, beta-blockade with 1-mg increments of propranolol or an infusion of esmolol may be added to this regimen. Alternatively, labetalol may be used in 10-mg increments to control blood pressure.

Tarlov E, Schmidek H, Scott RM et al: Reflex hypotension following carotid endarterectomy: Mechanism and management. J Neurosurg 39:323, 1973

Wade JD, Larson CP Jr, Hickey RF et al: Effect of carotid endarterectomy on carotid chemoreceptor and baroreceptor function in man. N Engl J Med 282:823, 1970

D.3. What immediate postoperative complications might you expect?

Immediate postoperative complications include hemodynamic instability, respiratory insufficiency, tension pneumothorax, and lack of chemoreceptor function.

Circulatory instability is common after carotid endarterectomy, with either hypotension or hypertension being observed. Hypotension may have any of several causes. These include hypovolemia, depression of the circulation by residual anesthetics, prolonged effect of intraoperatively administered antihypertensives, dysrhythmias, and myocardial ischemia. Each of these causes needs to be sought and, if present, treated appropriately. Another possible cause of hypotension is an excessive reflex response because of increased sensitivity of the carotid sinus after exposure of the baroreceptor mechanism to a higher pressure with removal of the plaque. If this is the cause, therapy needs to be instituted with fluids and inotropes.

Postoperative respiratory insufficiency is potentially life-threatening. This can be due to vocal cord paralysis from intraoperative traction on the laryngeal nerves. Should this present, the patient should be immediately reintubated. Airway obstruction can also occur from hematoma formation at the operative site, from either arterial or venous bleeding. The hematoma needs to be evacuated as quickly as possible and, depending on ventilatory status, the patient may need to be intubated. This is most easily done after evacuation of the hematoma, if the clinical condition allows.

Tension pneumothorax can result from air dissecting through the wound and the mediastinum to the pleura. This diagnosis is suggestive in all patients after carotid endarterectomy in whom is seen respiratory distress and no evidence of upper airway obstruction. Absence of breath sounds over half of the chest and hemodynamic instability strongly suggest this diagnosis.

Chemoreceptor function is irreversibly suspended in most patients after carotid endarterectomy for up to 10 months. Lack of chemoreceptor function means that there is a loss of circulatory response to hypoxia and an increase in resting $PaCO_2$ of approximately 6 mm Hg. This complication is potentially very serious, and one needs to be most concerned about its development in patients who have had a previous contralateral carotid endarterectomy, where function may be lost bilaterally. In all patients after carotid endarterectomy supplemental oxygen should be provided and opioids administered cautiously.

Rozier MF (ed): Anesthesia for Vascular Surgery, pp 131, 141–143. New York, Churchill Livingstone, 1990

Wade JC, Larson CP Jr, Hickey RF et al: Effect of carotid endarterectomy on carotid chemoreceptor and baroreceptor function in man. N Engl J Med 282:823, 1970

23 Spinal Cord Tumor

Elon H. Mehr
Alan Van Poznak

The patient was a 59-year-old man with melanoma. He had a recent onset of progressive quadriparesis and sensory loss. Magnetic resonance imaging (MRI) scan showed a large mass at C3 to C5 level with severe compression of the spinal cord. He was scheduled for emergent laminectomy C3 to C5 in the sitting position. He appeared short of breath at rest. He had only diaphragmatic breathing. His blood pressure was 90/50 mm Hg; pulse, 120 beats/min; temperature, 38.5°C.

A. Medical Disease and Differential Diagnosis

1. What is the differential diagnosis of spinal cord injury?
2. What radiographic techniques are used to evaluate spinal cord injury?
3. Discuss spinal cord perfusion in the presence of spinal cord injury.
4. Discuss the physiologic sequelae of acute spinal cord lesions.

B. Preoperative Evaluation and Preparation

1. What are your concerns in the preoperative evaluation of this patient?
2. How would you premedicate this patient?
3. Are there any preoperative maneuvers to decrease neurologic injury?

C. Intraoperative Management

1. How would you monitor this patient?
2. How could you detect air embolism?
3. What is the treatment of venous gas embolism?
4. How would you induce anesthesia and intubate the patient?
5. Is succinylcholine contraindicated in patients with acute paraplegia?
6. How would you maintain anesthesia?
7. What intraoperative complications may be reasonably expected from surgery near the upper cervical spinal cord?
8. What intravenous fluid would you give to this patient intraoperatively? Why?
9. Is hypothermia of value in managing these patients?

D. Postoperative Management

1. What is the principal complication peculiar to this type of surgery? How would you manage it?

E. Chronic Spinal Cord Injury

Postoperatively the patient progresses to a complete C3 quadriplegic. Two months later he returned to the operating room for an emergent exploratory laparotomy for perforated viscus.

1. **What are the physiologic sequelae of chronic spinal cord lesions?**
2. **What are some important factors in the preoperative evaluation of this patient?**
3. **Would you give anesthesia for this surgery because the patient is insensate at the surgical site?**
4. **What is the best method to treat the hypertension of autonomic hyperreflexia?**

A. Medical Disease and Differential Diagnosis

A.1. What is the differential diagnosis of spinal cord injury?

The differential diagnosis of spinal cord injury includes trauma, infection, tumor, and vascular malformations. Acute spinal cord injuries account for 11,000 patients each year. The most common cause is trauma, which occurs most frequently in young men.

Luce JM: Medical management of spinal cord injury. Crit Care Med 13:126, 1985

A.2. What radiographic techniques are used to evaluate spinal cord injury?

Radiographs of the neck are useful to evaluate possible cervical vertebral fracture in the emergency room setting. Myelograms and more commonly computed tomography (CT) myelograms are useful for assessing the flow of cerebrospinal fluid (CSF) and evaluating spinal cord masses. However, MRI remains the first line technique for evaluating spinal cord lesions.

Council on Scientific Affairs: Report of the Panel on Magnetic Resonance Imaging: Magnetic resonance imaging of the cardiovascular system. Present state of the art and future potential. JAMA 259:254, 1988

A.3. Discuss spinal cord perfusion in the presence of spinal cord injury.

Spinal cord perfusion is dependent on spinal cord perfusion pressure. This is analogous to the intracerebral perfusion pressure that perfuses the brain. Spinal cord perfusion pressure is defined as the mean spinal cord arterial pressure minus spinal cord venous pressure or spinal CSF pressure (whichever is greater).

In the setting of spinal cord injury all efforts should be made to preserve normal spinal cord perfusion pressure because injured spinal cord typically has diminished autoregulation of blood flow. In this patient, a mass was compressing the spinal cord causing the spinal cord perfusion pressure to be decreased. Arterial hypotension is thus best avoided to maintain spinal cord blood flow and to avoid further neurologic damage. Controlled hypotension would not be an attractive option in this patient.

Drummond JC, Oh Y, Cole DJ et al: Phenylephrine-induced hypertension decreases the area of ischemia following middle cerebral artery occlusion in the rat. Stroke 20:1538, 1989

Cole DJ, Drumond JC, Osborne TN et al: Hypertension and hemodilution during cerebral ischemia reduce brain injury and edema. Am J Physiol 259:H211, 1990

A.4. Discuss the physiologic sequelae of acute spinal cord lesions.

It depends on the level of the lesion. High lesions produce the most damage, including respiratory, cardiovascular, autonomic, sensory and motor functions. Lesions above C7 produces upper extremity paresis and sensory loss, whereas complete spinal cord damage produces loss of function of the spinal segments, thus abolishing sacral reflexes such as the anal wink.

Respiratory impairment includes loss of intercostal muscle activity if the lesion is at C5. These patients have vital capacities that are approximately 25% of normal. Because the phrenic nerve is innervated from C3 to C5, lesions above C3 will also abolish diaphragmatic ventilation, making artificial ventilation mandatory.

Hypotension and bradycardia following spinal cord injury, commonly called "spinal shock," can last from hours to days to even weeks. Circulating catecholamine levels are markedly depressed and increased sensitivity to exogenous catecholamines is present. Tachycardia is not seen because no sympathetic reflexes are present. In fact the only autonomic reflex present is the vagus nerve, which can produce dangerous levels of bradycardia. Left ventricular function is typically depressed following spinal cord injury. The decreased sympathetic outflow prevents increases in contractility, and increases in circulating blood volume can easily lead to pulmonary edema.

Autonomic impairment includes loss of thermal regulation so that body temperature will equilibrate with room temperature, leading easily to either hypo- or hyperthermia. In fact these patients are essentially poikilothermic. Hypothermia frequently exacerbates preexisting bradyarrhythmias.

These patients are at risk of gastric aspiration because gastric atony is common, and they must be treated as with a "full stomach" irrespective of their nothing per os (NPO) status.

Lemons VR, Wagner FC Jr: Respiratory complications after cervical spinal cord injury. Spine 19: 2315, 1994

Mackenzie CF, Shin B, Krishnaprasad D et al: Assessment of cardiac and respiratory function during surgery on patients with acute quadriplegia. J Neurosurg 62:842, 1985

Mathias CJ, Christensen NJ, Spalding JMK: Cardiovascular control in recently injured tetraplegics in spinal shock. Q J Med 48:273, 1979

Schneider RC, Crosby EC, Russo RH et al: Traumatic spinal cord syndromes and their management. Clin Neurosurg 20:424, 1973

B. Preoperative Evaluation and Preparation

B.1. What are your concerns in the preoperative evaluation of this patient?

One can suspect a possible pneumonia from the patient's vital signs. The temperature is elevated, the patient is short of breath, and only diaphragmatic breathing is apparent. Obviously, more information is needed. A chest x-ray film and preoperative blood gas values would be helpful, as well as pulmonary function tests. The source of the fever should be determined. It could be from causes other than pneumonia, and these should be sought. If possible, an antibiotic should be administered and another appropriate treatment should be carried out prior to surgery. If the urgency for decompression of the spinal cord will not allow a delay, then means to control the fever should be prepared for use during surgery. The low blood pressure and rapid pulse are also warnings of potential trouble. These can result from the anemia and hypovolemia that occur late in the course of many malignant diseases. In addition, there could be an expansion of the vascular tree caused by interruption of sympathetic nerve transmission from tumor compression of the spinal cord. In either case, the size of the vascular tree is disproportionate to its contents. Induction of further disproportion through cardiovascular effects of general anesthetics and head-up tilt could prove disastrous. For this reason, preoperative hypovolemia and anemia must be corrected. One should also remember that patients with chronic illness may have a reduced blood volume even though the hemoglobin and hematocrit values are not severely reduced.

Evans RH: The pharmacology of segmental transmission in the spinal cord. Prog Neurobiol 33:255–279, 1989

Goldman AL, George J: Postural hypoxemia in quadriplegic patients. Neurology 26:815, 1976

Hui KKP, Conolly ME: Increased numbers of beta receptors in orthostatic hypotension due to autonomic dysfunction. N Engl J Med 304:1473, 1981

B.2. How would you premedicate this patient?

Premedication, if used at all, should be limited to whatever dose of sedative is necessary to control the patient's anxiety. Often the preoperative visit by the anesthesiologist is the best medicine for this purpose. If physical pain is present, it should be controlled by an appropriately timed dose of analgesic narcotic. Opinions vary regarding the merits of preanesthetic anticholinergic agents. Because irritating inhalation agents are no longer used, the antisecretory effect is usually not needed. To accelerate the heart rate in this already tachycardic patient seems unwise. If, however, fiberoptic bronchoscopy is planned for intubation, a preoperative antisialagogue such as glycopyrolate is beneficial.

In addition, because this patient is at risk of gastric aspiration, premedication with an H_2-antagonist (e.g., ranitidine) and gastrointestinal motility stimulant (e.g., metoclopramide) is indicated.

B.3. Are there any preoperative maneuvers to decrease neurologic injury?

The best way to prevent further neurologic injury to the spinal cord is to surgically decompress the spinal cord as soon as possible.

High-dose methylprednisolone has recently been shown to be effective in decreasing neurologic injury when given in the first 8 hours after injury. In addition some people advocate local hypothermia to the damaged area of the spinal cord to lessen further injury. A recent study showed that ganglioside GM-1 possibly lessens neurologic injury after ischemic insult.

Bracken MB, Shepard MJ, Collins WF et al: A randomized, controlled trial of methylprednisolone or naloxone in the treatment of acute spinal cord injury: Results of the second national acute spinal cord injury study. N Engl J Med 322:1405, 1990

Geisler FH, Dorsey FC, Coleman WP: Recovery of motor function after spinal-cord injury—a randomized, placebo-controlled trial with GM-1 ganglioside. N Engl J Med 324:1829, 1991

Janssen L, Hansebout RR: Pathogenesis of spinal cord injury and newer treatments—A review. Spine 14:23, 1989

Veno T: Protection against ischemic spinal cord injury: One shot perfusion cooling and percutaneous topical cooling. J Vasc Surg 19:882–887, 1994

C. Intraoperative Management

C.1. How would you monitor this patient?

In addition to the routine monitors of noninvasive blood pressure, pulse oximetry, electrocardiogram, precordial stethoscope, and capnography, we would use a precordial Doppler bubble detector. We would also use a right atrial catheter to measure pressures and possibly to treat air embolism. Surgery in the sitting position invites air embolism if venous channels are opened in areas of negative venous pressure. Because the normal right atrial pressure is 8 to 10 cm H_2O, positive pressure is seen in veins that are not more than this height above the heart. In the sitting position, veins in the surgical field are easily >10 cm above the heart. In this surgery many veins in the surgical field are located in bones and thus may be noncollapsible in response to negative pressure, which greatly increases the risk of air embolism.

Monitoring spinal cord function can be accomplished with somatosensory or motor-evoked potentials. This is useful in surgeries that can produce spinal cord injuries such as Harrington rod placement for scoliosis correction.

Glassman SD, Zhang YP, Shields CB et al: An evaluation of motor-evoked potentials for detection of neurologic injury with correction of an experimental scoliosis. Spine 20:1765–1775, 1995

Yamada T: The anatomic and physiologic bases of median nerve somatosensory evoked potentials. Neurol Clin 6:705–733, 1988

C.2. How can you detect air embolism?

Many methods are available to diagnose venous gas embolism. The sensitivity of monitoring methods is shown in Table 23-1. Transesophageal echocardiography has the advantages of greatest sensitivity and noninvasiveness, but it is technically complex and expensive. Precordial Doppler ultrasound, when properly placed, is sensitive, noninvasive, and inexpensive, but its specificity is low. Inspired nitrogen deter-

Table 23-1. The Sensitivity of Monitoring Methods for Air Embolism

SENSITIVITY	MONITORING METHOD	MEAN QUANTITY OF AIR TO ELICIT POSITIVE RESPONSE (± SD) (ml/kg)
Greatest	Transesophageal Echocardiography	0.19 ± 0.25
	Precordial Doppler Ultrasound	0.24 ± 0.33
Intermediate	Pulmonary artery pressure	0.61 ± 0.37
	End-tidal CO_2 tension	0.63 ± 0.23
	Arterial oxygen tension	0.71 ± 0.54
	Tissue capillary oxygen tension	0.76 ± 0.58
Least	Arterial CO_2 tension	1.15 ± 0.76
	Mean arterial pressure	1.16 ± 0.76
	Tissue capillary CO_2 tension	1.54 ± 0.70

(Reprinted with permission from Glenski JA, Cucchiara RF, Michenfelder JD: Transesophageal echocardiography and transcutaneous O_2 and CO_2 monitoring for detection of venous air embolism. Anesthesiology 64:541–545, 1986)

mination by gas analysis is a sensitive and specific monitor. In the absence of anesthetic circuit leak, nitrogen is not usually found in the anesthetic circuit; therefore, the presence of inspired nitrogen indicates a sudden entrainment of air via the venous circulation. End-tidal carbon dioxide monitoring is also useful. A sudden decrease in the end-tidal CO_2 is an indication of an increased amount of pulmonary dead space produced by the interruption of capillary pulmonary blood flow by entrained air.

Our personal preference for the pulse oximeter is based on many years of experience. It is simple, safe, noninvasive, and it is the first portion of the circulatory system to shut down in the event of trouble. We have never had damage to the brain or myocardium from inadequate perfusion as long as the finger pulse monitor showed adequate perfusion. From this long experience comes another aphorism: if you are perfusing the finger, then you are perfusing the heart, brain, and other vital organs. Either we are correct in this assumption, or else we have been a lucky for a long time.

Gildenberg PC, O'Brien RP, Britt WJ: The efficacy of Doppler monitoring for the detection of venous air embolism. J Neurosurg 54:74–78, 1981

Glenski JA, Cucchiara RF, Michenfelder JD: Transesophageal echocardiography and transcutaneous O_2 and CO_2 monitoring for detection of venous air embolism. Anesthesiology 64:541–545, 1986

C.3. What is the treatment of venous gas embolism?

The best treatment is prevention. Avoidance of extreme positioning so that the surgical site is as low as possible is the first priority. Venous pressure in the neck can be elevated by raising the central venous pressure through fluid administration and positive end-expiratory pressure (PEEP). The clinical aphorism for judging the safety and adequacy of the system is simple. Look at the veins in the surgical field. If blood is coming out, then air cannot be going in. Spontaneous ventilation and especially bucking and sudden gasping can cause massive air entrainment secondary to generation of large negative thoracic venous pressures.

Treatment consists of immediately informing the surgeons to "flood the field," bathe the surgical site in irrigation fluid. Changing the patient to a less head-erect position may be desirable but not practical in neurosurgical work because of the complexities of neurosurgical fixation. Increasing venous pressure via jugular venous compression and PEEP is also beneficial.

In severe cases air can be aspirated via a right atrial catheter. A multilumen right atrial catheter positioned above the junction of the superior vena cava and right atrium has been shown to be the most effective way to aspirate air from the right atrium. In case of hypotension, an inotropic agent such as dopamine should be administered.

Bunegin L, Albin MS, Helsel PE et al: Positioning the right atrial catheter. Anesthesiology 55:343, 1981

Toung T, Ngeow YK, Long DL et al: Comparison of the effects of positive end-expiratory pressure and jugular venous compression on canine cerebral venous pressure. Anesthesiology 61:169–172, 1984

C.4. How would you induce anesthesia and intubate the patient?

The goals are for a smooth, controlled, hemodynamically stable anesthetic induction. The patient is at risk for gastric aspiration so a rapid-sequence intravenous induction with cricoid pressure or awake intubation is indicated.

Particular care should be given to avoidance of hypotension with anesthetic induction. In this patient with spinal shock and many risk factors for hypotension, a preinduction fluid bolus is strongly indicated. Large doses of thiobarbiturate or propofol can easily cause massive hypotension in this setting, so we would choose etomidate, because it has less hypotensive effects than these other induction agents.

With any question of cervical spine instability, a technique that allows neurologic function to be assessed after intubation is preferred. Awake intubation with a fiberoptic bronchoscope is an ideal method. After intubation a brief neurologic examination is conducted and then anesthetic induction is completed. If laryngoscopy is performed cervical stabilization must be performed until the head is securely fixed in a Mayfield pin head-holder or other suitable device.

Randolph H. Hastings, J Marks: Airway management for trauma patients with potential cervical spine injuries. Anesth Analg 73:471, 1991

C.5. Is succinylcholine contraindicated in patients with acute paraplegia?

No. If the injury is <24 to 48 hours old then succinylcholine can be used. The danger is acute hyperkalemia released from denervated muscle. After 6 to 8 months muscle atrophy occurs and the risk of hyperkalemia is reduced.

Gronert GA, Theye RA: Pathophysiology of hyperkalemia induced by succinylcholine. Anesthesiology 43:89, 1975

Tobey RE: Paraplegia, succinylcholine, and cardiac arrest. Anesthesiology 32:359, 1970

C.6. How would you maintain anesthesia?

The goals for anesthesia maintenance include stable hemodynamics, controlled ventilation, avoidance of low central venous pressure, and temperature control. In addition, anesthesia has to be planned so that postoperatively the patient can be awake and able to perform true, serial neurologic examinations. This can be accomplished with inhalation agents, a balanced technique such as a nitrous oxide-oxygen, narcotic and muscle relaxant mixture, or a propofol, oxygen-nitrous oxide technique.

The new inhalation agents, desflurane and sevoflurane, allow the patient to emerge from anesthesia faster than the isoflurane and halothane combination, thus providing earlier postoperative neurologic examinations.

C.7. What intraoperative complications may be reasonably expected from surgery near the upper cervical spinal cord?

The cervical spinal cord contains the motor neurons for the diaphragm at C3 to C5. Thus any dysfunction of the cord at this level will produce respiratory compromise. Edema of the spinal cord can produce dysfunction several dermatomes higher than the actual surgical site.

In addition, numerous autonomic pathways are involved in both sympathetic and parathsympathetic systems. Acute severe changes in hemodynamics, especially sudden bradyarrhythmias, can occur unexpectedly with surgical stimulation of certain areas of the upper spinal cord and brain stem. The surgical stimulation does not have to be profound; just slight retraction in certain areas can cause severe dysrhythmias.

Hunter AR (ed): Neurosurgical Anesthesia, 2nd ed, pp 309–323. New York, Oxford University Press, 1975

Oldfield EH, Doppman JL: Spinal arteriovenous malformations. Clin Neurosurg 34:161–183, 1988

Priestley JV: Neuroanatomy of the spinal cord: Current research and prospects. Paraplegia 25:198–204, 1987

C.8. What intravenous fluid would you give to this patient intraoperatively? Why?

A balanced salt solution such as lactated Ringer's solution, electrolyte solution *p*H 7.4, or even normal saline would be preferred over glucose-containing solutions. Hyperglycemia has been shown to worsen outcome in experimental conditions of neurologic ischemia.

Chopp M, Welch KMA, Tidwell CD et al: Global cerebral ischemia and intracellular *p*H during hyperglycemia and hypoglycemia in cats. Stroke 19:1383, 1988

Drummond JC, Moore SS: The influence of dextrose administration on neurologic outcome after temporary spinal cord ischemia in the rabbit. Anesthesiology 70:74, 1989

Sieber F, Smith DS, Kupferberg J: Effects of intraoperative glucose on protein catabolism and plasma glucose levels in patients with supratentorial tumors. Anesthesiology 74:453, 1986

C.9. Is hypothermia of value in managing these patients?

Hypothermia is the only way to reliably protect the central nervous system from ischemic insult. The more hypothermia the better the protection. Hypothermia is protective to the spinal cord during aortic cross-clamping for aneurysm surgery. However severe hypothermia itself causes problems such as dysrhythmias, delayed awakening, and coagulopathies. Mild hypothermia of 34° to 35°C is easily accomplished in the operating room setting, but complete rewarming may be difficult.

Baker KZ, Young WL, Stone JG et al: Deliberate mild intraoperative hypothermia for craniotomy. Anesthesiology 81:361, 1994

Salzano RP Jr, Ellison LH, Altonji PF et al: Regional deep hypothermia of the spinal cord protects against ischemic injury during thoracic aortic cross-clamping. Ann Thorac Surg 57:75–70, 1994

D. Postoperative Management

D.1. What is the principal complication peculiar to this type of surgery? How would you manage it?

Edema of the cervical spinal cord near the operative area may develop insidiously during the early postoperative period. If the patient has been extubated and is breathing spontaneously, gradual respiratory insufficiency may develop as edema spreads upward along the spinal cord to involve the respiratory centers. This condition can develop without initial significant impairment of consciousness. In addition, impairment of function of the ninth and tenth cranial nerves may occur, so that the patient has difficulty coughing and swallowing salivary secretions.

For these reasons, it is important to monitor brain stem function in terms of respiration and ability to cough and swallow. Should these brain stem functions become impaired, as evidenced clinically or by serial arterial blood gas determinations, consider reintubation or performing a tracheotomy until the period of postoperative edema has passed, which is usually 48 hours to 72 hours. Other useful measures to lessen edema during this period include steroids and hypertonic solutions such as mannitol.

Dommisse GF: The arteries, arterioles and capillaries of the spinal cord: Surgical guidelines for the prevention of postoperative paraplegia. Ann R Coll Surg Engl 62:369–375, 1980

McComish PB, Bodley PO: Anesthesia for Neurological Surgery. Chicago, Year Book Medical Publishers, 1971

E. Chronic Spinal Cord Injury

Postoperatively the patient progressed to a complete C3 quadriplegic. Two months later he returned to the operating room for an emergent exploratory laparotomy for perforated viscus.

E.1. What are the physiologic sequelae of chronic spinal cord lesions?

In addition to all the sequelae of acute lesions, chronic spinal cord lesions can manifest severe electrolyte abnormalities. Acute hyperkalemia after succinycholine administration can be life-threatening. Hypercalcemia from immobilization, which is common, can lead to dysrhythmias.

Pulmonary emboli due to these patients' intense immobility, pulmonary infections, and upper airway obstructions due to inability to cough and clear secretions are frequent causes of morbidity. Recent increases in life expectancy rates in these patients can be attributed to better pulmonary care.

Decubitus ulcers are invariably present and easily progress to further systemic infections.

Urinary calculus and infections are common; in fact, the leading cause of death in these patients is renal failure from chronic urinary tract infections.

Clause-Walker JL, Carter RE, Lipscomb HS et al: Daily rhythms of electrolytes and aldosterone excretion in men with cervical spinal cord section. J Clin Endocrinol Metab 29:300, 1969

Desmond J: Paraplegia: Problems confronting the anesthesiologist. Can Anaesth Soc J 17:435, 1970

DeVivo MJ: Life expectancy of ventilator-dependent patients. Chest 108:226–232, 1995

Reines HD, Harris RC: Pulmonary complications of acute spinal cord injuries. Neurosurgery 21:193, 1987

E.2. What are some important factors in the preoperative evaluation of this patient?

Many of the important considerations of acute spinal cord injury also pertain to chronic injury. Orthostasis is usually present; thus hypotension is always a risk because no sympathetic outflow is present to compensate for a reduction in blood volume or anesthetic-induced vasomotor tone.

Temperature considerations are important. As stated, these patients are essentially poikilothermic and become severely hypothermic in the usually frigid operating room suite.

In addition, all the preoperative considerations for a patient with a perforated viscus must be considered. These include emergent setting and increased risk of gastric aspiration, hypovolemia, and risk of postoperative septicemia.

Ditunno JF Jr, Formal CS: Chronic spinal cord injury. N Engl J Med 330:550–556, 1994

Schmidt KD, Chan CW: Thermoregulation and fever in normal persons and in those with spinal cord injuries. Mayo Clin Proc 67:469, 1992

E.3. Would you give anesthesia for this surgery because the patient is insensate at the surgical site?

Absolutely. This patient is at risk for autonomic hyperreflexia, the so-called "mass reflex." This syndrome produced usually by bowel or bladder stimulation produces a severe life-threatening hypertension and reflex bradycardia. Intense vasoconstriction below the spinal cord lesion produces this hypertension. Reflex vasodilatation above the lesion attempts to lessen the hypertension. Facial flushing, sweating, headache, and blurred vision are frequent symptoms. Severe episodes cause seizures, cerebral hemorrhages, and dysrhythmias. Autonomic hyperreflexia is not observed with spinal cord lesions below dermatome T7 because the splanchnic bed is still innervated and able to vasodilate, thus preventing hypertension from developing.

Either general anesthesia or regional anesthesia is effective in preventing autonomic hyperreflexia.

Lambert DH, Deane RS, Mazuzan JE: Anesthesia and the control of blood pressure in patients with spinal cord injury. Anesth Analg 61:344, 1982

Schonwald G, Fish KJ, Perkash I: Cardiovascular complications during anesthesia in chronic spinal cord injured patients. Anesthesiology 55:550, 1981

Thompson CE, Witham AC: Paroxysmal hypertension in spinal cord injuries. N Engl J Med 239:291, 1948

E.4. What is the best method to treat the hypertension of autonomic hyperreflexia?

Immediate withdrawal of the initial reflex trigger is the best treatment. Pharmacologic treatment includes vasodilators, sympathetic receptor blocking drugs, or deep levels of inhalational anesthesia.

Amzallag M: Autonomic hyperreflexia. Int Anesthesiol Clin 31:87–102, 1993

24 Head Injury

Robert F. Bedford

An 18-year-old man was brought to the emergency room after being extracted from the driver's side of an automobile that hit a telephone pole at high speed. He was semiconscious and combative. There was a suggestion that his right arm was stronger than his left. He had a temporal scalp laceration and a contusion on his chest where he had struck the steering wheel. Blood pressure, 180/100 mm Hg; heart rate, 120 beats/min; respiratory rate, 15 beats/min; hematocrit, 40%.

A. Medical Disease and Differential Diagnosis

1. What types of intracranial injuries are most likely to have occurred in this patient?
2. What is the effect of an expanding intracranial hematoma on intracranial pressure (ICP) and cerebral perfusion pressure?
3. What are the implications of arterial hypertension in a patient with a head injury?
4. What are the potential risks and benefits of empirically administering mannitol to this patient?
5. When is endotracheal intubation in the emergency room appropriate? What are the potential risks and benefits?
6. Should succinylcholine be used to facilitate endotracheal intubation. What are the risks of doing so? How can some of these risks be minimized?
7. Is nasal intubation appropriate in a patient who has blood visible behind one eardrum?

B. Preoperative Evaluation and Preparation

1. What is the role of computed tomography (CT) scanning in the initial evaluation of a patient with head injury?
2. Before going to the CT scanner, the trauma team wanted to perform peritoneal lavage. Is this appropriate? Does a normal venous hematocrit measurement mean blood volume is normal?
3. Why is a chest x-ray needed? Should cervical spine films be taken? Why?
4. The electrocardiogram (ECG) showed inverted T waves in the precordial leads. What is the probable cause? Is this indicative of myocardial injury? What changes would you expect if blood was found in the pericardium?

C. Intraoperative Management

1. What is appropriate hemodynamic monitoring during CT scanning and during craniotomy for removal of an intracranial hematoma?
2. What sort of sedation or anesthesia should be used during head CT scanning?
3. The patient was to undergo craniotomy for an acute epidural hematoma. Are there

492

anesthetic agents that should definitely not be used in this situation? Which ones? What agents might be preferred in this situation?

4. What should be done about intravenous (IV) fluid replacement during craniotomy for evacuation of an epidural hematoma? Should corticosteroids be given empirically?

5. In the middle of surgery, the blood pressure suddenly decreased, peak airway pressure and central venous pressure (CVP) increased, and the pulse oximeter indicated a decrease in oxygen saturation. What was the likely cause? What would be the likely cause if the CVP suddenly fell?

6. The patient was noted to be bleeding from vascular access sites. What are the possible causes of coagulopathy in this patient?

D. Postoperative Neurointensive Care Management

1. What specific measures should be used to control the patient's intracranial pressure?
2. What monitoring modalities might help assess the degree of residual injury and/or the chance for good recovery?
3. Outline the principles of respiratory and cardiovascular care for this patient.
4. Why would this patient develop diabetes insipidus in the postoperative period? How would you treat it?

A. Medical Disease and Differential Diagnosis

A.1. What types of intracranial injuries are most likely to have occurred in this patient?

In a patient without obvious signs of localizing neurologic defects, the most probable intracranial injury is cerebral contusion. This is usually a diffuse or multifocal process that results in disruption of the blood-brain barrier, causing widespread brain swelling due to edema. The diagnosis can be made with certainty only after ruling out other focal injuries, such as intracranial hematoma. Additionally, prior to any surgical interventions, one must be aware of potential concurrent injuries that threaten the neuraxis, such as basilar skull and cervical spine fractures. It is also important to consider that brain contusion does not occur only above the level of the tentorium. Evidence of brain stem whiplash injury may not be present at the beginning of emergent trauma surgery, but may become obvious postoperatively when the patient fails to awaken or cannot be weaned from mechanical ventilation.

Cohen W: Imaging and determination of posttraumatic spinal instability. In: Cooper PR (ed): Management of Post-Traumatic Spinal Instability: Neurosurgical Topics, Vol 2, p 19. Park Ridge, IL, AANS Publications, 1990

Eisenberg HM, Gary HE Jr, Aldrich EF et al: Initial CT findings in 753 patients with severe head injury. J Neurosurg 73:688, 1990

Lobato RD, Sarabia R, Cordobes F et al: Post-traumatic cerebral hemispheric swelling. J Neurosurg 49:530, 1988

A.2. What is the effect of an expanding intracranial hematoma on intracranial pressure (ICP) and cerebral perfusion pressure?

Intracranial hematomas, particularly those in the epidural space, create an expanding lesion that causes pressure on the brain, both locally and globally. This results in decreased cerebral perfusion pressure, decreased blood flow to the brain, and it ultimately leads to neuronal dysfunction and injury. In the case of epidural hematomas, the pathology usually results from laceration of the middle meningeal artery. Blood enters the cranial vault at arterial pressure, resulting in rapid and profound neurologic deficits. Subdural hematomas, by contrast, are the result of venous lacerations; they tend to develop slowly and more insidiously. Classically, the patient is described as having regained consciousness only to lose consciousness and deteriorate neurologically after a period of mental lucidness.

Eisenberg HM, Gary HE Jr, Aldrich EF et al: Initial CT findings in 753 patents with severe head injury. J Neurosurg 73:688, 1990

Seelig JM, Becker DP, Miller JD et al: Traumatic acute subdural hematoma: Major mortality reduction in comatose patients treated within four hours. N Engl J Med 304:1511, 1981

Yoshino E, Yamaki T, Higuchi T et al: Acute brain edema in fatal head injury: Analysis by dynamic CT scanning. J Neurosurg 63:830, 1985

A.3. What are the implications of arterial hypertension in a patient with head injury?

Hypertension is a common feature of head injury in patients who do not have massive blood loss associated with their injuries. Although the cause of the hypertension is thought to be primarily catecholamine related, considerable debate is found regarding its significance. Some authorities believe that cerebral perfusion is optimized when a high arterial pressure opposes the effects of elevated intracranial pressure. Others feel that, in the presence of a disrupted blood-brain barrier, arterial hypertension contributes only to extravasation of edema fluid and aggravation of brain swelling, resulting in further elevation of intracranial pressure. The management consensus at the present time is that arterial pressure should be maintained at approximately normal to slightly elevated levels. Above all, arterial hypotension is to be avoided, because it profoundly increases neuronal damage in the presence of elevated intracranial pressure.

Nagai H, Kamiya K, Ishii S (eds): Intracranial Pressure IX, pp 222–224. Tokyo, Springer-Verlag, 1994

A.4. What are the potential risks and benefits of empirically administering mannitol to this patient?

Traditionally, it was taught that mannitol could aggravate elevated ICP by diffusing across a disrupted blood-brain barrier and inducing additional brain edema. Indeed, this is seen in both normal animals and patients, where a small increase in ICP occurs after mannitol infusion. In intracranial mass lesions, however, mannitol has been found to induce a prompt decrease in ICP, without evidence of ICP rebound. Accordingly, most head injury protocols now call for empiric administration of intravenous mannitol in a dose range of 1 to 2 g/kg just as soon as the patient arrives at the hospital.

Hartwell RC, Sutton LN: Mannitol, intracranial pressure and vasogenic edema. Neurosurgery 32:444, 1993.

Ravussin P, Abou-Madi M, Archer D et al: Changes in CSF pressure after mannitol in patients with and without elevated CSF pressure. J Neurosurg 69:869, 1988

A.5. When is endotracheal intubation in the emergency room appropriate? What are the potential risks and benefits?

The primary advantages of endotracheal intubation in the emergency room are the protection and maintenance of the airway in the event that the patient deteriorates neurologically. If this should happen, two primary concerns are seen: (1) regurgitation and aspiration of stomach contents because of impaired protective airway reflexes, and (2) CO_2 retention due to impaired ventilatory drive and/or soft-tissue obstruction of the upper airway. In the former scenario, the patient is at risk for a protracted and complicated intensive care unit (ICU) course due to aspiration pneumonitis; in the latter scenario, the increased cerebral blood flow and blood volume resulting from hypercarbia will result in greater elevations in ICP than would have occurred otherwise. In addition, both conditions would result in hypoxemia, which has been identified as a leading cause of mortality in patients with head injury.

The process of intubating a combative patient with head injury, however, is not a simple undertaking. First, the cardiovascular responses to endotracheal intubation are likely to aggravate the ongoing intracranial pathology. In addition, it is likely that the patient may have a concurrent cervical spine injury. Accordingly, semielective intubation should be performed only after cervical spine films have documented the normal anatomy from C1 to C7. Finally, a strong, semiconscious young man will not be cooperative during this process.

The decision to intubate in the emergency room is a matter of judgment, because it may be possible to complete the necessary trauma workup without an endotracheal tube. On the other hand, many authorities feel that endotracheal intubation in this situation should be performed promptly, in much the same fashion as if it were being performed in the operating room: preoxygenation; defasciculation with a curariform nondepolarizing muscle relaxant; cricoid pressure to occlude the esophagus; a brief period of general anesthesia induced with intravenous thiopental (3 to 4 mg/kg) and lidocaine (1.5 mg/kg); and muscle relaxation accomplished by succinylcholine (1.5 mg/kg). Although this sequence does not guarantee that regurgitation and aspiration will not occur, it avoids many of the potential drawbacks of either awake intubation or "watchful waiting" while the remainder of the preoperative workup is completed. Once the airway is secured, modest hyperventilation to a $PaCO_2$ of approximately 30 mm Hg is instituted.

Bedford RF, Winn HR, Tyson G et al: Intracranial pressure response to endotracheal intubation: Efficacy of intravenous lidocaine pretreatment for patients with brain tumors. Intracranial Pressure IV, p 595. New York, Springer-Verlag, 1980

Gelb AW, Manninen PH, Mezon BJ, et al: The anaesthetist and the head-injured patient. Can J Anaesth 31:97, 1984

Miller RD (ed): Anesthesia, 4th ed, pp 2163–2164. New York, Churchill Livingstone, 1994

A.6. Should succinylcholine be used to facilitate endotracheal intubation? What are the risks of doing so? How can some of these risks be minimized?

The impact of succinylcholine on ICP has been controversial over the years, partly because the drug often is used concurrently with thiopental and just before endotracheal intubation. Because the former reduces ICP and the latter usually increases it, the conflicting results in the literature are not unexpected. In recent years, however, two studies have helped to clarify this issue. Lanier et al. clearly demonstrated in dogs that ICP increases in response to succinylcholine through increased neural input via muscle spindle activation at the time of depolarization. In humans, the same ICP response occurs, but it has been shown that it can be prevented by administering a defasciculating dose of curariform nondepolarizing muscle relaxant prior to giving succinylcholine.

Lanier WL, Milde JH, Michenfelder JD: Cerebral stimulation following succinylcholine in dogs Anesthesiology 64:551, 1986

Stirt JA, Grosslight KR, Bedford RF, et al: "Defasciculation" with metocurine prevents succinylcholine-induced increases in intracranial pressure. Anesthesiology 67:50, 1987

A.7. Is nasal intubation appropriate in a patient who has blood visible behind one eardrum?

The so-called "Battle" sign, or any other evidence of basal skull fracture (cerebrospinal fluid [CSF] rhinorrhea, for instance), is a contraindication to nasal intubation. Although this route is potentially useful for intubation in a combative patient, the risk of aggravating an intracranial injury far outweighs the advantages of this technique. In addition, a nasally placed endotracheal tube is likely to require replacement in any event, either because it is more difficult to keep patent or because of the risk of maxillary sinusitis.

Grindlinger GA, Neihoff J, Hughes L et al: Acute paranasal sinusitis related to nasotracheal intubation of head-injured patients. Crit Care Med 15:214, 1987

B. Preoperative Evaluation and Preparation

B.1. What is the role of computed tomography (CT) scanning in the initial evaluation of the patient with head injury?

Computed tomographic head scanning is the diagnostic test of choice in determining the extent of head injury and the necessity for immediate surgery, as opposed to more conservative neurointensive care unit management. After double-dose contrast tomography, evidence of an intracranial hematoma large enough to cause significant shift of brain structures is an indication for immediate surgical intervention. Conversely, conservative management would be indicated in the absence of a mass lesion or with no compression of the lateral ventricles or basal cisterns. At many centers, however, any patient who is unconscious will have an ICP monitor placed via a twist-drill craniectomy. If the ICP is >20 to 30 mm Hg despite maximal ICP control measures (hyperventilation to $PaCO_2$ = 20 to 25 mm Hg, mannitol treatment, and barbiturate anesthesia), then a decompressing craniectomy is performed in an attempt to control elevated ICP.

Cruz J: An additional therapeutic effect of adequate hyperventilation in severe acute brain trauma: Normalization of cerebral glucose uptake. J Neurosurg 82:379, 1995.

Saul TG, Ducker TB: Effect of intracranial pressure monitoring and aggressive treatment on mortality in severe head injury. J Neurosurg 56:498, 1982

B.2. *Before going to the CT scanner, the trauma team wanted to perform peritoneal lavage. Is this appropriate? Does a normal venous hematocrit measurement mean that blood volume is normal?*

Young, previously healthy patients have a remarkable ability to compensate for blood loss. Accordingly, even in a patient with normal vital signs, it is appropriate to perform peritoneal lavage whenever there is a chance of spleen or liver laceration, as is the case following a steering wheel injury. Furthermore, because the initial compensatory mechanism for acute blood loss is vasoconstriction, it is not unusual for a patient to have a normal hematocrit despite having lost more than a liter of blood into the peritoneal cavity or retroperitoneal space. Because the patient may decompensate later, either during diagnostic tests or during emergency neurosurgery, it is advisable to proceed with appropriate diagnostic testing prior to performing radiologic interventions.

Shoemaker WC, Corley RD, Liu M et al: Development and testing of a decision tree for blunt trauma. Crit Care Med 16:1199, 1988

B.3. *Why is a chest x-ray needed? Should cervical spine films be taken? Why?*

Probably the only intraoperative catastrophes that are even more devastating than occult intra-abdominal bleeding are unexpected intrathoracic derangements or a cervical spine injury. Because steering wheel trauma can also be responsible for cardiac or pulmonary contusion, laceration of great vessels or major airways, or hemopneumothorax, it is imperative that these entities be ruled out prior to surgery. Indeed, it is wise to perform these studies before the patient enters the CT scanner. Clearly, with any doubt regarding pulmonary contusion, a chest tube should be placed before tension pneumothorax occurs, particularly if the patient is going to receive positive pressure ventilation. Likewise with evidence of a widened mediastinum or other signs of great vessel injury, the operative management of the head injury may take second priority to the major vascular injury, which would be considered even more critical.

As discussed, a cervical spine injury, particularly at the C1 to C3 level, would have a profound impact on airway management, because routine endotracheal intubation risks inducing spinal cord injury. Accordingly, unless the patient is deeply comatose, it is wise to obtain lateral cervical spine x-rays before proceeding with routine endotracheal intubation. In the presence of cervical spine subluxation or fracture, head stabilization with skull fixation and traction should be initiated before any airway manipulation is undertaken. Indeed, many clinicians should argue for endotracheal intubation using either fiberoptic guidance or a transcricothyroid retrograde-directed catheter to place the endotracheal tube with minimal head and cervical spine motion. In the case of significant facial injury as well, most would opt for a semiemergent cricothyrotomy to eliminate most of the difficulties encountered by oral endotracheal intubation.

Barriot P, Riou B: Retrograde technique for tracheal intubation in trauma patients. Crit Care Med 16:713, 1988

Meschino A, Devitt JH, Koch JP et al: The safety of awake tracheal intubation in cervical spine injury. Can J Anaesth 39:114, 1992

Suderman VS, Crosby ET, Lui A: Elective oral tracheal intubation in cervical spine-injured adults. Can J Anaesth 38:785, 1991

B.4. The electrocardiogram (ECG) showed inverted T waves in the precordial leads. What is the probable cause? Is this indicative of myocardial injury? What changes would you expect if blood was found in the pericardium?

Inverted T waves are often seen in patients with neuropathologic processes, most typically ruptured intracranial aneurysms. However, severe head injury associated with blood in the ventricles or basal cisterns can also cause these abnormalities; they are not necessarily indicative of myocardial injury or ischemia. Cardiac contusion, often seen with steering wheel injuries, is characterized by ventricular arrhythmias or by ST segment elevation in the precordial leads. By contrast, blood in the pericardial cavity should be suspected whenever the ECG shows low voltage and the heart sounds are distant or muffled.

Clifton GL, Robertson CS, Kyper K et al: Cardiovascular responses to severe head injury. Neurosurgery 29:447, 1983

Mayfield W, Hurley EJ: Blunt cardiac trauma. Am J Surg 14:162, 1984

C. Intraoperative Management

C.1. What is appropriate hemodynamic monitoring during CT scanning and during craniotomy for removal of an intracranial hematoma?

It is axiomatic that hemodynamic monitoring should be commensurate with the anticipated changes in cardiovascular status during the planned procedure. Assuming that no evidence is seen of occult blood loss or major intrathoracic injury, the most aggressive monitoring during CT scanning should probably consist only of direct arterial pressure measurement. This is based on the requirement for arterial blood gas analysis and the possible need for vasoactive drugs to control hypertension. Conversely, with evidence of occult hemorrhage or major intrathoracic injury, then at least central venous pressure monitoring should be instituted; Swan-Ganz catheterization may be required if cardiac contusion is a consideration.

Once the decision is made to proceed with craniotomy, central venous cannulation should probably be added to direct arterial pressure monitoring. If, during the course of surgery, it becomes clear that blood pressure is difficult to maintain despite adequate fluid replacement, Swan-Ganz catheterization again should be considered to further delineate the nature of the myocardial dysfunction.

C.2. What sort of sedation or anesthesia should be used during head CT scanning?

Many combative and disoriented patients will lie quietly long enough to undergo a head CT scan without sedation or anesthesia. The decision to proceed in this fashion should be predicated on reasonable certainty that the patient's spontaneous ventilation is adequate to maintain normocapnea and that the level of coma is light enough that any regurgitated stomach contents can be handled by oropharyngeal reflexes. Finally, this decision demands that someone trained in airway management is observing the patient while the scan is being performed to ensure that adequate ventilation is maintained throughout the procedure. With any question regarding the patient's ability to breathe spontaneously in an unobstructed fashion and to handle secretions or stomach contents, then intubation should be instituted as described.

Given these caveats, it is obvious that "sedation" with benzodiazepines, opioids, or barbiturates probably should not be attempted in this clinical situation. Once the airway is secured and ventilation is controlled, then sedation and/or neuromuscular blockade can be instituted, if appropriate. This should be done with caution in a patient with multiple trauma because these agents can cause profound hypotension in patients rendered hypovolemic from occult hemorrhage.

Gelb AW, Manninen PH, Mezon BJ et al: The anaesthetist and the head-injured patient. Can J Anaesth 31:97, 1984

C.3. The patient was to undergo craniotomy for an acute epidural hematoma. Are there anesthetic agents that should definitely not be used in this situation? Which ones? What agents might be preferred in this situation?

The principles of anesthetic management for patients with rapidly expanding intracranial mass lesions are based on the ideal of maximizing intracranial compliance by minimizing the volume within the intracranial compartment. This means that any maneuver that increases cerebral blood volume should be avoided. Accordingly, hypercarbia should be avoided, and hyperventilation to the range of $PaCO_2 = 20$ to 25 mm Hg is desirable. Likewise, anesthetic agents such as ketamine and nitrous oxide cause significant increases in intracranial blood volume and ICP. In addition, evidence indicates that although hypocapnia may make it feasible to administer halothane, isoflurane, or enflurane to patients with slowly expanding brain tumors, these agents probably should be eschewed in patients with rapidly expanding intracranial hematoma, particularly if the patient is comatose prior to anesthesia. Finally, evidence indicates that the synthetic opioids, fentanyl, sufentanil and alfentanil, can also act as cerebral vasodilators and raise ICP.

Among the agents that act to decrease both cerebral blood volume and ICP, thiopental, etomidate, and propofol seem most feasible for emergency craniotomy. These agents must be administered cautiously to multiple trauma victims, in whom hypovolemia and hypotension are a possibility. If early awakening is not an issue, then thiopental infused at a rate of approximately 1 g/70 kg/h is sufficient to render an adult male insensible for craniotomy. With reasonable expectation that the patient will awaken quickly from operation, then propofol infused at approximately 50 μg/kg/min is a wise selection. The only gaseous agent required is sufficient inspired oxygen to maintain PaO_2 at approximately 100 mm Hg. Muscle relaxation can be maintained with whatever nondepolarizing neuromuscular blocking agent is appropriate to the patient's hemodynamic status. Arterial hypertension can be controlled with judicious administration of sympatholytic agents. By contrast, hypotensive agents that act by relaxing vascular smooth muscle (sodium nitroprusside, hydralazine, nitroglycerin) tend to elevate cerebral blood volume and ICP and have no place in the care of the patient with head injury.

Archer DP, Labrecque P, Tyler JL et al: Cerebral blood volume is increased in dogs during administration of nitrous oxide or isoflurane. Anesthesiology 67:642, 1987

Henricksen HT, Jogensen PB: The effect of nitrous oxide on ICP in patients with intracranial disorders. Br J Anaesth 45:486, 1973

Marsh ML, Shapiro HM, Smith RW et al: Changes in neurologic status and ICP associated with sodium nitroprusside. Anesthesiology 51:336, 1979

Marx W, Shah N, Long C et al: Sufentanil, alfentanil and fentanyl: Impact on cerebrospinal fluid pressure in patents with brain tumors. J Neurosurg Anesth 1:3, 1989

Scheller MS, Todd MM, Drummond JC et al: The ICP effects of isoflurane and halothane administered after cryogenic brain injury in rabbits. Anesthesiology 67:507, 1987

Shapiro HM, Galindo A, Whyte SR et al: Rapid intraoperative reduction of intracranial pressure with thiopentone. Br J Anaesth 45:1057, 1973

Sperry RJ, Bailey PL, Reichman MS et al: Fentanyl and sufentanil increase intracranial pressure in head trauma patients. Anesthesiology 77:416–420, 1992

C.4. What should be done about intravenous (IV) fluid replacement during craniotomy for evacuation of an epidural hematoma? Should corticosteroids be given empirically?

Rapid formation of brain edema is a common reaction associated with most neuropathologic processes, including epidural hematoma. Accordingly, it is important not to contribute to brain edema with excessive administration of crystalloid solutions. In the patient with multiple injuries, however, this approach must be tempered by the fact that resuscitation in the field and during transport to the hospital will consist almost exclusively of crystalloid solutions or plasma expanders (e.g., hetastarch) until albumin and/or whole blood is available. Once the patient arrives in the operating room, whole blood or packed cells should be administered along with colloid-containing solutions in quantities sufficient to replace intravascular blood volume (maintain a normal CVP) and to stabilize hematocrit at levels compatible with optimal oxygen transport (i.e, 30%). Because recent studies suggest that hyperglycemia is detrimental to neurologic outcome following ischemic insults, dextrose-containing solutions should be avoided, and, indeed, blood glucose determinations should be performed intraoperatively to ensure that hyperglycemia does not occur.

Corticosteroids have been shown to be effective in reducing cortical edema associated with brain tumors and abscesses, as well as in acute spinal cord injury. Prospective studies evaluating their efficacy in head trauma, however, have failed to demonstrate any benefit and, indeed, are occasionally associated with iatrogenic complications. Accordingly, most centers do not administer these agents to patients with head trauma.

Hypertonic saline (7.5%), although clinically used as a resuscitative fluid in Europe, is still considered experimental in the United States. Hypertonic saline draws water from the intracellular space; thus, in addition to restoring blood volume, it reduces brain edema and prevents elevation of the ICP as effectively as 20% mannitol. The intravascular volume expansion produced by hypertonic saline is transient and administration of hypertonic saline cannot be maintained for long periods of time. It may cause hypernatremia, hyperosmolality, and hyperchloremic acidosis; the latter probably results from renal bicarbonate loss secondary to the increased levels of Cl^-. Serum concentrations of Na^+ and Cl^- and the patient's acid-base status should be followed. Hypertonic saline administration should be discontinued if plasma Na^+ reaches 160 mEq/liter.

Albright AL, Latchaw RE, Robinson AG: Intracranial and systemic effects of hetastarch in experimental cerebral edema. Crit Care Med 12:496, 1984

Barash PG, Cullen BE, Stoelting RK (eds): Clinical Anesthesia, 3rd ed, pp 1181–1182. Philadelphia, Lippincott-Raven, 1997

Bracken MB, Shepard MJ, Collins WF Jr et al: Methylprednisolone or naloxone treatment after acute spinal cord injury: 1-year follow-up data: Results of the second National Acute Spinal Cord Injury Study. J Neurosurg 76:23, 1992

Deardon NM, Gibson JS, McDowell DC et al: Effect of high-dose dexamethasone on outcome from severe head injury. J Neurosurg 64:81, 1986

Freshman SP, Battistella FD, Matteucci M et al: Hypertonic saline (7.5%) versus mannitol: A comparison for treatment of acute head injuries. J Trauma 35:344, 1993

Kaieda R, Todd MM, Warner DS: Prolonged reduction in colloid osmotic pressure does not increase brain edema following cryogenic injury in rabbits. Anesthesiology 71:571, 1989

C.5. In the middle of surgery the blood pressure suddenly decreased, peak airway pressure and central venous pressure (CVP) increased, and the pulse oximeter indicated a decrease in oxygen saturation. What was the likely cause? What would be the likely cause if the CVP suddenly fell?

Although it is tempting to become fixated on the surgical problem at hand, the alert anesthesiologist must remain highly suspicious of additional delayed complications related to trauma. After blunt thoracic trauma, tension pneumothorax is always a potential complication, particularly in a patient receiving positive pressure ventilation. The hallmarks of tension pneumothorax are hypotension, hypoxemia, and elevations of both CVP and airway pressure. The diagnosis can usually be confirmed by auscultation of the chest; emergent chest tube placement is indicated immediately.

Another delayed complication following motor vehicle accidents is hepatic or splenic rupture, which may present from hours to days after the injury despite a previously "negative" peritoneal lavage. In this case, as in any other occult source of blood loss, cardiac filling pressures are diminished despite vigorous intravenous volume replacement. The diagnosis is confirmed by peritoneal tap, and treatment (i.e., laparotomy) needs to be undertaken promptly.

Miller RD (ed): Anesthesia, 4th ed, pp 2159–2169. New York, Churchill Livingstone, 1994

Reiss SJ, Raque GH Jr, Shields CB et al: Cervical spine fractures with major associated trauma. Neurosurgery 18:327, 1987

C.6. The patient was noted to be bleeding from vascular access sites. What are the possible causes of coagulopathy in this patient?

The most likely cause of coagulopathy in a patient with multiple injuries is dilution of labile clotting factors V and VIII and platelets when massive transfusion of banked blood is administered without specific clotting factor replacement. In the absence of massive blood replacement, an additional cause of coagulopathy in neurotrauma patients is release of brain thromboplastin into the circulation. Fortunately, only a small proportion of patients with head injury go on to develop symptoms of diffuse intravascular coagulopathy. Treatment should be directed toward debridement of nonviable brain tissue and specific therapy with appropriate clotting factors, according to the results of coagulation testing.

Clark JA, Finelli RD, Netsky MG: Disseminated intravascular coagulation following cranial trauma. J Neurosurg 52:266, 1980

D. Postoperative Neurointensive Care Management

D.1. What specific measures should be used to control the patient's intracranial pressure?

After removal of an intracranial hematoma, control of intracranial pressure is of paramount importance in the patient's recovery. Briefly, those patients whose ICP can be maintained <20 to 25 mm Hg tend to have significantly better outcomes than do patients whose ICP remains elevated. It has become common practice, therefore, to monitor ICP in head-injured patients during the postoperative period. This enables the intensivist to adjust treatment with hyperventilation, mannitol, CSF drainage, head-up tilt, and so forth, to achieve the desired ICP level. If these maneuvers fail, the next intervention is to maintain barbiturate coma to a level where the EEG shows burst suppression. This is continued until it is no longer required to control intracranial hypertension. After weaning from barbiturate therapy, the patient then can be weaned from diuretics and hyperventilation, as appropriate.

Centers that do not employ ICP monitoring must rely largely on the patient's level of consciousness to determine recovery from head injury. The patient must be awakened and muscle relaxation must be antagonized so that the patient can breathe spontaneously at the end of surgery. Although this is less aggressive than monitoring ICP and actively controlling it, risk is present of hypoventilation, hypercapnea, and worsening of neuropathology before therapeutic interventions are reinitiated. To date, however, the decision to which treatment regimen results in the best outcome remains controversial.

Marshall LF, Smith RW, Shapiro HM: Outcome with aggressive treatment in severe head injury. II. Acute and chronic barbiturate administration in the management of head injury. J Neurosurg 90:26, 1979

Narayan RJ, Kishore PRS, Becker DP et al: Intracranial pressure: To monitor or not to monitor: A review of our experience in severe head injury. J Neurosurg 56:650, 1982

Stuart GG, Merry GS, Smith JA et al: Severe head injury managed without intracranial pressure monitoring. J Neurosurg 59:601, 1983

D.2. What monitoring modalities might help assess the degree of residual injury and/or the chance for good recovery?

Somatosensory evoked potential monitoring is the most commonly used electrophysiologic modality for assessing neural function and prognosis in comatose patients with head injury. Brain stem auditory evoked potentials are useful to determine the integrity of the auditory pathways, but they tend to be resistant to the effects of moderately severe trauma, particularly above the level of the tentorium. Conversely, visually evoked potentials tend to be so exquisitely sensitive to sedatives and cortical injury that they are of relatively little use in the neurointensive care environment.

Cerebrovascular responsiveness to changes in $PaCO_2$ indicates a more favorable prognosis following head injury. Either direct measures of cerebral blood flow or indirect measures (e.g., ICP changes or changes in jugular venous-arterial PO_2 or glucose gradient) have been used effectively to predict improved outcome in neurotrauma intensive care units.

Cruz J: An additional therapeutic effect of adequate hyperventilation in severe acute brain trauma: Normalization of cerebral glucose uptake. J Neurosurg 82:379, 1995

Judson JA, Cant BR, Shaw NA: Early prediction of outcome from cerebral trauma by somatosensory evoked potentials. Crit Care Med 18:363, 1990

Yoshihara M, Bandoh K, Marmarou A: Cerebrovascular carbon dioxide reactivity assessed by intracranial pressure dynamics in severely head-injured patients. J Neurosurgery 82:386, 1995

D.3. Outline the principles of respiratory and cardiovascular care for this patient.

As indicated, controlled hyperventilation should be maintained into the postoperative period until such time as either the patient regains consciousness or the ICP remains <20 to 25 mm Hg. Hyperventilation can then be gradually withdrawn as long as the patient's neurologic status and ICP remain stable.

Cardiovascular care in the postoperative period is similar to that used before and during surgery. Hypertension is treated promptly with sympatholytics so that brain edema is not aggravated by elevated arterial pressure while the blood-brain barrier remains disrupted. Likewise, hypotension is treated aggressively with intravascular volume loading titrated as indicated by cardiac filling pressures. If this is not effective, vasopressors are administered as needed, to increase either peripheral vascular resistance or cardiac performance.

Marsh ML, Marshall LF, Shapiro HM: Neurosurgical intensive care. Anesthesiology 47:149, 1977

D.4. Why would this patient develop diabetes insipidus in the postoperative period? How would you treat it?

Diabetes insipidus is characterized by loss of free water from the kidneys because of insufficient amounts of antidiuretic hormone (ADH), vasopressin, being released from the posterior pituitary gland. Usually this occurs after severe head injury in association with a basilar skull fracture. Because vasopressin is produced in the hypothalamus and travels to the posterior pituitary gland, shearing of the pituitary stalk interrupts the ability of the hormone to the posterior pituitary gland. Accordingly, urine output can be reasonably normal during the immediate perioperative period, but then become dilute and excessive as the ADH stores in the posterior pituitary are exhausted. In neurotrauma patients, the differential diagnosis may be more difficult because of the need to induce osmotic diuresis with mannitol to control ICP. Treatment consists of water replacement and administration of desamino-D-arginine vasopressin (DDAVP), a synthetic analogue of ADH. DDAVP has minimal cardiovascular effects and a longer duration of action than ADH, which must be given in a continuous infusion to be effective.

Kern KB, Meislin HW: Diabetes insipidus: Occurrence after minor head trauma. J Trauma 24:69, 1984

Robinson AG: DDAVP in the treatment of central diabetes insipidus. N Engl J Med 294:507, 1976

Shucart W, Jackson I: Management of diabetes insipidus in neurosurgical patients. J Neurosurg 44:65, 1976

25 Cerebral Aneurysm

Patricia Fogarty Mack

A 43-year-old white woman presented to the emergency room 2 days ago, complaining of severe headache, nausea, and vomiting, followed by a witnessed 3-minute loss of consciousness. On regaining consciousness, the patient was noted by her family to be confused. Spinal tap showed subarachnoid blood. Angiogram revealed a small anterior communicating artery aneurysm.

She was scheduled for aneurysm clipping. At the present time, she was oriented only to person. She had no previous medical history; however, she had smoked one pack of cigarettes per day for the past 20 years. Blood pressure was 130/80 mm Hg, pulse 90 beats/min; respirations 18 beats/min. She had no focal neurologic deficits.

A. Medical Disease and Differential Diagnosis

1. What are the incidence, prevalence, and causes of subarachnoid hemorrhage (SAH) and what are the risk factors associated with rupture of intracranial aneurysms?
2. What are common sizes and locations of intracranial aneurysms?
3. What is the pathophysiology of aneurysmal rupture and SAH?
4. What are symptoms and signs of SAH?
5. How does one assess the severity of SAH?
6. What are the cardiovascular effects of SAH?
7. How is the diagnosis of SAH made?
8. What is the risk of rebleeding for a patient with subarachnoid hemorrhage?

B. Preoperative Evaluation and Preparation

1. How should the patient be managed prior to surgical clipping?
2. When is the ideal time after subarachnoid hemorrhage to perform surgical clipping of an aneurysm?
3. Should surgery be postponed due to the patient's elevated creatinine phosphokinase (CPK) MB fractions?
4. Would you premedicate this patient?

C. Intraoperative Management

1. What are the goals of the induction and maintenance of anesthesia for this patient?
2. What monitors should be used in this patient?
3. Why would a monitor of central venous pressure (CVP) be useful in this patient?
4. What other forms of monitoring would you consider?
5. What are your particular concerns during induction of anesthesia in this patient?
6. How would you accomplish a smooth and safe induction and intubation of this patient?
7. Would you perform a rapid-sequence induction and intubation on this patient?

8. What are the effects of hypoxemia and hypercapnea, such as would be seen with loss of the airway on induction, on cerebral blood flow?
9. What is optimal fluid management for aneurysm clipping? Would you use a dextrose containing solution?
10. After the bone plate was removed and as the dura was being opened the surgeon complained that the brain was "tight." What could you do to achieve better brain relaxations and facilitate surgical exposure?
11. What is the purpose of controlled hypotension and how is it achieved?
12. What are some of the potential drawbacks of controlled hypotension?
13. How else might transmural pressure be decreased to allow for aneurysm clip placement?
14. What methods of cerebral protection might you employ during this operation?
15. What are the advantages and disadvantages of intentional mild hypothermia as a means of cerebral protection?
16. What are the indications for deep hypothermic circulatory arrest?
17. What steps should be taken in the case of intraoperative rupture of an intracranial aneurysm?
18. How would you plan the emergence from an anesthetic for aneurysm clipping?

D. Postoperative Management

1. Would you extubate the patient postoperatively?
2. What would be the differential diagnosis if the patient did not return to her preoperative neurologic condition?
3. On postoperative day 2, the patient became disoriented and developed hemiplegia. A computed tomography (CT) scan was performed, which shows no new intracranial bleeding. What other diagnostic studies should be performed?
4. What is cerebral vasospasm and what causes it?
5. What are pathophysiologic changes seen in vasospasm?
6. How is the diagnosis of cerebral vasospasm made?
7. What steps can be taken to prevent cerebral vasospasm?
8. What treatments can be undertaken once a diagnosis of vasospasm is made?
9. What are other neurologic complications following SAH and aneurysm clipping?
10. What other organ systems may manifest problems postoperatively in aneurysm clipping patients?

A. Medical Disease and Differential Diagnosis

A.1. What are the incidence, prevalence, and causes of subarachnoid hemorrhage (SAH) and what are the risk factors associated with rupture of intracranial aneurysms?

The prevalence of SAH is 2% to 5% with an incidence of 10 to 28/100,000 people. There are 25,000 cases of SAH each year in the United States, comprising 10% of all cases of stroke. Sixty percent of the cases occur in young individuals between the ages of 40 and 60 years. Thus, a poor neurologic outcome is a devastating condition to be endured over a potentially long period of time.

Approximately one third of patients die as a result of the acute bleed. Of the two thirds who survive the acute bleed, one half (one third of total) later die or are severely disabled and one half (one third of total) have an acceptable outcome.

Cerebral aneurysms account for 75% to 80% of SAH; arteriovenous malformations are the cause in 4% to 5%, whereas no specific cause can be found in 15% to 20% of SAH. Other causes of SAH include trauma, mycotic aneurysm, sickle cell disease, cocaine use, and coagulation disorders.

Risk factors for rupture of cerebral aneurysms include hypertension, pregnancy, and vascular abnormalities (e.g., type III collagen deficiency and elastase abnormalities). One third of patients with polycystic kidney disease have been found to have intracranial aneurysms at autopsy. Genetic predisposition plays a role: 7% of berry aneurysms are familial, and 5% to 10% of patients with ruptured aneurysm have a first-order relative with ruptured aneurysm.

Smoking and alcohol abuse also appear to predispose to aneurysm formation and rupture. Cocaine abuse and resultant episodic hypertension may predispose to aneurysmal rupture at an early age.

Death and disability are primarily due to the initial bleed, vasospasm, and re-bleeding. Other causes include surgical complications, parenchymal hemorrhage, hydrocephalus, and complications of medical therapy.

Albin MS (ed): Textbook of Neuroanesthesia: With Neurosurgical and Neuroscience Perspectives, p 846. New York, McGraw-Hill, 1997

Barrow DL, Reisner A: Natural history of intracranial aneurysms and vascular malformations. Clin Neurol Neurosurg 40:3–39, 1993

Bekker AY, Baker KZ, Baker CJ et al: Anesthetic considerations for cerebral aneurysm surgery. Am J Anesthesiol 22:248–258, 1995

Cottrell JE, Smith DS (eds): Anesthesia and Neurosurgery, 3rd ed, pp 364–365. St. Louis, Mosby, 1994.

Guy J, McGrath BJ, Borel CO et al: Perioperative management of aneurysmal subarachnoid hemorrhage. Part 1. Operative management. Anesth Analg 81:1060–1072, 1995

A.2. What are common sizes and locations of intracranial aneurysms?

Small (<12 mm) aneurysms make up 78% of the total, whereas large (12–24 mm) are 20%, and giant (>24 mm) comprise 2%. Most aneurysms are located in the anterior circulation, with the junction of the anterior communicating and anterior cerebral arteries being the most common (39%). Thirty percent of aneurysms occur in the internal carotid artery, 22% in the middle cerebral artery, and 8% in the posterior circulation (posterior cerebral, basilar, and vertebral arteries).

Kasell NF, Torner JC, Haley C et al: The International cooperative study on the timing of aneurysm surgery. Part 1. Overall management results. J Neurosurg 73:18–32, 1990

Kasell NF, Torner JC, Haley C, et al: The International cooperative study on the timing of aneurysm surgery. Part 2. Surgical results. J Neurosurg 73:37–47, 1990

A.3. What is the pathophysiology of aneurysmal rupture and SAH?

Based on experimental models, aneurysmal rupture leads to the leakage of arterial blood and a rapid increase in intracranial pressure (ICP), approaching diastolic blood pressure in the proximal intracerebral arteries. This increase in ICP causes a decrease in cerebral perfusion pressure (CPP) and a fall in cerebral blood flow (CBF), leading to a loss of consciousness. The decrease in CBF diminishes bleeding and stops the

Table 25-1. Modified Hunt and Hess Clinical Grades

GRADE[a]	CRITERIA
0	Unruptured aneurysm
I	Asymptomatic or minimal headache and slight nuchal rigidity
II	Moderate to severe headache, nuchal rigidity, but no neurologic deficit other than cranial nerve palsy
III	Drowsiness, confusion, or mild focal deficit
IV	Stupor, mild to severe hemiparesis, possible early decerebrate rigidity, vegetative disturbance
V	Deep coma, decerebrate rigidity, moribund appearance

[a] Serious systemic disease such as hypertension, diabetes, severe arteriosclerosis, chronic pulmonary disease, and severe vasospasm seen on arteriography result in placement of the patient in the next less favorable category.

(Reprinted with permission from Hunt WE, Hess RM: Surgical risk as related to time of intervention in the repair of intracranial aneurysms. J Neurosurg 28:14–20, 1968)

SAH. A gradual reduction in ICP and an increase in CBF indicates improved cerebral function and possibly a return to consciousness. A persistent increase in ICP (perhaps due to thrombi in the cranial cisterns), however, indicates a persistent no-flow pattern with acute vasospasm, cell swelling, and death.

Asano T, Sano K: Pathogenic role of no-reflow phenomenon in experimental subarachnoid hemorrhage in dogs. J Neurosurg 46:446–453, 1977

A.4. What are symptoms and signs of SAH?

Headache occurs in 85% to 95% of patients. Often a brief loss of consciousness occurs, followed by diminished mentation; however, consciousness may be impaired to any degree or may be unaffected at the time of presentation. Symptoms may be similar to infectious meningitis (nausea, vomiting and photophobia) secondary to subarachnoid blood. The patient may also experience motor and sensory deficits, visual field disturbances, and cranial nerve palsies. Finally, blood in the subarachnoid space may cause an elevated temperature.

Albin MS (ed): Textbook of Neuroanesthesia: With Neurosurgical and Neuroscience Perspectives, p 847. New York, McGraw-Hill, 1997

Guy J, McGrath BJ, Borel CO et al: Perioperative management of aneurysmal subarachnoid hemorrhage. Part 1. Operative management. Anesth Analg 81:1060–1072, 1995

A.5. How does one assess the severity of SAH?

Two grading scales are commonly used to assess neurologic status following SAH, the Hunt and Hess Grade (Table 25-1) and the World Federation of Neurologic Surgeons' grade (Table 25-2), based on the Glasgow Coma Scale. The scales are useful in

Table 25-2. World Federation of Neurological Surgeons' (WFNS) Grading Scale

WFNS GRADE	GLASGOW COMA SCALE	MOTOR DEFICIT
I	15	Absent
II	14–13	Absent
III	14–13	Present
IV	12–7	Present or absent
V	6–3	Present or absent

(Reprinted with permission from Report of World Federation of Neurologic Surgeons Committee on a universal subarachnoid hemorrhage grading scale. J Neurosurg 68:985–986, 1988)

identifying a baseline neurologic status from which any acute changes should be assessed. In addition, the scales may correlate with physiologic status. Patients who are Hunt and Hess grades I and II have near normal cerebral autoregulation and ICP. Finally, failure of the patient to return to baseline following surgery warrants an investigation as to whether residual anesthetic effect or surgical mishap is the cause.

Hunt WE, Hess RM: Surgical risk as related to time of intervention in the repair of intracranial aneurysms. J Neurosurg 28:14–20, 1968

Report of World Federation of Neurologic Surgeons Committee on a universal subarachnoid hemorrhage grading scale. J Neurosurg 68:985–986, 1988

A.6. What are the cardiovascular effects of SAH?

Injury to the posterior hypothalamus from SAH causes the release of norepinephrine from the adrenal medulla and cardiac sympathetic efferents. Norepinephrine can cause an increase in afterload and direct myocardial toxicity leading to subendocardial ischemia. Pathologic analysis of myocardium of patients who have died acutely from SAH has revealed microscopic subendocardial hemorrhage and myocytolysis.

Electrocardiographic (ECG) abnormalities are present in 50% to 80% of patients with SAH. Most commonly these involve ST segment changes and T wave inversions; however, they also include prolonged QT interval, U waves, and P wave changes. ST-T wave changes are usually scattered and not related to a particular distribution.

Dysrhythmias occur in 80% of patients, usually in the first 48 hours. Premature ventricular contractions are the most common abnormality. However, any type of dysrhythmia is possible. They include severely prolonged QT interval, torsades de pointes, and ventricular fibrillation. In one series, 66% of the arrhythmias were considered mild, 29% moderate, and 5% severe. In addition to increased cathecholamine secretion, hypercortisolism and hypokalemia have been suggested as causes for the dysrhythmias seen with SAH.

Ventricular dysfunction, possibly leading to pulmonary edema, is present in about 30% of patients with SAH.

Albin, MS (ed): Textbook of Neuroanesthesia: With Neurosurgical and Neuroscience Perspectives, p 862. New York, McGraw-Hill, 1997

Cottrell JE, Smith DS (eds): Anesthesia and Neurosurgery, 3rd ed, pp 379–380. St. Louis, Mosby, 1994

Solenski NJ, Haley EC, Kassell NF et al: Medical complications of aneurysmal subarachnoid hemorrhage: A report of the multicenter Cooperative Aneurysm Study. Crit Care Med 23:1007–1017, 1995

A.7. How is the diagnosis of SAH made?

Noncontrast CT scan can determine the magnitude and location of the bleed. It may also be useful in assessing ventricular size and aneurysm location. High resolution CT with contrast can more precisely determine the location of the aneurysm. Magnetic resonance imaging (MRI) is not very useful assessing acute SAH, but it may determine the location of the aneurysm if it is >3 mm in diameter.

Lumbar puncture can be used to diagnose SAH if CT is negative, especially when the patient presents >1 week after an initial bleed. Xanthochromia, a yellow discoloration of the cerebrospinal fluid after centrifugation, is present from 4 hours to 3 weeks after SAH. The lumbar puncture itself can cause herniation or rebleeding. Therefore, a CT scan should be performed first if the patient presents within 72 hours of suspected SAH.

Four vessel angiography (right and left carotid and vertebral arteries) is used to visualize all intracranial vessels, to localize the source of bleeding, and to rule out multiple aneurysms (5% to 33% of patients).

Guy J, McGrath BJ, Borel CO et al: Perioperative management of aneurysmal subarachnoid hemorrhage. Part 1. Operative management. Anesth Analg 81:1060–1072, 1995

Kasell NF, Torner JC, Haley EC et al: The International Cooperative Study on the Timing of Aneurysm Surgery. Part 2. Surgical results. J Neurosurg 73:37–47, 1990

A.8. What is the risk of rebleeding for a patient with subarachnoid hemorrhage?

The risk of rebleeding from a ruptured aneurysm is highest, 4%, in the first 24 hours after the initial bleed and 1.5% per day thereafter. Cumulative risk is 19% in 14 days and 50% at 6 months. After 6 months, the rebleeding risk is 3% per year.

Kassell NF, Torner JC: Aneurysmal rebleeding: A preliminary report from the Cooperative Aneurysm Study. Neurosurgery 13:479–481, 1983

B. Preoperative Evaluation and Preparation

B.1. How should the patient be managed prior to surgical clipping?

Prior to surgical clipping medical therapy is aimed at avoiding increases in the transmural pressure of the aneurysm. This is accomplished by strict blood pressure control to maintain systolic blood pressure <160 mm Hg with esmolol, labetalol, or sodium nitroprusside; narcotics for pain management; lidocaine for tracheal suctioning, if the patient is intubated; and stool softeners.

Guy J, McGrath BJ, Borel CO et al: Perioperative management of aneurysmal subarachnoid hemorrhage. Part 1. Operative management. Anesth Analg 81:1060–1072, 1995

B.2. When is the ideal time after subarachnoid hemorrhage to perform surgical clipping of an aneurysm?

The ideal timing of aneurysm surgery was studied by the International Cooperative Study on the Timing of Aneurysm Surgery. The researchers found that during "early" surgery on day 0 or day 1 after SAH, the brain was "tight" but no increased incidence of brain contusion, laceration, or major brain resection was seen. Furthermore, no increased difficulty was found in dissection to expose the aneurysm, nor any difference in rate of intraoperative rupture in comparison with the later surgery group.

Late surgery, 11 to 14 days after SAH, patients had better outcome at 6 months than did the early surgery group; however, 30% of patients did not survive to have planned late surgery. During the 2-week wait for surgery findings were a 12% risk of

rebleeding and a 30% risk of vasospasm, defined as new-onset focal neurologic deficit without rebleeding or cerebral edema.

Mortality rate (20%) was similar in both groups, as was good outcome (60%).

The worst outcome was in the group operated on at 7 to 10 days, which was
coincident with the period with the highest incidence of vasospasm. Surgery timing
did not influence the incidence of vasospasm.

Kasell NF, Torner JC, Haley C et al: The International cooperative study on the timing of aneurysm
surgery. Part 2. Surgical results. J Neurosurg 73:37–47, 1990

B.3. Should surgery be postponed due to the patient's elevated creatinine phosphokinase (CPK) MB fractions?

Fifty percent of patients will have an increase in CPK-MB fractions; however, CPK-
MB per total CPK fraction is usually not consistent with transmural myocardial infarction (MI). In addition, although some patients (0.7%) do sustain a MI in the setting of SAH, little correlation is found between ECG abnormalities and ischemia in
this population.

The desire to delay surgery due to cardiac abnormalities must be weighed
against the risk of rebleeding and vasospasm. In most cases the risk of recurrent hemorrhage outweighs the risk of perioperative MI. Furthermore, even if coronary artery
disease is present, these patients are not candidates for myocardial revascularization,
which requires heparinization. If pulmonary edema or malignant dysrhythmias are
present, it may be prudent to postpone surgery until such problems are controlled
medically. However, if these problems are not present, then clipping of the aneurysm
may be indicated. If surgery is to be undertaken, a pulmonary artery catheter or
transesophageal echocardiography may be helpful in assessing ventricular function.

Albin MS (ed): Textbook of Neuroanesthesia: With Neurosurgical and Neuroscience Perspectives,
p 868. New York, McGraw-Hill, 1997

Guy J, McGrath BJ, Borel CO et al: Perioperative management of aneurysmal subarachnoid hemorrhage. Part 1. Operative management. Anesth Analg 81:1060–1072, 1995

Todd M: Anesthesia for intracranial vascular surgery. ASA Refresher Course No. 211, 1995

B.4. Would you premedicate this patient?

No. When the patient is in a Hunt and Hess grade III state, anxiety is unlikely. Furthermore, heavy sedation may decrease ventilation, raising $PaCO_2$ and increasing
CBF and ICP, which, at the very least, may hinder pre- and postoperative neurologic
evaluation. However, if the patient were Hunt and Hess grade I–II and after the preoperative visit concern existed that preoperative anxiety might lead to hemodynamic
instability, a small dose of benzodiazepine may be appropriate.

Medications such as calcium channel blockers (nimodipine), anticonvulsants, and
steroids should be continued preoperatively on the day of surgery.

If the patient is at risk for aspiration, medications to decrease gastric acidity and
volume are appropriate. Most patients will already be receiving an H_2-blocker if they
are on dexamethasone.

Albin MS (ed): Textbook of Neuroanesthesia: With Neurosurgical and Neuroscience Perspectives,
p 868. New York, McGraw-Hill, 1997

C. Intraoperative Management

C.1. What are the goals of the induction and maintenance of anesthesia for this patient?

The primary goal is to prevent aneurysm rupture on induction or intraoperatively while maintaining adequate cerebral perfusion pressure. The goal of matching anesthetic depth to surgical stimulation is more important than which specific drugs are used. In general, the anesthesiologist should provide for rapid and reversible titration of blood pressure, maintain CPP, and protect against cerebral ischemia. An additional goal is to provide a relaxed brain for ease of surgical exposure with minimal brain retraction. Finally, the anesthetic should be planned to achieve a rapid, smooth emergence, allowing prompt neurologic assessment. This can be accomplished with a combination of balanced anesthesia, muscle relaxation, and sympathetic blockers.

Cottrell JE, Smith DS (eds): Anesthesia and Neurosurgery, 3rd ed, p 384. St. Louis, Mosby, 1994

Guy J, McGrath BJ, Borel CO et al: Perioperative management of aneurysmal subarachnoid hemorrhage. Part 1. Operative management. Anesth Analg 81:1060–1072, 1995

Todd M: Anesthesia for intracranial vascular surgery. ASA Refresher Course No. 211, 1995

C.2. What monitors should be used in this patient?

In addition to ECG, pulse oximetry, and end-tidal CO_2, an arterial line should be placed, using local anesthesia, prior to induction. The arterial line should be zeroed at the level of the circle of Willis. This will allow close monitoring of the arterial blood pressure and prompt intervention if necessary to avoid sudden increases in transmural pressure at the critical times of induction and intubation as well as throughout the procedure.

C.3. Why would a monitor of central venous pressure (CVP) be useful in this patient?

Although not always directly monitored, CVP measurement may be useful in assessing volume replacement needs, especially because urine output will be affected by osmotic or loop diuretics administered to facilitate surgical exposure. If vasoactive medication becomes necessary, it can be most effectively administered via a central venous catheter.

One disadvantage of CVP monitoring is catheter placement. Some clinicians are concerned that placement of an internal jugular venous CVP will compromise venous outflow of the head, thus, predisposing to bleeding or brain swelling; however, this remains controversial. A "long-arm" or antecubital CVP line may be more difficult to insert and have a higher incidence of thrombophlebitis.

Finally, a poor correlation between CVP and left ventricular end-diastolic pressure has been documented in SAH, so a pulmonary artery (PA) catheter may be more useful in assessing volume status as well as providing a monitor of cardiac output in those patients who have had preoperative cardiac problems. Patients who are expected to be candidates for hypertensive hypervolemic hemodilution therapy (HHH) for vasospasm or for barbiturate coma may also benefit from placement of a PA catheter.

Central pressure monitoring is usually instituted after the patient is asleep to minimize stress to the patient. One should be careful to use the minimal degree of head-down tilt necessary to access the central circulation, as a severe Trendelenburg position may have deleterious effects on ICP and CPP.

Cottrell JE, Smith DS (eds): Anesthesia and Neurosurgery, 3rd ed, pp 386–387. St. Louis, Mosby, 1994

Guy J, McGrath BJ, Borel CO et al: Perioperative management of aneurysmal subarachnoid hemorrhage. Part 1. Operative management. Anesth Analg 81:1060–1072, 1995

Todd M, Drummond JC, Hoi SU: Hemodynamic effects of high dose pentobarbital: Studies in elective neurosurgical patients. Neurosurgery 20:559–563, 1987

C.4. What other forms of monitoring would you consider?

Electroencephalography (EEG) and somatosensory evoked potentials (SSEPs) have been advocated by some authors; however, they are not standard monitoring in most hospitals. Although EEG has been used to monitor cerebral ischemia, scalp electrodes may not reflect activity of brain areas most at risk. Cortical electrodes, such as those used in epilepsy surgery, may avoid the problem of attenuation of the scalp EEG signal by cerebrospinal fluid drainage and air between scalp electrodes and brain surface during surgery.

Somatosensory evoked potentials may detect reversible ischemia during temporary vessel occlusion; however, they may not detect ischemia in subcortical structures and motor cortex. Furthermore, SSEPs have relatively high false-positive (38% to 60%) and false-negative (5% to 34%) rates. Brain stem auditory evoked responses (BAERs) may be useful in monitoring during posterior circulation aneurysm clipping.

Monitoring of ICP is common, with the probability of increased ICP greatest 24 to 48 hours post SAH. An intraventricular catheter not only allows for ICP monitoring, but also for CSF drainage to improve operating conditions. If an intraventricular catheter is not present, lumbar spinal drains may be placed.

Intraoperative angiography, which we do not usually perform at our institution, is one means by which to assure complete obliteration of the aneurysm without clip occlusion of the parent artery or perforating branches.

Bekker AY, Baker KZ, Baker CJ et al: Anesthetic considerations for cerebral aneurysm surgery. Am J Anesthesiol 22:248–258, 1995

Manninen PH, Lam AM, Nantau WE: Monitoring of somatosensory evoked potentials during temporary arterial occlusion in cerebral aneurysm surgery. J Neurosurg Anesthesiol 2:97–104, 1990

Schramm J, Antou L, Gerhard S et al: Surgical and electrophysiological observations during clipping of 134 aneurysms with evoked potential monitoring. Neurosurgery 26:61–70, 1990

Young WL, Solomon RA, Pedley TA et al: Direct cortical EEG monitoring during temporary vascular occlusion for cerebral aneurysm surgery. Anesthesiology 71:794–799, 1989

C.5. What are your particular concerns during induction of anesthesia in this patient?

If an aneurysm ruptures during anesthetic induction, mortality is high (approximately 75%). Thus precise control of transmural pressure is important in preventing aneurysm rupture.

$$\text{Transmural pressure} = \text{cerebral perfusion pressure (CPP)} =$$

$$\text{MAP} - \text{ICP or CVP (whichever is greater)}$$

$$\text{Where MAP} = \text{mean arterial pressure}$$

On the other hand, one does not want CPP to be so low that ischemia develops, especially in areas of vasospasm.

Tsementzis SA, Hitchcock ER: Outcome from "rescue clipping" of ruptured intracranial aneurysms during induction of anesthesia and endotracheal intubation. J Neurol Neurosurg Psychiatry 48:160–163, 1985

C.6. How would you accomplish a smooth and safe induction and intubation of this patient?

Assuming that evaluation of the airway indicated that intubation would not be difficult, one would begin with preoxygenation. Thiopental (3 to 5 mg/kg), propofol (1.5 to 2.5 mg/kg), and etomidate (0.5 to 1.0 mg/kg) all have similar effects on cerebral blood flow and cerebral metabolic rate. Given that this woman had no other medical problems, I would select thiopental. One would want to avoid ketamine for induction because of its associated increase in CBF and ICP; recent evidence suggests that etomidate leads to an increase in infarct size after ischemic insults in animals.

After loss of consciousness and apnea, care must be taken to maintain a normal $PaCO_2$ and to avoid extreme hyperventilation. Vigorous hyperventilation will lower $PaCO_2$, decreasing CBF. This may lower ICP to such a degree that, if MAP is maintained or increased, transmural pressure may be increased, leading to rupture of the aneurysm.

A nondepolarizing muscle relaxant, which has no effect on ICP or CBF, should be added to facilitate intubation. The neuromuscular junction should be monitored to ensure that paralysis is adequate to avoid coughing with intubation.

Fentanyl (5 to 10 µg/kg) or sufentanil (0.5 to 1.0 µg/kg) can be added 3 to 5 minutes before laryngoscopy to blunt the hemodynamic response. Isoflurane (up to 1.0%) is added to deepen the anesthetic. Finally, approximately 90 seconds prior to laryngoscopy, lidocaine (1.5 to 2.0 mg/kg) or esmolol (0.5 mg/kg) or labetalol (10 to 20 mg) can be added to further blunt the hemodynamic response to intubation.

Lidocaine decreases both CBF and cerebral metabolic rate for oxygen, and at high concentrations it can cause seizures. Esmolol and labetalol have no effect on CBF and ICP, even in brain areas where autoregulation may not be intact. Extreme reductions in MAP (> 35%) may compromise CPP in patients with increased ICP.

Albin MS (ed): Textbook of Neuroanesthesia: With Neurosurgical and Neuroscience Perspectives, p 873. New York, McGraw-Hill, 1997

Cottrell JE, Smith DS (eds): Anesthesia and Neurosurgery, 3rd ed, pp 384-386. St. Louis, Mosby, 1994

Guy J, McGrath BJ, Borel CO et al: Perioperative management of aneurysmal subarachnoid hemorrhage. Part 1. Operative management. Anesth Analg 81:1060–1072, 1995

C.7. Would you perform a rapid-sequence induction and intubation on this patient?

No indication is seen for a rapid-sequence induction and intubation on this patient. Overall risk of aspiration during general anesthesia has been estimated at 0.05%; however, the risk of aneurysm rupture during induction is 1% to 2%. Therefore, unless a clear indication exists for rapid-sequence induction it is best avoided.

If rapid-sequence induction is indicated, one may consider using vecuronium

(0.15 to 0.20 mg/kg) or rocuronium (0.9 mg/kg) rather than succinylcholine. Succinyl-choline can cause an increase in ICP, although this increase can be attenuated or elim-inated by deep anesthesia or prior defasciculation. Furthermore, succinylcholine can lead to hyperkalemia and possibly ventricular fibrillation in those patients presenting with motor deficits following SAH.

In the case of a full stomach or an anticipated difficult airway, careful awake fi-beroptic intubation, with use of appropriate sedation and topical application of local anesthesia, is an appropriate alternative. Under such circumstances, it is necessary to have an assistant so that while one person is securing the airway, the other is solely focused on controlling the hemodynamics with titration of beta-blockers and sodium nitroprusside.

Cottrell JE, Smith DS (eds): Anesthesia and Neurosurgery, 3rd ed, pp 385–386. St. Louis, Mosby, 1994

Guy J, McGrath BJ, Borel CO et al: Perioperative management of aneurysmal subarachnoid hemor-rhage. Part 1. Operative management. Anesth Analg 81:1060–1072, 1995

Iwasuta N, Kuroda N, Amaha K et al: Succinylcholine induced hyperkalemia in patients with ruptured central aneurysms. Anesthesiology 53:64–67, 1980

Lanier WL, Milde JH, Michenfelder JD: Cerebral stimulation following succinylcholine in dogs. Anesthesiology 64:551–559, 1986

Olsson GL, Hullen B, Hambraeus-Johnzonk K: Aspiration during anesthesia: A computer-aided study of 185,838 anesthetics. Acta Anesthesiol Scand 30:84–92, 1986

Stirt JA, Grosslight KR, Bedford RF et al: Defasciculation with metocurine prevents succinylcholine associated increases in intracranial pressure. Anesthesiology 67:50–53, 1987

Tsementzis SA, Hitchcock ER: Outcome from "rescue clipping" of ruptured intracranial aneurysms during induction of anesthesia and endotracheal intubation. J Neurol Neurosurg Psychiatry 48:160–163, 1985

C.8. What are the effects of hypoxemia and hypercapnea, such as would be seen with loss of the airway on induction, on cerebral blood flow?

Each mm Hg increase in $PaCO_2$ increases CBF 3% to 4%, when $PaCO_2$ is in the range of 20 to 80 mm Hg. Additionally, the hypoxia that will ensue if the airway is not se-cured in a timely fashion will also cause an increase in CBF once PaO_2 is <60 mm Hg (Fig. 25-1).

Hunt WE, Hess RM: Surgical risk as related to time of intervention in the repair of intracranial aneurysms. J Neurosurg 28:14–20, 1968

C.9. What is optimal fluid management for aneurysm clipping? Would you use a dextrose containing solution?

It is useful in these patients to have a CVP or PA catheter to guide fluid replacement therapy. Maintenance fluid requirements and blood loss should be replaced. One wants to avoid profound hypovolemia not only for its detrimental cardiovascular ef-fects but also because it is associated with cerebral ischemia and perioperative neuro-logic deficits due to vasospasm. Some authors advocate mild hypervolemia to maxi-mize CBF and minimize vasospasm; however, one must keep in mind the possibility of cerebral edema.

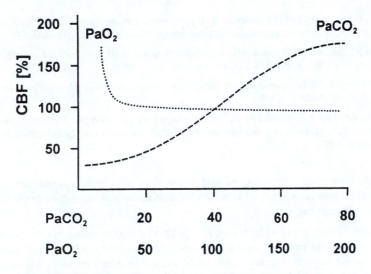

Figure 25-1. Change in cerebral blood flow as a function of arterial carbon dioxide ($PaCO_2$) and oxygen (PaO_2) tension. (Reprinted with permission from Albin MS [ed]: Textbook of Neuroanesthesia: With Neurosurgical and Neuroscience Perspectives, p 30. New York, McGraw-Hill, 1997)

In general, dextrose containing solutions should be avoided, as an increased incidence of neurologic deficits associated with hyperglycemia has been found in experimental models of focal cerebral ischemia. As many patients will be receiving dexamethasone, blood glucose should be monitored to detect hyperglycemia.

Use of crystalloid versus colloid for fluid management and which type of crystalloid solution, lactated Ringer's versus normal saline or Normosol, has long been a matter of controversy. Although some authors advocate colloid solutions to diminish the risk of brain swelling, no evidence exists that colloid use improves outcome. However, giving large amounts of hypo-osmolar (lactated Ringer's) solution may predispose to brain edema and contribute to hyponatremia, which may increase the incidence of delayed ischemic neurologic deficits.

As mannitol, which is hyperosmolar, is the preferred diuretic by which to achieve brain relaxation at our institution, Ringer's lactate has long been used without problems with brain edema or hypo-osmolality. If, however, large amounts of crystalloid are to be administered or used in any patient who has preoperative hyponatremia, normal saline would be the appropriate choice for crystalloid therapy.

A moderate degree of hemodilution to a hematocrit of 30% to 35% usually lowers blood viscosity, thus increasing cerebral blood flow. The goal is to increase oxygen delivery by increasing cerebral blood flow, without allowing the hematocrit to decrease to the degree that reduction in oxygen content negates the increase in CBF. Hematocrit, serum sodium, and serum osmolality measurements may be followed to guide fluid therapy.

Guy J, McGrath BJ, Borel CO et al: Perioperative management of aneurysmal subarachnoid hemorrhage. Part 1. Operative management. Anesth Analg 81:1060–1072, 1995

Hasan D, Wijdicks EFM, Vermuelen M: Hyponatremia is associated with cerebral ischemia in patients with aneurysmal subarachnoid hemorrhage. Ann Neurol 27:106–108, 1990

Maroon JC, Nelson PB: Hypovolemia in patients with subarachnoid hemorrhage: Therapeutic implications. Neurosurgery 4:223–226, 1979

Sieber FE, Smith DS, Traystman RJ et al: Glucose: A reevaluation of its intraoperative use. Anesthesiology 67:72–87, 1987

Solomon RA, Fink ME, Lennichon L: Early aneurysm surgery and prophylactic hypervolemic hypertensive therapy for the treatment of aneurysmal subarachnoid hemorrhage. Neurosurgery 23:669–704, 1988

C.10. *After the bone plate was removed and as the dura was being opened the surgeon complained that the brain was "tight." What could you do to achieve better brain relaxations and facilitate surgical exposure?*

Any method that rapidly decreases ICP prior to dural opening may suddenly increase transmural pressure and lead to aneurysm rupture. After dural opening, one of the fastest ways to decrease cerebral blood volume and improve exposure is through hyperventilation. Mild hypocarbia ($PaCO_2 = 30$ to 35 mm Hg can usually be established prior to dural opening, with moderate hypocarbia ($PaCO_2 = 25$ to 30 mm Hg) after dural opening. However, due to the risk of cerebral ischemia secondary to diminished CBF, normocarbia should be maintained whenever possible in patients with vasospasm, during induced hypotension, and after aneurysm clipping.

Mannitol is the most frequently used diuretic at our institution. It is given as an infusion for a total dose of 0.7 g/kg (0.25 to 1.0 g/kg). Its immediate effect is a transient rise in intravascular volume, which may pose problems in patients with impaired ventricular function. In addition, too rapid an infusion can lead to decreases in systemic vascular resistance. Its onset of diuretic action is in 10 to 15 minutes with peak effect occurring at 60 to 90 minutes. If mannitol does not produce the desired brain relaxation and the serum osmolality is >320 mOsm, additional mannitol is unlikely to produce additional effect. In those patients who may not tolerate the initial effects of mannitol, intravenous furosemide (0.25 to 0.5 mg/kg) can be substituted. Both medications can cause derangements in fluid status and serum electrolytes that require close monitoring.

Drainage of cerebrospinal from either a lumbar drain or an intraventricular catheter is usually effective in optimizing surgical exposure. One must be careful to avoid significant CSF drainage prior to dural opening to prevent either brain stem herniation or a sudden decrease in transmural pressure. Similarly, hemodynamic instability can ensue if CSF is drained too rapidly at any point in the operation.

If "tight" brain remains a problem, one must ascertain that there is no hypoxemia or hypercarbia. In addition, one should consider eliminating N_2O if it is in use and reducing the amount of volatile anesthetic, as all inhalational agents are cerebral vasodilators and may potentially increase ICP. Of course, if inhaled agents are reduced, appropriate intravenous agents should be substituted to ensure adequate anesthesia.

At the time of patient positioning, one must ensure that no impediment exists to venous outflow of the brain (i.e., that extreme flexion or rotation of the head is avoided and that no monitor cables [ECG leads] are draped across the neck).

Albin MS (ed): Textbook of Neuroanesthesia: With Neurosurgical and Neuroscience Perspectives, p 869. New York, McGraw-Hill, 1997

Guy J, McGrath BJ, Borel CO et al: Perioperative management of aneurysmal subarachnoid hemorrhage. Part 1. Operative management. Anesth Analg 81:1060–1072, 1995

Sullivan HG, Keenan RL, Isrow L: The critical importance of $PaCO_2$ during intracranial aneurysm surgery. J Neurol Neurosurg 52:426–431, 1980

C.11. What is the purpose of controlled hypotension and how is it achieved?

The goal of controlled hypotension is to decrease transmural pressure, making the aneurysm neck slack enough to allow placement of a clip without vessel rupture. Various agents have been used to achieve controlled hypotension, most commonly isoflurane, sodium nitroprusside, and esmolol. Labetalol, nitroglycerin, trimethaphan, and other agents can be used as well. The patient's preexisting medical conditions, especially coronary ischemia or poor ventricular function, should be considered when selecting agents for hypotension. In this patient, who is otherwise healthy, a sodium nitroprusside infusion is ideal for its rapid onset, easy titratability, and quick offset. An esmolol infusion can be added to augment hypotension and counteract the reflex tachycardia seen with nitroprusside. Other side-effects of nitroprusside include cyanide toxicity, rebound hypertension, and intrapulmonary shunting. Direct measurement of CVP is useful when planning to use controlled hypotension in these patients.

During controlled hypotension, MAP is usually maintained at a minimum of 50 mm Hg in previously normotensive individuals. Neurologic function monitors (EEG, SSEP, BAER) may be useful in guiding target level of MAP.

Albin MS (ed): Textbook of Neuroanesthesia: With Neurosurgical and Neuroscience Perspectives, pp 877–878. New York, McGraw-Hill, 1997

Ornstein E, Young WL, Ostapkovich N et al: Deliberate hypotension in patients with intracranial arteriovenous malformations: Esmolol compared with isoflurane and sodium nitroprusside. Anesth Analg 72:639–644, 1991

C.12. What are some of the potential drawbacks of controlled hypotension?

In the presence of vasospasm or in areas of brain retraction, cerebral perfusion pressure may be particularly compromised at low levels of mean arterial pressure. In addition, prolonged hypotension can lead to an increase in the amount of circulating vasoconstrictors so that when hypotensive agents are discontinued, rebound hypertension is dramatic. As no studies have shown that controlled hypotension reduces the incidence of intraoperative aneurysm rupture, it is reserved for brief periods around clip application and treatment following intraoperative rupture.

Ruta TS, Mutch WAC: Controlled hypotension for cerebral aneurysm surgery: Are the risks worth the benefits? J Neurosurg Anesthesiol 3:153–156, 1991

Todd M: Anesthesia for intracranial vascular surgery. ASA Refresher Course No. 211, 1995

C.13. How else might transmural pressure be decreased to allow for aneurysm clip placement?

An alternative method of producing a slack aneurysm to allow for clip placement is the use of temporary clip occlusion of one or more parent vessels. For example, to place a permanent clip on an anterior communicating artery aneurysm, a temporary clip can be placed on either the right or left anterior cerebral artery or both. Advantages of temporary clip use include a greater reduction in transmural pressure and greater ease in clipping, decreased incidence of intraoperative rupture, and less requirement for controlled hypotension.

The maximal duration of temporary clip application before a neurologic deficit occurs is unknown, but it is probably related to the location of the aneurysm and distribution of perforating vessels distal to the temporary clip. White matter and major deep nuclei are likely to be more susceptible than gray matter to temporary ischemia. Risk factors for neurologic deficit following temporary clip placement include poor preoperative neurologic condition, age >61 years, and distribution of perforating arteries in distal basilar and horizontal segments of middle cerebral artery.

Samson D, Hunt B, Bowman G et al: A clinical study of the parameters and effects of temporary arterial occlusion in the management of intracranial aneurysms. Neurosurgery 34:22–27, 1994

C.14. What methods of cerebral protection might you use during this operation?

Cerebral protection has long been a matter of much investigation and controversy. Barbiturate loading has been shown in animals to be protective against focal ischemia, but it has not been shown to improve outcome in humans. Barbiturates decrease both cerebral metabolic rate for glucose and oxygen and lower CBF and ICP. The dose is usually titrated to EEG silence or burst suppression. At doses used to suppress EEG activity, the patient may experience profound cardiovascular depression, making the presence of a PA catheter useful in guiding barbiturate administration. The dose of barbiturate necessary for cerebral protection may also prolong emergence and hinder postoperative neurologic evaluation.

Propofol is being investigated as an alternative to thiopental sodium. However, although propofol can cause EEG burst suppression, cerebral protection has not been confirmed in animal models.

Etomidate decreases cerebral metabolic rate at EEG burst suppression and prevents an increase in excitatory neurotransmitters during cerebral ischemia in animal models; however, it has been associated with a greater volume of injured brain than thiopental and control groups in focal ischemia in hypertensive rats.

Deliberate mild hypothermia (32.5° to 35.5°C) is used widely by many neuroanesthesiologists for cerebral protection, although randomized studies to assess outcome and identify side-effects are not completed. The practice at the New York Hospital-Cornell Medical Center is to allow the patient to spontaneously cool to 34.0°C, which is usually easily attained due to patient exposure to the cold operating room during induction and positioning. At this point the patient is warmed to maintain body temperature between 34.0° and 34.5°C. After the aneurysm is clipped, active rewarming is begun with the goal of achieving normothermia by the time of extubation and arrival to the intensive care unit/postanesthesia care unit. Active warming is achieved through the use of a warm-air convection blanket and fluid warmers.

Drummond JC, Cole DJ, Patel PM, Reynolds LW: Focal cerebral ischemia during anesthesia with etomidate, isoflurane, or thiopental: a comparison of the extent of cerebral injury. Neurosurgery 37:742–748, 1995

Guy J, McGrath BJ, Borel CO et al: Perioperative management of aneurysmal subarachnoid hemorrhage. Part 1. Operative management. Anesth Analg 81:1060–1072, 1995

Ravussin P, Detribolet N: Total intravenous anesthesia with propofol for burst suppression in cerebral aneurysm surgery—A preliminary report of 42 patients. Neurosurgery 32:236–240, 1990

Todd M: Anesthesia for intracranial vascular surgery. ASA Refresher Course No. 211, 1995

C.15. What are the advantages and disadvantages of intentional mild hypothermia as a means of cerebral protection?

Hypothermia causes a greater reduction in cerebral metabolic rate for glucose and oxygen than the level attained at EEG silence because its reduction of metabolism is caused by a reduction both in neuronal electrical activity and in enzyme activity related to maintenance of cellular function. Hypothermia also reduces the release of excitatory neurotransmitters. Significant reduction in infarct size after global and focal ischemia has been demonstrated in several animal studies.

Disadvantages of unintentional hypothermia documented in the literature include an increased incidence of myocardial ischemia in peripheral vascular surgery, increased incidence of postoperative wound infection in abdominal surgery, coagulopathy, prolonged drug clearance, and hyperglycemia. Studies to determine these risks and benefits of hypothermia during aneurysm surgery are planned.

Albin MS (ed): Textbook of Neuroanesthesia: With Neurosurgical and Neuroscience Perspectives, p 878. New York, McGraw-Hill, 1997

Frank SM, Beattie C, Christopherson R et al: Unintentional hypothermia is associated with postoperative myocardial ischemia. Anesthesiology 78:468–476, 1993

Kurz A, Sesler DI, Lenhardt R et al: Perioperative normothermia to reduce the incidence of surgical wound infection and shorten hospitalization. N Engl J Med 334:1209–1215, 1996

C.16. What are the indications for deep hypothermic circulatory arrest?

Hypothermic circulatory arrest at body temperature <22°C is reserved for giant aneurysms, difficult basilar artery aneurysms, and anatomically complex aneurysms that are not clippable without complete cessation of blood flow and are not amenable to the use of temporary clips. Deep hypothermic circulatory arrest requires cooperation between several services including anesthesiology, neurosurgery, cardiac surgery, and perfusionists. In addition to all the concerns mentioned regarding anesthesia for the person with an intracranial aneurysm and the need for prompt awakening for ease of neurologic assessment, deep hypothermic circulatory arrest adds the concerns regarding institution of and separation from cardiopulmonary bypass, systemic heparinization and protamine reversal, and, of course, rewarming from profound hypothermia.

Solomon RA, Smith CR, Raps EC et al: Deep hypothermic circulatory arrest for the management of complex anterior and posterior circulation aneurysms. Neurosurgery 29:732–738, 1991

C.17. What steps should be taken in the case of intraoperative rupture of an intracranial aneurysm?

The incidence of intraoperative rupture is 2% to 19%. The stage of the operation at which rupture occurs affects outcome, with rupture at induction being the worst. At any point in the operation a sudden, sustained increase in blood pressure with or without bradycardia is suggestive of rupture. If rupture is suspected on induction, one must institute measures to control ICP while maintaining CPP. Usually surgery is postponed to allow reassessment of status and prognosis.

If rupture occurs during surgical dissection, mortality is lower. The primary concern is to control bleeding while maintaining systemic perfusion. If bleeding cannot be controlled by placement of temporary clips then controlled hypotension to a MAP of 40 to 50 should be rapidly induced. Manual compression of the ipsilateral carotid artery for brief periods may be necessary. If bleeding is not controlled in a timely fashion and a significant amount of blood accumulates in the subarachnoid space, severe brain swelling that is refractory to all treatment may develop.

Guy J, McGrath BJ, Borel CO et al: Perioperative management of aneurysmal subarachnoid hemorrhage. Part 1. Operative management. Anesth Analg 81:1060–1072, 1995

Sundt TM, Whisnant JP: Subarachnoid hemorrhage from intracranial aneurysm: Surgical management and natural history of disease. N Engl J Med 299:116–122, 1978

C.18. How would you plan the emergence from an anesthetic for aneurysm clipping?

The goal is to have a patient comfortable and not coughing, straining, or subject to hypercarbia or wide variations in blood pressure.

After discontinuing all anesthetic agents and reversing neuromuscular blockade, the use of a lidocaine (1.5 mg/kg) bolus may minimize bucking and reaction to the endotracheal tube. Strict control of blood pressure must be observed especially in the presence of ischemic heart disease or in patients suspected of having multiple aneurysms. Keep the blood pressure within 20% of the patient's normal measurement.

D. Postoperative Management

D.1. Would you extubate the patient postoperatively?

Most patients who are in Hunt and Hess grades I and II can be extubated postoperatively with no need for airway support. Patients in grades IV and V usually require mechanical ventilation postoperatively, whereas grade III patients may or may not require intubation and mechanical ventilation. Patients with vertebral or basilar artery aneurysms may require airway protection secondary to cranial nerve damage and loss of protective reflexes.

If this patient was able to follow commands, was clinically recovered from the effects of muscle relaxants, and had established an adequate ventilatory pattern with return of protective airway reflexes, extubation would be appropriate.

Guy J, McGrath BJ, Borel CO et al: Perioperative management of aneurysmal subarachnoid hemorrhage. Part 1. Operative management. Anesth Analg 81:1060–1072, 1995

D.2. What would be the differential diagnosis if the patient did not return to her preoperative neurologic condition?

If the patient had a focal neurologic deficit on awakening in the operating room, the cause most likely would be a surgical one, although new-onset vasospasm is also a possibility.

If, however, the patient failed to awaken, the first step would be to ensure that all inhalational and infused anesthetics had been discontinued. Second, make sure that neuromuscular blockade was fully reversed. Make sure that the patient had been appropriately rewarmed, as hypothermia would prolong the duration of action of most intravenous medications. While considering reversal of benzodiazepines and narcotics, rule out other causes such as hypoxia, hypercarbia, hyponatremia, and hypoglycemia. Consider the possibility of intraoperative seizure, with delayed emergence being due to a postictal state. If after reversal of all anesthetic agents the patient had not awakened, a CT scan should be obtained to rule out subdural hematoma, intracranial hemorrhage, hydrocephalus, and pneumocephalus. An angiogram may also be obtained to rule out vascular occlusion.

Cottrell JE, Smith DS (eds): Anesthesia and Neurosurgery, 3rd ed, pp 392–393. St. Louis, Mosby, 1994

D.3. On postoperative day 2, the patient became disoriented and developed hemiplegia. A CT scan was performed which shows no new intracranial bleeding. What other diagnostic studies should be performed?

If transcranial Doppler is available, an increased value for cerebral arterial flow velocity would be suggestive for vasospasm. Angiography is the gold standard for the diagnosis of cerebral vasospasm and this should be obtained to confirm the diagnosis and characterize the number and location of the vessels involved. Cerebral vasospasm may be localized to the area of aneurysm rupture or in an area of the brain remote from the SAH. The worst prognosis is in those patients in whom vasospasm is diffuse. Of course, as these studies are being obtained, laboratory values should be checked to make sure no new or worsening metabolic derangement is contributing to the neurologic deterioration.

D.4. What is cerebral vasospasm and what causes it?

Vasospasm, which occurs in 35% of patients with SAH, is a segmental or diffuse narrowing of the lumen of one or more intracranial arteries. It is the most common cause of delayed cerebral ischemia, and may be seen angiographically in 60% of patients, even if clinical manifestations are not apparent.

The severity of vasospasm is apparently related to the amount and location of subarachnoid blood. Injection of blood into the subarachnoid space causes vasospasm in experimental animals and antifibrinolytics apparently worsen the spasm. On a molecular level one theory is that oxyhemoglobin causes the production of superoxide radicals which lead to a decrease in nitric oxide (NO) production in endothelial cells. This decrease in NO increases protein kinase C and an intracellular calcium, resulting in myofilament activation and vasospasm. Other theories involve prostaglandins and lipid peroxidases.

Findlay JM, Macdonald RL, Weir BKA: Current concepts of pathophysiology and management of cerebral vasospasm following aneurysmal subarachnoid hemorrhage. Cerebrovasc Brain Metab Rev 3:336–361, 1991

Kassell NF, Sasaki T, Colohan AR: Cerebral vasospasm following aneurysmal subarachnoid hemorrhage. Stroke 16:562–572, 1985

Mayberg M, Batjer H, Dacey R et al: Guidelines for management of aneurysmal subarachnoid hemorrhage. Special Report. Stroke 25:2315–2328, 1994

Mayberg MR, Okada T, Bark TH: The role of hemoglobin in arterial narrowing after subarachnoid hemorrhage. J Neurosurg 72:634–640, 1990

Vollrath AM, Weir BKA, Macdonald RL et al: Intracellular mechanisms involved in the responses of cerebrovascular smooth-muscle cells to hemoglobin. J Neurosurg 80:261–268, 1994

Wilkins RH: Cerebral vasospasm. Crit Rev Neurobiol 6:51–77, 1990

D.5. What are pathophysiologic changes seen in vasospasm?

Structurally, leukocytes, red blood cell, and macrophages are seen in arterial walls. Inflammatory mediators, such as eicosanoids, interleukin-1, and immune complexes are increased. Eventually, the vessel wall thickens, and smooth muscle proliferation and collagen deposition accompany degenerative changes in the tunica intima and media.

Functionally, autoregulation is often impaired, perhaps correlating to the degree of vasospasm. CBF in some areas appears to be pressure dependent, hence the reasoning behind hypertensive therapy.

McGrath BJ, Guy J, Borel CO et al: Perioperative management of aneurysmal subarachnoid hemorrhage. Part 2. Postoperative management. Anesth Analg 81:1295–1302, 1995

D.6. How is the diagnosis of cerebral vasospasm made?

The clinical diagnosis of cerebral vasospasm is made when the patient experiences an altered level of consciousness (drowsiness, disorientation) or a new focal neurologic deficit. These may be accompanied by increasing headache, meningismus, and fever. Vasospasm is rare in the first 3 days following SAH. It reaches peak incidence at 3 to 10 days, and usually resolves by 10 to 14 days after SAH. In this patient, the new onset of hemiplegia suggests that the middle cerebral artery is involved. If vessels in the posterior fossa are involved, respiratory and hemodynamic abnormalities may develop.

The differential diagnosis includes rebleeding, hydrocephalus, seizure, hyponatremia, and drug effects. Transcranial Doppler (TCD) cerebral blood flow velocity >120 cm/sec in association with a new focal neurologic deficit is usually sufficient to make the diagnosis of cerebral vasospasm; however, a change in TCD values over time may be more useful than an absolute value. Cerebral blood flow velocity >200 cm/sec is associated with a high risk of cerebral infarct, whereas a velocity <100 cm/sec indicates that cerebral vasospasm is unlikely.

Angiographic cerebral vasospasm can be found in 60% of patients following subarachnoid hemorrhage but only 50% of these patients will develop clinical focal neurologic deficits.

Albin MS (ed): Textbook of Neuroanesthesia: With Neurosurgical and Neuroscience Perspectives, p 852. New York, McGraw-Hill, 1997

McGrath BJ, Guy J, Borel CO et al: Perioperative management of aneurysmal subarachnoid hemorrhage. Part 2. Postoperative management. Anesth Analg 81:1295–1302, 1995

D.7. What steps can be taken to prevent cerebral vasospasm?

Calcium channel blockers are standard prophylactic therapy to prevent vasospasm. The mechanism is unknown, but presumably calcium channel blockers aid in maintaining cellular integrity by preventing calcium entry into ischemic cells. Nimodipine, taken orally, improves neurologic outcome. Patients given nimodipine have no change in overall incidence of vasospasm, but they have a lower incidence of severe narrowing. In addition, although no improvement is found in mortality, there is improvement in outcome for survivors.

Nicardipine, an intravenous agent, showed a lower incidence of vasospasm, but no improvement in outcome versus a placebo group; however, both groups received hypertensive, hypervolemic, hemodilution (HHH) therapy. The main complication of calcium channel blocker therapy is hypotension (0% to 8%), which may make it difficult to achieve HHH therapy.

Other steps to limit cerebral vasospasm include the removal of subarachnoid blood as quickly as possible, instillation of thrombolytic agents (e.g., urokinase) and use of pharmacologic agents to reduce inflammatory response, high-dose glucocorticoids, ibuprofen, and 21-amino-steroids (e.g., tirilizad), which inhibit iron-dependent lipid peroxidation. However, urokinase may increase likelihood of rebleeding.

Haley EC, Kassell NF, Torner JC et al: A randomized, controlled trial of high-dose intravenous nicardipine in aneurysmal subarachnoid hemorrhage. J Neurosurg 78:537–547, 1993

Jan M, Bucheit F, Tremoulet M: Therapeutic trial of intravenous nimodipine in patients with established cerebral vasospasm from rupture of intracranial aneurysms. Neurosurgery 23:154–157, 1988

Petruk KC, West M, Mohr G et al: Nimodipine treatment in poor-grade aneurysm patients. J Neurosurg 68:505–517, 1988

Pickard JD, Murray GD, Illingworth R et al: Effect of oral nimodipine on cerebral infarction and outcome after subarachnoid hemorrhage: British Aneurysm Nimodipine Trial. BMJ 298:636–642, 1989

D.8. What treatments can be undertaken once a diagnosis of vasospasm is made?

Treatment for cerebral vasospasm is multifactorial and includes continuation of prophylactic measures. HHH therapy is a plan to augment cerebral blood flow past the stenotic areas. It begins with hypervolemic hypertension, with intravascular volume expansion with crystalloid or colloid to increase cardiac output. Some recommended target values are CVP 10 to 12 mm Hg, pulmonary capillary wedge pressure (PCWP) 15 to 18 mm Hg, cardiac index 3.0 to 3.5 l/min/M^2, and hematocrit 30% to 35%. Various blood pressure targets have been reported but a reasonable plan is systolic blood pressure 160 to 200 mm Hg if the aneurysm is clipped, 120 to 150 mm Hg if unclipped. Vasoactive infusions are added if hypervolemia alone is inadequate. Endpoints of therapy are resolution of neurologic deficits or occurrence of complications of therapy, such as pulmonary edema (26%), myocardial ischemia, and rebleeding or rupture of a secondary aneurysm. A PA catheter is usually indicated.

Fluid used for HHH should be isotonic and have enough sodium to avoid hyponatremia. Vasopressin or fludrocortisone may be administered to counteract excessive sodium and fluid loss.

Other treatments for vasospasm, including intraarterial verapamil (or other vasodilator) infusions or angioplasty, are usually reserved for those cases that fail HHH therapy.

Kassell NF, Helm G, Simmons N et al: Treatment of cerebral vasospasm with intra-arterial papaverine. J Neurosurg 77:848–852, 1992

Livingston K, Hopkins LN: Intraarterial papaverine as an adjunct to transluminal angioplasty for vasospasm induced by subarachnoid hemorrhage. AJNR AM J Neuroradiol 14:346–347, 1993

McGrath BJ, Guy J, Borel CO et al: Perioperative management of aneurysmal subarachnoid hemorrhage. Part 2. Postoperative management. Anesth Analg 81:1295–1302, 1995

Newell DW, Eskridge JM, Mayberg MR et al: Angioplasty for the treatment of symptomatic vasospasm following subarachnoid hemorrhage. J Neurosurg 71:654–660, 1989

D.9. What are other neurologic complications following SAH and aneurysm clipping?

Hydrocephalus, manifesting with a gradual decrease in level of consciousness, occurs in 25% of patients surviving SAH. Diagnosis is confirmed by CT scan. Treatment is by ventricular drainage.

Seizures, which occur in 13% of patients with SAH, may herald rebleeding or vasospasm. Seizures cause an increase in MAP, CBF, ICP, and lactate production, predisposing to rebleeding in those patients with unclipped aneurysms and cerebral ischemia in those patients with vasospasm. Most patients receive prophylactic anticonvulsants.

Hyponatremia occurs in 10% to 34% of patients with SAH in a time course that parallels that of vasospasm. It may be due to syndrome of inappropriate antidiuretic hormone secretion (SIADH), "cerebral salt wasting," or prolonged or excessive mannitol use. Cerebral salt wasting syndrome is thought to be mediated by release of atrial natriuretic factor for the hypothalamus secondary to distention of the cerebral ventricles from hydrocephalus. In these patients, fluid restriction is not the treatment of choice, as hypovolemia may predispose to vasospasm. Instead patients should be treated with an isotonic salt containing fluid.

Finally, patients may experience brain swelling or edema, which is treated with mannitol and/or dexamethasone.

Albin MS (ed): Textbook of Neuroanesthesia: With Neurosurgical and Neuroscience Perspectives, p 861. New York, McGraw-Hill, 1997

Hart RG, Byer JA, Slaughter JR et al: Occurrence and implications of seizures in subarachnoid hemorrhage due to ruptured intracranial aneurysms. Neurosurgery 8:417–421, 1982

Heros RC: Acute hydrocephalus after subarachnoid hemorrhage. Stroke 20:715–717, 1989

Nelson PB, Seif SM, Maroon JC et al: Hyponatremia in intracranial disease: Perhaps not the syndrome in inappropriate secretion of antidiuretic hormone (SIADH). J Neurosurg 55:938–941, 1981

D.10. What other organ systems may manifest problems postoperatively in aneurysm clipping patients?

The lungs can be affected by pneumonia or neurogenic pulmonary edema, where disruption of the pulmonary capillary membrane occurs secondary to increased sympathetic nervous system activity. Because of inactivity, patients may be predisposed to developing deep venous thrombosis and pulmonary embolism. Patients may have fever secondary to subarachnoid blood, which may make workup of postoperative infection more difficult. In addition, as in most head injured patients, those with subarachnoid hemorrhage may have increased metabolic rate.

McGrath BJ, Guy J, Borel CO et al: Perioperative management of aneurysmal subarachnoid hemorrhage. Part 2. Postoperative management. Anesth Analg 81:1295–1302, 1995

Reflex Sympathetic Dystrophy

26

Vinod Malhotra

A 35-year-old man complained of diffuse burning pain in the left arm for the last 6 months following blunt trauma. His left hand felt colder than the right and occasionally the fingertips turned blue.

A. Medical Disease and Differential Diagnosis

1. What is the most likely diagnosis in this man?
2. What is reflex sympathetic dystrophy?
3. How does causalgia differ from neuralgia?
4. What is the pathophysiology of reflex sympathetic dystrophy?

B. Treatment

1. How would you treat this patient?
2. What is the sympathetic nerve supply to the arm?
3. Where is the stellate ganglion located? What are its important anatomic relationships?
4. What are the anatomic landmarks used in the stellate ganglion block?
5. What are the clinical signs of stellate ganglion block?
6. What is Horner's syndrome?
7. Following stellate ganglion block, this patient reports no significant change in pain in the arm despite Horner's syndrome. Is the pain psychogenic in this patient?
8. What type of nerve fibers are interrupted in a stellate ganglion block?
9. What are the two major classes of local anesthetics? Describe the major differences in their clinical pharmacology.
10. Describe some of the significant physiochemical properties of commonly available local anesthetics.
11. How does pH affect the action of local anesthetics?
12. How does the addition of epinephrine to commercially available premixed solutions affect the efficacy of local anesthetics?
13. Does increased concentration of the local anesthetic speed the induction of a block?
14. What are the effects of local anesthetic mixtures in clinical practice?

C. Complications

1. What are the possible complications of stellate ganglion block?
2. What is the systemic toxicity of local anesthetics?
3. How do you treat the systemic toxicity of local anesthetic drugs?

A. Medical Disease and Differential Diagnosis

A.1. What is the most likely diagnosis in this man?

The most likely diagnosis in this man is post-traumatic reflex sympathetic dystrophy (RSD). In recent years, this syndrome has been referred to as "sympathetic mediated pain" (SMP), then sympathetic maintained pain (SMP), and complex peripheral pain syndrome (CPPS). According to the most recent terminology, complex regional pain syndrome (CRPS) is divided into type I (RSD) and type II (causalgia).

International Association for the Study of Pain. Subcommittee on Taxonomy: Classification of chronic pain, description of chronic pain syndromes and definitions of pain terms. Pain 24:528–529, 1986

Stanton-Hicks M, Janis W, Hassenburch S: Reflex sympathetic dystrophy: Changing concepts and taxonomy. Pain 63:127–133, 1995

A.2. What is reflex sympathetic dystrophy?

Reflex sympathetic dystrophy is a syndrome characterized by diffuse burning pain, vasomotor and sudomotor changes, and hyperalgesia or hyperesthesia. It is usually aggravated by cold and emotional factors and follows trauma. It may progress to limb edema, muscular dysfunction and atrophy, and osteoporotic changes in the bones. Causalgia is one of the clinical entities included in this group of diseases and strictly the term should be used for the sympathetic dystrophy following blunt injury to a nerve trunk. Sympathetic dystrophies have been described under different names, as shown in Table 26-1, that have often been used interchangeably.

Abram SE: Pain Clinic Manual, pp 121–126. Philadelphia, JB Lippincott, 1990

Payne R: Neuropathic pain syndromes, with special reference to causalgia and reflex sympathetic dystrophy. Clin J Pain 2:59–73, 1986

Poacci P, Maresca M: Reflex sympathetic dystrophies and algodystrophies: Historical and pathogenic considerations. Pain 31:137–146, 1987

Raj PP: Practical Management of Pain, 2nd ed, pp 312–328. Chicago, Year Book Medical Publishers, 1992

A.3. How does causalgia differ from neuralgia?

The major differences are indicated in Table 26-2.

Raj PP: Practical Management of Pain, 2nd ed, pp 312–328. Chicago, Year Book Medical Publishers, 1992

Table 26-1. Names of Sympathetic Dystrophies

Causalgia — Minor / Major
Sudeck's atrophy
Post-traumatic pain syndrome
Sympathalgia
Shoulder-hand syndrome
Reflex sympathetic dystrophy

Table 26-2. The Differences Between Causalgia and Neuralgia

	CAUSALGIA	NEURALGIA
Time	Pain sustained	Usually paroxysmal
Distribution	Diffuse	Follows nerve distribution
Character	Burning	Sharp, shooting
Associated findings	Vasomotor changes	Usually absent
	Sudomotor changes	Usually absent
	Trophic changes	Disuse atrophy, may be seen

A.4. What is the pathophysiology of reflex sympathetic dystrophy?

As the name implies, the condition is characterized by sympathetic dysfunction, and sympathetic blockade alleviates pain in most of the patients. However, the cause of pain and hyperpathia in causalgia and reflex sympathetic dystrophy is not completely understood. Several hypotheses have been postulated to explain the phenomenon, but any single hypothesis fails to explain all the findings and responses to treatment in all the patients. These hypotheses include abnormal discharges in sympathetic and nociceptive afferents produced by trauma; sensitization of peripheral sensory receptors produced by sympathetic hyperactivity; formation of ephapses (artificial synapses) following peripheral nerve injury; and spontaneous neuronal ectopy at the site of demyelination or axonal injury. It is likely that more than one sequence of events takes place in a patient, giving rise to a mixed clinical picture. Finally, the psychological component and neuromodulation cannot be discernibly separated.

Abram SE: Pain Clinic Manual, pp 121–126. Philadelphia, JB Lippincott, 1990

Payne R: Neuropathic pain syndromes, with special reference to causalgia and reflex sympathetic dystrophy. Clin J Pain 2:59–73, 1986

Poacci P, Maresca M: Reflex sympathetic dystrophies and algodystrophies: Historical and pathogenic considerations. Pain 31:137–146, 1987

Raj PP: Practical Management of Pain, 2nd ed, pp 312–328. Chicago, Year Book Medical Publishers, 1992

B. Treatment

B.1. How would you treat this patient?

The recommended treatment is sympathetic blockade, which should be instituted early and in conjunction with physiotherapy. The two main factors that favorably affect the outcome of the treatment are early diagnosis and treatment and concomitant physiotherapy.

Treatment of choice in this patient is left stellate ganglion block with a local anesthetic. Other forms of therapy that have been tried with some success and may be considered are neurolytic or surgical sympathectomy; intravenous regional sympathetic block using guanethidine (10 to 20 mg), reserpine (1 to 2 mg), or bretylium (1 mg/kg) or lidocaine (0.5%); oral sympatholytic agents, such as propranolol, guanethidine, prazosin, and phenoxybenzamine; corticosteroids, tricyclic antidepressants, anticonvulsants and narcotic analgesics; and transcutaneous electrical nerve stimulation.

Ford SR, Forrest WH Jr, Eltherington L: The treatment of reflex sympathetic dystrophy with intravenous regional bretylium. Anesthesiology 68:137–140, 1988

Payne R: Neuropathic pain syndromes, with special reference to causalgia and reflex sympathetic dystrophy. Clin J Pain 2:59–73, 1986

Raj PP: Practical Management of Pain, 2nd ed, pp 312–328. Chicago, Year Book Medical Publishers, 1992

Wang JK, Johnson KA, Ilstrup DM: Sympathetic block for reflex sympathetic dystrophy. Pain 23:13–17, 1985

B.2. What is the sympathetic nerve supply to the arm?

The preganglionic sympathetic outflow to the upper extremity is derived from T2 to T9 and these fibers synapse with postganglionic fibers in the stellate ganglion. Therefore, a stellate ganglion block interrupts sympathetic outflow to the upper extremity.

Raj PP: Practical Management of Pain, 2nd ed, pp 312–328. Chicago, Year Book Medical Publishers, 1992

B.3. Where is the stellate ganglion located? What are its important anatomic relationships?

The stellate ganglion is a star-shaped (hence, the name) sympathetic ganglion formed by the fusion of the inferior cervical and the first thoracic ganglia. In some instances the fusion may not occur or the shape is different. It usually measures 2.5 cm × 1.5 cm × 0.5 cm and lies between the base of the transverse process of the seventh cervical vertebra and the neck of the first rib. It is situated behind the carotid sheath, ventral to the longus colli muscle, behind the vertebral artery, and lateral to the body of the vertebra. The subclavian, the inferior thyroid, and the first intercostal arteries are in close proximity to the ganglion and so is the recurrent laryngeal nerve. The left pleura is 1 to 2 cm below it, whereas the right pleura is in closer proximity. The efferent nerves from the stellate ganglion supply the sympathetics to the head, neck, and upper extremity.

Miller RD (ed): Anesthesia, 4th ed, p 2356. New York, Churchill Livingstone, 1994

Moore DC: Regional Block, p 123. Springfield, IL, Charles C Thomas, 1981

Raj PP: Practical Management of Pain, 2nd ed, pp 312–328. Chicago, Year Book Medical Publishers, 1992

B.4. What are the anatomic landmarks used in the stellate ganglion block?

The landmarks used in the stellate ganglion block are the jugular notch of the sternum, the sternocleidomastoid muscle, the cricoid cartilage, and Chassaignac's tubercle. In a supine patient with neck extended, a mark placed approximately 3.5 cm from the midline along the jugular notch and the same distance above the clavicle, should overlie the transverse process of the seventh vertebra and the medial border of the sternocleidomastoid muscle. This marking is further confirmed by palpating the cricoid cartilage, which lies at the level of the sixth cervical vertebra, and the anterior tubercle on the sixth vertebral transverse process, which is the most prominent tubercle in the neck (Chassaignac's tubercle).

Miller RD (ed): Anesthesia, 4th ed, p 2356. New York, Churchill Livingstone, 1994

Moore DC: Regional Block, p 127. Springfield, IL, Charles C Thomas, 1981

Raj PP: Practical Management of Pain, 2nd ed, pp 312–328. Chicago, Year Book Medical Publishers, 1992

B.5. What are the clinical signs of stellate ganglion block?

The clinical signs of a successful stellate ganglion block include the following on the ipsilateral side:

- Eye—ptosis, narrowing of palpebral fissure, miosis, enophthalmos, conjunctival injection, lacrimation
- Face and neck—anhidrosis, elevated local temperature, nasal stuffiness
- Arm—increased temperature, plethysmographic evidence of improved cutaneous blood flow

Miller RD (ed): Anesthesia, 4th ed, p 2356. New York, Churchill Livingstone, 1994

Moore DC: Regional Block, p 131. Springfield, IL, Charles C Thomas, 1981

Raj PP: Practical Management of Pain, 2nd ed, pp 312–328. Chicago, Year Book Medical Publishers, 1992

B.6. What is Horner's syndrome?

Horner's syndrome is a clinical entity characterized by the triad of ptosis, miosis, and anhidrosis. Usually seen in association with a disease process involving the cervical sympathetics, it is a classic sign of stellate ganglion block.

Miller RD (ed): Anesthesia, 4th ed, p 2356. New York, Churchill Livingstone, 1994

Moore DC: Regional Block, p 131. Springfield, IL, Charles C Thomas, 1981

Raj PP: Practical Management of Pain, 2nd ed, pp 312–328. Chicago, Year Book Medical Publishers, 1992

B.7. Following stellate ganglion block, this patient reports no significant change in pain in the arm despite Horner's syndrome. Is the pain psychogenic in this patient?

Not necessarily. Horner's syndrome indicates only the interruption of sympathetic supply to the head and neck. Unless it is accompanied by objective changes in the arm, it does not indicate sympathetic nerve block of the upper extremity.

Moore DC: Regional Block, p 131. Springfield, IL, Charles C Thomas, 1981

Raj PP: Practical Management of Pain, 2nd ed, pp 312–328. Chicago, Year Book Medical Publishers, 1992

B.8. What type of nerve fibers are interrupted in a stellate ganglion block?

The stellate ganglion block results in interruption of the preganglionic, thinly myelinated, type B fibers, as well as the postganglionic, unmyelinated, type C fibers.

Casale R, Glynn CJ, Buonocoe M: Autonomic variations after stellate ganglion block: Are they evidence of an autonomic afference? Journal of Functional Neurology 5:245–246, 1990

Raj PP: Practical Management of Pain, 2nd ed, pp 312–328. Chicago, Year Book Medical Publishers, 1992

B.9. What are the two major classes of local anesthetics? Describe the major differences in their clinical pharmacology.

The two major categories of clinically employed local anesthetics are esters and amides. The esters are hydrolyzed in the plasma by pseudocholinesterase; the amides are biotransformed in the liver. Although infrequent, local anesthetic toxicity is encountered more commonly in the ester group because of the para-aminobenzoic acid moiety. True allergic reactions to amides are rare. In most instances, they are caused by preservatives in the solution. Each of the two groups of local anesthetics contains drugs with varying degrees of rate of onset, duration of neural blockade, potency, and toxicity.

Raj PP (ed): Practical Management of Pain, 2nd ed, pp 685–700. Chicago, Year Book Medical Publishers, 1992

B.10. Describe some of the significant physiochemical properties of commonly available local anesthetics.

Ionization and protein binding are the two physiochemical properties of local anesthetics that are of most clinical significance. The commonly used local anesthetics are weakly basic tertiary amines that are lipid soluble and unstable in water. They are dispensed as acidic salts, because the ionized form, which is soluble in water, is stable. Therefore, the aqueous solution contains the ionized (cation) form of the local anesthetic in dissociation equilibrium with the unionized (free base) form depending on the pH of the medium.

$$R \equiv NH^+ \rightleftharpoons R \equiv N + H^+$$

Cation   Base

The degree of ionization is determined by the pH of the solution and the pKa of the local anesthetic.

$$pKa = pH - \log \frac{\text{nonionized base}}{\text{cation}}$$

The pKa of most local anesthetics is >7.4 (see Table 26-3). The free base, being lipid

Table 26-3. Physiochemical Properties of Commonly Used Local Anesthetics

LOCAL ANESTHETIC	pKa	PROTEIN BINDING (%)
Esters		
Procaine	8.9	5.8
Chloroprocaine	8.7	—
Tetracaine	8.5	75.6
Amides		
Lidocaine	7.9	64.3
Mepivacaine	7.6	77.5
Bupivacaine	8.1	95.6
Etidocaine	7.7	94

soluble, is important for diffusion of the anesthetic across membranes, whereas the cationic form is mainly responsible for neural blockade, owing to its binding to the neural membrane. Protein binding of the drug affects its local binding and diffusion as well as systemic elimination. With the exception of procaine and chloroprocaine, the commonly employed local anesthetics are highly protein bound (see Table 26-3).

Raj PP (ed): Practical Management of Pain, 2nd ed, pp 685–700. Chicago, Year Book Medical Publishers, 1992

B.11. *How does pH affect the action of local anesthetics?*

$$R \equiv NH \rightleftharpoons R \equiv N + H^+$$

Cation   Base

The degree of ionization of a local anesthetic is dependent on the pH of the solution. As the pH is lowered, more of the drug is ionized to the cationic form, which is poorly diffusible across the nerve membranes, thereby reducing the efficacy of the block. This is seen clinically when local anesthetics are injected into an infected region where the tissue pH is low. The concentration of local anesthetic base determines the quantity of local anesthetic that reaches the nerve membrane. The relative proportion of base is increased by raising the pH of the solution; alkalinizing a local anesthetic solution enhances drug penetration.

De Jong RH: Fundamentals of local anesthesia: Applied physiology. ASA Refresher Courses in Anesthesiology 2:49–64, 1974

Raj PP (ed): Practical Management of Pain, 2nd ed, pp 685–700. Chicago, Year Book Medical Publishers, 1992

B.12. *How does the addition of epinephrine to commercially available premixed solutions affect the efficacy of local anesthetics?*

The addition of epinephrine to a local anesthetic increases the duration and intensity of a block. However, in commercially available premixed solutions containing epinephrine, antioxidants are added to preserve epinephrine and the result is a lower buffered pH of the solution. This lowering of pH can result in decreased efficacy of the local anesthetic. Best results are achieved by adding the desired concentration of epinephrine to the local anesthetic solution just prior to injection.

Moore DC: The pH of local anesthetic solutions: Technical communication. Anesth Analg 60:833–834, 1981

Raj PP (ed): Practical Management of Pain, 2nd ed, pp 685–700. Chicago, Year Book Medical Publishers, 1992

B.13. *Does increased concentration of the local anesthetic speed the induction of a block?*

The rate of onset of local anesthesia bears a linear relationship to the logarithm of the dose. Therefore, an increase in concentration produces only a modest decrease in time of onset. However, a higher concentration of local anesthetic is more effective in blocking larger nerve fibers. For the same total volume, a higher concentration of local anesthetic results in an increase in the dose administered, thereby increasing the risk of systemic toxic effects.

De Jong RH: Fundamentals of local anesthesia: Applied physiology. ASA Refresher Courses in Anesthesiology 2:49–64, 1974

Raj PP (ed): Practical Management of Pain, 2nd ed, pp 685–700. Chicago, Year Book Medical Publishers, 1992

B.14. *What are the effects of local anesthetic mixtures in clinical practice?*

A combination of two local anesthetics can be used to try to achieve a decrease in time of onset and latency along with an increase in duration of the block. Depending on the site of the block, this may not be achieved each time.

The toxic effects of the two agents are essentially additive. It has also been shown that peak blood levels of two different agents, used concomitantly in a mixture, can occur at different intervals. The amide local anesthetics can inhibit the rate of hydrolysis of chloroprocaine. Occasionally, unsatisfactory anesthesia produced by chloroprocaine and bupivacaine has been attributed to the low *p*H of chloroprocaine (3.7) increasing the ionized fraction of bupivacaine.

Cohen SE: The rational use of local anesthetic mixtures. Regional Anesthesia 4(3):11–12, 1979

Raj PP, Rosenblatt R, Miller J: Dynamics of local anesthetic compounds in regional anesthesia. Anesth Analg 56:110–117, 1977

C. Complications

C.1. *What are the possible complications of stellate ganglion block?*

Although complications appear infrequently, the more common complications of this block are:

- Intra-arterial injection—toxic reaction, hematoma
- Recurrent laryngeal nerve paralysis—hoarseness of voice
- Brachial plexus block—motor weakness
- Pneumothorax—respiratory distress

A rare complication that can occur is an accidental subarachnoid injection.

Miller RD (ed): Anesthesia, 4th ed, p 2356. New York, Churchill Livingstone, 1994

Moore DC: Regional Block, pp 131–134. Springfield, IL, Charles C Thomas, 1981

Raj PP: Practical Management of Pain, 2nd ed, pp 312–328. Chicago, Year Book Medical Publishers, 1992

C.2. *What is the systemic toxicity of local anesthetics?*

The systemic toxic effects of local anesthetics are related to blood levels, and they are manifested mainly in the central nervous system and the cardiovascular system. As a rule, the central nervous system effects precede the cardiovascular system toxic manifestations.

Central Nervous System Effects
Light-headedness, dizziness, tinnitus, visual disturbances, drowsiness, disorientation, slurred speech, muscle twitching, generalized grand mal seizure, electroencephalographic changes. Blood levels of local anesthetics associated with central nervous system changes in man are:

- Procaine, 20 μg/ml
- Lidocaine, mepivacaine, prilocaine, 5 to 10 μg/ml

Table 26-4. Cardiovascular Effects of Lidocaine

BLOOD LEVEL µg/ml LIDOCAINE	ECG CHANGES	HEMODYNAMIC EFFECTS
<5	—	—
5–10	↑ PR interval ↑ QRS duration Sinus bradycardia	↓ Myocardial contraction ↓ Cardiac output Vasodilation
>10	↑ PR interval ↑ QRS duration Sinus bradycardia AV block Asystole	↓ Myocardial contraction ↓ Cardiac output Circulatory collapse

- Tetracaine, bupivacaine, etidocaine, 1.5 to 4 µg/ml
- Lowering the $PaCO_2$ by hyperventilation increases the convulsive threshold dose of a local anesthetic drug

Cardiovascular Effects

See Table 26-4.

Miller RD (ed): Anesthesia, 4th ed, pp 489–521. New York, Churchill Livingstone, 1994

Raj PP: Practical Management of Pain, 2nd ed, pp 685–700. Chicago, Year Book Medical Publishers, 1992

C.3. How do you treat the systemic toxicity of local anesthetic drugs?

The principles of treatment include the following:

- Secure and maintain airway
- Ensure adequate oxygenation and ventilation

Control seizures with the following:

- Diazepam, 0.1 to 0.2 mg/kg, intravenously
- Thiopental sodium, 1 to 2 mg/kg, intravenously
- Succinylcholine 1 mg/kg, intravenously (if the above measures fail)
- Provide circulatory support

Miller RD (ed): Anesthesia, 4th ed, pp 489–521. New York, Churchill Livingstone, 1994

27 Brachial Plexus Block

Vinod Malhotra

A 58-year-old machinist was brought for emergency repair of lacerated tendons and nerves in his right hand caused by a crush injury at work. He was given 75 mg of meperidine intramuscularly in the emergency room on arrival. No significant medical history was found other than current psychiatric treatment for depression.

A. Medical Disease and Differential Diagnosis

1. What were the presenting problems in this patient?
2. Do you have any concerns about the use of meperidine in the emergency room?
3. What are the possible drug interactions between meperidine and the commonly used psychotropic drugs?
4. What are the anesthetic implications of tricyclic antidepressants and monoamine oxidase (MAO) inhibitors?
5. In an elective case, would you discontinue the use of tricyclic or MAO inhibitors preoperatively?
6. What precautions should be taken to anesthetize a patient on MAO inhibitors?

B. Preoperative Evaluation and Preparation

1. What premedication would you order?

C. Intraoperative Management

1. What anesthetic technique would you employ?
2. Describe the formation and major branches of the brachial plexus.
3. What regional technique would you choose to block the brachial plexus in this patient?
4. What are the advantages and disadvantages of axillary, interscalene, subclavian, and supraclavicular nerve blocks?
5. Describe the landmarks and procedure of the axillary nerve block.
6. Describe the landmarks and the procedure of interscalene nerve block.
7. What are the most commonly missed nerves in axillary block and in interscalene nerve block? How can you circumvent this problem?
8. Following an axillary block, the patient complained of tourniquet pain. How would you manage this problem?
9. What local anesthetic agent would you use and why?
10. What is the maximal safe dose of the local anesthetics?
11. What would be your choice of technique if a bilateral block were required?

D. Postoperative Management

1. In the recovery room, the patient complained of shortness of breath. How would you manage this problem?

2. How do you treat a systemic reaction to local anesthetic?
3. On the second postoperative day the patient complained of persistent numbness and paresthesia in the right forearm and the hand. How would you manage this neurologic dysfunction?

A. Medical Disease and Differential Diagnosis

A.1. What were the presenting problems in this patient?

This patient presented for emergency surgery for a crush injury to the hand. Blood loss, which might be significant, was unknown. He probably had a full stomach. A possibility of recent ingestion of alcohol or a central nervous system (CNS) depressant drug should be entertained. It is important to determine the type of drug therapy he received for his psychiatric illness.

A.2. Do you have any concerns about the use of meperidine in the emergency room?

In this patient, meperidine presents several potential problems. Meperidine would potentiate the effects of recently ingested alcohol or any CNS depressant drug, which might lead to respiratory depression. If the patient has bled significantly, meperidine may induce hypotension. The emetic side-effects of meperidine, along with its effect on the gastroesophageal sphincter tone, may increase the likelihood of nausea and vomiting in this patient. It would be prudent to determine which psychotropic medication the patient was taking, because the potential for serious drug interaction exists.

Miller RD (ed): Anesthesia, 4th ed, pp 291–387. New York, Churchill Livingstone, 1994

A.3. What are the possible drug interactions between meperidine and the commonly used psychotropic drugs?

The psychotropic agents commonly employed and of concern to the anesthesiologist include antidepressants, antipsychotic agents, and lithium. This patient is most likely on antidepressants. Two types of antidepressants are available—tricyclics and MAO inhibitors. The commonly used tricyclics include imipramine, amitriptyline, desipramine, nortryptyline, doxepin, and protryptyline. Tricyclics enhance the effects of meperidine, namely analgesia, respiratory depression, and cholinergic side-effects. MAO inhibitors are usually the second line of antidepressants. They include tranylcypromine, phenelzine, pargyline, nialamide, furazolidone, and isocarboxazid. In the presence of MAO inhibitors, meperidine may cause profound respiratory depression, hypotension, agitation, excitement, restlessness, hypertension, headache, rigidity, convulsions, hyperpyrexia, and coma.

Miller RD (ed): Anesthesia, 4th ed, pp 291–387. New York, Churchill Livingstone, 1994

Wells DG, Bjorksten AR: Monoamine oxidase inhibitors revisited. Can J Anaesth 36:64–74, 1989

A.4. What are the anesthetic implications of tricyclic antidepressants and monoamine oxidase (MAO) inhibitors?

Tricyclic antidepressants block the re-uptake of norepinephrine and serotonin or dopamine at the presynaptic nerve endings. This predisposes the patients on chronic tri-

Table 27-1. Some Interactions Between Tricyclic Antidepressants and Drugs Used in Anesthesia

TRICYCLIC ANTIDEPRESSANTS	INTERACTION
Narcotics	↑ Analgesia
	↑ Respiratory depression
Barbiturates	↑ Sleep time
Anticholinergics	↑ Central activity
	↑ Peripheral activity
Sympathomimetics	↑ Effect of direct-acting agents

(Reprinted with permission from Smith NT, Corbascio AN [eds]: Drug Interactions in Anesthesia, 2nd ed, p. 268. Philadelphia, Lea & Febiger, 1986)

cyclic therapy to perioperative hypotension. The response to pressor agents is exaggerated two to ten times. Therefore, a possibility of hypertensive crisis exists with the usual doses of sympathomimetic amines. Other interactions are summarized in Table 27-1. It is conceivable that additive toxicity exists when drugs with similar effects on presynaptic nerve endings (cocaine, pancuronium, ketamine) are used concomitantly. Ventricular tachycardia and fibrillation have been described when halothane and pancuronium were used together in patients receiving tricyclic antidepressants.

Monoamine oxidase inhibitors prevent deamination of serotonin, norepinephrine, and dopamine. This causes an exaggerated response with the likelihood of hypertensive crisis, especially when indirect-acting pressors (e.g., ephedrine or metaraminol) are used. Potentially lethal interactions (although uncommon) occur with narcotics, especially meperidine. Other interactions with anesthetic drugs are summarized in Table 27-2.

El-Ganzouri AR, Ivankovich AD, Braverman E et al: Monoamine oxidase inhibitors: Should they be discontinued preoperatively? Anesth Analg 64:592, 1985

Miller RD (ed): Anesthesia, 4th ed, pp 291–387. New York, Churchill Livingstone, 1994

Stack CG, Rogers P, Linters PK: Monoamine oxidase inhibitors in anesthesia: A review. Br J Anaesth 60:222, 1988

Wells DG, Bjorksten AR: Monoamine oxidase inhibitors revisited. Can J Anaesth 36:64–74, 1989

Table 27-2. Some Interactions Between Monoamine Oxidase Inhibitors and Drugs Used in Anesthesia

MAOI	INTERACTION
Inhalation drugs	Muscle stiffness, hyperpyrexia (halothane in animals)
Narcotics	Meperidine → excitatory syndrome
	→ ↑ narcotic effect and coma
Barbiturates	↑ Sleep time
Anticholinergics	↑ Central activity
Sympathomimetics	↑↑ Effects of indirect-acting agents
	↑ Effects of direct-acting agents
	↑ Dopamine effects
Muscle relaxants	↑ Duration of block with succinylcholine
	(phenelzine decreases plasma cholinesterase)

(Reprinted with permission from Smith NT, Corbascio AN [eds]: Drug interactions in Anesthesia, 2nd ed, p 270. Philadephia, Lea & Febiger, 1986)

A.5. In an elective case, would you discontinue the use of tricyclic or MAO inhibitors pre-operatively?

Until recently, the common belief has been that MAO inhibitors should be discontinued for at least 2 weeks prior to surgery and that tricyclic antidepressants be substituted for therapy. A closer scrutiny of the literature reveals that the adverse drug reactions occur only in a few patients receiving MAO inhibitors and that anesthesia can be safely administered in these patients. Therefore, a 2-week discontinuation is not necessary if MAO inhibitor therapy is appropriate and properly monitored. Moreover, patients on MAO inhibitors often have severe depressive illness and run a major risk of suicide. Consequently, discontinuation of the drugs may be life-threatening. Direct adrenergic agonists or antagonists should be used to treat hypotension, hypertension, or arrhythmias. Tricyclics, on the other hand, can be continued to the day of surgery. Again, only direct adrenergic agonists or antagonists should be used in smaller than usual doses to treat any cardiovascular instability.

El-Ganzouri AR, Ivankovich AD, Braverman E et al: Monoamine oxidase inhibitors: Should they be discontinued preoperatively? Anesth Analg 64:592, 1985

Smith NT, Corbascio AN (eds): Drug Interactions in Anesthesia, 2nd ed, pp 261–281. Philadelphia, Lea & Febiger, 1986

Stack CG, Rogers P, Linters PK: Monoamine oxidase inhibitors in anesthesia: A review. Br J Anaesth 60:222, 1988

Wells DG, Bjorksten AR: Monoamine oxidase inhibitors revisited. Can J Anaesth 36:64–74, 1989

A.6. What precautions should be taken to anesthetize a patient on MAO inhibitors?

It is not possible to define those patients in whom adverse reactions are likely to occur. Therefore, all patients on MAO inhibitors should be assumed to be at potential risk of adverse drug reactions. The following precautions should be taken:

- Preoperative liver function test should be done because of the possibility of drug-induced abnormalities.
- Premedication should be generous to prevent overreaction to anxiety.
- Close monitoring of heart rate and blood pressure via an arterial cannula is recommended.
- Avoid sympathetic stimulation.
- Avoid meperidine. If narcotics are required, morphine or, preferably, fentanyl may be used.
- Avoid indirect-acting sympathomimetic amines such as ephedrine, methamphetamine, and mephentermine because they markedly increase the intraneuronal storage of norepinephrine. If needed, direct-acting sympathomimetics should be titrated carefully.
- Avoid cocaine because it inhibits re-uptake of endogenous norepinephrine, resulting in a buildup of norepinephrine.

Mangano DT (ed): Preoperative Cardiac Assessment, p 162. Philadelphia, JB Lippincott, 1990

Stack CG, Rogers P, Linters PK: Monoamine oxidase inhibitors in anesthesia: A review. Br J Anaesth 60:222, 1988

Wells DG, Bjorksten AR: Monoamine oxidase inhibitors revisited. Can J Anaesth 36:64–74, 1989

B. Preoperative Evaluation and Preparation

B.1. What premedication would you order?

No single premedication regimen has been shown to be consistently better than others. This patient has already received meperidine. If careful history rules out any significant problems or other drug intake, intravenous midazolam, carefully titrated in the operating room, may be beneficial if a plexus block with local anesthetics is planned. It has been shown that benzodiazepines elevate the patient's convulsion threshold to local anesthetics.

Cousins MJ, Bridenbaugh PO (eds): Neural Blockade in Clinical Anesthesia and Management of Pain, 2nd ed, p 194. Philadelphia, JB Lippincott, 1988

C. Intraoperative Management

C.1. What anesthetic technique would you employ?

Right brachial plexus block is preferred to a general anesthetic in this patient because it provides adequate anesthesia with good operating conditions while decreasing the likelihood of aspiration.

C.2. Describe the formation and major branches of the brachial plexus.

The brachial plexus supplies the nerves to the upper limb. It is formed by the ventral primary divisions of the fifth to eighth cervical and the first thoracic nerves, with contributions from the fourth cervical and the second thoracic roots. The roots join to form the superior, middle, and inferior trunks, which divide into anterior and posterior divisions (Fig. 27-1). The three posterior divisions form the posterior cord whose major branches are the radial and the axillary nerves. The upper two anterior divisions form the lateral cord whose major branches are the musculocutaneous nerve and the lateral root of the median nerve. The lowest anterior division forms the medial cord, which gives the medial root to the median nerve and terminates as the ulnar nerve. The sympathetic contributions to the brachial plexus are derived from the middle cervical ganglion and the stellate ganglion.

C.3. What regional technique would you choose to block the brachial plexus in this patient?

We would prefer an axillary perivascular technique of brachial plexus block. It is the easiest and the safest block to perform, and it provides adequate anesthesia for a surgical procedure on the hand.

C.4. What are the advantages and disadvantages of axillary, interscalene, subclavian, and supraclavicular nerve blocks?

Four classic routes were described for blocking the brachial plexus: paravertebral (Kappis); axillary (Hirschel); infraclavicular (Louis, Bazy); and supraclavicular (Kulenbampff). The first three techniques have been virtually abandoned and the supraclavicular technique is used only infrequently. The perivascular techniques of brachial plexus block (Winnie, Collins) by axillary, interscalene, or subclavian approach are

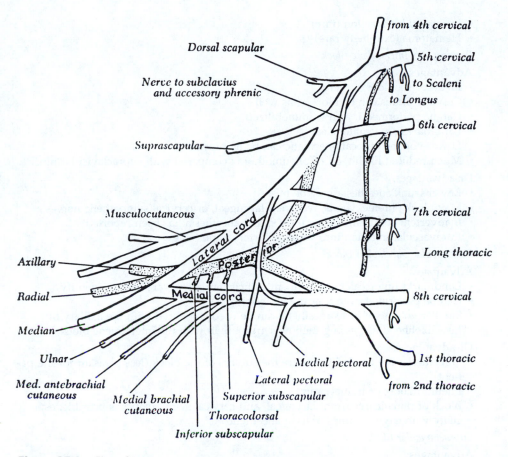

from 4th cervical

Dorsal scapular

5th cervical

Nerve to subclavius
and accessory phrenic

to Scaleni

to Longus

6th cervical

Suprascapular

Musculocutaneous

Lateral cord

7th cervical

Posterior

Axillary

Long thoracic

Radial

Medial cord

8th cervical

Median

Ulnar

Med. antebrachial
cutaneous

Medial brachial
cutaneous

Medial pectoral

1st thoracic

Lateral pectoral

from 2nd thoracic

Superior subscapular

Thoracodorsal

Inferior subscapular

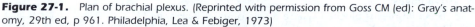

Figure 27-1. Plan of brachial plexus. (Reprinted with permission from Goss CM (ed): Gray's anatomy, 29th ed, p 961. Philadelphia, Lea & Febiger, 1973)

by far the most commonly employed techniques at present. The advantages and disadvantages of these techniques are described as follows:

Perivascular Axillary Block

Advantages:
- Provides excellent anesthesia of the forearm and hand
- Technique is easy
- Landmark (axillary artery) easy to identify
- Safest of all techniques
- Easiest of techniques to perform in children
- Paresthesias are not necessary

Disadvantages:
- Insufficient anesthesia for shoulder and upper arm
- Requires abduction of the arm to perform the technique (e.g., for painful shoulders or radius fractures)

- Intravascular injection (rare)
- Hematoma (extremely rare)

Perivascular Interscalene Block

Advantages:
- Ideal for shoulder surgery
- Cervical plexus can be blocked as well
- Can be performed if arm is immobilized
- Landmarks are usually clear
- Lower volume of local anesthetic can be employed
- Much reduced likelihood of pneumothorax compared with supraclavicular block

Disadvantages:
- Lower trunk anesthesia may be missed
- May block phrenic, vagus, recurrent laryngeal, or cervical sympathetic nerves
- Inadvertent epidural, subdural, or spinal anesthesia has been reported
- Intravascular injection into vertebral artery is possible

Perivascular Subclavian Block

Advantages:
- Landmarks (interscalene groove and subclavian artery) are easy to identify
- Can be performed even if arm is immobilized
- Smaller volume of local anesthetic can be used compared with the axillary block
- Less likelihood of missing the lower trunk than with the interscalene block

Disadvantages:
- Paresthesias are needed to ensure the success of the block (less pleasant for the patient)
- Pneumothorax (extremely rare)
- Block of phrenic, recurrent laryngeal, and cervical sympathetics is possible, especially with large volumes of local anesthetic

Supraclavicular Block

Advantages:
- Brachial plexus blocked where most compactly arranged
- Most intense block produced
- Smaller volume required
- Quick onset
- All of the nerves are reliably blocked
- Can be performed if arm is immobilized

Disadvantages:
- Paresthesias required (unpleasant for patient)
- Pneumothorax (0.5% to 6%)
- Phrenic nerve block (40% to 60%)
- Stellate ganglion block (70% to 90%)
- Possible neuritis

Adriani J (ed): Labat's Regional Anesthesia Techniques and Clinical Applications, 4th ed, pp 254–280. St. Louis, Warren H Green, 1985

Miller RD (ed): Anesthesia, 4th ed, pp 1535–1542. New York, Churchill Livingstone, 1994

Tetzlaff JE, Yoon HJ, Dilger J, et al: Subdural anesthesia as a complication of an interscalene brachial plexus block. Reg Anesth 19:357–359, 1994

Urmey WF, Talts KH, Sharrock NE: One hundred percent incidence of hemidiaphragmatic paresis associated with interscalene brachial plexus anesthesia as diagnosed by ultrasonography. Anesth Analg 72:498–503, 1991

Winnie AP: Plexus Anesthesia. Vol I. Perivascular Techniques of Brachial Plexus Block, pp 197–203. Denmark, Schultz, 1983

C.5. Describe the landmarks and procedure of the axillary block.

The major landmark for the axillary perivascular technique is the axillary artery. The patient lies supine with the arm abducted 75 to 90 degrees and the forearm flexed at the elbow. The axillary artery is palpated and followed as far proximally as possible under the pectoralis major. At this point, with the index finger directly over the pulse, a 1.5-inch, 21-gauge short bevel needle is inserted just above the fingertip and advanced toward the apex of the axilla at a 10- to 20-degree angle to the artery. (For the beginner, an easy procedure is to aim for the artery when advancing the needle, as if attempting to place an intra-arterial catheter.) When a "click" is felt, caused by penetration of the fascial sheath, 20 to 40 ml of the anesthetic solution is injected. The amount is determined by the patient's age. The finger over the pulse is pressed against the humerus to decrease the distal spread of the solution, thereby promoting the cephalad spread to anesthetize the entire brachial plexus. Repeated aspiration is a must during injection to prevent accidental injection of a large dose of a local anesthetic intravascularly.

Miller RD (ed): Anesthesia, 4th ed, pp 1535–1542. New York, Churchill Livingstone, 1994

Winnie AP: Plexus Anesthesia. Vol I. Perivascular Techniques of Brachial Plexus Block, pp 197–203. Denmark, Schultz, 1983

C.6. Describe the landmarks and the procedure of interscalene nerve block.

The landmarks for the interscalene block include the cricoid cartilage, the transverse process of C6 vertebra, the interscalene groove, and the external jugular vein.

The patient lies supine with head turned slightly to the contralateral side. The posterior border of the sternocleidomastoid muscle is palpated, and the fingers are rolled back to the interscalene groove at the level of C6 vertebra (cricoid cartilage). The needle is inserted at this point and directed caudad, mesiad, and posteriorly. Once paresthesia is elicited, 10 to 40 ml of solution is injected. In an adult, 20 ml of solution should anesthetize the brachial plexus (the lower trunk may often be spared with this volume). Increasing the volume to 40 ml blocks the cervical and brachial plexus effectively.

Miller RD (ed): Anesthesia, 4th ed, pp 1535–1542. New York, Churchill Livingstone, 1994

Winnie AP: Plexus Anesthesia. Vol I. Perivascular Techniques of Brachial Plexus Block. Denmark, Schultz, 1983

C.7. What are the most commonly missed nerves in axillary block and in interscalene nerve block? How can you circumvent this problem?

In axillary block, the nerves missed most often are the musculocutaneous and circumflex nerves because the exits from the sheath are higher up. Injecting a large volume (at least 40 ml in an adult male), keeping distal digital pressure to prevent distal spread of the solution, and avoiding abduction of the arm > 90 degrees during and after the injection can promote the cephalad spread of the solution to block these nerves. In addition, the musculocutaneous nerve can be blocked in the substance of coracobrachialis muscle by injecting 5 to 7 ml of the local anesthetic solution. The cutaneous branches can also be blocked at the lateral border of the biceps, just above the elbow crease. If a tourniquet is to be used, T2 must be blocked, which can be done easily by injecting 3 to 4 ml of local anesthetic subcutaneously as the needle is withdrawn after the axillary block.

In the interscalene approach, the most frequently missed nerves are the nerves derived from the lower trunk (C8, T1), namely, the ulnar, the medial brachial cutaneous, and the medial antebrachial cutaneous nerves. Use of a larger volume of anesthetic solution (40 ml in an adult male) and digital pressure proximal to the injection promotes distal spread of the solution, thus producing complete block of the brachial plexus. For surgery of the hand, the ulnar nerve can be blocked behind the medial epicondyle at the elbow. If surgery involves the forearm or if a tourniquet is to be used, the medial antebrachial nerve has to be blocked in the arm subcutaneously and T2 has to be blocked as described.

Winnie AP: Plexus Anesthesia. Vol I. Perivascular Techniques of Brachial Plexus Block, pp 197–203. Denmark, Schultz, 1983

C.8. Following an axillary block, the patient complained of tourniquet pain. How would you manage this problem?

Tourniquet pain seems to be mediated by the somatic and the sympathetic nerves. This entity is not completely understood and occasionally may be refractory to the usual means of management. Several steps can be taken to manage tourniquet pain—the intercostobrachial nerves can be blocked by injecting 3 to 5 ml of the local anesthetic subcutaneously in the axilla; the musculocutaneous nerve can be blocked in the substance of coracobrachialis using 5 to 7 ml of the local anesthetic solution; a circumferential subcutaneous infiltration with local anesthesia may be used, although its use has been questioned by many; intravenous analgesic sedation may be added; nitrous oxide analgesia may be added to the regimen; and if conditions allow, the tourniquet can be released temporarily and reinflated after a rest period; occasionally, the surgeon may be able to finish the rest of the procedure without the tourniquet. If none of these steps is helpful or practical, general anesthesia may have to be induced, with intubation of the trachea to protect the airway. Each of the above measures can be instituted separately or in combination with others, depending on the individual demands of each situation.

Table 27-3. Duration of Procedure and Selection of Local Anesthetics[a]

ANTICIPATED DURATION OF OPERATION	LOCAL ANESTHETIC RECOMMENDED
20–30 min	2% procaine
30–60 min	2% procaine with epinephrine or 2% chloroprocaine[b]
60–90 min	2% chloroprocaine with epinephrine or 1% lidocaine
2–3 h	1% lidocaine with epinephrine or 1% mepivacaine
3–4 h	1% mepivacaine with epinephrine or 1% prilocaine or mixture of mepivacaine and tetracaine with epinephrine
5–6 h	0.15% to 0.2% tetracaine with epinephrine
10–12 h	0.5% bupivacaine or 0.5% ropivacaine

[a] All durations are approximate guidelines at best, because fairly wide standard deviations exist when durations of local anesthetic actions are measured clinically.
[b] Epinephrine is recommended in 1:200,000 concentrations.

Table 27-4. Maximum Safe Doses of Local Anesthetics for Infiltration and Blocks

LOCAL ANESTHETIC	DOSE PLAIN (mg)	DOSE WITH EPINEPHRINE (mg)
Lidocaine	400	500 (7 mg/kg)
Prilocaine	400	600
Mepivacaine	400	500
Etidocaine	300	400
Bupivacaine	175	250 (3 mg/kg)
Procaine	500	750 to 1000
Chloroprocaine	600	800 to 1000
Tetracaine	100	150 to 200

C.9. What local anesthetic agent would you use and why?

A wide spectrum of local anesthetics is available and the choice is dictated primarily by the duration of the procedure (see Table 27-3).

Miller RD (ed): Anesthesia, 4th ed, pp 489–521. New York, Churchill Livingstone, 1994

Thompson GE: Upper and lower extremity blocks. 1996 Annual Refresher Course Lectures No. 143. New Orleans, American Society of Anesthesiologists, 1996

Winnie AP: Plexus Anesthesia. Vol I. Perivascular Techniques of Brachial Plexus Block, pp 197–203. Denmark, Schultz, 1983

C.10. What is the maximal safe dose of the local anesthetics?

The maximal safe doses of the commonly used local anesthetics for infiltration and blocks are shown in Table 27-4.

Miller RD (ed): Anesthesia, 4th ed, pp 489–521. New York, Churchill Livingstone, 1994

C.11. What would be your choice of technique if a bilateral block were required?

Bilateral blocks in the neck (interscalene, subclavian, supraclavicular) should not be performed because of the potentially fatal complications of bilateral phrenic nerve block, recurrent laryngeal nerve block, and pneumothorax. Bilateral blocks in the axilla would require a total local anesthetic dose in excess of the maximal safe dose; hence they should be avoided. To circumvent this problem, it seems prudent to perform one block in the axilla and the other in the neck to reduce the total dose of local anesthetic used. Alternatively, the two blocks can be spaced to allow for biodegradation of the drug. General anesthesia should also be considered and its risks and benefits weighed against bilateral brachial plexus block.

D. Postoperative Management

D.1. In the recovery room, the patient complained of shortness of breath. How would you manage this problem?

Pneumothorax should always be ruled out if the patient has shortness of breath following brachial plexus block. The presence of subcutaneous emphysema is indicative of pneumothorax. Supportive therapy, including oxygen, should be instituted immediately and a chest x-ray film obtained to determine the extent of the pneumothorax. Pneumothorax resolves spontaneously in most cases. Patients with >50% pneumothorax invariably require treatment. Air can be aspirated by means of a wide-bore needle through the second intercostal space, or a chest tube may need to be inserted and connected to underwater drainage.

D.2. How do you treat a systemic reaction to local anesthetic?

Refer to Chapter 26, question C.3.

D.3. On the second postoperative day the patient complained of persistent numbness and paresthesia in the right forearm and the hand. How would you manage this neurologic dysfunction?

Persistent neurologic dysfunction following brachial plexus block has been reported to be from 0.1% to 1.9%. However, before assuming anesthetic technique or neurotoxicity of local anesthetic to be the cause other causes must be carefully ruled out. In this patient they include the crush injury to the hand and lacerated nerves, tourniquet pressure, retractors used during surgery, a tight cast or dressing, positioning of the arm during surgery and in the immediate postoperative period while the neural block is still present, and any undiagnosed preexisting conditions such as previous injury, diabetes, or alcoholic neuropathy.

A detailed history for preexisting conditions must be sought. Assuming none exists, a careful history of current anesthetic technique including eliciting of paresthesia should be obtained. Anesthetic drugs, their concentration, dose, and any additives should be documented. A review of pattern of onset of regional block and its regression is necessary.

A detailed focused physical examination is helpful in localizing the nerve injury and therefore useful in differential diagnosis. For example, a glove and stocking type distribution may suggest tourniquet-induced injury, whereas a neurologic injury in the dermatomal distribution where paresthesia was obtained might indicate a needle-induced nerve lesion.

Most nerve injuries resolve within days or weeks; however, some may persist and become permanent. Therefore, a neurologic consult is recommended for initial evaluation and follow-up. Electromyograph and nerve conduction studies may or may not be abnormal initially but will become abnormal in subsequent weeks if symptoms persist. Reassuring the patient and effective communication between the anesthesiologist, the neurologist, and the surgeon is a must.

Cooper K, Kelley H, Carrithers J: Perception of side-effects following axillary block used for outpatient surgery. Reg Anesth 20:212–216, 1995

Kroll DA, Caplan RA, Posner K: Nerve injury associated with anesthesia. Anesthesiology 73:202–207, 1990

Selander D: Neurotoxicity of local anesthetics: Animal data. Reg Anesth 18:461–468, 1993

Winchell SW, Wolfe R: The incidence of neuropathy following upper extremity blocks. Reg Anesth 10:12–15, 1985

Nerve Blocks of the Lower Extremity 28

Jeffrey Y.F. Ngeow

A 35-year-old man was scheduled for drainage of an abscess in his left big toe. He also had an effusion in his right knee that might need arthroscopy, pending Gram stain result of intraoperative needle aspiration. His medical history was significant for heavy smoking and recurrent attacks of lower extremity pain, which were associated with sloughing of the pulp tissues of the digits. He had a previous magnetic resonance angiogram that was read as abnormal.

A. Medical Disease and Differential Diagnosis

1. **What are the possible causes of abscess in the digits?**
2. **What is a Charcot joint?**
3. **What is Charcot-Marie-Tooth disease?**
4. **What is thromboangiitis obliterans?**

B. Preoperative Evaluation and Preparation

1. **How would you assess the status of the local perfusion in the foot? Why would you be concerned?**
2. **Would you be concerned with the status of neurologic function in this patient?**
3. **What other information would you gather in evaluating this patient?**
4. **What anesthetic options would you discuss with the patient?**

C. Intraoperative Management

1. **What monitoring would you employ during the surgery?**
2. **Which anesthetic technique would you select for this operation?**
3. **What are the landmarks for the ankle block?**
4. **What are the advantages and disadvantages of an ankle block?**
5. **Are there other options in providing a unilateral lower extremity block?**
6. **Neuraxial anesthesia was refused for the arthroscopy. Are there alternatives?**

D. Postoperative Management

1. **How would you handle the postoperative pain management of this patient?**
2. **Why would you follow the neurovascular status of the patient subsequently?**

A. Medical Disease and Differential Diagnosis

A.1. What are the possible causes of abscess in the digits?

The possible causes of abscess may be local, regional, or systemic.

Local causes include acute infection from traumatic contamination, foreign bod-

545

ies such as splinters or inclusion cysts, and chronic infections such as osteomyelitis with sequestrum. Also diseases such as gout may cause local conditions that predispose to infection.

Regional conditions that produce local neurovascular insufficiency can lead to eventual infection. They include venous stasis disease, previous surgery or trauma that resulted in denervation and fibrosis, Charcot joint, syringomyelia, Hansen's disease, and tabes dorsalis.

Systemic causes may include generalized vascular insufficiency such as Buerger's disease (thromboangiitis obliterans), Raynaud's disease, disseminated lupus erythematosis, sickle cell disease, and neurologic deficiencies caused by conditions such as chemical or nutritional neuropathies, multiple sclerosis, and cerebral vascular accidents. Other causes, which may come from a distant part of the anatomy, include thromboemboli such as from valvular vegetation in subacute bacterial endocarditis, mycotic aneurysms, and carcinomatosis.

Baker AB (ed): Clinical Neurology, 2nd ed, pp 1565–1582. New York, Harper and Brothers, 1962

LeFrock JL, Joseph WS: Bone and soft tissue infections of the lower extremity in diabetics. Clin Podiatr Med Surg 12:87–103, 1995

A.2. What is a Charcot joint?

A Charcot joint is a neurogenic destructive arthropathy. Severe joint disorganization is associated with a diminished sensory perception to pain, temperature, and position. The underlying condition is neurologic dysfunction. Neurogenic arthropathy can result from a wide range of diseases including metabolic disturbances such as diabetes mellitus, chronic uremia, and chronic alcoholism.

Conditions specifically resulting in destruction of dorsal column fibers such as in syringomyelia or tabes dorsalis (tertiary syphilis) are also included. For the extremes of age groups, spina bifida with meningomyelocele in children or spinal cord tumors and degenerative diseases with nerve root compression in the elderly may be responsible. A sizable group of hereditary neuropathic conditions can also cause a Charcot joint.

Lee MM, Noeller KR: Charcot arthropathy of the first metatarsophalangeal joint. J Foot Surg 30:564–567, 1991

A.3. What is Charcot-Marie-Tooth disease?

Charcot-Marie-Tooth disease is one of the most common forms of hereditary sensory motor neuropathies. In about half of the afflicted, the condition has a progressive weakening and atrophy of the peroneal muscles as its early manifestation. It is transmitted as an autosomal dominant trait. Symptoms typically present in middle childhood with gradual footdrop and pes cavus. Later a mild sensory loss may occur in a stocking glove distribution. The histopathology is usually segmental demyelination and remyelination.

Holmes JR, Hansen ST: Foot and ankle manifestations of Charcot-Marie-Tooth disease. Foot Ankle 14:476–486, 1993

A.4. What is thromboangiitis obliterans?

Also known as Buerger's disease, thromboangiitis obliterans is a condition in which an inflammatory, nonatherosclerotic obliteration of medium and small blood vessels is found in the extremities. Ischemic changes may affect neural functions. Superficial thrombophlebitis is characteristic. The victims are usually young adult males who are heavy smokers. The condition is sometimes reversible when smoking ceases.

Olin JW: Thromboangiitis obliterans. Curr Opin Rheumatol 6:44–49, 1994

B. Preoperative Evaluation and Preparation

B.1. How will you assess the status of the local perfusion in the foot? Why would you be concerned?

Local perfusion in an extremity can be evaluated at the bedside by palpating for arterial pulses, observing the skin temperature and color, and estimating the adequacy of capillary refill. If tissue edema due to inflammation, infection, or gangrene is present, a zone of demarcation may be apparent.

When arterial pulses cannot be found by palpation, the Doppler ultrasound flow detector can be used to locate the blood vessel. In this patient who has an abnormal magnetic resonance angiogram, a high likelihood exists that arterial blood flow to the foot is decreased. Therefore any intervention that may further compromise the perfusion of the extremity (e.g., injection of solutions containing a vasoconstrictor or prolonged use of a tourniquet) should be avoided.

B.2. Would you be concerned with the status of neurologic function in this patient?

When infection is severe enough to cause cell death and tissue loss a loss of neurologic functions will occur locally. This finding naturally needs to be documented before any anesthetic intervention, be it regional or general. One must not forget, however, to also perform a brief overall neurologic examination of the patient to seek out sensory or motor deficits in the other parts of the body, especially when a systemic cause for the local neurologic deficit is suspected. From a medicolegal point of view, caution dictates that an intraspinal anesthetic technique be avoided when active central nervous system disease is present, unless the advantage clearly outweighs the risks.

B.3. What other information would you gather in evaluating this patient?

Routine preoperative workups should include a review of chest x-ray film and biochemistry as well as the coagulation profile. Blood glucose level will help to rule out diabetes mellitus. Abnormal coagulation studies will preclude neuraxial anesthetic injections. Chest x-ray may show unsuspected immobile or elevated hemidiaphragm in a demyelination condition. Pulmonary scarring or even pericardial effusion may suggest intravenous drug abuse. Such findings can have a bearing on postoperative analgesic requirements. It may be helpful to look at x-rays of the foot itself. If necrotic bone is present and sequestrum excision is part of the surgical plan, bone graft may need to be harvested either around the ankle or in the iliac crest. This possibility certainly needs to be considered in the anesthetic plan.

B.4. What anesthetic options would you discuss with the patient?

For an operative procedure that involves one and maybe both lower extremities, the anesthesiologist can offer the patient the choice of a single regional anesthetic or a combination of different techniques. For many patients the mere mention of nerve blocks evokes fear of the painful needle and anxiety from being awake but helpless on the operating table. Therefore, regardless of the kind of anesthetic techniques finally chosen, the patient must be assured of adequate relief from anxiety and pain during both the anesthesia induction time and the subsequent operation.

To this reassurance can be added another reinforcement by mentioning that, to many patients and surgeons, regional anesthesia has been found to be simple, safe, reliable, acceptable, and well tolerated.

Even when the patient does prefer a regional method, however, the preoperative discussion must also include discussion of the nature of the drugs involved (e.g., any sedatives or tranquilizers, as well as the local anesthetic agents to be used) with possible side-effects from each of them.

In addition, the patient should be told that when a regional anesthetic is used, as is in the case of general anesthesia, neither complete anesthesia nor total oblivion can be assured at all stages of the operation.

Moerman N, Bonk B, Oosting J: Awareness and recall during general anesthesia. Facts and feelings. Anesthesiology 79:454–464, 1993

Myerson MS, Ruland CM, Allon SM: Regional anesthesia for foot and ankle surgery. Foot Ankle 13:282–288, 1992

C. Intraoperative Management

C.1. What monitoring will you employ during the surgery?

Monitoring of the patient should include all routine vital sign measurements such as electrocardiogram (ECG), blood pressure, pulse oximetry, and body temperature in addition to specific items for monitoring that the patient or surgical situation demands. In our case, where there is significantly reduced regional blood flow, a Doppler ultrasound flow detector probe may be used on the operated limb before and after induction of anesthesia. In most cases, an increase in blood flow occurs after successful neural blockade. Any change, or lack of a change, in the perfusion status of the foot should be documented. When continued intraoperative blood flow monitoring is needed, a sterile probe for a pulse oximeter with plethysmographic display can be attached to a nearby digit if the operating condition permits. If a tourniquet is necessary, which is usually the case when blood flow is not severely compromised, the tourniquet pressure and acceptable ischemia time must be discussed with the surgeon beforehand and carefully followed. In noncritical cases of vascular insufficiency, a simple preoperative test noting the reperfusion time following a brief period of ischemia can be used as a guide for tourniquet acceptability.

Couse NF, Delaney CP, Horgan PG et al: Pulse oximetry in the diagnosis of non-critical peripheral vascular insufficiency. J R Soc Med 87:511–512, 1994

C.2. Which anesthetic techniques would you select for this operation?

As with all surgical cases the simplest anesthetic method that is compatible with requirements of the surgery and patient acceptance should be used. In this situation a spinal anesthetic is certainly a simple and straightforward choice.

If a strictly unilateral anesthetic is desired at the start of surgery and because the possibility exists that the opposite leg will be operated on, the anesthetic technique chosen must provide the flexibility for bilateral as well as unilateral blockade. Here, a reasonable choice may include an ankle block for the left foot and placement of an epidural catheter in anticipation of the need of arthroscopy of the opposite knee or bone graft harvesting from the right pelvis. Alternatively, peripheral nerve blocks for the knee and the iliac crest can be done for the right leg.

C.3. What are the landmarks for an ankle block?

"Classic" ankle block calls for injections above the ankle joint as originally described by Labat. For complete anesthesia of the foot each of the five foot nerves must be individually blocked (Fig. 28-1). The technique has been modified slightly by many authors and the exact landmarks chosen also have varied somewhat with each author. Essentially the two major nerves, the posterior tibial and the deep peroneal, require

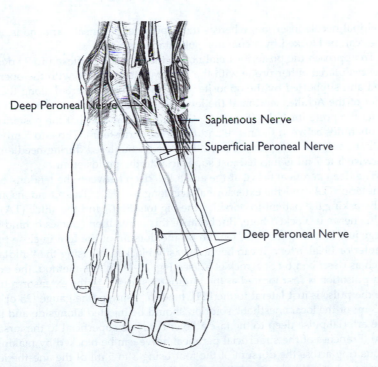

Deep Peroneal Nerve

Saphenous Nerve

Superficial Peroneal Nerve

Deep Peroneal Nerve

Figure 28-1.   Position of needle for deep peroneal nerve block in right foot.

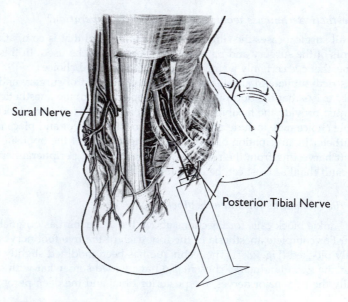

Sural Nerve

Posterior Tibial Nerve

Figure 28-2.   Position for left posterior tibial nerve block.

individual needle insertion, whereas the superficial peroneal, saphenous, and sural nerves can be blocked by a common subcutaneous ring.

To approach the posterior tibial nerve, the foot is dorsiflexed to 90 degrees. The patient is placed either prone with the leg straight or supine with the operated leg flexed and supported by the opposite leg. The needle is inserted along the medial border of the Achilles tendon at the level of the medial malleolus and advanced to contact the posterior tibia (Fig. 28-2). One must be aware that the posterior tibial artery often lies between the nerve and the tibial periosteum. Three to 5 ml of the local anesthetic solution is injected if paresthesia is encountered during needle insertion, otherwise 5 to 7 ml is injected just superficial to the periosteum.

The deep peroneal nerve at the ankle lies deep between the tendons of the tibialis anterior (TA) and the extensor hallucis longus (EHL). These tendons are identified by asking the patient to dorsiflex the big toe (EHL) and the ankle (TA). Traditionally the nerve is blocked here. But because this nerve then courses behind the EHL to emerge just lateral to the EHL tendon on the dorsum of the foot in close proximity to the anterior tibial artery, it can be more easily blocked by using the "midtarsal" approach as described by Sharrock et al (see Fig. 28-1). In this method, the dorsalis pedis pulsation is first located at the midfoot just distal to the extensor retinaculum. Here the pulse is just lateral to the EHL tendon. Using a fine gauge (25 or 27) needle, 2 to 3 ml of the local anesthetic solution should be injected alongside and just lateral to the arterial pulse deep to the fascia layer (i.e., just superficial to the tarsal periosteum). Branches of the superficial peroneal nerve can be blocked by making a subcutaneous ring across the dorsum of the foot using 3 to 5 ml of the anesthetic solution. This ring wheal will also block the terminal saphenous nerve medially and the sural nerve laterally.

Adriani J: Labat's Regional Anesthesia Techniques and Clinical Applications, 4th ed, pp 373–384. St. Louis, Warren Green, 1985

Scott DB: Techniques of Regional Anesthesia, pp 134–137. Appleton & Lange, Mediglobe S. A., 1989

Sharrock NE, Waller JF, Fierro LE: Midtarsal block for surgery of the forefoot. Br J Anaesth 58:37–40, 1986

C.4. What are the advantages and disadvantages of an ankle block?

The main advantage of an ankle block lies in its relative safety compared with other regional methods. Because only a small part of the extremity is anesthetized, no major hemodynamic changes similar to a spinal or epidural block will occur. Short of direct intravascular injections, systemic toxic effect from the usual volume (about 15 to 20 ml) of local anesthetic agents rarely occurs. This may be due to slower uptake and distribution of the local anesthetic into the central compartment. With adequate explanation of the procedure and expressed caution to avoid intense paresthesia, the patient is usually less apprehensive about this anesthetic technique and often requires little sedation while receiving the block. This block can therefore be done while the patient is in the "holding area" before entering the operating room, thus saving significant operating room time otherwise needed to establish the nerve block.

The main disadvantage is that the pneumatic tourniquet, unless placed just supramalleolarly around the well-padded ankle, is poorly tolerated. In addition, the long tendons of the foot continue to work because the muscles have their nerve supply more proximally. The patient must be reminded not to move the foot during surgery.

When prolonged numbness can be tolerated by the patient and is acceptable by the surgeons, the patient can be relieved of postsurgical pain for many hours with long-acting local anesthetic agents such as bupivacaine. Thus if only one extremity is involved, the patient may be discharged ambulating with crutches. Both the patient and the surgical team must be forewarned of the anticipated delay in sensory and motor recovery, however, to alley anxiety during the immediate postoperative period.

Lichtenfeld NS: The pneumatic ankle tourniquet with ankle block anesthesia for foot surgery. Foot Ankle 13:344–349, 1992

Mineo R, Sharrock NE: Venous levels of lidocaine and bupivacaine after midtarsal ankle block. Reg Anesth 17:47–49, 1992

C.5. Are there other options in providing a unilateral lower extremity block?

Progressing up the leg from the ankle, we have the option of using an intravenous regional block, when venous access is available. For anesthesia of the lower leg when the tourniquet is placed on the calf, 30 ml of a local anesthetic solution injected after exsanguination usually suffices. If the tourniquet is placed on the thigh then 50 to 60 ml will be needed.

Alternatively, the tibial, common peroneal, and saphenous nerve blocks can be done around the knee joint. At this level the exact location of the saphenous nerve is more variable. It may be blocked easily, however, by a transverse skin wheal just infe-

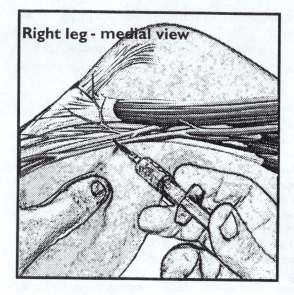

Figure 28-3.   Saphenous nerve block.

rior to the medial tibial condyle (Fig. 28-3). The tibial nerve on the other hand, can be consistently found at the top center of the popliteal fossa just lateral to the popliteal pulse (Fig. 28-4). The common peroneal nerve is also consistent in its location in the popliteal fossa just medial to the biceps femoris tendon or just below the neck of the fibula (Fig. 28-5).

   Using anesthetic solutions in higher concentrations such as 2% lidocaine or 0.75% bupivacaine with these nerve blocks, the motor nerves to the long tendons of

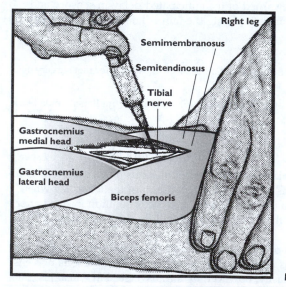

Figure 28-4.   Tibial nerve block.

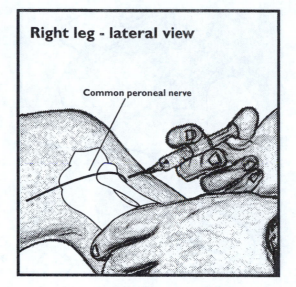

Right leg - lateral view

Common peroneal nerve

Figure 28-5. Common peroneal nerve block.

the ankle as well as the sensory supply to the lower leg and foot are anesthetized. Patient movements during foot surgery are thus minimized.

Mcleod DH, Wond DH, Vaghadia H: Lateral popliteal sciatic nerve block compared with ankle block for analgesia following foot surgery. Can J Anaesth 42:765–769, 1995

Rogers JN, Ramamurthy S: Lower extremity blocks. In Brown DL (ed): Regional Anesthesia and Analgesia, pp 279–291. Philadelphia, WB Saunders, 1996

C.6. Neuraxial anesthesia was refused for the arthroscopy. Are there alternatives?

An alternative to spinal or epidural anesthesia to anesthetize a knee joint would be the combined femoral and sciatic nerve blocks. Although the obturator nerve also innervates the knee, its sensory terminals supply only a small area of skin just medial and superior to the knee joint. The area involved (usually just beyond the medial portal for the arthroscopy) can easily be anesthetized, if necessary, by the surgeon with local infiltration.

The femoral nerve supplies most of the anterior knee and can be blocked easily in the supine patient by injecting at the femoral triangle (see question D.1. below).

The sciatic nerve can be blocked using the classic posterior approach described by Labat. This approach does require placing the patient on his side with the intended side up and the hip and knee flexed. The landmark is determined by first drawing two lines from the greater trochanter, one to the sacral hiatus and the other to the posterior superior iliac spine (PSIS).

Secondly from the midpoint of the PSIS line another line is drawn perpendicularly to meet the sacral hiatus line. The intersection of the perpendicular line and the sacral hiatus line is the needle insertion point. When a needle is inserted here to a depth of 6 to 8 cm, paresthesia may be elicited. Ideally, the paresthesia should be below the knee. If bone is contacted first then the needle should be redirected along

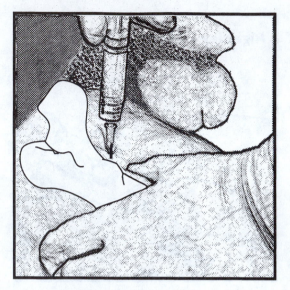

Figure 28-6.   Anterior approach for right sciatic nerve block.

the sacral hiatus line. A volume of 20 to 25 ml of the anesthetic solution will be needed to cover the nerve adequately.

Alternately, if the patient cannot be turned laterally, an anterior approach to the sciatic nerve can be used. In the supine patient, a line is drawn along the inguinal ligament from the anterior superior iliac spine to the pubic tubercle. This line is trisected. Another line is drawn from the tip of the greater trochanter inferomedially parallel to the inguinal line. At the junction of the medial and second third of the trisected line a perpendicular line is drawn to meet the trochanteric line. The intersection is the point of needle entry. A needle inserted vertically here will contact the medial border of the femur at the lesser trochanter (Fig. 28-6). The needle is then directed slightly medially to pass the medial femoral surface. Paresthesia should be sought about 5 cm deep to the femur. The posterior femoral cutaneous nerve, which leaves the main trunk early, may be missed by this approach.

Bridenbaugh P: The lower extremity: Somatic blockade in neural blockade. In Cousins MJ, Bridenbaugh PO (eds): Neural Blockade in Clinical Anesthesia and Management of Pain, 2nd ed, pp 417–441. Philadelphia, JB Lippincott, 1988

Sharrock N, Pinchot H: Anesthetic considerations in arthroscopy. In Scott WN (ed): Arthroscopy of the Knee: Diagnosis and Treatment, pp 37–42. Philadelphia, WB Saunders, 1990

D. Postoperative Management

D.1. *How would you handle the postoperative pain management of this patient?*

With a nerve block in place, the patient will have a gradual return of sensations as the local anesthetic wears off. In our patient, if he had received synovectomy for inflammatory conditions during the knee arthroscopy, he is likely to experience severe pain in the knee joint after the epidural anesthesia subsides. Because some evidence suggests that preemptive analgesia can reduce the intensity or duration of postsurgical pain, it is important that adequate analgesia be given. The patient should therefore be advised to ask for whatever the prescribed analgesic in the anesthesia care unit before sensations fully recover and pain becomes severe.

In the event when conventional doses of orally or parenterally administered analgesics prove to be insufficient we can offer the patient a femoral nerve block for pain control. This is conveniently done in the outstretched, operated leg by inserting a small-gauge short bevelled needle to the depth of 1.5 inches, a finger's breadth lateral to the femoral pulse. In obese persons where the femoral pulse is hard to find, a 4-inch nerve stimulator needle can be used to elicit paresthesia to the anterior thigh. Injection of 10 ml of 0.25% bupivacaine here usually provides adequate relief so that ambulation can still be allowed.

D.2. Why would you follow the neurovascular status of the patient subsequently?

It is important to follow the neurovascular function of the lower extremity for a period of 24 to 36 hours because a relatively higher incidence of persistent paresthesia is found following foot and ankle surgery. This may be a result of the nerve blocks or the dressings. During this period, the patient should be encouraged to report any abnormal sensations, and the surgical dressing should be carefully examined to ensure no excessive pressure is present that could reduce circulation or cause nerve compression. In the longer term, the patient should be followed for possible neuroma formation at both the needle insertion and surgical sites. The natural history of any preexisting neurologic dysfunction should be considered when evaluating any reported complications.

Kofoed H: Peripheral nerve blocks at the knee and ankle in operations for common foot disorders. Clin Orthop 168:97–101, 1982

29 Cancer Pain

Mindy Lyn Nestampower
Samyadev Datta
Subhash Jain

The patient was a 62-year old woman with a history of adenocarcinoma of the rectum which extended distally into the anus. She had been treated with chemotherapy, including 5-fluoro-uracil. She presented with severe lower abdominal and perineal pain. The patient was taking sustained-release morphine sulfate (MS Contin) 60 mg by mouth every 8 hours, and immediate-release morphine sulfate (MSIR) 15 mg by mouth every 2 to 3 hours for breakthrough pain. The patient was admitted to the hospital for management of intractable lower abdominal and perineal pain.

A. Medical Disease and Differential Diagnosis

1. What further information would you obtain in regard to this patient's pain?
2. Define pain.
3. What is nociception?
4. What is neuropathic pain?
5. What is allodynia? Is this different from hyperalgesia?
6. What is the differential diagnosis of lower abdominal and perineal pain?
7. Why is it important to obtain a complete history, including chemotherapeutic agents used in the patient's treatment?
8. Discuss common toxic effects of the commonly used chemotherapeutic agents adriamycin, mitomycin, and cyclophosphamide.
9. Is it important to understand the psychological effects of this patient's disease, and is this important in her pain management?

B. Pharmacologic Treatment of Pain

1. What classes of medications are used in the treatment of cancer pain?
2. How are opioids classified?
3. Would you use a mixed agonist/antagonist for treatment of this patient's pain?
4. What is the mechanism of action of opioids?
5. Discuss common side-effects of opioid therapy.
6. How would you treat opioid-induced respiratory depression?
7. What is the mechanism of opioid-induced nausea and vomiting?
8. How would you treat constipation occurring secondary to opioids?
9. How would you control this patient's pain crisis?
10. For long-term pain management, what is the preferred route of administration of opioids? What are the alternative routes available?
11. If this patient has inadequate analgesia and dose-limiting side-effects from opioid therapy via the above routes, what can you offer?
12. The patient decided to have an epidural catheter placed. What are the risks of this procedure?

13. What symptoms should alert you to the diagnosis of an epidural abscess?
14. How do you treat an established epidural abscess?
15. Why are tricyclic antidepressants (TCAs) used for the treatment of pain?
16. What are common side-effects of the tricyclic antidepressants (TCAs)?

C. Nonpharmacologic Therapies

1. Would you consider neuraxial neurolysis for the relief of this patient's pain?
2. What is the basis of subarachnoid neurolysis?
3. What are the potential complications of subarachnoid neurolysis?
4. Would you consider neurolytic subarachnoid block in this patient?
5. Would you consider epidural neurolysis?
6. In a patient with normal bowel and bladder function, what other block may be considered?
7. Would you consider superior hypogastric plexus blockade in this patient?
8. List the complications of superior hypogastric plexus blockade?

A. Medical Disease and Differential Diagnosis

A.1. What further information would you obtain in regard to this patient's pain?

The physician should ask the patient to try to locate the pain, and define its quality, intensity, onset, and duration. Understanding the nature and characteristics of the pain is important in making a pain diagnosis. It is also necessary to distinguish between long-standing and recent pain. Is this pain relieved by taking additional doses of MSIR? How long does the relief last? Determine whether any aggravating or relieving factors are present as well as any other associated signs or symptoms.

Bonica JJ (ed): The Management of Pain, 2nd ed, pp 1166–1171. Philadelphia, Lea & Febiger, 1990

A.2. Define pain.

Pain, as defined by the International Association for the Study of Pain, is "an unpleasant sensory and emotional experience associated with actual or potential tissue damage or described in terms of such damage." Pain is always subjective.

International Association for the Study of Pain, Subcommittee on Taxonomy. Pain terms: A current list with definitions and notes on usage. Pain 6:249, 1979; 14:205, 1982

A.3. What is nociception?

Nociception is the activity produced in the nervous system by potentially tissue-damaging stimuli. Nociceptive pain is the term used when the perceived pain is associated with tissue damage from an identifiable somatic or visceral lesion. When this pain originates from somatic structures, it is usually well localized and characterized as sharp, aching, throbbing, or pressurelike. Visceral pain is typically more diffuse. When it occurs in conjunction with obstruction of a hollow viscus, it is often gnawing or cramping in nature. With involvement of organ capsules or mesenteric structures, it tends to be aching, sharp, or throbbing. Nociceptive pains tend to be responsive to opioids and therapies that obliterate or denervate the peripheral lesion. In contrast, pain associated with visceral distention may not be responsive to opioids.

Wall PD, Melzack R (eds): Textbook of Pain, 3rd ed, pp 787–788. Edinburgh, Churchill Livingstone, 1994

A.4. What is neuropathic pain?

Neuropathic pain is a term used to describe pain that occurs as a result of aberrant somatosensory processing secondary to injury to the peripheral or central nervous system (CNS). It is most often associated with a dysesthesia, an abnormal discomfort, or unfamiliar pain. Dysesthetic pain is typically unpleasant and may be burning, numbing, tingling, pressurelike, or pruritic. Neuropathic pain can be continuous with episodic lancinating or shocklike sensations. Neuropathic pain can be further classified as deafferentation or sympathetically maintained pain. Deafferentation pain is due to aberrant processing that occurs in the CNS. Sympathetically maintained pain occurs after insult to the sympathetic chain. Neuropathic pains are generally not as responsive to opioid therapy as nociceptive pains. However, recent studies suggest that neuropathic pain may actually respond to high-dose opioids.

Patt RB (ed): Cancer Pain, pp 6–8. Philadelphia, JB Lippincott, 1993

Portenoy RK, Foley KM, Inturrisi CF: The nature of opiate responsiveness and its implication for neuropathic pain: New hypothesis derived from studies of opiate infusions. Pain 43:273–286, 1990

Wall PD, Melzack R (eds): Textbook of Pain, 3rd ed, pp 787–790. Edinburgh, Churchill Livingstone, 1994

A.5. What is allodynia? Is this different from hyperalgesia?

Allodynia is the sensation of pain in response to a stimulus that is not normally painful. Hyperalgesia is the sensation of pain of greater severity than that which would be expected from a painful stimulus.

Bonica JJ (ed): The Management of Pain, 2nd ed, pp 20–21. Philadelphia, Lea & Febiger, 1990

Wall PD, Melzack R (eds): Textbook of Pain, 3rd ed, pp 202–204. Edinburgh, Churchill Livingstone, 1994

A.6. What is the differential diagnosis of lower abdominal and perineal pain?

This patient had a known source of pain from adenocarcinoma of the rectum and anus. However, it is important to rule out any coexisting abdominal and perineal pathology. Other possible causes for her pain should include bowel obstruction, perforation, constipation, appendicitis, diverticular disease, ischemic bowel, renal or ureteral process (colic, infection, stone), gynecologic disease or dysfunction, abscess, pancreatitis, porphyria, gastritis, disease of the urinary bladder, urinary retention, myofascial syndromes, and diabetic ketoacidosis.

Bonica JJ (ed): The Management of Pain, 2nd ed, pp 1171–1185. Philadelphia, Lea & Febiger, 1990

A.7. Why is it important to obtain a complete history, including chemotherapeutic agents used in the patient's treatment?

Each chemotherapeutic agent has actions, interactions, and toxic effects of which it is important for the clinician to be aware. This patient has been treated with 5-fluorouracil, an antimetabolite. Common complications associated with fluorouracil include bone marrow suppression and gastrointestinal disturbances, ranging from nausea, vomiting, and diarrhea to ulcers, hemorrhagic enteritis, and bowel perforation.

Desiderio DP: Cancer chemotherapy: Complications and interactions with anesthesia. Hospital Formulary 25:176–185, 1990

A.8. Discuss common toxic effects of the commonly used chemotherapeutic agents adriamycin, mitomycin, and cyclophosphamide.

Adriamycin is an anthracycline antibiotic chemotherapeutic agent. It has dose-limiting cardiotoxic effects, including electrocardiographic (ECG) changes, supraventricular and ventricular arrhythmias, and heart block. Cardiomyopathy can occur, especially when the total dose exceeds 550 mg/m^2. Mitomycin, another antibiotic chemotherapeutic agent, can cause myelosuppression and severe interstitial pneumonitis. Cyclophosphamide, an alkylating agent, is associated with hemorrhagic cystitis, water retention, nausea, vomiting, and myelosuppression. It also inhibits plasma cholinesterase synthesis, and may prolong the action of succinylcholine.

Desiderio DP: Cancer chemotherapy: Complications and interactions with anesthesia. Hospital Formulary 25:176–185, 1990

A.9. Is it important to understand the psychological effects of this patient's disease, and is this important in her pain management?

To treat a patient effectively, the physician must understand that pain is not just a physical experience. Rather, it affects the patient's personality, behavior, mood, cognition, and interpersonal relations. The cancer patient will have many fears. Her level of psychological distress could have profound effects on her perception of pain. In recent years, a great deal of emphasis has been placed on addressing the psychological and psychosocial aspects of the patient's disease and its associated pain.

Breitbart WS: Role of psychological assessment and intervention in patients with cancer pain. In: Current Concepts in Acute, Chronic and Cancer Pain Management '95. Syllabus of the Postgraduate Course at Memorial Sloan-Kettering Cancer Center, pp 245–250. New York, The World Foundation for Pain Relief and Research, Inc., 1995

B. Pharmacologic Treatment of Pain

B.1. What classes of medications are used in the treatment of cancer pain?

The World Health Organization recommended an "analgesic ladder," a stepwise approach to the administration of pain medications. Nonopioid analgesics, including aspirin and other nonsteroidal anti-inflammatory drugs (NSAIDs), are the first line of treatment with or without use of adjuvant drugs. If pain persists or increases, a weak opioid is added, with or without adjuvants. If pain relief continues to be inadequate, a strong opioid is substituted along with NSAIDs and adjuvant medications. The commonly used adjuvant medications include corticosteroids, tricyclic antidepressants, anxiolytics, phenothiazines, and other centrally acting agents, such as antiepileptic medications and central nervous system stimulants.

Bonica JJ (ed): The Management of Pain, 2nd ed, pp 421–425. Philadelphia, Lea & Febiger, 1990

B.2. How are opioids classified?

Classification of opioids is based on their relative efficacy in treating pain. Weak opioids are limited in their analgesic effect by their associated side-effects at higher dosages. Drugs classified as weak opioids are propoxyphene, codeine, oxycodone, and hydrocodone. Strong opioids can be used in escalating doses, as necessary, to relieve severe pain. These include morphine, hydromorphone, fentanyl, methadone, levorphanol, and meperidine.

Patt RB (ed): Cancer Pain, pp 130–132. Philadelphia, JB Lippincott, 1993

Wall PD, Melzack R (eds): Textbook of Pain, 3rd ed, pp 943–944. Edinburgh, Churchill Livingstone, 1994

B.3. Would you use a mixed agonist/antagonist for treatment of this patient's pain?

Mixed agonists/antagonists are not recommended for patients on chronic opioid therapy because the antagonist effects may precipitate a withdrawal reaction. Drugs in this class include pentazocine, butorphanol, and nalbuphine. In the opioid-naive patient, they produce analgesia with minimal respiratory depression and have less potential for physical dependence than pure opioid agonists. These drugs have a ceiling effect, above which escalating dosages will not produce an increased analgesic response.

Inturrisi CE: Principles of opioid therapy. In: Current Concepts in Acute, Chronic and Cancer Pain Management '95. Syllabus of the Postgraduate Course at Memorial Sloan-Kettering Cancer Center, pp 191–195. New York, The World Foundation for Pain Relief and Research, Inc, 1995

Stoelting RK(ed): Pharmacology and Physiology in Anesthetic Practice, 2nd ed, pp 72–73. Philadelphia, JB Lippincott, 1991

B.4. What is the mechanism of action of opioids?

Opioids bind to stereospecific and saturable receptor sites in the brain stem and spinal cord as well as other tissues, including peripheral receptor sites. Three main receptor subtypes involved in pain modulation exist: the mu, delta, and kappa receptors. The frequently used exogenous opioid agonists act at the mu receptors. Some opioids act on a variety of receptors.

The mu-1 receptors are the primary receptors involved in supraspinal analgesia. Mu-2 receptors mediate hypoventilation, bradycardia, physical dependence, and euphoria. Delta receptors modulate mu receptor activity. Stimulation of kappa receptors causes analgesia and miosis with minimal respiratory depression. Many of the opioid agonist/antagonists act at the kappa receptors. Sigma receptor activation is associated with dysphoria and excitatory symptoms such as hypertonia, tachycardia, and tachypnea.

Kolesnikov YA, Jain S, Wilson R et al: Peripheral K1-opioid receptor mediated analgesia in mice. Eur J Pharmacol 310:141–143, 1996

Kolesnikov YA, Jain S, Wilson R et al: Peripheral morphine analgesia: Synergy with central sites and a target of morphine tolerance. J Pharmacol Exp Ther 279(2):502–506, 1996

Patt RB (ed): Cancer Pain, pp 131–132. Philadelphia, JB Lippincott, 1993

Stoelting RK (ed): Pharmacology and Physiology in Anesthetic Practice, 2nd ed, pp 72–73. Philadelphia, JB Lippincott, 1991

B.5. Discuss common side-effects of opioid therapy.

Constipation is the most common side-effect of opioid therapy. Central nervous system effects include euphoria, dysphoria, cough suppression, sedation, confusion, delirium, and hallucinations. Nausea, vomiting, and pruritus are frequently seen. All narcotics can cause respiratory depression or respiratory arrest. This is the most serious side-effect of opioid therapy. Pain is a significant respiratory stimulant and counters this opioid effect if used carefully. Myoclonus is a dose-related effect that can occur with any opioid administered in high doses. Urinary retention can occur secondary to increased urinary sphincter tone.

Bonica JJ (ed): The Management of Pain, 2nd ed, pp 428–429. Philadelphia, Lea & Febiger, 1990

Wall PD, Melzack R (eds): Textbook of Pain, 3rd ed, pp 1447–1451. Edinburgh, Churchill Livingstone, 1994

B.6. How would you treat opioid-induced respiratory depression?

Mild respiratory depression, without any other associated signs can be treated by reducing the dosage of the drug or holding the next scheduled dose. However moderate to severe ventilatory depression associated with excessive sedation, cyanosis, or lack of arousability, must be treated with naloxone. Rapid reversal of the narcotic with a large bolus of naloxone is undesirable, especially in an opioid-dependent patient, as it may precipitate severe withdrawal symptoms, seizures, or a pain crisis. A dilute solution of naloxone, such as 0.04 mg/ml, may be given in 0.5- to 1-ml increments. The half-life of naloxone is about 30 minutes. Thus, repeated doses or a continuous infusion with the patient in a monitored setting may be appropriate for continued management. For severe respiratory depression, intubation and controlled ventilation may be necessary. If respiratory depression is associated with inadequate relief of pain, the patient should be given a trial with another opioid.

Bonica JJ (ed): The Management of Pain, 2nd ed, pp 428–429. Philadelphia, Lea & Febiger, 1990

Patt RB (ed): Cancer Pain, pp 186–187. Philadelphia, JB Lippincott, 1993

B.7. What is the mechanism of opioid-induced nausea and vomiting?

Both central and peripheral mechanisms are involved in opioid-induced nausea and vomiting. Opioids stimulate the medullary vomiting center and chemoreceptor trigger zone, and they can increase vestibular sensitivity. Peripherally, they increase gastric antral tone, reduce gastrointestinal motility, and delay gastric emptying. Some commonly used antiemetics oppose these actions, including phenothiazines, gastric motility agents, anticholinergics, antihistamines, butyrophenones, cannabinoids, and benzodiazepines.

Patt RB (ed): Cancer Pain, pp 188–190. Philadelphia, JB Lippincott, 1993

Wall PD, Melzack R (eds): Textbook of Pain, 3rd ed, pp 1449–1450. Edinburgh, Churchill Livingstone, 1994

B.8. How would you treat constipation occurring secondary to opioids?

Constipation should be prevented in patients taking opioids. Patients should be encouraged to consume fluids and bulk-forming foods. Contact cathartics, such as senna preparations and bisacodyl (Dulcolax), can be started on an around-the-clock basis. The bulk-forming laxatives, Metamucil and bran, or osmotic cathartics, including milk of magnesia and magnesium citrate, can be added if constipation persists. Enemas and disimpaction are generally reserved for situations unresponsive to the above therapies.

Patt RB (ed): Cancer Pain, pp 188–189; 200–203. Philadelphia, JB Lippincott, 1993

B.9. How would you control this patient's pain crisis?

After a full history, physical examination, and evaluation, if other reversible causes of pain are ruled out, her pain can be rapidly controlled by intravenous administration of opioids, titrated to effect. As the patient had been on morphine, we can commence treatment with the same medication. With appropriate monitoring, intravenous morphine might be given as repeated bolus injections until the pain is controlled. Once the pain is tolerable, the patient may continue receiving opioid therapy via intravenous morphine patient controlled analgesia (PCA). The settings on the PCA should take into consideration the total daily dose of morphine the patient was receiving, including the rescue doses of MSIR. The conversion ratio for oral to intravenous morphine is 3:1. The basal hourly rate should reflect this total daily dose. The rescue dose should be about 25% to 50% of the hourly dose, and it should be available every 15 minutes. Provided the patient's pain is controlled and she has no contraindication to taking oral medication, she could be converted to oral morphine in about 24 to 48 hours.

Patt RB (ed): Cancer Pain, pp 134–137. Philadelphia, JB Lippincott, 1993

B.10. For long-term pain management, what is the preferred route of administration of opioids? What are the alternative routes available?

For chronic opioid therapy, oral opioid administration is the preferred route because of its relative ease and convenience. Approximately 70% to 80% of patients will have their pain effectively controlled via the oral route. Thus, if no contraindication is seen to oral administration, this route must be given an adequate trial. Often, patients experience side-effects with the initiation of oral opioid therapy. However, in many cases, the side-effects are transient and subside over the first week of use. If side-effects persist, another opioid can be substituted. It is preferable to use long-acting opioids.

Transdermal administration of fentanyl is a convenient method of delivering opioid therapy, especially for patients unable to tolerate medications orally. At the site of application of the transdermal patch, a drug reservoir is created. This system establishes relatively constant plasma levels of the drug. The patient is required to change the patch once every 48 to 72 hours.

The parenteral route may be considered for patients who cannot absorb sufficient amounts of medications by mouth because of nausea, vomiting, or gastrointestinal intolerance or obstruction. This route is generally more expensive than the oral route, and it requires intravenous access and attachment to an infusion pump, which may limit the ambulatory patient. Intravenous PCA allows the patient the ability to titrate the analgesic to the desired effect, and to control pain management.

Morphine, hydromorphone, and oxymorphone can be given as rectal suppositories for patients intolerant of oral analgesics. Subcutaneous infusion or PCA are alternatives when the gastrointestinal tract cannot be used. A theoretic concern is that irregular absorption from the subcutaneous tissues may occur due to differences in skin perfusion. At times of greater perfusion, absorption may be heightened.

Sublingual, buccal, and intranasal administration are being evaluated. Due to the high vascularity in these areas, drugs may be absorbed rapidly into the blood without first-pass hepatic metabolism.

Foley KM: The treatment of cancer pain. N Engl J Med 313:84–95, 1985

Inturrisi C: Principles of opioid therapy. In: Current Concepts in Acute, Chronic and Cancer Pain Management '95. Syllabus of the Postgraduate Course at Memorial Sloan-Kettering Cancer Center, pp 26–28. New York, The World Foundation for Pain Relief and Research, Inc, 1995

Patt RB (ed): Cancer Pain, pp 161–180. Philadelphia, JB Lippincott, 1993

B.11. *If this patient has inadequate analgesia and dose-limiting side-effects from opioid therapy via the above routes, what can you offer?*

Intraspinal opioid therapy via the epidural or intrathecal route may be considered in patients with intractable pain or dose-limiting side-effects of medications. This is particularly useful for cancer patients who have or will develop pain in multiple areas. Intraspinal opioids are most effective for treatment of continuous somatic pain, but can be useful for intermittent, visceral, or neuropathic pains, as well as superficial cutaneous pains.

The basis of this delivery system is the administration of small amounts of medication near its site of action in the spinal cord. In the epidural space, only a fraction of the medication given systemically is needed to achieve the same degree of analgesia. An even smaller fraction of this dose is needed in the intrathecal space, especially when hydrophilic drugs are used.

To determine if the patient is a candidate for this mode of therapy, a trial of the opioid can be given via the epidural or intrathecal route. If successful, the patient can then have a permanent implanted catheter placed and attached to an infusion device. Some patients may not achieve adequate analgesia with an opioid alone. A low concentration of local anesthetic can be added to the opioid for administration via the epidural or intrathecal route. This may improve pain control and decrease opioid requirements and side-effects, especially in patients with refractory pain.

Patt RB (ed): Cancer Pain, pp 285–306. Philadelphia, JB Lippincott, 1993

Sjoberg M, Appelgren L, Einarsson S et al: Long-term intrathecal morphine and bupivacaine in refractory cancer pain. I. Results from the first series of 52 patients. Acta Anaesthesiol Scand 35:30–43, 1991

B.12. *The patient decided to have an epidural catheter placed. What are the risks of this procedure?*

Risks of epidural catheter placement include inadvertent dural puncture, total spinal blockade, postdural puncture headache, subdural placement of catheter, epidural hematoma, epidural abscess, anterior spinal artery syndrome, backache, and possible neurologic sequelae.

Cousins MJ, Bridenbaugh PO (eds): Neural Blockade in Clinical Anesthesia and Management of Pain, 2nd ed, pp 339–341. Philadelphia, JB Lippincott, 1988

B.13. What symptoms should alert you to the diagnosis of an epidural abscess?

Common findings associated with an epidural abscess include severe back pain, local back tenderness, fever, elevated white blood cell count, and neurologic deficits. A culture of the epidural aspirate helps to confirm the diagnosis. Magnetic resonance imaging of the spine is useful in the evaluation for an epidural abscess.

Cousins MJ, Bridenbaugh PO (eds): Neural Blockade in Clinical Anesthesia and Management of Pain, 2nd ed, pp 339–341. Philadelphia, JB Lippincott, 1988

DuPen SL, Peterson DG, Williams A: Infection during chronic epidural catheterization: Diagnosis and treatment. Anesthesiology 73:905–909, 1990

Jain S, Datta S, Kolesnikov Y: Culture of epidural fluid is beneficial in diagnosing infection of temporary epidural catheter. Abstracts of the 8th World Congress on Pain, p 486. Vancouver, Canada, 1996

B.14. How do you treat an established epidural abscess?

Management of an epidural abscess includes aggressive intravenous antibiotic therapy, removal of the catheter, and, in severe cases, laminectomy. Prior to removing the catheter, one may irrigate the epidural space with saline to try to evacuate some of the infective material. Epidural catheters should not be removed unless the diagnosis has been confirmed, especially in the terminally ill cancer pain patient.

Cousins MJ, Bridenbaugh PO (eds): Neural Blockade in Clinical Anesthesia and Management of Pain, 2nd ed, pp 339–341. Philadelphia, JB Lippincott, 1988

DuPen SL, Peterson DG, Williams A: Infection during chronic epidural catheterization: Diagnosis and treatment. Anesthesiology 73:905–909, 1990

B.15. Why are tricyclic antidepressants (TCAs) used for the treatment of pain?

Neuropathic pain is infrequently relieved by opioids, but it may respond to high-dose opioids. Tricyclic antidepressant drugs have been found to be useful in the treatment of continuous, dysesthetic, burning or lancinating neuropathic pain. They potentiate the analgesic action of opioids. Often used as adjuvants in cancer pain management, TCAs are especially helpful in managing pain secondary to tumor invasion of neural structures. Tricyclic antidepressants also improve nighttime sleep and elevate the patient's mood. These drugs act by blocking presynaptic re-uptake of norepinephrine (NE) and serotonin (5-HT), thus increasing the amount of NE and 5-HT available at the receptors.

Bonica JJ (ed): The Management of Pain, 2nd ed, p 424. Philadelphia, Lea & Febiger, 1990

Hardman JG, Limbird LE, Molinoff PB et al (eds): Goodman and Gilman's The Pharmacological Basis of Therapeutics, 9th ed, pp 432–439. New York, McGraw-Hill, 1996

Portenoy RK, Foley KM, Inturrisi CF: The nature of opiate responsiveness and its implications for neuropathic pain: New hypothesis derived from studies of opiate infusions. Pain 43: 273–286, 1990

Wall PD, Melzack R (eds): Textbook of Pain, 3rd ed, p 1454. Edinburgh, Churchill Livingstone, 1994

B.16. What are common side-effects of the tricyclic antidepressants (TCAs)?

The TCAs have anticholinergic (antimuscarinic) effects, including constipation, urinary retention, blurred vision, dry mouth, and worsening of narrow angle glaucoma. Amitriptyline has the greatest anticholinergic potency and desipramine the least.

These drugs must be used cautiously in patients with a cardiac history, as they can increase heart rate. Their use has been associated with arrhythmias, orthostatic hypotension, and ECG changes, such as T-wave inversion and flattening, and altered cardiac conduction (prolonged QT interval). Sedation and confusion may be seen, especially in the elderly. An early evening dosing schedule is recommended to reduce the chance of daytime somnolence.

Hardman JG, Limbird LE, Molinoff PB et al (eds): Goodman and Gilman's The Pharmacological Basis of Therapeutics, 9th ed, pp 436–440. New York, McGraw-Hill, 1990

C. Nonpharmacologic Therapies

C.1. Would you consider neuraxial neurolysis for the relief of this patient's pain?

Neurolytic blocks are most effective in relieving pain that is primarily somatic in origin and less beneficial in management of neuropathic and visceral pain. Neuraxial neurolytic blocks, including intrathecal and epidural blocks, are indicated for severe intractable pain caused by advanced or terminal cancer. The patient is considered a candidate for neurolysis when the pain is felt to be intractable after adequate trials of analgesics or when therapy has been limited by unacceptable side-effects. Pain that is unilateral and well-localized to two to three dermatomes is most amenable to this therapy. There must be careful assessment of the patient and the potential risks must be weighed against the benefits of the procedure. The ultimate goal is to relieve suffering and improve the quality of life without causing any significant long-lasting side-effects.

Patt RB (ed): Cancer Pain, pp 275–281. Philadelphia, JB Lippincott, 1993

Waldman SD, Winnie AP (eds): Interventional Pain Management, pp 167–171. Philadelphia, WB Saunders, 1996

C.2. What is the basis of subarachnoid neurolysis?

Most of the nociceptive input to the spinal cord from the skin, subcutaneous tissue, deep somatic structures, and viscera is carried via the posterior roots. By proper patient positioning, hypobaric alcohol or hyperbaric phenol in glycerin can diffuse mainly to the axons of the posterior roots. Here, the neurolytic agents cause demyelination and degeneration of the dorsal nerve roots. This posterior root chemical rhizotomy can last from weeks to months and possibly longer. Because the cell bodies are not destroyed, axon regeneration will likely occur at some point in time. Using the smallest volume of neurolytic that will give the desired result allows for the maximal benefit with the least side-effects. If the block is effective, the patient's systemic opioid therapy will need to be reduced.

Bonica JJ (ed): The Management of Pain, 2nd ed, pp 1999–2001. Philadelphia, Lea & Febiger, 1990

Waldman SD, Winnie AP (eds): Interventional Pain Management, pp 167–171. Philadelphia, WB Saunders, 1996

C.3. What are the potential complications of subarachnoid neurolysis?

Serious complications can occur as a result of this procedure. The incidence of complications can be reduced by proper patient selection, preparation, positioning, and technique.

Diffusion of the neurolytic agent to anterior rootlets of the spinal cord can interrupt motor function and lead to paresis or paralysis of the muscles supplied by these fibers. At the sacral level, neurolytic spread to the anterior roots can cause interruption of the parasympathetic fibers to the bladder, rectum, and lower colon, resulting in loss of sphincter function, urinary retention, and bowel incontinence. Dysesthesias and loss of proprioception and touch can occur because of involvement of the posterior rootlets.

Tumor infiltration within the spinal canal at the level of injection is a relative contraindication to the procedure. Tumor can limit the contact area between the neurolytic agent and the targeted roots, thereby decreasing its efficacy. A much higher risk exists that bleeding or pressure from the injection may cause spinal cord compression and neurologic compromise. Complete obstruction of the subarachnoid space by tumor is an absolute contraindication to intrathecal neurolysis. Placement of a needle below the obstruction can cause downward coning and herniation of the cord. Thus, it is important to have radiologic studies of the spine performed prior to undertaking the procedure.

Postspinal headache can occur. Mechanical nerve damage, and aseptic and septic meningitis are uncommon complications that have been reported.

Bonica JJ (ed): The Management of Pain, 2nd ed, pp 2008–2009. Philadelphia, Lea & Febiger, 1990

Patt RB (ed): Cancer Pain, pp 427–430. Philadelphia, JB Lippincott, 1993

Warfield CA (ed): Principles and Practice of Pain Management, pp 389–393. New York, McGraw-Hill, 1993

C.4. Would you consider neurolytic subarachnoid block in this patient?

This is a fairly simple procedure with consistently good results. However, at the sacral level it should generally be reserved for patients with preexisting bowel and bladder dysfunction and surgical diversions of the bowel and bladder because of the high risk of causing incontinence. Another significant risk associated with the procedure is muscular paresis. Therefore, one must weigh the risks versus the benefits of this treatment, especially in this ambulatory, continent patient. This therapy should be reserved for consideration after all other modalities have been exhausted and with the patient's complete understanding of all potential outcomes.

Patt RB (ed): Cancer Pain, pp 371–372. Philadelphia, JB Lippincott, 1993

Warfield CA (ed): Principles and Practice of Pain Management, pp 389–393. New York, McGraw-Hill, 1993

C.5. Would you consider epidural neurolysis?

Some potential advantages of epidural neurolysis over intrathecal block include pain relief over a larger anatomic area. With this procedure less risk is seen of meningeal irritation, less cephalad spread, decreased bowel and bladder problems, less motor weakness, and fewer headaches. However, in the past, subarachnoid block had better results in terms of pain relief and thus most physicians performed spinal in preference to epidural neurolysis. Recent trials using repeated administration of phenol via a temporary epidural catheter over a period of several days have shown good results.

Bonica JJ (ed): The Management of Pain, 2nd ed, pp 2009–2011. Philadelphia, Lea & Febiger, 1990

Patt RB (ed): Cancer Pain, pp 439–441. Philadelphia, JB Lippincott, 1993

C.6. In a patient with normal bowel and bladder function, what other block may be considered?

Selective sacral root blocks may be performed to decrease perineal, rectal, and lower limb pain. Continence and muscle strength are usually not affected. The roots are injected where they emerge from the sacral foramina on the posterior sacral plate on the side of the predominant pain. This is best done under radiologic guidance. The procedure can first be performed using local anesthetic, and if successful, neurolysis may be performed.

Patt RB (ed): Cancer Pain, pp 371–372. Philadelphia, JB Lippincott, 1993

C.7. Would you consider superior hypogastric plexus blockade in this patient?

The superior hypogastric plexus is part of the sympathetic nervous system located bilaterally at the lower third of the fifth lumbar vertebral body and the upper third of the first sacral vertebral body. It is retroperitoneal and near the bifurcation of the common iliac blood vessels. Many of the structures in the pelvis and perineum have complex mixed sympathetic and somatic innervation. Superior hypogastric plexus block may help relieve visceral cancer pain that is sympathetically mediated. Pain in the perineal region is often vague, poorly localized, and often burning in nature. If this pain originates from the descending colon, rectum, vagina, bladder, prostate, testes, uterus, or ovary, it may be palliated by superior hypogastric plexus blockade.

Patt RB (ed): Cancer Pain, pp 411–417. Philadelphia, JB Lippincott, 1993

Waldman SD, Winnie AP (eds): Interventional Pain Management, pp 384–391. Philadelphia, WB Saunders, 1996

C.8. List the complications of superior hypogastric plexus blockade?

Risks of superior hypogastric plexus block include intravascular injection, hemorrhage, hematoma, and intramuscular and intraperitoneal injection. Less common complications include subarachnoid and epidural injection, somatic nerve injury, and renal and ureteral puncture.

Patt RB (ed): Cancer Pain, pp 411–417. Philadelphia, JB Lippincott, 1993

Waldman SD, Winnie AP (eds): Interventional Pain Management, pp 384–391. Philadelphia, WB Saunders, 1996

The Endocrine System

V

Thyrotoxicosis

30

Dana L. Oster
Su-Pen Bobby Chang

A 48-year-old man presented with diffuse neck swelling. History of present illness was significant for dyspnea, dysphagia, weight loss, paroxysmal palpitations, and heat intolerance. Vital signs were blood pressure 160/100 mm Hg; heart rate 120 beats/min; hematocrit was 29%.

A. Medical Disease and Differential Diagnosis

1. What diagnosis is compatible with these symptoms?
2. Describe the synthesis, release, and peripheral conversion of triiodothyronine (T_3) and thyroxine (T_4).
3. What is the role of the hypothalamic-pituitary axis in thyroid function?
4. Describe the effects of thyroid hormone.
5. What are the causes of hyperthyroidism?
6. What are the clinical signs and symptoms of thyrotoxicosis?
7. How would you distinguish thyroid storm from thyrotoxicosis?
8. What can precipitate thyroid storm?

B. Preoperative Evaluation and Preparation

1. Are there anatomic problems associated with an enlarged thyroid gland?
2. Describe the signs and symptoms of superior vena cava syndrome.
3. How would you assess the possibility of airway obstruction?
4. Discuss the laboratory assessment of thyroid function.
5. Describe medical strategies for achieving an euthyroid state.
6. What are the benefits of adrenergic blockade?
7. When is the hyperthyroid patient ready for elective surgery?
8. How would you premedicate this patient?
9. How would you prepare the thyrotoxic patient for emergent surgery?

C. Intraoperative Management

1. How would you monitor this patient?
2. How would you induce anesthesia?
3. Is endotracheal intubation necessary for this operation? Discuss the type and length of tube you would use.
4. How would you maintain anesthesia?
5. Intraoperatively the patient became hyperthermic and tachycardic. Discuss the differential diagnosis of malignant hyperthermia and thyroid storm. How would you intervene?
6. How would you extubate this patient?

571

D. Postoperative Management

1. **The patient became stridorous and dyspneic in the recovery room. What was your differential diagnosis and intervention strategy?**
2. **When does thyroid storm most often present?**
3. **Discuss innervation of the larynx.**

A. Medical Disease and Differential Diagnosis

A.1. What diagnosis is compatible with these symptoms?

These signs and symptoms are classic for hyperthyroidism. Differential diagnosis includes other hypermetabolic states such as pheochromocytoma, carcinoid, carcinoma, chronic infection, and anxiety states.

Rakel RE (ed): Saunders Manual of Medical Practice, pp 638–641. Philadelphia, WB Saunders, 1996

A.2. Describe the synthesis, release, and peripheral conversion of triiodothyronine (T_3) and thyroxine (T_4).

The synthesis of thyroid hormone is dependent on iodine. Sufficient amounts of iodine must come from dietary intake or from the deiodination of preexisting thyroid hormone. Iodine is actively transported into thyroid cells. Organification occurs as iodine binds to tyrosine residues of thyroglobulin, the receptor protein for iodine. Coupling of iodinated tyrosine residues results in the formation of T_4 and T_3. Once cleaved from thyroglobulin, thyroid hormone is released into the circulation. Ninety percent of the hormone secreted from the thyroid gland is T_4, whereas only 10% is T_3, the biologically active form. However, in the peripheral tissues, most of the T_4 is converted to T_3. T_4 can also be converted to reverse T_3, an inactive metabolite. In the circulation most of the T_4 and T_3 bind to plasma proteins; 80% with thyroxine-binding globulin, 10% to 15% with thyroxine-binding prealbumin, and the rest with albumin.

Goldman D: Surgery in patients with endocrine dysfunction. Med Clin North Am 71:502–504, 1987

Guyton A, Hall J: Textbook of Medical Physiology, 9th ed, pp 945–948. Philadelphia, WB Saunders, 1996

Mitchell J: Thyroid disease in the emergency department. Emerg Med Clin North Am 7:885–888, 1989

A.3. What is the role of the hypothalamic-pituitary axis in thyroid function?

The hypothalamus secretes thyroid-releasing hormone, which in turn stimulates the synthesis and release of thyroid-stimulating hormone (TSH) by the anterior pituitary gland. TSH stimulates the synthesis and secretion of thyroid hormones by the thyroid gland. Within pituitary cells, T_4 is converted to T_3. The intracellular level of T_3 within pituitary cells regulates the pituitary release of thyroid-stimulating hormone. Low levels of T_3 stimulates the release of TSH, whereas increased levels of thyroid hormone decreases TSH secretion.

Guyton A, Hall J: Textbook of Medical Physiology, 9th ed, pp 951–953. Philadelphia, WB Saunders, 1996

A.4. Describe the effects of thyroid hormone.

Thyroid hormone has effects at the cellular, organ, and systemic levels.

Cellular Effects

- Thyroid hormone regulates the nuclear transcription of messenger RNA in all cells. T_3 binds to a DNA domain named the "thyroid response element." Once bound, T_3 initiates the transcription of an array of biochemical enzymes which regulate tissue metabolism. T_3 is also postulated to bind to mitochondrial T_3 binding proteins with resultant transcription and synthesis of cytochromes. Basal metabolic rate can increase as much as 60% to 100% when large quantities of thyroid hormones are secreted. One ubiquitous enzyme that is transcribed in response to thyroid hormone stimulation is Na, K-ATPase.
- In addition to its role in enzyme transcription, thyroid hormone regulates cellular energy utilization. It stimulates cellular glucose utilization by increasing glucose absorption from the gastrointestinal tract, glycogenolysis, gluconeogenesis, insulin secretion, and cellular uptake of glucose. Thyroid hormone increases free fatty acid availability by increasing lipid mobilization from adipocytes. Conversely, thyroid hormone decreases plasma levels of cholesterol, phospholipids, and triglycerides by increasing the rate of cholesterol secretion into the bile.

Organ Effects

- Thyroid hormone is believed to have a direct effect on the heart by increasing heart rate and contractility with resultant increased cardiac output.
- Thyroid hormone increases oxygen consumption and carbon dioxide production with a compensatory increase in respiratory rate and tidal volume.
- Thyroid hormone increases bone formation and catabolism with resultant changes in parathyroid hormone levels.

Systemic Effects

- Increased cellular metabolism and production of metabolic end products result in vasodilatation and enhanced tissue blood flow.

Guyton A, Hall J: Textbook of Medical Physiology, 9th ed, pp 948–951. Philadelphia, WB Saunders, 1996

Mitchell J: Thyroid disease in the emergency department. Emerg Med Clin North Am 7:885–888, 1989

Smallridge R: Metabolic and anatomic thyroid emergencies. Crit Care Med 20:276–291, 1992

Tietgens S, Leinung M: Thyroid storm. Med Clin North Am 79:169–178, 1995

A.5. What are the causes of hyperthyroidism?

Graves' disease accounts for 90% of all cases of hyperthyroidism. The next most common cause is thyroiditis. Less commonly, toxic multinodular goiter, toxic solitary nodule, and excessive exogenous iodide consumption can cause hyperthyroidism. Trophoblastic tumors (e.g., hydatidiform mole and choriocarcinoma) are infrequent causes of hyperthyroidism.

de los Santos E, Mazzaferri E: Thyrotoxicosis results and risks of current therapy. Postgrad Med 87:277–294, 1990

Smallridge R: Metabolic and anatomic thyroid emergencies. Crit Care Med 20:276–291, 1992

A.6. What are the clinical signs and symptoms of thyrotoxicosis?

Nonspecific constitutive signs such as sweating, heat intolerance, weakness, and restlessness are common clinical signs and symptoms of thyrotoxicosis. Weight loss occurs despite a normal or increased appetite due to the increased caloric requirements.

Cardiovascular involvement is a prominent feature of thyrotoxicosis. Alterations include tachyarrythmias, increased stroke volume, increased cardiac output, increased oxygen consumption, and decreased systemic and pulmonary vascular resistance. Pulse pressure can be widened with an increase in systolic blood pressure. In patients with coronary atherosclerosis, angina may be precipitated or worsened. Young adults usually tolerate hyperthyroidism without cardiovascular decompensation. However, high output congestive heart failure can occur in older patients. Thyrotoxic patients may present with sinus tachycardia, atrial fibrillation, complete heart block, or ventricular dysrhythmias.

Hypercarbia and increased oxygen consumption due to the hypermetabolic state results in a compensatory increased minute ventilation with tachypnea and elevated tidal volumes.

Neurologic manifestations include anxiety, agitation, tremors, insomnia, muscle weakness, and changes in cognition such as confusion and delirium. This can progress in severe cases to stupor, obtundation, and coma. Other manifestations include myopathies, periodic paralysis, seizures, chorea, and a fine resting tremor.

Thyrotoxicosis shortens gastrointestinal transit time and a secretory diarrhea may develop. Weight loss caused by increased caloric requirements is often observed.

Hematologic derangements include anemia, neutropenia, and thrombocytopenia.

Pronovost P, Parris K: Perioperative management of thyroid disease. Postgrad Med 98:83–96, 1995

Smallridge R: Metabolic and anatomic thyroid emergencies. Crit Care Med 20:276–291, 1992

A.7. How would you distinguish thyroid storm from thyrotoxicosis?

Thyrotoxicosis refers to all disorders of increased thyroid hormone concentrations. The clinical spectrum ranges from asymptomatic biochemical abnormalities to life-threatening crisis with multisystem dysfunction and a high mortality rate. Thyroid storm exists when a patient's metabolic, thermoregulatory, and cardiovascular compensatory mechanisms fail. No laboratory test differentiates between thyroid storm and thyrotoxicosis. Thyroid function tests should be given. However, once thyroid storm is suspected treatment should be immediately instituted and not delayed for test results.

Smallridge R: Metabolic and anatomic thyroid emergencies. Crit Care Med 20:276–291, 1992

A.8. What can precipitate thyroid storm?

Thyroid storm is triggered by conditions that cause a rapid rise in thyroid hormone levels such as thyroid surgery, withdrawal of antithyroid drug therapy, radioiodine therapy, iodinated contrast dyes, and vigorous thyroid manipulation. Nonthyroid illnesses such as nonthyroid surgery, infection, cerebral vascular accident, congestive heart failure, bowel infarction, pulmonary embolism, pregnancy, parturition, diabetic ketoacidosis, or trauma can also precipitate thyroid storm. It is the acute change of thyroid hormone levels rather than the absolute levels that precipitates thyroid storm.

Burch H, Wartofsky L: Life threatening thyrotoxicosis. Endocrinol Metab Clin North Am 22:263–274, 1993

Nicoloff J: Thyroid storm and myxedema coma. Med Clin North Am 69:1005–1012, 1985

B. Preoperative Evaluation and Preparation

B.1. Are there anatomic problems associated with an enlarged thyroid gland?

The thyroid gland incompletely encircles the trachea and esophagus. Glandular enlargement can cause tracheoesohageal compression. The anatomic location of the thyroid, suprasternal versus substernal, has important implications. Airway involvement can include deviation, compression, or luminal narrowing. With muscle relaxation an enlarged substernal thyroid can cause unanticipated tracheal compression following the administration of agents that result in loss of respiratory muscle tone. Tracheal invasion or intratracheal hemorrhage can occur with thyroid carcinomas.

The anatomic position of the superior vena cava in the thorax makes it vulnerable to compression by mediastinal masses.

Acute respiratory insufficiency secondary to bilateral vocal cord paralysis from recurrent laryngeal nerve compression has been reported in patients with intrathoracic goiter.

Fauci AS, Braunwald E, Isselbacher K et al (eds): Harrison's Principles of Internal Medicine, 14th ed, pp 2024–2025. New York, McGraw-Hill, 1998

Peters K, Nance P, Wingard D: Malignant hyperthyroidism or malignant hyperthermia. Anesth Analg 60:613–615, 1981

Smallridge R: Metabolic and anatomic thyroid emergencies. Crit Care Med 20:276–291, 1992

Steenerson R, Barton R: Mediastinal goiter and superior vena cava syndrome. Laryngoscope 88:1688–1690, 1978

B.2. Describe the signs and symptoms of superior vena cava syndrome.

Superior vena cava syndrome has an insidious onset and a slow progression. The low flow, low pressure, thin-walled superior vena cava is susceptible to compression from expanding mediastinal masses. The obstruction of venous drainage from the upper thorax produces face, neck, and upper extremity edema, dilatation of collateral veins of the upper thorax and neck, and symptoms of headache and vertigo. Due to the predominance of right-sided thyromegaly, compression of the right innominate vein is more common. As the superior vena cava becomes obstructed, collaterals such as the azygous, internal mammary, vertebral, and lateral thoracic venous plexuses form. Venography is the "gold standard" for anatomic delineation.

Ulreich S, Lowman R, Stern H: Intrathoracic goiter: A cause of the superior vena cava syndrome. Clin Radiol 28:663–665, 1977

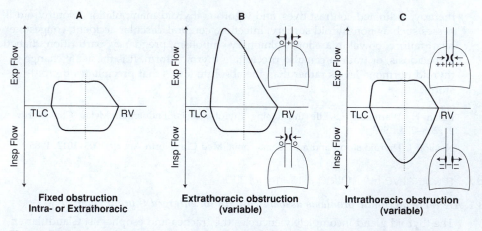

Figure 30-1. Flow-volume curves in fixed and variable obstruction. **(A)** Fixed obstruction, intra- or extrathoracic. **(B)** Extrathoracic obstruction (variable). **(C)** Intrathoracic obstruction (variable). (Reprinted with permission from Benumof J: Anesthesia for Thoracic Surgery, 2nd ed, p 536. Philadelphia, WB Saunders, 1995)

B.3. How would you assess the possibility of airway obstruction?

Chest x-ray and computed tomography scanning of the neck are helpful in evaluating tracheal position and airway obstruction.

Pulmonary function testing is a noninvasive method used to evaluate patients with airway obstruction. Flow-volume loop analysis determines the extent and location of airway obstruction. Flow-volume loops are generated by inhaling to total lung capacity, exhaling to residual volume, and then inhaling back to total lung capacity. Differing patterns in flow-volume loops can distinguish intrathoracic versus extrathoracic airway obstructions (Fig. 30-1).

Fixed lesions of the upper airway, which include tracheal tumors, subglottic stenosis, and goiters, will produce plateaus in both the inspiratory and expiratory cycle of the flow-volume loop (see Fig. 30-1A).

Variable intrathoracic lesions, which include endobronchial tumors, tracheal tumors, and tracheomalacia, produce plateau of the expiratory cycle only. Inhalation is unimpaired because negative intrathoracic pressure will stent the airway. During exhalation, positive intrathoracic pressure narrows the airway and results in plateau of the expiratory limb of the flow-volume loop (see Fig. 30-1C). These patients will have preserved forced vital capacity but marked reductions of forced expiratory volume in 1 second (FEV_1).

Variable extrathoracic lesions are most often caused by vocal cord paralysis, vocal cord neoplasms, and neoplasms in the neck. The inspiratory limb of the flow-volume loop is plateaued. During inhalation, the generation of negative intrathoracic pressure pulls the extrathoracic airway closed. During exhalation airflow maintains the patency of the airway.

Benumof J: Anesthesia for Thoracic Surgery, 2nd ed, p 536. Philadelphia, WB Saunders, 1995

Lunn W, Sheller J: Flow volume loops in the evaluation of upper airway obstruction. Otolaryngol Clin North Am 28:721–729, 1995

Table 30-1. Serum Thyroid Hormone Tests in Health and Disease

	TOTAL T$_4$	T$_3$U	FT$_4$INDEX	FREE T$_4$	T$_3$	rT$_3$	TSH
Euthyroid	N	N	N	N	N	N	N
Hyperthyroid	↑	↑	↑	↑	↑	↑	↓
Hypothyroid	↓	↓	↓	↓	N, ↓	↓	↑
TBG excess	↑	↓	N	N	↑	↑	N
TBG deficiency	↓	↑	N	N, ↓	↓	↓	N
Nonthyroidal illness	N,↓	↑	N, ↓	↑, N, ↓	↓	↑	N, ↓
FDH	↑	N	↑	↑	N	N	N

Abbreviations: TBG, Thyroxine-binding globulin; FDH, familial dysalbuminemic hyperthyroxinemia; T$_3$U, T$_3$ uptake; FT$_4$, free T$_4$; rT$_3$, reverse T$_3$; TSH, thyroid-stimulating hormone; N, normal; ↑, increased; ↓ decreased.
  (Reprinted with permission from Smallridge RC: Metabolic and anatomic thyroid emergencies: A review. Crit Care Med 20: 276, 1992)

B.4. Discuss the laboratory assessment of thyroid function.

Thyroid function tests are divided into three categories:

- Direct tests of thyroid function
- Tests related to concentration and binding of thyroid hormones
- Tests of homeostatic control of thyroid function

Direct tests of thyroid function involve administration of radioactive iodine and measurement of its uptake by the thyroid. Radioactive iodine uptake is measured 24 hours after administration of the isotope. Uptake will vary inversely with the plasma iodide concentration and vary directly with thyroid function.

Tests related to hormone concentration and binding in serum include measurements of T$_4$ and T$_3$. Radioimmunoassays of both free and total T$_3$ and T$_4$ are available. Although some centers measure the percent of T$_4$ or T$_3$ that is dialyzable or free, most use an *in vitro* uptake test. Serum is enriched with labeled T$_4$ or labeled T$_3$ and is then incubated with a resin that binds free hormone. Labeled T$_3$ will bind to unoccupied hormone binding sites. If these sites are already occupied by endogenous thyroid hormone, such as during hyperthyroidism, labeled T$_3$ will be picked up by the resin. T$_3$ uptake will also be elevated when thyroid binding sites are decreased as in low protein states such as malnutrition, nephrotic syndrome, and cirrhosis. T$_3$ uptake is low during hypothyroidism or when thyroid-binding globulin sites are increased as during pregnancy, with use of oral contraceptives, and in infectious hepatitis.

Although nonspecific, serum creatinine phosphokinase, lactate dehydrogenase, and aspartate aminotransferase levels are slightly depressed in hyperthyroidism.

Tests of homeostatic control include measurement of serum TSH and thyrotropin-releasing hormone stimulating test. TSH levels will vary inversely with thyroid hormone levels. Thyrotropin-releasing hormone stimulation test assesses the hypothalamic-pituitary-thyroid axis.

Serum thyroid hormone tests in health and disease are listed in Table 30-1.

de los Santos E, Mazzaferri E: Thyrotoxicosis results and risks of current therapy. Postgrad Med 87:277–294, 1990

Fauci AS, Braunwald E, Isselbacher K et al (eds): Harrison's Principles of Internal Medicine, 14th ed, p 2025. New York, McGraw-Hill, 1998

Goldman D: Surgery in patients with endocrine dysfunction. Med Clin North Am 71:502–504, 1987

Mitchell J: Thyroid disease in the emergency department. Emerg Med Clin North Am 7:885–888, 1989

Smallridge RC: Metabolic and anatomic thyroid emergencies: A review. Crit Care Med 20:276, 1992

Surks M, Chopra I, Mariash C et al: American Thyroid Association guidelines for use of laboratory tests in thyroid disorders. JAMA 263:1529–1532, 1990

B.5. Describe medical strategies for achieving an euthyroid state.

Medical strategy is directed at blocking the production of thyroid hormone, the release of thyroid hormone, and the adrenergic effects of excessive hormonal levels.

Initial therapy is directed at blocking thyroid hormone synthesis using antithyroid drugs such as methimazole and propylthiouracil. These drugs are iodinated within the thyroid gland, thus diverting iodine away from new thyroid hormone synthesis. They do not block the release of thyroid hormone and are not effective until thyroid hormone stores are depleted. Propylthiouracil also inhibits peripheral conversion of T_4 to T_3. Side-effects of antithyroid medications include fever, urticaria, arthralgias, arthritis, leukopenia, agranulocytosis, and, rarely, toxic hepatitis. Glucocorticoids inhibit peripheral conversion of T_4 to T_3, and they have an additive effect when given with propylthiouracil.

Iodine will inhibit the release of T_3 and T_4 from the thyroid gland. Onset of action occurs within 24 hours. Iodine can also be given for 8 to 10 days preoperatively to decrease the vascularity of the thyroid gland. Iodine therapy requires 2 weeks for maximal effect. An euthyroid state should be achieved with antithyroid drugs before initiating iodine therapy, otherwise the exogenous iodine can be used as substrate for the synthesis of new thyroid hormone. Exogenous iodine administration blocks the binding of intrinsic iodine. This Wolff-Chaikoff effect lasts only a few days. Thereafter formation of thyroid hormone resumes despite the continued high intake of iodine. Iodides are mainly useful for thyroid crisis and for emergency surgery in hyperthyroid patients. In parturients iodine is contraindicated, as it can cross the placenta.

Beta-antagonists are useful to block the peripheral adrenergic manifestations of hyperthyroidism. Patients become clinically euthyroid; however, without additional intervention they will remain chemically hyperthyroid. Propranolol is the most commonly used beta-adrenergic antagonist because it additionally inhibits peripheral conversion of T_4 to T_3. In thyrotoxic patients larger doses of beta-antagonists may be required due to accelerated metabolism. Centrally acting adrenergic antagonists such as reserpine or guanethidine can be used in patients who cannot take beta-blockers.

de los Santos E, Mazzaferri E: Thyrotoxicosis results and risks of current therapy. Postgrad Med 87:277–294, 1990

Falk S: The management of hyperthyroidism. Otolaryngol Clin North Am 23:361–362, 1990

Smallridge R: Metabolic and anatomic thyroid emergencies. Crit Care Med 20:276–291, 1992

B.6. What are the benefits of adrenergic blockade?

Catecholamines contribute to the symptoms of thyrotoxicosis. Pharmacologic agents that deplete stores or block the action of catecholamines will decrease heart rate, cardiac output, and cardiac irritability. Drugs used in the treatment of thyrotoxic symptoms include beta-antagonists, combined alpha-beta antagonists, and centrally acting agents such as reserpine and guanethidine. Side-effects associated with use of these drugs include hypotension, sedation, depression, myocardial depression, bronchospasm, and diarrhea.

Ingbar S: Management of emergencies, thyrotoxic storm. N Engl J Med 274:1252–1254, 1966

B.7. When is the hyperthyroid patient ready for elective surgery?

Emphasis should be placed on relief of symptoms. The patient should demonstrate a return of normal heart rate, pulse pressure, and sinus rhythm, and a resolution of recent onset cardiac murmurs. Tremors, anxiety, palpitations, dyspnea, and heat intolerance should be relieved.

B.8. How would you premedicate this patient?

The goal of premedication of the thyrotoxic patient is to relieve anxiety and prevent the activation of the sympathetic nervous system. Benzodiazepines such as oral (po) diazepam (5 to 10 mg) or central adrenergic blockers such as clonidine (3 to 5 μg/kg po) are appropriate. Antimuscarinics such as atropine and scopolamine are not recommended as they cause tachycardia and interfere with normal heat regulation.

Smallridge R: Metabolic and anatomic thyroid emergencies. Crit Care Med 20:276–291, 1992

Stoelting R, Dierdorf S, McCammon R: Anesthesia and Coexisting Disease, 3rd ed, pp 349–350. New York, Churchill Livingstone, 1993

B.9. How would you prepare the thyrotoxic patient for emergent surgery?

When surgery is emergent, measures should be taken to prevent thyroid storm. Reduction of the hyperadrenergic state along with decreased conversion of T_4 to T_3 can be attempted with propranolol. Esmolol, as an alternative, may offer some advantages due to its $beta_1$-specificity and short half-life. However, esmolol has not been shown to decrease peripheral conversion. Antithyroid drugs should be given to prevent further thyroid hormone synthesis. Either propylthiouracil (200 to 400 mg po every 6 hours) or methimazole (20 to 40 mg po every 6 hours) should be administered as soon as possible. Methimazole in an aqueous solution, but not propylthiouracil, can be administered rectally. Propylthiouracil and glucocorticoids can also block peripheral conversion of T_4 to T_3 and together they have an additive effect. Intravenous (IV) dexamethasone (2 mg every 6 hours) or hydrocortisone (40 mg IV every 6 hours) can be administered. Saturated solution of potassium iodide (5 drops po every 6 hours) or Lugol's solution (30 drops po every 6 to 8 hours) can be given to acutely inhibit release of T_4 and T_3. Parasympatholytics such as atropine and pancuronium should be avoided, as unopposed sympathetic activity may result.

Therapy should also be directed at correcting systemic decompensation. Fluids and electrolytes need to be replaced. Invasive monitoring may be needed to guide the administration of inotropes and vasopressors when hypotension is unresponsive to fluids.

Gavin L: Thyroid crises. Med Clin North Am 75:179–190, 1991

Pronovost P, Parris K: Perioperative management of thyroid disease. Postgrad Med 98:83–96, 1995

Shoemaker W, Ayres S, Grenvik A et al (eds): Textbook of Critical Care, 3rd ed, pp 1073–1081. Philadelphia, WB Saunders, 1995

Tietgens S, Leinung M: Thyroid storm. Med Clin North Am 79:169–178, 1995

C. Intraoperative Management

C.1. How would you monitor this patient?

Once blood pressure, end tidal carbon dioxide, pulse oximetry, electrocardiogram, and core temperature monitors are in place, the thyrotoxic patient is monitored to manage any cardiac decompensation and to recognize increased thyroid and adrenergic activity. If the patient presents to the operating room in thyroid storm, large-bore peripheral intravenous lines and an arterial line should be placed. If the patient is presently in or has a history of congestive heart failure, myocardial ischemia, renal failure, or hypotension, placement of central venous or pulmonary artery catheter is warranted. Invasive monitors should be placed before skin incision. Once surgery has begun, access for placement of monitors will be difficult.

C.2. How would you induce anesthesia?

Induction and intubation can proceed with standard techniques if airway obstruction is not suspected. Patients with orthopnea, dyspnea, stridor, wheezing, or hoarseness require further preoperative evaluation. Preoperative studies as described above (question B.3.) need to be reviewed. At minimum, the chest x-ray film needs to be evaluated by the anesthesiologist. Airway obstruction necessitates awake fiberoptic intubation or spontaneous inhalation induction. Inhalational induction using halothane or ethrane will maintain spontaneous respiration and airway patency. Isoflurane and desflurane may be too irritating to the airway for inhalation induction. Intubation should be attempted only after a deep plane of anesthesia is achieved. Patients with severe obstruction may require awake intubation, which will require anesthetizing the glossopharyngeal, superior laryngeal, and recurrent laryngeal nerves. Judicious use of small amounts of amnestic or anxiolytic agents may be necessary to prevent the precipitation of thyroid storm.

A rigid bronchoscope should be available in the event of airway collapse. Emergency tracheotomies are difficult to perform because of anatomic distortion and increase in tissue vascularity. Small reinforced endotracheal tubes should be available.

C.3. Is endotracheal intubation necessary for this operation? Discuss the type and length of tube you would use.

Endotracheal intubation is necessary for thyroid surgery. If tracheal obstruction is suspected a reinforced anode endotracheal tube should be used to prevent airway collapse. The length of the tube should be sufficient to extend beyond the thyroid gland.

C.4. How would you maintain anesthesia?

Maintenance of anesthesia should avoid sympathetic nervous system activation. Muscle relaxants are not necessary. Narcotics such as fentanyl or morphine should be given only in small amounts to ensure an alert patient who can maintain the airway after extubation. Treatment of hypotension with sympathomimetic drugs must take into account possible exaggerated responses. Because of the high level of circulating endogenous catecholamines, direct sympathomimetics such as epinephrine or norepinephrine or alpha-agonists such as phenylephrine are more appropriate than indirect sympathomimetics such as ephedrine or metaraminol.

C.5. Intraoperatively the patient became hyperthermic and tachycardic. Discuss the differential diagnosis of malignant hyperthermia and thyroid storm. How would you intervene?

Differential diagnosis includes hyperthyroid storm, malignant hyperthermia, pheochromocytoma, and carcinoid crisis. Many of the clinical manifestations of malignant hyperthermia and thyroid storm are compensatory mechanisms for hyperthermia. However, malignant hyperthermia will result in metabolic acidosis, profound hypercarbia, and muscle rigidity, which are not present during thyroid storm. Hyperthyroidism decreases the level of creatinine phosphokinase to about half normal, whereas creatinine phosphokinase levels are increased during malignant hyperthermia. Both disorders progress rapidly and intervention is urgent.

Once thyroid storm is suspected, treatment must start immediately. Goals of intervention include:

- Diagnosis and treatment of inciting event—Without treatment of the underlying cause, therapy will be less effective.
- Supportive measures—Replace fluids, glucose, and electrolytes. Reduce temperature with acetaminophen, cold lavage of body cavities, cooling blankets, ice packs, and reduction of ambient temperature. Aspirin should not be used as an antipyretic. It displaces thyroid hormones from binding proteins, thus raising free hormone levels. Inotropes, diuretics, and supplemental oxygen may be needed for acute congestive heart failure.
- Reduce secretion and production of thyroid hormones—Antithyroid drugs prevent iodide binding in the thyroid within the hour. One hour after the administration of methimazole or propylthiouracil, iodide can be started.
- Block the metabolic effects of thyroid hormones—Metabolic manifestations can be treated with beta-adrenergic blockers such as propranolol or catecholamine depleting agents such as reserpine or guanethidine.

Peters K, Nance P, Wingard D: Malignant hyperthyroidism or malignant hyperthermia. Anesth Analg 60:613–615, 1981

C.6. How would you extubate this patient?

If tracheomalacia is suspected, direct visualization of airway patency is suggested. The fiberoptic bronchoscope can be used to assess for airway collapse and vocal cord movement as the endotracheal tube and bronchoscope together are slowly pulled back. If tracheal collapse is noted, the endotracheal tube and bronchoscope should be immediately readvanced. Vocal cord assessment must be done. If any question exists of the patient's ability to protect his airway, leave the endotracheal tube in place. A tracheostomy set, endotracheal tubes, and laryngoscope should be readily available at bedside.

D. Postoperative Management

D.1. The patient became stridorous and dyspneic in the recovery room. What was your differential diagnosis and strategy of intervention?

Causes of respiratory failure include hemorrhage, respiratory obstruction, recurrent laryngeal nerve palsies, tracheomalacia, pneumothorax, and hypocalcemia.

Signs of airway obstruction require emergent evaluation. Hematomas can cause compressive airway obstruction and also restrict venous and lymphatic drainage of tracheal mucosa. Hematoma evacuation requires opening and drainage of incisional sites. However, tracheal obstruction from mucosal edema may still persist. Patients should be intubated early before airway edema from compromised lymphatic and venous return occurs. Initially patients should be seated upright at 45 degrees to facilitate venous drainage. Steroids and racemic epinephrine via nebulization should be used to decrease laryngeal edema. If dyspnea worsens, the patient should be intubated.

Injury to bilateral recurrent laryngeal nerves results in respiratory obstruction. Patients demonstrate paramedian position of both of the true vocal cords. These patients require emergent airway intervention including intubation or tracheotomy. Patients with unilateral recurrent laryngeal nerve paralysis present with hoarseness and minimal signs of airway obstruction.

If dissection is carried down to the mediastinum, pneumothorax must be ruled out as a cause of postoperative respiratory deterioration.

Hypocalcemia secondary to inadvertent excision of parathyroid tissue manifests within the first 3 days postoperatively. Acute airway obstruction in the immediate postoperative period is uncommon. The patient will complain of circumoral numbness and tingling of the hands and feet. If calcium is not supplemented, the patient can develop stridor and airway obstruction secondary to muscle weakness. Severe hypocalcemia can also be associated with seizures and tetany.

Netterville J, Aly A, Ossoff R: Evaluation and treatment of complications of thyroid and parathyroid surgery. Otolaryngol Clin North Am 23:529–550, 1990

D.2. When does thyroid storm most often present?

Thyroid storm most often occurs postoperatively rather than intraoperatively. Treatment with the same regimen as outlined for emergency surgery is indicated (see question B.9.). Supportive measures with fluids, oxygen, and a cooling blanket are important. Aspirin should not be used as an antipyretic, as it displaces thyroid hormones from binding proteins and thus raises free hormone levels.

D.3. Discuss innervation of the larynx.

Innervation of the larynx is from two branches of the vagus nerve, the superior laryngeal and recurrent laryngeal. The superior laryngeal nerve divides just superficial to the thyrohyoid membrane into the internal laryngeal nerve (sensory and autonomic) and external laryngeal nerve (motor). The internal laryngeal nerve pierces the thyrohyoid membrane and supplies sensory fibers to the larynx superior to the vocal cords. The external laryngeal nerve remains superficial to the thyrohyoid membrane to supply the cricothyroid muscle and a portion of the transverse arytenoid muscle.

The recurrent laryngeal nerve supplies motor innervation to all of the remaining intrinsic muscles of the larynx and sensory innervation to the larynx inferior to the vocal cords.

The cricothyroid muscle is the only tensor muscle of the larynx. Bilateral recurrent laryngeal nerve injury will result in motor paralysis of all the intrinsic muscles of the larynx except the cricothyroid muscle and part of the transverse arytenoid muscle. Respiratory obstruction occurs as the vocal cords become approximated at midline. However, the cords are flaccid, not tense. The cricothyroid muscle requires resistance from the other intrinsic muscles to tense the cords. Unilateral recurrent laryngeal nerve injury results in one midline, flaccid cord with the other cord being normal. Hoarseness and risk of aspiration are more problematic than respiratory obstruction.

Barash P, Cullen B, Stoelting R (eds): Clinical Anesthesia, 3rd ed, pp 1067–1069. Philadelphia, JB Lippincott, 1997

Moore KL: Clinically Oriented Anatomy, 2nd ed, pp 1061–1062. Baltimore, Williams & Wilkins, 1985

31 Pheochromocytoma

Gregory E. Kerr

The patient was a 28-year-old woman with a 10-day history of recurrent headaches. The headaches were unresponsive to medical therapy and increasing in frequency. Therefore, she was admitted to her local hospital. On admission, her heart rate was 84 beats/min with a systolic blood pressure of 210 mm Hg. The patient had no previous history of medical problems. Further studies were obtained to evaluate the cause of her high blood pressure and headaches.

A. Medical Disease and Differential Diagnosis

1. What are some common causes of hypertension?
2. What is a pheochromocytoma?
3. Trace the embryology of the adrenal gland and describe its normal anatomy.
4. What substances are secreted by the adrenal medulla?
5. What are the mechanisms of action of epinephrine and norepinephrine?
6. What is the pathway for synthesis and breakdown of catecholamines?
7. What substances are secreted by the adrenal cortex?
8. What are the metabolic actions of the glucocorticoids and the mineralocorticoids?
9. What are some clinical features associated with a pheochromocytoma?
10. In whom do we find it?
11. How is a pheochromocytoma diagnosed and localized?

B. Preoperative Evaluation and Preparation

1. How would you pharmacologically prepare the patient with a pheochromocytoma for surgery?
2. What other aspects of preoperative management are important?

C. Intraoperative Management

1. What drugs should be avoided during the operation?
2. How would you monitor this patient?
3. Describe acceptable options for administering anesthesia to this patient.
4. What are some methods of controlling the effects of catecholamine release during surgical manipulation?
5. What hemodynamic changes would you expect following removal of the tumor?
6. If a pheochromocytoma is found complicating pregnancy, does magnesium sulfate have a role in managing the hypertension?

D. Postoperative Management

1. What is the significance of postoperative hypotension? How is it treated?
2. What other problems can arise in the postoperative period?

A. Medical Disease and Differential Diagnosis

A.1. What are some common causes of hypertension?

The causes of hypertension are:

- Essential hypertension—unknown cause
- Primary renal disease—nephritis, renal artery stenosis, renal infarction
- Endocrine—adrenocortical hyperfunction, thyroid disease, pheochromocytoma, acromegaly
- Hemodynamic alterations—increased peripheral vascular resistance, increased intravascular volume
- Sympathetic stimulation—light anesthesia, hypoxia, hypercarbia
- Neurogenic—seizure activity, elevated intracranial pressure, denervation of the carotid sinus
- Miscellaneous—malignant hyperthermia, neuroleptic malignant syndrome, carcinoid syndrome, toxemia of pregnancy

Fauci AS, Braunwald E, Isselbacher KJ, et al (eds): Harrison's Principles of Internal Medicine, 14th ed, pp 1380–1381. New York, McGraw-Hill, 1998

Hickler R, Vandam LD: Hypertension. Anesthesiology 33:219, 1970

A.2. What is a pheochromocytoma?

Pheochromocytomas are catecholamine-secreting tumors of chromaffin tissue. They are usually located in the adrenal medullae or sympathetic paraganglia, but can be found anywhere chromaffin tissue exists. These locations extend from the base of the skull to the anus. Although most pheochromocytomas are found in the medulla portion of the adrenal gland, 10% of these tumors are located elsewhere.

Pheochromocytomas are entities that account for only 0.1% of the cases of hypertension. When unsuspected or improperly managed during surgery, the physiologic effects of the released catecholamines can be profound.

Hull CJ: Pheochromocytoma. Br J Anaesth 58:1453–1468, 1986

Malhotra V (ed): Anesthesia for Renal and Genito-Urologic Surgery, p 80. New York, McGraw-Hill, 1996

Pullerits J, Ein S, Balfe JW: Anesthesia for pheochromocytoma. Can J Anesth 35:526–534, 1988

A.3. Trace the embryology of the adrenal gland and describe its normal anatomy.

The adrenal cortex and medulla have separate embryologic origins. The medullary portion is derived from the chromaffin ectodermal cells of the neural crest. These cells are split off early from the sympathetic ganglion cells and migrate further ventrally, to lie ventrolateral to the aorta, where they form the paraganglia. Several such nodules near the cranial end of the gonads combine into a larger mass of cells lying between the dorsal aorta and the dorsomedial border of the mesonephros. Here they come into approximation with a group of mesodermal cells destined to become the adrenal cortex. These latter cells are derived principally from a narrow strip of coelomic mesothelium lying between the dorsal mesentery and the genital ridge. These cells, arising in numerous places in the suprarenal ridge, lose their connection with the mesothelium and form a complete layer of mesoderm around the ectodermal cells derived from the sympathetic ganglia. The chromaffin cells become enclosed within the adrenal cortex to form the medulla. The organs of Zuckerkandl are paraganglia around the aorta at the level of the kidney anterior to the inferior aorta. Accessory areas for the occurrence of pheochromocytoma are in the mediastinum, in the bladder, occasionally in the neck, in the sacrococcygeal region, or in the anal or vaginal areas.

Schwartz SI, Shires GT, Spencer FC et al (eds): Principles of Surgery, 6th ed, pp 1561–1603. New York, McGraw-Hill, 1994

A.4. What substances are secreted by the adrenal medulla?

The adrenal medulla primarily secretes three substances, all of which are catecholamines. They are epinephrine, norepinephrine, and dopamine. These three compounds are found in the chromaffin cells of the sympathetic nervous system, which includes the adrenal medulla, aberrant tissue along the sympathetic chain, and paraganglia. Both norepinephrine and dopamine are found at the endings of the postganglionic fibers of the sympathetic nervous system and in the central nervous system.

Schwartz SI, Shires GT, Spencer FC (eds): Principles of Surgery, 6th ed, pp 1561–1603. New York, McGraw-Hill, 1994

A.5. What are the mechanisms of action of epinephrine and norepinephrine?

These catecholamines exert their effects by acting on alpha- and beta-adrenergic receptors. It is believed that the results of beta-receptor stimulation are largely mediated by the stimulation of adenylate (adenyl) cyclase, which results in the production and activation of cyclic adenosine monophosphate (cAMP). The stimulation of cAMP eventually leads to an increased inward calcium (Ca^{2+}) flux, thus increasing cytoplasmic Ca^{2+} concentrations. The increased availability of Ca^{2+} ultimately results in enhanced actin and myosin interactions. The stimulation of alpha$_1$-receptors creates an increased inward flux of Ca^{2+} and also affects the formation of inositol triphosphate. The stimulation of alpha$_2$-receptors inhibits the action of adenylate cyclase (Fig. 31-1).

The pharmacologic response is dependent on the location of the receptors throughout the body. The distribution and density of the receptors determine the predominant response to each catecholamine.

Hardman JG, Lilnbird LE, Molinoff PB et al (eds): Goodman and Gillman's the Pharmacologic Basis of Therapeutics, 9th ed, pp 127–130; 105–139. New York, Macmillan, 1996

Stoelting RK: Pharmacology and Physiology in Anesthetic Practice, 2nd ed, pp 264–284. Philadelphia, JB Lippincott, 1991

A.6. What is the pathway for synthesis and breakdown of catecholamines?

The synthesis of endogenous catecholamines begins with the active transport of the amino acid tyrosine from the circulation into postganglionic sympathetic nerve endings. The hydroxylation of tyrosine is generally regarded as the rate-limiting step of the pathway (Fig. 31-2.) Any drug containing the 3,4-dihydroxy benzene (catecholamine) structure is rapidly inactivated by catechol-o-methyl transferase (COMT) or

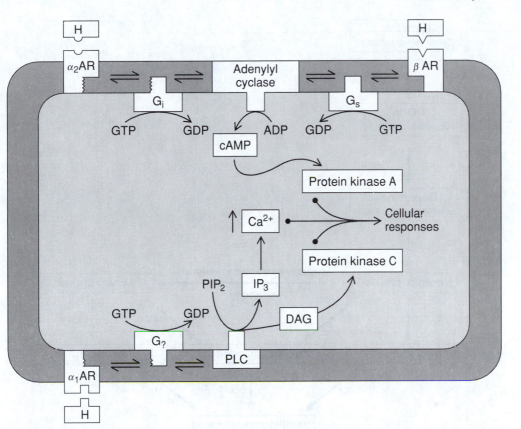

Figure 31-1. H, neurotransmitter or hormone; AR, adrenergic receptor; G_i, regulatory protein that, along with GTP, inhibits adenylate cyclase; G_s, regulatory protein that interacts with liganded beta-adrenergic receptor to stimulate adenylate cyclase; GTP, guanosine triphosphate; GDP, guanosine diphosphate; cAMP, cyclic adenosine monophosphate; Ca^{2+}, calcium; DAG, diacylglycerol; IP_3, inositol triphosphate; PIP_2, phosphatidyl inositol biphosphate. (Reprinted with permission from Goodman AG, Rall TW, Nies AS et al [eds]: The Pharmacologic Basis of Therapeutics, 8th ed, p 109. New York, Macmillan, 1993)

monoamine oxidase (MAO). The most important aspect of the termination of the biologic activity of these catecholamines is re-uptake into the nerve endings.

A.7. What substances are secreted by the adrenal cortex?

The adrenal cortex secretes more than 30 different corticosteroids. These can be divided into two major classes, the mineralocorticoids and the glucocorticoids. The precursor of all corticosteroids is cholesterol. Aldosterone is the most important mineralocorticoid secreted by the adrenal cortex, whereas cortisol is the most important glucocorticoid secreted. The adrenal cortex is also responsible for secreting sex steroids. Each of these substances is secreted by different zones: the mineralocorticoids

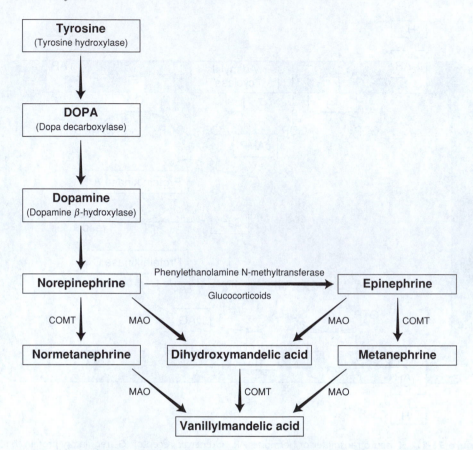

Figure 31-2.   *Synthesis and metabolism of endogenous catecholamine. (Reprinted with permission from Pullerits J, Ein S, Balfe JW: Anesthesia for phaeochromocytoma. Can J Anesth 35:526–534, 1988)*

are secreted by the zona glomerulosa, the glucocorticoids by the zona fasciculata, and the sex steroids (the androgens and estrogens) by the zona reticularis.

Hardman JG, Lilnbird LE, Molinoff PB et al (eds): Goodman and Gillman's the Pharmacologic Basis of Therapeutics, 9th ed, pp 1465–1481. New York, Macmillan, 1996

Stoelting RK: Pharmacology and Physiology in Anesthetic Practice, 2nd ed, pp 264–284. Philadelphia, JB Lippincott, 1991

A.8. ***What are the metabolic actions of the glucocorticoids and the mineralocorticoids?***

The glucocorticoids have their predominant mechanism of action on intermediary metabolism. These effects include increased gluconeogenesis, fatty acid mobilization, protein catabolism, and anti-inflammatory effects. About 95% of the glucocorticoid activity is from the secretion of cortisol. The mineralocorticoids have their predominant action on the body minerals, sodium and potassium. By conserving sodium ions they sustain extracellular fluid volume. They also help maintain normal potassium plasma concentrations.

Goodman AG, Rall TW, Nies AS et al (eds): The Pharmacologic Basis of Therapeutics, 8th ed, pp 1431–1462. New York, Macmillan, 1993

Stoelting RK: Endocrine System, Pharmacology and Physiology in Anesthetic Practice, 2nd ed, pp 752–768. Philadelphia, JB Lippincott, 1991

A.9. What are some clinical features associated with a pheochromocytoma?

The classic triad is severe headache, diaphoresis, and palpitations. One or more of the following often signals the presence of a pheochromocytoma: sudden severe headaches, perspiration, weight loss, paroxysmal hypertension, pallor, palpitations, diabetes-like syndrome with elevated fasting blood sugar, nausea, vomiting, fever, and encephalopathy. Although hypertension can be paroxysmal, 65% of adults with pheochromocytomas demonstrate sustained hypertension. The aforementioned symptoms are usually paroxysmal in nature. These attacks can last from a few moments to hours.

A pressor response to particular drugs suggests the presence of a pheochromocytoma. These drugs include histamine, glucagon, droperidol, tyramine, metoclopramide, cytotoxic drugs, saralasin, tricyclic antidepressant, and phenothiazines.

Hull CJ: Phaeochromocytoma. Br J Anaesth 58:1453–1468, 1986

Malhotra V (ed): Anesthesia For Renal and Genito-Urologic Surgery, p 80. New York, McGraw-Hill, 1996

A.10. In whom do we find it?

Pheochromocytomas occur in both genders with peak incidence in the third to fifth decades of life. Approximately 5% of cases of pheochromocytomas are inherited as an autosomal dominant trait either alone or as part of the neoplastic syndrome, which is called "multiple endocrine adenomatosis." See Table 31-1.

Malhotra V (ed): Anesthesia for Renal and Genito-Urologic Surgery, p 80. New York, McGraw-Hill, 1996

Pullerits J, Ein S, Balfe JW: Anesthesia for pheochromocytoma. Can J Anesth 35:526–534, 1988

Table 31-1. Multiple Endocrine Adenomatosis (MEA)

Type IIa (Sipple's syndrome)	• Parathyroid adenoma/hyperplasia • Medullary carcinoma of thyroid • Pheochromocytoma
Type IIb	• Medullary carcinoma of the thyroid • Mucosal adenomas • Marfanoid appearance • Pheochromocytoma
Von Hippel-Landau syndrome	• Hemangioblastoma of the retina, cerebellum or other parts of the central nervous system • Pheochromocytoma

Table 31-2.   Laboratory Tests for Pheochromocytoma

DIAGNOSTIC TEST	NORMAL VALUES	PHEOCHROMOCYTOMA
Blood		
Plasma catecholamines	<1000 pg/ml	>2000 pg/ml
Urine (24-hour collection)		
Catecholamines	<125 μg	>1200 μg
Norepinephrine	<100 μg	Increased
Epinephrine	<1 μg	Increased
Metanephrines	<1.6 mg	>2.5 mg
Vanillylmandelic acid	<8 mg	>10 mg
Confirmation if tests are equivocal		
Clonidine suppression of norepinephrine secretion	Suppressed in essential hypertensive patients	Not suppressed
Localization of tumor		
Magnetic resonance imaging		
Computed tomography		
Scintigraphy with metaiodobenzyl guanidine (MIBG)		
Selective adrenal venous catheterization and sampling		

(Reprinted with permission from Artusio J: Anesthesiology for pheochromocytoma. In Malhotra V [ed]: Anesthesia for Renal and Genito-Urologic Surgery, p 84. New York, McGraw-Hill, 1996)

A.11. How is a pheochromocytoma diagnosed and localized?

The laboratory tests for pheochromocytoma are shown in Table 31-2.

The biochemical diagnosis is based on the fact that pheochromocytomas release an excessive amount of catecholamines and metabolites. The diagnosis is made by measuring 24-hour urinary catecholamines and their structure metabolites, which include urinary norepinephrine, epinephrine, dopamine, total metanephrines, and vanillylmandelic acid (VMA), which are collected during a 24-hour period. The total metanephrines have given the highest true-positive results, about 98% to 99%.

In theory, the hydroxy-methoxy-mandelic acid (often misnamed VMA) level should be the most reliable laboratory test because it is the final common product of both catecholamine metabolic pathways. In practice, however, the intermediate metanephrines have proved to be better discriminators of pheochromocytomas. Some authors suggest that plasma catecholamine concentrations are the best single indicator of pheochromocytomas. High-pressure liquid chromatographic and radioenzyme methods for measuring catecholamine levels in the plasma have added to diagnostic accuracy.

The clonidine-suppression test is still occasionally used. It may be helpful in distinguishing the patient with a pheochromocytoma whose hypersecretion of norepinephrine does not respond to the drug from the patient without the tumor whose high basal plasma concentration is decreased to normal by the drug.

Computed tomography (CT) with or without ^{131}I-labeled metaiodobenzyl guanadine (MIBG) is extremely accurate in diagnosing and localizing the tumor. Arteriography, once popular, should be performed cautiously because dye can stimulate catecholamine release. Magnetic resonance imaging (MRI) scanning and CT scanning are the only imaging techniques that visualize normal adrenal glands when the diagnosis is equivocal. For extra-adrenal locations and in pregnant patients, MRI scanning may be a more desirable choice.

Bravo EL, Gifford RW: Pheochromocytoma: Diagnosis, localization and management. N Engl J Med 311:1298–1302, 1984

Hull CJ: Phaeochromocytoma. Br J Anaesth 58:1453–1468, 1986

Malhotra V (ed): Anesthesia for Renal and Genito-Urologic Surgery, p 84. New York, McGraw-Hill, 1996

Sheps SG, Jiang N, Klee GG et al: Recent developments in the diagnosis and treatment of pheochromocytoma. Mayo Clin Proc 65:88–95, 1990

B. Preoperative Evaluation and Preparation

B.1. How would you pharmacologically prepare the patient with a pheochromocytoma for surgery?

The major goal is both to partially block the responses to catecholamines and to avoid their pressor effects. Although surgery remains the only definitive therapy, the above goals must be obtained by using pharmacologic methods as soon as the diagnosis is made.

Administration of alpha-adrenergic blockers has been the cornerstone of management of patients with pheochromocytoma. The most commonly used agents have been phenoxybenzamine (Dibenzyline) starting at 10 to 20 mg, twice daily orally (po), prazosin (2 to 5 mg twice daily po), and phentolamine (5 mg) intravenously 2 hours before surgery. Phenoxybenzamine has been most widely used because of its relatively long duration of action and ease of administration. It irreversibly alkylates alpha$_1$-adrenergic receptors on vascular smooth muscle, thereby making them nonfunctional. It can cause postural hypotension and reflex tachycardia, which can be avoided with the careful administration of fluid volume as well as beta-blockers. Be sure not to start beta-blockade until the alpha-blockers have been started, otherwise congestive heart failure may be precipitated. Many feel that beta-blockers should only be used when tachycardia or arrhythmias exist.

Prazosin has been used but it does not seem to adequately prevent perioperative hypertensive episodes. Prazosin as well as magnesium sulfate, beta-blockers, angiotensin converting enzyme (ACE) inhibitors, and calcium channel blockers have been used in combination with phenoxybenzamine to attain hemodynamic stability.

Alpha-Methyl paratyrosine inhibits tyrosine hydroxylase. It can be given orally, gradually increasing the dose from 0.5 g/d to 4 g/d. This may decrease the catecholamine synthesis by 40% to 80%. It is effective, but it can cause diarrhea, sedative fatigue, anxiety or agitated depression, or tumors.

However, a study from the Cleveland Clinics suggests that preoperative use of alpha-blocking agents may not necessarily decrease the incidence of intraoperative hypertension or tachycardia. In fact, patients who did not receive preoperative phenoxybenzamine had a few advantages. Eighty percent of these patients did not require vasopressors in the postanesthesia care unit (PACU), whereas the rest did so for a very short period of time. Similarly, 79% of patients received no vasodilators in the PACU. No difference was found in intensive care unit length of stay between those patients who received preoperative alpha-blockers versus those who did not.

It is possible that advances in anesthetic and monitoring techniques as well as the availability of fast-acting drugs capable of correcting sudden changes in hemodynamics has eliminated the need to use alpha-blockers in the preoperative period for those patients who are about to undergo surgery for a pheochromocytoma resection.

Boutros AR, Bravo EL, Zanettin G et al: Perioperative management of 63 patients with pheochromocytoma. Cleve Clin J Med 57:613–617, 1990

Bravo EL, Gifford RW: Pheochromocytoma: Diagnosis, localization and management. N Engl J Med 311:1298–1302, 1984

Hull CJ: Phaeochromocytoma. Br J Anaesth 58:1453–1468, 1986

Malhotra V (ed): Anesthesia for Renal and Genito-Urologic Surgery, p 80. New York, McGraw-Hill, 1996

Pullerits J, Balfe JW: Anesthesia for phaeochromocytoma. Can J Anesth 35:526–534, 1988

B.2. What other aspects of preoperative management are important?

The circulating blood volume is decreased in many patients with pheochromocytomas. Therefore, many clinicians support the idea of administering volume (frequently blood) prior to surgery while patients receive alpha-blockers. One must be careful with patients who have decreased myocardial function to avoid congestive heart failure. Many other clinicians feel volume loading is not necessary. They feel that if the patient has been on alpha-blockers for 2 weeks or more, then the volume has been restored.

Sedation for the preoperative period is considered by many clinicians to be important prior to surgery. Sedation may obviate the need to use high doses of antihypertensive agents prior to surgery.

Boutros AR, Bravo EL, Zanettin G et al: Perioperative management of 63 patients with pheochromocytoma. Cleveland Clin J Med 57:613–617, 1990

Bravo EL, Gifford RW: Pheochromocytoma: Diagnosis, localization and management. N Engl J Med 311:1298–1302, 1984

Hull CJ: Phaeochromocytoma. Br J Anaesth 58:1453-1468, 1986

Malhotra V (ed): Anesthesia for Renal and Genito-Urologic Surgery, p 80. New York, McGraw-Hill, 1996

Pullerits J, Balfe JW: Anesthesia for phaeochromocytoma. Can J Anesth 35:526-534, 1988

C. Intraoperative Management

C.1. What drugs should be avoided during the operation?

Because many agents are available from which to choose, the controversial agents should be avoided (Table 31-3). Droperidol, although used by many, has been associated with pressor responses. This appears to be secondary to the inhibition of catecholamine re-uptake. Atropine exacerbates the chronotropic effects of epinephrine by vagal inhibition. All drugs that release histamine (e.g., morphine, curare, atracurium) might be avoided because histamine has been known to provoke pheochromocyto-

Table 31-3. Suggested Drugs to Avoid in Patients with Pheochromocytoma

Cocaine	Pancuronium	Halothane	Morphine
Droperidol	Ketamine	Metoclopramide	Curare
	Ephedrine		Atracurium

(Reprinted with permission from Artusio J: Anesthesiology for pheochromocytoma. In: Malhotra V [ed]: Anesthesia for Renal and Genito-Urologic Surgery, p 84. New York, McGraw-Hill, 1996)

mas. Agents that cause an indirect increase in catecholamine levels (e.g., pancuronium, ketamine, ephedrine) should be avoided. It should be noted that morphine, curare, atracurium, and pancuronium have all been used with clinical reports documenting their safe use.

Hull CJ: Phaeochromocytoma. Br J Anaesth 58:1453–1468, 1986

Malhotra V (ed): Anesthesia for Renal and Genito-Urologic Surgery, p 80. New York, McGraw-Hill, 1996

Pullerits J, Balfe JW: Anesthesia for phaeochromocytoma. Can J Anesth 35:526–534, 1988

C.2. How would you monitor this patient?

Monitoring in these patients should include an electrocardiogram with a V_5 lead, core temperature, pulse oximetry, end-tidal CO_2, intra-arterial blood pressure, central venous pressure, and a urinary catheter. For patients with known or suspected myocardial dysfunction, a pulmonary artery catheter should be considered.

Desmonts M, Marty J: Anesthetic management of patients with phaeochromocytoma. Br J Anaesth 56:781, 1984

C.3. Describe acceptable options for administering anesthesia to this patient.

Either general anesthesia, regional anesthesia, or a combination of the two are considered acceptable. For all techniques, it is important to avoid wide swings in blood pressure.

For general anesthesia, induction with thiopental has been most commonly used, but induction with propofol has recently been reported to be a safe technique. One can lessen the response to intubation by administering 1.5 mg/kg lidocaine intravenously 2 minutes prior to laryngoscopy. Other measures to attenuate hemodynamic responses to intubation are described in Chapter 14, Hypertension, questions C.5 and C.6. General anesthesia has been maintained with most of the inhalation agents, but most commonly with isoflurane. Clinicians seem also to like the concomitant use of narcotics with the inhalation agent. Some authors advocate the avoidance of halothane because of its ability to increase the incidence of arrhythmias. Recently, the safety of desflurane was demonstrated. It was effective at controlling hypertensive surges in well-prepared patients, although it is known to cause sympathetic stimulation.

Hull CJ: Phaeochromocytoma. Br J Anaesth 58:1453–1468, 1986

Lippman M, Ford M, Lee C et al: Use of desflurane during resection of phaeochromocytoma. Br J Anaesth 72:707–709, 1994

Pullerits J, Ein S, Balfe JW: Anesthesia for phaeochromocytoma. Can J Anesth 35:526–534, 1988

Strebel S, Schendigger S: Propofol-fentanyl anesthesia for pheochromocytoma resection. Acta Anaesthesiol Scand 35:375–377, 1991

C.4. What are some methods of controlling the effects of catecholamine release during surgical manipulation?

Massive catecholamine secretion during surgery causes hypertension, tachycardia, and arrhythmias. Drugs used to control intraoperative hypertension are listed in

Table 31-4. Drugs to Manage High Blood Pressure

DRUG	ROUTE	DOSE
Nitroprusside	IV	Infuse initially with 0.5–1.5 μg/kg/min to maximum of 8 μg/kg/min over 1–3 h
Phentolamine	IV	1–5 mg every 5 minutes or infuse initially with 1 mg/min
Propanolol	IV	1 mg boluses up to total 10 mg
Labetalol	IV	10 mg boluses to total 150 mg
Esmolol	IV	5–10 boluses or infusion
Hydralazine	IV	5–10 mg boluses every 30 min
Magnesium sulfate	IV	2 g boluses; be cautious in patients with renal failure and neuromuscular blockade

Table 31-4. Phentolamine, a short-acting alpha-blocking agent, can be given as a continuous infusion to control blood pressure. Phentolamine along with isoflurane may maintain an appropriate blood pressure. However, sodium nitroprusside (solution 0.01%) has become the most commonly used agent for control of high blood pressure during pheochromocytoma surgery because it is faster and shorter acting than phentolamine. Greater familiarity with the drug and a decreased incidence of reflex tachycardia are additional advantages.

Magnesium sulfate ($MgSO_4$) is another agent that is commonly used as an adjunct vasodilator. Beta-blockers are helpful during the perioperative period to control blood pressure as well as heart rate and possible arrhythmias. Lidocaine should also be considered for the control of arrhythmias.

Bravo EL, Gifford RW: Pheochromocytoma: Diagnosis, localization and management. N Engl J Med 311:1298–1302, 1984

Hull CJ: Phaeochromocytoma. Br J Anaesth 58:1453–1468, 1986

Pullerits J, Ein S, Balfe JW: Anesthesia for phaeochromocytoma. Can J Anesth 35:526–534, 1988

C.5. What hemodynamic changes would you expect following removal of the tumor?

It is important to be aware of the fact that blood pressure can fall very quickly after the blood supply of the tumor is interrupted. Blood pressure can be maintained by administering norepinephrine drip (8 mg in 250 ml solution) as well as fluids. Blood should be administered if the blood loss is substantial.

Bravo EL, Gifford RW: Pheochromocytoma: Diagnosis, localization and management. N Engl J Med 311:1298–1302, 1984

Hull CJ: Phaeochromocytoma. Br J Anaesth 58:1453–1468, 1986

Pullerits J, Ein S, Balfe JW: Anesthesia for phaeochromocytoma. Can J Anesth 35:526–534, 1988

C.6. If a pheochromocytoma is found complicating pregnancy, does magnesium sulfate have a role in managing the hypertension?

Reports indicate that magnesium sulfate can be used in conjunction with several potent inhalation anesthetics to control blood pressure. Hypomagnesemia may be present in the pregnant patient and it should be corrected preoperatively. Magnesium is an ideal adjunct to the anesthetic management because its use to control blood pressure is not deleterious to the fetus.

Michael FM, Huddle RL: Use of magnesium sulphate in the management of pheochromocytoma in pregnancy. Can J Anesth 35:178–182, 1988

D. Postoperative Management

D.1. What is the significance of postoperative hypotension? How is it treated?

Postoperative hypotension is often seen after the excision of the tumor, and it may be caused by hypovolemia and/or persistent fatigue of the vasoconstrictor mechanism. Once the excess catecholamines are diminished after tumor removal, the response by the vascular bed to maintain pressure may be sluggish. Hypotension is rarely seen in patients who have received adequate volume-expansion and alpha-blockade preoperatively. If it does occur, it should be treated with volume administration and, if needed, norepinephrine. Be cognizant of the fact that persistent hypotension may be secondary to bleeding, which necessitates a prompt return to the operating room.

Hull CJ: Phaeochromocytoma. Br J Anaesth 58:1453–1468, 1986

Malhotra V (ed): Anesthesia for Renal and Genito-Urologic Surgery, p 80. New York, McGraw-Hill, 1996

Pullerits J, Ein S, Balfe JW: Anesthesia for phaeochromocytoma. Can J Anesth 35:526–534, 1988

D.2. What other problems can arise in the postoperative period?

For the first 48 hours after surgery, these patients may be very somnolent, possibly because of the sudden removal of activating catecholamines. Frequently, this results in decreased narcotic requirements.

Be aware that these patients are also prone to significant hypoglycemia, which alone can make a patient somnolent. In more severe cases, hypoglycemia can cause loss of consciousness and respiratory arrest. The hypoglycemia results from the fact that the suppression of beta-cell function disappears after removal of the tumor. Hence the plasma insulin level rises. Neoglycogenesis and glycogenolysis, which had sustained the high blood sugar, are no longer present. Therefore, one should consider switching to a glucose-containing intravenous fluid after tumor removal and monitor the glucose levels closely for at least 24 hours in the postoperative period.

Persistent hypertension after removal of a pheochromocytoma occasionally signifies that a residual pheochromocytoma tumor is present. Be aware that plasma catecholamine levels may not decrease to normal levels for many days after removal of the tumor.

Bravo L, Gifford RW: Pheochromocytoma: Diagnosis, localization and management. N Engl J Med 311:1298, 1984

Bravo EL, Tarazl RC, Gifford RW et al: Circulating and urinary catecholamines in pheochromocytoma: Diagnostic and pathophysiologic implications. N Engl J Med 301:682–686, 1979

Lippman M, Ford M, Lee C et al: Use of desflurane during rejection of pheochromocytoma. Br J Anaesth 72:707–709, 1994

Sheps S, Jiang N, Klee GG et al: Recent developments in the diagnosis and treatment of pheochromocytoma. Mayo Clin Proc 65:88–95, 1990

Streibel S, Scheidegger D: Propofol-fentanyl anesthesia for pheochromocytoma resection. Acta Anaesth Scand 35:275–277, 1991

32 Diabetes

Vinod Malhotra

A 45-year-old woman had a known history of diabetes for 30 years. Her diabetes was controlled with regular crystalline insulin, 35 units daily. She was scheduled for emergency surgery for tubo-ovarian abscess. Blood glucose was 350 mg/dl.

A. Medical Disease and Differential Diagnosis

1. What is the incidence of diabetes mellitus in the general population?
2. What are the factors in the cause of the disease?
3. How do you classify diabetes mellitus?
4. What are the complications of diabetes mellitus?
5. How would you treat the different forms of this illness?
6. How do you adequately monitor the control of the disease?
7. What are some of the factors that alter insulin requirement?
8. What are the principles of management of diabetic ketoacidosis?

B. Preoperative Evaluation and Preparation

1. How would you evaluate this patient preoperatively?
2. How would stiff joint syndrome affect her airway management?
3. What are the signs and implications of autonomic neuropathy in the diabetic patient?
4. How would you prepare this patient for anesthesia and surgery?
5. For elective surgery, how do you manage the insulin and glucose requirements on the day of surgery?
6. How would you premedicate this patient? Why?

C. Intraoperative Management

1. What is the effect of anesthesia and surgery on insulin and glucose metabolism?
2. What anesthetic techniques would you employ?
3. How would you monitor this patient?
4. How would you treat hyperglycemia intraoperatively?
5. How would you recognize and treat hypoglycemic shock intraoperatively?

D. Postoperative Management

1. How would you control diabetes in this patient postoperatively?
2. What are the common postoperative complications you expect in a diabetic patient?
3. Does diabetes increase perioperative risk? Is it necessary to achieve tight perioperative control of blood glucose?

A. Medical Disease and Differential Diagnosis

A.1. What is the incidence of diabetes mellitus in the general population?

The estimated incidence of diabetes mellitus in the United States varies depending on the criteria used to define the disease. The National Commission on Diabetes reported an incidence of 5% in 1976. The National Diabetes Data Group used the diagnostic criterion of a fasting plasma glucose in excess of 140 mg/dl on two separate occasions or an impaired glucose tolerance with two values of plasma glucose of 200 mg/dl during the 2 hours following glucose ingestion. On the basis of these two criteria, they reported the prevalence of the disease at 6.6% and an impaired glucose tolerance in nearly twice that population. It is estimated that by the year 2000, nearly 10% of all Americans may be affected by diabetes mellitus. Of the approximately 14 million diabetics in America, >90% are non–insulin-dependent. Most of these patients tend to be elderly and overweight.

Fauci AS, Braunwald E, Isselbacher KJ et al (eds): Harrison's Principles of Internal Medicine, 14th ed, pp 2061–2062. New York, McGraw-Hill, 1998

Report of the National Commission on Diabetes of the Congress of the United States. Vol. 1: The Long Range Plan to Combat Diabetes. DHEW publication no. (NIH) 76–1018, 1976

Roizen MF: Perioperative Management of the Diabetic Patient. ASA Annual Refresher Course Lectures No.245. 1996

A.2. What are the factors in the cause of the disease?

Three main factors have received widespread recognition in the cause of diabetes mellitus; these include genetics, immune response, and viruses. The role of genetic factors in the development of the disorder is undisputed, although the mode of inheritance still remains controversial. Studies on monozygotic twins show a concordance rate for the disease to be <50% if the age at onset in the index twin is <40 years. The rate approaches 100% if the age at onset is >40 years in the index twin. In the offspring of conjugal diabetic parents, the incidence of the overt disease is 6% to 10% and that of chemical diabetes 25% to 40%, based on the glucose tolerance test. In view of such diverse findings, it is reasonable to assume a polygenic transmission modified by environmental factors.

Histopathologic studies, elevated titers of histocompatibility antigens (notably human leukocyte antigen [HLA]), presence of insulin antibodies, and association of juvenile-onset diabetes with certain well-known autoimmune diseases (e.g., thyroiditis and myasthenia gravis) underline the significance of immune factors in the pathogenesis of this entity. Virus beta-cell interactions have been postulated in the pathogenesis of juvenile diabetes in recent years, with supportive evidence of antiviral antibody titers implicating several common RNA and DNA viruses.

A possible scenario then for a type I diabetic could be a genetically susceptible individual who is exposed to a virus that causes inflammation of the pancreatic islet cells and lymphocytic infiltration with subsequent triggering of the autoimmune response, ultimately destroying beta-cells.

Craighead JE: Current views on the etiology of insulin-dependent diabetes mellitus. N Engl J Med 299:1439–1445, 1978

Fauci AS, Braunwald E, Isselbacher KJ et al (eds): Harrison's Principles of Internal Medicine, 14th ed, pp 2062–2065. New York, McGraw-Hill, 1998

Ganda OP, Soeldner SS: Genetic, acquired, and related factors in the etiology of diabetes mellitus. Arch Intern Med 137:461–469, 1977

Miller RD (ed): Anesthesia, 4th ed, pp 905–907. New York, Churchill-Livingstone, 1994

A.3. How do you classify diabetes mellitus?

Although several classifications exist for diabetes mellitus, the best way to classify the disease is to differentiate the two different forms of the clinical entity. Type I, then, is the insulin-dependent diabetes. It is more severe, and the onset is usually in the young. A gene-virus interaction and immune disturbance are believed to be the main causative factors. Type II, on the other hand, is non–insulin-dependent, mild, and affects all ages, the incidence increasing with age. Genetic factors probably predominate in the cause of this form.

Fauci AS, Braunwald E, Isselbacher KJ et al (eds): Harrison's Principles of Internal Medicine, 14th ed, pp 2061–2062. New York, McGraw-Hill, 1998

Miller RD (ed): Anesthesia, 4th ed, pp 905–907. New York, Churchill-Livingstone, 1994

Roizen MF: Perioperative Management of the Diabetic Patient. ASA Annual Refresher Course Lectures No. 245. 1996

A.4. What are the complications of diabetes mellitus?

The long-term complications of diabetes mellitus are the result of end-organ pathology due to chronic hyperglycemia. Cardiovascular changes include coronary artery disease, hypertension, cardiac autonomic neuropathy, and microangiopathic myocardiopathy. Myocardial infarction is the most common cause of death in the elderly diabetic. Diabetic retinopathy, neuropathy, nephropathy, and vascular changes are other well-known complications of the long-standing disease. In the case of a juvenile diabetic such as this patient, however, the common life-threatening complications are mainly caused by poor control and include hypoglycemia, hyperglycemia, diabetic ketoacidosis, and coma. Long-term complications of diabetes are believed to be due to poor glycemic control and hyperglycemia. Recent literature clearly indicates that a tight control of blood glucose levels reduces the risk of chronic complications in the type I diabetic.

Clark CM Jr, Lee DA: Prevention and treatment of the complications of diabetes mellitus. N Engl J Med 332:1210–1217, 1995

The Diabetic Control and Complications Trial Research Group: The effect of intensive treatment of diabetes on the development and progression of long-term complications for insulin dependent diabetes mellitus. N Engl J Med 329:977–987, 1993

Fauci AS, Braunwald E, Isselbacher KJ et al (eds): Harrison's Principles of Internal Medicine, 14th ed, pp 2071–2077. New York, McGraw-Hill, 1998

Winegrad AI: Banting Lecture 1986: Does a common mechanism induce the diverse complications of diabetes? Diabetes 36:396–409, 1986

A.5. How would you treat the different forms of this illness?

The type I diabetic, who has the severe form of the disease, is insulin-dependent and susceptible to diabetic ketoacidosis. Two preparations of insulin in common use

Table 32-1. Onset and Duration of Action of Subcutaneous Insulin Injection in Diabetic Patients

TYPE	ONSET (HOURS)	PEAK ACTIVITY (HOURS)	DURATION (HOURS)
Regular insulin (crystalline insulin)	1	6	16
NPH Insulin (Isophane insulin)	2.5	11	25

today include the regular crystalline insulin and the NPH (Neutral Protamine Hagedorn) insulin. Most insulins are of animal origin. However, in recent years human insulin (Humulin) produced by recombinant DNA has been used increasingly because of its improved efficacy and lower incidence of allergic reactions. The onset and duration of action of these agents in diabetic patients by subcutaneous injection are shown in Table 32-1. However, in normal persons the onset of regular insulin is within minutes, maximal action is around 2 hours, and duration is only 6 to 8 hours; with NPH, the onset, peak, and duration of action are approximately the same for both normal persons and diabetic patients.

The type II patient is a mild diabetic and is usually obese. The rationale for treatment in these patients centers around weight loss and diet control. Weight reduction and diet control together can control most of these patients' diabetes. Patients whose diabetes is not controlled well on this regimen require oral hypoglycemics or insulin. The University Group Diabetes Program study revealed a higher incidence of cardiovascular deaths in patients treated with tolbutamide, with no significant difference in efficacy of treatment compared with placebo. Since the first report in 1970, this study has been a subject of major controversy regarding the toxicity of oral hypoglycemics. Both tolbutamide and phenformin have been shown to be inadequate in sustained lowering of blood sugar in treated populations. The question of efficacy of other agents is still open. The newer sulfonyl ureas, namely glyburide (Micronase) and glipizide (Glucotrol), have a longer effect in lowering blood sugar and are frequently used. However, the role for oral hypoglycemics is still questionable, except in selected individuals where insulin control poses problems in a maturity-onset diabetic. Most maturity-onset diabetics can be treated with diet and exercise, and if that fails to control the disease adequately, insulin should be added to the regimen.

Newer drugs and other therapies currently being studied include:

- Amino guanidine—prevents glucose from binding to tissues and causing damage
- Metformin—improves cellular sensitivity to insulin
- Miglitol—slows the breakdown of carbohydrates
- Pancreas transplants
- Transplant of islet cells

Availability of a noninvasive meter to measure blood glucose will further facilitate tight control.

The Diabetic Control and Complications Trial Research Group: The effect of intensive treatment of diabetes on the development and progression of long-term complications for insulin dependent diabetes mellitus. N Engl J Med 329:977–987, 1993

Fauci AS, Braunwald E, Isselbacher KJ et al (eds): Harrison's Principles of Internal Medicine, 14th ed, pp 2066–2068. New York, McGraw-Hill, 1998

University Group Diabetes Program: A study of the effects of hypoglycemic agents on vascular complications with adult-onset diabetes. II. Mortality results. Diabetes 19(Suppl):787–830, 1970

A.6. How do you adequately monitor the control of the disease?

Mild diabetics and well-controlled diabetics are usually self-monitored by daily urine test for reducing sugars and ketones. In acute management of hyperglycemia or in situations where insulin requirement is altered (as in the above patient secondary to infection), the best control is achieved with regular crystalline insulin and frequent monitoring of blood sugars, because the changes in urinary sugar appear after a lag period. A quick bedside method of blood sugar assessment involves the use of Dextrostix and the Ames dextrometer.

Increasing evidence indicates that most of the end-organ complications of diabetes are the result of chronic hyperglycemia. Therefore maintaining as close to a euglycemic state as possible is the goal. Most patients who follow their blood glucose level can do so at home using the readily available kits. Diabetologists frequently measure HbA_{1c} to monitor long-term control. HbA_{1c} (normal value 6%) is increased in poorly controlled diabetics because its synthesis depends on nonenzymatic glycosylation.

Ammon JR: Perioperative management of the diabetic patient. ASA Annual Refresher Course Lectures No. 144. 1994

Fauci AS, Braunwald E, Isselbacher KJ et al (eds): Harrison's Principles of Internal Medicine, 14th ed, pp 2068–2069. New York, McGraw-Hill, 1998

A.7. What are some of the factors that alter insulin requirement?

Factors commonly known to increase the insulin requirement include a high-carbohydrate diet, infection, sepsis, stress, and certain frequently employed drugs, namely, corticosteroids, thyroid preparations, oral contraceptives, and thiazide diuretics. Exercise and alcohol commonly result in decreased requirements, as do certain drugs, such as phenylbutazone, dicumarol, and salicylates, which mainly interfere with the pharmacodynamics of oral hypoglycemics.

Fauci AS, Braunwald E, Isselbacher KJ et al (eds): Harrison's Principles of Internal Medicine, 14th ed, pp 2079–2080. New York, McGraw-Hill, 1998

Shen SW, Bressler R: Clinical pharmacology of oral antidiabetic agents. N Engl J Med 296:493–497, 1977

A.8. What are the principles of management of diabetic ketoacidosis?

Diabetic ketoacidosis is an acute medical emergency characterized by an absolute or relative deficiency of insulin resulting in an accumulation of ketone acids in the blood. The main disturbances are hyperglycemia, glycosuria, intracellular dehydration, acidosis, and electrolyte imbalance. Conventionally, severe ketoacidosis implies levels of ketone acids in the blood generally >7 mM/liter, a decrease in serum bicarbonate to <10 mEq/liter or a decrease in pH to <7.25. Initial physical examination should be supported with urinalysis, venous blood analysis for glucose, electrolytes, urea nitrogen, complete blood count, and serum ketone estimation. Reagent strips can be used to determine the blood glucose (Dextrostix) and ketones (Ketostix) quickly, and therapy can be initiated. An arterial blood gas sample should be analyzed to determine acid-base imbalance. The mainstay of treatment includes fluids, insulin, bicarbonate, and potassium.

• Fluids—Most patients are dehydrated and the loss of water exceeds that of salt.

Therefore, a hypotonic saline solution (0.45% sodium chloride) is considered optimal. Five percent glucose should be instituted once the serum glucose falls below 300 mg per 100 ml. A central venous pressure measurement and urine output are good guidelines for fluid therapy.

- Insulin—All patients in ketoacidosis are in immediate need of insulin. Therefore, a rapid-onset short-acting insulin should be employed to attain better control. Insulin (10 to 20 units) is given intravenously initially and an infusion of insulin at a rate of 1 to 2 units per hour is started depending on blood glucose levels. Initial bolus dose can be repeated depending on the severity of ketoacidosis and hyperglycemia, and the glucose lowering response to the initial dose.
- Bicarbonate—Sodium bicarbonate should be used to correct severe metabolic acidosis (with pH 7.20) as guided by determinations of arterial blood pH, PCO_2, and bicarbonate. Overcorrection should be avoided.
- Potassium—Following acidosis, osmotic diuresis, and vomiting, body potassium stores are depleted by 5 to 10 mEq per kilogram of body weight. Serum potassium, although initially normal, usually decreases because the correction of hyperglycemia and acidosis results in movement of potassium from extracellular space to intracellular space. Therefore, potassium should be added to the intravenous infusion 3 to 4 hours after initiating the therapy, provided the renal function is adequate. Frequent laboratory data and clinical findings should dictate the dose and frequency regimen of the treatment. Supportive therapy for associated problems should continue, and overcorrection should be avoided.

Fauci AS, Braunwald E, Isselbacher KJ et al (eds): Harrison's Principles of Internal Medicine, 14th ed, pp 2071–2073. New York, McGraw-Hill, 1998

Hirsh IB, McGill JB, Cryer PE et al: Perioperative management of surgical patients with diabetes mellitus. Anesthesiology 74:346–359, 1991

Kitabchi AE: Low dose insulin therapy in diabetic ketoacidosis: Fact or fiction? Diabetes Metab Rev 5:337–363, 1989

Roizen MF: Perioperative Management of the Diabetic Patient. ASA Annual Refresher Course Lectures No. 245. 1996

Walker M, Marshall SM, Alberti KGMM: Clinical aspects of diabetic ketoacidosis. Diabetes Metab Rev 5:651–663, 1989

B. Preoperative Evaluation and Preparation

B.1. How would you evaluate this patient preoperatively?

A complete preoperative evaluation includes a history and physical examination supported by the following laboratory data:

- Electrocardiogram
- Urinalysis for detecting sugar and ketones
- Venous blood estimation of complete blood count, serum electrolytes, urea nitrogen, sugar, and ketones (serum osmolality if available)
- Arterial blood gas analysis to determine acid-base status

Of great pertinence is the history of the last intake of meal and the last dose of insulin. Nausea and vomiting in this patient will affect her state of hydration, acid-base status, and electrolyte balance significantly. The patient should be questioned and examined for stiff joint syndrome, which can render the intubation difficult.

Alberti KGMM, Thomas DJB: The management of diabetes during surgery. Br J Anaesth 51:693–710, 1979

Ammon JR: Perioperative management of the diabetic patient. ASA Annual Refresher Course Lectures No. 144. 1994

Hirsh IB, McGill JB, Cryer PE et al: Perioperative management of surgical patients with diabetes mellitus. Anesthesiology 74:346–359, 1991

B.2. How would stiff joint syndrome affect her airway management?

Stiff joint syndrome has been reported as frequently as in approximately one of four adolescent diabetics. As the name implies, it is characterized by stiff joints due to non-enzymatic glycosylation of the collagen tissues. This is the same phenomenon that results in an increase in HbA_{1c}, frequently used to monitor the adequacy of diabetes control. If this process involves the atlanto-occipital joint, the resultant limitation of extension of the head may make endotracheal intubation difficult.

Ammon JR: Perioperative management of the diabetic patient. ASA Annual Refresher Course Lectures No. 144. 1994

Salzarulo HH, Taylor LA: Diabetic "stiff joint syndrome" as a cause of difficult endotracheal intubation. Anesthesiology 64:366–368, 1986

B.3. What are the signs and implications of autonomic neuropathy in the diabetic patient?

Autonomic neuropathy occurs in approximately 1 of every 10 diabetics. In the older population, especially those with coexisting hypertension, the incidence increases four to fivefold. Signs of autonomic neuropathy include lack of sweating, early satiety, orthostatic hypotension, gastric reflux, and lack of change in pulse rate with deep inspiration. Impotence and urinary symptoms of dysautonomic bladder may be evident.

The implication of autonomic neuropathy is increased morbidity and mortality. Orthostatic hypotension in the perioperative period is common, and it may be severe immediately postoperatively. Myocardial ischemia would be painless with risks of cardiorespiratory arrest. Gastroparesis predisposes these patients to nausea, vomiting, regurgitation, and aspiration.

Charleson MC, Mackenzie CR, Gold JP: Preoperative autonomic function abnormalities in patients with diabetes mellitus and patients with hypertension. J Am Coll Surg 179:1–10, 1994

Roizen MF: Perioperative management of the diabetic patient. ASA Annual Refresher Course Lectures No. 245. 1996

B.4. How would you prepare this patient for anesthesia and surgery?

The preoperative evaluation will determine the preparation of this patient, the principles of which are as follows:

Hydration
• Poor oral intake secondary to malaise and abdominal pain, concomitant vomiting, if present, and osmotic diuresis owing to glycosuria make dehydration likely in

this patient. Any dehydration that is present, therefore, should be rapidly corrected. Normal or half-normal saline is a preferred intravenous solution because the blood glucose level is already elevated in this instance.

Insulin

- Infection and stress are known to increase insulin requirements, which explains hyperglycemia in this patient. Insulin can be given to this patient either in small doses (5 to 10 units intravenously) every hour or as a continuous infusion at 1 to 2 units per hour using a pump. Hourly blood and urine glucose and acetone measurements should be used to adequately monitor this therapy. Acid-base and electrolyte correction should be carried out as dictated by blood tests. Antibiotics should be instituted once appropriate culture samples are obtained.

Alberti KGMM, Thomas DJB: The management of diabetes during surgery. Br J Anaesth 51:693–710, 1979

Ammon JR: Perioperative management of the diabetic patient. ASA Annual Refresher Course Lectures No. 144. 1994

Hirsh IB, McGill JB, Cryer PE et al: Perioperative management of surgical patients with diabetes mellitus. Anesthesiology 74:346–359, 1991

Roizen MF: Perioperative management of the diabetic patient. ASA Annual Refresher Course Lectures No. 245. 1996

B.5. For elective surgery, how do you manage the insulin and glucose requirements on the day of surgery?

A large number of protocols exist for managing insulin and glucose requirements in the insulin-dependent diabetic. For the non–insulin-dependent diabetic, the morning dose of oral hypoglycemic agent is omitted, and for most surgical procedures, the glucose-containing intravenous solutions can be avoided. Based on blood sugar determinations, regular insulin can be used to treat hyperglycemia. For extensive procedures and when the patient is not expected to resume oral intake for a few days, glucose should be given in the intravenous solution as a substrate for the increased metabolic demand, thus providing protein-sparing effect. Parenteral regular insulin is best suited to control hyperglycemia in that situation. For the insulin-dependent diabetic, the problem is more acute and none of the commonly followed protocols offers a complete solution (see Table 32-2).

Frequent blood sugar estimation is the key to tailoring insulin therapy for each individual. It is recommended that blood glucose be measured the morning of surgery. For cases scheduled for surgery later in the day, this can be repeated prior to anesthesia. Intraoperatively, blood sugar should be measured every 2 hours, or more frequently, if necessary. Glucose can be infused by a steady continuous drip providing 50 g every 8 hours. Insulin infusion is started at 1 to 2 units per hour. Small doses of insulin (5 to 10 units) can be given intravenously to treat hyperglycemia >250 mg/dl, if necessary.

Ammon JR: Perioperative management of the diabetic patient. ASA Annual Refresher Course Lectures No. 144. 1994

Hirsh IB, McGill JB, Cryer PE et al: Perioperative management of surgical patients with diabetes mellitus. Anesthesiology 74:346–359, 1991

Table 32-2. Perioperative Insulin Therapy Protocols in the Diabetic Patient

PROTOCOL	LIMITATIONS	COMMENTS
No insulin or glucose on the day of surgery	Not suitable for the juvenile diabetic Patient's stores of glucose are used to meet increased metabolic demands Unacceptable in severe diabetics for even a short period Patients on long-acting oral hypoglycemics predisposed to hypoglycemia	Acceptable for maturity-onset diabetes and minor surgical procedures Frequent blood sugar monitoring and insulin therapy, as necessary, are recommended
Partial dose NPH insulin in AM of surgery, 5% dextrose solution IV, 125 cc/h	Insulin requirements vary in perioperative period Onset and peak effect may not correlate with glucose administration or start of surgery Predisposes to hypoglycemia, especially in afternoon	Has been shown to have the lowest therapeutic ratio in a controlled study Frequent blood glucose monitoring recommended
Constant intravenous infusion of insulin using special pumps, DSW given	Insulin requirements vary greatly intraoperatively Insulin is adsorbed to bottles, IV tubing Predisposes to hypoglycemia Setting up pump or drips is a tedious process	Frequent blood glucose monitoring recommended
Intravenous bolus injection of regular insulin	Difficult to control preoperatively on patient floors Best suited for intraoperative and immediate postoperative period	Frequent blood glucose monitoring recommended
Subcutaneous regular insulin based on sliding scale	Perioperative changes in regional blood flow owing to heating, cooling, anesthesia, intrinsic or extrinsic catecholamines; vasconstriction owing to pain, hypovolemia, anxiety, shivering, caused by unpredictable absorption of subcutaneous insulin	Frequent blood sugar monitoring and appropriate IV insulin therapy

Roizen MF: Perioperative management of the diabetic patient. ASA Annual Refresher Course Lectures No. 245. 1996

Walts LF, Miller J, Davidson MB et al: Perioperative management of diabetes mellitus. Anesthesiology 55:104–109, 1981

B.6. How would you premedicate this patient? Why?

I would premedicate this patient with 10 mg of metoclopramide given orally about 1 hour before surgery. Metoclopramide has been shown to be effective in improving gastric emptying manifold in the diabetic with gastroparesis. This should decrease the likelihood of regurgitation and aspiration as well as nausea and vomiting.

Roizen MF: Perioperative management of the diabetic patient. ASA Annual Refresher Course Lectures No. 245. 1996

C. Intraoperative Management

C.1. What is the effect of anesthesia and surgery on insulin and glucose metabolism?

Anesthesia alone, in the normal human, is unaccompanied by a significant change in plasma insulin level during halothane, methoxyflurane, enflurane, thiopental-nitrous oxide, and spinal anesthesia. Glucose levels have been shown to rise significantly during halothane, methoxyflurane, and thiopental-nitrous oxide anesthesia, thereby resulting in a decreased plasma insulin to blood glucose ratio. The insulin to glucose ratio has been reported to be unchanged during enflurane and spinal anesthesia. The earlier studies were done with ether and cyclopropane, both of which are not in use today, and, hence, these results are not clinically significant. Overall, the metabolic effects of modern anesthetics are minor compared with the stress of surgery itself. Muscle relaxants and premedicant drugs in common use today are of little concern to diabetics.

Surgery provides a classic stress situation with catabolic response. The extent of the metabolic response is related to the severity of the operation and other concomitant factors, such as sepsis and shock, if present in this patient. The well-recognized hormonal changes include increased catecholamines, adrenocorticotrophic hormone, and cortisol secretions, as well as plasma cyclic adenosine monophosphate and glucagon levels. Despite unaltered plasma insulin levels, blood glucose levels are known to increase during and after surgery. Also a phase of relative insulin resistance follows surgery. All these changes increase the insulin requirement acutely in a diabetic.

Alberti KGMM, Thomas DJB: The management of diabetes during surgery. Br J Anaesth 51:693–710, 1979

Ammon JR: Perioperative management of the diabetic patient. ASA Annual Refresher Course Lectures No. 144. 1994

Hirsh IB, McGill JB, Cryer PE et al: Perioperative management of surgical patients with diabetes mellitus. Anesthesiology 74:346–359, 1991

C.2. What anesthetic techniques would you employ?

A general anesthetic with intubation of the trachea will be a satisfactory choice. After adequate preoxygenation, a rapid-sequence induction and intubation with cricoid compression should be used to prevent aspiration for emergency surgery in the diabetic patient. No significant difference is found among the commonly employed general anesthetics regarding their effect on diabetic control. Close monitoring is necessary to provide cardiovascular stability and adequate control of diabetes.

Ammon JR: Perioperative management of the diabetic patient. ASA Annual Refresher Course Lectures No. 144. 1994

Hirsh IB, McGill JB, Cryer PE et al: Perioperative management of surgical patients with diabetes mellitus. Anesthesiology 74:346–359, 1991

C.3. How would you monitor this patient?

In addition to continuous monitoring of electrocardiogram, blood pressure, temperature, pulse oximeter, capnogram, and precordial stethoscope, frequent determinations of both blood and urine glucose should be made. The blood glucose can be estimated easily in the operating room with the use of Dextrostix and the Ames dextrometer, which will dictate further insulin therapy.

Ammon JR: Perioperative management of the diabetic patient. ASA Annual Refresher Course Lectures No. 144. 1994

Hirsh IB, McGill JB, Cryer PE et al: Perioperative management of surgical patients with diabetes mellitus. Anesthesiology 74:346–359, 1991

Roizen MF: Perioperative management of the diabetic patient. ASA Annual Refresher Course Lectures No. 245. 1996

Walts LF, Miller J, Davidson MB et al: Perioperative management of diabetes mellitus. Anesthesiology 55:104–109, 1981

C.4. How would you treat hyperglycemia intraoperatively?

Intraoperative hyperglycemia (blood sugar >250 mg/dl) should be treated with intravenous regular insulin. Small doses (up to 10 units) of insulin can be used as single injections intravenously for the ease, controllability, and reliability of this method of administration. A useful rule of thumb is that each unit of regular insulin lowers the blood sugar by approximately 30 mg/dl in an adult. Blood sugars monitored every 1 to 2 hours further dictate the continuation of therapy. Although the half-life of intravenous insulin is short, hypoglycemia has been observed as late as 3 hours after an injection.

Another way to control hyperglycemia intraoperatively is with a continuous infusion of insulin, starting at 1 unit per hour if preoperatively the patient required 20 units or less of NPH insulin daily. In this patient, a starting rate of 2 units per hour, further dictated by frequent blood and urine glucose estimations, will be an adequate regimen. Use of an infusion pump with a plastic syringe affords a 90% recovery of insulin. The keystone to intraoperative diabetes management is the measurement of blood glucose concentration.

Ammon JR: Perioperative management of the diabetic patient. ASA Annual Refresher Course Lectures No. 144. 1994

Hirsh IB, McGill JB, Cryer PE et al: Perioperative management of surgical patients with diabetes mellitus. Anesthesiology 74:346–359, 1991

Roizen MF: Perioperative management of the diabetic patient. ASA Annual Refresher Course Lectures No. 245. 1996

Walts LF, Miller J, Davidson MB et al: Perioperative management of diabetes mellitus. Anesthesiology 55:104–109, 1981

C.5. How would you recognize and treat hypoglycemic shock intraoperatively?

It is virtually impossible to differentiate hypoglycemic shock from other forms of shock intraoperatively unless supported by low blood glucose concentrations measured concomitantly. Treatment lies in administration of glucose, which can be given as a bolus of 50% glucose followed by a 10% glucose-insulin infusion. Blood sugar increases approximately 30 mg/dl for each 7.5-g bolus of dextrose in a 70-kg adult.

Alberti KGMM, Thomas DJB: The management of diabetes during surgery. Br J Anaesth 51:693–710, 1979

Roizen MF: Perioperative management of the diabetic patient. ASA Annual Refresher Course Lectures No. 245. 1996

D. Postoperative Management

D.1. How would you control diabetes in this patient postoperatively?

Infusions of 10% glucose-insulin-potassium, as determined by blood glucose and potassium every 4 to 6 hours, should be continued. NPH insulin should be replaced by regular insulin in divided doses. An additional 20% of insulin can be given because infection is present. As the patient totally resumes her controlled diet, the original preoperative regimen should be restored.

Ammon JR: Perioperative management of the diabetic patient. ASA Annual Refresher Course Lectures No. 144. 1994

Hirsh IB, McGill JB, Cryer PE et al: Perioperative management of surgical patients with diabetes mellitus. Anesthesiology 74:346–359, 1991

Roizen MF: Perioperative management of the diabetic patient. ASA Annual Refresher Course Lectures No. 245. 1996

D.2. What are the common postoperative complications you expect in a diabetic patient?

In addition to the usual complications, the common problems in a diabetic include poor diabetes control and infection. A higher incidence of cardiovascular and renal problems and autonomic neuropathy, resulting in postural hypotension and urinary retention, may be encountered. Overall morbidity and mortality are increased.

Ammon JR: Perioperative management of the diabetic patient. ASA Annual Refresher Course Lectures No. 144. 1994

Hirsh IB, McGill JB, Cryer PE et al: Perioperative management of surgical patients with diabetes mellitus. Anesthesiology 74:346–359, 1991

Roizen MF: Perioperative management of the diabetic patient. ASA Annual Refresher Course Lectures No. 245. 1996

D.3. Does diabetes increase perioperative risk? Is it necessary to achieve tight perioperative control of blood glucose?

The two principal causes of death in the diabetic patient are sepsis and complications of arteriosclerosis. It has been questioned whether the diabetes in itself, segregated from its end-organ complications, increases the perioperative risk. But to the clinician who is to attend to the patient as a whole with a spectrum of attendant end-organ changes or complications, a diabetic patient presents an increased perioperative risk. Obesity, a frequent accompaniment of diabetes, carries its own risks (see Chapter 57 Morbid Obesity). Attendant cardiovascular changes are a leading cause of death in these patients. Other changes, such as nephropathy and autonomic neuropathy (gastric atonia, urinary retention, painless myocardial ischemia), contribute to increased morbidity. Episodes of hyperglycemia, hypoglycemia, and diabetic ketoacidosis (conditions not encountered in the normal population) carry a higher than normal risk of perioperative morbidity.

Care of the diabetic patient (especially the insulin-dependent diabetic) is a critical factor in the perioperative outcome. Although controversy has existed in the past to how tightly blood sugar levels should be controlled chronically in diabetic patients, the preponderance of recent data suggests that the long-term benefits of such tight control include delayed onset and limitation of complications of diabetes. It is also known that hyperglycemia can worsen neurologic outcome after intraoperative cerebral ischemia. Studies suggest that hyperglycemia >250 mg/dl inhibits polymorphonuclear cell activity. Increased incidence of infection, decreased wound healing, and a higher incidence of transplant rejections may prompt us to achieve tight perioperative control of blood sugar level in these patients. A lack of controlled data exists to support this belief, but if short-term perioperative control is viewed as a continuation of chronic long-term therapy, then it follows that adequate control of the blood sugar level (until more data are available) is probably beneficial.

Clark CM Jr, Lee DA: Prevention and treatment of the complications of diabetes mellitus. N Engl J Med 332:1210–1217, 1995

The Diabetic Control and Complications Trial Research Group: The effect of intensive treatment of diabetes on the development and progression of long-term complications for insulin dependent diabetes mellitus. N Engl J Med 329:977–987, 1993

Miller RD (ed): Anesthesia, 4th ed, pp 905–907. New York, Churchill-Livingstone, 1994

Roizen MF: Perioperative management of the diabetic patient. ASA Annual Refresher Course Lectures No. 245. 1996

The Genitourinary System

VI

Transurethral Resection of the Prostate **33**

Isaac Azar
Fun-Sun F. Yao

A 79-year-old man with benign prostatic hypertrophy was scheduled for transurethral prosta-tectomy (TURP). Past medical history included myocardial infarction complicated by conges-tive heart failure 7 months earlier. The patient had been on diuretics and calcium channel blockers.

A. Medical Disease and Differential Diagnosis

1. Are there differences in morbidity and mortality rates between TURP and suprapu-bic or retropubic prostatectomy?
2. What chronic medical conditions are common in TURP patients?
3. Does a history of prior myocardial infarction increase the patient's risk of periopera-tive reinfarction?
4. In patients with history of recent myocardial infarction, would you recommend that the surgery be postponed for a certain period of time? If so, why?

B. Preoperative Evaluation and Preparation

1. How would you evaluate the patient's cardiac condition? What laboratory tests would you like to have done? Would you recommend the patient to undergo coro-nary angiography prior to surgery?
2. Are patients with a Q-wave infarction at a greater risk of reinfarction than those with a non–Q-wave infarction?
3. Would you discontinue any antihypertensives or any medications for angina?
4. How would you premedicate this patient?

C. Intraoperative Management

1. What monitors would you use for this patient?
2. What anesthetic technique is preferable for TURP patients and why?
3. Is regional anesthesia associated with a lower incidence of perioperative reinfarction than general anesthesia?
4. What intravenous (IV) fluid would you use during TURP?
5. After premedication with midazolam (2 mg IV) a patient scheduled for TURP re-ceived spinal anesthesia with tetracaine (10 mg). The level of anesthesia was T10. About 20 minutes after surgery had started, the patient became restless, his blood pressure started to rise, and the heart rate decreased. Two more milligrams of mida-zolam were given. Shortly thereafter, the patient became cyanotic and obtunded, his blood pressure fell precipitously, and his pupils became dilated and unresponsive to light. What is the differential diagnosis of this set of clinical signs during TURP?
6. What are the important characteristics of irrigation solutions used during TURP?

7. Why is plain distilled water rarely used for irrigation during TURP? What types of irrigation solutions are presently available?
8. What is the effect of continuous bladder irrigation during TURP on body temperature?
9. What are the definition and signs and symptoms of the TURP syndrome?
10. How does the patient absorb irrigation solution during TURP? How much irrigation solution is typically absorbed?
11. How can one estimate the volume of irrigation solution absorbed during TURP?
12. What is the relationship between the duration of surgery and the incidence of TURP syndrome?
13. What factors increase the incidence of TURP syndrome?
14. What is the effect of excessive absorption of irrigation solution during TURP on cardiopulmonary, renal, and central nervous system (CNS) functions?
15. What is the cause of water intoxication in TURP patients?
16. What is the physiologic role of sodium ions in the body? What is the effect of excessive absorption of irrigation solution on serum sodium level?
17. What is the relationship between serum sodium level and the incidence of neurologic symptoms in TURP patients?
18. What is the effect of acute hyponatremia on the cardiovascular system?
19. What prophylactic measures may reduce the incidence of TURP syndrome?
20. What therapeutic measures are recommended for patients with TURP syndrome?
21. Is saline administration always necessary to correct hyponatremia? What are the risks of rapid correction of hyponatremia?
22. What are the toxic effects of glycine? Is there an antidote to glycine toxicity? What are the metabolic byproducts of glycine?
23. What are the symptoms and clinical course of TURP-induced hyperammonemia?
24. Why do some TURP patients develop hyperammonemia and others do not? Is there a preventive treatment against hyperammonemia in TURP patients?
25. What are the clinical characteristics, causes, and prognosis of TURP blindness?
26. What gynecologic procedure has been associated with a syndrome similar to TURP syndrome?
27. What are the symptoms and signs of acute hemolysis?
28. What are the causes of excessive bleeding during TURP?
29. What triggers disseminated intravascular coagulopathy in TURP patients? How would you treat it?
30. What are the causes, signs, and treatment of bladder perforation during TURP?
31. What are the causes, symptoms, and preventive measures of bladder explosion during TURP?
32. What are the causes of hypotension during TURP?

D. Postoperative Management

1. What is the source of postoperative bacteremia in TURP patients? What factors increase the incidence of bacteremia?
2. What are the signs of post-TURP septicemia? What preventive measures are recommended?
3. What bacteria-related cause may possibly lead to sudden postoperative shock in TURP patients?

4. **Is postoperative hypothermia a risk factor for myocardial ischemia?**
5. **How would you make a diagnosis of perioperative myocardial infarction?**

A. Medical Disease and Differential Diagnosis

A.1. Are there differences in morbidity and mortality rates between TURP and suprapubic or retropubic prostatectomy?

TURP is considered by many to be a simpler and safer procedure than "open" prostatectomy. However, despite many improvements in anesthesia and surgery, 7% of TURP patients sustain major complications and about 1% die perioperatively. No differences are seen in mortality rates between TURP and retropubic or suprapubic prostatectomy patients.

Fox M, Hammonds JC, Copland RF: Prostatectomy in patients of 70 and over. Eur Urol 7:27–30, 1981

Melchior J, Valk WL, Foret JD et al: Transurethral prostatectomy: Computerized analysis of 2,223 consecutive cases. J Urol 112:634–642, 1974

Nanninga JB, O'Coner VJ Jr: Suprapubic prostatectomy: A review, 1966–1970. J Urol 108:453–454, 1972

Rhymer JC, Bell TJ, Perry KC et al: Hyponatremia following transurethral resection of the prostate. Br J Urol 57:450–452, 1985

A.2. What chronic medical conditions are common in TURP patients?

TURP patients are often elderly and suffer from cardiac, pulmonary, vascular, and endocrinologic disorders. The incidence of cardiac disease is 67%, cardiovascular disease 50%, abnormal electrocardiogram (ECG) 77%, chronic obstructive pulmonary disease 29%, and diabetes mellitus 8%. On occasion, these patients are dehydrated and depleted of essential electrolytes because of long-term diuretic therapy and restricted fluid intake.

Desmond J: Serum osmolality and plasma electrolytes in patients who develop dilutional hyponatremia during transurethral resection. Can J Surg 13:116–121, 1970

Fox M, Hammonds JC, Copland RF: Prostatectomy in patients of 70 and over. Eur Urol 7:27–30, 1981

Harrison RH, Boren JS, Robinson JR: Dilutional hyponatremia: Another concept of the transurethral prostatic resection reaction. J Urol 75:95–110, 1956

Mebust WK, Brady TW, Valk WL: Observations on cardiac output, blood volume, central venous pressure, fluid and electrolyte changes in patients undergoing transurethral prostatectomy. J Urol 103:632–636, 1970

A.3. Does a history of prior myocardial infarction increase the patient's risk of perioperative reinfarction?

Yes, the incidence of perioperative reinfarction depends on the time interval between myocardial infarction and operation. See Chapter 18, Ischemic Heart disease and Noncardiac Surgery, question A.2, for details.

A.4. In patients with history of recent myocardial infarction, would you recommend that the surgery be postponed for a certain period of time? If so, why?

It is generally recommended to delay elective surgery 6 months after a myocardial infarction. However, the validity of this practice has recently been questioned. The functional status of the patient's cardiac disease may play a more important role in determining the acceptability of surgery. See Chapter 18, question A.3 for details.

B. Preoperative Evaluation and Preparation

B.1. How would you evaluate the patient's cardiac condition? What laboratory tests would you like to have done? Would you recommend the patient to undergo coronary angiography prior to surgery?

In addition to the routine history and physical examination of all organ systems, special attention should be paid to circulatory functions. Minimally, routine ECG and chest x-ray should be obtained to evaluate the presence of myocardial ischemia and/or infarction, and congestive heart failure. Functional capacity of the patient is best evaluated by initial history. If the patient presents with signs and symptoms of congestive heart failure, further cardiac testing should be considered.

B.2. Are patients with a Q-wave infarction at a greater risk of reinfarction than those with a non–Q-wave infarction?

Recent studies suggest that patients who survive a non–Q-wave infarction are at greater risk of reinfarction than those who survive a Q-wave infarction. See also Chapter 18, question B.4.

B.3. Would you discontinue any antihypertensives or any medications for angina?

All antihypertensive and antianginal drugs should be continued until the time of surgery to prevent rebound hypertension and tachycardia due to sudden withdrawal of these drugs.

B.4. How would you premedicate this patient?

The patient with ischemic heart disease should be sedated before surgery to avoid anxiety-induced tachycardia and hypertension, which can cause adverse myocardial ischemic events. However, this patient was 79 years old. I would premedicate with low doses of lorazepam (0.5 to 1 mg) orally to achieve sedation without significant cardiopulmonary depression.

C. Intraoperative Management

C.1. What monitors would you use for this patient?

The following monitors would be used for this patient.

- ECG—Simultaneous leads V_5 and II, multiple-lead ST segment analysis if available
- Blood pressure—Noninvasive automatic Doppler sphygmomanometric technique
- Swan-Ganz catheter—Pulmonary capillary wedge pressure (PCWP), pulmonary artery pressure (PAP), and hemodynamic study only for patients with ventricular dysfunction

- Continuous venous pressure (CVP) line—If the patient has good left ventricular function
- Temperature
- End-tidal CO_2 analyzer—If general anesthesia is administered
- Pulse oximeter for arterial oxygenation

C.2. What anesthetic technique is preferable for TURP patients and why?

Regional anesthesia is the anesthetic technique of choice for TURP patients because:

- It allows monitoring of the patient's mentation and thus early detection of signs of TURP syndrome
- It promotes vasodilatation and peripheral pooling of blood and thus reduces the severity of circulatory overloading
- It reduces blood loss by reducing the blood pressure during surgery
- It provides postoperative analgesia and, thus, reduces the incidence of postoperative hypertension and tachycardia that often accompanies recovery from general anesthesia

Cunningham AJ, McKenna JA, Skene DS: Single injection spinal anaesthesia with amethocaine and morphine for transurethral prostatectomy. Br J Anaesth 55:423–427, 1983

Madsen RE, Madsen PO: Influence of anesthesia on blood loss in transurethral prostatectomy. Anesth Analg 46:330–332, 1967

C.3. Is regional anesthesia associated with a lower incidence of perioperative reinfarction than general anesthesia?

Yes, the reinfarction rate for spinal anesthesia has been reported to be <1%, versus 2% to 8% for general anesthesia. Therefore, regional anesthesia may benefit patients with prior myocardial infarction undergoing TURP.

Erlik D, Valero A, Birkhan J, Gersh I: Prostatic surgery and the cardiovascular patient. Br J Urol 40:53–61, 1968

McGowen SW, Smith GFN: Anesthesia for transurethral prostatectomy: A comparison of spinal intradural analgesia with two methods of general anaesthesia. Anaesthesia 35:847–853, 1980

C.4. What intravenous (IV) fluid would you use during TURP?

Because hyponatremia commonly occurs in patients undergoing TURP, the IV fluid of choice perioperatively should contain sodium. Any sodium-containing crystalloid solution would be acceptable. It is important, however, to remember that circulatory overloading is common in TURP patients and, therefore, only a minimal amount of IV fluid should be administered during surgery.

C.5. After premedication with midazolam (2 mg IV) a patient scheduled for TURP received spinal anesthesia with tetracaine (10 mg). The level of anesthesia was T10. About 20 minutes after surgery had started, the patient became restless, his blood pressure started to rise, and the heart rate decreased. Two more milligrams of midazolam were given. Shortly thereafter, the patient became cyanotic and obtunded, his blood pressure fell precipitously, and his pupils became dilated and unresponsive to light. What is the differential diagnosis of this set of clinical signs during TURP?

Restlessness and incoherence during TURP are particularly ominous signs of TURP syndrome. These are often caused by subtle pulmonary edema, hypoxemia, and cerebral edema. It is particularly important not to misinterpret these as signs of inadequate anesthesia. The administration of sedatives or general anesthesia in the presence of TURP syndrome is often fraught with severe complications and even death.

Aasheim GM: Hyponatremia during transurethral surgery. Can Anaesth Soc J 20:274–280, 1973

Gravenstein D: Transurethral resection of the prostate (TURP) syndrome: A review of the pathophysiology and management. Anesth Analg 84:438–446, 1997

C.6. What are the important characteristics of irrigation solutions used during TURP?

TURP irrigation solutions are either isotonic or nearly isotonic, electrically inert, nontoxic, and transparent. Hypotonic solutions are avoided because they can cause hemolysis. Electrolyte-containing solutions are also avoided because they can conduct electrical current from the resectoscope to the surrounding tissues and cause burns. Because significant absorption of irrigation solution occurs during TURP, only solutions with nontoxic solutes are used. Also, the solution must be transparent to allow the surgeon to visualize the surgical site.

Gravenstein D: Transurethral resection of the prostate (TURP) syndrome: A review of the pathophysiology and management. Anesth Analg 84:438–446, 1997

Madsen PO, Madsen RE: Clinical and experimental evaluation of different irrigating fluids for transurethral surgery. Invest Urol 3:122–129, 1965

C.7. Why is plain distilled water rarely used for irrigation during TURP? What types of irrigation solutions are presently available?

Distilled water is totally transparent and electrically inert and in the past was regularly used for irrigation during TURP. However, because it is extremely hypotonic, when absorbed by the patient it may cause hemolysis, shock, and renal failure.

Over the years, a number of isotonic and nearly isotonic irrigation solutions have been introduced and they almost totally replaced plain distilled water. The more commonly used solutions today are glycine (1.2% and 1.5%). Mannitol (3%), glucose (2.5% to 4%), Cytal (a mixture of sorbitol 2.7% and mannitol 0.54%), and urea (1%) solutions are also occasionally used. To maintain their transparency, these solutions are purposely prepared moderately hypotonic.

Gravenstein D: Transurethral resection of the prostate (TURP) syndrome: A review of the pathophysiology and management. Anesth Analg 84:438–446, 1997

Madsen PO, Madsen RE: Clinical and experimental evaluation of different irrigating fluids for transurethral surgery. Invest Urol 3:122–129, 1965

Marx GF, Orkin LR: Complications associated with transurethral surgery. Anesthesiology 23:802–813, 1962

C.8. What is the effect of continuous bladder irrigation during TURP on body temperature?

Several liters of irrigation solution pass through the bladder during TURP, which can reduce body temperature at the rate of 1°C per hour (Fig. 33-1). About half of all TURP patients become hypothermic and shiver at the conclusion of surgery.

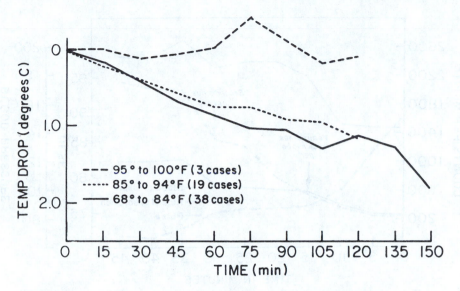

Figure 33-1. The fall in body temperature during TURP is related to the temperature of the irrigating solution and to the duration of surgery. (Reprinted with permission from Allen TD: Body temperature changes during prostatic resection as related to the temperature of the irrigating solution. J Urol 110:433–435, 1973)

Allen TD: Body temperature changes during prostatic resection as related to the temperature of the irrigating solution. J Urol 110:433–435, 1973

C.9. What are the definition and signs and symptoms of the TURP syndrome?

Rapid absorption of a large volume irrigation solution during TURP can lead to one or more of the following complications: pulmonary edema, water intoxication, hyponatremia, glycine toxicity, hyperammonemia, visual disturbances, and hemolysis. Usually, several of these complications occur concurrently; when this happens the constellation of signs and symptoms observed is called "TURP syndrome."

The TURP syndrome can occur as early as a few minutes after surgery has started and as late as several hours after surgery. The patient begins to complain of dizziness, headaches, nausea, tightness in the chest and throat, and shortness of breath. He then becomes restless, confused, and starts to retch. Some patients complain of abdominal pain. The blood pressure rises (both systolic and diastolic) and the heart rate decreases (Fig. 33-2). If not treated promptly, the patient becomes cyanotic and hypotensive, and ultimately sustains cardiac arrest.

Occasionally, the TURP syndrome starts with neurologic signs. The patient first becomes lethargic and then unconscious and his pupils dilate and react sluggishly to light. This can be followed by short episodes of tonic-clonic seizures and then coma that lasts from a few minutes to many hours.

If the patient is under general anesthesia, the presenting signs of the TURP syndrome are typically a rise and then a fall in blood pressure, respiratory arrest, and severe refractory bradycardia. The ECG may show nodal rhythm, ST changes, U waves, and widening of the QRS complex. Recovery from general anesthesia is usually delayed.

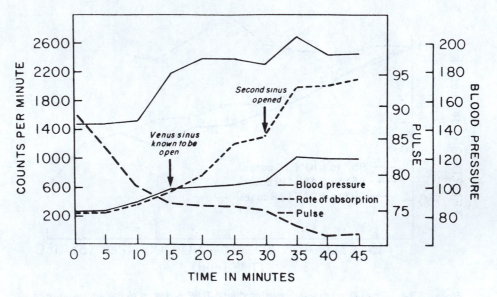

Figure 33-2.   The blood pressure, heart rate, and absorption rate of radioactively tagged irrigation solution during TURP. (Reprinted with permission from Taylor RO, Maxson ES, Carter FH et al: Volumetric gravimetric and radioisotopic determination of fluid transference in transurethral prostatectomy. J Urol 79:490–499, 1958)

Charlton AJ: Cardiac arrest during transurethral prostatectomy after absorption of 1.5% glycine. A case report and review of the literature. Anaesthesia 35:804–806, 1980

Day JO: Acute water intoxication complicating transurethral resection of the prostate. J Med Assoc Ga 72:845–846, 1983

Gravenstein D: Transurethral resection of the prostate (TURP) syndrome: A review of the pathophysiology and management. Anesth Analg 84:438–446, 1997

Henderson DJ, Middleton RG: Coma from hyponatremia following transurethral resection of prostate. Urology 15:267–271, 1980

Hurlbert BJ, Wingard DW: Water intoxication after 15 minutes of transurethral resection of the prostate. Anesthesiology 50:355–356, 1979

Melchior J, Valk WL, Foret JD et al: Transurethral prostatectomy: Computerized analysis of 2,223 consecutive cases. J Urol 112:634–642, 1974

Norris HT, Aasheim GM, Sherrad DJ et al: Symptomatology, pathophysiology, and treatment of the transurethral resection of the prostate syndrome. Br J Urol 45:420–427, 1973

Roesch RP, Stoelting RK, Lingeman JE et al: Ammonia toxicity resulting from glycine absorption during a transurethral resection of the prostate. Anesthesiology 58:577–579, 1983

Still AJ, Modell JA: Acute water intoxication during transurethral resection of the prostate using glycine solution for irrigation. Anesthesiology 38:98–99, 1973

C.10. How does the patient absorb irrigation solution during TURP? How much irrigation solution is typically absorbed?

The irrigation solution enters the blood stream directly through open prostatic venous sinuses and also accumulates in the periprostatic and retroperitoneal spaces. The latter occurs primarily when the prostatic capsule is violated during surgery.

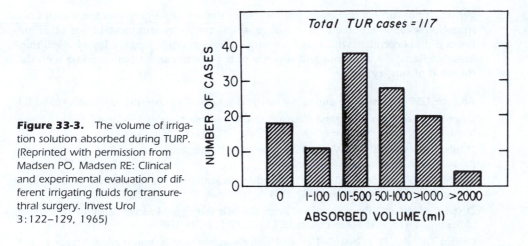

Figure 33-3. The volume of irrigation solution absorbed during TURP. (Reprinted with permission from Madsen PO, Madsen RE: Clinical and experimental evaluation of different irrigating fluids for transurethral surgery. Invest Urol 3:122–129, 1965)

Reports in the literature suggest that as many as 8 liters of irrigation solution can be absorbed by the patient during TURP. The average rate of absorption is 20 ml/min and the average weight gain by the end of surgery is 2 kg (Fig. 33-3).

Masloff JI, Milam JH, Bunts RC: Fluid and electrolyte changes associated with transurethral prostatic resection. South Med J 59:1203–1208, 1966

Oester A, Madsen PO: Determination of absorption of irrigating fluid during transurethral resection of the prostate by means of radioisotope. J Urol 102:714–719, 1969

C.11. How can one estimate the volume of irrigation solution absorbed during TURP?

A practical method to estimate the absorbed volume of irrigation solution during TURP is based on the following equation:

$$\text{Volume absorbed} = \frac{\text{preoperative } [Na^+]}{\text{postoperative } [Na^+]} \times ECF - ECF$$

To use this equation, serum sodium level ($[Na^+]$ is determined at the beginning of surgery and again at the time of estimation of the volume absorbed. The extracellular fluid (ECF) volume is assumed to be 20% to 30% of body weight. For example: If the patient's preoperative body weight is 60 kg and the ECF is assumed to constitute 20% of his body weight, then a fall in serum sodium level from 140 to 100 mEq/liter would suggest an absorption of 4.8 liters:

$$140/100 \times ECF - ECF = 1.4\ ECF - ECF = 0.4\ ECF = 0.4 \times 60 \times 20\% = 4.8 \text{ liters}$$

Henderson DJ, Middleton RG: Coma from hyponatremia following transurethral resection of prostate. Urology 15:267–271, 1980

C.12. What is the relationship between the duration of surgery and the incidence of the TURP syndrome?

Many believe that the duration of surgery is the most important determinant of incidence of TURP syndrome. However, several studies in the literature report severe TURP syndrome occurring as early as 15 to 20 minutes after surgery has started. In general, poor correlation is seen between the duration of surgery and the amount of irrigation solution absorbed. In one large series, morbidity and mortality of TURP patients did not correlate with length of surgery, except when surgery lasted >150 minutes. Similarly, the incidence and severity of hyponatremia did not correlate with the duration of surgery.

Aasheim GM: Hyponatremia during transurethral surgery. Can Anaesth Soc J 20:274–280, 1973

Desmond J: Serum osmolality and plasma electrolytes in patients who develop dilutional hyponatremia during transurethral resection. Can J Surg 13:116–121, 1970

Hurlbert BJ, Wingard DW: Water intoxication after 15 minutes of transurethral resection of the prostate. Anesthesiology 50:355–356, 1979

Melchior J, Valk WL, Foret JD et al: Transurethral prostatectomy: Computerized analysis of 2,223 consecutive cases. J Urol 112:634–642, 1974

Oester A, Madsen PO: Determination of absorption of irrigating fluid during transurethral resection of the prostate by means of radioisotope. J Urol 102:714–719, 1969

Osborn DE, Rao PN, Green MJ et al: Fluid absorption during transurethral resection. BMJ 281:1549–1550, 1980

C.13. What factors increase the incidence of the TURP syndrome?

TURP syndrome is more likely to occur if the prostatic gland is particularly large, the prostatic capsule is violated during surgery, or the hydrostatic pressure of the irrigation solution is excessively high. Large prostatic glands have rich venous networks that promote intravascular absorption of irrigation solution. The violation of the prostatic capsule during surgery promotes entry of irrigation solution into the periprostatic and retroperitoneal spaces. The hydrostatic pressure of the irrigation solution is an important determinant of the solution absorption rate of the patient. This pressure depends primarily on the height of the irrigation solution pole. When the height of the pole exceeds 60 cm, the absorption of irrigation solution is greatly enhanced. Also, excessively distended bladder during surgery facilitates absorption.

Hulte'n J, Bengtsson M, Engberg A et al: The pressure in the prostatic fossa and fluid absorption. Scand J Urol Nephrol 82(Suppl):33–43, 1984

Logie JRC, Keenan RA, Whiting PH et al: Fluid absorption during transurethral prostatectomy. J Urol 52:526–528, 1980

Madsen PO, Naber KG: The importance of the pressure in the prostatic fossa and absorption of irrigation fluid during transurethral resection of prostate. J Urol 109:446–452, 1973

Walsh RC, Gittes RE, Perlmutter AD et al: Campbell's Urology, pp 2815–2834. Philadelphia, WB Saunders, 1986

C.14. What is the effect of excessive absorption of irrigation solution during TURP on cardiopulmonary, renal, and central nervous system functions?

Excessive absorption of irrigation solution during TURP causes hypervolemia and hypertension and may provoke angina and pulmonary edema (Fig. 33-4). It may also have an adverse effect on renal function. Inverse relationship has been observed between the amount of irrigation solution absorbed during surgery and postoperative urinary output.

Some patients with TURP syndrome exhibit neurologic signs due to water intoxi-

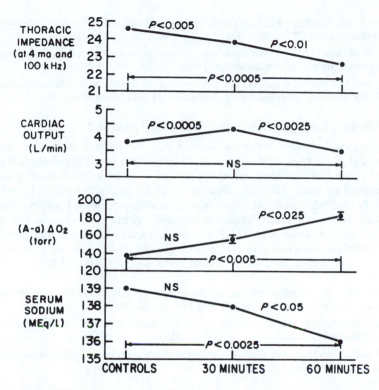

Figure 33-4. Mean changes in thoracic impedance, cardiac output, alveolar-arterial oxygen tension difference, and in serum sodium level during TURP. (Reprinted with permission from Casthely P, Ramanathan S, Chalon J et al: Decrease in electric impedance during transurethral resection of the prostate: An index of early water intoxication. J Urol 125:347–349, 1981)

cation. They assume a decerebrate posture, exhibit clonus and positive Babinski reflex, and eventually convulse and lapse into coma. Examination of the eyes reveals papilledema and dilated and sluggishly reacting pupils. The EEG shows low voltage bilaterally. The patients remain in coma from a few hours to several days.

Casthely P, Ramanathan S, Chalon J et al: Decrease in electric impedance during transurethral resection of the prostate: An index of early water intoxication. J Urol 125:347–349, 1981

Charlton AJ: Cardiac arrest during transurethral prostatectomy after absorption of 1.5% glycine. A case report and review of the literature. Anaesthesia 35:804–806, 1980

Desmond J: Serum osmolality and plasma electrolytes in patients who develop dilutional hyponatremia during transurethral resection. Can J Surg 13:116–121, 1970

Gravenstein D: Transurethral resection of the prostate (TURP) syndrome: A review of the pathophysiology and management. Anesth Analg 84:438–446, 1997

Hahn R, Berlin T, Lewenhaupt A: Rapid massive irrigating fluid absorption during transurethral resection of the prostate. Acta Chir Scand 530(Suppl):63–65, 1986

Henderson DJ, Middleton RG: Coma from hyponatremia following transurethral resection of prostate. Urology 15:267–271, 1980

Oester A, Madsen PO: Determination of absorption of irrigating fluid during transurethral resection of the prostate by means of radioisotope. J Urol 102:714–719, 1969

Taylor RO, Maxson ES, Carter FH et al: Volumetric gravimetric and radioisotopic determination of fluid transference in transurethral prostatectomy. J Urol 79:490–499, 1958

C.15. What is the cause of water intoxication in TURP patients?

The exact mechanism of water intoxication in TURP patients is not clear. However, the crucial physiologic derangement of CNS function is not hyponatremia per se, but acute hypo-osmolality. Cerebral edema caused by acute hypo-osmolality can increase intracranial pressure, which results in bradycardia and hypertension by the Cushing reflex. Furthermore, cerebral edema is not caused by decreased serum colloid oncotic pressure, but by decreased osmolality. Apparently, the hypervolemia and hyponatremia that often accompany TURP promote cerebral edema and this, in turn, raises intracranial pressure and provokes neurologic symptoms. The rise in intracranial pressure is directly related to the gain in body weight during TURP.

Gravenstein D: Transurethral resection of the prostate (TURP) syndrome: A review of the pathophysiology and management. Anesth Analg 84:438–446, 1997

Harrison RH, Boren JS, Robinson JR: Dilutional hyponatremia: Another concept of the transurethral prostatic resection reaction. J Urol 75:95–110, 1956

Maluf NSR, Boren JS, Brandes GE: Absorption of irrigating solution and associated changes upon transurethral electroresection of prostate. J Urol 75:824–835, 1956

C.16. What is the physiologic role of sodium ions in the body? What is the effect of excessive absorption of irrigation solution on serum sodium level?

Sodium is an ubiquitous electrolyte that is essential for proper function of excitatory cells, particularly those of the heart and brain. Extreme reduction in serum sodium level alters brain function, as well as cardiac and renal function.

During TURP, serum sodium level typically falls 3 to 10 mEq/liter. However, the correlation between the severity of the hyponatremia and the amount of irrigation solution absorbed during surgery is inconsistent. Apparently, the fall in serum sodium level depends primarily on the rate at which the irrigation solution is absorbed rather than the total amount absorbed.

Ceccarelli FE, Mantell LK: Studies on fluid and electrolyte alterations during transurethral prostatectomy. I. J Urol 85:75–82, 1961

Desmond J: Serum osmolality and plasma electrolytes in patients who develop dilutional hyponatremia during transurethral resection. Can J Surg 13:116–121, 1970

Hahn RG: Relations between irrigation absorption rate and hyponatraemia during transurethral resection of the prostate. Acta Anaesthesiol Scand 32:53–60, 1988

Mebust WK, Brady TW, Valk WL: Observations on cardiac output, blood volume, central venous pressure, fluid and electrolyte changes in patients undergoing transurethral prostatectomy. J Urol 103:632–636, 1970

Pierce JM: The treatment of water intoxication following transurethral prostatectomy. J Urol 87:181–183, 1962

Rhymer JC, Bell TJ, Perry KC et al: Hyponatremia following transurethral resection of the prostate. Br J Urol 57:450–452, 1985

Surawicz B: Relationship between electrocardiogram and electrolytes. Am Heart J 73:814–834, 1967

C.17. What is the relationship between serum sodium level and the incidence of neurologic symptoms in TURP patients?

Acute severe hyponatremia is often associated with abnormal neurologic symptoms, and it can lead to irreversible brain damage. The neurologic signs may be accompanied by electroencephalographic (EEG) abnormalities such as loss of alpha-wave activity and irregular discharge of high-amplitude slow wave activity. However, the correlation between the severity of the hyponatremia and the incidence of neurologic symptoms is inconsistent. In some cases, moderate hyponatremia is associated with severe neurologic symptoms, in others severe hyponatremia causes no symptoms at all. Apparently, the determining factor is the rate at which serum sodium level falls rather than the total fall. The faster the fall in serum sodium level, the greater the incidence of neurologic symptoms. A slow fall in serum sodium level apparently allows the CNS to adapt to the hyponatremia.

Epstein FH, Levitin H, Glasser G et al: Cerebral hyponatremia. N Engl J Med 265:513–518, 1961

Henderson DJ, Middleton RG: Coma from hyponatremia following transurethral resection of prostate. Urology 15:267–271, 1980

Maluf NSR, Boren JS, Brandes GE: Absorption of irrigating solution and associated changes upon transurethral electroresection of prostate. J Urol 75:824–835, 1956

Raskind M: Psychosis, polydipsia, and water intoxication: Report of a fatal case. Arch Gen Psychiatry 30:112–114, 1974

C.18. What is the effect of acute hyponatremia on the cardiovascular system?

When serum sodium level falls below 120 mEq/liter, signs of cardiovascular depression can occur. A fall below 115 mEq/liter causes bradycardia, widening of the QRS complex, ventricular ectopic beats, and T-wave inversion. Patients with serum sodium level <100 mEq/liter can develop respiratory and cardiac arrest.

Logie JRC, Keenan RA, Whiting PH et al: Fluid absorption during transurethral prostatectomy. J Urol 52:526–528, 1980

Mebust WK, Brady TW, Valk WL: Observations on cardiac output, blood volume, central venous pressure, fluid and electrolyte changes in patients undergoing transurethral prostatectomy. J Urol 103:632–636, 1970

Osborn DE, Rao PN, Green MJ et al: Fluid absorption during transurethral resection. BMJ 281:1549–1550, 1980

Surawicz B: Relationship between electrocardiogram and electrolytes. Am Heart J 73:814–834, 1967

C.19. What prophylactic measures may reduce the incidence of TURP syndrome?

The incidence of TURP syndrome depends primarily on the surgeon's technical skills. However, if the patient is properly prepared before surgery and closely monitored during surgery, the incidence and severity of the syndrome can be reduced.

Fluid and electrolyte imbalance should be corrected preoperatively and special attention paid to serum sodium level during surgery. Patients with preoperative congestive heart failure should be treated vigorously with diuretics and fluid restriction. A conservative surgical approach should be considered in critically ill patients. A simple canalization or balloon dilation of the urethra or a staged TURP is less likely to provoke TURP syndrome.

The most important preventive measure during surgery is preservation of the prostatic capsule. Another preventive measure is limiting the hydrostatic pressure of the irrigation solution to 60 cm H_2O. This can be accomplished by limiting the height of the irrigation pole to 60 cm. Also, the bladder should not be allowed to overdistend and the duration of surgery should be restricted.

If a sudden significant fall in serum sodium level occurs, the surgeon should be informed and therapeutic measures immediately instituted. If sodium blood level falls below 120 mEq/liter, surgery should be terminated as soon as possible.

Intravenous fluids should be cautiously administered during TURP. A microdrip is recommended particularly in patients with cardiac or renal disease. If regional anesthesia causes hypotension, a small dose of a vasoconstrictor is recommended to raise the blood pressure rather than rapid infusion of intravenous fluids.

Gale DW, Notley RG: TURP without TURP syndrome. Br J Urol 57:708–710, 1985

Madsen PO, Naber KG: The importance of the pressure in the prostatic fossa and absorption of irrigation fluid during transurethral resection of prostate. J Urol 109:446–452, 1973

Maluf NSR, Boren JS, Brandes GE: Absorption of irrigating solution and associated changes upon transurethral electroresection of prostate. J Urol 75:824–835, 1956

Watkins-Pitchford JM, Payne SR, Rennie CD et al: Hyponatremia during transurethral resection—Its practical prevention. Br J Urol 56:676–678, 1984

C.20. *What therapeutic measures are recommended for patients with TURP syndrome?*

When symptoms of TURP syndrome appear, the following therapeutic measures are recommended:

- Terminate surgery as soon as possible.
- Administer furosemide (20 mg IV).
- Administer oxygen by nasal cannula or face mask.
- If the patient develops pulmonary edema, consider tracheal intubation and positive pressure ventilation with oxygen.
- Draw a sample of arterial blood for blood gas and serum sodium analysis.
- If serum sodium level is abnormally low and clinical signs of hyponatremia are seen, intravenous administration of hypertonic saline (3% to 5%) is recommended. The hypertonic solution should be given at a rate no faster than 100 ml/h. In most cases, no more than 300 ml of saline is needed to correct the hyponatremia.
- If the patient develops seizures, a short-acting anticonvulsant agent such as diazepam (5 to 20 mg) or midazolam (2 to 10 mg) can be administered intravenously. If this does not stop the seizures, a barbiturate or phenytoin can be added. As a last resort, a muscle relaxant may also be used.
- If pulmonary edema or hypotension develops, invasive hemodynamic monitoring is recommended. This will serve as a guide for pharmacologic support and fluid administration.
- If significant blood loss is suspected, the administration of packed red blood cells

should be considered. In general, IV fluids should be administered cautiously because of the propensity of these patients to develop pulmonary edema.

C.21. Is saline administration always necessary to correct hyponatremia? What are the risks of rapid correction of hyponatremia?

The administration of saline to correct hyponatremia is not always necessary and sometimes it can be detrimental. Unless the patient develops clinical signs of hyponatremia, saline administration is not recommended. Spontaneous or induced diuresis usually corrects the hyponatremia within a few hours.

TURP patients often sustain circulatory overloading during surgery and, therefore, saline administration in these patients can provoke pulmonary edema. In addition, rapid administration of hypertonic saline has been associated with central pontine myelinolysis—a poorly understood and fatal neurologic complication.

To reduce the hazards of saline administration, it has been recommended that the hyponatremia be corrected at a rate no faster than 0.5 mEq/liter per hour.

Bird D, Slade N, Feneley RCL: Intravascular complications of transurethral resection of the prostate. Br J Urol 54:564–565, 1982

Day JO: Acute water intoxication complicating transurethral resection of the prostate. J Med Assoc Ga 72:845–846, 1983

Desmond J: Serum osmolality and plasma electrolytes in patients who develop dilutional hyponatremia during transurethral resection. Can J Surg 13:116–121, 1970

Hantman D, Rossier B, Zohlman R: Rapid correction of hyponatremia in the syndrome of inappropriate secretion of antidiuretic hormone: An alternative treatment to hypertonic saline. Ann Intern Med 78:870–875, 1973

Henderson DJ, Middleton RG: Coma from hyponatremia following transurethral resection of prostate. Urology 15:267–271, 1980

Pierce JM: The treatment of water intoxication following transurethral prostatectomy. J Urol 87:181–183, 1962

Rothenberg DM, Berns AS, Ivankovich AD: Isotonic hyponatremia following transurethral prostate resection. J Clin Anesth 2:48–53, 1990

Sterns RH, Riggs JE, Schochet SS Jr: Osmotic demyelinization syndrome following correction of hyponatremia. N Engl J Med 314:1535–1542, 1986

C.22. What are the toxic effects of glycine? Is there an antidote to glycine toxicity? What are the metabolic byproducts of glycine?

When absorbed by the patient in large amounts, glycine has direct toxic effects on the heart and retina. In TURP patients, glycine absorption has been shown to cause an average fall of 17.5% in cardiac output. In animal studies, the administration of the amino acid arginine reversed the myocardial depressing effect of glycine. Neither the mechanism by which glycine depresses cardiac function nor the one by which arginine protects the heart is known.

Glycine toxicity in TURP patients is uncommon, probably because most of the absorbed glycine is retained in the periprostatic and retroperitoneal spaces where access to the circulation is limited.

The most common metabolites of glycine are ammonia and glyoxylic and oxalic

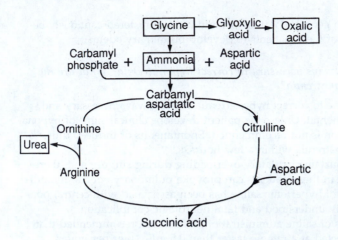

Figure 33-5. Metabolic pathways of glycine. (Reprinted with permission from McGilvery RW, Goldstein GW: Biochemistry: A Functional Approach, 3rd ed, p 584. Philadelphia, WB Saunders, 1983)

acids (Fig. 33-5). In some patients, excessive absorption of glycine during TURP leads to hyperammonemia.

Handler P, Kamin H, Harris JS: The metabolism of parenterally administered amino acid. I. Glycine. J Biol Chem 179:283–301, 1949

McGilvery RW, Goldstein GW: Biochemistry: A Functional Approach. 3rd ed, p 584. Philadelphia, WB Saunders, 1983

Mebust WK, Brady TW, Valk WL: Observations on cardiac output, blood volume, central venous pressure, fluid and electrolyte changes in patients undergoing transurethral prostatectomy. J Urol 103:632–636, 1970

Ovassapian A, Joshi CW, Brumer EA: Visual disturbances: An unusual symptom of transurethral prostatic resection reaction. Anesthesiology 57:332–334, 1982

Wang JM, Wong KC, Creel DJ et al: Effects of glycine on hemodynamic responses and visual evoked potentials in the dog. Anesth Analg 64:1071–1077, 1985

C.23. What are the symptoms and clinical course of TURP-induced hyperammonemia?

The signs and symptoms of hyperammonemia usually appear within 1 hour after surgery. Typically, the patient becomes nauseated, vomits, and then becomes comatose. Blood ammonia level rises to >500 mmol/liter. The patient remains comatose for 10 to 12 hours and eventually awakens when ammonia blood level falls to <150 mmol/liter. The hyperammonemia tends to linger postoperatively, probably because glycine absorption from the periprostatic space continues after surgery.

Oester A, Madsen PO: Determination of absorption of irrigating fluid during transurethral resection of the prostate by means of radioisotope. J Urol 102:714–719, 1969

C.24. Why do some TURP patients develop hyperammonemia and others do not? Is there a preventive treatment against hyperammonemia in TURP patients?

Because ammonia is metabolized primarily in the liver, it has been speculated that hyperammonemia after TURP is a result of liver dysfunction. However, no liver dys-

AMMONIA CONCENTRATIONS

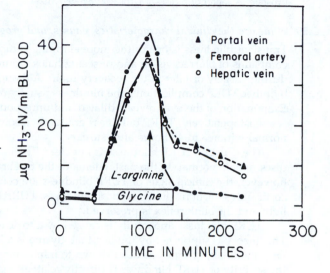

Figure 33-6. *Ammonia blood levels during glycine administration in dogs before and after arginine supplementation. (Reprinted with permission from Nathans D, Fahey JL, Ship AG: Sites of origin and removal of blood ammonia formed during glycine infusion: Effect of L-arginine. J Lab Clin Med 51:124–133, 1958)*

function has been found in these patients. Nor is there evidence that patients with a known liver dysfunction are susceptible to hyperammonemia after TURP.

A more plausible explanation for the hyperammonemia is arginine deficiency. Normally, the ornithine cycle in the liver converts ammonia to urea (see Fig. 33-5). Arginine is an important intermediate product of this cycle. Apparently, TURP patients with arginine deficiency cannot detoxify the excess ammonia produced from glycine metabolism and, thus, develop hyperammonemia.

Several studies support this hypothesis. In dogs, the administration of arginine concurrently with glycine reduced the secretion of ammonia by the liver (Fig. 33-6). In humans, prophylactic administration of arginine or ornithine prevents hyperammonemia that otherwise follows rapid intravenous administration of glycine. Routine administration of arginine in TURP patients, however, is not recommended because they rarely develop hyperammonemia.

Fahey JL: Toxicity and blood ammonia rise resulting from intravenous amino acid administration in man: The protective effect of L-arginine. J Clin Invest 36:1647–1655, 1957

Fahey JL, Perry RS, McCoy PF: Blood ammonia elevation and toxicity from intravenous L-amino acid administration to dogs: The protection role of L-arginine. Am J Physiol 192:311–317, 1958

McGilvery RW, Goldstein GW: Biochemistry: A Functional Approach, 3rd ed, p 584. Philadelphia, WB Saunders, 1983

Nathans D, Fahey JL, Ship AG: Sites of origin and removal of blood ammonia formed during glycine infusion: Effect of L-arginine. J Lab Clin Med 51:124–133, 1958

Oester A, Madsen PO: Determination of absorption of irrigating fluid during transurethral resection of the prostate by means of radioisotope. J Urol 102:714–719, 1969

Roesch RP, Stoelting RK, Lingeman JE et al: Ammonia toxicity resulting from glycine absorption during a transurethral resection of the prostate. Anesthesiology 58:577–579, 1983

Ryder KW, Olson JF, Khanoski RJ et al: Hyperammonemia after transurethral resection of the prostate: A report of 2 cases. J Urol 132:995–997, 1984

C.25. What are the clinical characteristics, causes, and prognosis of TURP blindness?

Transient blindness is one of the more alarming complications of TURP. The patient complains of blurred vision and of seeing halos around objects. This can occur either during surgery or later in the recovery room. Although it is sometimes accompanied by other TURP complications, the blindness usually occurs as an isolated symptom. Examination of the eyes reveals dilated and unresponsive pupils.

Postoperatively, TURP blindness gradually resolves and the eyesight returns to normal within 8 to 48 hours after surgery.

The cause of TURP blindness is not clear. The intraocular pressure and optic discs remain normal. In the past, edema of the cerebral optical cortex was suspected; however, the clinical signs of TURP blindness are consistent with retinal rather than cortical dysfunction. Unlike cortical blindness, TURP blindness allows perception of light and the blink reflex is preserved.

TURP blindness apparently is caused by a toxic effect of glycine on the retina. This theory is supported by the fact that glycine is a known inhibitory neurotransmitter. In animals, glycine has been shown to inhibit neuronal visual pathways. Also, the severity of TURP blindness is directly related to glycine blood level. Postoperatively, the vision gradually improves as the glycine blood level declines.

Appelt GL, Benson GS, Corrier JN Jr: Transient blindness: Unusual initial symptom of transurethral prostatic resection reaction. Urology 13:402–404, 1979

Defalque RJ, Miller DW: Visual disturbances during transurethral resection of the prostate. Can Anaesth Soc J 22:620–621, 1975

Gooding JM, Holcomb MC: Transient blindness following intravenous administration of atropine. Anesth Analg 56:872–873, 1977

Kaiser R, Adragna MG, Weis FR Jr et al: Transient blindness following transurethral resection of the prostate in an achondroplastic dwarf. J Urol 133:685–686, 1985

Korol S, Leunberger PM, Englert U et al: In vivo effects of glycine on retinal ultrastructure and averaged electroretinogram. Brain Res 97:235–251, 1975

Ovassapian A, Joshi CW, Brumer EA: Visual disturbances: An unusual symptom of transurethral prostatic resection reaction. Anesthesiology 57:332–334, 1982

Peters KR, Muir J, Wingard DW: Intraocular pressure after transurethral prostatic surgery. Anesthesiology 55:327–329, 1981

Wang JM, Wong KC, Creel DJ et al: Effects of glycine on hemodynamic responses and visual evoked potentials in the dog. Anesth Analg 64:1071–1077, 1985

C.26. What gynecologic procedure has been associated with a syndrome similar to TURP syndrome?

Hysteroscopy has been associated with symptoms not unlike those of TURP syndrome. The procedure involves visualization of the interior lining of the uterus for diagnostic purposes and, on occasion, for transcervical resection of the endometrium or submucous myomectomy. The latter often requires electrical cauterization. As is the case of TURP, hysteroscopy requires irrigation with nonionic isotonic solutions. Commonly used solutions contain either glucose or glycine. Side-effects such as hyponatremia, hyperglycemia, circulatory overloading, and coagulopathy have been reported.

Carson SA, Hubert GD, Schriock ED et al: Hyperglycemia and hyponatremia during operative hysteroscopy with 5% dextrose in water distention. Fertil Steril 51:341–343, 1989

Goldenberg M, Zolti M, Seidman DS et al: Transient blood oxygen desaturation, hypercapnia, and coagulopathy after operative hysteroscopy with glycine used as the distending medium. Am J Obstet 170:25–29, 1994

C.27. What are the symptoms and signs of acute hemolysis?

In the past, when plain water was used for irrigation, acute hemolysis was a common complication of TURP. Presently, no significant hemolysis occurs. However, occasionally, plain water is still used when other irrigation solutions are contraindicated.

   The clinical signs of acute hemolysis are sudden prostration, chills, clammy skin, tight chest, and bronchospasm. Massive hemolysis reduces the oxygen-carrying capacity and raises the potassium and free hemoglobin blood levels. Some believe that the cause of death in these patients is ventricular fibrillation caused by the hyperkalemia. The free hemoglobin in the blood tends to precipitate in renal tubuli and cause renal failure.

Maluf NSR, Boren JS, Brandes GE: Absorption of irrigating solution and associated changes upon transurethral electroresection of prostate. J Urol 75:824–835, 1956

Marx GF, Orkin LR: Complications associated with transurethral surgery. Anesthesiology 23:802–813, 1962

C.28. What are the causes of excessive bleeding during TURP?

TURP patients commonly bleed perioperatively. One possible cause is dilutional thrombocytopenia resulting from excessive absorption of irrigation solution. Another possible cause is local release fibrinolytic agents (plasminogen and urokinase) from the mucosa of the lower urinary tract. During and immediately after TURP these agents cause local fibrinolysis and promote bleeding from the raw surfaces of the prostatic gland. The existence of a local fibrinolytic mechanism is supported by the observation that prophylactic administration of epsilon-aminocaproic acid (an antifibrinolytic agent) reduces bleeding from the prostatic bed.

   Systemic coagulopathy can also occur during TURP. Contrary to common misconception, the coagulopathy is due to disseminated intravascular coagulation (DIC) rather than primary fibrinolysis. Characteristically, the platelet count and fibrinogen blood level are abnormally low. At autopsy, multiple microthrombi are observed in various parts of the body. The high level of fibrin degradation products found in the blood of these patients is caused by secondary fibrinolysis, which commonly accompanies DIC.

Friedman NJ, Hoag MS, Robinson AJ et al: Hemorrhagic syndrome following transurethral prostatic resection for benign adenoma. Arch Intern Med 124:341–349, 1969

Ladehoff AA, Rasmussen J: Fibrinolysis and thromboplastic activities in relation to hemorrhage in transvesical prostatectomy. Scand J Clin Lab Invest 13:231–244, 1961

Ljungner H, Bergquist D, Isacson S: Plasminogen activator activity in patients undergoing transvesical and transurethral prostatectomy. Eur Urol 9:24–27, 1983

Smith RB, Riach P, Kaufman JJ: Epsilon aminocaproic acid and the control of post-prostatectomy bleeding: A prospective double blind study. J Urol 131:1093–1095, 1984

C.29. What triggers disseminated intravascular coagulopathy in TURP patients? How would you treat it?

Apparently DIC is triggered during TURP by prostatic particles rich in thromboplastin that enter the blood stream during surgery. The recommended treatment for DIC is replacement of blood loss and administration of platelets, cryoprecipitates, and fresh-frozen plasma. Heparin administration is controversial.

Friedman NJ, Hoag MS, Robinson AJ et al: Hemorrhagic syndrome following transurethral prostatic resection for benign adenoma. Arch Intern Med 124:341–349, 1969

Ladehoff AA, Rasmussen J: Fibrinolysis and thromboplastic activities in relation to hemorrhage in transvesical prostatectomy. Scand J Clin Lab Invest 13:231–244, 1961

Malhotra V (ed): Anesthesia for Renal and Genito-Urologic Surgery, p 108. New York, McGraw-Hill, 1996

C.30. What are the causes, signs, and treatment of bladder perforation during TURP?

The incidence of bladder perforation during TURP is about 1%. The causes are trauma by surgical instrumentation, overdistention of the bladder, and rarely, explosion of traces of hydrogen gas inside the bladder.

An early sign of bladder perforation is a sudden decrease in return of irrigation solution from the bladder. This sign often goes unnoticed until a significant amount of irrigation solution accumulates in the abdomen and causes abdominal distress. Other clinical signs are hypotension followed by hypertension and nausea. Reflex-type movements of the limbs have been observed under both general and regional anesthesia. When the perforation is intraperitoneal, the symptoms develop faster; they include severe shoulder pain caused by diaphragmatic irritation.

Diagnosis of bladder perforation is confirmed using cystourethrography. Treatment is immediate suprapubic cystotomy.

Hansen RI, Iverson P: Bladder explosion during uninterrupted transurethral resection of the prostate: A case report and experimental model. Scand J Urol Nephrol 13:211–212, 1979

C.31. What are the causes, symptoms, and preventive measures of bladder explosion during TURP?

A rare but extremely dangerous complication of TURP is gas explosion inside the bladder during surgery. Various explosive gases, particularly hydrogen, are generated by the cauterization of prostatic or bladder tissue during TURP. The explosion is triggered by the hot metal loop of the resectoscope. Following a loud thump, the patient complains of a sudden abdominal pain. This is accompanied by abrupt decline in return of irrigation solution. Usually, the concentration of oxygen in the bladder is too low to support combustion or explosion. However, if air is allowed to enter the irrigation system during surgery, the oxygen concentration in the bladder will rise and this, in turn, may support an explosion.

Strict precautions should be taken to prevent entry of air into the bladder during TURP. If air is observed in the bladder at the beginning of surgery, it must be evacuated before cauterization starts. The bladder should be emptied often to avoid accumulation of explosive gases during surgery.

Hansen RI, Iverson P: Bladder explosion during uninterrupted transurethral resection of the prostate: A case report and experimental model. Scand J Urol Nephrol 13:211–212, 1979

C.32. What are the causes of hypotension during TURP?

The more common causes of hypotension during TURP are circulatory overloading with congestive heart failure, myocardial infarction or myocardial ischemia, severe anemia due to blood loss, and severe hyponatremia and water intoxication.

D. Postoperative Management

D.1. What is the source of postoperative bacteremia in TURP patients? What factors increase the incidence of bacteremia?

The prostatic gland often harbors large amounts of various bacteria. TURP facilitates the entry of these bacteria into the blood stream, leading to postoperative bacteremia. Also, a preoperative indwelling catheter promotes bacterial growth in the urethra. About 30% of TURP patients have infected urine preoperatively and half of them sustain bacteremia postoperatively.

Surgical disruption of the prostatic venous sinuses and excessive hydrostatic pressure of the irrigation solution facilitate the entry of bacteria into the blood stream.

Biorn CL, Browning WH, Thompson L: Transient bacteremia immediately following transurethral prostatic resection. J Urol 63:155–161, 1950

Creevy CD, Feeney MJ: Infection following transurethral resection of the prostate gland. Bulletin of the University of Minnesota Hospital 20:314–327, 1949

Grey PN: The incidence and the type of bacteremia at the time of various prostatectomy procedures. J Urol 73:709–711, 1955

Kidd EE, Kennedy B: Bacteremia, septicemia, and intravascular haemolysis during transurethral resection of the prostate gland. Br J Urol 37:551–559, 1965

Murphy DM, Stassen L, Carr ME et al: Bacteremia during prostatectomy and other transurethral operations: Influence of timing of antibiotic administration. J Clin Pathol 37:673–676, 1984

D.2. What are the signs of post-TURP septicemia? What preventive measures are recommended?

The signs of septicemia usually appear postoperatively in the postanesthesia care unit. They include fever, chills, low blood pressure, and tachycardia.

Antibiotics administered prophylactically before TURP do not sterilize the urine because they do not easily penetrate the prostatic gland. Nevertheless, the preoperative administration of antibiotics is recommended to render the blood stream hostile to bacteria. The prophylactic administration of antibiotics in TURP patients is particularly important because of the grave prognosis of septicemia in these patients.

If sepsis is suspected postoperatively in a TURP patient, broad spectrum antibiotics should be immediately started without waiting for blood cultures.

Robinson MRG, Cross RJ, Shetty MB et al: Bacteriaemia and bacteriogenic shock in district hospital urological practice. Br J Urol 52:10–14, 1980

D.3. What bacteria-related cause may possibly lead to sudden postoperative shock in TURP patients?

On occasion, TURP patients develop postoperatively a short episode of hypotension, severe chills, and fever. These symptoms last only a few hours and then the patient recovers uneventfully. The cause of these symptoms is not clear; however, absorption of bacterial endotoxins has been suspected. Experimentally, the administration of bacterial endotoxins in humans provoked symptoms similar to those described above.

Bennett IL: Pathogenesis of fever. Bull NY Acad Med 37:440–447, 1961

Calapinto V, Armstrong DJ, Finlayson DC: Red cell mass and plasma volume changes during transurethral resection of the prostate. Can J Surg 16:143–151, 1973

D.4. Is postoperative hypothermia a risk factor for myocardial ischemia?

Yes. Unintentional hypothermia is associated with a significantly higher incidence of postoperative myocardial ischemia. Therefore, it is important to maintain normothermia during the perioperative period. See also Chapter 18, question D.4.

D.5. How would you make a diagnosis of perioperative myocardial infarction?

An intraoperative myocardial infarction can be totally silent or it may be called to the attention of the anesthesiologist by a sudden fall in blood pressure. The sudden fall in blood pressure may be accompanied by tachycardia, which is indistinguishable from the hypovolemic hypotension resulting from acute blood loss.

The electrocardiogram is a good monitor of the adequacy of the coronary circulation. Only the appearance of Q waves >0.03 second in width is diagnostic of definite myocardial infarction. However, the Q waves usually appear postoperatively instead of intraoperatively. Postoperative measurements of the myocardial isoenzymes of creatine phosphokinase (CPK-MB) may confirm the diagnosis. See also Chapter 18 question D.5.

Kidney Transplant

34

Fun-Sun F. Yao

A 35-year-old man with a long-standing history of chronic glomerulonephritis had end-stage renal disease (ESRD). He had been on hemodialysis for 3 years. He was scheduled for emergency renal transplantation using a cadaver kidney.

A. Medical Disease and Differential Diagnosis

1. What are the common causes of chronic renal failure?
2. What are the common problems related to end-stage renal disease?
3. What hemoglobin level would you expect to find in this patient? Why?
4. What is the patient's oxygen-carrying capacity? How can you improve it?
5. How do uremic patients compensate for anemia? Are there any changes in 2,3-diphosphoglycerate (2,3-DPG) levels?
6. What are the effects of severe anemia on the speed of induction with potent inhalation anesthetics?
7. When are you going to transfuse the patient? What kind of blood would you use? Why?
8. What kind of bleeding disorder would you expect?
9. Do these patients have electrolyte imbalances? Discuss Na, K, Mg, Ca, P, and CO_2 content.
10. How would you treat the hyperkalemia?
11. When would you correct the metabolic acidosis? What are the dangers of overzealous correction?
12. Discuss the cardiovascular disorders of ESRD and their treatment.
13. What are the problems related to chronic hemodialysis?
14. What are the contraindications to kidney transplantation?
15. Describe operative procedure of kidney transplantation.

B. Preoperative Evaluation and Preparation

1. What medication might the patient have been receiving? What steroid preparation would you order?
2. What preoperative workup would you order?
3. What are the normal values of blood urea nitrogen (BUN), serum creatinine, and creatinine clearance?
4. How would you differentiate prerenal, renal, and postrenal oliguria?
5. What kind of immunosuppressive therapy would be given to the transplant recipient?
6. What premedication would you choose? Why?

C. Intraoperative Management

1. What anesthesia equipment and monitors would you use? Why?
2. How would you conduct the anesthesia induction?

3. Is succinylcholine dangerous for this patient?
4. What anesthetic agents would you use for maintenance? Discuss the advantages and disadvantages of inhalation and intravenous (IV) agents.
5. Would you use sevoflurane for renal transplantation? Why?
6. What percentage of the halogenated inhalation anesthetics are metabolized in the body? What concentrations of inorganic fluoride would you consider nephrotoxic?
7. What are the serum inorganic fluoride levels after 2 to 4 hours of anesthesia with halothane, isoflurane, enflurane, methoxyflurane, desflurane, and sevoflurane?
8. What are the effects of halothane, enflurane, isoflurane, and fentanyl on renal blood flow (RBF), glomerular filtration rate (GFR), and urine output?
9. Would you consider using regional anesthesia? Why?
10. What muscle relaxants would you choose? Discuss the excretion of *d*-tubocurarine, pancuronium, gallamine, atracurium, cisatracurium, rocuronium, vecuronium, doxacurium, pipecuronium, mivacurium, and succinylcholine.
11. How would you handle intraoperative fluid therapy?
12. The case proceeded without complication until the conclusion of the transplantation. Before the donor kidney was unclamped, the electrocardiogram (ECG) showed normal sinus rhythm with a rate of 90 beats/min. Blood pressure was 120/80 mm Hg. On release of the vascular clamps, multifocal premature ventricular contractions developed immediately and rapidly progressed to ventricular tachycardia. Blood pressure increased to 160/115 mm Hg and pulse rate to 150 beats/min. What are the possible causes? How would you treat it?
13. At the end of surgery, the patient is apneic. What are you going to do?
14. How much neostigmine would you use? Are there any limits? Why?
15. What are the other unusual situations that cause prolonged neuromuscular blockade?
16. What is apneic oxygenation? Who did the pioneer study?
17. What is diffusion hypoxia? How do you prevent it?

D. Postoperative Management

1. What are the early postoperative complications?
2. How would you make the diagnosis of rejection?

A. Medical Disease and Differential Diagnosis

A.1. What are the common causes of chronic renal failure?

The common causes of chronic renal failure are diabetic nephropathy (27.7%), hypertension (24.5%), glomerulonephritis (21.2%), polycystic kidney (3.9%), and diseases (22.7%) such as pyelonephritis, lupus erythematosus, vasculitis, Wegener's granulomatosis, and congenital anomalies. Generally, the particular cause of chronic renal failure has little effect on the decisions of the anesthesiologists or surgeons.

Fauci AS, Braunwald E, Isselbacher KJ et al (eds): Harrison's Principles of Internal Medicine, 14th ed, pp 1274–1275. New York, McGraw-Hill, 1998

A.2. What are the common problems related to end-stage renal disease?

The common problems related to ESRD include:

• Water, electrolyte, and acid-base imbalances

- Hematologic abnormalities—anemia and coagulopathies
- Cardiovascular abnormalities—hypertension, pericarditis, atherosclerosis
- Infections
- Osteodystrophy—hyperparathyroidism
- Neuropathy
- Myopathy
- Treatment with steroids and immunosuppressants
- Chronic hemodialysis

Fauci AS, Braunwald E, Isselbacher KJ et al (eds): Harrison's Principles of Internal Medicine, 14th ed, pp 1514–1518. New York, McGraw-Hill, 1998

Linke CL: Anesthesia considerations for renal transplantation. Cont Anesth Practice 10:183–231, 1987

Yao FS: Anesthesia for renal transplantation. In: Malhotra V (ed): Anesthesia for Renal and Genito-Urological Surgery, pp 45–59. New York, McGraw-Hill, 1996

A.3. What hemoglobin level would you expect to find in this patient? Why?

It is not uncommon for uremic patients to have hemoglobin concentrations of 5 to 7 g/100 ml, corresponding to hematocrits of 15% to 25%. Erythropoiesis is depressed in ESRD, owing both to the effects of retained toxins on bone marrow and to diminished biosynthesis of erythropoietin by the diseased kidney or to the presence of erythropoietin inhibitors. The primary cause of anemia in ESRD is a deficiency of erythropoietin normally produced in the kidney. This may be the result of destruction of renal parenchyma, the presence of circulating inhibitors, or protein deprivation. Other factors may contribute to anemia. The anemia of ESRD may also be caused in part by aluminum intoxication, which causes a microcytic anemia; fibrosis of the bone marrow due to hyperparathyroidism; and occasionally inadequate replacement of folic acid. Iron absorption from the gut is decreased in patients with ESRD. Chronic hemodialysis can cause folate deficiency due to folate dialyzability and iron deficiency because of frequent blood sampling and loss of blood in hemodialysis coils. In addition, patients with ESRD have the following intrinsic erythrocytic factors contributing to anemia: decreased Na^+, K^+-ATPase activity, pentose phosphate dysfunction, and microangiopathic hemolysis. Clinical trials with recombinant human erythropoietin show this agent to be extremely effective in correcting anemia of ESRD.

Fauci AS, Braunwald E, Isselbacher KJ et al (eds): Harrison's Principles of Internal Medicine, 14th ed, p 1518. New York, McGraw-Hill, 1998

A.4. What is the patient's oxygen-carrying capacity? How can you improve it?

The oxygen-carrying capacity is equivalent to the oxygen content, which consists of the amount of oxygen carried by hemoglobin and the amount of dissolved oxygen in plasma. O_2 content (ml/100 ml blood) = $1.34 \times Hb \times O_2$ saturation + $0.0031 \times PaO_2$. Normal oxygen content is 20.3 ml/100 ml blood. Dissolved oxygen, 0.3 ml/100 ml blood, normally is only 1.5% of the total oxygen content, but in severely anemic patients with a hemoglobin of 5 g/100 ml, the dissolved oxygen is 4.5% of the total oxygen content in room air. If the patient breathes 100% oxygen, the PaO_2 is normally >600 mm Hg. The dissolved oxygen will be 1.86 ml/100 ml blood, which is 21.7% of the total oxygen content. This is why a high inspired-oxygen concentration during anesthesia can significantly increase the patient's oxygen-carrying capacity. We can improve this capacity by increasing hemoglobin, oxygen saturation, and oxygen tension.

A.5. How do uremic patients compensate for anemia? Are there any changes in 2,3-diphosphoglycerate (2,3-DPG) levels?

A uremic patient's oxygen-carrying capacity is decreased to less than half normal. This is tolerated because of increased cardiac output. Although the 2,3-DPG is significantly higher in patients with renal disease than in normal subjects, it is below that expected for the degree of anemia present, because acidemia associated with ESRD decreases the production of 2,3-DPG. Oxygen transport at the tissue level is improved by increased 2,3-DPG and acidemia, both shifting the oxygen dissociation curve to the right with resultant easy release of oxygen from hemoglobin to tissue.

Bastron RD: Anesthetic considerations for patients with end-stage renal disease. ASA Refresher Courses in Anesthesiology 13:33–41, 1985

Zauder HL: Anesthesia for patients who have terminal renal disease. ASA Refresher Courses in Anesthesiology 4:163–173, 1976

A.6. What are the effects of severe anemia on the speed of induction with potent inhalation anesthetics?

Severe anemia has been reported to decrease the blood-gas partition coefficients for potent inhalation agents by 15% to 25%. Therefore, the rate of induction and emergence from anesthesia is increased.

Ellis DE, Stoelting RK: Individual variations in fluroxene, halothane, and methoxyflurane blood-gas partition coefficients, and the effect of anemia. Anesthesiology 42:748, 1975

A.7. When are you going to transfuse the patient? What kind of blood would you use? Why?

Well-controlled anemic patients usually tolerate hematocrits of 15% to 25% well. Preoperative transfusion is usually not indicated.

At a time when it appeared that transfusion-induced sensitization against a random lymphocyte panel was predictive of a high graft failure rate, a number of transplantation centers undertook a policy of withholding blood from as many dialysis patients as possible. However, in the 1970s it was found that the nontransfused patients were at the highest risk for graft failure and that multitransfused patients had the best transplantation results. Therefore, deliberate transfusions of five or more units of blood have become a policy at many dialysis centers. Since the early 1980s, however, a progressive loss of the transfusion effect has been seen, with little or no detriment now remaining in the nontransfused patients. This may be attributed to the early recognition and treatment of rejection and the introduction of cyclosporine.

Current practice is to use little or no blood in preparation for transplantation because of concerns regarding human immunodeficiency virus (HIV) transmission. The efficacy of recombinant erythropoietin in sustaining red blood cell mass in patients with ESRD further reduces the clinical need for blood transfusion. During surgery, blood can be administered for hypotension from blood loss or a hematocrit below 15%. When indicated, packed, washed red cells (leuckocyte-poor blood) are transfused, because the introduction of leukocytic antigens can induce production of additional antibodies, predisposing to rejection of a subsequently implanted kidney.

Belani KG, Palahniuk RJ: Kidney transplantation. Int Anesthesiol Clin 29:17–39, 1991

Fauci AS, Braunwald E, Isselbacher KJ et al (eds): Harrison's Principles of Internal Medicine, 14th ed, pp 1518, 1525. New York, McGraw-Hill, 1998

Linke CL: Anesthesia considerations for renal transplantation. Cont Anesth Practice 10:183–231, 1987

Yao FS: Anesthesia for renal transplantation. In Malhotra V (ed): Anesthesia for Renal and Genito-Urological Surgery, pp 45–59. New York, McGraw-Hill, 1996

A.8. What kind of bleeding disorder would you expect?

Although the platelet count is often low, the primary effect is platelet dysfunction. Prolonged bleeding time, decreased platelet adhesiveness, and abnormal prothrombin consumption and thromboplastin generation are the clinical manifestations of platelet dysfunction. Increased plasma levels of guanidinosuccinic acid cause a decline in platelet factor 3 availability, thereby inhibiting secondary platelet aggregation. Hemodialysis effectively eliminates the offending compounds and usually restores adequate platelet function. In addition to platelet dysfunction, certain coagulation factors, primarily the vitamin K-dependent factors (II, VII, IX, X) and factor V, tend to be low in patients with ESRD. Subclinical diffuse intravascular coagulation occasionally occurs in chronic renal disease patients. Fresh-frozen plasma, cryoprecipitate, deamino-8-D-arginine vasopressin (DDAVP), conjugated estrogen, and erythropoietin have been shown to correct the bleeding tendency in uremic patients.

Fauci AS, Braunwald E, Isselbacher KJ et al (eds): Harrison's Principles of Internal Medicine, 14th ed, p 1518. New York, McGraw-Hill, 1998

A.9. Do these patients have electrolyte imbalances? Discuss Na, K, Mg, Ca, P, and CO_2 content.

In most patients with stable chronic renal failure, a modest increase in total body sodium and water content can be documented. On the other hand, hyponatremia and weight gain are the consequence of excessive ingestion of water. In most patients, hyponatremia is relatively mild or asymptomatic. Hyponatremia is commonly found in patients with ESRD and is caused by urinary loss, salt restriction, vomiting, and diarrhea.

The serum potassium level can also rise to dangerous levels when oliguria supervenes and urinary output falls below 500 to 1000 ml daily in patients with renal decompensation. Potassium-sparing diuretics such as spironolactone, triamterene, or amiloride should be used with extreme caution. Likewise, angiotensin-converting enzyme inhibitors, beta-blockers, and cyclosporine can cause hyperkalemia. Hyperkalemia can also be induced by abrupt lowering of arterial blood pH, because acidosis is associated with efflux of potassium from intracellular to extracellular fluids. As a general rule, for every 0.1 unit change in blood pH, a reciprocal change occurs in serum potassium concentration of approximately 0.6 mEq/liter.

Hypermagnesemia can accompany chronic renal failure, especially when the glomerular filtration rate (GFR) declines below 10 ml/min. It is usually controlled by dialysis. Hypermagnesemia may enhance the effects of depolarizing and nondepolarizing muscle relaxants.

Phosphate is excreted by glomerular filtration. As the GFR diminishes, phosphate is retained, thereby depressing the serum calcium level.

Both protein-bound and ionized calcium are reduced in uremic patients. Hypocalcemia results from hyperphosphatemia and impaired intestinal absorption of calcium secondary to decreased activity of vitamin D. Decreased vitamin D activity emphasizes the fact that the kidneys are responsible for the final step in conversion of vitamin D to its highly active metabolite, 1,25-dihydroxyvitamin D.

The kidneys normally excrete 40 to 60 mEq of hydrogen ion every day. Moderate metabolic acidosis is frequently present in patients with ESRD because the kidneys are unable to excrete hydrogen ions. Therefore, plasma CO_2 content is decreased.

Fauci AS, Braunwald E, Isselbacher KJ et al (eds): Harrison's Principles of Internal Medicine, 14th ed, pp 1515–1516. New York, McGraw-Hill, 1998

Stoelting RK, Dierdorf SF, McCammon RL (eds): Anesthesia and Co-Existing Disease, 3rd ed, p 298. New York, Churchill Livingstone, 1993

Yao FS: Anesthesia for renal transplantation. In: Malhotra V (ed): Anesthesia for Renal and Genito-Urological Surgery, pp 45–59. New York, McGraw-Hill, 1996

A.10. *How would you treat the hyperkalemia?*

No patient should be anesthetized who has a serum K^+ in excess of 5.5 mEq/liter. Hyperkalemia should be controlled by dialysis prior to operation. Serial electrolyte determinations should be taken during the operative procedure. Should a significant increase in potassium occur, 500 ml of 10% glucose, deliberate hyperventilation, and 50 mEq $NaHCO_3$ may be given to a 70-kg patient to shift extracellular potassium intracellularly. One-half to 1.0 g of calcium gluconate or calcium chloride can be given to counteract the effect of hyperkalemia on the myocardial conduction system. Because glucose evokes release of endogenous insulin, we give insulin only to patients with diabetes. One unit of insulin for every 2 to 5 g glucose should be given for a diabetic patient. If possible, patients should undergo preoperative dialysis 12 to 24 hours before anesthesia and surgery.

Fauci AS, Braunwald E, Isselbacher KJ et al (eds): Harrison's Principles of Internal Medicine, 14th ed, p 1516. New York, McGraw-Hill, 1998

Stoelting RK, Dierdorf SF, McCammon RL (eds): Anesthesia and Co-Existing Disease, 3rd ed, p 298. New York, Churchill Livingstone, 1993

Vandam LD (ed): To Make the Patient Ready for Anesthesia: Medical Care of the Surgical Patient, 2nd ed, pp 100–101. Menlo Park, CA, Addison-Wesley, 1984

A.11. *When would you correct the metabolic acidosis? What are the dangers of overzealous correction?*

Moderate metabolic acidosis (HCO_3^- of 10 to 20 mEq/liter) is frequently seen in uremia and may not require correction. More severe acidosis (pH <7.20) reflects a need for repeated dialysis. If dialysis is not possible because of the emergency nature of the surgical procedure, sodium bicarbonate therapy is indicated. We tend to correct the extracellular base deficit only. HCO_3^- required = $0.2 \times$ body weight (kg) $\times$ base deficit. Only half of the calculated HCO_3^- is given. Repeated HCO_3^- analyses are critical to titrate the amount of HCO_3^- needed for each patient. Overzealous use of $NaHCO_3$ may cause volume overload, precipitation of tetany in uremic patients with preexisting hypocalcemia, and overshoot alkalosis.

Vandam LD (ed): To Make the Patient Ready for Anesthesia: Medical Care of the Surgical Patient, 2nd ed, p 91. Menlo Park, CA, Addison-Wesley, 1984

Yao FS: Anesthesia for renal transplantation. In: Malhotra V (ed): Anesthesia for Renal and Genito-Urological Surgery, pp 45–59. New York, McGraw-Hill, 1996

A.12. Discuss the cardiovascular disorders of ESRD and their treatment.

Hypertension is almost always present at some stage of chronic renal failure. In most patients, hypertension is the result of fluid overload. Adequate dialysis, sodium depletion, and fluid restriction usually control hypertension in this group. In a few patients, plasma renin levels are high and potent antihypertensive drugs, such as methyldopa, propranolol, hydralazine, diazoxide, minoxidil, captopril, enalapril, or guanethidine may be needed. Congestive heart failure, pulmonary edema, pericarditis, and pericardial effusion may exist in uremic patients. The best initial therapy for uremic pericarditis is daily dialysis for approximately 1 week. If pericarditis is refractory to dialysis, intrapericardial injection of nonabsorbable steroids may prove therapeutic. Partial pericardiectomy may be needed if there is no response to medical treatment.

A unique form of pulmonary congestion and edema may occur even in the absence of volume overload and is associated with normal or mildly elevated intracardiac and pulmonary wedge pressures. This entity, characterized radiologically by perihilar vascular congestion giving rise to a "butterfly wing" distribution, is due to increased permeability of the alveolar capillary membrane. This low pressure pulmonary edema usually responds promptly to vigorous dialysis.

Fauci AS, Braunwald E, Isselbacher KJ et al (eds): Harrison's Principles of Internal Medicine, 14th ed, pp 1517–1518. New York, McGraw-Hill, 1998

A.13. What are the problems related to chronic hemodialysis?

Hepatitis B may be found in 19% to 50% of patients. A higher rate of non-A, non-B hepatitis and cytomegalovirus infection is found, but these are usually of mild degree. Plasma cholinesterase levels were significantly depressed when the relatively crude cellophane membranes were used. The newer types of membranes now in use apparently cause less decrease in pseudocholinesterase levels. Prolonged apnea owing to reduced pseudocholinesterase titers has not been any more prevalent in patients with ESRD than in the general population.

Gastric emptying times are prolonged during dialysis. The half-time for gastric emptying is nearly 300 minutes in uremic patients and can be as long as 700 minutes during dialysis.

The "dialysis disequilibrium" syndrome may occur when fluid electrolyte shifts are too rapid. This syndrome is characterized by headache, nausea, and vomiting, and it can progress to muscle twitching, convulsion, and coma. This syndrome can be prevented by the use of more frequent and shorter initial dialysis.

Bastron RD: Anesthetic considerations for patients with end-stage renal disease. ASA Refresher Courses in Anesthesiology 15:33–41, 1985

Desmond JW, Gordon RA: The effect of hemodialysis on blood volume and plasma cholinesterase levels. Can Anaesth Soc J 16:292–301, 1969

Fauci AS, Braunwald E, Isselbacher KJ et al (eds): Harrison's Principles of Internal Medicine, 14th ed, pp 1274–1275. New York, McGraw-Hill, 1998

Lutterman RD: Renal transplantation. N Engl J Med 301:1038–1048, 1979

A.14. *What are the contraindications to kidney transplantation?*

Among the contraindications to kidney transplantation are:

Absolute Contraindications
- Reversible renal involvement
- Ability of conservative measures to maintain useful life
- Advanced forms of major extrarenal complications (cerebrovascular or coronary disease, neoplasia)
- Active infection
- Active glomerulonephritis
- Previous sensitization to donor tissue

Relative Contraindications
- Age >60 to 65 years
- Presence of vesical or urethral abnormalities
- Iliofemoral occlusive disease
- Psychiatric Problems
- Oxalosis

Fauci AS, Braunwald E, Isselbacher KJ et al (eds): Harrison's Principles of Internal Medicine, 14th ed, p 1524. New York, McGraw-Hill, 1998

A.15. *Describe the operative procedure of kidney transplantation?*

The cadaveric kidney is most often placed extraperitoneally, in the lower abdomen on either the right side or left side depending on which kidney is used; the right kidney is placed in the left groin and vice versa. The inferior epigastric vessels are divided and the round ligament in the female is divided but the spermatic cord in the male is usually preserved. The usual anastomoses are the renal artery end-to-end to the internal iliac artery, renal vein end-to-end to the external iliac vein, and the ureter is inserted into the bladder via a tunneling technique. In the event that the patient weighs <20 kg, the kidney is placed intra-abdominally, at which time the aorta and vena cava may be the major vessels employed. In this instance, the wound is not irrigated with the antibiotic solution and the kidney is usually placed on the right side posterior to the right colon.

Kidneys from living related donors are flushed immediately after removal from the donor with iced Ringer's lactate solution containing heparin and mannitol. The ischemic time during implantation is usually about 20 to 30 minutes. In cadaver kidney transplants, prior to release of the arterial clamp and following completion of the anastomosis, an intra-arterial injection of verapamil is given (10 mg) by direct push into the kidney. In addition, furosemide (200 mg) is usually given immediately to all transplant recipients.

Yao FS: Anesthesia for renal transplantation. In: Malhotra V (ed): Anesthesia for Renal and Genito-Urological Surgery, pp 45–59. New York, McGraw-Hill, 1996

B. Preoperative Evaluation and Preparation

B.1. What medication might the patient have been receiving? What steroid preparation would you order?

Many patients require centrally acting antihypertensive agents (methyldopa), beta-adrenergic blockers (propranolol), direct arterial dilators (minoxidil), or calcium channel blockers (verapamil) to decrease peripheral vasoconstriction. The antihypertensive drugs should be continued up until the time of surgery. Transplant recipients might have been receiving steroids or immunosuppressants. Steroids should be given to prevent rejection and possible adrenal insufficiency secondary to chronic administration of steroids. The usual preoperative preparation is 250 mg methylprednisolone (Solu-Medrol) before the induction of anesthesia. Postoperatively methylprednisone (250 mg IV) is given twice daily for 2 days followed by 125 mg IV twice daily for 1 day. Then the steroid is tapered and maintained for 6 months.

Fauci AS, Braunwald E, Isselbacher KJ et al (eds): Harrison's Principles of Internal Medicine, 14th ed, p 1517. New York, McGraw-Hill, 1998

The New York Hospital-Cornell Medical Center Protocol, New York, NY

Yao FS: Anesthesia for renal transplantation. In: Malhotra V (ed): Anesthesia for Renal and Genito-Urological Surgery, pp 45–59. New York, McGraw-Hill, 1996

B.2. What preoperative workup would you order?

In addition to the routine systemic tests, such as ECG, chest radiograph, blood counts, urinalysis, electrolytes, blood sugar, BUN, creatinine, platelet count, prothrombin time, partial thrombin time, serum glutamic oxaloacetic transaminase (SGOT), serum glutamic pyruvic transaminase (SGPT), bilirubin, albumin, and globulin, I would like to have arterial blood gases to determine the acid-base balance.

B.3. What are the normal values of blood urea nitrogen (BUN), serum creatinine, and creatinine clearance?

Normal BUN is 10 to 20 mg/100 ml. Normal serum creatinine is 0.6 to 1.3 mg/100 ml. Normal values for creatinine clearance are 85 to 125 ml/min for women and 95 to 140 ml/min for men (average 120 ml/min).

Stoelting RK, Dierdorf SF, McCammon RL (eds): Anesthesia and Co-Existing Disease, 3rd ed, pp 291–292. New York, Churchill Livingstone, 1993

Vandam LD (ed): To Make the Patient Ready for Anesthesia: Medical Care of the Surgical Patient, 2nd ed, pp 68–69. Menlo Park, CA, Addison-Wesley, 1984

B.4. *How would you differentiate prerenal, renal, and postrenal oliguria?*

The diagnosis of postrenal obstruction is characteristically established by complete anuria, as opposed to the oliguria found in patients with hypovolemic and acute tubular necrosis. It must be emphasized that all collection tubing should be checked to be sure it is properly connected, patent, and not kinked.

Careful examination of urine sediment is of major importance in determining the cause of oliguria. The presence of renal tubular cells, casts, and many pigmented granular casts is strong evidence of acute tubular necrosis. A normal sediment suggests a diagnosis of hypovolemic prerenal failure. In prerenal hypovolemia oliguria, a decrease is seen in glomerular filtration rate (GFR) and an increase in water, sodium, and urea reabsorption, resulting in concentration of nonresorbable solute. Usually urine sodium is <20 mEq/liter; urine:plasma creatinine is >30; BUN: serum creatinine is >20. The response to mannitol is brisk when blood pressure and hydration are adequate. In renal failure, the nephrons that continue to function do so in a state of osmotic diuresis. Creatinine is not concentrated in urine. BUN and serum creatinine are both increased and their ratio is normal, 10:1, because the urea reabsorption is not potentiated. Mannitol is uniformly ineffective in promoting diuresis.

The most sensitive indices are fractional excretion of sodium (FeNa) and renal failure index. FeNa relates sodium clearance (Una/Pna) to creatinine clearance (Ucr/Pcr). Sodium is reabsorbed avidly from glomerular filtrate in prerenal azotemia in an attempt to restore intravascular volume but not in renal failure because of epithelial injury. In contrast, creatinine is reabsorbed less efficiently than sodium in both situations. Therefore, patients with prerenal azotemia typically have a FeNa <1.0% (frequently <0.01%), whereas in patients with renal failure the FeNa is usually >1.0%. The renal failure index, Una/(Ucr/Pcr), provides similar information (see Table 34-1).

Bastron RD: Pathophysiology of acute renal failure. ASA Refresher Courses in Anesthesiology 8:1–12, 1980

Fauci AS, Braunwald E, Isselbacher KJ et al (eds): Harrison's Principles of Internal Medicine, 14th ed, pp 1508–1510. New York, McGraw-Hill, 1998

Thadhani R, Pascual M, Bonventure JV: Acute renal failure. N Engl J Med 334:1448–1460, 1996

B.5. *What kind of immunosuppressive therapy would be given to the transplant recipient?*

At present, immunosuppressive therapy in clinical use or under investigation includes corticosteroids, azathioprine, cyclosporine, cyclophosphamide, retroplacental

Table 34-1.   Differentiation of Prerenal and Renal Failure

	PRERENAL	RENAL
Urinary sediment	Hyaline casts	Tubular cells, granular casts
Urinary specific gravity	>1.018	<1.012
Urinary osmolality (mOsm/kg)	>500	<250
Urinary Na (mEq/liter)	<10	>20
Urine: plasma creatinine ratio	>40	<20
Blood urea nitrogen (BUN): Serum creatinine ratio	>20	<10–15
Mannitol response	Brisk	None
Renal failure index Una/(Ucr/Pcr)	<1	>1
Fractional excretion of sodium (%) (Una/Pna)/(Ucr/Pcr)	<1	>1

gamma globulin (RPGG), antithymocyte globulin (ATG) or antilymphocyte globulin (ALG), monoclonal antibodies, total lymphoid irradiation, and plasma leukapheresis.

At The New York Hospital-Cornell Medical Center, all kidney transplant recipients receive corticosteroids, azathioprine, and cyclosporine. A corticosteroid, such as methylprednisolone (250 mg IV), is given 1 hour before and 6 hours after surgery for all transplant recipients. Then the steroid is tapered and maintained for 6 months. Cyclosporine is started 7 days before transplantation of a living-donor kidney but 1 day after transplantation of a cadaveric kidney. Azathioprine is begun 2 days before transplantation of a living-donor kidney but on the day of transplantation of a kidney of cadaveric origin. Mycophenolate mofetil (1 g twice daily) starting 1 day before surgery for 6 months may replace azathioprine for both living donor and cadaveric kidney transplantation. All three immunosuppressives are maintained for 6 months.

All transplant recipients receive a calcium channel blocker as part of their immunosuppressive protocol. It is believed that the addition of such a family of drugs allows us to use relatively higher doses of cyclosporine without adversely affecting renal function. Nifedipine is most commonly used, because diltiazem, verapamil, and nicardipine can interfere with the P450-mediated degradative metabolism of cyclosporine, thus increasing its half-life. Nifedipine (Procardia 30 XL) is given orally prior to surgery. Intraoperatively, 10 mg of verapamil is given intra-arterially following arterial anastomosis. All recipients are to receive nifedipine as soon as oral medications are allowed in the immediate postoperative period.

Fauci AS, Braunwald E, Isselbacher KJ et al (eds): Harrison's Principles of Internal Medicine, 14th ed, pp 1526–1528. New York, McGraw-Hill, 1998

The New York Hospital-Cornell Medical Center Protocol, New York, NY

B.6. What premedication would you choose? Why?

Numerous combinations of sedatives, tranquilizers, and narcotics, with or without vagolytic agents, have been used satisfactorily. We usually give pentobarbital (Nembutal) (100 mg) and atropine (0.4 mg) intramuscularly 1 hour prior to surgery for a 70-kg patient. Pentobarbital will achieve adequate sedation without significant respiratory and circulatory depression. Atropine is given to prevent a vagal reflex from tracheal intubation. A nonparticulate antacid, such as 30 ml of 0.3 M sodium citrate, can be given about half an hour before surgery to prevent aspiration pneumonitis.

Yao FS: Anesthesia for renal transplantation. In: Malhotra V (ed): Anesthesia for Renal and Genito-Urological Surgery, pp 45–59. New York, McGraw-Hill, 1996

C. Intraoperative Management

C.1. What anesthesia equipment and monitors would you use? Why?

Because of a high incidence of serum hepatitis from chronic hemodialysis and low resistance to infection from steroid and immunosuppressant therapy, a sterile disposable anesthetic circuit, endotracheal tube, and laryngoscope are used to prevent cross-infection from patient to patient. The anesthesiologist is required to use gloves and gown to protect the patient and himself or herself. We routinely monitor blood pressure and ECG; use a pulse oximeter, end-tidal CO_2 analyzer, and nerve stimulator; monitor rectal or esophageal temperature; and record urine output and central venous pressure. Electrolytes, blood gases, and hematocrit are determined when necessary. Sudden increase in body temperature is an important sign of superacute rejection of the transplanted kidney. Unless evidence is seen of left ventricular failure, we do not recommend pulmonary wedge pressure monitoring. Simple central venous pressure monitoring is usually sufficient to guide the fluid therapy.

Yao FS: Anesthesia for renal transplantation. In: Malhotra V (ed): Anesthesia for Renal and Genito-Urological Surgery, pp 45–59. New York, McGraw-Hill, 1996

C.2. How would you conduct the anesthesia induction?

Rapid-sequence induction of anesthesia is required. Kidney transplantation is often emergency surgery. In addition, the gastric emptying time is prolonged in uremic patients, especially during hemodialysis. After pretreatment with 3 mg of *d*-tubocurarine and denitrogenation with 100% oxygen for 3 minutes, anesthesia is induced with an ultrashort-acting barbiturate, such as thiopental sodium (250 mg for a 70-kg patient). Endotracheal intubation is facilitated with 100 mg of succinylcholine. If serum potassium is elevated, a nondepolarizing muscle relaxant such as rocuronium, cisatracurium, or vecuronium can be given with the priming technique to facilitate rapid tracheal intubation. Ketamine or etomidate can be used for induction if the patient's hemodynamic status is unstable. If the patient has uremia with ischemic heart disease, fentanyl (5 μg/kg) can be given before rapid-sequence induction to blunt circulatory responses to tracheal intubation.

Bastron RD: Anesthetic considerations for patients with end-stage renal disease. ASA Refresher Courses in Anesthesiology 13:33–41, 1985

Cook DR: Anesthetic considerations for organ transplantation. ASA Refresher Courses in Anesthesiology 18:97–115, 1990

Linke CL: Anesthesia considerations for renal transplantation. Cont Anesth Practice 10:183–231, 1987

Randall CC, Weiss JL, Hameroff SR et al: Fentanyl preloading for rapid-sequence induction of anesthesia. Anesth Analg 63:60, 1984

Yao FS: Anesthesia for renal transplantation. In: Malhotra V (ed): Anesthesia for Renal and Genito-Urological Surgery, pp 45–59. New York, McGraw-Hill, 1996

C.3. Is succinylcholine dangerous for this patient?

When serum potassium is within the normal range (3.5 to 5.0 mEq/liter) a regular clinical dose of succinylcholine can be used without difficulty. Potassium flux after administration of succinylcholine in patients with renal failure does not differ from that seen in patients with normal renal function. The mean maximal increase in serum potassium was 0.5 mEq/liter. When serum potassium is close to or above 5.5 mEq/liter, we try to avoid succinylcholine. The pseudocholinesterase levels were significantly depressed when the relatively crude cellophane membranes were used for hemodialysis, but the newer types of membranes now in use cause less decrease in pseudocholinesterase. Prolonged apnea owing to reduced pseudocholinesterase has not been any more prevalent than in the general population.

Cook DR: Anesthetic consideration for organ transplantation. ASA Refresher Courses in Anesthesiology 18:97–115, 1990

Desmond JW, Gordon RA: The effect of hemodialysis on blood volume and plasma cholinesterase levels. Can Anaesth Soc J 16:292–301, 1969

Koide M, Ward BE: Serum potassium concentration after succinylcholine in patients with renal failure. Anesthesiology 36:142–145, 1972

Linke CL: Anesthesia considerations for renal transplantation. Cont Anesth Practice 10:183–231, 1987

Yao FS: Anesthesia for renal transplantation. In: Malhotra V (ed): Anesthesia for Renal and Genito-Urological Surgery, pp 45–59. New York, McGraw-Hill, 1996

C.4. What anesthetic agents would you use for maintenance? Discuss the advantages and disadvantages of inhalation and intravenous (IV) agents.

The current choice for maintenance of anesthesia is desflurane or isoflurane-oxygen with or without supplementary N_2O or fentanyl. Desflurane and isoflurane have little biotransformation (only 0.02% and 0.2%, respectively) and less cardiac depression than halothane or enflurane. Although the halothane-oxygen sequence has also been used successfully, we rarely use halothane because of a high incidence of serum hepatitis in those patients under chronic hemodialysis. In addition, halothane depresses the cardiovascular system more than isoflurane, and it may cause hepatic dysfunction. Enflurane is avoided for renal transplantation. Although the biotransformation of enflurane with liberation of inorganic fluoride is low, postoperative transplant renal failure has been reported with enflurane use. Methoxyflurane is contraindicated because of a high concentration of free fluoride from biotransformation. For surgery other than renal transplantation, methoxyflurane is a good choice for the anephric patient because the target organ of nephrotoxicity is absent. Potent inhalation anesthetics provide a steady depth of anesthesia and are useful in controlling intraoperative hypertension and reducing the doses of muscle relaxants needed for adequate surgical exposure.

Nitrous oxide-oxygen with neuroleptic agents (fentanyl-droperidol) can be used when the anemia is not severe enough to seriously impair the oxygen-carrying capacity. Narcotic agents do not depress cardiac and renal function, whereas most potent inhalation agents do. More muscle relaxants may be needed because narcotic agents offer no muscle relaxation. Using a narcotic technique, a high concentration of N_2O is needed to keep the patient unconscious. Therefore, very high concentrations of oxygen cannot be given to improve oxygen-carrying capacity by increasing the dissolved oxygen in plasma.

Barash PG, Cullen BF, Stoelting RK (eds): Clinical Anesthesia, 3rd ed, pp 370–371. Philadelphia, Lippincott-Raven, 1997

Belani KG, Palahniuk RJ: Kidney transplantation. Int Anesthesiol Clin 29:17–39, 1991

Cook DR: Anesthetic considerations for organ transplantation. ASA Refresher Courses in Anesthesiology 18:97–115, 1990

Linke CL: Anesthesia considerations for renal transplantation. Cont Anesth Practice 10:183–231, 1987

Yao FS: Anesthesia for renal transplantation. In Malhotra V (ed): Anesthesia for Renal and Genito-Urological Surgery, pp 45–59. New York, McGraw-Hill, 1996

C.5. Would you use sevoflurane for renal transplantation? Why?

I would not use sevoflurane because of its potential nephrotoxicity. Sevoflurane undergoes biodegradation to inorganic fluoride and degradation by carbon dioxide absorbents to a vinyl ether called "compound A." Both inorganic fluoride and compound A can produce renal injury. Although several reports indicate that inorganic fluoride produced by prolonged sevoflurane anesthesia does not cause renal injury, one report did indicate a link, prompting an editorial suggesting caution when administering sevoflurane to patients with renal disease. Recently, Eger et al compared the nephrotoxicity of 8 hours of 1.25 minimum alveolar concentration (MAC) of sevoflurane versus desflurane in volunteers using fresh gas flow rate of 2 liters/min. Desflurane did not produce renal injury, whereas sevoflurane was associated with transient injury to:

- Glomerulus, as revealed by albuminuria
- Proximal tubule, as revealed by glucosuria and increased urinary alpha-GST
- Distal tubule, as revealed by increased urinary π-GST

However, neither anesthetic affected serum creatinine or BUN nor changed the ability of the kidney to concentrate urine in response to vasopressin. Their results support the theory that renal toxicity results from exposure to compound A. Therefore, to decrease renal toxicity, they recommended high fresh gas flow rates to decrease the concentration of inspired compound A. However, Higuchi et al found that renal injury correlated with increased inorganic fluoride levels produced by sevoflurane biodegradation. Therefore, even the use of high fresh gas flow rates may not eliminate all risk of renal injury. However, two recent clinical studies of low-flow sevoflurane reported no evidence of nephrotoxicity. The two studies compared low-flow sevoflurane with low-flow isoflurane and high-flow sevoflurane and found no differences in a variety of experimental enzymatic markers and established clinical indices and renal function.

Bito H, Ikeuchi Y, Ikeda K: Effects of low-flow sevoflurane anesthesia on renal function: Comparison with high-flow sevoflurane anesthesia and low-flow isoflurane anesthesia. Anesthesiology 86:1231–1237, 1997

Eger EI II, Koblin DD, Bowland T et al: Nephrotoxicity of sevoflurane anesthesia in volunteers. Anesth Analg 84:160–168, 1997

Higuchi H, Sumikura H, Sumita S et al: Renal function in patients with high serum fluoride concentration after prolonged sevoflurane anesthesia. Anethesiology 83:449–448, 1995

Kharasch ED, Frink EJ Jr, Zager R et al: Assesment of low-flow sevoflurane and isoflurane effects on renal function using sensitive markers of tubular toxicity. Anesthesiology 86:1238-1254, 1997

C.6. What percentage of the halogenated inhalation anesthetics are metabolized in the body? What concentrations of inorganic fluoride would you consider nephrotoxic?

Desflurane (0.02%); isoflurane (0.2%); enflurane (2%); sevoflurane (3%); halothane (12% to 20%); and methoxyflurane (20% to 40%) are metabolized in the body (rule of 2). When serum inorganic fluoride reaches 50 to 80 mM/liter, subclinical renal toxicity (laboratory abnormalities) occurs. Clinical nephrotoxicity usually becomes apparent when serum fluoride is >80 mM/liter. The high-output renal failure is dose-related and characterized by vasopressin-resistant polyuria, hypernatremia, serum hyperosmolarity, increased serum urea nitrogen, and inorganic fluoride concentration.

Barash PG, Cullen BF, Stoelting RK (eds): Clinical Anesthesia, 3rd ed, pp 370–371. Philadelphia, Lippincott-Raven, 1997

Cohen EN: Metabolism of the volatile anesthetics. ASA Refresher Courses in Anesthesiology 5:21–32, 1977

Mazze RI: Renal toxicity of anesthetics. ASA Refresher Courses in Anesthesiology 1:85–99, 1973

C.7. What are the serum inorganic fluoride levels after 2 to 4 hours of anesthesia with halothane, isoflurane, enflurane, methoxyflurane, desflurane, and sevoflurane?

The inorganic fluoride levels after 2 to 4 hours of anesthesia with halothane, isoflurane, and enflurane are 1 to 2 mM/liter, 3 to 5 mM/liter, and approximately 20 mM/liter, respectively. Methoxyflurane has a dose-dependent renal toxicity. The serum fluoride levels are 50 to 80 and 90 to 120 mM/liter after 2.5 to 3, and 5 MAC-hours of methoxyflurane anesthesia. Desflurane extremely resists biodegradation because fluorine is the only halogen in the desflurane molecule. Serum fluoride levels do not increase with desflurane, whereas they often peak above 50 mM/liter even when sevoflurane is administered during surgery of average duration. The average fluoride concentrations for 10 MAC hours of desflurane and sevoflurane anesthesia plus 4 hours recovery periods are 1.5 ± 0.5 mM/liter and 71 ± 13 mM/liter, respectively. Sevoflurane increased serum fluoride concentrations to >100 mM/liter in 6 of 10 volunteers; the highest value was 125 mM/liter. Obesity itself increases biotransformation of all the above-mentioned inhalation agents, resulting in increased serum fluoride levels.

Eger EI II, Koblin DD, Bowland T et al: Nephrotoxicity of sevoflurane anesthesia in volunteers. Anesth Analg 84:160–168, 1997

Mazze RI, Sievenpiper TS, Stevenson J: Renal effects of enflurane and halothane in patients with abnormal renal function. Anesthesiology 60:161, 1984

Miller RD (ed): Anesthesia, 4th ed, pp 169–171. New York, Churchill Livingstone, 1994

Young SR, Stoelting RK, Peterson C et al: Anesthesia biotransformation and renal function in obese patients during and after methoxyflurane and halothane anesthesia. Anesthesiology 42:451, 1975

C.8. What are the effects of halothane, enflurane, isoflurane, and fentanyl on renal blood flow (RBF), glomerular filtration rate (GRF), and urine output?

Halothane does not decrease RBF, because it decreases renal vascular resistance and perfusion pressure proportionally. Enflurane decreases RBF. Isoflurane minimally alters RBF with light levels of anesthesia (i.e., 1 MAC) and significantly decreases renal vascular resistance. As the depth of anesthesia with isoflurane is increased, RBF decreases because of a greater decrease in perfusion pressure than in vascular resistance. Fentanyl was found to decrease RBF and increase renal vascular resistance in the anesthetized dog, but to mildly increase RBF and renal vascular resistance in the conscious dog. All anesthetic agents and techniques decrease GFR, with subsequent decrease in urine output.

Priano LL: The effects of anesthesia on renal blood flow and function. ASA Refresher Courses in Anesthesiology 13:143–156, 1985

C.9. Would you consider using regional anesthesia? Why?

Because of possible uremic neuropathy and coagulopathy, epidural or spinal anesthesia is not recommended at The New York Hospital-Cornell Medical Center. However, regional anesthesia has been used successfully for transplantation. Intubation of the trachea and potential pulmonary infections are avoided in the immunosuppressed patient.

Cook DR: Anesthetic considerations for organ transplantation. ASA Refresher Courses in Anesthesiology 18:97–115, 1990

Zauder HL: Anesthesia for patients who have terminal renal disease. ASA Refresher Courses in Anesthesiology 4:163–173, 1976

C.10. What muscle relaxants would you choose? Discuss the excretion of d-tubocurarine, pancuronium, gallamine, atracurium, cisatracurium, rocuronium, vecuronium, doxacurium, pipecuronium, mivacurium, and succinylcholine.

Atracurium, cisatracurium, rocuronium, vecuronium, and possibly mivacurium are the preferred muscle relaxants used in patients with ESRD. However, *d*-tubocurarine and pancuronium have been widely and successfully used in the presence of renal failure.

The dependence of various muscle relaxants on the kidney for their elimination is shown in Table 34-2. Atracurium and cisatracurium are broken down by enzymatic ester hydrolysis and nonenzymatic alkaline hydrolysis (Hoffmann elimination) to inactive products, and they are not dependent on renal or hepatic excretion for termination of action. Therefore, the elimination half-lives of atracurium and cisatracurium are the same in patients with normal renal function and in those with absent renal function. Vecuronium and rocuronium appear to be excreted mostly by the liver with about 40% excreted by the kidneys. Therefore, the duration of neuromuscular blockade by vecuronium and rocuronium are associated with little prolongation in patients with ESRD. Mivacurium, a short-acting muscle relaxant, is rapidly hydrolyzed by plasma cholinesterase at a rate of 70% of that of succinylcholine. It also may be partly metabolized by the liver, and only <5% of mivacurium is eliminated by the

Table 34-2. Dependence (Percentage of Injected Dose) of Various Muscle Relaxants on the Kidney for Their Elimination

DRUG	RENAL EXCRETION (%)	ELIMINATION HALF-LIFE (h)	
		Normal	ESRD
Gallamine	100	1.5	12.5
Metocurine	>98	5.0	11.4
Doxacurium	>90	1.7	3.7
Pipecurium	>90	2.3	4.4
Pancuronium	85	2.2	4.3
d-Tubocurarine	60–80	1.4	2.2
Rocuronium	40	1.2	1.6
Vecuronium	40–50	0.9–1.3	1.4–1.6
Atracurium	10–40	0.3	0.4
Mivacurium	<5	2 min	2 min
Sucinylcholine	<2	2 min	2 min

ESRD, end-stage renal disease.

kidneys. *D*-tubocurarine is eliminated in large part by the kidneys (45% excreted in 24 hours) and to a lesser extent by the liver (12% in 24 hours). The excretion of *d*-tubocurarine is delayed in patients with renal failure. Studies in humans indicate that doxacurium, pipecuronium, and pancuronium are more dependent on renal excretion than is *d*-tubocuraine. Pancuronium is largely excreted in the urine, but a significant portion of this is after biotransformation to the less active 3-hydroxy and 3,17-dihydroxy-pancuronium. The elimination half-life of pancuronium is prolonged by >95%, compared with 57% for *d*-tubocurarine, in patients with ESRD. Therefore, *d*-tubocurarine is preferred to pancuronium. Gallamine, decamethonium, and probably metocurine are almost totally excreted by the kidneys. Their use in anephric patients is contraindicated. Succinylcholine is hydrolyzed by pseudocholinesterase to succinylmonocholine and then to succinic acid and choline. Succinylmonocholine is excreted by the kidney and has nondepolarizing blocking activity. Theoretically, large doses of succinylcholine, as might occur with an IV drip administration, should be avoided in patients with renal failure. However, succinylcholine has been used without difficulty.

Barash PG, Cullen BF, Stoelting RK (eds): Clinical Anesthesia, 3rd ed, pp 388–397, 953. Philadelphia, Lippincott-Raven, 1997

Miller RD (ed): Anesthesia, 4th ed, pp 432; 458–459. New York, Churchill Livingstone, 1994

C.11. *How would you handle intraoperative fluid therapy?*

Probably the most important determinant of immediate renal function and avoidance of postoperative acute tubular necrosis is the adequacy of perfusion of the transplanted kidney at the time when the vascular clamps are released. Central venous pressure or pulmonary artery pressure (only in patients with left ventricular dysfunction) should be used to guide fluid therapy. Patients undergoing kidney transplantation tend to have a hypovolemic state despite abnormally increased total body fluid. In addition, a cadaveric kidney seems to require higher arterial blood pressure and larger plasma volume to initiate diuresis than a normal kidney. Systolic blood pressure is kept around 130 to 160 mm Hg and central venous pressure around 10 to 15 cm H_2O. Five percent albumin or normal saline can be used to expand plasma volume. Potassium-containing solutions are avoided. Normal saline can be used to replace blood loss. Hemodialysis can be used effectively to remove excess fluid postoperatively.

Beebe DS, Belani KG, Mergens P et al: Anesthetic management of infants receiving an adult kidney transplant. Anesth Analg 73: 725–730, 1991

Carlier M, Souifflet JP, Pirson Y et al: Maximal hydration during anesthesia increases pulmonary arterial pressures and improves early function of human renal transplants. Transplantation 34:201–204, 1982

Cook DR: Anesthetic considerations for organ transplantation. ASA Refresher Courses in Anesthesiology 18:97–115, 1990

C.12. *The case proceeded without complication until the conclusion of the transplantation. Before the donor kidney was unclamped, the electrocardiogram (ECG) showed normal sinus rhythm with a rate of 90 beats/min. Blood pressure was 120/80 mm Hg. On release of the vascular clamps, multifocal premature ventricular contractions developed immediately and rapidly progressed to ventricular tachycardia. Blood pressure increased to 160/115 mm Hg and pulse rate to 150 beats/min. What are the possible causes? How would you treat it?*

The acute hemodynamic changes following the release of vascular clamps from the transplanted kidneys have been reported to be associated with the effect of the intact adrenal glands on donor kidneys. The hypertension can be mediated by the release of catecholamines from the intact adrenal gland of the donor kidney or by release of renin from the donor graft. The arrhythmias may be caused by hyperkalemia associated with washout of potassium-containing Collins solution used to perfuse the donor kidney before transplantation. Furthermore, reperfusion of the ischemic leg on release of the vascular clamps causes transient systemic acidosis, which further increases hyperkalemia by shifting potassium from intracellular to extracellular fluids.

Lidocaine should be given to treat ventricular arrhythmia. Direct current (DC) cardioversion may be used if necessary. The surgeon should be notified immediately and the adrenal vein should be ligated. The adrenal gland should be drained and excised. Usually the hemodynamics return to normal within 3 to 10 minutes. Hypertension and tachycardia can be treated with vasodilators and beta-blockers.

Freilich JD, Waterman PM, Rosenthal JT: Acute hemodynamic changes during renal transplantation. Anesth Analg 63:158, 1984

Hirshman CA, Edelstein G: Intraoperative hyperkalemia and cardiac arrest during renal transplantation in an insulin-dependent diabetic patient. Anesthesiology 51:161–162, 1979

C.13. At the end of surgery, the patient is apneic. What are you going to do?

The possible causes of apnea must be identified and specific treatment established accordingly. Apnea can result from central depression or peripheral neuromuscular blockade. The respiratory center may be depressed by hypocarbia and anesthetics, including both inhalation and intravenous agents, such as narcotics and barbiturates. Peripheral blockade is usually the result of residual muscle relaxants. Hypocarbia can be corrected by hypoventilation with high inspired-oxygen concentration to prevent hypoxia. When respiration is depressed by narcotics, the pupils are usually miotic. Naloxone in 0.1-mg increments may be titrated to reverse narcotic depression. Potent inhalation agents should be terminated to decrease respiratory depression.

Neuromuscular blockade can be evaluated with a peripheral nerve stimulator. Nondepolarizing blockade is characterized by fade from single twitch stimulations to tetanic stimulation, and by post-tetanic facilitation. Neostigmine or pyridostigmine may be given with atropine to reverse the blockade. Normally, neostigmine and atropine can be administered concomitantly because the vagolytic effects of atropine precede the cardiac muscarinic effects of neostigmine by 1 to 2 minutes. However, in cardiac patients or in patients with electrolyte or acid-base imbalance, we recommend careful titration of atropine in 0.1- to 0.2-mg increments and neostigmine in 0.25- to 0.5-mg increments in separate syringes to keep the heart rate change within 10% to 15% of its control value. Cardiac response to atropine and neostigmine may be unpredictable in patients with irritable hearts or electrolyte imbalance. Sinus arrest and severe tachycardia have been experienced by those patients after concomitant administration of atropine and neostigmine.

Miller RD (ed): Anesthesia, 4th ed, pp 461–468. New York, Churchill Livingstone, 1994

C.14. How much neostigmine would you use? Are there any limits? Why?

The dose of neostigmine depends on the intensity of the neuromuscular blockade, which is determined by the total amount of muscle relaxant given, the frequency of administration, and the time of the last dose. Usually 1.5 to 3.0 mg of neostigmine will antagonize most nondepolarizing blocks in the average adult patient. If the blockade is not reversed adequately, a total dose of up to 5 mg (60 to 80 μg/kg) can be given. Larger doses of neostigmine may reinforce the neuromuscular blockade by causing its own nondepolarizing blockade. Other unusual situations have to be studied.

Miller RD (ed): Anesthesia, 4th ed, p 468. New York, Churchill Livingstone, 1994

C.15. What are the other unusual situations that cause prolonged neuromuscular blockade?

Other unusual situations causing prolonged neuromuscular blockade include:

Electrolyte Imbalance
- Hypokalemia and hypernatremia can increase the transmembrane potential and postjunctional membrane threshold for depolarization, and thus increase the action of a nondepolarizing muscle relaxant. However, the increase of transmembrane potentials also increases release of neurotransmitter from the nerve terminal and decreases the action of a nondepolarizing relaxant. Clinically, the net effect is unpredictable.
- Hypermagnesemia enhances the action of a nondepolarizing relaxant by decreasing the release of acetylcholine from the nerve terminal and reducing the sensitivity of the postjunctional membrane to acetylcholine.
- Calcium has various effects at the neuromuscular junction. It enhances the release of acetylcholine from the nerve terminal, decreases the sensitivity of the postjunctional membrane to acetylcholine, and enhances excitation-contraction coupling in the muscle. Calcium appears to be effective in antagonizing neuromuscular blockade associated with muscle relaxants, magnesium, and antibiotics.

Acid-Base Imbalance
- Respiratory acidosis enhances the nondepolarizing relaxants.
- The effects of respiratory alkalosis, metabolic alkalosis, and metabolic acidosis are inconsistent.

Drug Interactions
- Antibiotics—Certain antibiotics, alone or in combination with nondepolarizing relaxants, cause apnea by neuromuscular blockade. The aminoglycosides (neomycin, gentamicin, kanamycin, and streptomycin), as well as tetracycline, decrease acetylcholine release by blocking the influx of calcium ions necessary for transmitter release. Penicillin V, erythromycin, clindamycin, polymyxin, and tetracycline produce partial paralysis by directly decreasing muscle contractility. Paromomycin, viomycin, colistin, lincomycin, amikacin, and netilmicin also produce neuromuscular blockade.
- Local anesthetics—Both the ester and amide types of local anesthetics enhance the effects of *d*-tubocurarine. In addition, local anesthetics directly depress the respiratory center.

- Antiarrhythmic agents—Lidocaine, procainamide, and quinidine enhance the effects of *d*-tubocurarine.
- Furosemide (Lasix) enhances *d*-tubocurarine by inhibiting the cyclic AMP system and reducing neurotransmitter output.
- Ketamine enhances the effects of *d*-tubocurarine, but not pancuronium.
- The hypotensive agents trimethaphan, pentolinium, nitroglycerin, and nitroprusside enhance *d*-tubocurarine in very high doses, but not in clinical doses.
- Hypothermia—Hypothermia reduces serum clearances as well as renal and biliary excretion of both *d*-tubocurarine and pancuronium. The metabolism of pancuronium to less active metabolites is reduced. The neuromuscular effects of relaxants are prolonged. Hypothermia can have a direct mechanical effect on the muscle, slowing contraction and relaxation and thus enhancing the blockade.
- Atypical pseudocholinesterase causing prolonged apnea after administration of succinylcholine.

Ham J: Factors affecting administration of nondepolarizing neuromuscular blocking agents. ASA Refresher Courses in Anesthesiology 8:61–78, 1980

Miller RD (ed): Anesthesia, 4th ed, pp 461–470. New York, Churchill Livingstone, 1994

Sokoll MD, Gergis SD: Antibiotics and neuromuscular function. Anesthesiology 55:148–159, 1981

C.16. What is apneic oxygenation? Who did the pioneer study?

Draper and Whitehead conducted the pioneer study on apneic oxygenation in 1944. Apneic oxygenation (formerly known as diffusion respiration) is actually caused by mass movement oxygenation. When the lungs are completely denitrogenized with oxygen and the airway is connected to an oxygen source, continuous oxygenation takes place by mass movement. Normally, every minute, 250 ml of oxygen is removed from the alveoli for metabolism and 200 ml of CO_2 is produced and eliminated from the lungs. When a person is apneic, only 10% of CO_2 accumulates in the alveoli, and 90% of CO_2 stays in the blood as bicarbonate. Consequently, 250 ml of oxygen is removed from the lungs and 20 ml of CO_2 accumulates in the lungs, creating a 230 ml vacuum effect and sucking in oxygen. Carbon dioxide tension continues to rise because no elimination occurs during apnea. The total pressure in the alveoli is constant, so the fall in P_{O_2} equals the rise in P_{CO_2}, ranging from 3 to 6 mm Hg per minute. If the patient had been breathing 100% oxygen prior to respiratory arrest, the starting alveolar P_{O_2} would be about 650 mm Hg, and therefore the patient could theoretically survive about 100 minutes of apnea provided that his airway remained clear and connected to 100% oxygen. This does, in fact, happen and has been demonstrated in both animals and humans. However, as seen in suffocation, gross hypoxia supervenes after about 90 seconds if apnea with airway occlusion follows air breathing at the functional residual capacity. When the airway is patent and the ambient gas is air, gross hypoxia supervenes after about 2 minutes of apnea as seen during intubation without preoxygenation. However, if the patient is preoxygenated for 3 minutes, gross hypoxia will not occur until 6 minutes of apnea for the normal weight patients and until about 3 minutes of apnea for morbidly obese patients.

Jense HG, Dubin SA, Silverstein PL et al: Effect of obesity on safe duration of apnea in unanesthetized humans. Anesth Analg 2:89–93, 1991

Nunn JF: Nunn's Applied Respiratory Physiology, 4th ed, pp 241–244. Oxford, Butterworth-Heinemann, 1993

C.17. What is diffusion hypoxia? How do you prevent it?

Fink and associates in 1954 first reported diffusion hypoxia during recovery from nitrous oxide-oxygen anesthesia. A mild degree of hypoxia can develop for >10 minutes when nitrous oxide-oxygen anesthesia is concluded and the patient is allowed to breathe room air. The arterial oxygen saturation can fall 5% to 10% and often reaches values <90% (PaO_2 <60 mm Hg). This occurs at the times when nitrous oxide is eliminated rapidly through the lungs. Nitrous oxide is 35 times more soluble in blood than nitrogen. Therefore, the amount of nitrous oxide diffused from blood to alveoli is much more than the amount of nitrogen diffused from alveoli to blood. Hence, alveolar oxygen is diluted by nitrous oxide. Diffusion hypoxia can be prevented by the inhalation of high concentrations of oxygen for several minutes before the patient is allowed to breathe room air.

Fink BR: Diffusion anoxia. Anesthesiology 16:511–519, 1955

Fink BR, Carpenter SL, Holaday DA et al: Diffusion anoxia during recovery from nitrous oxide-oxygen anesthesia. Fed Proc 13:354, 1954

Sheffer L, Steffenson JL, Birch AA: Nitrous-oxide-induced diffusion hypoxia in patients breathing spontaneously. Anesthesiology 37:436, 1972

D. Postoperative Management

D.1. What are the early postoperative complications?

The early postoperative complications are acute renal failure, renal artery occlusion, hyperacute rejection, graft rupture, urinary fistula, wound infection, and lymphoceles.

Guttmann RD: Renal transplantation. N Engl J Med 301:1038–1048, 1979

Schwartz SI (ed): Principles of Surgery, 6th ed, pp 444–447. New York, McGraw-Hill, 1984

D.2. How would you make the diagnosis of rejection?

The signs of rejection are fever, decreased urine output, and increased serum creatinine. Often renal enlargement and tenderness are found. Unfortunately, without renal biopsy, rejection cannot be distinguished from acute pyelonephritis or recurrent glomerulopathy.

Fauci AS, Braunwald E, Isselbacher KJ et al (eds): Harrison's Principles of Internal Medicine, 14th ed, pp 1528–1529. New York, McGraw-Hill, 1998

Schwartz SI (ed): Principles of Surgery, 6th ed, pp 445–447. New York, McGraw-Hill, 1984

35 Placenta Previa/Placenta Accreta

Howard D. Koff

A 32-year-old female, gravida 4 para 3, was admitted with painless vaginal bleeding at 37 weeks gestation. The patient had a history of three prior cesarean sections. An emergency cesarean section was planned. The patient's vital signs were heart rate 110 beats/min, blood pressure (BP) 85/45 mm Hg, respirations 24 per minute. Spun hematocrit was 26%.

A. Medical Disease and Differential Diagnosis

1. What are the leading causes of maternal mortality?
2. What is the differential diagnosis for third-trimester bleeding in a pregnant patient?
3. What is placenta previa and what are the different types?
4. How is the diagnosis of placenta previa made?
5. What is a double set-up, and how does one prepare a patient for it?
6. What is the treatment for placenta previa?
7. What is placenta accreta and how many types exist?
8. What are some of the causes of placenta accreta?
9. What is the association between placenta accreta and placenta previa?
10. How is placenta accreta diagnosed?
11. What is the treatment of placenta accreta?
12. What are the maternal respiratory changes at term?
13. Of what significance are the changes in respiratory function to the anesthesiologist?
14. When do the maternal respiratory changes return to prepregnancy values?
15. What are the maternal cardiovascular changes of pregnancy?
16. When do the maternal cardiovascular changes return to prepregnancy values?
17. What is the relative anemia of pregnancy?
18. What are the maternal gastrointestinal changes of pregnancy?
19. When do the maternal gastrointestinal changes return to prepregnancy values?
20. What is the supine hypotensive syndrome?

B. Preoperative Evaluation and Preparation

1. Would you transfuse this patient preoperatively?
2. How can you evaluate fetal maturity preoperatively?
3. Would evaluation of fetal maturity be indicated in this patient?
4. What preoperative medications would you give this patient?

C. Intraoperative Management

1. What monitors would you use for this patient?
2. Discuss the anesthetic management for a patient with placenta previa.
3. Was this patient at high risk for a placenta accreta?

4. Discuss the anesthetic management for a patient with a high risk for placenta accreta.
5. What type of anesthesia would you administer to this patient?
6. What are the absolute and relative contraindications of regional anesthesia?
7. Would a history of low-dose aspirin use in a patient contraindicate a regional anesthesia?
8. How would you induce and maintain anesthesia in this patient?
9. What are the determinants of placental transfer of drugs to the fetus?
10. What is the importance of preoxygenation?
11. What are the effects of maternal hyperventilation?
12. Sudden preoperative blood loss necessitates the use of type O Rh negative (universal donor) uncrossmatched blood. How should intraoperative blood transfusions be managed?
13. Significant intraoperative blood loss required the transfusion of 10 U of type-specific, crossmatched packed red blood cells. Generalized oozing into the surgical field and hematuria were noted. What is your differential diagnosis?
14. What is dilutional thrombocytopenia?
15. Should fresh-frozen plasma be administered?
16. What causes disseminated intravascular coagulation (DIC)?
17. What laboratory tests could be used to diagnose the cause of this hemorrhagic diathesis and why?
18. What are the signs and symptoms of a hemolytic transfusion reaction?
19. How is a hemolytic transfusion reaction treated?
20. What is a delayed hemolytic reaction?
21. What are nonhemolytic transfusion reactions?
22. What is the current infectious risk from red cell transfusion?
23. What are various methods of autologous transfusion, and how useful would they be in this patient?
24. What are the advantages and disadvantages of epidural versus spinal anesthesia for elective cesarean section?
25. How does one administer an epidural test dose?
26. What are the possible complications of epidural anesthesia and how are they treated?

D. Postoperative Management

1. When should this patient be extubated?
2. If this patient decided to have a tubal ligation during her postpartum course, would she still be at risk for aspiration?
3. Two days following epidural cesarean section, a patient with no significant past medical history complains of a postural headache. What is your differential diagnosis?
4. What are the symptoms of a postdural puncture headache?
5. When do postdural puncture headaches usually present?
6. What causes the pain and discomfort associated with a postdural puncture headache?
7. What is the treatment of a postdural puncture headache?
8. How does one perform an epidural blood patch?

A. Medical Disease and Differential Diagnosis

A.1. What are the leading causes of maternal mortality?

The maternal mortality rate is traditionally defined as the number of maternal deaths divided by the number of live births during the same reporting period. The current maternal mortality rate is 1/10,000. The three leading causes are pulmonary embolism, preeclampsia or eclampsia, and anesthesia, in that order. Causes of maternal deaths attributed to anesthesia (in order of decreasing incidence) include aspiration of stomach contents, hypoxia due to esophageal or failed intubation, misuse of drugs, accidents with apparatus, and inadvertent intrathecal injection of anesthetic during attempted epidural block. It should be noted that three of the four most common causes of anesthetic-related maternal mortality are related to general anesthesia.

Maternal mortality caused by hemorrhage is the fourth most common cause of maternal mortality. Hemorrhage accounted for 18% of maternal deaths among women who had a live birth in the United States between 1979 and 1986. Postpartum hemorrhage is still the leading cause of maternal mortality in underdeveloped countries.

Chestnut DH (ed): Obstetric Anesthesia: Principles and Practice, p 699. St. Louis, Mosby, 1994

James DK, Steer PJ, Weiner CP (eds): High Risk Pregnancy Management Options. Philadelphia, WB Saunders, 1994

Lehman KD, Mabie WC, Miller JM et al: The epidemiology and pathology of maternal mortality. Charity Hospital of Louisiana in New Orleans, 1965–1984. Obstet Gynecol 69:833–839, 1987

Sachs BP, Oriol NE, Ostheimer GW et al: Anesthetic-related maternal mortality 1954–1985. J Clin Anesth 1:333–338, 1989

Schnider SM, Levinson G (eds): Anesthesia for Obstetrics, 3rd ed, pp 455–458. Baltimore, Williams & Wilkins, 1993

A.2. What is the differential diagnosis for third-trimester bleeding in a pregnant patient?

Two major causes are found for third-trimester antepartum hemorrhage:

• Placenta previa—encroachment of the placenta on the internal cervical os
• Abruptio placenta—premature separation of the placenta from the wall of the uterus.

The absence of pain is often regarded as a significant distinguishing factor between placenta previa and abruptio placenta. In general, placenta previa presents as painless vaginal bleeding without uterine hyperactivity or tenderness. In contrast, bleeding from an abruptio placenta is often associated with contractions, and it can appear per vagina or remain concealed. The clinical presentation is a function of the location of the separation and its severity. Placenta previa and abruptio placenta account for one half to two thirds of all cases of antepartum hemorrhage. The remainder are caused by cervical pathology, polyps, carcinoma, vaginal and valvular varicosities, circumvallate placenta, and vasopravia.

James DK, Steer PJ, Weiner CP (eds): High Risk Pregnancy Management Options, pp 119–122. Philadelphia, WB Saunders, 1994

Schnider SM, Levinson G (eds): Anesthesia for Obstetrics, 3rd ed, pp 385–391. Baltimore, Williams & Wilkins, 1993

A.3. What is placenta previa and what are the different types?

Placenta previa is caused by placental implantation in the lower uterine segment; the type is determined by the degree to which the placenta encroaches on the internal cervical os. Four types of placenta previa are seen:

- Complete placenta previa—the placenta totally covers the internal cervical os
- Partial placenta previa—the placenta extends partially into the cervical os and only a portion of the lateral os is covered
- Marginal placenta previa—the placental edge is at the margin of the cervical os
- Low-lying placenta—the placenta is implanted in the lower uterine segment but the placental edge does not encroach at all on the internal cervical os

Chamberlain G (ed): Turnbull's Obstetrics, 2nd ed, pp 315–319. Hong Kong, Churchill Livingstone, 1995

Dunnihoo DR (ed): Fundamentals of Gynecology and Obstetrics, pp 474–475. Philadelphia, JB Lippincott, 1990

A.4. How is the diagnosis of placenta previa made?

Although placenta previa is the cause of vaginal bleeding in only about one third of antepartum hemorrhages, all patients with third trimester bleeding should be considered to have placenta previa until disproved.

Various methods have been used to confirm the diagnosis of placenta previa. Some methods, such as soft tissue placentography (using x-rays), radioisotope radiography, pelvic angiography, and thermography are no longer used. Magnetic resonance imaging (MRI) may be a technique of the future, but at present high cost limits its availability.

The mainstay for diagnosis is ultrasound. Ultrasound allows for a safe, simple diagnosis of placenta previa, with a 95% accuracy rate.

Posterior or lateral placental implantation and maternal obesity can make placental visualization under ultrasound more difficult. Color Doppler ultrasonography can be helpful in these cases.

Occasionally in patients whose ultrasound examinations have demonstrated marginal or low-lying placentas, direct examination of the cervical os is indicated. This is the definitive way to confirm the diagnosis, and it allows one to determine the degree of placenta encroachment on the internal cervical os. This procedure should be conducted only in a double set-up.

Moore TR, Reiter RC, Rebas RW (eds): Gynecology and Obstetrics: A Longitudinal Approach, pp 483–484. New York, Churchill Livingstone, 1993

Schnider SM, Levinson G (eds): Anesthesia for Obstetrics, 3rd ed, pp 385–386. Baltimore, Williams & Wilkins, 1993

A.5. What is a double set-up, and how does one prepare a patient for it?

In a double set-up examination, a vaginal examination is performed by the obstetrician in an operating room with everything prepared to proceed with immediate cesarean section and the management of sudden hemorrhage should it occur.

The double set-up examination provides the most accurate assessment of the relationship of the lower edge of the placenta to the cervical os. It should only be done when delivery is going to be undertaken. It is contraindicated in the presence of active profuse hemorrhage, fetal malposition precluding vaginal delivery, fetal distress, or clear ultrasonographic evidence of complete placenta previa. It can be considered when ultrasonographic evidence of placenta previa is inconclusive.

A double set-up should be performed only after the patient's cardiovascular status has been stabilized and she has been prepared for general anesthesia and possible sudden massive blood loss. Insertion of a central venous pressure (CVP) line is especially useful in evaluating and treating hypovolemia.

Hemorrhage severity prior to the procedure should be estimated by the observed blood loss, the patient's vital signs, hematocrit, and CVP level, and her resuscitation should take place rapidly.

During the vaginal examination for the diagnosis of placenta previa, sudden severe maternal hemorrhage may occur, necessitating immediate emergency cesarean section. In preparation for anesthesia, the patient should have two large-bore intravenous lines. Blood pumps and warmers should be in the operating room. The patient's blood must be crossmatched, and at least 2 units of blood must be present in the operating room prior to examination of the patient.

In preparation for general anesthesia, the patient should receive 30 ml of nonparticulate oral antacid 15 to 30 minutes before the examination. The patient should be placed in the lithotomy position with left lateral displacement. One hundred percent oxygen should be administered. The usefulness of this defasciculation dose of nondepolarizing muscle relaxant is controversial and may be omitted. An assistant should be present to provide cricoid pressure. The patient's abdomen should be prepared and draped. Only when the obstetric, anesthesia, pediatric, and nursing teams are ready should the cervical os be examined.

Datta S (ed): Anesthesia and Obstetric Management of High Risk Pregnancy 2nd ed, pp 99–100. St. Louis, Mosby, 1996

James DK, Steer PJ, Weiner CP (eds): High Risk Pregnancy Management Options, pp 126–127. Philadelphia, WB Saunders, 1994

Shnider SM, Levinson G (eds): Anesthesia for Obstetrics, 3rd ed, pp 385–386. Baltimore, Williams & Wilkins, 1993

A.6. What is the treatment for placenta previa?

Obstetric management is based on the severity of vaginal bleeding and the maturity of the fetus. The goal is to achieve maximal fetal maturity while minimizing the risks to both mother and fetus. If fetal maturity is >36 weeks, immediate delivery (i.e., cesarean section or double set-up) is indicated.

If the diagnosis of placenta previa is confirmed without inducing bleeding and immediate delivery of a premature fetus is not indicated, the patient is usually managed with bed rest in the hope that the bleeding will cease spontaneously. Once the patient is near term, fetal maturity is assessed by amniocentesis and the fetus is delivered by cesarean section.

If the conservative approach is pursued, the following criteria must be met:

- The mother should remain hospitalized.
- Adequately crossmatched blood should always be available.
- The fetus should definitely be premature.

- Neither mother nor fetus is in jeopardy.
- Any repetitive hemorrhages are infrequent and mild.

Considerable debate is found over whether or not conservative management obligates the patient to remain hospitalized, with bed rest, until the end of the pregnancy. The main disadvantages of continuous hospitalization are the cost and the psychological effect on families. The advantages include easy access to resuscitation and delivery, and ensuring bed rest and activity limitation.

A significant number of patients with placenta previa have preterm labor. Because vaginal examinations to confirm cervical dilation are contraindicated, it is difficult to document the diagnosis of preterm labor. Obstetricians must balance the potential cardiovascular consequences of tocolytic therapy in the presence of maternal hemorrhage versus the consequences of preterm delivery. Tocolytic therapy is commonly used in the hope that pregnancy can be lengthened. Tocolytic therapy is not recommended for patients with uncontrolled hemorrhage or those suspected of having placental abruption. The choice of tocolytic drug is controversial. Magnesium sulfate is often chosen because it may be less likely to cause maternal hypotension during hemorrhage than beta-adrenergic drugs. In addition, the beta-adrenergic agents produce maternal tachycardia, which makes it more difficult to assess maternal intravascular volume.

Chestnut DH (ed): Obstetric Anesthesia: Principles and Practice, p 701. St. Louis, Mosby, 1994

Datta S (ed): Anesthesia and Obstetric Management of High Risk Pregnancy 2nd ed, pp 95–98. St. Louis, Mosby, 1996

James DK, Steer PJ, Weiner CP (eds): High Risk Pregnancy Management Options, pp 126–127. Philadelphia, WB Saunders, 1994

Norris MC (ed): Obstetric Anesthesia, pp 587–589. Philadelphia, JB Lippincott, 1993

A.7. What is placenta accreta and how many types exist?

Placenta accreta is defined as an abnormally adherent placenta. It can be defined histopathologically based on the absence or deficiency of the decidua basalis between the villi and the myometrium causing abnormal adherence of the placenta and preventing normal separation of placenta from myometrium.

Placenta accreta can also be categorized by the degree of placental penetration; three types exist:

- Placenta accreta vera—implies adherence of the placental villi directly to the myometrium, without invasion into the uterine muscle.
- Placenta increta—involves actual invasion into the myometrium.
- Placenta percreta—erosion of villi through the myometrium to involve uterine serosa or other pelvic structures.

Chestnut DH (ed): Obstetric Anesthesia: Principles and Practice, p 711. St. Louis, Mosby, 1994

James DK, Steer PJ, Weiner CP (eds): High Risk Pregnancy Management Options, p 1175. Philadelphia, WB Saunders, 1994

A.8. What are some of the causes of placenta accreta?

Etiology of placenta accreta includes:

- Uterine abnormalities (fibroids, bicornuate uterus, and so forth)
- Previous cesarean section

- Manual removal of placenta
- Placenta previa and uterine curettage
- Sepsis or surgery

Previous scarring of the endometrium (uterine trauma) interferes with placental implantation in subsequent pregnancies. The incidence of placenta accreta may be increasing because of the increased incidence of cesarean section. The combination of one or more prior cesarean sections and a current placenta previa or low-lying placenta should raise suspicion regarding the presence of a placenta accreta.

Chestnut DH (ed): Obstetric Anesthesia: Principles and Practice, pp 711–712. St. Louis, Mosby, 1994

A.9. What is the association between placenta accreta and placenta previa?

The risk of placenta accreta is directly related to the number of prior cesarean sections. Placenta accreta is also commonly associated with placenta previa probably because of a deficiency of decidua in the lower uterine segment.

A 5% risk of placenta accreta is seen in a patient with a history of placenta previa and no prior cesarean sections. This risk rises sharply to >50% risk in a patient with placenta previa and two or more previous cesarean sections.

Chestnut DH (ed): Obstetric Anesthesia: Principles and Practice, pp 711–712. St. Louis, Mosby, 1994

James DK, Steer PJ, Weiner CP (eds): High Risk Pregnancy Management Options, pp 114–120. Philadelphia, WB Saunders, 1994

A.10. How is placenta accreta diagnosed?

Placenta accreta is rarely diagnosed prior to the delivery of the placenta, but it is possible to identify the patients at risk. In some cases the condition is first suspected at vaginal delivery when the obstetrician notes difficulty in separating the placenta. The definitive diagnosis is often made at laparotomy. Ultrasonography use may help identify those patients with placenta previa and previous cesarean section who are at risk for placenta accreta. If the placenta appears to extend anteriorly in the region of the old uterine scar, a high likelihood of placenta accreta is expected. Transvaginal color Doppler sonography and MRI have correctly identified placenta accreta and placenta percreta.

Chestnut DH (ed): Obstetric Anesthesia: Principles and Practice, p 712. St. Louis, Mosby, 1994

Finberg HJ, Williams JL: Placenta accreta: Prospective sonographic diagnosis in patients with placenta previa and prior cesarean section. J Ultrasound Med 11:333–343, 1992

Weckstein LN, Masserman JSH: Placenta accreta: A problem of increasing clinical significance. Obstet Gynecol 69:480–482, 1986

A.11. What is the treatment of placenta accreta?

The treatment of placenta accreta is primarily to control bleeding and restore hemodynamic stability. It is important for the obstetrician to recognize the problem and make a prompt decision to proceed with definitive therapy (i.e., hysterectomy).

Placenta accreta is now the most common indication for obstetric hysterectomy.

Between 30% and 72% of patients with placenta accreta require cesarean hysterectomy. Blood loss in these cases is often substantial. Reported average blood loss ranges from 2000 to 5000 ml with some patients requiring >40 U of blood. Appropriate preparations should be made for this potential blood loss (large gauge intravenous (IV) lines, blood in the room, and so forth).

Chestnut DH (ed): Obstetric Anesthesia: Principles and Practice, p 712. St. Louis, Mosby, 1994

James DK, Steer PJ, Weiner CP (eds): High Risk Pregnancy Management Options, p 1175. Philadelphia, WB Saunders, 1994

A.12. What are the maternal respiratory changes at term?

A number of maternal respiratory changes are seen at term:

- Capillary engorgement of the mucosa throughout the respiratory tract, causing swelling of the vocal cord and oral pharynx, larynx, and trachea
- Increased minute ventilation (50%), tidal volume (40%), respiratory rate (15%), and oxygen consumption (20%)
- Chest wall compliance decrease (45%)
- Arterial P_{CO_2} decrease (10 to 11 mm Hg)
- Functional residual capacity decrease (20%)
- Expiratory reserve volume decrease (20%)
- Residual volume decrease (20%)

No change occurs in dead space, lung compliance, arterial pH, vital capacity, or closing volume.

Shnider SM, Levinson G (eds): Anesthesia for Obstetrics, 3rd ed, pp 3–6. Baltimore, Williams & Wilkins, 1993

A.13. Of what significance are the changes in respiratory function to the anesthesiologist?

These changes in respiratory function during pregnancy have great significance to the anesthesiologist. The decrease in functional residual capacity combined with the increased minute ventilation increases the rapidity of anesthesia induction, emergence from anesthesia, and changes in the depth of anesthesia. In addition, the minimum alveolar concentration (MAC) of inhalational drugs has been found to be decreased in pregnancy. This combination of accelerated onset and decreased anesthetic requirements makes parturients susceptible to anesthetic overdose. The decrease in functional residual capacity, increased oxygen consumption, and increased A-a gradient lower the maternal oxygen reserve, making the pregnant patient more susceptible to hypoxia. This is the reason for administering supplemental oxygen to high-risk labor parturients or parturients undergoing general anesthesia. The apnea associated with induction of anesthesia rapidly causes a decrease in PaO_2 in the parturient. Administration of 100% oxygen for at least 3 minutes of tidal volume breathing produces nitrogen washout from the mother, and maximal maternal oxygen reserves are achieved.

Russell GN, Smith CL, Snowdon SK et al: Pre-oxygenation and the parturient patient. Anaesthesia 42:346–351, 1987

Stoelting RK, Dierdorf SF, McCammon RL: Anesthesia and Co-Existing Disease, 3rd ed, pp 541–543. New York, Churchill Livingstone, 1993

A.14. When do the maternal respiratory changes return to prepregnancy values?

The functional residual capacity increases after delivery but remains below the prepregnant value for 1 to 2 weeks. Oxygen consumption, tidal volume, and minute ventilation remain elevated until at least 6 to 8 weeks after delivery. The alveolar and mixed venous P_{CO_2} increase slowly after delivery and are still slightly below prepregnant levels at 6 to 8 weeks postpartum.

Chestnut DH (ed): Obstetric Anesthesia: Principles and Practice, p 20. St. Louis, Mosby, 1994

A.15. What are the maternal cardiovascular changes of pregnancy?

Cardiovascular changes of pregnancy at term include the following:

- Intravascular fluid volume   up 35%
- Plasma volume   up 45%
- Red blood cell volume   up 20%
- Cardiac output   up 40%
- Stroke volume   up 30%
- Heart rate   up 15%
- Systolic blood pressure   down 0 to 15 mm Hg
- Systemic vascular resistance   down 15%
- Diastolic blood pressure   down 10 to 20 mm Hg
- CVP   no change

The changes listed are in relation to nonpregnancy values. Cardiac output increases 40% during the first trimester over prelabor values. During labor, cardiac output rises 15% during the latent phase, 30% during the active phase, and 45% during the expulsive phase, compared with prelabor values. Each uterine contraction increases cardiac output an additional 10% to 25%. The greatest increase in cardiac output occurs immediately after delivery, when the cardiac output is 60% to 80% above prelabor values.

Stoelting RK, Dierdorf SF, McCammon RL: Anesthesia and Co-Existing Disease, 3rd ed, pp 539–541. New York, Churchill Livingstone, 1993

A.16. When do the maternal cardiovascular changes return to prepregnancy values?

Cardiac output falls to just below prelabor values at 48 hours postpartum. It subsequently decreases to 10% above the prepregnant level after 2 weeks, and then gradually returns to the prepregnant level between 12 and 24 weeks postpartum. Heart rate falls after delivery, reaches the prepregnant rate by 2 weeks postpartum, and remains slightly below the prepregnant rate for the next several months. Stroke volume remains above prelabor values at 48 hours and declines slowly through 24 weeks postpartum at which time it is still 10% above the prepregnant values.

Chestnut DH (ed): Obstetric Anesthesia: Principles and Practice, p 23. St. Louis, Mosby, 1994

A.17. What is the relative anemia of pregnancy?

With pregnancy, plasma volume increases about 45% and red blood cell volume increases about 20%. This disproportionate increase in plasma volume accounts for the relative anemia of pregnancy.

Stoelting RK, Dierdorf SF, McCammon RL: Anesthesia and Co-Existing Disease, 3rd ed, p 1539. New York, Churchill Livingstone, 1993

A.18. What are the maternal gastrointestinal changes of pregnancy?

Gastrointestinal changes during pregnancy make parturients vulnerable to regurgitation of gastric contents and to the development of acid pneumonitis should pulmonary aspiration occur. The enlarged uterus displaces the pylorus upward and backward, which retards gastric emptying and changes the angle of the gastroesophageal junction. This frequently results in incompetence of the lower esophageal sphincter (the gastroesophageal pinchcock mechanism), which allows gastric reflux. It makes the parturient more susceptible to regurgitation. Gastrin is produced by the placenta, which raises the acid, chloride, and enzyme content of the stomach. Progesterone further decreases gastrointestinal motility. The changes emphasize that parturients are susceptible to silent regurgitation, even in the absence of sedative drugs or general anesthesia.

Shnider SM, Levinson G (eds): Anesthesia for Obstetrics, 3rd ed, pp 13–14. Baltimore, Williams & Wilkins, 1993

Stoelting RK, Dierdorf SF, McCammon RL: Anesthesia and Co-Existing Disease, 3rd ed, pp 544–545. New York, Churchill Livingstone, 1993

A.19. When do the maternal gastrointestinal changes return to prepregnancy values?

Gastric emptying in women on their first and third postpartum day is comparable to that in nonpregnant women. Gastric volume and *p*H are also similar in fasting women who are 1 to 42 hours postpartum and nonpregnant individuals undergoing elective surgery.

Chestnut DH (ed): Obstetric Anesthesia: Principles and Practice, p 27. St. Louis, Mosby, 1994

Somwanshi M, Tripathi A, Singh B: Effect of preoperative oral fluids on gastric volume and *p*H on postpartum patients. Middle East J Anesthesiol 13:197–203, 1995

A.20. What is the supine hypotensive syndrome?

Supine hypotensive syndrome, or aortocaval obstruction, is caused by the pregnant patient in the supine position. The gravid uterus can completely obstruct the inferior vena cava, causing blood to return to the heart in part via the paravertebral (epidural) veins emptying into the azygos system. The symptoms of supine hypotensive syndrome (hypotension, pallor, sweating, nausea, vomiting) are caused by lack of venous return to the heart.

Compression of the aorta by the gravid uterus can cause arterial hypotension in the lower extremities and uterine arteries without associated maternal symptoms. Prevention of aortocaval compression (supine hypotensive syndrome) is preferred to treatment. The parturient at term should never be allowed to assume the supine position. Prevention of aortocaval compression consists of left uterine displacement, which can be accomplished by positioning the patient on her left side and by tilting the delivery table 15 degrees to the left, or by placing sheets or a pillow under the patient's right side.

Shnider SM, Levinson G (eds): Anesthesia for Obstetrics, 3rd ed, pp 9–12. Baltimore, Williams & Wilkins, 1993

B. Preoperative Evaluation and Preparation

B.1. *Would you transfuse this patient preoperatively?*

Fluid resuscitation with blood, plasmanate, and crystalloid should be started immediately and as rapidly as possible. The fact that this patient was tachycardic and hypotensive implies that she was already severely volume depleted and probably in hemorrhagic shock. Because normal pregnancy is characterized by a state of hypervolemia, tachycardia and hypotension may not be apparent in the parturient until blood loss exceeds 2 liters.

The ideal replacement blood product is obviously type-specific crossmatched whole blood, but if massive blood loss does not allow for waiting for typing and crossmatching, O-negative packed blood cells can be given in emergencies until blood typing is completed.

If the mother is bleeding copiously, it may not be possible to correct the blood loss completely prior to surgery because the hemorrhaging will continue until the placenta is removed. Massive hemorrhage necessitates immediate surgical intervention. In these situations, adequate volume replacement can be difficult or impossible until the placenta is removed.

Concerns regarding blood-borne infectious diseases have led to re-evaluation of indications for red cell transfusion, particularly during the perioperative period. This increased awareness by physicians and patients about infectious risks from blood products has led to a decline in transfusion rates. This decrease in transfusion use would only have significance in patients who have had mild hemorrhage, but this patient shows signs of moderate hemorrhage (25% to 35% blood loss), and red cell transfusion is imperative. The physical findings in relation to percent of blood loss are listed in Table 35-1.

Table 35-1.   The Physical Findings in Relation to Percentage of Blood Loss

% BLOOD LOSS	PHYSICAL FINDINGS
<15%	None
20%–25%	Tachycardia (>100 beats/min)
	Mild hypotension
	Peripheral vasoconstriction
25%–35%	Tachycardia (100–120 beats/min)
	Hypotension (systolic BP 80–100 mm Hg)
	Restlessness
	Oliguria
>35%	Tachycardia (>120 beats/min)
	Hypotension (systolic BP <60 mm Hg)
	Altered consciousness
	Anuria

Berkowitz RL (ed): Critical Care of the Obstetric Patient, pp 107–109. New York, Churchill Living-stone, 1983

Chestnut DH (ed): Obstetric Anesthesia: Principles and Practice, p 700. St. Louis, Mosby, 1994

Naef RW, Washburne JF, Martin RW: Hemorrhage associated with cesarean delivery: When is transfusion needed. J Perinatol 15:32–35, 1995

B.2. *How can you evaluate fetal maturity preoperatively?*

Many methods are available to evaluate fetal size, fetal weight, fetal age, and fetal lung maturity, but only ultrasound and amniotic fluid analysis can be done quickly with immediate results.

Ultrasound can be used to assess fetal age, fetal growth, fetal weight, and placental location. Fetal age is determined by the fetal biparietal diameter. Ultrasound can often locate fetal anomalies.

Amniotic fluid analysis is most commonly used to assess fetal lung maturity by evaluating surfactant activity, which can be measured directly using the amniotic fluid foam test (shake test) or by measuring the major phospholipids lecithin and sphingomyelin (L:S) ratio. Additional information can be gained by measuring the levels of the minor lipids, phosphatidylinositol and phosphatidylglycerol.

The foam test is based on the ability of lecithin to stabilize foam produced by mechanical agitation of a solution of amniotic fluid and alcohol. Amniotic fluid in three dilutions with saline is mixed with 95% ethanol. When the solution is shaken with air, stable bubbles form if significant lecithin levels exist. The foam test is based on the ability of lecithin to stabilize the foam produced by mechanical agitation of the solution. More bubbles means increased lecithin, which means increased lung maturity. The advantage of the foam test is its rapidity and simplicity; the disadvantage is a high level of false-negative results and the fact that it cannot be performed if specimens are contaminated by meconium or blood.

The surfactant complex is made primarily of phospholipids, the most abundant of which is lecithin. Lecithin, which is secreted by type II alveolar cells, is excreted into the fetal trachea and therefore into the amniotic fluid. The L:S ratio is measured using chromatography. An L:S ratio of >2.0 to 3.5 minimizes the risk of fetal lung immaturity. The higher the ratio, the higher the concentration of lecithin and the greater the maturity of the fetal lungs.

Other tests of fetal maturity and placental function are as follows:

- Urinary and plasma maternal estrogens (estriol E-3), to assess fetal well-being and placental abnormalities
- Maternal plasma levels of human placental lactogen correlating well with placental and fetal weight
- Oxytocin challenge or stress test, to assess fetal well-being
- Fetal nonstress test

Queenan J (ed): Management of High Risk Pregnancy, 2nd ed, pp 657–667. Oradell, Medical Economics Books, 1987

Shnider SM, Levinson G (eds): Anesthesia for Obstetrics, 3rd ed, pp 645–655. Baltimore, Williams & Wilkins, 1993

B.3. Would evaluation of fetal maturity be indicated in this patient?

In a patient with placenta previa who is bleeding profusely, fetal maturity is of secondary importance. In this situation, an emergency cesarean section is carried out despite the gestational age of the fetus. Patients not bleeding profusely and having a premature fetus can be treated conservatively with bed rest. Once a patient is near term, fetal maturity is assessed by amniocentesis and the baby is delivered via cesarean section. If a cesarean section is performed prior to 30 weeks gestation, fetal and neonatal mortality is in the range of 60% to 70%. This patient has a term baby and shows signs of hypovolemic shock. Emergency cesarean section without testing fetal maturity is indicated.

James DK, Steer PJ, Weiner CP (eds): High Risk Pregnancy Management Options, pp 121–127. Philadelphia, WB Saunders, 1994

Shnider SM, Levinson G (eds): Anesthesia for Obstetrics, 3rd ed, pp 385–386. Baltimore, Williams & Wilkins, 1993

B.4. What preoperative medications would you give this patient?

This patient should be given 30 ml of a nonparticulate oral antacid (e.g., 0.3 M sodium citrate) 15 to 30 minutes prior to the anesthesia induction in an attempt to minimize the risk of aspiration pneumonitis. Premedication with sedatives or narcotics is not indicated before cesarean section because the neonatal depressant effects outweigh any possible maternal benefits.

Shnider SM, Levinson G (eds): Anesthesia for Obstetrics, 3rd ed, pp 214, 225–226. Baltimore, Williams & Wilkins, 1993

C. Intraoperative Management

C.1. What monitors would you use for this patient?

One would use the following monitors: electrocardiogram (ECG), BP cuff, pulse oximeter, end-tidal CO_2, temperature probe, CVP line and transducer, F_IO_2 analyzer, precordial stethoscope, and Foley catheter.

Barash PPG, Cullen BF, Stoelting RK (eds): Clinical Anesthesia 3rd ed, pp 1069–1070; 1074–1075. Philadelphia, JB Lippincott, 1997

C.2. Discuss the anesthetic management for a patient with placenta previa.

The choice of anesthetic technique depends on the indication and urgency for cesarean section, and the degree of maternal hypovolemia. All patients with placenta previa are at risk for increased intraoperative blood loss for three reasons:

- The obstetrician may inadvertently cut into the placenta during uterine incision.
- After delivery the lower uterine segment implantation site does not contract as well as the normal fundal implantation site.
- A patient with placenta previa is at increased risk for placenta accreta, especially with a history of previous cesarean section.

Some anesthesiologists feel that because of this potential for sudden massive blood loss, general anesthesia should always be used. Others believe that patients who are not bleeding and are hemodynamically stable can safely receive a regional technique.

Bleeding patients represent a greater challenge for the anesthetic care team. Because the placental site is the source of bleeding, bleeding may continue until the placenta is removed, and the uterus contracts. Rapid sequence induction of general anesthesia is the preferred technique for actively bleeding patients.

Chestnut DH (ed): Obstetric Anesthesia: Principles and Practice, pp 701–703. St. Louis, Mosby, 1994

Datta S (ed): Anesthesia and Obstetric Management of High Risk Pregnancy, 2nd ed, pp 99–100. St. Louis, Mosby, 1996

Shnider SM, Levinson G (eds): Anesthesia for Obstetrics, 3rd ed, pp 387–388. Baltimore, Williams & Wilkins, 1993

C.3. Was this patient at high risk for a placenta accreta?

The combination of placenta previa and three prior cesarean sections gives this patient a 40% risk of placenta accreta.

Chestnut DH (ed): Obstetric Anesthesia: Principles and Practice, p 712. St. Louis, Mosby, 1994

Clark SL, Koonings PP, Phelan JP: Placental previa/accreta and prior cesarean sections. Obstet Gynecol 66:90, 1985

C.4. Discuss the anesthetic management for a patient with a high risk for placenta accreta.

Between 30% and 72% of patients with placenta accreta require cesarean hysterectomy to control blood loss. Controversy exists regarding the type of anesthesia: What should be administered to the patient who is scheduled for an elective cesarean hysterectomy or is a high risk for emergency hysterectomy during elective cesarean section?

As stated, a regional technique can be considered in a normovolemic patient undergoing an elective, repeat cesarean section for placenta previa, despite the risk for placenta accreta and emergency hysterectomy.

Many anesthesiologists would avoid regional anesthesia. The combination of risk of massive blood loss in a patient with regional induced sympathetic block, along with prolonged surgical duration would make general anesthesia more desirable.

Either technique can be safely administered to a hemodynamically stable patient. Regardless of the anesthetic technique used, the following preparations should be made for massive blood loss:

- Insertion of at least two large-gauge IV catheters
- At least 2 units of packed red blood cells present in the operating room
- Additional blood should be available without delay
- Invasive monitoring should be immediately available
- Vasoactive drugs should be immediately available
- Blood pumps and warmer should be in the operating room
- Assistance should be present to help establish invasive monitoring or help pump blood as needed

Chestnut DH (ed): Obstetric Anesthesia: Principles and Practice, p 714. St. Louis, Mosby, 1994

James DK, Steer PJ, Weiner CP (eds): High Risk Pregnancy Management Options, pp 125–129. Philadelphia, WB Saunders, 1994

C.5. What type of anesthesia would you administer to this patient?

General endotracheal anesthesia is indicated in this patient because this parturient had a recent vaginal bleed and was hypotensive due to hypovolemia. Regional anesthesia would only lower her blood pressure further. In addition, this was an emergency cesarean section, where the quicker she could have her definitive treatment, the less the total blood loss would be.

Chestnut DH (ed): Obstetric Anesthesia: Principles and Practice pp 701–703. St. Louis, Mosby, 1994

Datta S (ed): Anesthesia and Obstetric Management of High Risk Pregnancy, 2nd ed, pp 99–100. St. Louis, Mosby-Year Book, 1996

C.6. What are the absolute and relative contraindications of regional anesthesia?

Absolute Contraindications
• Patient refusal
• Infection at site of needle injection
• Hypovolemic shock (active bleeding)
• Coagulopathies

Relative Contraindications
• Preexisting neurologic diseases of the spinal cord or peripheral nerves
• Systemic infection or infection not at the site of needle injection (e.g., genital herpes)
• Spinal deformities (e.g., spina bifida)
• Sensitivity to local anesthetics
• Certain cardiac conditions (e.g., pericarditis, pulmonary stenosis, idiopathic hypertrophic subaortic stenosis)

Cousins MJ, Bridenbaugh PO (eds): Neural Blockade, 2nd ed, p 192. Philadelphia, JB Lippincott, 1988

Shnider SM, Levinson G (eds): Anesthesia for Obstetrics, 3rd ed, p 150. Baltimore, Williams & Wilkins, 1993

C.7. Would a history of low-dose aspirin use in a patient contraindicate a regional anesthetic?

Multiple studies concerning patients ingesting chronic doses of aspirin and nonsteroidal anti-inflammatory drugs (NSAIDS) have not shown significant effects on the incidence of spinal or epidural hematoma formations, particularly in a large series of pregnant women ingesting low-dose aspirin for preeclampsia management.

Horlocker TT, Wedel DJ, Schroeder DR: Preoperative blood platelet therapy does not increase the risk of spinal hematoma associated with regional anesthesia. Anesth Analg 80:303–309, 1995

Sibai BM, Caritis SN, Thom E: Low dose aspirin in nulliparous women: Safety of continuous epidural block and correlation between bleeding time and maternal-neonatal bleeding complications. Am J Obstet Gynecol 172:1553–1557, 1995

Vandermeulen EP, Van Aken H, Vermylen J: Anticoagulants and spinal-epidural anesthesia. Anesth Analg 79:1165–1177, 1994

C.8. How would you induce and maintain anesthesia in this patient?

Anesthetic induction for an emergency cesarean section is done via a rapid-sequence technique. The choice of IV induction agents depends on the degree of cardiac stability. The patient is positioned on the operating table with left uterine displacement. She is given 100% oxygen to breathe for at least 3 minutes while the abdomen is prepared and draped. Ketamine and etomidate represent the best choices for bleeding patients. Ketamine (0.5 to 1.0 mg/kg) can cause myocardial depression in patients with severe hypovolemia. Etomidate (0.3 mg/kg) is an acceptable alternative to ketamine. A reduced dose is appropriate in patients with severe hemorrhage.

When the surgeon is ready to operate, anesthesia induction is accomplished with either ketamine (0.5 to 1.0 mg/kg) or etomidate (0.3 mg/kg), immediately followed by succinylcholine (1.0 to 1.5 mg/kg) to facilitate intubation. A precurarization dose of nondepolarizing muscle relaxant is controversial and subjective. The induction drugs are rapidly pushed intravenously, while an assistant applies cricoid pressure (Sellick maneuver), and no positive pressure ventilation should be given until the trachea is secured by a cuffed endotracheal tube. Prior to the delivery of the fetus, the agents used to maintain anesthesia will depend on the status of the mother. Nitrous oxide may be added to oxygen in concentrations up to 50%. The concentration of nitrous oxide can be reduced (or omitted) in cases of fetal distress. Inhalational anesthetic agents (halothane 0.5%, ethrane 0.75%, forane 0.75%) can be added to prevent maternal awareness if vital signs are stable. Neuromuscular blockade can be used as necessary. Once the fetus and placenta are delivered, blood loss should be controlled and hemodynamic stability restored. Anesthesia can then be deepened and maintained with nitrous oxide, narcotic, or barbiturate, with discontinuation of the inhalational anesthetic. Oxytocin (20 U/liter) should be infused immediately after delivery. The lower uterine segment does not contract as well as the fundus.

If the placenta does not easily separate, a placenta accreta may exist. In such cases, massive blood loss and the need for cesarean hysterectomy should be expected. Of greatest importance is the ability to be prepared for these events as follows:

- Blood pumps and warmers in the operating room
- Presence of large-gauge IV catheters
- Presence of at least 2 units of blood in the operating room
- Availability of additional blood without delay
- Availability of invasive monitoring
- Availability of assistance to help pump blood, and so forth

Norris MC (ed): Obstetric Anesthesia, pp 587–589. Philadelphia, JB Lippincott, 1993

Shnider SM, Levinson G (eds): Anesthesia for Obstetrics, 3rd ed, pp 225–229. Baltimore, Williams & Wilkins, 1993

C.9. What are the determinants of placental transfer of drugs to the fetus?

Passive diffusion is the principal mechanism for transfer of substances across the placenta. Diffusion of substances across the placenta depends on maternal-to-fetal concentration gradients, molecular weight, protein binding, lipid solubility, and degree of ionization. Interaction of these factors is described by Fick's equation of passive diffusion.

Miller RD (ed): Anesthesia, 4th ed, pp 2039–2040. New York, Churchill Livingstone, 1994

Shnider SM, Levinson G (eds): Anesthesia for Obstetrics, 3rd ed, pp 71–77. Baltimore, Williams & Wilkins, 1993

Stoelting RK, Dierdorf SF, McCammon RL (eds): Anesthesia and Co-Existing Disease, 3rd ed, pp 545–549. New York, Churchill Livingstone, 1993

C.10. What is the importance of preoxygenation?

The combination of 20% increase in oxygen consumption and 20% decrease in functional residual capacity in the parturient means that such patients are at increased risk for hypoxia during induction of general anesthesia. During a 1-minute period of apnea after preoxygenation, a parturient will sustain a 150 mm Hg reduction in PaO_2, compared with a 50 mm Hg reduction in a nonpregnant patient. If the patient is preoxygenated, denitrogenation occurs and maximal oxygen is stored in the lungs, which allows more reserve for preventing hypoxia.

The usual method of preoxygenation is to have the patient breathe 100% oxygen for 3 to 5 minutes prior to the induction of anesthesia. It has been demonstrated that having parturients take four maximally deep breaths of 100% oxygen immediately prior to the induction of anesthesia is also effective.

Bone ME, May AE: Preoxygenation techniques in the obstetric patient. Anesth Rev 15:37–41, 1988

Carmichael FJ, Cruise CJ, Crago RR et al: Preoxygenation: A study of denitrogenation. Anesth Analg 68:406–409, 1989

Norris MC, Kirkland MR, Thomas MC: Denitrogenation in pregnancy. Can J Anaesth 36:525, 1989

Shnider SM, Levinson G (eds): Anesthesia for Obstetrics, 3rd ed, pp 228–229. Baltimore, Williams & Wilkins, 1993

C.11. What are the effects of maternal hyperventilation?

Maternal hyperventilation via excessive positive pressure ventilation should be avoided because maternal $PaCO_2$ <20 mm Hg can cause fetal hypoxemia and acidosis. The etiology includes reduced uterine and umbilical blood flow from decreased cardiac output secondary to increased intrathoracic pressure, uterine vasoconstriction secondary to maternal hypocarbia, and increased affinity of maternal hemoglobin for oxygen due to alkalosis (Bohr effect). The results are less placental transfer of oxygen, which can lead to fetal hypoxia, and acidosis. Therefore, the recommendation is to maintain normal $PaCO_2$ of 30 to 33 mm Hg (normal $PaCO_2$ is 35 to 45 mm Hg for nonpregnant patients).

Shnider SM, Levinson G (eds): Anesthesia for Obstetrics, 3rd ed, pp 228–229. Baltimore, Williams & Wilkins, 1993

C.12. Sudden preoperative blood loss necessitates the use of type O Rh negative (universal donor) uncrossmatched blood. How should intraoperative blood transfusions be managed?

Type O blood has been termed the universal donor and can be used in emergency transfusion when typing or crossmatching is not available. However, some type O donors produce high titers of hemolytic IgG, IgM, anti-A, and anti-B antibodies. High titers of these hemolysins in donor units are capable of causing destruction of A or B red blood cells of a non-type O recipient. Thus, type O Rh negative un-crossmatched packed red blood cells should be used in preference to type O Rh negative whole blood, because packed erythrocytes will have smaller volumes of plasma and are almost free of hemolytic anti-A and anti-B antibodies. If type O Rh negative whole blood is to be used, the blood bank must supply type O blood that is free of hemolytic anti-A and anti-B antibodies.

After emergency transfusion of >2 units of type O Rh negative uncrossmatched whole blood, the patient probably cannot be switched to her blood type (A, B, or AB) once the blood bank determines the correct blood type. Switching could cause major intravascular hemolysis of donor red cells by increasing titers of transfused anti-A and anti-B. Continued use of type O Rh negative whole blood results only in minor hemolysis of recipient red cells, with hyperbilirubinemia as the only complication. The patient must not receive a transfusion of her correct blood type until the blood bank determines that the transfused anti-A and anti-B has fallen to levels that permit safe transfusion of type-specific blood.

Miller RD (ed): Anesthesia, 4th ed, p 1623. New York, Churchill Livingstone, 1994

C.13. Significant intraoperative blood loss has required the transfusion of 10 U of type-specific, crossmatched packed red blood cells. Generalized oozing into the surgical field and hematuria were noted. What is your differential diagnosis?

- Dilutional thrombocytopenia
- Low factors V and VIII
- Disseminated intravascular coagulation (DIC)
- Hemolytic transfusion reaction

Miller RD (ed): Anesthesia, 4th ed, pp 1629–1631. New York, Churchill Livingstone, 1994

C.14. What is dilutional thrombocytopenia?

Dilutional thrombocytopenia is a possible cause of hemorrhagic diathesis in any patient who has received multiple units of banked blood. Platelets in stored blood have reduced survival time and viability. After 24 to 48 hours of storage, platelet activity is 5% to 10% of normal. Platelet counts >100,000/mm^3 are ideal for adequate surgical hemostasis. This patient was transfused with packed red blood cells, not whole blood, so the dilutional effect would be exaggerated. Dilutional coagulopathy results from the replacement of blood loss with crystalloid and packed cells, which dilute concentrations of coagulate factors and/or platelets.

Platelet transfusion should not be given prophylactically with various transfusions until platelet counts reveal a definitive thrombocytopenia (50 to 100 $\times$ 10^3/mm^3).

ASA Task Force: Practice guideline for blood component therapy. Anesthesiology 84:732–747, 1996

Miller RD (ed): Anesthesia, 4th ed, pp 1626–1627. New York, Churchill Livingstone, 1994

Pillai M: Platelets and pregnancy. Br J Obstet Gynaecol 100:201–204, 1993

C.15. Should fresh-frozen plasma be administered?

Most of the factors are stable in stored blood except factors V and VIII. These factors gradually decrease to 15% and 50% of normal, respectively, after 21 days of storage. However, only 5% to 20% of factor V and 30% of factor VIII are needed for adequate hemostasis during surgery. Fresh-frozen plasma is rarely indicated because despite even massive blood transfusion, factors V and VIII rarely decrease below those levels required by hemostasis.

ASA Task Force: Practice guideline for blood component therapy. Anesthesiology 84:732–747, 1996

Miller RD (ed): Anesthesia, 4th ed, pp 1640–1741. New York, Churchill Livingstone, 1994

C.16. What causes disseminated intravascular coagulation (DIC)?

The specific reasons for the development of DIC are usually not apparent. However, hypoxic acidic tissues with stagnant blood flow probably release tissue thromboplastin through liberation of a toxin. This triggers the coagulation process resulting in the consumption of factors I, II, V, VII, and platelets. Supposedly, thrombi and fibrin are deposited in the microcirculation of vital organs interrupting their blood flow. In an attempt to counteract the hypercoagulable state, the fibrinolytic system is activated to lyse the excessive fibrin. This secondary fibrinolysis activates plasminogen to plasmin. With fulminant DIC and subsequent rapid depletion of coagulation factors, plasmin is formed from plasminogen at a rapid rate. This fibrinolysis contributes to the severity of the bleeding diathesis.

Plasmin digests fibrinogen, and this results in the formation of fibrin-split products in the serum.

Disseminated intravascular coagulation should not be considered a distinct disease entity but rather a sign of another disease. DIC has been associated with nearly all life-threatening diseases.

Miller RD (ed): Anesthesia, 4th ed, pp 1627–1628. New York, Churchill Livingstone, 1994

C.17. What laboratory tests could be used to diagnose the cause of this hemorrhagic diathesis and why?

- Platelet count
- Partial thromboplastin time
- Plasma fibrinogen level

Platelet count is necessary to rule out dilutional thrombocytopenia. Try to maintain levels >100,000/mm^3. A partial thromboplastin time >1.5 times normal probably reflects low levels of factors V and VIII. Low plasma fibrinogen levels (<150 mg/100 ml) reflect DIC.

Miller RD (ed): Anesthesia, 4th ed, pp 1629–1631. New York, Churchill Livingstone, 1994

C.18. What are the signs and symptoms of a hemolytic transfusion reaction?

The classic signs and symptoms—chills, fever, chest, and flesh pain, and nausea—are masked by anesthesia. Under general anesthesia, the only signs may be hemoglobinuria, bleeding diathesis, or hypotension.

Miller RD (ed): Anesthesia, 4th ed, pp 1633–1635. New York, Churchill Livingstone, 1994

C.19. How is a hemolytic transfusion reaction treated?

- Stop the transfusion
- Maintain urine output (1 to 2 ml/kg/h) by the following methods:
  - Generous IV fluids (crystalloid)
  - Mannitol 12.5 to 50 g
  - Consider furosemide 20 to 40 mg
- Alkalinize the urine to prevent precipitation of acid hematin ($NaHCO_3$, 40 to 70 mEq/70 kg)
- Return unused blood to blood bank for recrossmatch
- Send patient blood sample to blood bank for antibody screen and direct antiglobulin test
- Send to the laboratory urine and plasma hemoglobin levels, platelet count, partial thromboplastin time, and serum fibrinogen levels
- Supportive care: Prevent hypotension to ensure adequate renal blood flow.

Miller RD (ed): Anesthesia, 4th ed, pp 1634–1635. New York, Churchill Livingstone, 1994

C.20. What is a delayed hemolytic reaction?

In many cases of hemolytic transfusion reaction, the transfused donor cells may survive well initially but after a variable delay (2 to 21 days) will be hemolyzed. This type of reaction occurs mainly in recipients sensitized to red cell antigens by previous blood transfusions or pregnancy. As a result, this type of delayed reaction is more common in women who have a known disposition of alloimmunization. These reactions are delayed hemolytic transfusion reactions—those in which the level of antibody at the time of transfusion is too low to be detected or too low to cause red cell destruction. These delayed reactions are often manifested only by a decrease in the post-transfusion hematocrit. However, jaundice and/or hemoglobinuria can occur in these patients. Hemolytic reactions can also cause some impairment in renal function, but only rarely do they lead to the demise of the patient.

Although impairment of renal function is not common, the surgical team should include in their differential diagnosis a delayed hemolytic transfusion reaction in any patient who has an unexplained decrease in hematocrit 2 to 21 days after a transfusion, even without obvious manifestation of hemolysis. This is especially important in a postoperative patient when the decrease in hematocrit is thought to be from blood loss and may be an important criterion to whether additional surgery is necessary.

Miller RD (ed): Anesthesia, 4th ed, p 1635. New York, Churchill Livingstone, 1994

C.21. What are nonhemolytic transfusion reactions?

Nonhemolytic transfusion reactions to blood transfusions usually are not serious, and they are either febrile or allergic. The most common adverse reactions to blood transfusions are the febrile reactions. Symptoms consist of chills, fever, headache, myalgia, nausea, and nonproductive cough occurring shortly after blood transfusion. Less frequently the patient may have hypotension, chest pain, vomiting, and dyspnea. Because febrile reactions involve fever, they can be easily confused with a hemolytic transfusion reaction. A direct antiglobulin test readily differentiates a hemolytic reaction from a febrile reaction, because this test rules out the attachment of a red cell antibody to transfused donor red cells.

Most allergic transfusion reactions are mild (anaphylactoid), and they are considered to be caused by foreign protein in the transfused blood. The most common symptom is urticaria associated with itching. Occasionally, the patient will have facial swelling. Allergic reactions occur in about 3% of all transfusions. Antihistamines are used to relieve the symptoms of the allergic reaction. Infrequently a more severe form of allergic reaction involving anaphylaxis will occur in which the patient has dyspnea, hypotension, laryngeal edema, chest pain, and shock. These are anaphylactic reactions caused by the transfusion of IgA to patients who are IgA-deficient, and they have formed anti-IgA. This type of reaction does not involve red cell destruction, and it occurs very rapidly. The patients who experience these anaphylactic reactions must be given transfusions with washed red blood cells from which all traces of donor IgA have been removed.

Miller RD (ed): Anesthesia, 4th ed, p 1635. New York, Churchill Livingstone, 1994

C.22. What is the current infectious risk from red cell transfusion?

The incidence of hepatitis B transmission is 1:200,000 per unit of blood. The incidence of hepatitis C is 0.03% per unit (1:3300). The current risk of human immunodeficiency virus (HIV) infection is 1:450,000 to 1:660,000 per transfused unit of blood.

The most common viral agent transmitted by blood transfusion is cytomegalovirus. Most of these infections are subclinical but infection in the immunocompromised patient and fetal transmission can produce serious sequelae.

ASA Task Force: Practice guideline for blood component therapy. Anesthesiology 84:732–747, 1996

C.23. What are various methods of autologous transfusion, and how useful would they be in this patient?

Three methods of autologous transfusion exist: preoperative antepartum donation, intraoperative blood salvage, and normovolemic hemodilution.

Preoperative donation and normovolemic hemodilution are useful techniques when blood loss can be predicted before surgery. Preoperative donation does not exist for emergency surgery, and normovolemic hemodilution would have limited application in pregnant patients because of the relative anemia of pregnancy.

Intraoperative blood salvage (autotransfusion) is a technique of scavenging blood lost during surgery, processing it by centrifugation and washing, then transfusing the scavenged, autologous red cells. Red cells that are salvaged, processed, and transfused have an excellent survival rate. Malignancy, infection, the presence of old hemolyzed blood, and the use of collagen or hemostatic material are relative contraindications to the use of intraoperative blood salvage. It is of concern that blood processing and washing may not adequately remove amniotic fluid and fetal debris. The autotransfusion may precipitate amniotic fluid embolism. Few published data are available regarding the use of this technique in obstetric patients.

In conclusion, none of these three techniques offers any usefulness in this hypovolemic, anemic, pregnant patient for emergency surgery.

Chestnut DH (ed): Obstetric Anesthesia: Principles and Practice, p 715. St. Louis, Mosby, 1994

C.24. What are the advantages and disadvantages of epidural versus spinal anesthesia for elective cesarean section?

The choice of anesthesia for cesarean section depends on the indication for the operation, the degree of urgency, the desire of the patient, and the judgment of the anesthesiologist.

Both epidural and spinal anesthesia allow the mother to be awake, minimize the problems of maternal aspiration, and avoid the neonatal drug depression caused by general anesthesia.

Spinal (subarachnoid) anesthetics are easily administered and require much lower doses of local anesthetics. The high doses used for epidural anesthetics can produce a systemic effect after uptake from the injection site, in contrast to the much smaller doses used in spinal anesthesia, which has little or no systemic effect. Spinal anesthetics create a rapid sympathetic blockade that can cause hypotension. With epidural anesthesia, sympathetic blockade occurs less precipitously; consequently hypotension is easier to prevent or treat. The anesthetic level is also more controllable with epidural anesthesia because if the initial dose does not produce a satisfactory sensory block, more drug can be injected through the epidural catheter. Postspinal headaches are rarely a problem with epidural anesthesia, as opposed to spinal anesthesia.

Recent advances in spinal needle design have reduced the risk of postspinal headaches, leading to a resurgence in the use of spinal anesthetics for cesarean section. Spinal anesthesia appears to have a lower rate of complications and significantly lower cost than epidural anesthesia. These factors account for its desirability for elective cesarean section in uncomplicated patients.

Miller RD (ed): Anesthesia, 4th ed, pp 2056–2057. New York, Churchill Livingstone, 1994

Riley E, Cohen S, Macario A: Spinal versus epidural anesthesia for cesarean section: A comparison of time, efficiency, costs, charges and complications. Anesth Analg 80:709–712, 1995

Shnider SM, Levinson G (eds): Anesthesia for Obstetrics, 3rd ed, pp 143–151; 214–219. Baltimore, Williams & Wilkins, 1993

C.25. How does one administer an epidural test dose?

The purpose of the test dose is to help recognize unintentional cannulation of a blood vessel or the subarachnoid space. The test dose should contain a dose of local anesthetic and/or another marker, sufficient to allow recognition of intravenous or subarachnoid injection, but not so large as to cause systemic toxicity or total spinal anesthesia. The test dose is a trial injection of local anesthetic followed by a waiting period of 3 to 5 minutes to ensure that the injection is neither intravascular nor intrathecal. During the waiting period, the patient should be meticulously monitored. A test dose is recommended before administering the initial dose and before each subsequent dose as a safeguard against accidental subarachnoid or intravenous injection.

Many ways are available to administer test dosing. The current way is to administer 3 ml of 1.5% lidocaine with 1:200,000 epinephrine (5 μg/ml). If this test dose is injected intravenously, an epinephrine response will occur within 45 seconds: an increase in heart rate and blood pressure, circumoral pallor, palpitations, and tremulousness. The increase in heart rate of ≥20 beats/min might only last 15 seconds, so continuous ECG monitoring is mandatory. Be sure to administer the test dose after a uterine contraction because a uterine contraction can increase heart rate on its own. The effects of an intrathecal injection may not be apparent for 3 to 5 minutes, so this is the minimal time that should be spent before administering more local anesthetic. Other test dose regimens designed to detect intravascular injections include isoproterenol, ephedrine, fentanyl, and air.

Abraham RA, Harris AP, Maxwell LG et al: The efficacy of 1.5% lidocaine with 7.5% dextrose and epinephrine as an epidural test dose for obstetrics. Anesthesiology 64:116–119, 1986

Baker BW, Longmire S, Jones MM et al: The epidural test dose in obstetrics reconsidered [Abstract]. Anesthesiology 67:A625, 1987

Cherala SR, Greene R, Mehta D: Ephedrine as a marker of intravascular injection in laboring parturients. Reg Anesth 15:15–18, 1990

Chestnut DH (ed): Obstetric Anesthesia: Principles and Practice, pp 197–198. St. Louis, Mosby, 1994

Leighton BL, DeSimone CA, Norris MC, et al: Isoproterenol is an effective marker of intravenous injection in laboring women. Anesthesiology 71:206–209, 1989

Leighton BL, Gross JB: Air: An effective indicator of intravenously located epidural catheters. Anesthesiology 71:848–851, 1989

Leighton BL, Norris MC, DeSimone CA et al: The air test as a clinically useful indicator of intravenously placed epidural catheters. Anesthesiology 73:610–613, 1990

Rottman RL, Miller M, Yoshii WY et al: Fentanyl as an epidural intravascular test dose in obstetrics [Abstract]. Anesth Analg 70:S336, 1990

Van Zundert AA, Vaes LE, Soetens M et al: Every dose given in epidural analgesia for vaginal anesthesia can be a test dose. Anesthesiology 67:436–440, 1987

C.26. What are the possible complications of epidural anesthesia and how are they treated?

The most serious life-threatening complications include severe hypotension, local anesthetic convulsions, and total spinal anesthesia.

Hypotension remains the most common side-effect of major conduction anesthesia because of the sympathetic blockade. Treatment includes administration of oxygen, applications of more left uterine displacement, placing the patient in the Trendelenburg position, and increasing administration of IV fluids. If the blood pressure is not restored within 1 to 2 minutes, give ephedrine 5 to 15 mg IV.

Local anesthetic convulsions occur when a large dose of local anesthetic is inadvertently injected into the intravascular compartment and produces systemic toxicity. Frank convulsions can result, and the dangers to the patient are hypoxia, aspiration, and/or cardiovascular collapse. If the patient begins to show signs of systemic toxicity (tingling of mouth or lips, tremulousness, ringing in the ears), first administer 100% oxygen, and then titrate small doses of central nervous depressants, either diazepam in doses of 1 to 5 mg or sodium thiopental, 25 to 50 mg. This approach usually prevents the toxic reaction to progress to convulsions. If convulsions do occur, the first priority is maintenance of oxygenation. Convulsions are not lethal, but the anoxia and acidosis that they produce may be. Tracheal intubation with a cuffed endotracheal tube and ventilation with 100% oxygen may be necessary. Support the circulation with Trendelenburg position, left uterine displacement, IV fluids, and vasopressors as necessary. Treat possible cardiac arrest with complete cardiopulmonary resuscitation, external cardiac massage, ventilation with 100% oxygen, and appropriate pharmacologic life support.

Total spinal anesthesia may occur from excessive spread of local anesthetic administered intrathecally, extradurally, or even subdurally. Treatment consists of establishing an airway and ventilating with oxygen. Endotracheal intubation should be performed as early as possible to protect the airway from aspiration. Blood pressure should be supported with left uterine displacement, Trendelenburg position, IV fluids, and vasopressors.

Other possible complications of epidural anesthesia include the following:

- Postspinal headache
- Broken catheter remnants left in the epidural space
- Epidural hematomas and abscesses

Postspinal headaches are due to persistent cerebrospinal fluid (CSF) leaks through a needle hole in the dura. In its milder forms, the headache is usually self-limiting and will resolve spontaneously after conservative treatment with bed rest and fluids (either IV or oral). However, for those refractory headaches that are incapacitating, an epidural blood patch should be considered. Broken catheter remnants can be left in the epidural space by being sheared off by inappropriate withdrawal through the epidural needle. Attempted removal of an inert piece of Teflon catheter is probably far more traumatic and potentially harmful than a policy of reassurance and noninterference.

Epidural hematomas and epidural abscesses consistently present with a symptom of back pain. The onset of back pain and tenderness should raise the possibility of a space-occupying lesion, especially if fever and bacteremia are present. Definitive diagnosis is made with a myelogram, computerized tomography, or magnetic resonance imaging. Once the diagnosis of a space-occupying lesion is made, emergency decompression laminectomy and drainage of the lesion must be performed. Antibiotic therapy should be instituted immediately and coagulation abnormalities corrected. Note that epidural abscesses and hematomas are very rare lesions. No more than 31 cases of epidural lesions reported in the world literature to date can be considered to have been caused by an epidural technique.

Bromage PR: Epidural Anesthesia, pp 650–683. Philadelphia, WB Saunders, 1978

Chestnut DH (ed): Obstetric Anesthesia: Principles and Practice, pp 367–372. St. Louis, Mosby, 1994

Miller RD (ed): Anesthesia, 4th ed, pp 2053–2055. New York, Churchill Livingstone, 1994

Shnider SM, Levinson G (eds): Anesthesia for Obstetrics, 3rd ed, pp 135–143. Baltimore, Williams & Wilkins, 1993

D. Postoperative Management

D.1. When should this patient be extubated?

This patient should be extubated when she is awake, can protect her airway against aspiration, and is breathing adequately.

Shnider SM, Levinson G (eds): Anesthesia for Obstetrics, 3rd ed, p 225. Baltimore, Williams & Wilkins, 1993

D.2. If this patient decided to have a tubal ligation during her postpartum course would she still be at risk for aspiration?

It is not known precisely when the physiologic gastrointestinal changes of pregnancy (decreased gastric emptying, increased gastric acid production, and so forth) that predispose these pregnant patients to increased risk of aspiration return to normal. As stated in question A.19, gastric emptying, gastric volume, and gastric pH, all appear to return to prepregnancy values within the first 3 days postpartum. No one time interval absolutely guarantees that a specific patient is free of risk. Therefore, the following preventative measures should be taken for postpartum surgery:

- Attempt to use regional anesthesia (spinal or epidural).
- If general anesthesia is selected, a rapid-sequence induction, as outlined in question C.8 should be followed to minimize the risk of aspiration.

Blouw R, Scatliff J, Craig DB, et al: Gastric volume and pH in the postpartum period. Anesthesiology 45:456–457, 1976

Chestnut DH (ed): Obstetric Anesthesia: Principles and Practice, p 27. St. Louis, Mosby, 1994

Gin T, Cho AMW, Lew JKL: Gastric emptying in the postpartum period. Anesth Intens Care 19: 521–524, 1991

Shnider SM, Levinson G (eds): Anesthesia for Obstetrics, 3rd ed, pp 248–250. Baltimore, Williams & Wilkins, 1993

D.3. Two days following epidural cesarean section, a patient with no significant past medical history complains of a postural headache. What is your differential diagnosis?

Postpartum patients frequently suffer from headaches. Often the cause is unrelated to anesthesia. Possible causes of postpartum headaches include postdural puncture headache, nonspecific headache, migraine, hypertension, brain tumor, subdural hematoma, subarachnoid hemorrhage, cortical vein thrombosis, pseudotumor cerebri, sinusitis, meningitis, pneumocephalus, caffeine withdrawal, and lactation headache. The fact that this patient had an epidural anesthetic does not rule out the possibility of an inadvertent dural puncture. The cause of a postural headache in the postpartum period is almost always due to a postdural puncture headache.

Chestnut DH (ed): Obstetric Anesthesia: Principles and Practice, pp 606–609. St. Louis, Mosby, 1994

McSwiney M, Phillips J: Postdural puncture headache. Acta Anaesthesiol Scand 39:990–995, 1995

Shnider SM, Levinson G (eds): Anesthesia for Obstetrics, 3rd ed, pp 436–439. Baltimore, Williams & Wilkins, 1993

D.4. What are the symptoms of a postdural puncture headache?

Patients with a postdural puncture headache usually complain of pain in the front occipital region that radiates to the neck, which may be stiff. Some patients have a mild headache, others have severe and incapacitating headache. Nausea and vomiting are unusual. Symptoms are worse in the upright position and are relieved somewhat in the horizontal position.

Chestnut DH (ed): Obstetric Anesthesia: Principles and Practice, p 608. St. Louis, Mosby, 1994

D.5. When do postdural puncture headaches usually present?

Postdural puncture headaches usually appear on the first or second day after a dural puncture, and rarely after 7 days. Most headaches last less than a week, but there are several reports of symptoms lasting for months or even years.

Chestnut DH (ed): Obstetric Anesthesia: Principles and Practice, p 608. St. Louis, Mosby, 1994

Lybecker H, Djernes M, Schmidt JF: Postdural puncture headache: onset, duration, severity, and associated symptoms. Acta Anaesthesiol Scand 39:606–612, 1995

D.6. What causes the pain and discomfort associated with a postdural puncture headache?

Leakage of cerebrospinal fluid (CSF) through the puncture hole in the dura causes diminished hydraulic support for intracranial structures. Tension on these structures results in headache as a symptom and rarely oculomotor or trigeminal nerve paresis as a sign. Severity of the headache is related to the rate of loss of CSF. This in turn is determined by the degree of pressure exerted by distended veins inside and outside the dural tube, and by the size of the puncture hole through which CSF escapes.

Chestnut DH (ed): Obstetric Anesthesia: Principles and Practice, pp 608–609. St. Louis, Mosby, 1994

Shnider SM, Levinson G (eds): Anesthesia for Obstetrics, 3rd ed, p 437. Baltimore, Williams & Wilkins, 1993

D.7. What is the treatment of a postdural puncture headache?

Patients with a postdural puncture headache should rest in the horizontal position and receive psychological support. Mild headache often responds to oral analgesics and/or caffeine. If the headache is severe, the physician should either try caffeine or proceed directly to a blood patch. In most cases, at least 24 hours have elapsed after dural puncture before therapeutic blood patch is performed. However, it is appropriate to perform a therapeutic blood patch earlier if the headache is severe. A second blood patch can be performed if the first patch fails. If the second blood patch fails, alternative diagnoses should be excluded before performance of a third patch or a trial of an epidural saline infusion.

Autologous blood patch has become recognized as the definitive treatment for postdural headache. Three requirements are necessary for success:

- Normal clotting profile.
- The blood should be introduced close to or at the site of puncture.
- A sufficient volume of blood must be injected to seal the hole, and to exert enough pressure around the dural tube to restore CSF pressure and immediately relieve the headache. The instant relief characteristics of a successful blood patch depend on the administration of 15 to 20 ml of autologous blood.

Chestnut DH (ed): Obstetric Anesthesia: Principles and Practice, pp 614–617. St. Louis, Mosby, 1994

Shnider SM, Levinson G (eds): Anesthesia for Obstetrics, 3rd ed, p 223. Baltimore, Williams & Wilkins, 1993

D.8. How does one perform an epidural blood patch?

The anesthesiologist should provide a thorough explanation of risks and benefits. The patient should give written consent to the procedure, which can be done as an outpatient if necessary.

If the anesthesiologist is uncertain of the location of the dural puncture, the more caudal interspace should be chosen. The anesthesiologist identifies the epidural space in the usual manner. Using meticulous sterile technique, an assistant then withdraws 15 to 20 ml of blood. Approximately 15 ml of this blood is injected slowly, but the injection is terminated if pain occurs.

After the procedure the patient rests quietly in the horizontal position for 1 to 2 hours. Subsequently, the patient may resume ambulation.

Chestnut DH (ed): Obstetric Anesthesia: Principles and Practice, p 613. St. Louis, Mosby, 1994

Pregnancy-Induced Hypertension

36

Edwina Sia-Kho

A 40-year-old primigravida, at 33 weeks gestation, was admitted to the hospital because of persistent headaches, rapid weight gain (> 7 kg = 15 lbs in 3 weeks), with blood pressure elevated to 150/100 mm Hg, and proteinuria (>2 g daily).

A. Medical Disease and Differential Diagnosis

1. What is the upper limit of normal blood pressure as recommended by the American Obstetric Committee? What is the classification of hypertension during pregnancy given by the American College of Obstetricians and Gynecologists?
2. What is pregnancy-induced hypertension (PIH)? What is toxemia of pregnancy?
3. Define gestational hypertension and chronic hypertension.
4. Compare the clinical manifestations and laboratory data of different degrees of preeclampsia.
5. What is eclampsia? Discuss the characteristics of convulsions in eclampsia.
6. Why is the diagnosis of PIH frequently made early in its evolution before proteinuria occurs? Is edema a reliable diagnostic feature of preeclampsia?
7. What is the incidence of PIH?
8. What are the etiology and the precipitating factors of preeclampsia?
9. Discuss the pathophysiologic alterations of preeclampsia in different organs.
10. What is the prognosis for patients with preeclampsia and eclampsia?
11. What are the maternal and perinatal mortality rates from PIH?

B. Preoperative Evaluation and Preparation

1. What are the important physical examinations for PIH patients?
2. What laboratory tests are needed for PIH patients?
3. What are the important routine monitors for PIH patients? When is a central venous pressure (CVP) monitor indicated?
4. What is the significance of the supine pressor response or roll-over test?
5. What is the contraction stress test (oxytoxin stress test)?
6. Discuss the treatment of preeclamptic patients.
7. Why should every incidence of acute hypertension be managed as preeclampsia with the threat of convulsions?
8. In the United States, what is the first line of treatment for preeclampsia? Discuss its actions.
9. What is the suggested regimen using magnesium sulfate?
10. How would you judge the therapeutic effects of magnesium sulfate?
11. What precautions should be taken in using magnesium sulfate?
12. How would you avoid magnesium toxicity?
13. What are the effects of increasing plasma magnesium levels?
14. Discuss the treatment of magnesium toxicity.

15. What are the effects of magnesium sulfate on the fetus?
16. When is diazepam useful in preeclamptic patients?
17. What are the side-effects of diazepam on neonates?
18. If the patient is having an eclamptic fit, what is the immediate therapy?
19. When is an antihypertensive agent indicated? How much can the diastolic blood pressure be lowered? Why?
20. What are the most common antihypertensive agents used to lower blood pressure?

C. Intraoperative Management

1. What is your choice of anesthesia for PIH patients?
2. Is epidural anesthesia advisable for patients with high blood pressure? What are the advantages?
3. What is the advantage of prehydration?
4. How should patients be hydrated before epidural anesthesia?
5. What precautions should be taken when a patient who is receiving an antihypertensive drug is also going to have an epidural block?
6. What level of epidural anesthesia should be reached in preeclamptic patients?
7. What local anesthetics are used in obstetric anesthesia? Discuss their advantages and disadvantages.
8. Is the addition of epinephrine to local anesthetics advisable in preeclamptic patients?
9. What is the treatment for the asphyxic fetal heart rate pattern seen with maternal hypotension after epidural anesthesia is instituted?
10. What would you do after an inadvertent spinal tap? How do you treat spinal headache?
11. How would you manage total spinal anesthesia?
12. When and how would you give spinal anesthesia?
13. What is HELLP syndrome and what is its importance?
14. What are the modifications of a standard general anesthesia technique in PIH patients?
15. How would you control intraoperative hypertension during general anesthesia for cesarean section?
16. What are the disadvantages of trimethaphan?
17. What are the advantages and disadvantages of nitroglycerin and nitroprusside?
18. Should ergometrine (Ergotrate) be given to preeclamptic patients?

D. Postoperative Management

1. Discuss the postpartum care of preeclamptic patients.

A. Medical Disease and Differential Diagnosis

A.1. What is the upper limit of normal blood pressure as recommended by the American Obstetric Committee? What is the classification of hypertension during pregnancy given by the American College of Obstetricians and Gynecologists?

A blood pressure of 130/80 mm Hg is the upper limit of normal at any time during pregnancy.

The three types of hypertension during pregnancy are:

- Pregnancy-induced hypertension (PIH)
  - Preeclampsia
  - Eclampsia
  - Gestational hypertension (late or transient hypertension of the third trimester)
- Coincidental hypertension (chronic hypertension preceding pregnancy)
- Chronic hypertension with superimposed PIH
  - Superimposed preeclampsia
  - Superimposed eclampsia

Chesley L: History and epidemiology of preeclampsia-eclampsia. Clin Obstet Gynecol 27:801–835, 1984

A.2 What is pregnancy-induced hypertension (PIH)? What is toxemia of pregnancy?

Pregnancy-induced hypertension is diagnosed when a pregnant woman has a blood pressure of ≥140/90 mm Hg, or a rise of 30 mm Hg systolic or 15 mm Hg diastolic over baseline, or an increase in mean arterial pressure (MAP) of 20 mm Hg, or a MAP >105 mm Hg. Blood pressure has to be taken at least twice, ≥6 hours apart. This patient also has abnormal edema or proteinuria or both after 20 weeks of gestation.

Toxemias of pregnancy are synonymous with preeclampsia and eclampsia; recently these conditions have been referred to as "PIH."

Chestnut DH (ed): Obstetric Anesthesia: Principles and Practice pp 846–847. New York, Churchill Livingstone, 1994

Shnider SM, Levinson G (eds): Anesthesia for Obstetrics, 3rd ed, p 305. Baltimore, Williams & Wilkins, 1993

A.3 Define gestational hypertension and chronic hypertension.

Gestational hypertension is hypertension without proteinuria or generalized edema during the last weeks of pregnancy or immediately after delivery.

Chronic hypertension is persistent hypertension, regardless of cause, before the 20th week of gestation or beyond 6 weeks after delivery.

Shnider SM, Levinson G (eds): Anesthesia for Obstetrics, 3rd ed, p 305. Baltimore, Williams & Wilkins, 1993

A.4. Compare the clinical manifestations and laboratory data of different degrees of preeclampsia.

See Table 36-1.

Burrow GN, Ferris TF: Medical Complications during Pregnancy, 3rd ed, p 22. Philadelphia, WB Saunders, 1988

Table 36-1.   Clinical Manifestations and Laboratory Data of Different Degrees of Preeclampsia

	MILD	MODERATE	SEVERE
Blood pressure	140/95	150/100–160/110	>160/110
Clinical	1 + edema	1 to 2 + edema	3 to 4 + edema
	Normal reflexes	1 to 2 + hyperreflexia	3 to 4 + hyperreflexia
	No visual signs	Early visual signs	Convulsion (eclampsia)
			Congestive heart failure
			Visual signs
LABORATORY VALUES			
BUN mg/100 ml	<10	10–20	>20
Serum creatinine mg/100 ml	<1	1–1.6	>1.6
Urate mg/100 ml	<4.5	4.5–6	>6
Urinary protein	1 + (0.5)	2 to 3 + (0.5–2 g/24 h)	3 to 4 + (>2 g/24 h)
Thrombocytopenia	Absent	Mild	Present
Decreased clotting factors	Absent	Absent	Present occasionally
Delivery	If fetus at term, delivery indicated; delay delivery if BP and renal function stable	Delivery usually indicated	Delivery indicated as soon as cardiovascular and CNS signs stable

Datta S (ed): Anesthetic and Obstetric Management of High-Risk Pregnancy, p 424. St. Louis. Mosby-Year Book, 1991

A.5. What is eclampsia? Discuss the characteristics of convulsions in eclampsia.

The occurrence of convulsions not caused by coincidental neurologic disease (e.g., epilepsy) in a pregnant woman who fulfills the criteria for preeclampsia is called "eclampsia." Eclampsia can develop in the presence of either mild or severe preeclampsia.

The convulsion is grand mal in character and appears before, during, or after delivery. Any seizure that occurs >48 hours postpartum is due to other central nervous system (CNS) lesions.

Cunningham FG, MacDonald PG, Gant NF: Williams' Obstetrics, 20th ed, p 657. Stamford, CT, Appleton & Lange, 1997

Shnider SM, Levinson G (eds): Anesthesia for Obstetrics, 3rd ed, p 305. Baltimore, Williams & Wilkins, 1993

A.6. Why is the diagnosis of PIH frequently made early in its evolution before proteinuria occurs? Is edema a reliable diagnostic feature of preeclampsia?

The diagnosis of PIH is made early before proteinuria occurs because of the following:

- Proteinuria and alterations of glomerular histology develop late in the course of PIH.
- Perinatal mortality rate begins to rise with the appearance of hypertension alone, even before proteinuria occurs.
- Eclampsia can occur in women with PIH (5% to 10%) who do not have proteinuria.

Edema is not a reliable diagnostic feature because many preeclampsia patients do not have edema and many normal patients with large babies can have considerable edema. Pedal edema may be caused by inferior vena cava compression. Sixty-four percent of pregnant women may have edema in a nondependent portion of the body. The first sign of impending preeclampsia is often a rapid weight gain of ≥2.25 kg in 1 week before any noted increased edema. Edema of upper and lower extremities is usually seen.

Chestnut DH (ed): Obstetric Anesthesia: Principles and Practice, p 847. New York, Churchill Livingstone, 1994

Datta S (ed): Anesthetic and Obstetric Management of High-Risk Pregnancy, 2nd ed, p 387. St. Louis, Mosby-Year Book, 1996

Worley R: Pathophysiology of pregnancy-induced hypertension. Clin Obstet Gynecol 27:821, 1984

A.7. What is the incidence of PIH?

Preeclampsia affects 6% to 8% of all pregnancies in the United States. Incidence of severe preeclampsia has increased from 2.4/1000 deliveries to 5.2/1000 deliveries. It is typically a disease of the young (age <20) women, affecting about 85% of nulliparae, although mortality increases with age.

Eskenazi B, Fenster L, Sidney S: A multivariate analysis of risk factors for preeclampsia. JAMA 266:237–241, 1991

Malinow AM: Preeclampsia and Eclampsia: Anesthetic Management. ASA Annual Refresher Course Lectures #511, American Society of Anesthesiologist, 1996

Saftlas AF, Olson DR, Franks AL et al: Epidemiology of preeclampsia and eclampsia in the United States, 1979–1986. Am J Obstet Gynecol 163:460–465, 1990

Zuspan FP: New concepts in the understanding of hypertensive diseases during pregnancy: an overview. Clin Perinatol 18:653–659, 1991

A.8. What are the etiology and the precipitating factors of preeclampsia?

The etiology of PIH is unknown. There are two theories: that of immunologic injury and that of uteroplacental ischemia. The prevalence in primigravidae can be explained by insufficient development of the uterine vasculature as well as lack of effective immunization to factors inherent in the pregnant state.

Immunologic disorders may arise from abnormal maternal-fetal antigen-antibody response or from the contents of seminal fluids; spermatozoa may produce antibody formation or prostagalandins may initiate uterine vasoconstriction. The fetus acquires 50% of its genes from the father, which represents in part a paternal allograft that interacts with maternal tissue as fetal trophoblast migrates into the maternal decidua after implantation. Migration normally occurs in two phases. Trophoblasts displace the muscular structure of the maternal spiral arteries before the 20 weeks gestation, causing their adrenergic denervation and converting them from high-resistance to low-resistance vessels. At the same time, biochemical adaptations occur in the maternal vasculature, with an increased dominance of endothelium-dependent vasodilators, prostacyclin (PGI), and nitric oxide. In preeclampsia, the second wave of trophoblastic migration fails and arteries retain their adrenergic innervation. Their myometrial segments remain intact, and they do not dilate. The hallmark is vaso-

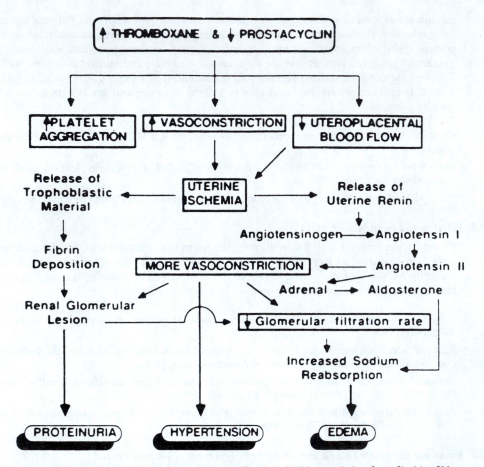

Figure 36-1. Pathogenesis of preeclampsia. (Reprinted with permission from Shnider SM, Levinson G [eds]: Anesthesia for Obstetrics, 2nd ed, p 227. Baltimore, Williams & Wilkins, 1987)

spasm that produces pathologic changes in organ systems throughout the body. These changes may be related to disruption and damage to three major cell types: endothelial cells, platelets, and trophoblasts. The current concept is shown in Figure 36-1. Preeclampsia and other chronic placental insufficiency syndromes are the result of prostacyclin deficiency in the mother and in fetomaternal tissues and an overproduction of thromboxane A_2 in the placenta. These changes cause vasoconstriction and platelet hyperactivity, which are pathognomonic for hypertensive pregnancies. PGI (also called epoprostenol or prostaglandin I_2) was first identified from the vessel wall. It is chemically a bicyclic allylic ether prostaglandin. It can be synthesized by other vessel wall components, such as smooth muscle cells and even nonvascular tissues. Thromboxane A_2 is formed from cyclic endoperoxides through thromboxane synthetase, particularly in the platelets and in other tissues, such as the vascular wall. In preeclamptic pregnancy, an imbalance occurs in placental prostacyclin and thromboxane production, with the placenta producing seven times more thromboxane than prostacyclin. Thromboxane causes increased vasoconstriction, platelet aggregation, and uterine activity, and decreased uteroplacental blood flow. All these contribute to the signs and symptoms of preeclampsia. A familial factor in preeclapmsia also appears to exist in some populations because of a recessive genetic inheritance.

The precipitating factors of preeclampsia are as follows:
- Adolescent and elderly primigravidae
- Obesity
- Diabetes
- Multiple pregnancy
- Essential hypertension
- Hydatidiform mole
- Renal disease
- Polyhydramnios

Chestnut DH (ed): Obstetric Anesthesia: Principles and Practice, pp 847–848. New York, Churchill Livingstone, 1994

Datta S (ed): Anesthetic and Obstetric Management of High-Risk Pregnancy, 2nd ed, p 387. St. Louis, Mosby-Year Book, 1996

Walsh SW: Preeclampsia: An imbalance in placental prostacyclin and thromboxane production. Am J Obstet Gynecol 152:335–340, 1985

Worley R: Pathophysiology of pregnancy-induced hypertension. Clin Obstet Gynecol 27:821, 1984

A.9. Discuss the pathophysiologic alterations of preeclampsia in different organs.

The underlying condition is vasoconstriction caused by circulating levels of renin, angiotensin, aldosterone, and catecholamines.

Hematologic Changes
- A decrease in circulating blood volume, primarily plasma, occurs in spite of excess total body sodium and water, resulting in hemoconcentration.
- Increased blood viscosity aggravates the existing decreased perfusion.
- Despite increased hematocrit and hemoglobin, relative anemia usually exists; these patients tolerate blood loss poorly.
- A disseminated intravascular coagulopathy (DIC) is characterized initially by reduction in platelet count to <150,000/mm^3 in 11% to 50% of patients secondary to platelet adherence at the sites of disrupted endothelium, later by a rise in fibrin degradation product, a fall in fibrinogen level, and prolongation of partial thromboplastin time (PTT) and prothrombin time (PT).
- About 10% to 25% of preeclamptic patients with normal platelet count have prolonged bleeding times, more so when platelet count drops below 100,000/mm^3.

Cerebral Changes
- The classic manifestations of preeclampsia include severe headache, visual disturbance, CNS, hyperexcitability, and hyperreflexia
- In 45% of eclamptic patients, some computed tomographic (CT) abnormality will be demonstrated and 90% will have electroencephalographic (EEG) abnormality
- Coma can occur without eclampsia.
- Increased intracranial pressure can be exacerbated by hypercarbia, metabolic acidosis, and hypoxia.

Respiratory Changes
- Upper airway and laryngeal edema occurs. Edema of face and distortion of glottic architecture may make intubation and airway management difficult.
- Overloading with fluid can lead to pulmonary edema with left ventricular failure.
- The oxyhemoglobin dissociation curve may shift to the left, decreasing the availability of oxygen to the fetus.

Cardiovascular Changes
- Preeclamptic women typically develop (but not always) a high cardiac output, high systemic resistance, decreased circulating volume, and increased left ventricular work. CVP measurements vary significantly. Poor correlation is seen between CVP and pulmonary capillary wedge pressure (PCWP) in severe cases. PCWP is usually not increased, yet volume expansion may cause left ventricular overloading and pulmonary edema.

Ophthalmic Changes
- Retinal arteriolar spasm occurs. Bilateral retinal detachment, owing to massive edema in the retina, is seen in severe cases, and it can result in blindness.

Uterine Changes
- The uterus is hyperactive and markedly sensitive to oxytocin. Rapid labor and painful contractions are common. The placenta shows signs of premature aging and has infarcts, fibrin deposits, calcifications, and/or abruption.

Renal Changes
- Decreased urate clearance results in the well-recognized increase in serum uric acid concentration. This occurs earlier than reduction of the glomerular filtration rate.
- A reduction occurs in filtration fraction (glomerular filtration rate/renal plasma flow).
- Renal lesions consist of glomerular capillary endothelial swelling with narrowing of glomerular capillaries owing to severe swelling of endothelial cells. Fibrin deposits are found in glomeruli, which is pathognomonic of the disease.
- Proteinuria results from increased permeability of damaged renal glomeruli.

Hepatic Changes
- In severe cases, hepatocellular damage occurs because of periportal hemorrhage from vasospasm, and subcapsular hematomas have been seen. Rupture of the liver is a rare occurrence. The hepatic swelling produces epigastric pain.
- Serum transaminase levels frequently increase in mild preeclampsia.
- Hemolysis occurs as jaundice secondary to hepatocellular damage and heme pigment deposited in body stores. This can progress to fatty metamorphosis of the liver and ultimately to death.

Chestnut DH (ed): Obstetric Anesthesia: Principles and Practice, p 852. New York, Churchill Livingstone, 1994

Malinow AM: Preeclampsia and Eclampsia: Anesthetic Management. ASA Annual Refresher Course Lectures #511, American Society of Anesthesiologists, 1996

Shnider SM, Levinson G (eds): Anesthesia for Obstetrics, 3rd ed, pp 313–314. Baltimore, Williams & Wilkins, 1993

A.10. What is the prognosis for patients with preeclampsia and eclampsia?

Maternal Complications
Maternal complications include DIC, convulsion, congestive heart failure with

pulmonary edema, postpartum hemorrhage, acute renal failure, rupture of the liver, cerebrovascular accident, and septic shock. The leading cause of death is intracranial hemorrhage.

Fetal Complications
Complications for the fetus include prematurity with respiratory distress, intrauterine growth retardation, oligohydramnious, intracranial hemorrhage, small size for gestational age, and aspiration of meconium.

    The leading cause of intrauterine mortality is placental infarcts followed by retardation of placental growth, placental abruption, and acute infection of amniotic fluid.

Datta S (ed): Anesthetic and Obstetric Management of High-Risk Pregnancy, 2nd ed, pp 388–390. St. Louis, Mosby-Year Book, 1996

Shnider SM, Levinson G (eds): Anesthesia for Obstetrics, 3rd ed, p 314. Baltimore, Williams & Wilkins, 1993

A.11. What are the maternal and perinatal mortality rates from PIH?

Preeclampsia and eclampsia are the leading causes (accounting for 20%; perhaps as high as 40%) of the maternal mortality recorded in the United States, England, and Scandinavia. The maternal mortality rate is 0.4% to 11.9%. The perinatal death rate is 20% to 30%.

Shnider SM, Levinson G (eds): Anesthesia for Obstetrics, 3rd, p 305. Baltimore, Williams & Wilkins, 1993

B. Preoperative Evaluation and Preparation

B.1. What are the important physical examinations for PIH patients?

- Frequent blood pressure determinations
- Fundoscopic examination for headache and visual disturbances
- Neurologic examination for knee reflex
- Daily weight measurement
- Check for edema and epigastric pain
- Cervical examination
- Check of fetal weight, fundal measurement, and fetal heart rate
- Amniocentesis for fetal maturity

Shnider SM, Levinson G (eds): Anesthesia for Obstetrics, 3rd ed, p 323. Baltimore, Williams & Wilkins, 1993

B.2. What laboratory tests are needed for PIH patients?

- Blood studies—complete blood count (CBC), electrolytes, magnesium level, clotting studies, PT, PTT, platelets, fibrinogen, and fibrin-split products. Platelets are the most important feature of the CBC. If platelet count is $>100,000/mm^3$ then the routine coagulation assessment is unnecessary. The admission platelet count is an excellent predictor of subsequent thrombocytopenia.
- Urine studies—protein, creatinine clearance, 24-hour protein

- Renal function tests—blood urea nitrogen (BUN), creatinine, uric acid plus albumin
- Liver function tests—serum glutamate pyruvate transaminase (SGPT), serum glutamic-oxaloacetic transaminase (SGOT), lactate dehydrogenase (LDH), alkaline phosphatase, total bilirubin
- Fetal well-being—estriol or human placental lactogen, ultrasound, nonstress test, contraction stress test

Chestnut DH (ed): Obstetric Anesthesia: Principles and Practice, p 858. New York, Churchill Livingstone, 1994

Leduc L, Wheeler JM, Kirshon B, et al: Coagulation profile in severe preeclampsia. Obstet Gynecol 79:14–18, 1992

B.3. What are the important routine monitors for PIH patients? When is a central venous pressure (CVP) monitor indicated?

A CVP monitor is indicated in severe preeclampsia with the following conditions:

- Diastolic pressure >105 mm Hg after magnesium treatment
- Persistent oliguria
- Extended use of oxytoxin >10 mU/min to determine if hypertension is caused by pregnancy or oxytoxin antidiuretic hormone (ADH)-like effect
- Receiving antihypertensive in addition to magnesium
- Difficulty in fluid management during delivery and postpartum period. In the immediate postpartum period, the autotransfusion of uterine involution can increase blood volume and cause relative fluid overload.

The important routine monitors are as follows:

- Urine output monitor by Foley catheter
- Noninvasive electronic monitoring of arterial blood pressure
- Invasive intra-arterial line when frequent blood gas analysis is needed such as in pulmonary edema, when using rapid-acting vasodilators such as continuous infusion of nitroprusside, or when using a mechanical ventilator
- Electrocardiogram (ECG) for maternal heartbeat
- Magnesium level 2 hours after starting magnesium sulfate therapy
- Maternal ventilation, deep tendon reflex, and muscle strength
- Uterine contraction monitoring
- Continuous fetal heart rate with cardioscope or internal monitor, or fetal scalp pH

Datta S (ed): Anesthetic and Obstetric Management of High-Risk Pregnancy, 2nd ed, pp 391–393. St. Louis, Mosby-Year Book, 1996

Shnider SM, Levinson G (eds): Anesthesia for Obstetrics, 3rd ed, pp 318–319. Baltimore, Williams & Wilkins, 1993

B.4. What is the significance of the supine pressor response or roll-over test?

The supine pressor response (roll-over) test is noninvasive, simple, reliable, and the only test to predict the clinical course of mild preeclamptic disease. Women who are susceptible to develop severe preeclampsia show an increase of >30 mm Hg of diastolic blood pressure in the supine position after lying in the lateral recumbent position. The test is taken twice. It shows an intrinsic vascular hypersensitivity in these women. Those who have a mild pressor response (between 20 and 29 mm Hg diastolic) develop only mild preeclampsia in the later part of pregnancy. Those who show an elevation of <20 mm Hg diastolic blood pressure are considered negative.

Gant NF: A clinical test useful for predicting the development of acute hypertension in pregnancy. Am J Obstet Gynecol 120:1, 1974

Yemini M: Predictive value of roll-over test in women with mild preeclampsia. Am J Obstet Gynecol 153:77–78, 1985

B.5. What is the contraction stress test (oxytoxin stress test)?

Oxytoxin is given to mimic labor. Three uterine contractions in 10 minutes without fetal rate decelerations related to the contractions is considered a negative test. Three consecutive contractions followed by a "late" deceleration is evidence of uteroplacental insufficiency and delivery is indicated.

Datta S (ed): Anesthetic and Obstetric Management of High-Risk Pregnancy, 2nd ed, p 380. St. Louis. Mosby-Year Book, 1996

B.6. Discuss the treatment of preeclamptic patients.

The aim of therapy is to minimize vasospasm. Treatment is symptomatic, but the definitive treatment is delivery of the fetus and placenta. Treatment is as follows:

- Prevent convulsion by giving magnesium sulfate.
- Improve circulation to the uterus, placenta, and kidneys.
- Administer oxygen and monitor the fetal heart rate.
- Keep the patient in the left lateral decubitus position to prevent aortocaval compression.
- Treat increased blood pressure (to a level not <150/100 mm Hg) to provide adequate perfusion.
- Improve intravascular volume.
- Administer isotonic crystalloid or lactated Ringer's solution at a rate of 75 to 150 ml/h until the urine output is 20 to 30 ml/h. For mild preeclampsia, adequate fluids, a high-protein diet, and adequate salt intake promote diuresis and decrease blood pressure.
- Avoid dextrose in water alone if oxytocin is added to the intravenous solution, to prevent water intoxication and convulsion. When oxytocin is given over 20 mU/min or in lower doses for >24 hours, the antidiuretic effect may be seen. A balanced salt solution such as lactated Ringer's or normal saline is recommended. Rapid infusion of dextrose-containing solution may result in maternal hyperglycemia and neonatal hypoglycemia with hyperbilirubinemia. However, 7 to 10 ml/h of 5% dextrose in 0.45% normal saline is not associated with neonatal hypoglycemia, and it will supply sufficient calories for maternal metabolic needs to prevent maternal ketoacidosis.
- Transfuse blood when the hematocrit is <27%; give blood components when the platelet count is <20,000/mm^3 and when the fibrinogen is <100 mg/dl.

Datta S (ed): Anesthetic and Obstetric Management of High-Risk Pregnancy, 2nd ed, pp 403–405. St. Louis. Mosby-Year Book, 1996

Kenepp NB, Shelley WC, Steven GG et al: Fetal and neonatal hazards of maternal hydration with 5% dextrose before cesarean section. Lancet 1:1150, 1982

Shnider SM, Levinson G (eds): Anesthesia for Obstetrics, 3rd ed, p 319. Baltimore, Williams & Wilkins, 1993

B.7. Why should every incidence of acute hypertension be managed as preeclampsia with the threat of convulsions?

Because 22% of eclamptic patients reported had their first convulsion with a systolic blood pressure that had not even exceeded 140 mm Hg.

Chesley L: History and epidemiology of preeclampsia-eclampsia. Clin Obstet Gynecol 27:801–820, 1984

B.8. In the United States, what is the first line of treatment for preeclampsia? Discuss its actions.

Magnesium sulfate is the initial therapy used to prevent convulsions and hypertension. Eclamptic convulsions are prevented at a plasma magnesium level of 4 to 6 mEq/liter. The actions of magnesium are as follows:

- It is a CNS system depressant and anticonvulsant.
- It inhibits the release of acetylcholine at the neuromuscular junction, decreases the sensitivity of the motor endplate to acetylcholine, and decreases muscle membrane excitability.
- It decreases uterine hyperactivity by its mild relaxant effect on vascular and uterine smooth muscle, thereby improving uterine blood flow.
- It diminishes fibrin deposition and improves renal and hepatic circulation, therefore relieving hepatic pain.
- It is a mild vasodilator in vascular beds (including small diameter cerebral vessels) by a direct or indirect (Ca^{2+} competing) effect; and it has a mild antihypertensive effect.

B.9. What is the suggested regimen using magnesium sulfate?

An initial bolus of 4 to 6 g in a 20% solution is given intravenously over 5 to 20 minutes or 8 to 10 ml of 50% magnesium sulfate in 100 to 250 ml of normal saline over 30 to 45 minutes followed by continuous infusion of 1 to 2 g/h. If the initial treatment of 4 g does not control convulsions, an additional 2 to 4 g can be administered intravenously. If seizures persist, 10 mg of diazepam or 200 mg of thiopental should be slowly infused intravenously.

Datta S (ed): Anesthetic and Obstetric Management of High-risk Pregnancy, 2nd ed, p 405. St. Louis. Mosby-Year Book, 1996

B.10. How would you judge the therapeutic effects of magnesium sulfate?

Clinical signs such as knee jerks (present but hypoactive) and respiratory rate (>10 to 12 per minute) are helpful in monitoring the administration of magnesium sulfate. The absence of deep tendon reflex indicates impending magnesium toxicity, which occurs at about 10 mEq/liter. If urine output is <30 ml/h, decrease or stop magnesium administration. The therapeutic range of plasma level of magnesium is 4 to 8 mEq/

liter. (Normal plasma level is 1.5 to 2 mEq/liter.) The presence of deep tendon reflexes assures the anesthesiologist that the serum magnesium level is <10 mEq/liter.

Datta S (ed): Anesthetic and Obstetric Management of High-Risk Pregnancy, 2nd ed, p 405. St. Louis. Mosby-Year Book, 1996

B.11. What precautions should be taken in using magnesium sulfate?

Magnesium is excreted by the kidneys. It must be used cautiously in patients with preexisting renal disease. Intake and urine output must be monitored with an indwelling Foley catheter.

Magnesium potentiates nondepolarizing and depolarizing muscle relaxants. A nerve stimulator must be used. During surgery, muscle relaxants must be used in smaller doses. Nondepolarizing agents are not necessary prior to administration of succinylcholine because magnesium sulfate attenuates the fasciculations of succinylcholine by its curariform action. It is to be noted that patients with PIH have greater reductions in plasma cholinesterase activity than those in normal pregnancy, resulting in potentiation of succinylcholine independent of magnesium therapy.

Magnesium potentiates the effect of sedatives and narcotics; therefore, their doses must be reduced.

Chestnut DH (ed): Obstetric Anesthesia: Principles and Practice, pp 866–867. New York, Churchill Livingstone, 1994

Kambam JR, Moriton S et al: Effect of preeclampsia on plasma cholinesterase action. Can J Anaesth 34:509–511, 1987

Malinow AM: Preeclampsia and Eclampsia: Anesthetic Management. ASA Annual Refresher Course Lectures #511, American Society of Anesthesiologists, 1996

Miller RD (ed): Anesthesia, 4th ed, pp 2061–2062. New York, Churchill Livingstone, 1994

B.12. How would you avoid magnesium toxicity?

Parenterally administered magnesium is cleared almost totally by the kidneys. Toxicity is avoided by ensuring, before administering the next dose, that urine flow was at least 100 ml during the previous 4 hours, the patellar reflex is present, and there is no respiratory depression. Magnesium level must be measured 2 hours after starting magnesium therapy.

Chestnut DH (ed): Obstetric Anesthesia: Principles and Practice, pp 875–878. New York, Churchill Livingstone, 1994

Cunningham LG, MacDonald PG, Gant NF: Williams' Obstetrics, 18th ed, pp 680–682. Norwalk, CT, Appleton & Lange, 1989

B.13. What are the effects of increasing plasma magnesium levels?

Magnesium causes a transient decrease in uterine contraction frequency during and immediately after the initial loading dose. With high concentrations, it has been demonstrated to depress myometrial contractility both in vivo and in vitro. At 5 to 10 mEq/liter, prolonged P-Q intervals and widened QRS complexes are seen; at 10 mEq/liter, a loss of deep tendon reflexes occurs; at 15 mEq/liter, sinoatrial and atrioventricular block and respiratory paralysis occurs; and at 25 mEq/liter, cardiac arrest ensue.

Miller RD (ed): Anesthesia, 4th ed, p 2062. New York, Churchill Livingstone, 1994

B.14. Discuss the treatment of magnesium toxicity.

Magnesium sulfate should be withheld. However, a risk is seen in giving calcium to the mother because it will antagonize the anticonvulsant effect of magnesium. Except in cases of gross magnesium overdosing and cardiac depression, it is probably safer to support the mother's depressed respiration with a respirator and to avoid calcium. For respiratory arrest, prompt endotracheal intubation and ventilation are lifesaving.

McCubbin JH, Sibai BM, Abdella TN et al: Cardiopulmonary arrest due to acute maternal hypermagnesemia. Lancet 1:1058, 1981

Shnider SM, Levinson G (eds): Anesthesia for Obstetrics, 3rd ed, p 316. Baltimore, Williams & Wilkins, 1993

B.15. What are the effects of magnesium sulfate on the fetus?

Magnesium sulfate crosses the placenta. If given as a large single IV, magnesium sulfate can transiently cause a loss of beat-to-beat variability in the fetal heart rate. Hypermagnesemia results in a drowsy neonate with decreased muscle tone and hypoventilation requiring assisted ventilation. Intravenous calcium may partially overcome these effects. It is given in a dose of 20 mg/kg of 10% calcium chloride or 60 mg/kg of 10% calcium gluconate.

Chestnut DH (ed): Obstetric Anesthesia: Principles and Practice, pp 866–867. New York, Churchill Livingstone, 1994

Cunningham LG, MacDonald PG, Gant NF: Williams' Obstetrics, 18th ed, p 683. Norwalk, CT, Appleton & Lange, 1989

Gregory GA (ed): Pediatric Anesthesia, 2nd ed, p 600. New York, Churchill Livingstone, 1989

Miller RD (ed): Anesthesia, 4th ed, pp 2061–2062. New York, Churchill Livingstone, 1994

B.16. When is diazepam useful in preeclamptic patients?

When the patient shows premonitory signs of CNS irritability, such as headache, tremulousness or hyperreflexia, abdominal pain unrelated to uterine activity, or a sharp increase in blood pressure, diazepam should be given IV in a dose of 5 to 10 mg. It is used as an anticonvulsant throughout much of the world.

Chestnut DH (ed): Obstetric Anesthesia: Principles and Practice, p 875. New York, Churchill Livingstone, 1994

Crawford JS: Principles and Practice of Obstetric Anaesthesia, 5th ed, p 360. Oxford, Blackwell, 1984

B.17. What are the side-effects of diazepam on neonates?

Diazepam crosses the placenta rapidly. Although the neonate is capable of metabolizing small doses of diazepam, when the total maternal dosage during labor exceeds 30 mg, the newborn can manifest neonatal hypotonia, poor feeding, lethargy, apneic spells, hypothermia, and loss of heat regulation.

Chestnut DH (ed): Obstetric Anesthesia: Principles and Practice, pp 70–232. New York, Churchill Livingstone, 1994

B.18. If the patient is having an eclamptic fit, what is the immediate therapy?

- Initially, intravenous administration of 50 to 100 mg thiopental to terminate the convulsion. Further convulsions are treated with diazepam or magnesium sulfate.
- Maintain adequate airway. Give oxygen to prevent hypoxia. Turn the patient to her left side, with head-down tilt, and elevate the chin. An endotracheal tube should be placed following administration of succinylcholine and cricoid pressure.
- Bicarbonate may be needed after arterial blood gases and *p*H are determined, because convulsions are often associated with metabolic acidosis.

Chestnut DH (ed): Obstetric Anesthesia: Principles and Practice, pp 70–232. New York, Churchill Livingstone, 1994

Crawford JS: Principles and Practice of Obstetric Anaesthesia, 5th ed, p 360. Oxford, Blackwell, 1984

B.19. When is an antihypertensive agent indicated? How much can the diastolic blood pressure be lowered? Why?

An antihypertensive agent is indicated when the maternal blood pressure is 170/100 mm Hg or when the diastolic is >110 mm Hg despite treatment with magnesium or diazepam. It is given to lessen the risk of maternal CNS hemorrhage.

The goal is to maintain the diastolic blood pressure at 95 to 100 mm Hg. Therefore, it should not be lowered to <90 mm Hg. Fetal distress will result from a sudden drop in the maternal blood pressure, leading to inadequate perfusion to the fetus.

The aim of an antihypertensive agent is to produce a partial return of blood pressure to the patient's normal level or to obtain a diastolic pressure <110 mm Hg until after delivery.

Shnider SM, Levinson G (eds): Anesthesia for Obstetrics, 3rd ed, p 316. Baltimore, Williams & Wilkins, 1993

B.20. What are the most common antihypertensive agents used to lower blood pressure?

Hydralazine is the most common antihypertensive agent used because of its rapid onset, short duration, and direct vasodilating effect that increases renal and uterine blood flow. Any blood pressure >170/110 mm Hg requires treatment with an antihypertensive agent. The full extent of its effect is evident in 20 minutes; therefore, if sufficient time is not allowed between injections, severe hypotension will be seen. It is used in 5 to 10 mg increments IV every 20 to 30 minutes until the diastolic blood pressure is lowered. The maximal dose is 200 mg/d. Blood pressure should be maintained at a level not <120/90 mm Hg during therapy.

Hydralazine directly decreases peripheral vascular resistance. Reflex sympathetic activity can result in tachycardia and in increased stroke volume and cardiac output. This can be corrected with propranolol, providing the mother does not have asthma. Propranolol given to the mother can result in fetal bradycardia. Therefore, caution should be exercised. Hydralazine can also cause fetal hypotension if maternal blood pressure suddenly drops. The patient may complain of headache and flushing of face during its therapy.

Labetalol is the next commonly used drug. When given in an initial IV bolus dose of 10 to 20 mg, it has a faster onset of action than hydralazine. It is useful in the management of refractory hypertension. If necessary, the dose is doubled every 10 minutes to a maximal dose of 220 to 300 mg. It can be administered by continuous IV infusion, starting at 40 mg/h, with the dose doubled every 30 minutes until a satisfactory response is achieved, up to a maximal dose of 160 mg/h.

Chestnut DH (ed): Obstetric Anesthesia: Principles and Practice, p 860. New York, Churchill Livingstone, 1994

Ramanathan S (ed): Obstetric Anesthesia, p 151. Philadelphia, Lea & Febiger, 1988

Shnider SM, Levinson G (eds): Anesthesia for Obstetrics, 3rd ed, pp 316–317. Baltimore, Williams & Wilkins, 1993

C. Intraoperative Management

C.1. What is your choice of anesthesia for PIH patients?

Continuous lumbar epidural anesthesia is the best technique for managing patients with PIH, provided that the coagulation profile is acceptable, circulating volume is adequately maintained, maternal blood pressure is controlled, and aortocaval compression is avoided.

Chestnut DH (ed): Obstetric Anesthesia: Principles and Practice, p 867. New York, Churchill Livingstone, 1994

Malinow AM: Preeclampsia and Eclampsia: Anesthetic Management. ASA Annual Refresher Course Lectures #511, American Society of Anesthesiologists, 1996

C.2. Is epidural anesthesia advisable for patients with high blood pressure? What are the advantages?

Epidural anesthesia should not be used to correct hypertension, but its use provides the following advantages:

- Epidural analgesia can produce complete pain relief and negate the need for maternal narcotics, which depress ventilation and adversely affects the premature fetus.
- It prevents the increase in blood pressure associated with bearing down, avoiding increased CSF pressure, which can climb >50 mm Hg with expulsive efforts.
- Epidural anesthesia can abolish the neurally imposed vasoconstrictor tone of placental spiral arteries, and it reduces the circulating catecholamines that occur with anxiety and labor pain. Intervillous blood flow and renal blood flow are improved.
- It can provide excellent conditions for forceps delivery, which avoids prolonged maternal pushing accompanied by marked fluctuations in cardiovascular functions.
- In epidural anesthesia without hypotension, the condition of the newborn at birth is better, even if uterine-incision delivery time is prolonged.

- Epidural anesthesia results in a slower onset of sympathetic blockade and hypotension, avoiding the sudden drop in blood pressure seen in spinal anesthesia. In preeclamptic patients, who already have reduced uteroplacental perfusion, a sudden drop in blood pressure of 30% below preblock value may not be tolerated by the fetus. Epidural anesthesia lowers the baseline blood pressure of the patient only moderately.
- It prevents precipitous delivery of a preterm or small neonate which is associated with neonatal intracerebral hemorrhage.
- It can result in stable cardiac output. Because preeclamptic women are at increased risk for cesarean section, early administration of epidural analgesia facilitates the subsequent administration of epidural anesthesia for emergency cesarean section.

Newsome LR, Bramwell RS, Curling PE: Severe preeclampsia: Hemodynamic effects of lumbar epidural anesthesia. Anesth Analg 65:31–36, 1986

Shnider SM, Levinson G (eds): Anesthesia for Obstetrics, 3rd ed, p 321. Baltimore, Williams & Wilkins, 1993

C.3. What is the advantage of prehydration?

Prehydration improves urinary output and prevents dramatic falls in blood pressure. Volume loading is a short-term therapy to enable the patient to tolerate the trespasses of anesthesia. Care must be taken to prevent cardiovascular volume excess, which can lead to pulmonary edema, ascites, and pleural effusion.

Katz J, Benumof J, Kadis LB (eds): Anesthesia and Uncommon Diseases: Pathophysiologic and Clinical Correlations, 3rd ed, p 162. Philadelphia, WB Saunders, 1990

C.4. How should patients be hydrated before epidural anesthesia?

In mild preeclampsia, prehydration is accomplished with 10 to 15 ml/kg crystalloid. In severe preeclampsia, the patient should be prehydrated to a central venous pressure of 3 to 4 cm H_2O or a PCWP of 5 to 12 mm Hg. Without CVP monitoring, prehydrate with a 500 ml solution containing 250 ml of plasmanate and 250 ml of lactated Ringer's solution. Crystalloid should be limited to 1 liter, and if more fluid is required, colloid in the form of 25% albumin in <50 ml should be infused.

Chestnut DH (ed): Obstetric Anesthesia: Principles and Practice, p 872. New York, Churchill Livingstone, 1994

Shnider SM, Levinson G (eds): Anesthesia for Obstetrics, 3rd ed, pp 321–324. Baltimore, Williams & Wilkins, 1993

C.5. What precautions should be taken when a patient who is receiving an antihypertensive drug is also going to have an epidural block?

The dose of antihypertensive drug, such as hydralazine, should be reduced before epidural block is instituted and before each top-up epidural dose, because of the dangers of a superimposition of a fall in blood pressure on a level already considerably lowered by the antihypertensive medication.

Chestnut DH (ed): Obstetric Anesthesia: Principles and Practice, p 872. New York, Churchill Livingstone, 1994

C.6. What level of epidural anesthesia should be reached in preeclamptic patients?

The level of epidural anesthesia for preeclamptic patients is not different from that for normotensive patients. For labor pain, the segmental band of T10 to L1 provides analgesia for uterine contractions. As the second stage of labor is entered, the block can be extended to the perineum (S1–S5). Fentanyl, 50 to 75 μg, is added to the local anesthetic. For cesarean section, the block is extended gradually to T2 to T4; the blood pressure must not drop suddenly. Left uterine displacement should be maintained at all times until delivery. When the epidural level reaches T8, it can denervate the uterus, kidneys, and adrenal glands, thereby facilitating blood pressure control and improving uterine perfusion.

Chestnut DH (ed): Obstetric Anesthesia: Principles and Practice, p 867. New York, Churchill Livingstone, 1994

Jouppila P, Jouppila R, Hollman A et al: Lumbar epidural analgesia to improve intervillous blood flow during labor in severe preeclampsia. Obstet Gynecol 59:159, 1982

C.7. What local anesthetics are used in obstetric anesthesia? Discuss their advantages and disadvantages.

Three local anesthetics commonly used in obstetric anesthesia are 2-chloroprocaine, lidocaine, and bupivacaine.

2-Chloroprocaine
2-Chloroprocaine (Nesacaine) is an ester type of local anesthetic. It is hydrolyzed by plasma cholinesterase, and it has a rapid plasma metabolism, making it the drug of choice whenever fetal local anesthetic plasma concentrations are of concern (e.g., acid trapping of local anesthetics across the placenta causing fetal acidosis). It is used in a 1.5% to 2% solution for labor pain and a 3% solution for cesarean section. It has a fast onset, low toxicity, and is a high quality block. Its duration of action is 40 to 60 minutes.

Lidocaine
Lidocaine (Xylocaine) is an amide type of local anesthetic, which is 65% maternal plasma protein-bound, and it is metabolized by the liver microsomes. It is used in a 1% to 1.5% solution for labor pain, and a 2% solution for cesarean section. Tachyphylaxis occurs with three to five repeated doses. Lidocaine used without epinephrine has a higher systemic absorption rate, increased toxicity, and shorter duration of action. Lidocaine 2% with 1:200,000 epinephrine is an excellent epidural anesthetic for cesarean section, with reliability of onset and spread of anesthetic similar to 2-chloroprocaine, but with a longer duration of action (70 to 90 minutes). With epinephrine, a 500 mg epidural injection results in a plasma concentration of 2 to 4 μg/ml, which is below the convulsive threshold (10 to 12 μg/ml).

Bupivacaine
Bupivacaine (Marcaine) is another amide type of local anesthetic that has a long duration of action (90 to 180 minutes) when used in the epidural space. It is four times more potent than lidocaine. It is 90% to 95% bound to maternal plasma protein.

The intravascular injection of bupivacaine 0.75% has caused cardiac arrest and resulted in 15 maternal deaths and 4 cases of permanent brain damage since 1973. It is known to be more cardiotoxic than lidocaine. The mechanism relates to its action on cardiac sodium channels. Bupivacaine and lidocaine both block sodium channels to the nerves and heart. They are similar in that they both cause a rapid block of cardiac sodium channels on depolarization. They differ in their recovery from block. The lidocaine block is complete within less than a second, whereas bupivacaine takes five times longer. Bupivacaine is a "fast-in, slow-out" agent. Its main advantage is that it has a longer duration and a weak motor block when given in analgesic concentrations. Perineal anesthesia can be obtained after two to three repeated doses without the patient sitting up. The incidence of hypotension is lower because of its slow onset, but the time to reach surgical anesthesia is longer too. The 0.25% solution is used for labor pain; a 0.5% solution is used for cesarean section. Bupivacaine has become the choice of local anesthetic in labor. It provides potent analgesia with less motor block when used in dilute solutions (i.e., 0.0625% or 0.125%) plus fentanyl (2 to 4 µg/ml, a total dose of 100 µg) through the continuous epidural infusion at an initial rate of 10 ml/h.

Albright GA, Ferguson JE II, Joyce TH III et al (eds): Anesthesia in Obstetrics: Maternal, Fetal, and Neonatal Aspects, 2nd ed, pp 123–127. Boston, Butterworth, 1986

Chestnut DH (ed): Obstetric Anesthesia: Principles and Practice, p 867. New York, Churchill Livingstone, 1994

C.8. Is the addition of epinephrine to local anesthetics advisable in preeclamptic patients?

The addition of epinephrine to reduce the blood level of local anesthetics and to intensify the epidural block is not advisable in preeclamptic patients. These patients are unusually sensitive to its chronotropic properties, and they respond with acute severe hypertension if there is an inadvertent intravascular injection during the epidural procedure. However, available data indicate that preeclampsia does not increase the incidence of adverse reactions to anesthetic with epinephrine when injected into the epidural space. Therefore, most local anesthetics are now added with 1:400,000 epinephrine.

Datta S (ed): Anesthetic and Obstetric Management of High-Risk Pregnancy, 2nd ed, p 396. St. Louis, Mosby-Year Book, 1996

Miller RD (ed): Anesthesia, 4th ed, pp 2057, 2063. New York, Churchill Livingstone, 1994

C.9. What is the treatment for the asphyxic fetal heart rate pattern seen with maternal hypotension after epidural anesthesia is instituted?

- Administration of oxygen with face mask
- Left uterine displacement
- Increase in hydration
- Elevation of lower extremities to facilitate venous return
- Administration of small increments of ephedrine (2.5 mg IV) if the blood pressure falls significantly, resulting in late deceleration or decreases by >20% of control, and all conservative measures fail

Miller RD (ed): Anesthesia, 4th ed, p 2053. New York, Churchill Livingstone, 1994

C.10. What would you do after an inadvertent spinal tap? How do you treat spinal headache?

Inadvertent spinal tap is treated by repositioning the epidural needle in another interspace, preferably the higher space, and cautiously administering the local anesthetic by means of a catheter. This can result in confusing signs of partial spinal anesthesia from leakage of the epidural drug through the dural hole. After delivery of the fetus, when anesthesia wears off, 30 ml increments of preservative-free normal saline can be injected epidurally to a total of 100 to 120 ml or until the patient has a sensation of neck pressure. This is a prophylactic measure to prevent postspinal tap headache. The incidence of spinal headache is 70% with an 18-gauge epidural needle. If headache occurs, the patient should be well hydrated with 6 liters of fluid daily. Analgesics and an abdominal binder can be used. If headache persists after 24 to 48 hours, epidural blood patch (12 to 15 ml) has given good results. The blood patch can be repeated. The best result occurs when it is injected at the same level as the dural tap. The patient is instructed to lie supine for 60 minutes before ambulation. Immediate relief occurs in 80% to 100% of patients. Transient side-effects are backache, neck ache, paresthesia of legs and toes, and a crampy abdominal sensation.

Albright GA, Ferguson JE II, Joyce TH III et al (eds): Anesthesia in Obstetrics: Maternal, Fetal, and Neonatal Aspects, 2nd ed, pp 257–344. Boston, Butterworth, 1986

C.11. How would you manage total spinal anesthesia?

- Maintain venous return by left uterine displacement, Trendelenburg position and crystalloid IV fluids.
- Ventilate with oxygen and intubate after oxygenating.
- Give ephedrine for hypotension.
- Give anesthesia when stable (if necessary).
- Within 10 to 20 minutes after stabilization of ventilation and circulation, withdraw CSF using the epidural catheter (twice the volume of local anesthetic that was accidentally injected). At least 10 ml should be withdrawn; replace with two to three times the volume of preservative-free normal saline or lactated Ringer's solution.

Covino BG, Marx GF, Finster M, et al: Prolonged sensory motor deficits following inadvertent spinal anesthesia. Anesth Analg 59:399, 1980

Shnider SM, Levinson G (eds): Anesthesia for Obstetrics, 3rd ed, p 142. Baltimore, Williams & Wilkins, 1993

C.12. When and how would you give spinal anesthesia?

Spinal anesthesia can be used in a mild case or in women with incipient coagulopathy, because the technique does not involve the use of a catheter, which can lacerate a vein. To prevent sudden hypotension, the crystalloid preload (10 to 15 ml/kg) is added to 250 to 500 ml of 5% albumin. Hyperbaric bupivacaine 0.75% in dose of 1.5 to 1.6 ml (11.25 to 12 mg) added with 12.5 to 25 µg of fentanyl and 0.25 to 0.3 mg of morphine.

Chestnut DH (ed): Obstetric Anesthesia: Principles and Practice, p 872. New York, Churchill Livingstone, 1994

C.13. What is HELLP syndrome and what is its importance?

HELLP is the syndrome of hemolysis, elevated liver enzyme, and low platelets presented by a unique group of preeclamptic/eclamptic patients with or without the usual clinical findings of PIH. It is often misdiagnosed as a disorder unrelated to pregnancy. It can occur antepartum or postpartum. Recognizing this syndrome is important to prevent maternal and neonatal death. Findings include:

- Hemolysis (H)—The peripheral blood smear shows microangiopathic hemolytic anemia with "burr" cells (crenated, contracted, distorted red blood cells (RBC) with spiny projections along the periphery); schistocytes (small, irregularly shaped RBC fragments; polychromasia. There is normal PT, PTT and fibrinogen in 96% of patients.
- Elevated liver enzymes (EL)—abnormal function tests with elevated SGOT, SGPT, and hyperbilirubinemia (especially indirect bilirubin); elevated BUN and creatinine in half the cases.
- Low platelets (LP)—thrombocytopenia of <100,000/mm^3. The main symptoms are malaise, nausea, epigastric pain, and edema. Hypertension may not be seen. One maternal death occurred with a maximal elevation of blood pressure recorded as 140/95 mm Hg. Once the diagnosis is made, expedite delivery. Prolonged induction of labor should be avoided. The patient who has excessive bleeding should receive platelet transfusion if the platelet count is <20,000/mm^3. Because of continued hemolysis with a hematocrit drop during the postpartum period, packed RBC transfusions are necessary.

Weinstein L: Preeclampsia/eclampsia with hemolysis, elevated liver enzymes and thrombocytopenia. Obstet Gynecol 66:657, 1985

Weinstein L: Syndrome of hemolysis, elevated liver enzymes, and low platelet count: A severe consequence of hypertension in pregnancy. Am J Obstet Gynecol 142:159, 1982

C.14. What are the modifications of a standard general anesthesia technique in PIH patients?

- Use a smaller endotracheal tube because of the exaggerated edema of the upper airway.
- Defasciculation prior to succinylcholine is not necessary if the patient is receiving magnesium sulfate.
- Administer lidocaine (100 mg IV) 3 to 5 minutes before induction to prevent rise of blood pressure during intubation.
- Administer succinylcholine (1.5 mg/kg) to ensure rapid complete relaxation for intubation.
- Titrate the dose of muscle relaxants, nondepolarizing and depolarizing, because of the interactions with magnesium sulfate. Use a nerve stimulator before injecting additional muscle relaxant.
- Avoid potentiating nephrotoxic or hypertensive drugs, such as methoxyflurane or ketamine, exceeding 0.75 mg/kg.
- Use a low dose (i.e., two thirds minimal alveolar concentration) of desflurane, sevoflurane, enflurane, or isoflurane to prevent intraoperative hypertension, but remember to discontinue early to prevent uterine relaxation.
- Magnesium sulfate should not be discontinued during the intraoperative and postoperative period.

- Antihypertensive drugs can be given as required.

Shnider SM, Levinson G (eds): Anesthesia for Obstetrics, 3rd ed, p 325. Baltimore, Williams & Wilkins, 1993

C.15. How would you control intraoperative hypertension during general anesthesia for cesarean section?

One of the following methods can be used to prevent or control hypertension:

- Hydralazine (5 to 10 mg IV) is given 10 to 15 minutes before the induction of anesthesia.
- Lidocaine (100 mg) is given 3 to 5 minutes before induction of anesthesia.
- Trimethaphan can be used for hypertensive crisis (1 to 4 mg) IV boluses or infusions (500 mg in 250 ml of 5% dextrose). It does not decrease autoregulation of cerebral blood flow and its greater molecular weight can limit placental transfer. It is hydrolyzed by plasma cholinesterase.
- Labetalol (10 to 20 mg), followed by increments of 10 mg up to a maximum of 1 to 3 mg/kg may attenuate hypertensive response to intubation without adverse neonatal effects.
- Nitroglycerin can be used at 5 to 50 μg/min just before direct laryngoscopy.
- Sodium nitroprusside can be used if an arterial line is present.

Shnider SM, Levinson G (eds): Anesthesia for Obstetrics, 3rd ed, pp 326–329. Baltimore, Williams & Wilkins, 1993

C.16. What are the disadvantages of trimethaphan?

- It is associated with histamine release, tachycardia, and tachyphylaxis.
- It causes vasodilatation, resulting in reduced venous return.
- It inhibits plasma pseudocholinesterase and can prolong the action duration of succinylcholine, but this is not a problem clinically.

Datta S (ed): Anesthetic and Obstetric Management of High-Risk Pregnancy, 2nd ed, p 403. St. Louis, Mosby-Year Book, 1996

C.17. What are the advantages and disadvantages of nitroglycerin and nitroprusside?

The advantages of nitroglycerin and nitroprusside are their rapid onset and short duration of action, providing minute-to-minute control of blood pressure. They do not decrease uterine blood flow despite a 20% decrease in perfusion pressure.

The disadvantage is that prolonged use of nitroprusside can result in fetal cyanide intoxication.

Shnider SM, Levinson G (eds): Anesthesia for Obstetrics, 3rd ed, pp 316–317. Baltimore, Williams & Wilkins, 1993

C.18. Should ergometrine (Ergotrate) be given to preeclamptic patients?

Only under the most unusual circumstances of uterine atony that is unresponsive to all other therapeutic measures should ergometrine be given. It can induce vomiting, further increase in blood pressure, and initiate eclampsia.

Crawford JS: Principles and Practice of Obstetric Anaesthesia, 5th ed, p 352. Oxford, Blackwell, 1984

D. Postoperative Management

D.1. Discuss the postpartum care of preeclamptic patients.

- Continue magnesium sulfate for 24 hours and, for eclamptic patients, for another 24 hours after the last postpartum convulsion. Twenty-five percent of eclampsia occurs in the puerperium; therefore, continuous monitoring is required.
- Continue hydralazine or substitute with another long-acting antihypertensive agent, such as methyldopa.
- Pain medications are required to avoid further convulsions; avoid Ergotrate or aspirin. Epidural narcotic (e.g., morphine) can provide sustained postoperative analgesia.
- Maintain IV fluids—lactated Ringer's solution with 5% dextrose at 60 to 150 ml/h, unless there is unusual fluid loss from vomiting, diarrhea, and diaphoresis, or excessive blood loss. An appreciable fall in blood pressure soon after delivery is due to excessive blood loss and not to miraculous dissolution of the vasospastic disease. When oliguria follows and the hematocrit decreases, then blood transfusion is indicated.

Shnider SM, Levinson G (eds): Anesthesia for Obstetrics, 3rd ed, p 327. Baltimore, Williams & Wilkins, 1993

37 Breech Presentation, Fetal Distress, and Mitral Stenosis

Jill Fong

A 25-year-old unregistered primigravida at 38 weeks gestation presented to the labor room in labor. The patient had a history of rheumatic fever with no subsequent medical follow-up and had a diastolic murmur. She was attached to an external fetal heart rate (FHR) monitor and tocodynamometer; severe variable deceleration was noted. Simultaneously, the patient was found to have ruptured membranes, meconium-stained amniotic fluid, a fetal foot in her vagina, and a prolapsed umbilical cord. She was rushed to the operating room for an emergency cesarean section. Blood pressure, 100/60 mm Hg; regular pulse, 100 beats/min; respiratory rate, 18 breaths/min.

A. Medical Disease and Differential Diagnosis

1. How are fetal lie, presentation, and position defined and determined?
2. What is the approximate frequency of the various lies and presentations at or near term?
3. What are the different types of breech presentation, and what is their incidence?
4. What is the cause of breech presentation?
5. What are the problems associated with breech presentation?
6. What is the incidence of heart disease in pregnancy?
7. What are maternal and fetal mortality rates with maternal cardiac disease?
8. What is the functional classification of heart disease by the New York Heart Association (NYHA)?
9. What are the cardiovascular changes of pregnancy?
10. What changes can normally occur in heart sounds during pregnancy?
11. What are the physiologic consequences of mitral stenosis?
12. What are the auscultation findings associated with mitral stenosis?
13. What may be seen on the electrocardiogram in patients with mitral stenosis?
14. What is the effect of the physiologic changes of pregnancy on patients with mitral stenosis?
15. What are the determinants of fetal oxygenation?
16. What are the determinants of uterine blood flow?

B. Preoperative Evaluation and Preparation

1. How is fetal well-being assessed during labor?
2. How are FHR and maternal contractions monitored?
3. What is the normal FHR with beat-to-beat variability?
4. What are transient or periodic decelerations?
5. How accurate is FHR monitoring in predicting fetal well-being?

6. What is the significance of the fetal scalp capillary blood sample? What are the normal values of fetal blood gases?
7. Can fetal scalp capillary blood pH sampling give false signals?
8. What are the causes of acute fetal distress?
9. What is the significance of meconium-stained amniotic fluid?
10. What is meconium aspiration syndrome?
11. What is the proposed cause of meconium aspiration syndrome?
12. What are the usual noninvasive tests used to evaluate the pregnant cardiac patient?
13. What preoperative medications would you give this patient?

C. Intraoperative Management

1. What monitors would you use in the NYHA class II patient during her cesarean section?
2. When would one use invasive monitoring in a pregnant patient with cardiac disease?
3. What are the hemodynamic goals of intraoperative management of the pregnant patient with mitral stenosis?
4. What anesthetic technique would you use for this emergency cesarean section?
5. What technique could you use for this general anesthesia?
6. Would this patient benefit from the use of beta-blockade?
7. What is the effect of the inhalation agents on uterine contractility?
8. What is the Apgar scoring system?
9. What is the significance of Apgar scores?
10. At birth, what should be done to minimize the infant's risk of meconium aspiration syndrome?
11. The Apgar score of the newborn was 3 at 1 minute. How would you treat the newborn?

D. Postoperative Management

1. Immediately after the baby was delivered, the patient's oxygen saturation decreased. What is the differential diagnosis?
2. If you had been unable to intubate this patient, how would you have managed the airway?

A. Medical Disease and Differential Diagnosis

A.1. How are fetal lie, presentation, and position defined and determined?

Fetal lie is the relation of the long axis of the fetus to the long axis of the mother. Longitudinal, transverse, and oblique lies exist. Longitudinal lies are either cephalic or pelvic (breech), depending on which fetal structure enters the maternal pelvis. Oblique lie results when the long axis of the fetus is at an acute angle to that of the mother. It is usually only transitory and converts to a transverse or longitudinal lie when labor begins.

Presentation describes the part of the fetus that is lowermost in the pelvis: cephalic, breech, or shoulder. Cephalic presentations are further subdivided into vertex, brow, and face presentations.

Position of the presenting part is described as a relationship between a certain pole of the presenting part and the surrounding pelvis.

Fetal lie, presentation, and position can often be determined by manual pelvic and abdominal examinations. Ultrasonography is also useful, especially when palpation is inconclusive, as with multiple gestations, placenta preavia, and hydramnios.

Cunningham FG, MacDonald PC, Gant NF et al: Williams' Obstetrics, 20th ed, pp 251–260. Stamford, CT, Appleton & Lange, 1997

A.2. What is the approximate frequency of the various lies and presentations at or near term?

Vertex presentation, 96%; breech presentation, 3% to 5%; transverse lie, 0.3%; and face presentation, 0.3%.

Cunningham FG, MacDonald PC, Gant NF et al: Williams Obstetrics, 20th ed, p 436. Stamford, CT, Appleton & Lange, 1997

A.3. What are the different types of breech presentation, and what is their incidence?

- Frank breech—Both fetal lower extremities are flexed at the hips and extended at the knees. The incidence is 60%.
- Complete breech—The knees are flexed, as are the hips. The incidence is 10%.
- Incomplete or footling breech—One or both hips are extended and a foot or knee hangs below the breech. The incidence is 30%.

Shnider SM, Levinson G (eds): Anesthesia for Obstetrics, 3rd ed, pp 297, 298. Baltimore, Williams & Wilkins, 1993

A.4. What is the cause of breech presentation?

The cause is unknown, but certain factors are associated with this presentation including prematurity, hydramnios, oligohydramnios, multiparity, multiple fetuses, hydrocephalus, anencephalus, myomas, placenta previa, cornual-fundal placenta implantation, and previous breech delivery.

Cunningham FG, MacDonald PC, Gant NF et al: Williams' Obstetrics, 20th ed, p 435. Stamford, CT, Appleton & Lange, 1997

A.5. What are the problems associated with breech presentation?

With breech presentation is found an increased incidence of prolapsed cord, perinatal morbidity and mortality due to difficult delivery, low birth weight, fetal anomalies, placenta previa, uterine anomalies, and operative intervention.

Chestnut DH (ed): Obstetric Anesthesia: Principles and Practice, p 671. St. Louis, Mosby, 1994

Cunningham FG, MacDonald PC, Gant NF et al: Williams' Obstetrics, 20th ed, p 435. Stamford, CT, Appleton & Lange, 1997

A.6. What is the incidence of heart disease in pregnancy?

The incidence of heart disease in pregnancy varies from 1.6% to 3.6%. Rheumatic heart disease accounts for approximately 75% of the heart disease in pregnancy. Of the patients with rheumatic heart disease, 90% have mitral stenosis. Congenital heart disease comprises the other 25% of heart disease in pregnancy.

Shnider SM, Levinson G (eds): Anesthesia for Obstetrics, 3rd ed, pp 485, 486. Baltimore, Williams & Wilkins, 1993

A.7. What are maternal and fetal mortality rates with maternal cardiac disease?

Both maternal and fetal mortality rates are increased in patients with cardiac disease. The incidence varies depending on the severity of maternal cardiac disease. With rheumatic heart disease the incidence of mortality varies from 1% in asymptomatic patients to 17% in those patients with mitral stenosis and atrial fibrillation. Fetal mortality is approximately 3.5%. Additionally, 5% to 10% of pregnant cardiac patients fall into NYHA class III or IV. These patients have a 75% to 90% maternal mortality rate and high fetal loss.

James FM, Wheeler AS, Dewan DM (eds): Obstetric Anesthesia: The Complicated Patient, 2nd ed, p 162. Philadelphia, FA Davis, 1988

Shnider SM, Levinson G (eds): Anesthesia for Obstetrics, 3rd ed, pp 485, 486. Baltimore, Williams & Wilkins, 1993

A.8. What is the functional classification of heart disease by the New York Heart Association?

The New York Heart Association classification of a complete diagnosis of cardiovascular disease has changed since 1973. Prior to 1973 the categories were etiology, anatomy, physiology, functional capacity, and therapeutic. The new categories are etiology, anatomy, physiology, cardiac status, and prognosis. For patients with angina pectoris, the Canadian Cardiovascular Society classification is used commonly to describe the amount of effort needed to produce angina. The grading of dyspnea and fatigue caused by heart failure is often still classified using the old functional NYHA classification.

Class I—No limitation of physical activity.
Class II—Slight limitation of physical activity. Symptoms with ordinary activity.
Class III—Marked limitation of physical activity. Symptoms with less than ordinary activity.
Class IV—Unable to carry on any physical activity without discomfort. Symptoms may be present at rest.

Cunningham FG, MacDonald PC, Gant NF et al: Williams' Obstetrics, 20th ed, p 1081. Stamford, CT, Appleton & Lange, 1997

Hurst JW et al (eds): The Heart, 8th ed, pp 201–203. New York, McGraw-Hill, 1994

A.9. What are the cardiovascular changes of pregnancy?

During the first trimester of pregnancy, the cardiac output increases to 30% to 40% above normal and plateaus at approximately 28 weeks gestation. It remains stable until the traditional stresses imposed by labor increase it further. The increase in cardiac output is due to a 30% increase in stroke volume and a 15% increase in heart rate. During labor and immediately postpartum, cardiac output increases 30% to 40% and 60% to 80%, respectively. Blood pressure, however, is not elevated because peripheral vascular resistance decreases.

James FM, Wheeler AS, Dewan DM (eds): Obstetric Anesthesia: The Complicated Patient, 2nd ed, p 166. Philadelphia, FA Davis, 1988

Walters WAW, MacGregor WG, Hill M: Cardiac output at rest during pregnancy and the puerperium. Clin Sci 30:1–11, 1966

A.10. *What changes may normally occur in heart sounds during pregnancy?*

In a study of 50 normal pregnant women at varying stages in pregnancy, a phonocardiographic study found that the first heart sound may have an exaggerated split with increased loudness of both components. In up to 84% of pregnant patients, a third heart sound is also evident. Functional systolic murmurs, which disappear shortly after delivery, occur in >90% of pregnant women. Soft transient diastolic murmurs occur in 20% of these women, and 10% have continuous murmurs apparently arising from the breast vasculature. These murmurs alone, therefore, are not indicative of organic heart disease. Similarly, venous distention, tachycardia, edema, and breathlessness, which may be seen with pregnancy, are not signs of heart disease.

Cutforth R, MacDonald CB: Heart sounds and murmurs in pregnancy. Am Heart J 71:741, 1966

A.11. *What are the physiologic consequence of mitral stenosis?*

The normal mitral valve orifice area is 4 to 6 cm^2. With mitral stenosis the valve area is reduced. When the valve area reaches 2 cm^2, cardiovascular hemodynamics become impaired. As the area decreases further to 1 cm^2, left atrial pressure increases to about 25 mm Hg to maintain an adequate cardiac output. Left ventricular diastolic pressure is usually normal, and the diastolic atrioventricular pressure gradient is the hemodynamic hallmark of this condition. Pulmonary venous and capillary pressures increase, leading to exertional dyspnea. If pulmonary capillary pressure exceeds blood oncotic pressure, pulmonary edema can develop. Pulmonary hypertension can result from elevated left atrial pressure and pulmonary arteriolar constriction. If severe pulmonary hypertension develops, right-sided heart failure can occur. Factors that may increase pulmonary pressure include tachycardia, increased cardiac output, and atrial fibrillation.

Brady K, Duff P: Rheumatic heart disease in pregnancy. Clin Obstet Gynecol 32:21, 1989

Burrow GN, Ferris TF: Medical Complications During Pregnancy, p 110. Philadelphia, WB Saunders, 1975

A.12. *What are the auscultation findings associated with mitral stenosis?*

The first heart sound is increased. An opening snap may be heard along the left sternal border. A diastolic rumbling murmur is present at the mitral area and may be best heard with the patient in the left lateral decubitus position.

Bates B: A Guide to Physical Examination, 5th ed, p 319. Philadelphia, JB Lippincott, 1991

A.13. What may be seen on the electrocardiogram in patients with mitral stenosis?

Broadened diphasic P waves may be seen in lead V_1; they are indicative of left atrial enlargement. Signs may be seen of right-axis deviation and right ventricular hypertrophy. Atrial fibrillation may be present.

Dubin D: Rapid Interpretation of EKGs, 4th ed, pp 188; 198–212. Tampa, Cover Publishing, 1989

A.14. What is the effect of the physiologic changes of pregnancy on patients with mitral stenosis?

The increased physiologic cardiovascular load of pregnancy can cause patients to deteriorate and advance from one NYHA classification to another.

A.15. What are the determinants of fetal oxygenation?

Fetal oxygenation is dependent on uteroplacental blood flow, oxygen-carrying capacity, oxygen affinity, arterial oxygen tension, placental diffusion capacity, placental vascular geometry, and placental oxygen consumption.

Shnider SM, Levinson G (eds): Anesthesia for Obstetrics, 3rd ed, pp 24–26. Baltimore, Williams & Wilkins, 1993

A.16. What are the determinants of uterine blood flow?

Uterine blood flow is derived from Ohm's law, which states that pressure equals flow times resistance. Therefore, uterine blood flow is shown as follows:

$$\text{Uterine blood flow} = \frac{\text{uterine arterial pressure} - \text{uterine venous pressure}}{\text{uterine arterial resistance}}$$

Normally, 10% of the maternal cardiac output goes to the uterus. Of this, the placenta receives 80%, and the myometrium receives the rest. Uterine blood flow is directly related to blood pressure; the uterine vessels do not autoregulate.

Shnider SM, Levinson G (eds): Anesthesia for Obstetrics, 3rd ed, pp 1–23. Baltimore, Williams & Wilkins, 1993

B. Preoperative Evaluation and Preparation

B.1. How is fetal well-being assessed during labor?

Fetal well-being is dependent on an intact uteroplacental unit. Simultaneous monitoring of FHR and uterine contractions aids in the detection of fetal distress.

B.2. How are FHR and maternal contractions monitored?

Fetal heart rate can be monitored noninvasively by using the Doppler technique or invasively using a fetal scalp electrode. Uterine contractions can be monitored noninvasively by a tocodynamometer, which measures the tightening of maternal abdominal muscles, or invasively by a transcervical pressure catheter hooked to a strain gauge.

Shnider SM, Levinson G (eds): Anesthesia for Obstetrics, 3rd ed, pp 657–660. Baltimore, Williams & Wilkins, 1993

B.3. What is the normal FHR with beat-to-beat variability?

The normal FHR is 120 to 160 beats/min with beat-to-beat variability. Abnormalities in FHR such as bradycardia, tachycardia, dysrhythmias, decreased or absent beat-to-beat variability, or transient decelerations can be a sign of fetal asphyxia.

Shnider SM, Levinson G (eds): Anesthesia for Obstetrics, 3rd ed, p 660. Baltimore, Williams & Wilkins, 1993

B.4. What are transient or periodic decelerations?

Transient or periodic decelerations in fetal heart rate fall into three categories depending on their shape and timing with respect to maternal contractions (Fig. 37-1).

Early or type 1 decelerations are uniform FHR decreases that coincide with the onset, peak, and end of uterine contraction. This is a vagal response due to fetal head compression, and it is usually not associated with fetal hypoxia.

Late or type 2 decelerations are gradual decreases in fetal heart rate that begin after the onset of a contraction and last beyond the end of the contraction. They indicate uteroplacental insufficiency and require prompt evaluation and treatment.

Variable or type 3 decelerations occur variably and usually abruptly in relationship to contractions. They usually result from umbilical cord compression. Variable decelerations are further classified, depending on degree and duration, into mild, moderate, and severe categories.

Mild Variable Decelerations
- Usually insignificant
- FHR >80 beats/min
- Any FHR deceleration lasting <30 seconds

Moderate Variable Decelerations
- May signify mild hypoxia
- FHR <70 beats/min for 30 to 60 seconds
- FHR 70 to 80 beats/min lasting >30 seconds

Severe Variable Decelerations
- Can indicate frank fetal acidosis
- FHR <70 beats/min lasting >60 seconds

Cunningham FG, MacDonald PC, Gant NF et al: Williams' Obstetrics, 20th ed, pp 404–410. Stamford, CT, Appleton & Lange, 1997

James FM, Wheeler AS, Dewan DM (eds): Obstetric Anesthesia: The Complicated Patient, 2nd ed, pp 37–44. Philadelphia, FA Davis, 1988

Shnider SM, Levinson G (eds): Anesthesia for Obstetrics, 3rd ed, pp 661–669. Baltimore, Williams & Wilkins, 1993

B.5. How accurate is FHR monitoring in predicting fetal well-being?

If the FHR tracing is normal, 99% of the time the fetus is not depressed, as exhibited by a 5-minute Apgar score of >6. In contrast, however, if the FHR tracing is abnormal, in 50% of cases the infants are normal and have no umbilical cord acidosis.

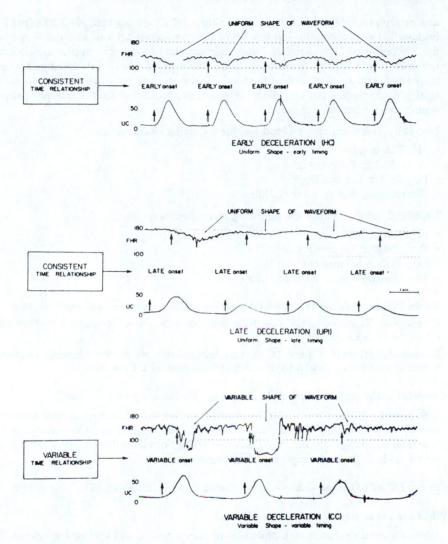

Figure 37-1.   Fetal heart rate decelerations in relation to the time of onset of uterine contractions. (Reprinted with permission from Hon EH: *An Atlas of Fetal Heart Rate Patterns*. New Haven, CT, Harty Press, 1968)

Brown DC (ed): Risk and Outcome in Anesthesia, p 330. Philadelphia, JB Lippincott, 1988

B.6. What is the significance of the fetal scalp capillary blood sample? What are the normal values of fetal blood gases?

The fetal scalp capillary blood pH is considered a sensitive indicator of perinatal asphyxia. Significant fetal hypoxia leads to anaerobic metabolism and systemic fetal acidosis. A positive correlation is seen between fetal scalp blood pH with umbilical vein and artery pH. Fetal capillary blood pH values $\geq$7.25 are normal; pH 7.20 to pH 7.24 is classified as preacidotic, and a pH <7.20 is considered acidotic and delivery of the fetus is performed immediately. Fetal scalp capillary blood pH samples are obtained when FHR tracings are abnormal, because ominous fetal heart rate tracings are only associated with acidosis 48% of the time. Obviously, one must have access to the fetal scalp for fetal scalp sampling; therefore, this tool is not useful in abnormal presentations or placenta previa.

Normally, umbilical artery blood has the following characteristics:

- pH, 7.28 $\pm$ 0.05
- P_{CO_2}, 49.2 $\pm$ 8.4 mm Hg
- P_{O_2}, 18.0 $\pm$ 6.2 mm Hg
- Bicarbonate, 22.3 $\pm$ 2.5 mEq/liter

Umbilical vein blood has the following characteristics:

- pH, 7.35 $\pm$ 0.05
- P_{CO_2}, 38.2 $\pm$ 5.6 mm Hg
- P_{O_2}, 29.2 $\pm$ 5.9 mm Hg
- Bicarbonate, 20.4 $\pm$ 2.1 mEq/liter

Brown DC (ed): Risk and Outcome in Anesthesia, p 332. Philadelphia, JB Lippincott, 1988

Cunningham FG, MacDonald PC, Gant NF et al: Williams Obstetrics, 20th ed, pp 402–403. Stamford, CT, Appleton & Lange, 1997

Yeomans ER, Hauth JC, Gilstrap LC III et al: Umbilical cord pH, P_{CO_2} and bicarbonate following uncomplicated term vaginal deliveries. Am J Obstet Gynecol 151:798, 1985

B.7. Can fetal scalp capillary blood pH sampling give false signals?

Yes. Sometimes neonates can be depressed neonates despite a normal fetal scalp capillary blood pH because of maternal alkalosis and/or drug effects. Conversely, with a low fetal scalp capillary blood pH, infants can be normal and well oxygenated if maternal acidosis or local scalp effects are present.

Brown DC (ed): Risk and Outcome in Anesthesia, p 330. Philadelphia, JB Lippincott, 1988

B.8. What are the causes of acute fetal distress?

Uteroplacental dysfunction, umbilical cord compression, and uterine hypertonus are causes of acute fetal distress. Some causes of uteroplacental insufficiency include maternal hypotension, placental abruption, and pregnancy-induced hypertension. Umbilical cord compression can be secondary to umbilical cord prolapse and/or oligohydramnios. Uterine hypertonus or tetany may signify dehydration or hyperstimulation by parental oxytocin.

James FM, Wheeler AS, Dewan DM (eds): Obstetric Anesthesia: The Complicated Patient, 2nd ed, p 386. Philadelphia, FA Davis, 1988

B.9. What is the significance of meconium-stained amniotic fluid?

The physiology of meconium passage and its adverse sequelae are incompletely understood. Umbilical cord compression and hypoxia may trigger meconium passage. Meconium-stained amniotic fluid has been associated with an increased risk of neonatal depression at birth, and it occurs more frequently with intrauterine growth retardation and postdate pregnancies. Although meconium staining occurs in 10% to 15% of all deliveries, not all of the infants are depressed; a high false-positive rate and low sensitivity for acidemia are seen.

Chestnut DH (ed): Obstetric Anesthesia: Principles and Practice, p 130. St. Louis, Mosby, 1994

B.10. What is meconium aspiration syndrome?

Of the 5% to 15% of births with meconium-stained amniotic fluid, 5% of the infants develop meconium aspiration pneumonia. Thirty percent of these infants require mechanical ventilation, and 5% to 10% may die.

Meconium is a combination of swallowed amniotic fluid, fetal hair, and gastrointestinal cells and secretions. Meconium aspiration syndrome is characterized by respiratory distress with a low lung compliance and a marked mismatch of ventilation to perfusion ratio. Pneumothorax and pneumomediastinum are complications. With severe disease, pulmonary hypertension leading to persistent fetal circulation can occur.

Nelson WE, Behrman RE, Kliesman RM et al (eds): Nelson Textbook of Pediatrics, 15th ed, pp 485–486. Philadelphia, WB Saunders, 1996

B.11. What is the proposed cause of meconium aspiration syndrome?

Two causes are proposed for meconium aspiration syndrome. One is that the aspiration of meconium directly causes the injury resulting in this syndrome. The other is that intrauterine hypoxia leads to the pulmonary changes.

Chestnut DH (ed): Obstetric Anesthesia: Principles and Practice, p 149. St. Louis, Mosby, 1994

B.12. What are the usual noninvasive tests used to evaluate the pregnant cardiac patient?

Physical examination, exercise tolerance test, chest roentgenograph, electrocardiogram, pulse oximeter oxygen saturation, serial vital capacities, Holter monitoring, and echocardiography may all be useful in evaluating these patients.

James FM, Wheeler AS, Dewan DM (eds): Obstetric Anesthesia: The Complicated Patient, 2nd ed, p 163. Philadelphia, FA Davis, 1988

B.13. What preoperative medications would you give this patient?

The patients should receive prophylaxis against endocarditis and rheumatic fever. The standard regimen is ampicillin (2 g) given intramuscularly (IM) or intravenously (IV) and gentamicin (1.5 mg/kg) IM or IV, given 30 minutes to 1 hour before the procedure or at the start of labor and continuing for 2 days after delivery, as recommended by the American Heart Association.

In addition, by the 12th to 14th week of gestation, gastric emptying is prolonged. Gastric content increases, gastric acidity increases, gastric motility decreases, lower esophageal sphincter tone decreases, and the gastroesophageal junction angle changes. These changes put the pregnant patient at increased risk for aspiration pneumonitis. Patients are considered at risk for aspiration pneumonitis if gastric volume exceeds 25 ml (0.4 ml/kg) and the *p*H is <2.5. In this patient presenting for emergency cesarean, an oral nonparticulate antacid such as 15 to 30 ml of 0.3 M sodium citrate given immediately prior to anesthesia induction reduces the risk of developing aspiration pneumonitis. Ranitidine, cimetidine, and metoclopramide may also decrease this risk, but they require more time to be effective.

Hurst JW et al (eds): The Heart, 8th ed, p 1704. New York, McGraw-Hill, 1994

James FM, Wheeler AS, Dewan DM (eds): Obstetric Anesthesia: The Complicated Patient, 2nd ed, p 164. Philadelphia, FA Davis, 1988

Kaplan EL, Bisplo A, Derrick W et al: Prevention of rheumatic fever. Circulation 55:1, 1977

Simpson KH, Stakes AF, Miller M: Pregnancy delays paracetamol absorption and gastric emptying in patients undergoing surgery. Br J Anaesth 60:24–27, 1988

C. Intraoperative Management

C.1. What monitors would you use in the NYHA class II patient during her cesarean section?

All pregnant cardiac patients should be monitored with an electrocardiogram, blood pressure monitoring, pulse oximetry, precordial or esophageal stethoscope, temperature monitor, Foley catheter, end-tidal carbon dioxide monitor (if general anesthesia), and neuromuscular blockage monitor (if general anesthesia).

C.2. When would one use invasive monitoring in a pregnant patient with cardiac disease?

Patients in n NYHA class I and II do not routinely require invasive hemodynamic monitoring. However, patients with class III and IV status are usually monitored with an intra-arterial line for serial arterial blood gas determinations and continuous blood pressure monitoring. Additionally, central venous pressure (CVP) monitoring and Swan-Ganz catheter placement are often used. Unlike CVP monitoring, the Swan-Ganz catheter allows you to obtain added information on pulmonary artery pressure, pulmonary capillary wedge pressure, and thermodilution cardiac output.

James FM, Wheeler AS, Dewan DM (eds): Obstetric Anesthesia: The Complicated Patient, 2nd ed, pp 166–167. Philadelphia, FA Davis, 1988

C.3. What are the hemodynamic goals of intraoperative management of the pregnant patient with mitral stenosis?

- Avoid tachycardia
- Maintain sinus rhythm
- Avoid marked decreases in systemic vascular resistance
- Avoid marked increases in central blood volume
- Avoid increases in pulmonary vascular resistance

Increased heart rates should be avoided because decreases in the amount of diastolic time for blood to flow across the stenotic mitral valve can lead to pulmonary edema and a decreased cardiac output. Atrial fibrillation with a rapid ventricular response similarly can result in cardiac decompensation, and the loss of atrial contraction is also detrimental. Marked decreases in systemic vascular resistance should be avoided because compensatory increases in heart rate can result. Elevation of pulmonary vascular resistance, as can occur with hypercarbia, hypoxia, and acidosis, is also poorly tolerated by these patients.

Burrow GN, Ferris TF: Medical Complications during Pregnancy, pp 111–112. Philadelphia, WB Saunders, 1975

Shnider SM, Levinson G (eds): Anesthesia for Obstetrics, 3rd ed, pp 489–492. Baltimore, Williams & Wilkins, 1993

C.4. What anesthetic technique would you use for this emergency cesarean section?

The choices of anesthetic techniques for cesarean section are regional, spinal, or epidural anesthesia, or general anesthesia. In this case, a general anesthetic would be the anesthetic of choice. General anesthesia has a rapid onset, which is necessary because of fetal distress. In addition, if the patient has not been adequately hydrated with an IV crystalloid solution prior to a rapid regional anesthetic induction, the resulting decrease in systemic vascular resistance, hypotension, and reflex tachycardia can exacerbate fetal distress and lead to maternal cardiac decompensation in the patient with mitral stenosis.

C.5. What technique could you use for this general anesthesia?

- Intravenous crystalloid solution via large-bore cannula (if not already present).
- Place the patient on the table in the supine position with left lateral tilt to avoid aortocaval compression.
- Preoxygenate the mother and place monitors on her quickly. Preoxygenation can be accomplished by allowing her to breathe 100% oxygen by mask for 3 to 5 minutes or to take four maximally deep inspirations if time is limited.
- After abdominal preparation and draping, perform a rapid-sequence induction using thiopental sodium (4.0 mg/kg) and succinylcholine (1.0 mg/kg). Ketamine should be avoided because it can increase heart rate. Pregnant women do not experience severe fasciculations, so a defasciculatory dose of nondepolarizing muscle relaxant is not necessary to prevent a rise in intragastric pressure.
- Endotracheal intubation cricoid pressure is maintained until the endotracheal tube cuff is inflated and the position checked. Cricoid pressure effectively prevents regurgitation with gastric pressures as high as 50 to 94 cm H_2O.
- Maintenance of anesthesia before the baby is delivered involves the following: N_2O with 50% oxygen, volatile anesthetic agent (e.g., 0.5% halothane or 0.75% to 1% enflurane), and muscle relaxant as needed (succinylcholine drip, vecuronium, or atracurium). Isoflurane probably should be avoided in this patient because it can cause tachycardia.
- Maintenance of anesthesia after the baby is delivered no longer requires fetal consideration. A narcotic technique can be implemented using, for instance, fentanyl, midazolam, muscle relaxant, nitrous oxide, and oxygen.
- Extubation of the patient is done after her protective laryngeal reflexes have returned.

Fanning GL: The efficacy of cricoid pressure in regurgitation of gastric contents. Anesthesiology 32:553, 1970

Norris MC, Dewan DM: Preoxygenation for cesarean section. A comparison of two techniques. Anesthesiology 62:827, 1985

Thind GS, Bryson THL: Single dose suxamethonium and muscle pain in pregnancy. Br J Anaesth 55:743, 1983

C.6. Would this patient benefit from the use of beta-blockade?

This patient is asymptomatic, and beta-blockade is unnecessary at this point. However, if compromising tachycardia should occur, beta-blockade with inderal or esmolol may be useful, as may cardioversion, digitalis, or verapamil, depending on her dysrhythmia.

In patients with mitral stenosis it is important to prevent tachycardia. Al Kasab et al. have shown that pregnant patients with symptomatic mitral stenosis who receive beta-blockade with inderal or atenolol have a significant decrease in the incidence of pulmonary edema with no adverse neonatal side-effects.

Al Kasab SM, Sabag T, Zaibag MA et al: B-adrenergic receptor blockage in the management of pregnant women with mitral stenosis. Am J Obstet Gynecol 163:37–40, 1990

C.7. What is the effect of the inhalation agents on uterine contractility?

If <1 MAC of a potent volatile inhalation agent, such as halothane, isoflurane, or enflurane, is used no increase in blood loss or decrease in uterine contractility should be seen because at these low concentrations the uterus still responds to oxytocin. At higher concentrations, the uterine contractility is decreased and blood loss is increased.

Munson ES, Embro WJ: Enflurane, isoflurane and halothane and isolated human uterine muscle. Anesthesiology 46:11, 1977

Tjeuw MTB, Yao FS, Van Poznak A: Depressant effects of anesthetics on isolated human gravid and nongravid uterine muscle. Chin Med J 99:235–242, 1986

Warren TM, Datta S, Ostheimer GW et al: Comparison of the maternal and neonatal effects of halothane, enflurane and isoflurane for cesarean delivery. Anesth Analg 62:516, 1983

C.8. What is the Apgar scoring system?

The Apgar scoring system is used in the delivery room to assess the neonate's condition at 1 minute and 5 minutes. Each of five categories is given a rating of 0 to 2, and the final score at each time is the sum of the individual category scores. Ten points is the best possible neonatal Apgar score (see Table 37-1).

Table 37-1. Apgar Scoring System

MNEMONIC	SIGN	SCORE 0	SCORE 1	SCORE 2
A	Appearance (color)	Blue, pale	Body pink, extremities blue	Pink
P	Pulse	Absent	<100/min	>100/min
G	Grimace (reflex irritability; response to catheter in the nose)	Absent	Grimace	Cough, sneeze
A	Activity (muscle tone)	Limp	Some extremity flexion	Active motion
R	Respiratory effect	Absent	Slow, irregular	Good cry

Apgar V: A proposal for a new method of evaluation of the newborn infant. Curr Res Anesth Analg 32:260, 1953

C.9. What is the significance of the Apgar scores?

Overall, Apgar scores qualitatively measure basic neurologic reflexes and correlate with generalized neonatal depression. They correlate only loosely with acidosis and asphyxia. Apgar scores aid in predicting mortality but poorly predict morbidity; the longer the Apgar score is low, the higher the neonatal mortality.

Brown DC (ed): Risk and Outcome in Anesthesia, pp 333–334. Philadelphia, JB Lippincott, 1988

C.10. At birth, what should be done to minimize the infant's risk of meconium aspiration syndrome?

It is agreed that the obstetrician should suction the mouth and nose of the newborn before the infant's first breath and the delivery of its shoulders. Depressed newborns and those with signs of airway obstruction should have endotracheal intubation and suctioning. Many experts also recommend that vigorous newborns or those with light meconium exposure not be intubated and suctioned.

Chestnut DH (ed): Obstetric Anesthesia: Principles and Practice, pp 148–151. St. Louis, Mosby, 1994

Linder N, Aranda JV, Tsur M, et al: Need for endotracheal intubation and suction in meconium-stained neonates. J Pediatr 112:613–615, 1988

C.11. The Apgar score of the newborn was 3 at 1 minute. How would you treat the newborn?

In addition to minimizing heat loss and upper airway suctioning, this newborn is moderately depressed with the Apgar score of 3 or 4 and requires oxygen with positive pressure ventilation via facemask and rebreathing bag. If clinical improvement is not prompt, then endotracheal intubation should be undertaken. If ventilation with 100% oxygen does not lead to improvement, umbilical vessel catheterization and appropriate fluid and drug administration are required.

Levthner SR, Jansen RD, Hageman JR: Cardiopulmonary resuscitation of the newborn. Pediatr Clin North Am 41:893–907, 1994

Schnider SM, Levinson G (eds): Anesthesia for Obstetrics, 3rd ed, pp 700–702. Baltimore, Williams & Wilkins, 1993

D. Postoperative Management

D.1. Immediately after the baby was delivered, the patient's oxygen saturation decreased. What is the differential diagnosis?

- Mechanical problems with the endotracheal tube
- Cardiac decompensation with pulmonary edema
- Pulmonary venous embolism: air, amniotic, thrombotic

Brady K, Dugg P: Rheumatic heart disease in pregnancy. Clin Obstet Gynecol 32:21, 1989

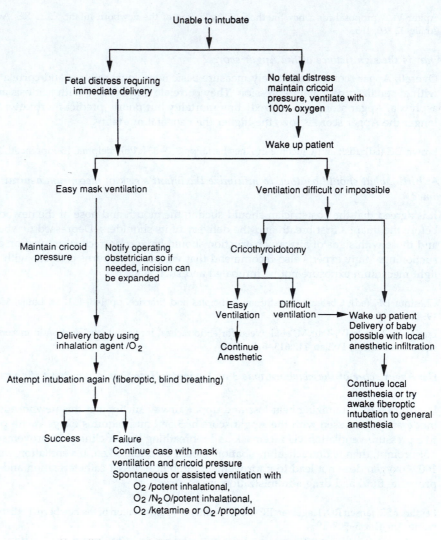

Unable to intubate

Fetal distress requiring immediate delivery

No fetal distress maintain cricoid pressure, ventilate with 100% oxygen

Wake up patient

Easy mask ventilation

Ventilation difficult or impossible

Maintain cricoid pressure

Notify operating obstetrician so if needed, incision can be expanded

Cricothyroidotomy

Easy Ventilation

Difficult ventilation

Wake up patient Delivery of baby possible with local anesthetic infiltration

Continue Anesthetic

Continue local anesthesia or try awake fiberoptic intubation to general anesthesia

Delivery baby using inhalation agent /O$_2$

Attempt intubation again (fiberoptic, blind breathing)

Success

Failure Continue case with mask ventilation and cricoid pressure Spontaneous or assisted ventilation with O$_2$ /potent inhalational, O$_2$ /N$_2$O/potent inhalational, O$_2$ /ketamine or O$_2$ /propofol

Note: If the surgeon infiltrates region with local anesthetic, it will decrease your general anesthetic requirement.

Figure 37-2. *Algorithm for management of difficult intubation. Note: Some have added the laryngeal mask airway to the failed intubation and difficult mask ventilation arm of the algorithm. However, its use is not time tested in the obstetric patient.*

Fong J, Gadalla R, Pierri MK et al: Are Doppler-detected venous emboli during cesarean section air emboli? Anesth Analg 71:254, 1990

D.2. If you had been unable to intubate this patient, how would you have managed the airway?

See Figure 37-2.

This is one way to deal with the failed intubation in the obstetric patient. However, other anesthetic techniques can be used. For instance, some would paralyze the patient and continue mask ventilation in an attempt to decrease the likelihood of bucking and regurgitation. Laryngeal mask airway use has also been added to the failed intubation and difficult mask ventilation arm of the algorithm. Its use, however, in the obstetric population has not been time tested.

However, it is important to remember that the mother's life should not be endangered to deliver a distressed fetus. Also a call for help when difficulties arise is wise.

Benumof JL: The ASA Difficult Airway Algorithm: New Thoughts/Considerations. ASA Refresher Course Lectures, no. 253, 1995

Chestnut DH: Fetal monitoring. ASA Refresher Courses in Anesthesiology 17:29–38, 1989

Shnider SM, Levinson G (eds): Anesthesia for Obstetrics, 3rd ed, p 420. Baltimore, Williams & Wilkins, 1993

38 Appendectomy for a Pregnant Patient

Farida Gadalla

A 25-year-old woman at 32 weeks' gestation presented to the emergency room with vague right abdominal pain. She had lost her appetite and had had two episodes of vomiting. Temperature 37.5°C; pulse 100 beats/min; hematocrit 34%; white blood cell count (WBC) 15,000/mm³.

A. Medical Disease and Differential Diagnosis

1. What is the differential diagnosis for this patient?
2. How would you attempt to make the diagnosis of acute appendicitis clinically?
3. What is the incidence of appendicitis during pregnancy?
4. Why is the incidence of gangrenous appendix higher in pregnant than in nonpregnant women?
5. What is Alders' sign?
6. What is the incidence of perforation of the appendix and in which trimester is it most likely to occur?
7. What is the incidence of surgery during pregnancy?
8. What are the main concerns associated with nonobstetric surgery in the pregnant patient?
9. What are the factors influencing teratogenicity in mammals? Discuss the teratogenicity of anesthetic agents.
10. How would you prevent intrauterine fetal asphyxia?
11. Although this patient presented with an acute abdomen, what is the major reason for nonobstetric surgical intervention in the pregnant patient?

B. Preoperative Evaluation and Preparation

1. What would you discuss with this patient preoperatively?
2. Is there a difference in the aim of anesthesia for delivery and for nonobstetric surgery in a pregnant patient?
3. How would you premedicate this patient?

C. Intraoperative Management

1. What factors would alter your anesthetic technique from that used for a nonpregnant patient?
2. Describe your technique and dosage if you choose epidural anesthesia.
3. If the patient is in need of supplemental medication, what would be your choice?
4. What vasopressor would you choose to improve uteroplacental perfusion?
5. When this patient arrived in the operating room she was panic-stricken and desired a general anesthetic. Describe your technique.
6. Does any controversy exist surrounding the use of nitrous oxide?

7. What is the incidence of fetal loss and what factors influence it?
8. If the patient was having surgery on her hand, what would you do differently?
9. What would you expect to see on the fetal monitor during an enflurane- or isoflurane-nitrous oxide-oxygen anesthetic?

D. Postoperative Management

1. When would you extubate this patient?
2. What monitors would you use postoperatively?
3. What other precautions would you take postoperatively?
4. What is the incidence of preterm delivery following nonobstetric surgery during pregnancy?
5. The next day the patient went into premature labor having "failed" tocolytic therapy. She now needed a cesarean section for prematurity and breech presentation. She required another general anesthetic. In what way would your technique differ from your previous anesthetic technique?

A. Medical Disease and Differential Diagnosis

A.1. What is the differential diagnosis for this patient?

The differential diagnosis includes the following:

Medical Conditions
- Sickle cell disease
- Porphyria
- Glomerulonephritis
- Pyelonephritis
- Pneumonia
- Withdrawal from drug addition

Obstetric Conditions
- Labor
- Abruptio placentae
- Chorioamnionitis

Gynecologic Conditions
- Salpingitis
- Degenerating myoma
- Ovarian cyst or tumor, either torted or ruptured
- Tubo-ovarian abscess

Surgical Conditions
- Appendicitis
- Cholecystitis
- Pancreatitis
- Mesenteric adenitis
- Intestinal obstruction

Baden JM, Brodsky JB (eds): The Pregnant Surgical Patient, pp 165–166. Mt Kisco, NY, Futura Publishing, 1985

Chestnut DH (ed): Obstetric Anesthesia: Principle and Practice, p 286. St. Louis, Mosby, 1994

Weinold AB: Appendicitis in pregnancy. Clin Obstet Gynecol 26:801, 1983

A.2. How would you attempt to make the diagnosis of acute appendicitis clinically?

Diagnosis is based on a detailed history and the following symptoms:

- Vague abdominal pain, variable in position owing to the growing uterus
- Anorexia
- Vomiting

The signs are:

- Abdominal tenderness
- Rebound pain
- Abdominal guarding
- Rectal tenderness
- Mildly elevated temperature, 37° to 38°C
- Mildly elevated pulse rate
- An increase in WBC, although this is not useful owing to the already existing relative leukocytosis in pregnancy

Baden JM, Brodsky JB (eds): The Pregnant Surgical Patient, p 150. Mt Kisco, NY, Futura Publishing, 1985

Weingold AB: Appendicitis in pregnancy. Clin Obstet Gynecol 26:801, 1983

A.3. What is the incidence of appendicitis during pregnancy?

Appendicitis is the most common surgical emergency during pregnancy. Incidence varies from 1:350 to 1:10,000. Appendicitis is the reason for approximately two thirds of the laparotomies performed during pregnancy.

Babaknia A, Parsa H, Woodruff JD: Appendicitis during pregnancy. Obstet Gynecol 50:40, 1977

Weingold AB: Appendicitis in pregnancy. Clin Obstet Gynecol 26:801, 1983

A.4. Why is the incidence of gangrenous appendix higher in pregnant than in nonpregnant women?

The incidence of gangrenous appendix is higher during pregnancy because the enlarging uterus pushes the appendix away from the abdominal wall (Fig. 38-1), thereby causing the diseased appendix to produce little pain. This will delay the diagnosis and allow the appendix time to become gangrenous. Another factor contributing to the delay in diagnosis of a nonobstetric abdominal crisis is that useful diagnostic procedures such as radiography and laparoscopy are postponed because of concern for the fetus.

Baden JM, Brodsky JB (eds): The Pregnant Surgical Patient, p 150. Mt Kisco, NY, Futura Publishing, 1985

Weingold AB: Appendicitis in pregnancy. Clin Obstet Gynecol 26:802, 1983

A.5. What is Alders' sign?

Alders' sign is a clinical sign used to differentiate between uterine and appendiceal pain.

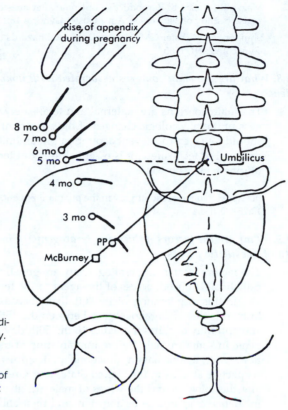

Figure 38-1. Changes in position and direction of the appendix during pregnancy. (Reprinted with permission from Baer JL, Reis RA, Arens RA: Appendicitis in pregnancy with changes in position and axis of normal appendix in pregnancy. JAMA 98: 1359, 1932)

The pain is localized with the patient supine. The patient then lies on her left side. If the area of pain shifts to the left, it is presumed to be uterine.

Alders N: A sign for differentiating uterine from extrauterine complications of pregnancy. BMJ 2: 1194, 1951

A.6. What is the incidence of perforation of the appendix and in which trimester is it most likely to occur?

The incidence of perforation of the appendix is approximately 15%. Thirty percent of these occur in the first and second trimesters and 70% during the third trimester.

Weingold AB: Appendicitis in pregnancy. Clin Obstet Gynecol 26:801, 1983

A.7. What is the incidence of surgery during pregnancy?

The incidence of surgery is estimated at between 0.75% and 2.2%.

Baden JM, Brodsky JB (eds): The Pregnant Surgical Patient, p 223. Mt Kisco, NY, Futura Publishing, 1985

Mazze RI, Kallen B: Reproductive outcome after anesthesia and operations during pregnancy: A registry study of 5405 cases. Am J Obstet Gynecol 16:1178–1185, 1989

Shnider SM, Webster GM: Maternal and fetal hazards of surgery during pregnancy. Am J Obstet Gynecol 92:891, 1965

A.8. What are the main concerns associated with nonobstetric surgery in the pregnant patient?

The main concerns are maternal and fetal safety. To ensure maternal safety, awareness of the physiologic changes of the parturient is of great importance. Special care should be taken to prevent aspiration pneumonitis and supine hypotension syndrome. For fetal safety, it is essential to avoid teratogenic anesthetic agents and intrauterine fetal asphyxia.

Blass NH: Nonobstetric surgery in the pregnant patient. ASA Refresher Courses in Anesthesiology 12:25–32, 1984

A.9. What are the factors influencing teratogenicity in mammals? Discuss the teratogenicity of anesthetic agents.

The factors influencing teratogenicity are genetic factors, nature and dosage of the anesthetic agent used, access of the agent to the fetus, and fetal developmental stage.

In this case, teratogenicity is unlikely because the most susceptible time in the human is that of organogenesis, between the 15th and the 30th day postconception; susceptibility declines thereafter to the 50th day. Almost all anesthetics are teratogenic in some animals. Before implantation of the ovum, teratogenicity leads to abortion. Later, malformation, functional deficiencies, and even death can occur. Large retrospective studies in the United States and Great Britain suggest that female anesthesiologists and the wives of male anesthesiologists had significantly increased incidence of spontaneous abortion, and their children were more likely to have congenital anomalies than those of non–operating-room physicians. It has been suggested that chronic exposure to trace anesthetic gases was the causative factor. However, no documented reports are found of teratogenicity in humans ascribed to any anesthetic agent used during pregnancy. Nevertheless, we recommend that only time-tested anesthetics, instead of new agents, be used for the pregnant patient, especially in the first trimester of pregnancy.

Blass NH: Nonobstetric surgery in the pregnant patient. ASA Refresher Courses in Anesthesiology 12:25–32, 1984

Chestnut DH (ed): Obstetric Anesthesia: Principles and Practice, pp 275–283. St. Louis, Mosby, 1994

Cohen EN, Bellville WJ, Brown BW Jr: Anesthesia, pregnancy, and miscarriage: A study of operating room nurses and anesthetists. Anesthesiology 35:343, 1971

A.10. How would you prevent intrauterine fetal asphyxia?

It is essential to maintain maternal homeostasis to ensure fetal well-being. Fetal oxygenation is directly dependent on maternal oxygen tension, oxygen saturation, hemoglobin content, oxygen affinity, and uteroplacental perfusion. Maternal hypoxia will result in fetal hypoxia, and if uncorrected, fetal abnormalities or death. Factors that decrease uterine blood flow must be avoided. Uterine blood flow is determined by uterine vascular resistance and uterine perfusion pressure. Uterine blood flow may be decreased by the following: maternal hypotension, stress (which releases maternal catecholamines), pain, anxiety, hypoxia, hypercarbia, hyperventilation, positive pressure ventilation, and pressor agents.

The following principles govern the administration of anesthesia to parturients:

- Delay elective surgery until after delivery.
- Try to avoid surgery during the first trimester.
- Use regional anesthesia where feasible.
- Attach greater importance to anesthetic management than to agents used.
- Change anesthetic management to conform to changes in maternal physiology.

No anesthetic technique is truly precluded for surgery in the pregnant patient. The avoidance of maternal hypoxia, hypotension, and hypovolemia is of greater importance than the choice of anesthetic technique.

Blass NH: Nonobstetric surgery in the pregnant patient. ASA Refresher Courses in Anesthesiology 12:25–32, 1984

Shnider SM, Levinson G (eds): Anesthesia for Obstetrics, 3rd ed, pp 23–28. Baltimore, Williams & Wilkins, 1993

A.11. Although this patient presented with an acute abdomen, what is the major reason for nonobstetric surgical intervention in the pregnant patient?

Trauma, particularly blunt trauma to the abdomen, is the most common occasion for nonobstetric surgical intervention in the pregnant patient. Blunt trauma results in 61% of unsuccessful pregnancies. If admitted in shock, 80% of these patients miscarry. Uterine rupture can follow blunt trauma, particularly if the patient has had a previous cesarean section.

Rothenberger D, Quattlebaum FW, Perry JF Jr et al: Blunt maternal trauma. A view of 103 cases. J Trauma 18:173, 1978

B. Preoperative Evaluation and Preparation

B.1. What would you discuss with this patient preoperatively?

It is important to discuss her options concerning regional versus general anesthesia, emphasizing that statistically the fetal outcome is similar, but regional anesthesia is the technique of choice for the mother.

Shelley WC: Anesthetic considerations for nonobstetric surgery. Clin Perinatol 9:149, 1982

B.2. Is there a difference in the aim of anesthesia for delivery and for nonobstetric surgery in a pregnant patient?

Yes. The aim of obstetric anesthesia is to permit pain-free labor and delivery without interfering with the progress of labor, whereas the aim of surgical anesthesia is to provide maternal anesthesia without stimulating uterine activity and precipitating premature labor. Second, obstetric anesthesia should provide maternal analgesia without fetal neurologic depression and delayed neonatal breathing. Surgical anesthesia, on the other hand, is designed to maintain uteroplacental perfusion but without consideration for fetal neurologic or respiratory depression.

Diaz JH: Perioperative management of the pregnant patient undergoing non-obstetric surgery. Anesth Rev 18(1):21–27, 1991; 18(2):27–34, 1991

B.3. How would you premedicate this patient?

Premedication may be avoided by reassurance and support. If necessary, barbiturates can be given for sedation. Glycopyrrolate, which does not cross the placental barrier, can be used as a vagolytic and antisialagogue.

A nonparticulate antacid, such as 30 ml of 0.3 M sodium citrate, is given about half an hour before surgery to prevent aspiration pneumonitis.

Chestnut DH (ed): Obstetric Anesthesia: Principles and Practice, p 287. St. Louis, Mosby, 1994

Shelley WC: Anesthetic considerations for non-obstetric surgery. Clin Perinatol 9:149, 1982

C. Intraoperative Management

C.1. What factors would alter your anesthetic technique from that used for a nonpregnant patient?

The anatomic and physiologic changes of pregnancy alter the anesthetic technique.

Cardiovascular System
- Increased blood volume (more increase in plasma than in red blood cell count [RBC])
- Increased cardiac output (stroke volume and heart rate)
- Decreased peripheral resistance
- Decreased mean arterial blood pressure
- Vena caval and aortic compression in the supine position as shown in Figure 38-2. (Therefore, the pregnant patient should be tilted by a wedge under her right hip.)

Respiratory System
- Increased minute ventilation
- Increased oxygen consumption
- Decreased functional residual capacity as shown in Figure 38-3

Gastrointestinal System
- Decreased gastrointestinal motility and increased gastric emptying time.
- Decreased volume of gastrointestinal secretions.
- Increased gastric acidity.
- Decreased lower esophageal tone owing to increased progesterone levels For these reasons, a pregnant patient beyond the first trimester should always be considered as having a full stomach and must be considered at risk for regurgitation and aspiration.

Central Nervous System
- Decreased minimal alveolar capacity (MAC)
- Increased sensitivity to local anesthesia
- Decreased volume of epidural anesthetic required, owing to engorgement of epidural veins and consequent decrease in size of epidural space

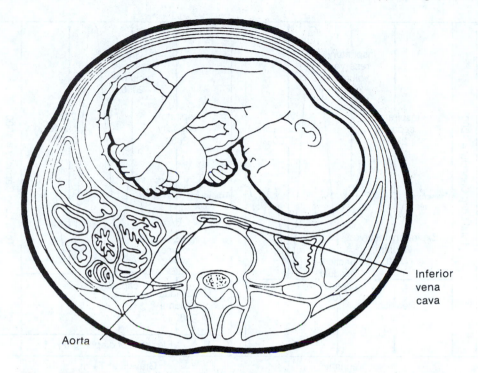

Aorta

Inferior
vena
cava

Figure 38-2.   The pregnant uterus compressing the aorta and the inferior vena cava (aortocaval compression) in supine position. (Reprinted with permission from Ostheimer GW: *Regional Anesthesia Techniques in Obstetrics.* New York, Breon Laboratories, 1980)

Skin and Mucous Membranes
• More friable mucous membranes and engorged mucosal capillaries. (Therefore, avoid insertion of nasal airways and nasotracheal and nasogastric tubes.)

Metabolic
• Increase in oxygen consumption by 20%

Chestnut DH: Obstetric Anesthesia: Principles and Practice, pp 17–35. St. Louis, Mosby, 1994

James FM, Wheeler AS: Obstetric Anesthesia: The Complicated Patient, 2nd ed, p 533. Philadelphia, FA Davis, 1988

C.2. Describe your technique and dosage if you choose epidural anesthesia.

The patient is placed in the left lateral decubitus position and is hydrated with 1000 to 1500 ml of crystalloid solution. She is then placed on her side or in the sitting position and prepared and draped. The epidural block is placed at L2–L3 or L3–L4 using the loss-of-resistance or hanging-drop technique. After testing for inadvertent spinal or intravascular placement, the local anesthetic is given in divided doses to attain a T4 level. This takes between one half and two thirds of the dose used for a nonpregnant patient (between 18 and 24 ml average volume). An inadvertent spinal injection

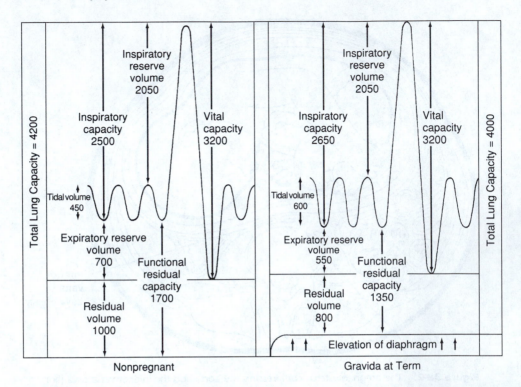

Figure 38-3. Pulmonary volumes and capacities during pregnancy. (Reprinted with permission from Bonica JJ: Principles and Practice of Obstetric Analgesia and Anesthesia. Philadelphia, FA Davis, 1967)

is detected by the rapid onset of a solid motor block following a 2 to 5 ml test dose; and an intravascular injection is evidenced by signs of systemic toxicity (e.g., dizziness, tinnitus, or circumoral numbness).

The patient is once again placed in the left lateral decubitus position, oxygen is delivered by mask, and her blood pressure is monitored closely.

My choices of local anesthetics are either 2% lidocaine or 0.5% bupivacaine. These agents afford good analgesia with a degree of motor blockade that provides muscular relaxation.

Shnider SM, Levinson G (eds): Anesthesia for Obstetrics, 3rd ed, pp 143–144; 215. Baltimore, Williams & Wilkins, 1993

C.3. If the patient is in need of supplemental medication, what would be your choice?

It is best to use the narcotics that have been tried by time and appear to be safe, such as morphine and meperidine. Small doses of ketamine (0.25 mg/kg intravenously [IV]) may also be given.

Barion WM: Medical evaluation of the pregnant patient requiring non-obstetric surgery. Clin Perinatol 12:488, 1985

Shnider SM, Levinson G (eds): Anesthesia for Obstetrics, 3rd ed, p 221. Baltimore, Williams & Wilkins, 1993

C.4. What vasopressor would you choose to improve uteroplacental perfusion?

Pure alpha-agonists such as phenylephrine cause uterine vasoconstriction with uterine hypoperfusion, and they are contraindicated in the management of maternal hypotension. Epinephrine and norepinephrine, mixed agonists, also reduce uterine blood flow, constrict placental vascular beds, and cause fetal hypoperfusion and hypoxia. Ephedrine appears to be the safest vasopressor because it increases mean arterial pressure and uterine artery blood flow without a concomitant decrease in uteroplacental perfusion. The overall increase in cardiac output from the beta-adrenergic stimulation of ephedrine will maintain uterine artery perfusion and compensate for its mild adrenergic vasoconstriction.

Chestnut DH (ed): Obstetric Anesthesia: Principles and Practice, pp 51–52. St. Louis, Mosby, 1994

Diaz JH: Perioperative management of the pregnant patient undergoing non-obstetric surgery. Anesth Rev 18(1):21–27, 1991; 18(2):27–34, 1991

C.5. When this patient arrived in the operating room she was panic-stricken and desired a general anesthetic. Describe your technique.

- Check the adequacy of the IV.
- Preoxygenate for at least 3 minutes to ensure denitrogenation and to avoid maternal and fetal hypoxemia during induction and intubation.
- Carry out induction using a rapid-sequence technique (precurarization, thiopental sodium, succinylcholine, cricoid pressure, and intubation using a cuffed endotracheal tube with a 7 mm internal diameter).
- Carry out maintenance using agents with a long history of safety, including morphine, meperidine, succinylcholine, nondepolarizing muscle relaxants isoflurane, enflurane, halothane, and nitrous oxide:oxygen 50:50. (The inhalation anesthetics have the added advantage of relaxing the uterus in the hope of preventing premature labor.)
- Avoid hyperventilation and hypoventilation.
- Extubate when the patient is awake and has regained laryngeal reflexes.

Chestnut DH (ed): Obstetric Anesthesia: Principles and Practice, p 288. St. Louis, Mosby, 1994

James FM, Wheeler AS, Dewar DM (eds): Obstetric Anesthesia: The Complicated Patient, 2nd ed, pp 538–540. Philadelphia, FA Davis, 1988

Pedersen H, Finster M: Anesthetic risk in the pregnant surgical patient. Anesthesiology 51:439–451, 1979

C.6. Does any controversy exist surrounding the use of nitrous oxide?

Yes, especially during early pregnancy. This is because nitrous oxide inhibits methionine synthetase potentially affecting DNA synthesis.

Nitrous oxide also increases adrenergic tone and decreases uterine blood flow. This, however, can be prevented by the addition of a volatile agent.

Nitrous oxide can cause teratogenic effects in animals during prolonged exposure at critical times. However, teratogenicity has not been demonstrated in humans.

In addition, omission of nitrous oxide can result in a drop in maternal blood pressure because of the need to use higher concentration of volatile agents.

Chestnut DH (ed): Obstetric Anesthesia: Principles and Practice, pp 280–281. St. Louis, Mosby, 1994

Hawkins JL: Anesthesia for the pregnant patient undergoing nonobstetric surgery. ASA Annual Refresher Course Lectures #156, 1996

C.7. What is the incidence of fetal loss and what factors influence it?

Prenatal loss may be caused by premature labor, but it also can be caused by generalized peritonitis and sepsis. Fetal loss is more related to the severity of the disease than to the surgical procedure or the anesthetic. The perinatal mortality rate in cases of prematurity owing to generalized peritonitis is 200 to 350 per 1000. The perinatal mortality rate for nonperforated appendicitis is approximately 50 per 1000 women.

Duncan PG, Pope WDB, Cohen MM et al: Fetal risk of anesthesia and surgery during pregnancy. Anesthesiology 64:790–794, 1986

Shnider SM, Webster GM: Maternal and fetal hazards of surgery during pregnancy. Am J Obstet Gynecol 92:891, 1965

Weingold AB: Appendicitis in pregnancy. Clin Obstet Gynecol 26:801, 1983

C.8. If the patient was having surgery on her hand, what would you do differently?

Initially, offer the patient the choice of a brachial plexus block or an IV regional technique. You should also monitor the fetal heart continuously during surgery and monitor for uterine contractions using a tocodynamometer. Continuous fetal heart monitoring using transabdominal Doppler is possible at about 18 weeks gestation.

Biehl DR: Foetal monitoring during surgery unrelated to pregnancy. Can Anaesth Soc J 32:455–459, 1985

Shnider SM, Levinson G (eds): Anesthesia for Obstetrics, 3rd ed, p 276. Baltimore, Williams & Wilkins, 1993

C.9. What would you expect to see on the fetal monitor during an enflurane- or isoflurane-nitrous oxide-oxygen anesthetic?

One would expect to see a decrease in beat-to-beat variability during anesthesia using inhalation agents.

Liu PL: Clinical reports: Fetal monitoring in patients undergoing surgery unrelated to pregnancy. Can Anaesth Soc J 32:525–532, 1985

D. Postoperative Management

D.1. When would you extubate this patient?

The patient can be extubated when she is fully awake and in command of her airway reflexes and able to avoid pulmonary aspiration.

Shnider SM, Levinson G (eds): Anesthesia for Obstetrics, 3rd ed, p 225. Baltimore, Williams & Wilkins, 1993

D.2. What monitors would you use postoperatively?

- ECG
- Foley catheter
- Intermittent monitoring of pulse, blood pressure, and temperature
- Tocodynamometer to detect premature labor
- Fetal heart monitor to ensure fetal well-being

Shnider SM, Levinson G (eds): Anesthesia for Obstetrics, 3rd ed, p 276. Baltimore, Williams & Wilkins, 1993

D.3. What other precautions would you take postoperatively?

- Provide adequate hydration
- Continue left uterine displacement
- Administer supplemental oxygen

Many obstetricians use heavy sedation plus a course of beta-agonist drugs to prevent premature labor. In our institution, all pregnant patients are observed in the obstetric floor for a minimum of 12 hours following nonobstetric surgery. Magnesium sulfate is given intravenously if labor occurs.

Ostheimer GW (ed): Manual of Obstetric Anesthesia, 2nd ed, pp 245–248. New York, Churchill Livingstone, 1992

D.4. What is the incidence of preterm delivery following nonobstetric surgery during pregnancy?

In a study of 778 women who underwent appendectomy while pregnant, 22% delivered during the following week if surgery occurred between 24 and 36 weeks' gestation.

Mazza RI, Källen B: Appendectomy during pregnancy. A Swedish registry study of 778 cases. Obstet Gynecol 77:835–840, 1991

D.5. The next day the patient went into premature labor having "failed" tocolytic therapy. She now needed a cesarean section for prematurity and breech presentation. She required another general anesthetic. In what way would your technique differ from your previous anesthetic technique?

Do not precurarize the patient—magnesium sulfate prevents the muscle fasciculations that normally occur following the administration of succinylcholine.

Use smaller doses of muscle relaxants—less is required owing to the interaction between relaxants and magnesium.

Avoid the use of narcotics until after delivery; then stop the inhalation agent and begin using a narcotic technique.

Ostheimer GW (ed): Manual of Obstetric Anesthesia, 2nd ed, pp 247–248. New York, Churchill Livingstone, 1992

Shnider SM, Levinson G (eds): Anesthesia for Obstetrics, 3rd ed, pp 348–350. Baltimore, Williams & Wilkins, 1993

39 Laparoscopic Surgery

Judith Weingram

A 72-year-old man with biopsy-proved carcinoma of the prostate had a prostate-specific antigen (PSA) of 22 ng/ml, but negative pelvic computed tomography (CT) and bone scans. He weighed 100 kg. Despite hypertension and a 50 pack-year smoking history, he was vigorous and active, and he was anxious to begin definitive treatment. First, he was scheduled for laparoscopic pelvic lymph node dissection.

A. Medical Disease and Differential Diagnosis

1. What is the incidence of carcinoma of the prostate?
2. How is prostate cancer diagnosed?
3. Our patient is scheduled for pelvic lymph node dissection. What are the indications for this procedure and by which techniques can it be performed? What are the advantages and disadvantages of each technique?
4. What other types of cancer can be staged by laparoscopic lymph node dissection?
5. Define laparoscopy.
6. What are the three major forces that uniquely alter the patient's physiology during laparoscopy?
7. What are the advantages and disadvantages of laparoscopy?
8. What are the contraindications to laparoscopic surgery?
9. What other specialties commonly perform laparoscopic or minimally invasive surgery? Where are the frontiers?
10. What are the differences in pulmonary function after laparoscopic cholecystectomy compared with open cholecystectomy?
11. Why is carbon dioxide the gas of choice for laparoscopy? What are its disadvantages?
12. How much endogenous CO_2 is produced at basal level and at maximal exercise?
13. How much CO_2 is stored in the body? Where is it stored? Of what significance is this to laparoscopy?
14. Describe the diffusion and solubility properties of CO_2 and their significance in laparoscopy.
15. Describe the equilibration processes that occur after CO_2 is insufflated into the peritoneal cavity.
16. Is CO_2 soluble in blood? Why?

B. Preoperative Evaluation and Preparation

1. What do you want to know about this patient's history and physical condition that may affect whether or not you clear him for laparoscopic surgery?
2. What factors increase this patient's risk of pulmonary complications?
3. What laboratory tests should be performed preoperatively?

4. What specific information should the patient be given about laparoscopic surgery prior to obtaining informed consent?
5. What additional procedures should be done prior to surgery?
6. What three general areas should you be concerned about in your attempts to minimize or prevent complications during laparoscopy?

C. Intraoperative Management

1. What monitors and devices would you apply to the patient? Why?
2. What intravenous (IV) solution and how much fluid volume do you plan to deliver?
3. How would the patient be positioned?
4. What are the respiratory and circulatory effects of the Trendelenburg position?
5. What is the anesthetic technique of choice for laparoscopy? Why?
6. What anesthetic agents or adjuvant drugs are recommended for laparoscopy? Are any anesthetic agents contraindicated?
7. Should N_2O be used during laparoscopy? What are the pros and cons? Does N_2O cause bowel distention during laparoscopy? Does N_2O cause nausea and vomiting after laparoscopy?
8. Can laparoscopy be performed under local anesthesia or regional anesthesia?
9. What two techniques are available for initial laparoscopic access to the peritoneal cavity? What anesthetic problems can arise during insufflation?
10. What is the purpose of the heparinized saline irrigation-suction device used by the surgeon and why should you be concerned with it?
11. Under what circumstances should laparoscopy be converted to laparotomy?
12. What is the mechanism of increase in shunting due to embolization?
13. What are the arterial to end-tidal CO_2 gradients ($PaCO_2 - P_{ET}CO_2$) in the normal awake patient? What is the cause of the gradient? Does the gradient change during laparoscopy? Why?
14. Is an arterial line necessary? Why? Does end-tidal CO_2 tension accurately reflect arterial CO_2 tension? Under what circumstances may the $P_{ET}CO_2$ exceed the $PaCO_2$? Why?
15. What are the possible causes of hypercarbia?
16. What factors play a role in the unusually rapid and marked elevation of CO_2 that is sometimes seen in laparoscopy?
17. How rapidly does the $PaCO_2$ rise in the apneic patient (endogenous CO_2)? How rapidly does the $PaCO_2$ rise if 5% CO_2 gas is inhaled (exogenous)? How rapidly can the CO_2 rise during laparoscopy? What factors explain the differences?
18. What are the direct and indirect effects of hypercarbia on the cardiovascular system? How are these effects altered by increased intra-abdominal pressure and patient position?
19. What are the direct and indirect effects of hypercarbia on the respiratory system? How does the Trendelenburg position and the increased intra-abdominal pressure of pneumoperitoneum alter these effects?
20. What are the direct and indirect effects of hypercarbia on the central nervous system?
21. What are the direct and indirect effects of CO_2 on the renal system?
22. What is the effect of hypercarbia and laparoscopy on the bowel and gastrointestinal system?

23. How would you recognize CO_2 embolism during laparoscopy? How does this differ from air embolism? Why should N_2O be discontinued during suspected embolization? Will N_2O increase the size of the CO_2 emboli?
24. How is gas embolism (CO_2 or air) treated?
25. What are the causes of pneumothorax or pneumomediastinum during laparoscopy? How would you diagnose it? How would you treat it?
26. How would you decide when to extubate?

D. Postoperative Management

1. What are some of the unique complications of laparoscopy?
2. What postoperative orders will you write? When would you remove the Foley catheter and arterial line? Under what circumstances would you order a chest x-ray?
3. What is the incidence of postoperative nausea and vomiting?

A. Medical Disease and Differential Diagnosis

A.1. What is the incidence of carcinoma of the prostate?

Carcinoma of the prostate is the most common nonskin cancer (surpassing carcinoma of the lung in 1994) and the second most common cause of death from cancer in American men. In 1983 the incidence of carcinoma of the prostate was about 75,000 new cases, along with 25,000 deaths of "old" cases. In 1996, the American Cancer Society estimates that the incidence will be 317,000 new cases, (far > 184,000 expected new cases of breast cancer), along with 43,000 deaths, (nearly as many as for breast cancer). Thus, carcinoma of the prostate is expected to account for nearly 25% of all new nonskin cancers diagnosed in 1996.

This "epidemic" increase in carcinoma of the prostate is believed to result from new methods for early detection, rather than from a true rise in incidence of the disease. Undetected microscopic prostate cancer cells are believed to be present in 30% to 40% of men over age 50, but it is estimated that only about 8% of these will become clinically significant. In fact, it has been stated that more men die with prostate cancer than from it. Therefore it is not yet known whether early detection of subclinical disease, much of which may have remained clinically insignificant, will improve survival.

Carcinoma of the prostate is rare in Asian men, whereas African-American men have about twice the incidence as white American men.

Dugan JA, Bostwick DG, Myers RP et al: The definition and preoperative prediction of clinically insignificant prostate cancer. JAMA 275:288–294, 1996

Potosky AL, Miller BA, Albertsen PC et al: The role of increasing detection in the rising incidence of prostate cancer. JAMA 273:548–552, 1995

A.2. How is prostate cancer diagnosed?

The most reliable methods for diagnosis include digital rectal examination plus the serum PSA level. Palpation of a tumor or indurated area and finding an elevated PSA should be followed by prostatic needle biopsies, perhaps under transrectal ultrasound (TRUS) guidance.

Gann PH, Hennekens CH, Stampfer MJ: A prospective evaluation of plasma prostate-specific antigen for detection of prostatic cancer. JAMA 273:289–294, 1995

Oesterling JE: Prostate-specific antigen: Improving its ability to diagnose early prostate cancer [Editorial]. JAMA 267:2236–2238, 1992

A.3. Our patient is scheduled for pelvic lymph node dissection. What are the indications for this procedure and by which techniques can it be performed? What are the advantages and disadvantages of each technique?

Histologic examination of the pelvic lymph nodes is necessary to accurately stage the tumor and select the appropriate treatment. Our patient is elderly, has multisystem disease, a suspiciously high PSA, and has chosen to be treated nonsurgically.

Pelvic lymph node dissection can be performed by several techniques. Before laparoscopic surgery was introduced, each patient underwent major open abdominal surgery. Currently, open lymphadenectomy is done when it is expected that the nodes will be negative, and it is followed by immediate radical retropubic prostatectomy through the same incision.

In patients who do not select retropubic surgery or in whom surgery would be inappropriate treatment, a minimally invasive (i.e., laparoscopic) operation may be chosen. In much the same way that a breast lump can be locally excised and a biopsy performed on 1 day and treated definitively at another time, laparoscopic staging permits the patient to avoid a major incision and to have more options in choosing his own treatment.

Treatment choices vary not just with the stage of the disease, but also with the patient's age and life-expectancy, associated medical conditions, and life style. A patient with positive lymph nodes can choose to be treated with radiation or hormones, other nonsurgical options, or even to have no treatment.

The laparoscopic approach to the pelvic lymph nodes can be transabdominal (i.e., entering the peritoneum anteriorly, then opening the posterior peritoneum for access), or it can be done directly extraperitoneally. In either case, laparoscopy avoids a large incision, is less painful, has less morbidity and quicker recovery, and offers about the same nodal yield as open surgery. The chief disadvantages of the laparoscopic approach are the longer duration and higher cost, especially if disposable instruments are used. These disadvantages, however, may be offset by a shorter hospitalization.

Guidelines for patient selection for laparoscopic rather than open lymphadenectomy include:

- Patients should have no radiologic evidence of metastases.
- PSA should be >20 ng/ml or there should be suspicion of extracapsular or lymph node spread.
- Patient is too old or too ill to choose surgical treatment even if nodes are negative.
- Patient is not old or ill but will choose radical perineal (not retropubic) prostatectomy, radiation, or other treatment if nodes are negative.

Donohue RE, Mani JH, Whitesel JA et al: Pelvic lymph node dissection: Guide to patient management for clinically locally confined adenocarcinoma of prostate. Urology 20:559–565, 1982

Gershman A, Daykhovsky L, Chandra M et al: Laparoscopic pelvic lymphadenectomy. J Laparoendosc Surg 1:63–67, 1990

Jarrard DF, Chodak GW: Prostate cancer staging after radiation utilizing laparoscopic pelvic lymphadenectomy. Urology 46:538–541, 1995

Stock RG, Stone NN, Ianuzzi C et al: Seminal vesicle biopsy and laparoscopic pelvic lymph node dissection: Implications for patient selection in the radiotherapeutic management of prostate cancer. Int J Radiat Oncol Biol Phys 33:815–821, 1995.

A.4. What other types of cancer can be staged by laparoscopic lymph node dissection?

Laparoscopic lymph node dissections have been performed in association with carcinomas of the prostate, bladder, urethra, and penis. In addition, laparoscopic dissections of bilateral aortic and pelvic lymph nodes for staging of gynecologic malignancies (especially cervical and ovarian) have recently become popular.

Childers JM, Lang J, Surwit EA et al: Laparoscopic surgical staging of ovarian cancer. Gynecol Oncol 59:25–33, 1995

Melendez TD, Childers JM: Laparoscopic lymphadenectomy. Curr Opin Obstet Gynecol 7:307–310, 1995

Plante M, Roy M: The use of operative laparoscopy in determining eligibility for pelvic exenteration in patients with recurrent cervical cancer. Gynecol Oncol 59:401–404, 1995

Spirtos NM, Schlaerth JB, Spirtos TW: Laparoscopic bilateral pelvic and paraaortic lymph node sampling: An evolving technique. Am J Obstet Gynecol 173:105–111, 1995

A.5. Define laparoscopy.

Laparoscopy (or peritoneoscopy) is a "minimally invasive" procedure allowing endoscopic access to the peritoneal cavity after insufflation of a gas (CO_2) to create space between the anterior abdominal wall and the viscera. The space is necessary for the safe manipulation of instruments and organs. Laparoscopic surgery can also be extraperitoneal and, more recently, gasless with abdominal wall retraction.

Etwaru D, Raboy A, Ferzli G et al: Extraperitoneal endoscopic gasless pelvic lymph node dissection. J Laparoendosc Surg 4:113–116, 1994

Weingram J: Laparoscopic and laser surgery. In: Malhotra V (ed): Anesthesia for Renal and Genito-Urologic Surgery, pp 151–176. New York, McGraw-Hill, 1996

A.6. What are the three major forces that uniquely alter the patient's physiology during laparoscopy?

- The increase in intra-abdominal pressure and volume, (which are transmitted to the thorax).
- The effects of patient positioning, (obviously Trendelenburg or lateral positions will have effects different from the head-up position).
- Carbon dioxide, which acts as both a drug and a waste product. It is not inert. It has profound effects at the local tissue level and at the overall systemic level. It has contradictory roles as an endogenous chemical and as an exogenous foreign substance. Changes in its concentration and tensions have enormous biochemical and physiologic consequences. The marvel of the human body is that it can safely handle this waste by-product of metabolism in seemingly toxic doses (i.e., in amounts far greater than what the most strenuous exercise or hypermetabolic situation can produce).

These three forces, separately or in combination, have profound effects on the patient's hemodynamic, respiratory, and metabolic functions. The early gynecologic laparoscopies were usually brief, and they were performed on young healthy females who tolerated these physiologic trespasses with nearly insignificant changes. These same three forces, however, may produce significant physiologic changes in long complex laparoscopies in older sicker patients unable to compensate.

Cullen DJ, Coyle JP, Teplick R et al: Cardiovascular, pulmonary, and renal effects of massively increased intra-abdominal pressure in critically ill patients. Crit Care Med 17:118–121, 1989

Sosa RE, Weingram J: Physiologic considerations in laparoscopic surgery. J Endourol 6:285–287, 1992

A.7. What are the advantages and disadvantages of laparoscopy?

The advantages include the cosmetic results of small, nonmuscle-splitting incisions, decreased blood loss, less postoperative pain and ileus, shorter hospitalization and convalescence, and ultimately lower cost. Postoperative respiratory muscle function returns to normal more quickly than in open surgery, especially in laparoscopic cholecystectomy and other upper abdominal procedures. Wound complications such as infection and dehiscence are less frequent, and host defense mechanisms may be greater in laparoscopic than in open surgery.

The disadvantages include the long learning curve for the surgeon (most complications occur during the first ten laparoscopies), the narrowed two-dimensional visual field on video, the need for general anesthesia, and the often longer duration. Although the costs are sometimes higher (especially with disposable instruments), it is recaptured by shorter hospitalizations. Ideally, surgeons should have more advanced laparoscopic skills, especially in knot tying, suturing, and working two instruments simultaneously.

Collet D, Vitale GC, Reynolds M et al: Peritoneal host defenses are less impaired by laparoscopy than by open operation. Surg Endosc 9:1059–1064, 1995

Rovina N, Bouros D, Tzanakis N et al: Effects of laparoscopic cholecystectomy on global respiratory muscle strength. Am J Respir Crit Care Med 153:458–461, 1996

A.8. What are the contraindications to laparoscopic surgery?

Increasing experience with the laparoscopic technique has made most contraindications relative, not absolute. However it is probably best to avoid or to use extreme caution in patients with coagulopathy, diaphragmatic hernia, severe cardiovascular or pulmonary disease (including bullae), increased intracranial pressure or space occupying masses, impending renal shutdown, a history of extensive surgery or adhesions, morbid obesity, sickle cell disease (because sickle crisis may be precipitated by acidosis), peritonitis, a large intra-abdominal mass, tumor of the abdominal wall, hypovolemic shock, a beta-blocked patient, or patient refusal. The strongest contraindication may be a surgeon who is inexperienced in the technique.

Cunningham AJ, Schlanger M: Intraoperative hypoxemia complicating laparoscopic cholecystectomy in a patient with sickle hemoglobinopathy. Anesth Analg 75:838–843, 1992

A.9. What other specialties commonly perform laparoscopic or minimally invasive surgery? Where are the "frontiers?"

Laparoscopic gynecologic surgery includes tubal surgery (sterilization, treatment of ectopic pregnancy, and so forth), cystectomies, hysterectomies, various ablations (endometriosis), and so on. Laparoscopy has even been performed in pregnancy. Complications include bladder and ureteral injuries and fistulae, but apparently these are not more prevalent than in standard surgery.

Laparoscopic general surgery includes cholecystectomy, hernia repair, antireflux procedures, splenectomy, appendectomy, bowel surgery, and various upper and lower abdominal procedures. Newer techniques including abdominal wall lift have obviated the need for pneumoperitoneum.

Thoracoscopic surgery and neurosurgical intracranial surgery using modified laparoscopic instruments, but without the need for gas insufflation, are two of the more recent areas of "minimally invasive surgery." Lumbar discectomies and other types of spinal surgery have also been done laparoscopically via an anterior approach. Even autopsies have been attempted laparoscopically! The list continues to grow, and it is patient-driven. Some say that the era in which surgery is performed with the surgeon's hands in the patient's body will soon be past.

Lindgren L, Koivusalo AM, Kellokumpu I: Conventional pneumoperitoneum compared with abdominal wall lift for laparoscopic cholecystectomy. Br J Anaesth 75:567–572, 1995

Mage G, Masson FM, Canis M et al: Laparoscopic hysterectomy. Curr Opin Obstet Gynecol 7:283–289, 1995

Saidi MH, Sadler RK, Vancaillie TG et al: Diagnosis and management of serious urinary complications after major operative laparoscopy. Obstet Gynecol 87:272–276, 1996

Zelko JR, Misko J, Swanstrom L et al: Laparoscopic lumbar discectomy. Am J Surg 169:496–498, 1995

A.10. What are the differences in pulmonary function after laparoscopic cholecystectomy compared with open cholecystectomy?

Pulmonary function is substantially impaired after a large upper abdominal incision, as in open cholecystectomy. Marked diaphragmatic dysfunction occurs postoperatively, caused by both reflex diaphragmatic changes and incisional pain. Vital capacity and functional residual capacity (FRC) may be reduced by 20% to 40% of preoperative values, and they may not return to normal until 2 to 3 days after surgery. The mini incision of laparoscopic cholecystectomy results in far less pulmonary and diaphragmatic loss of function, as well as less ileus.

Cunningham AJ, Brull SJ: Laparoscopic cholecystectomy: Anesthetic implications [Review]. Anesth Analg 76:1120–1133, 1993

Frazee RC, Roberts JW, Okeson GC et al: Open versus laparoscopic cholecystectomy: A comparison of postoperative pulmonary function. Ann Surg 213:651–653, 1991

A.11. Why is carbon dioxide the gas of choice for laparoscopy? What are its disadvantages?

Carbon dioxide is the insufflating gas of choice because it is nonflammable, does not support combustion, readily diffuses across membranes, is rapidly removed in the lungs, and is highly soluble due to rapid buffering in blood. The risk of CO_2 embolization is small. As much as 200 ml of CO_2 injected directly into a peripheral vein may not be lethal, whereas only 20 ml of air may prove to be so. In addition, CO_2 levels in blood and expired air can easily be measured, and its elimination can be augmented by increasing ventilation. As long as oxygen requirements are met, a high concentration of blood CO_2 can be tolerated. Also, medical grade CO_2 is readily available and inexpensive.

The disadvantages mainly stem from the fact that CO_2 is not inert. It causes direct peritoneal irritation and pain during laparoscopy under local anesthesia because it forms carbonic acid when in contact with the moist peritoneum. In addition, CO_2 is not very soluble in the absence of red blood cells, and therefore it can remain intraperitoneally after laparoscopy, causing referred shoulder pain. Hypercarbia and respiratory acidosis occur when the buffering capacity of blood is temporarily exceeded. In addition, CO_2 exerts widespread local and (often contradictory) systemic effects that may manifest overall as hypertension, tachycardia, cerebral vasodilation, increased cardiac output, hypercarbia, and respiratory acidosis.

Weingram J: Laparoscopic and laser surgery. In: Malhotra V (ed): Anesthesia for Renal and Genito-Urologic Surgery, p 157. New York, McGraw-Hill, 1996

A.12 How much endogenous CO_2 is produced at basal level and at maximal exercise?

Carbon dioxide and water are the major end products of aerobic metabolism in the mitochondria of the cells. Carbonic acid, the major acid produced in the body, is uniquely volatile, and therefore it must be largely eliminated by the lungs. (Other acids are eliminated by the kidney.)

At basal rate, an average adult manufactures about 200 ml of CO_2 per minute (while consuming 250 ml of O_2), or 12 liters of CO_2 (35 g) per hour. At maximal metabolic rate, it is estimated that the body can produce, transport, and excrete 90 to 100 liters per hour, an increase of 800% over basal rate.

Kinney JM: Transport of carbon dioxide in the blood. Anesthesiology 21:615–619, 1960

A.13 How much CO_2 is stored in the body? Where is it stored? Of what significance is this to laparoscopy?

The body contains about 120 liters of carbon dioxide. (This is about 100 times the amount of stored oxygen). CO_2 in the blood is in equilibrium with CO_2 in different tissues. The rate of uptake and distribution of CO_2 from the blood depends on the perfusion and storage capacity of those different tissues. The well-perfused tissues, including blood, brain, and kidney, come to rapid equilibrium. The medium-perfused compartment consists mainly of resting skeletal muscle. The slowly perfused compartment, mainly fat and bone, has the largest CO_2 storage capacity. In contrast to rapidly changing oxygen levels, CO_2 levels reach equilibrium more slowly.

These storage sites serve to buffer and stabilize blood CO_2 levels because they provide a place for excess CO_2 to "park" until ventilation can catch up and restore equilibrium. The increase in CO_2 storage during laparoscopy is illustrated clinically by the decelerating rate of rise in $P_{ET}CO_2$ despite continuing insufflation. Blood or end-tidal CO_2 levels increase rapidly at first, then plateau at between 15 and 35 minutes, despite continuing low flow insufflation. At constant ventilation, CO_2 levels increase, but not as much as if no simultaneous storage processes were occurring. But if ventilation is increased to keep CO_2 constant, then the increase needed is only about 40% of the predicted volume of ventilation because of the drain-off of CO_2 into the storage sites.

Farhi LE, Rahn H: Dynamics of changes in carbon dioxide stores. Anesthesiology 21:604–614, 1960

Nunn JF: Nunn's Applied Respiratory Physiology, 4th ed, pp 228–242. Oxford, Butterworth-Heinemann, 1993

Seed RF, Shakespeare TF, Muldoon MJ: Carbon dioxide homeostasis during anaesthesia for laparoscopy. Anaesthesia 25:223–231, 1970

A.14 Describe the diffusion and solubility properties of CO_2 and their significance in laparoscopy.

Residual carbon dioxide gas trapped in the abdomen after laparoscopy must first travel through the peritoneal membrane, ride through the blood stream, and, finally, travel through the alveolar-capillary membrane of the lung to leave the body. The ability to do this depends on the water solubility and diffusing capacity of CO_2.

Diffusion describes the process by which gases travel from an area of higher partial pressure to one of lower partial pressure. For a gaseous environment, Graham's law states that the rate of diffusion of a gas is inversely proportional to the square root of its density (i.e., the smaller the molecule the more easily it will diffuse).

When that same gas molecule arrives at an aqueous membrane (e.g., a gas-liquid interface), the solubility of that gas in water now becomes the major factor in determining its diffusing capacity, as shown in Table 39-1. The water solubility of CO_2 is 24 times that of O_2, whereas the diffusion capacity of CO_2 is 20.5 times that of O_2. The capacity of a gas to diffuse across a membrane is directly proportional to its solubility in water and inversely proportional to its molecular weight. However, the actual movement of that gas across the aqueous membrane depends not only on its diffusing capacity, but, more importantly, on the pressure gradient across that membrane.

Nunn JF: Nunn's Applied Respiratory Physiology, 4th ed, p 211. Oxford, Butterworth-Heinemann, 1993

A.15. Describe the equilibration processes that occur after CO_2 is insufflated into the peritoneal cavity.

The fate of CO_2 gas insufflated into the peritoneal cavity is the same that would occur in any other closed but distensible cavity. The pressure obtained within the cav-

Table 39-1. Influence of Physical Properties on the Diffusion of Gas through a Gas/Liquid Interface

GAS	MOLECULAR WEIGHT	DENSITY RELATIVE TO O_2	WATER SOLUBILITY RELATIVE TO O_2	DIFFUSION CAPACITY RELATIVE TO O_2
O_2	32	1.0	1.0	1.0
N_2	28	0.88	0.515	0.55
CO_2	44	1.37	24.0	20.5
N_2O	44	1.37	16.3	14.0
He	4	0.125	0.37	1.05

ity varies directly with the volume of gas insufflated and indirectly with the compliance of the closed cavity. CO_2 moves out of the closed cavity at a rate that is dependent on its intrinsic diffusion and solubility properties, the rate of continuing CO_2 insufflation, the surface area of the cavity, and the partial pressure difference across membranes. Insufflation of 100% CO_2 gas should result in an initial pressure differential from intraperitoneal to intracapillary CO_2 of 760 mm Hg minus 47 mm Hg for H_2O, minus 46 mm Hg for venous CO_2, or 667 mm Hg at standard temperature and pressure.

A.16. Is CO_2 soluble in blood? Why?

Carbon dioxide is relatively insoluble in plasma, interstitial fluid, and water. The solubility of CO_2 in water at 37°C is 0.03 mmol/liter/mm Hg. This must be contrasted to the very high solubility of CO_2 in blood. This extremely important distinction exists because of a zinc-containing enzyme, carbonic anhydrase, that exists only within the erythrocyte, and not at all in plasma.

$$H_2O + CO_2 \xrightarrow{\text{carbonic anhydrase}} H_2CO_3 \rightarrow H^+ + HCO_3^-$$

In the equation shown above, carbonic anhydrase catalyzes only the left side of the equation (i.e., the hydration of CO_2 to H_2CO_3). Once formed, carbonic acid is unstable and quickly dissociates into H^+ and HCO_3^-. It is estimated that without carbonic anhydrase it takes 200 seconds at 38°C for the above reaction to come to 10% equilibrium. Because blood travels through the pulmonary capillaries in < 1 second, carbonic anhydrase speeds up the reaction by a factor of 7500 times.

Christian G, Greene NM: Blood carbonic anhydrase activity in anesthetized man. Anesthesiology 23:179–186, 1962

B. Preoperative Evaluation and Preparation

B.1. What do you want to know about this patient's history and physical condition that may affect whether or not you clear him for laparoscopic surgery?

Because of his advanced age we want to make a judgment about his general physical condition. Despite written reports from other specialists (who may have never seen and do not understand the actual rigors and duration of the operation this patient will undergo), it is best to form one's own observations of his mental and physical condition. Is he confused, short of breath, kyphoscoliotic, and so forth? A glimpse at where and how this patient's body weight is distributed means more than just knowing that he weighs 100 kg. Ask about wheezing or any change in exercise tolerance, cough, or recent upper respiratory infection. Consult with the surgeon regarding the need for preoperative antibiotics. If you have any doubts, acquire the history and perform the physical examination yourself, or get consultations.

B.2. What factors increase this patient's risk of pulmonary complications?

- *The laparoscopic procedure itself.* The basic laparoscopic Trendelenburg position and the increased intraperitoneal volumes and pressures in a paralyzed, mechanically ventilated patient cause respiratory dysfunction. Additionally, an increased CO_2

load might call for respiratory minute volumes that are so large that further cardiopulmonary compromise occurs.

- *Age.* Pulmonary function declines with age, especially in a patient past age 70.
- *Smoking/Chronic obstructive pulmonary disease (COPD).* Smokers have increased tracheobronchial secretions with decreased ciliary transport function. They may already have significant pulmonary dysfunction, which may be manifested by diminished exercise tolerance. The forced vital capacity (FVC) may be diminished in restrictive pulmonary disease, whereas the forced expired volume in 1 second (FEV_1) is likely to be decreased in obstructive pulmonary disease.
- *Obesity.* Obesity compounds the problems of increased intra-abdominal pressure in the Trendelenburg position. Excessive weight and pressure on the diaphragm and lung bases can lead to marked ventilation and perfusion abnormalities, difficulty in inserting trochars, upward displacement of the carina (leading to possible endobronchial intubation), barotrauma, and so forth.
- *Overhydration.* Patients often experience oliguria during laparoscopy. This may be interpreted as insufficient hydration, and a relative overtransfusion may ensue. Unless frank pulmonary edema occurs, this cause of mild or moderate respiratory distress in the postanesthesia care unit (PACU) may not be recognized without a chest film.

B.3. What laboratory tests should be performed preoperatively?

Basic tests should include complete blood count (CBC), urinalysis, clotting functions, electrocardiogram (ECG), and blood typing and screening. In addition, baseline electrolytes, chemistries, and renal function tests (blood urea nitrogen [BUN], creatinine) should be obtained because of the possibility of oliguria during a long laparoscopy. Baseline pulmonary function tests, arterial blood gas measurement, and oxygen saturation values while breathing room air would be helpful in this patient. Markedly abnormal values might suggest the need for bronchodilators, antibiotics, postural drainage, and delay in surgery until pulmonary function is optimal for this particular patient. Baseline chest films are necessary not only to rule out active disease, but also for postoperative comparison of acute changes such as subcutaneous or mediastinal emphysema, pneumothorax, or interstitial or pulmonary edema. The presence of bullae on preoperative chest films may represent a contraindication to laparoscopic surgery because of the accompanying large tidal volumes and high intrathoracic pressures.

B.4. What specific information should the patient be given about laparoscopic surgery prior to obtaining informed consent?

In addition to the usual general complications of the planned surgery and anesthesia, the patient must also be told of the complications unique to laparoscopy, and consent for possible laparotomy must be obtained. Emergency laparotomy may be required in the event of such complications as hemorrhage or organ perforation, or because of anatomic or technical reasons. The patient should also be advised of the possibility of postoperative referred shoulder pain.

B.5. What additional procedures should be done prior to surgery?

Although the surgery is described as "minimally invasive," the patient must be ready for maximally invasive surgery if necessary. Therefore the patient must comply with preoperative orders regarding:

- Diet—It should consist of clear liquids the day before surgery. Nothing orally after midnight.
- A complete bowel preparation is necessary.
- Preoperative antibiotics, as per surgeon.

B.6. What three general areas should you be concerned about in your attempts to minimize or prevent complications during laparoscopy?

- Pneumoperitoneum, and problems related to its creation, maintenance, and consequences.
- Carbon dioxide, including its chemical and physical properties, and its local and systemic effects.
- Position on the operating table, which in this case will be Trendelenburg with alternating side elevations.

C. Intraoperative Management

C.1. What monitors and devices would you apply to the patient? Why?

The usual intraoperative monitors including standard 5-lead ECG with ST trending, systemic blood pressure using automated oscillometry, pulse oximetry, capnography, a nerve stimulator, and indicators of inspired oxygen fraction, minute ventilation, and peak airway pressures are necessary. An esophageal probe may be used for both temperature monitoring (optimal at the distal esophagus) and for breath, heart, and murmur sound monitoring (at heart level). Rarely, continuous venous pressure (CVP), pulmonary artery pressure, pulmonary capillary wedge pressure (PCWP), and cardiac output may be measured in severely deranged patients. Other possibilities include Doppler, transesophageal echocardiography, and noninvasive assessment of cardiac output by thoracic bioimpedance or thoracic ultrasound. An arterial line is used almost routinely.

Sequential compression antiembolic stockings should be applied. Shoulder braces are used for support in the Trendelenburg position. After the patient is asleep, a naso- or orogastric tube and a Foley catheter is inserted for decompression of stomach and bladder. Use of an orogastric tube is not optional. In addition to the danger of regurgitation from the increased abdominal pressure, reports have been made of stomach perforation by trochars. The orogastric tube should not be clamped after initial placement, and intermittent suctioning should continue because CO_2 gas continues to diffuse into the stomach and distend it.

In addition to mechanical monitoring, visual and tactile monitoring are necessary during laparoscopy. Skin color, skin turgor, and capillary refill should be monitored periodically, as they can change abruptly. The head, neck, and upper chest may assume a purplish color in the dependent position, especially during hypercarbia. The upper chest wall should be checked periodically for subcutaneous emphysema. The cornea and conjunctiva should be checked periodically for edema, especially in the Trendelenburg position, and also whenever oliguria occurs because the extent of the edema may influence your decision on when to extubate.

It is extremely important to maintain accurate data on the volume of fluids infused, and the patient's hourly or half-hourly urine output, along with observations on its color and concentration.

Weingram J: Laparoscopic and laser surgery. In: Malhotra V (ed): Anesthesia for Renal and Genito-Urologic Surgery, pp 166–168. New York, McGraw-Hill, 1996

C.2. What intravenous (IV) solution and how much fluid volume do you plan to deliver?

Two large bore angiocatheters should be placed because of the possibility of major hemorrhage. The amount of IV fluid infused is of vital importance, especially in the elderly. In our early cases, we increased our infusion rate in response to waning urine output, and we hydrated intraperitoneal laparoscopic cases as if they were open intraperitoneal cases. After several cases of "unexplained" pulmonary edema in the PACU, we concluded that the oliguria seen in laparoscopy is not related to volume depletion, and we have decreased our fluid replacement to 2.5 to 4 ml/kg/h of Ringer's lactate solution, depending on the patient's condition and the volume of intraperitoneal irrigation fluid used by the surgeon. In calculating fluid requirements during laparoscopy, it is important to remember that much less "third-spacing" occurs than in open surgery; no fluid loss is caused by evaporation; and the volume of retained intraperitoneal saline (used for irrigation by the surgeon) should be added to the final total volume of infused intravenous fluids.

Tittel A, Schippers E, Grablowitz V et al: Intraabdominal humidity and electromyographic activity of the gastrointestinal tract. Laparoscopy versus laparotomy. Surg Endosc 9:786–790, 1995

Weingram J, Sosa RE, Stein B: Oliguria during laparoscopic pelvic lymph node dissection. Anesth Analg 82:S484, 1996

C.3. How would the patient be positioned?

Our patient will be in the supine Trendelenburg position with both arms tucked in at the sides. The side to be worked on is usually elevated, enabling gravity to assist in separating the organs, and allowing blood to pool away from the operative field. Thus, the patient may be supine, in the Trendelenburg position (with possible lateral rotation) for urology; in dorsolithotomy for gynecology; in the head-up position for upper gastrointestinal and biliary tract surgery, and in the lateral decubitus position for thoracoscopy, nephrectomy, and adrenalectomy.

C.4. What are the respiratory and circulatory effects of the Trendelenburg position?

Respiratory
Vital capacity and FRC are reduced. The abdominal contents restrict movement of the diaphragm, especially in the obese and elderly. Decreased compliance, increased ventilation-perfusion abnormalities, and cephalad displacement of the mediastinum commonly occur.

Circulatory
In healthy patients, Trendelenburg position results in minimal circulatory changes. Venous return and cardiac output are increased, whereas central venous pressure (CVP), PCWP, systemic vascular resistance (SVR), and heart rate are essentially unchanged. In patients with cardiovascular disease, the Trendelenburg position may result in increased CVP, PCWP, and decreased cardiac output. The increase in venous return and myocardial oxygen demand that occurs in severe cardiovascular disease can precipitate acute heart failure.

Battillo JA, Hendler MA: Effects of positioning during anesthesia. Int Anesthesiol Clin 31:67–86, 1993

C.5. What is the anesthetic technique of choice for laparoscopy? Why?

The technique of choice for laparoscopy is general anesthesia with a cuffed endotracheal tube and controlled positive pressure ventilation, because of the following reasons:

- Duration may be long.
- Patient may be anxious.
- The Trendelenburg position may cause respiratory compromise and dyspnea in the awake or in the spontaneously breathing patient with abdominal contents under pressure. The obese patient may be especially uncomfortable in this position.
- A naso- or orogastric tube, difficult to insert in a conscious patient, is necessary to decompress the stomach and minimize the risk of aspiration or perforation by trochars. Carbon dioxide, as with N_2O, diffuses into the stomach.
- But perhaps the most important reason relates to muscle relaxation. Muscle relaxation and paralysis are necessary because the increase in intra-abdominal pressure and splinting of the diaphragm make spontaneous breathing difficult. It provides a quieter surgical field and better surgical exposure. "Bucking" increases negative pressure in the chest, increasing the risk of pneumothorax or gas dissection. Coughing can further increase pressure in the abdomen and cause movement of, and perforation by, intra-abdominal instruments. Moreover, muscle relaxation is necessary to control and augment ventilation to compensate for the hypercarbia and respiratory acidosis that results from absorption of CO_2.

Brull SJ: Anesthetic considerations for laparoscopic procedures. ASA Refresher Courses in Anesthesiology 23:15–28, 1995

Chassard D, Berrada K, Tournadre J-P et al: The effects of neuromuscular block on peak airway pressure and abdominal elastance during pneumoperitoneum. Anesth Analg 82:525–527, 1996

Chui PT, Gin T, Oh TE: Anaesthesia for laparoscopic general surgery. Anaesthesia and Intensive Care 21:163–171, 1993

DeGrood PMRM, Harbers JBM, VanEgmond J et al: Anaesthesia for laparoscopy. A comparison of five techniques including propofol, etomidate, thiopentone and isoflurane. Anaesthesia 42:815–823, 1987

C.6. What anesthetic agents or adjuvant drugs are recommended for laparoscopy? Are any anesthetic agents contraindicated?

Almost any combination that provides amnesia, analgesia, and paralysis is suitable. Because closure of a laparoscopic procedure may be abrupt, because patients may be discharged soon after surgery, and because a large painful (stimulating) incision is absent, the most common combination probably includes an inhalation agent, a medium duration narcotic, and an intermediate acting muscle relaxant.

Droperidol (or other antiemetic) is recommended to counteract the nausea resulting from peritoneal distention (secondary to insufflation) and bowel distention (secondary to diffusion of CO_2 into the bowel). Droperidol should be given early in the procedure because it potentiates sedation, it is long acting, and as an alpha-blocker it helps counteract the hypertensive effects of systemic CO_2.

A vagolytic drug should be at hand because acute stretching of the peritoneum may cause reflex bradycardia. This is more likely to occur in young females than in the elderly.

Halothane is the only anesthetic that should probably be avoided because it can cause arrhythmias in the presence of hypercarbia. Hypnotics and sedatives should be used cautiously in the elderly because their duration is often prolonged.

Seed RF, Shakespeare TF, Muldoon MJ: Carbon dioxide homeostasis during anaesthesia for laparoscopy. Anaesthesia 25:223–231, 1970

C.7. Should N_2O be used during laparoscopy? What are the pros and cons? Does N_2O cause bowel distention during laparoscopy? Does N_2O cause nausea and vomiting after laparoscopy?

The use of N_2O has been considered controversial. The controversies surrounding laparoscopic use of N_2O center on the causes of bowel distention during surgery, and nausea and vomiting postoperatively.

In examining the issue of bowel distention with N_2O, we note the following. The diffusion capacity of N_2O is about 15 times that of O_2 and 30 times that of nitrogen. Therefore, in a closed space that contains air, N_2O enters faster than N_2 can leave, thereby increasing the size of the closed space. It has been calculated that the volume of an enclosed air pocket can be doubled by inhalation of 50% N_2O, and quadrupled by inhalation of 75% N_2O after several hours.

However, during laparoscopy, we are concerned about CO_2 pockets, not air pockets. N_2O, which has a diffusion capacity almost as great as CO_2, will diffuse from the blood stream into the intraperitoneal pocket of 100% CO_2 at a rate determined by its solubility in water, its diffusing capacity through an aqueous membrane, and its pressure gradients, as discussed in question A.14. Similarly, CO_2 will leave the peritoneal cavity according to its pressure gradients and solubility and diffusion characteristics. Eventually, the amount of N_2O found in the peritoneal cavity can be significant, and theoretically it can form an ignition hazard. (However, Hunter states that it is necessary for methane or hydrogen to occupy at least 5.5% of the gas volume for nitrous oxide to support combustion, a condition that does not naturally occur.)

In the situation of an air pocket in the bowel, it is well known that N_2O will diffuse in more rapidly than O_2 is displaced or consumed, thus enlarging the pocket. However, few realize that even in the absence of N_2O, CO_2 will also diffuse into this pocket and expand it in a manner that is clinically indistinguishable from N_2O.

Surgeons frequently blame N_2O for a distended bowel during laparoscopy, unaware that CO_2 is equally capable of diffusing into and distending the bowel. In a double-blinded study of bowel distention in patients undergoing laparoscopic cholecystectomy with either isoflurane 70%-N_2O-O_2 or isoflurane-air-O_2, the surgeon was able to identify the use of N_2O correctly only 44% of the time. In addition, postoperative nausea and vomiting was independent of the use of N_2O, because the incidence was similar in both groups. Another study found no difference in the incidence of postoperative nausea and vomiting between groups receiving propofol-air-O_2 or propofol-N_2O-O_2 in gynecologic laparoscopy. In fact, the propofol-N_2O-O_2 group had the advantages of significantly more rapid emergence, use of 30% less propofol, additional analgesia, and less risk of awareness.

Eger EI II, Saidman LJ: Hazards of nitrous oxide anesthesia in bowel obstruction and pneumothorax. Anesthesiology 26:61–66, 1965

Hunter JG, Staheli J, Oddsdottir M et al: Nitrous oxide pneumoperitoneum revisited. Is there a risk of combustion? Surg Endosc 9:501–504, 1995

Munson ES, Merrick HC: Effect of nitrous oxide on venous air embolism. Anesthesiology 27: 783–787, 1966

Munson ES: Transfer of nitrous oxide into body air cavities. Br J Anaesth 46:202–209, 1974

Neuman GG, Sidebotham G, Negoianu E et al: Laparoscopic explosion hazards with N_2O. Anesthesiology 78:875–879, 1993

Sukhani R, Lurie J, Jabamoni R: Propofol for ambulatory gynecologic laparoscopy: Does omission of nitrous oxide alter postoperative emetic sequelae and recovery? Anesth Analg 78:831–835, 1994

Taylor E, Feinstein R, White PF et al: Anesthesia for laparoscopic cholecystectomy. Is nitrous oxide contraindicated? Anesthesiology 76:541–543, 1992

C.8. Can laparoscopy be performed under local anesthesia or regional anesthesia?

Yes. However, under local anesthesia, CO_2 causes pain intraperitoneally and in the shoulder. It is for this reason that N_2O, which is nonirritating to the peritoneum, has been used as the insufflating gas for laparoscopy under local anesthesia. However, rapid peritoneal distention causes nausea, which may be worsened without a nasogastric tube. Also the possibility, although remote, of having to open the abdomen speaks against local anesthesia.

Regional anesthesia can be used for laparoscopy. However, it too has serious drawbacks. It requires a high level of sensory block, possibly causing dyspnea in the Trendelenburg position. A nasogastric tube may not be tolerated. Hyperventilation in response to hypercarbia may cause too much movement in the surgical field. Because the systemic response to hypercarbia is mediated primarily through sympathetic stimulation, the sympathetic denervation of high regional anesthesia will result in hypotension and decreased cardiac output rather than the opposite.

Fishburne JI: Anesthesia for laparoscopy: Considerations, complications and techniques. J Reprod Med 21:37–40, 1978

C.9. What two techniques are available for initial laparoscopic access to the peritoneal cavity? What anesthetic problems can arise during insufflation?

Pneumoperitoneum can be achieved by a "blind" or closed technique of percutaneous insertion of the 2 mm diameter hollow Veress needle, which after verification of correct positioning is connected to the CO_2 insufflator. (After Veress needle insertion, the first trochar is also inserted blindly).

Alternatively, if previous surgery or adhesions are to be avoided, an "open" approach is taken. A mini incision is created, and the blunt-tipped Hasson cannula is inserted without prior pneumoperitoneum. The laparoscope is then inserted through the trocar to verify the intra-abdominal position before insufflation begins.

During insufflation, abdominal distention should be evenly distributed in all four quadrants. Respiratory variations of intraperitoneal pressure should be visible, and peak inspiratory pressures will gradually increase as the abdomen distends. It is at this time that the anesthesiologist should be alert to the possibility of vagally mediated reflexes. Bronchospasm, bradycardia, and even sinus arrest have been reported, especially in young women. Visceral and vascular perforations are also well-reported complications, especially with the blind technique. Cardiovascular collapse and gas emboli have been reported when CO_2 has been inadvertently insufflated directly into a blood vessel.

Dingfelder JR: Direct laparoscope trochar insertion without prior pneumoperitoneum. J Reprod Med 21:45–47, 1978

Mori T, Bhoyrul S, Way LW (eds): Fundamentals of Laparoscopic Surgery, pp 79–154. New York, Churchill Livingstone, 1995

C.10. What is the purpose of the heparinized saline irrigation-suction device used by the surgeon and why should you be concerned with it?

The heparinized saline solution (2000 to 5000 U/liter delivered by a bag pressurized to 300 mm Hg) is used by the surgeons to retard clot formation in the abdomen, to remove blood from the field, and to remove smoke from electrocautery. It takes the place of lap pads and sponges in open surgery. If the tip of the suction device is not kept under the fluid level, CO_2 gas will be aspirated, and exposure of the field will be lost.

Its further significance to the anesthesiologist is twofold. First, the difference between the volume of saline missing from the irrigation bag and the volume in the suction collection bottle must be considered as part of the patient's fluid intake. Second, the temperature of the saline solution intraperitoneally can alter the patient's body temperature.

C.11. Under what circumstances should laparoscopy be converted to laparotomy?

Laparotomy should be performed immediately in cases of bleeding or major organ damage. Other circumstances include persistent problems with inadequate exposure, procedure beyond the surgeon's capability, procedure taking too long, inability to create or maintain pneumoperitoneum, patient deterioration, equipment failure, and discovery of other unsuspected disease.

Tabboush ZS: When hypotension during laparoscopic cholecystectomy indicates termination of the laparoscopy [Letter]. Anesth Analg 79:195–196, 1994

C.12. What is the mechanism of increase in shunting due to embolization?

Emboli in the pulmonary capillaries cause an increase in pulmonary vascular resistance (vasoconstriction), which leads to increased pulmonary artery, right ventricle, and right atrium pressures and opening of pulmonary precapillary arteriovenous anastomoses, resulting in shunt and hypoxemia.

C.13. What are the arterial to end-tidal CO_2 gradients ($PaCO_2 - P_{ET}CO_2$) in the normal awake patient? What is the cause of the gradient? Does the gradient change during laparoscopy? Why?

In the awake person at rest, the normal arterial to end-tidal P_{CO_2} difference is small, perhaps ranging from 2 to 6 mm Hg. The gradient and its variations are measures of the alveolar dead space. The gradient is the sum of the difference between the arterial and alveolar CO_2 plus the difference between the alveolar and end-tidal CO_2. It is commonly increased in emphysema. The difference is increased when underperfused alveoli are ventilated, as often occurs during hyperventilation in laparoscopy.

The total physiologic dead space consists of the anatomic dead space (passageways that do not participate in gas exchange, about 150 ml) and the alveolar dead space (i.e., underperfused alveoli). The alveolar dead space gas is expired at the same time as the alveolar ideal gas from well-perfused alveoli in equilibrium with pulmonary capillary blood. The dilution of the ideal alveolar gas by the alveolar dead space gas is represented by the end-tidal CO_2.

Some of the factors resulting in a relative increase in ventilation-to-perfusion ratio include mechanical ventilation, hyperventilation, rapid or shallow ventilation, and Trendelenburg or lateral decubitus position.

Some of the factors resulting in a relative decrease in perfusion-to-ventilation ratio include hypotension, decreased cardiac output, anesthesia and myocardial depression, pulmonary emboli, high positive airway pressure, and ablation of the hypoxic pulmonary vasoconstriction reflex.

Christensen MA, Bloom J, Sutton KR: Comparing arterial and end-tidal carbon dioxide values in hyperventilated neurosurgical patients. Am J Crit Care 4:116–121, 1995

Nunn JF: Nunn's Applied Respiratory Physiology, 4th ed, p 236. Oxford, Butterworth-Heinemann, 1993

C.14. Is an arterial line necessary? Why? Does end-tidal CO_2 tension accurately reflect arterial CO_2 tension? Under what circumstances may the $P_{ET}CO_2$ exceed the $PaCO_2$? Why?

An arterial line is recommended whenever the laparoscopic procedure is unusually complex or long, or when the patient has significant cardiopulmonary disease. In such cases, ventilation-perfusion abnormalities, intraoperative hypoxemia, marked hypercarbia, or high airway pressures may be expected. During these situations, and possibly in all laparoscopies, an unsteady state exists with respect to CO_2, and the assumption that $P_{ET}CO_2$ may accurately reflect a predictable relationship to $PaCO_2$ is not valid.

End-tidal CO_2 tension can either estimate $PaCO_2$ or, more frequently, it may underestimate $PaCO_2$ or, less frequently, it may even exceed $PaCO_2$. Furthermore, the values for these two measurements do not always change proportionally, nor do they always change in the same direction. The relationship between $P_{ET}CO_2$ and $PaCO_2$ varies during the course of the procedure. At the beginning of insufflation, $P_{ET}CO_2$ can be used as a rough estimate of $PaCO_2$. However, when redistribution of the excess CO_2 from the well-perfused tissues to the less well perfused tissues begins, $P_{ET}CO_2$ begins to underestimate the $PaCO_2$. Characteristically, the arterial to end-tidal CO_2 difference progressively increases as hyperventilation (and dead space) increases.

Especially during strenuous exercise when metabolic CO_2 production is increased and during laparoscopy when excess exogenous CO_2 must be excreted, the $P_{ET}CO_2$ may be found to exceed the $PaCO_2$. This condition has also been reported in a hyperventilating patient at cesarean section. This occurs because the $PaCO_2$ fluctuates during each deep breath and may not represent the highest value at that instant, whereas the $P_{ET}CO_2$ shows the maximal value (i.e., because of tidal ventilation and pulsatile blood flow in exercise, $P_{ET}CO_2$ may exceed mean alveolar and arterial CO_2).

Gravenstein JS (ed): Gas Monitoring and Pulse Oximetry, pp 106–116. Boston, Butterworth-Heinemann, 1990

Jones NL, Robertson DG, Kane JW: Difference between end-tidal and arterial P_{CO_2} in exercise. J Appl Physiol 47(5):954–960, 1979

Lee T-S: End-tidal partial pressure of carbon dioxide does not accurately reflect $PaCO_2$ in rabbits treated with acetazolamide during anaesthesia. Br J Anaesth 73:225–226, 1994

Scheid P, Meyer M, Piper J: Arterial-expired P_{CO_2} differences in the dog during acute hypercapnia. J Appl Physiol 47(5):1074–1078, 1979

Shankar KB, Moseley H, Kumar Y et al: Arterial to end-tidal carbon dioxide tension difference during Caesarean section anaesthesia. Anaesthesia 41:698–702, 1986

C.15. What are the possible causes of hypercarbia?

- Hypoventilation.
- CO_2 in the inspired gas—Rebreathing endogenous CO_2 will increase $PaCO_2$ by 3 to 6 mm Hg per minute.
- Increased CO_2 supply or production—Occurring in the hypermetabolic states of malignant hyperpyrexia, fever, and hyperthyroidism; laparoscopy; or following administration of bicarbonate or lactate (1 ampule of 50 mEq of bicarbonate liberates >1 liter of CO_2).
- Increased dead space (rare)—As in pulmonary embolism, ventilation of a lung cyst, or in advanced COPD

Nunn JF: Nunn's Applied Respiratory Physiology, 4th ed, p 238. Oxford, Butterworth-Heinemann, 1993

Wolf JS Jr, Clayman RV, Monk TG et al: Carbon dioxide absorption during laparoscopic pelvic operation. J Am Coll Surg 180:555–560, 1995

C.16. What factors play a role in the unusually rapid and marked elevation of CO_2 that is sometimes seen in laparoscopy?

- Patients with significant cardiopulmonary disease.
- Intra-abdominal pressure is >15 mm Hg.
- Presence of subcutaneous emphysema.
- Retroperitoneal rather than intraperitoneal approach.
- Long duration of laparoscopy

Liem KS, Kallewaard JW, deSmet AM et al: Does hypercarbia develop faster during laparoscopic herniorrhaphy than during laparoscopic cholecystectomy? Assessment with continuous blood gas monitoring. Anesth Analg 81:1243–1249, 1995

C.17. How rapidly does the $PaCO_2$ rise in the apneic patient (endogenous CO_2)? How rapidly does the $PaCO_2$ rise if 5% CO_2 gas is inhaled (exogenous)? How rapidly can the CO_2 rise during laparoscopy? What factors explain the differences?

In the apneic patient, $PaCO_2$ rises at the rate of 3 to 6 mm Hg/min. Rebreathing, or inhalation of 5% CO_2 in oxygen, causes a much more rapid rise in $PaCO_2$, up to 8 to 10 mm Hg/min. The difference in rate of rise between endogenous and exogenous CO_2 is explained by the presence of large body stores of CO_2. About 120 liters of CO_2 exist in the body (100 times the amount for O_2), distributed among well-perfused tissue (e.g., blood, brain), moderately perfused tissue (e.g., muscle), and poorly perfused tissue (e.g., fat, bone). These storage places adjust slowly to acute CO_2 changes. In the steady state, the amount of CO_2 produced metabolically in the body is equal to the amount expired via the lungs, and there is no change in the body stores of CO_2. During laparoscopy an unsteady state exists, with the rate of rise of P_{CO_2} being greatest during the first 20 to 30 minutes. After that time, new equilibrium levels are reached between the different compartments, and the P_{CO_2} rate of rise is slower.

Frumin et al. studied the hypercarbic state during their classic study of apneic oxygenation. In paralyzed apneic intubated denitrogenated patients receiving only thiopental for amnesia, Frumin demonstrated at least a 3 mm average rise in $PaCO_2$ per minute, and an ultimate $PaCO_2$ as high as 250 mm Hg (*p*H 6.72) with 98% to 100% O_2 saturation after 53 minutes of apnea. They also found that the hypercarbia was accompanied by hypertension (mean arterial pressure rise of 26%, followed by fall of 14% on return of respirations and normocarbia). Other features accompanying apneic hypercarbic hypertension included normal sinus rhythm with an essentially unchanged rate, rising arterial epinephrine and norepinephrine concentrations, and rising arterial potassium levels (which rose still further after ventilation and normocarbia resumed) with unchanged sodium levels.

Frumin J, Epstein RM, Cohen G: Apneic oxygenation in man. Anesthesiology 20:789–798, 1959

Nunn JF: Nunn's Applied Respiratory Physiology, 4th ed, pp 237–238. Oxford, Butterworth-Heinemann, 1993

C.18. *What are the direct and indirect effects of hypercarbia on the cardiovascular system? How are these effects altered by increased intra-abdominal pressure and patient position?*

Hypercarbia's effects on the circulatory system are complex and often contradictory. At the cellular level, hypercarbia is a direct depressor of myocardial contractility and rate of contraction, and a direct stimulant of myocardial irritability and arrhythmicity, all of which probably result from the reduced *p*H caused by hypercarbia rather than directly from the hypercarbia itself.

The direct effect of hypercarbia on isolated or denervated blood vessels is a diminished responsiveness to catecholamines, and vasodilation, especially on the venous side, leading to peripheral pooling, decreased venous return, and decreased cardiac output. The exception to the dilatory effect of hypercarbia and acidosis on blood vessels exists in the pulmonary vessels, which undergo vasoconstriction. It appears, however, that the effects on the pulmonary vessels are actually due to acidosis rather than hypercarbia because if the *p*H is kept constant while the P_{CO_2} rises, then pulmonary vascular resistance does not change.

In the patient, however, the direct or local effects of CO_2 can be overshadowed by a variety of systemic effects. Simultaneous with these local or direct effects, hypercarbia causes profound systemic changes secondary to stimulation of the central nervous system and sympathoadrenal system. The net effect usually includes an increase in cardiac output, heart rate, force of myocardial contraction, blood pressure, CVP, vasoconstriction in the pulmonary (capacitance) vessels, and decreased peripheral resistance. The rise in cardiac output of up to 50% exceeds the rise in blood pressure, owing to the drop in peripheral resistance and increase in blood flow primarily in the cerebral and coronary circulations. This net stimulatory effect accompanies the elevation of P_{CO_2} up to about 90 mm Hg. Above this level, further increases in CO_2 cause a marked drop in response.

In a normal anesthetized human breathing 7% to 15% inspired CO_2, these stimulatory changes were shown to correspond primarily to rising plasma concentrations of epinephrine and norepinephrine. When the sympathoadrenal response was prevented by subarachnoid block, ganglioplegics, or beta-adrenergic blockers, the cardiovascular response to inhaled CO_2 was hypotension and decreased cardiac output. The stimulatory response is also diminished by general anesthesia.

Hypercarbia can cause arrhythmias during epinephrine infiltrations or in the presence of halothane but not other anesthetics. Other than in these two circumstances, hypercarbia is not arrhythmogenic unless hypoxia is also present.

The full range of possible effects of hypercarbia on the cardiovascular system are subject to many influences. Healthy (American Society of Anesthesiologists [ASA] class I) patients are less likely than ASA class III patients to undergo extreme changes. Similarly, a brief surgical duration, head-up positioning, low intra-abdominal pressures, and intraperitoneal (rather than extraperitoneal) surgery can limit the range of physiologic and metabolic responses to near-normal.

Arrhythmias such as bradycardia, nodal rhythm, or even asystole can follow rapid peritoneal distention and vagal stimulation. In general, blood pressure (BP), pulse, cardiac output (CO), and CVP will increase up to an intra-abdominal pressure of 15 mm Hg. At pressures of 20 to 30 mm Hg, a decrease in BP, CO, and CVP will occur because of pressure on the inferior vena cava and decreased venous return.

Lenz RJ, Thomas TA, Wilkens DG: Cardiovascular changes during laparoscopy. Studies of stroke volume and cardiac output using impedance cardiography. Anaesthesia 31:4–12, 1976

Marshall RL, Jebson PJR, Davie IT et al: Circulatory effects of carbon dioxide insufflation of the peritoneal cavity for laparoscopy. Br J Anaesth 44:680–684, 1972

Nunn JF: Nunn's Applied Respiratory Physiology, 4th ed, p 525. Oxford, Butterman-Heinemann, 1993

C.19. What are the direct and indirect effects of hypercarbia on the respiratory system? How does the Trendelenburg position and the increased intra-abdominal pressure of pneumoperitoneum alter these effects?

Hypercarbia and acidosis stimulate the respiratory center both directly, and indirectly via chemoreceptors, hormones, and autonomic nerves. In the conscious patient breathing oxygen, the maximal stimulating effect occurs at 100 to 150 mm Hg, producing minute volumes of up to 75 liters. Above these levels, CO_2 becomes a respiratory depressant. Current anesthetics blunt the stimulatory respiratory response to CO_2. (Diethyl ether, however, the only volatile anesthetic known to stimulate respiration, is reported to have caused a patient to continue to breathe spontaneously at an inadvertent P_{CO_2} of 234 mm Hg).

In the awake patient, each mm Hg increase in $PaCO_2$ increases ventilation by 2 to 3 liters per minute (if PaO_2 is constant). This response is diminished by anesthesia. Hypercarbia also produces bronchodilatation; acidosis, rather than hypercarbia per se, causes pulmonary vascular constriction.

General anesthesia with intubation and mechanical ventilation results in a decrease in FRC, which is caused by loss of muscle tone, diaphragmatic displacement, and loss of thoracic volume. Lung compliance drops, airway pressures increase, and $\dot{V}/\dot{Q}$ abnormalities occur. However, most patients have no difficulty tolerating these changes. These changes are exaggerated in the Trendelenburg position, especially in the elderly, the obese, and those with preexisting cardiopulmonary disease. Intrathoracic, peak inspiratory, and plateau pressures increase, then increase even further when pneumoperitoneum creates an increase in pressure and volume. Endobronchial intubation can occur as a result of cephalad movement of the carina, and it should be ruled out if hypoxemia occurs.

Bardoczky GI, Engelman E, Levarlet M et al: Ventilatory effects of pneumoperitoneum monitored with continuous spirometry. Anaesthesia 48:309, 1993

Brimacombe JR, Orland H, Graham D: Endobronchial intubation during upper abdominal laparoscopic surgery in the reverse Trendelenburg position [Letter]. Anesth Analg 78:601, 1994

Gunnarsson L, Lindberg P, Tokics L et al: Lung function after open versus laparoscopic cholecystectomy. Acta Anaesthesiol Scand 39:302–306, 1995

Kendall AP, Bhatt S, Oh TE: Pulmonary consequences of carbon dioxide insufflation for laparoscopic cholecystectomies. Anaesthesia 50:286–289, 1995

Nunn JF: Nunn's Applied Respiratory Physiology, 4th ed, p 523. Oxford, Butterworth-Heinemann, 1993

Obeid F, Saba A, Fath J et al: Increases in intra-abdominal pressure affect pulmonary compliance. Arch Surg 130:544–547, 1995

Wittgen CM, Andrus CH, Fitzgerald SD et al: Analysis of the hemodynamic and ventilatory effects of laparoscopic cholecystectomy. Arch Surg 126:997–1001, 1991

C.20. What are the direct and indirect effects of hypercarbia on the central nervous system?

The brain is particularly sensitive to changes in P_{CO_2}. Slight elevations of CO_2 cause direct cortical depression, and increase the threshold for seizures. Higher levels of CO_2 (25% to 30%) stimulate subcortical hypothalamic centers, resulting in increased cortical excitability and seizures. This hyperexcitability level is enhanced by adrenal cortical and medullary hormones released secondary to hypercarbia-induced stimulation of the hypothalamus. Further elevations of CO_2 cause an anesthetic-like state of cortical and subcortical depression.

Carbon dioxide was first used as an anesthetic by Hickman in 1824 and reintroduced by Leake and Waters in 1928. CO_2 caused an N_2O-like narcosis at about 90 to 120 mm Hg. However, hypercarbia also causes increased excitability of neurons so that seizures occurred shortly afterward. In dogs, however, general anesthesia is achieved at the higher level of P_{CO_2}—about 245 mm Hg—probably by intracellular derangements caused by low pH.

Carbon dioxide, not H^+, crosses the blood-brain barrier and the brain cell membrane, and affects the cell metabolism. Therefore a change in P_{CO_2} also causes a rapid change in cerebrospinal fluid (CSF) pH. CO_2 is the most important factor in regulating cerebral blood flow (CBF). The relation between cerebral blood flow and P_{CO_2} is essentially linear from 20 to 100 mm Hg, with maximal vasodilatation at about 120 mm Hg. Normal CBF is approximately 20% of cardiac output, or 50 ml/100 g/min. For each 1 mm Hg increase in P_{CO_2} between 25 and 100 mm Hg, CBF increases by

2% to 4%. Hypercarbia decreases cerebral vascular resistance, causing cerebral blood flow to increase.

Hypercarbia causes an increase in intracranial pressure, probably secondary to vasodilatation. When the patient is placed in the Trendelenburg position, venous congestion of the head and neck occurs. Additional increases in intra-abdominal and intrathoracic pressures contribute to further increases in intracranial and CSF pressures.

Irgau I, Koyfman Y, Tikellis JI: Elective intraoperative intracranial pressure monitoring during laparoscopic cholecystectomy. Arch Surg 130:1011–1013, 1995

Kirkinen P, Hirvonen E, Kauko M et al: Intracranial blood flow during laparoscopic hysterectomy. Acta Obstet Gynecol Scand 74:71–74, 1995

Nunn JF: Nunn's Applied Respiratory Physiology, 4th ed, p 518. Oxford, Butterworth-Heinemann, 1993

C.21. What are the direct and indirect effects of CO_2 on the renal system?

Oliguria has been frequently observed during laparoscopy despite adequate hydration. Although prerenal causes such as hypovolemia, positive pressure ventilation, and positive end-expiratory pressure (PEEP) contribute to oliguria, it is believed that neurohumoral changes (e.g., antidiuretic hormone [ADH] secretion) secondary to hypercarbia, and increased intra-abdominal pressure secondary to insufflation may be responsible. Sympathetic stimulation causes a release of catecholamines, resulting in decreased renal cortical blood flow with shunting of blood to the adrenal medulla, constriction of glomerular afferent arterioles, and decreased glomerular filtration rate. It has recently been shown that when intraperitoneal insufflation reaches a pressure of 15 mm Hg, renal cortical blood flow decreases about 60%, and a reversible 50% drop in urine volume occurs. In contrast, no decrease in urine output occurred when the abdominal wall was lifted with a force of 15 mm Hg during the new "gasless laparoscopy." It has also been shown that pneumoretroperitoneum, which causes a more gradual increase in intra-abdominal pressure, also caused a more gradual decrease in renal perfusion. Finally, it has been shown that unilateral retroperitoneal insufflation causes decreased renal cortical perfusion of only the ipsilateral kidney if the intra-abdominal pressure is not elevated.

Chiu AW, Chang LS, Birkett DH: The impact of pneumoperitoneum, pneumoretroperitoneum, and gasless laparoscopy on the systemic and renal hemodynamics. J Am Coll Surg 181:397–406, 1995

Hunter JG: Laparoscopic pneumoperitoneum: The abdominal compartment syndrome revisited [Editorial]. J Am Coll Surg 181:469–470, 1995

Nunn JF: Nunn's Applied Respiratory Physiology, 4th ed, p 526. Oxford, Butterworth-Heinemann, 1993

C.22. What is the effect of hypercarbia and laparoscopy on the bowel and gastrointestinal system?

Although CO_2 directly causes vasodilatation of the splanchnic capillary beds, the increased intra-abdominal pressure of laparoscopy decreases perfusion, increases SVR, and may cause bowel hypoxia at high pressures. On release of intra-abdominal pressure, residual CO_2 causes vascular dilation, allowing additional CO_2 to enter the blood stream. Myoelectric activity and recovery from ileus is faster after laparoscopic than after open surgery. The combined effect of the increase in abdominal pressure, stretching of the peritoneum by insufflation, and diffusion of CO_2 into bowel is probably responsible for any postoperative nausea.

Bohm B, Milsom JW, Fazio VW: Postoperative intestinal motility following conventional and laparoscopic intestinal surgery. Arch Surg 130:415–419, 1995

Eleftheriadis E, Kotzampassi K, Papanotas K et al: Gut ischemia, oxidative stress, and bacterial translocation in elevated abdominal pressure in rats. World J Surg 20:11–16, 1996

C.23. How would you recognize CO_2 embolism during laparoscopy? How does this differ from air embolism? Why should N_2O be discontinued during suspected embolization? Will N_2O increase the size of CO_2 emboli?

Insufflation of a large amount of CO_2 directly into a blood vessel can occur initially after blind Veress needle insertion, especially at high pressures. This should be suspected if the abdominal cavity does not distend equally in all four quadrants despite insufflation of several liters of CO_2. Hypotension, hypoxia, cyanosis, or cardiac arrest can occur. If the gas volume is large enough, a "mill-wheel" murmur may be heard through a precordial or esophageal stethoscope. If ventilation is kept constant, a sudden decrease in end-tidal CO_2 may be noted. The most sensitive means to detect gas emboli are the precordial and transesophageal Doppler and transesophageal echocardiography. Aspiration of foamy blood from a central venous catheter is diagnostic.

Carbon dioxide embolism, however, must be distinguished from air embolism, a far more ominous event, as shown in Table 39-2. Carbon dioxide, being extremely soluble in the presence of red blood cells, is much less life-threatening than an identically sized intravascular bolus of air. It has been reported that the lethal volume of intravascular CO_2 gas in cats is 30 times greater than the lethal volume of intravascular air.

Air emboli are likely to be entrained in open veins above the level of the heart, a condition that can exist during head and neck or neurosurgery. Other gases that are present, nitrous oxide, for example, will diffuse into that air space according to their diffusion capacities and pressure gradients. Therefore nitrous oxide will diffuse in, oxygen will be consumed and/or diffuse out, and the size or pressure of the bubble will increase. It is estimated that inhalation of 50% N_2O will double the size of an air (i.e., nitrogen) bubble in 10 minutes, whereas inhalation of 75% N_2O will quadruple its size. A gas bubble composed of 100% CO_2, however, will not enlarge in a patient inhaling 50% or even 75% N_2O because more CO_2 will move out or be absorbed or buffered (also more quickly) than N_2O moving in. This is not to deny that CO_2 gas

Table 39-2.   Differences Between Air and Carbon Dioxide Emboli

EMBOLISM	AIR	CO$_2$
Composition	79% N$_2$, 21% O$_2$	100% CO$_2$
Position	Sitting, upright	Any
Origin	Vein open to air	No contact with air
Pressure source	Hydrostatic	Insufflator
Solubility	Negligible	Large
Effect of N$_2$O	Enlarged	Not enlarged

has caused fatal embolisms or that N_2O should be discontinued if embolism is suspected. A recent study using transesophageal echocardiography in 16 patients undergoing laparoscopic cholecystectomy reported gas embolism in 11 of the 16 patients (5 during peritoneal insufflation and 6 during gallbladder dissection), but all were subclinical with no signs of cardiorespiratory instability. In addition, conditions for creating CO_2 embolism differ from conditions for air embolism. Other than direct insufflation of CO_2 into a vein, as during Veress needle insufflation, the capillaries and veins within the abdomen are collapsed by the positive pressure within the abdomen.

Derouin M, Couture P, Boudreault D et al: Detection of gas embolism by transesophageal echocardiography during laparoscopic cholecystectomy. Anesth Analg 82:119–124, 1996

Kunkler A, King H: Comparison of air, oxygen, and carbon dioxide embolization. Ann Surg 449:95–99, 1959

Ostman PL, Pantle-Fisher FH, Faure EA: Circulatory collapse during laparoscopy. J Clin Anesth 2:129–132, 1990

C. 24. How is gas embolism (CO_2 or air) treated?

- Nitrous oxide should be discontinued, and the F_IO_2 should be increased to 1.0.
- Identify and occlude the air entrainment site. Insufflation (in the case of CO_2) should be halted.
- An increase in the rate and volume of controlled ventilation with PEEP has been suggested as a method of minimizing air entrainment. However, this may decrease the cardiac output and excessively increase the airway pressure and pulmonary vascular resistance (and can lead to paradoxical air embolization).
- If possible, the patient should be placed in steep left lateral decubitus Trendelenburg position to prevent obstruction of the pulmonary outflow tract and right ventricular failure.
- A CVP catheter is useful for diagnosis and for therapeutic aspiration of air. Radial artery cannulation is useful to track improvement or deterioration.
- Therapy is essentially supportive and may include fluids, vasopressors, and Swan-Ganz catheterization. A large bolus of gas may form a gas lock in the right atrium, decreasing the cardiac output. Smaller bubbles can lodge in the lungs, causing pulmonary hypertension, right ventricular failure, and pulmonary edema. Venous gas emboli may also enter the arterial circulation through an atrial septal defect or open foramen ovale, a condition that may exist in 20% of patients.

Beck DH, McQuillan PJ: Fatal carbon dioxide embolism and severe haemorrhage during laparoscopic salpingectomy. Br J Anaesth 72:243–245, 1994

Gravenstein N (ed): Manual of Complications During Anesthesia, pp 332–345. Philadelphia, Lippincott, 1991

C. 25. What are the causes of pneumothorax or pneumomediastinum during laparoscopy? How would you diagnose it? How would you treat it?

Pneumothorax can result from migration of the laparoscopic gas under pressure or from direct pulmonary barotrauma.

During laparoscopy, CO_2 under pressure can pass from the abdominal cavity into the pleural and pericardial spaces through anatomic or congenital paths (as the hiatus around the esophagus) or through acquired defects in the diaphragm. (Embryologically, before formation of the diaphragm, the peritoneal and pleural cavities derived from one sac.) CO_2 gas insufflated retroperitoneally gains rapid direct access to a vast space.

Pneumothorax can be diagnosed by a sudden decrease in pulmonary compliance, an increase in airway pressure, an increase in $P_{ET}CO_2$ and $PaCO_2$, an unchanged or decreased PaO_2, an unchanged or decreased BP, abnormal motion of the involved side hemidiaphragm, and absence of breath sounds without wheezing on the affected side. The shape of the capnogram is usually unchanged. Fiberoptic bronchoscopy will rule out endobronchial intubation, and intraoperative chest fluoroscopy or x-ray will confirm the diagnosis.

Pneumothorax caused by laparoscopic gas is easily treated or it can resolve spontaneously. One study reports an incidence of pneumothorax in 7 of 46 patients undergoing laparoscopic fundoplication for repair of hiatus hernia. In these cases, intraoperative treatment consisted of PEEP and increased minute ventilation to reinflate the lung, and increased pressure to decrease the gradient from abdomen to pleural cavity, and possibly to seal the tear.

Alternatively, pneumothorax may be undetected until the patient wakes up and exhibits respiratory distress and restlessness, which can be misinterpreted as pain or inadequate reversal of the muscle relaxant. Treatment consists of 100% oxygen by mask. CO_2 will quickly diffuse out, as can be easily seen by serial blood gases and x-rays, and invasive treatment is unnecessary.

Because of the increased volumes and pressures in the lung during laparoscopy, pneumothorax can also result from barotrauma. This cause of pneumothorax is far more serious, and may require tube thoracostomy. Attempts at hyperventilating to decrease the $P_{ET}CO_2$ can result in overdistention and rupture of alveoli, with subsequent dissection of the anesthetic gases into the perivascular sheaths, mediastinum, pleura, and fascial planes of the head and neck. Large tidal volumes and rapid ventilator rates can be especially dangerous in patients with COPD or bullae because insufficient emptying time may increase air trapping.

Batra MS, Driscoll JJ, Coburn WA et al: Evanescent nitrous oxide pneumothorax after laparoscopy. Anesth Analg 62:1121–1123, 1983

Joris JL, Chiche J-D, Lamy ML: Pneumothorax during laparoscopic fundoplication: Diagnosis and treatment with positive end-expiratory pressure. Anesth Analg 81:993–1000, 1995

C.26. How would you decide when to extubate?

In addition to the usual criteria for extubation, prolonged laparoscopy in the Trendelenburg position requires other considerations.

Delay extubation if the patient has edema, venous congestion, and duskiness of the head and neck. Sometimes the tongue becomes edematous. If unsure, check the eyes for conjunctival and lid edema, and keep the patient in head-up position until the conjunctivae no longer seem raised or watery.

Causes of edema include dependent stasis from the Trendelenburg position, resistance from elevated abdominal and thoracic pressures, and temporary fluid overload from oliguria or anuria. In some cases it is best to leave the patient intubated until diuresis has begun, especially because "PACU pulmonary edema" is not rare.

D. Postoperative Management

D. 1. What are some of the unique complications of laparoscopy?

Injuries from Instruments
Improper placement of Veress needle or trochars can cause abdominal wall bleeding, blood vessel or visceral puncture, subcutaneous emphysema, peritonitis, wound infections, hernia at the trochar site, and hemorrhage. Thermal injuries may occur from cautery or laser use. Staples and clips can cause nerve entrapment.

Complications of Pneumoperitoneum
Increased intra-abdominal pressure can result in bowel ischemia, omental or bowel herniation, gastric regurgitation, excessive compression of vena cava, decreased venous return, venous stasis in legs, hypotension, increased intrathoracic pressure, mediastinal and subcutaneous emphysema, pneumothorax, barotrauma, CO_2 gas embolism, atelectasis, nausea and vomiting, bradyarrhythmias from peritoneal distention, and shoulder pain from retained CO_2.

Systemic Effects of CO_2 Absorption
Among the systemic effects of CO_2 absorptions are hypercarbia, acidosis, increased sympathoadrenal stimulation, hypertension, tachycardia, increased intracranial pressure, and sickle cell crisis. Arrhythmias can occur from hypercarbia, hypoxia, catecholamines, and in combination with halothane

Trendelenburg Position
Venous congestion of head and neck, increased venous pressure, increased intracranial pressure, retinal hemorrhage, retinal detachment, increased intraocular pressure and glaucoma attack, endobronchial intubation and hypoxemia, ventilation-perfusion mismatch and hypoxia, neuropathy, corneal and conjunctival edema, edema of airway including larynx, airway obstruction and closure, brachial plexus injury from shoulder braces, femoral nerve and peroneal neuropathies, and an assortment of respiratory complications have been reported with use of the Trendelenburg position.

Late Complications
Among the late complications are bowel obstruction from injury; cautery burn; intestine or omentum herniation through the trochar site; adhesions; deep vein thrombosis; and nerve injury due to improper padding. Fever may indicate infection from bowel necrosis. Cutaneous metastasis can occur at the port site.

Bangma CH, Kirkels WJ, Chadha S et al: Cutaneous metastasis following laparoscopic pelvic lymphadenopathy for prostatic carcinoma. J Urol 153:1635–1636, 1995

Bolder PM, Norton ML: Retinal hemorrhage following anesthesia. Anesthesiology 61:595–597, 1984

Chapin JW, Hurlbert BJ, Scheer K: Hemorrhage and cardiac arrest during laparoscopic tubal ligation. Anesthesiology 53:342–343, 1980

Childers JM, Caplinger P: Spontaneous pneumothorax during operative laparoscopy secondary to congenital diaphragmatic defects. A case report. J Reprod Med 40:151–153, 1995

Querleu D, Chapron C: Complications of gynecologic laparoscopic surgery. Curr Opin Obstet Gynecol 7:257–261, 1995

D.2. What postoperative orders will you write? When would you remove the Foley catheter and arterial line? Under what circumstances would you order a chest x-ray?

Immediate chest x-ray is ordered if respiratory distress, subcutaneous emphysema, and actual or suspected pneumothorax occurred; or if the case was prolonged and retroperitoneal, the patient was oliguric despite adequate hydration, intra-abdominal pressure was >15 mm Hg, or if the patient has a history of cardiac or pulmonary disease.

Do not remove the arterial line until the patient is stable and blood gases are normal.

Check urine volumes. Expect an immediate diuresis. Do not remove the Foley catheter until the patient is stable, with fluid intake and volume output stable. Order IV fluids. Check voiding after the catheter is removed.

D.3. What is the incidence of postoperative nausea and vomiting?

The incidence of nausea and vomiting after laparoscopy has been reported to be as high as 42%. It is the most important factor in causing an overnight admission after ambulatory surgery. Intravenous droperidol or ondansetron should be given, preferably during surgery. The cause of nausea and vomiting is believed to be rapid peritoneal distention. Neurogenic pathways are activated by traction reflexes and by splanchnic pressure and manipulation.

Green G, Jonsson L: Nausea: the most important factor determining length of stay after ambulatory anaesthesia. A comparative study of isoflurane and/or propofol techniques. Acta Anaesthesiol Scand 37:742–746, 1993

Sukhani R, Lurie J, Jabamoni R: Propofol for ambulatory gynecologic laparoscopy: Does omission of nitrous oxide alter postoperative emetic sequelae and recovery? Anesth Analg 78:831–835, 1994

The Hematologic System

VII

Hemophilia and Coagulation Disorders   **40**

Robert E. Kelly
Fun-Sun F. Yao

A 28-year-old man was a known hemophiliac and human immunodeficiency virus (HIV) positive. He fractured his left radial head while rollerblading. The orthopedic surgeon scheduled a surgical repair of the fracture for the following morning.

A. Medical Disease and Differential Diagnosis

1. Describe the differences between hemophilia A and B.
2. Describe the pathophysiology associated with von Willebrand's disease.
3. Discuss the different components of factor VIII.
4. Describe the normal physiology of hemostasis.
5. What prevents the extension of a clot beyond the site of injury?
6. Describe the procoagulant factors involved in the extrinsic, intrinsic, and common coagulation cascade.
7. Describe the levels of factor VIII necessary for hemostasis.
8. Describe the various laboratory tests that evaluate the coagulation cascade and the specific components measured by each.

B. Preoperative Evaluation and Preparation

1. What steps would you take to correct this patient's coagulation status?
2. What is meant by 1 U of factor VIII clotting activity and how much does 1 U of factor VIII clotting activity per kilogram of body weight increase factor VIII concentrations?
3. Would you administer factor VIII using a bolus or infusion technique?
4. Can a hemophilic patient fail to mount an appropriate coagulation response following factor VIII infusion?
5. If a patient with hemophilia does not respond to a bolus injection of factor VIII can an infusion technique be effective?
6. How much factor VIII activity is present in fresh-frozen plasma (FFP)?
7. How much factor VIII activity is present in cryoprecipitate?
8. Describe the products that are available for transfusion of factor VIII activity and their advantages and disadvantages.
9. Would you use DDAVP (desmopressin) preoperatively for hemostatic management of this patient?

C. Intraoperative Management

1. Would you administer an intramuscular (IM) premedicant to this patient prior to surgery?

2. What type of anesthetic would you plan for this patient?
3. Is it safe to intubate this patient for general anesthesia?
4. Would you use any special precautions for this patient who is HIV positive?
5. Are there special considerations in choosing anesthetic drugs for this patient?
6. During the operative procedure, the surgeon indicated that significant blood loss had occurred. Would you transfuse this patient with packed red blood cells or whole blood?
7. During the transfusion of the first unit of whole blood, the patient's temperature rose from 36.8° to 37.9°C. What immediate steps should be taken by the anesthesiologist at this time?
8. Does giving blood intraoperatively increase the potential for the development of factor VIII inhibitors?
9. Can factor VIII be safely administered to patients who have developed circulating inhibitors?
10. Is it appropriate to suction the endotracheal tube and oropharynx of this patient prior to extubation?

D. Postoperative Management

1. If the patient is to be discharged 7 hours following the surgical procedure, should any special instructions be given regarding pain management or the use of over-the-counter medications?
2. What steps should be taken to enhance the coagulation status of this patient in the postoperative period while at home?

A. Medical Disease and Differential Diagnosis

A.1. Describe the differences between hemophilia A and B?

Hemophilia A is an X-linked recessive genetic disorder caused by deficient or defective factor VIII. This results in a hemorrhagic tendency that, in its most severe form, can be life-threatening. A screening test for hemophilia A is the partial thromboplastin time (PTT), which will be prolonged in all but those with mild disease. Measuring factor VIII activity provides a definitive diagnosis.

Hemophilia B is an X-linked genetic disorder with an inheritance pattern and clinical features indistinguishable from those of hemophilia A. However, this disease is a result of a defective or deficient factor IX molecule. As in the patient with hemophilia A, the PTT will be prolonged and the diagnosis for hemophilia B will require the demonstration of a low or absent plasma factor IX concentration.

Stoelting RK, Dierdorf SF (eds): Anesthesia and Co-existing Disease, 3rd ed, pp 411–412. New York, Churchill Livingstone, 1993

A.2. Describe the pathophysiology associated with von Willebrand's disease?

Von Willebrand's disease is inherited as an autosomal dominant trait (type 1 and 2) or, rarely, as an autosomal recessive trait (type 3). This coagulation disorder is caused by a quantitative abnormality of factor VIII: von Willebrand's factor (type 1) or a qualitative abnormality of this complex (type 2). Type 3 involves a markedly defective synthesis of factor VIII that results in a bleeding pattern similar to that seen in severe hemophilia A. Patients with von Willebrand's disease often have a life-long history of bruising and mild epistaxis from mucosal services, but can be unaware of having the disease. They have a bleeding disorder until they undergo surgery or experience trauma. Diagnosis of von Willebrand's disease is suggested by the patient's history and the presence of a prolonged bleeding time, despite a normal platelet count.

Miller RD (ed): Anesthesia, 4th ed, p 251. New York, Churchill Livingstone, 1994

Stoelting RK, Dierdorf SF (eds): Anesthesia and Co-existing Disease, 3rd ed, pp 412–413. New York, Churchill Livingstone, 1993

A.3. Discuss the different components of factor VIII.

Factor VIII is a procoagulant complex that consists of two portions, factor VIII:vWF and factor VIII:C. In hemophilia A factor VIII:C production is different in both amount and quality, whereas in von Willebrand's disease (type 1) a decrease is seen in both factor VIII:C and factor VIII:vWF. In type 2 von Willebrand's disease factor VIII:C levels are normal, whereas factor VIII:vWF levels are depressed.

Miller RD (ed): Anesthesia, 4th ed, p 251. New York, Churchill Livingstone, 1994.

A.4. Describe the normal physiology of hemostasis.

When the circulatory system is interrupted, coagulation proceeds in three phases.

- The vascular contraction of smooth muscle resulting in vasoconstriction occurs as a result of the release of thromboxane A_2 from platelets that have adhered to the injury site.
- The formation of a platelet plug. Platelet membrane receptors bind at the site of injury and release adenosine diphosphate (ADP), which causes other platelets to aggregate.
- Activation of the clotting cascade. The tissue under the vascular injury site initiates the activation of circulating procoagulants. The platelets interact with both fibrin and thrombin to fuse the platelet plug, whereas activation of factor XIII produces cross-polymerization of the loose fibrin to produce a firm clot.

Ellison N: Hemostasis and hemotherapy. In: Miller RD (ed): Anesthesia, 4th ed, p 251. New York, Churchill Livingstone, 1994

Stoelting RK, Dierdorf SF (eds): Anesthesia and Co-existing Disease, 3rd ed, p 407. New York, Churchill Livingstone, 1993

A.5. What prevents the extension of a clot beyond the site of injury?

Localization of the coagulation process to the site of injury due to many factors, which include:

- Dilution of procoagulants in the flowing blood.
- Removal of activated factors by the liver.
- Action of circulating procoagulant inhibitors such as antithrombin III and protein C.

- The release of tissue plasminogen activator (tPA) to convert plasminogen to plasmin, a serene protease that digests fibrinogen and factors V and VIII. This process initiates the physiologic function of fibrinolysis, which digests fibrin into small segments known as "fibrin degradation" (split) products, which are removed by the mononuclear phagocyte system.

Ellison N: Hemostasis and hemotherapy. In: Miller RD (ed): Anesthesia, 4th ed, pp 251–254. New York, Churchill Livingstone, 1994

Stoelting RK, Dierdorf SF (eds): Anesthesia and Co-existing Disease, 3rd ed, p 407. New York, Churchill Livingstone, 1993

A.6. Describe the procoagulant factors involved in the extrinsic, intrinsic, and common coagulation cascade.

The common coagulation cascade is shown in Figure 40-1.

The rigid division of the coagulation cascade into an intrinsic and extrinsic system has lost absolute validity because of the crossover of many factors. For instance, factor VIIa can activate factor IX, but factors IXa, Xa, thrombin, and XIIa can activate factor VII. Effective homeostasis requires both systems to function together.

Ellison N: Hemostatis and hemotherapy. In: Miller RD (ed): Anesthesia, 4th ed, p 253. New York, Churchill Livingstone, 1994

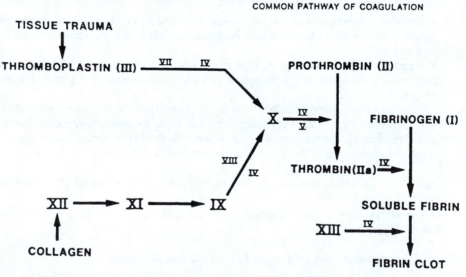

Figure 40-1. Schematic diagram of the procoagulant phase of coagulation depicting the cascade sequence in three steps, designated as the intrinsic, extrinsic, and common coagulation pathways. (Reprinted with permission from Stoelting RK, Dierdorf SF, McCammon RL [eds]: Anesthesia and Co-Existing Disease, 2nd ed, p 577. New York, Churchill Livingstone, 1988)

Table 40-1. The Levels of Factor VIII Necessary for Hemostasis

CLINICAL PRESENTATION	FACTOR VIII CONCENTRATION (% OF NORMAL)
Spontaneous hemorrhage	1%–3%
Moderate trauma	4%–8%
Hemarthrosis and deep skeletal muscle hemorrhage	10%–15%
Major surgery	>30%

Stoelting RK, Dierdorf SF (eds): Anesthesia and Co-existing Disease, 3rd ed, p 409. New York, Churchill Livingstone, 1993

A.7. Describe the levels of factor VIII necessary for hemostasis.

See Table 40-1.

Jamco RL, McClean WE, Terrin JM et al: A prospective study of patterns of bleeding in boys with hemophilia. Haemophilia 2:202–206, 1996

Stoelting RK, Dierdorf SF (eds): Anesthesia and Co-existing Disease, 3rd ed, p 411. New York, Churchill Livingstone, 1993

A.8. Describe the various laboratory tests that evaluate the coagulation cascade and the specific components measured by each.

Laboratory evaluation of the coagulation cascade can be defined as shown in Table 40-2.

A prolongation of the prothrombin time (PT) or PTT can be caused by either a circulating anticoagulant or a coagulation factor deficiency. If the test is repeated with equal volumes of control plasma and patient plasma compared with a 9 to 1 patient:control plasma dilution, the diagnosis is made of an inhibitor with continued prolongation in the former, although shortening with the latter indicates a coagulation factor deficiency.

Miller RD (ed): Anesthesia, 4th ed, p 255. New York, Churchill Livingstone, 1994

Stoelting RK, Dierdorf SF (eds): Anesthesia and Co-existing Disease, 3rd ed, p 409. New York, Churchill Livingstone, 1993

B. Preoperative Evaluation and Preparation

B.1. What steps would you take to correct this patient's coagulation status?

Orthopedic surgical procedures require more factor replacement than other types of surgery when a raw bone surface must heal, or when a small amount of bleeding

Table 40-2. Specific Components Measured by Different Coagulation Tests

LABORATORY TESTS	COMPONENTS MEASURED
Bleeding time	Platelet count, vascular integrity
Prothrombin time	I, II, V, VII and X
Partial prothrombin time (PTT)	I, II, V, VII, IX, X, XI and XII
Thrombin time	I, II

into or around a prosthetic joint will lead to infection and destruction of the surrounding tissue. When the extremity or operative site is to be held firm with plaster, or if good surgical apposition of tissues can be achieved with sutures, less factor replacement is required. Factor VIII levels 30% of normal usually provide adequate hemostasis; however, most clinicians will correct factor VIII levels to near normal. This overcompensation allows for adequate homeostasis to continue, even when factor VIII levels may diminish if a bolus technique is used.

For a major orthopedic procedure, the patient's plasma factor VIII levels should be corrected to 100% approximately 1 to 2 hours prior to the procedure. For the first 4 postoperative days, the levels should be maintained at 80% of normal, whereas during the subsequent 4 days the factor VIII level should be maintained at 40% of normal. Finally, for the patient with severe disease a level of 10% should be maintained for the following 3 weeks.

Hilgartner MW: Factor replacement. In Hilgartner MW (ed): Hemophilia in the Child and Adult, p 76. New York, Masson Publishers, 1983

Inwood MJ, Meltzer DB: The female carrier of hemophilia: A problem for the anesthetist. Can Anaesth Soc J 25(4):266–269, 1978

B.2. What is meant by 1 U of factor VIII clotting activity and how much does 1 U of factor VIII clotting activity per kilogram of body weight increase factor VIII concentrations?

One unit of factor VIII clotting activity is defined as the amount present in 1 ml of fresh normal, pooled plasma. A single unit of factor VIII clotting activity per kilogram of body weight will increase plasma factor VIII levels approximately 2%. Therefore, to prescribe the factor VIII activity necessary to correct a 70 kg hemophilia patient with 5% factor VIII activity to 95% of normal, one would calculate as follows:

$$\frac{95\% - 5\%}{2\%} \times 70 \text{ kg} = 3150 \text{ U of factor VIII to be infused}$$

Ellison N: Diagnosis and management of bleeding disorders. Anesthesiology 47:17–80, 1977

Pisciotto PT (ed): Blood Transfusion Therapy, a Physician's Handbook, 3rd ed, Arlington, VA, AABB, 1989

B.3. Would you administer factor VIII using a bolus or infusion technique?

Factor VIII requirements can be reduced while maintaining a desired hemostatic level if given by continuous infusion. This eliminates the high peak concentration observed following bolus injections, as well as the trough when the concentration may fall below a desired level. Fortunately, factor VIII concentrates are stable after reconstitution during storage at room temperature and thus lend themselves well to continuous infusion techniques.

Schulman S, Gitel S, Martinowitz U: The stability of factor VIII concentrates after reconstitution. Am J Hematol 45:217–223, 1994

Schulman S, Martinowitz U: Continuous infusion instead of bolus injections of factor concentrate? Haemophilia 2:189–191, 1996

B.4. Can a hemophilic patient fail to mount an appropriate coagulation response following factor VIII infusion?

Approximately 7% to 10% of hemophiliacs will develop an antibody inhibitor against factor VIII, and they do not achieve the anticipated response following factor VIII infusion.

Schulman S, Martinowitz U: Continuous infusion instead of bolus injections of factor concentrate? Haemophilia 2:189–191, 1996

Stoelting RK, Dierdorf SF (eds): Anesthesia and Co-existing Disease, 3rd ed, p 412. New York, Churchill Livingstone, 1993

B.5. If a patient with hemophilia does not respond to a bolus injection of factor VIII can an infusion technique be effective?

Some patients who do not respond well to bolus injections may have measurable low titers of inhibitors. A continuous infusion has proved to be effective in stopping hemorrhage in this situation because appropriate levels of the missing factor can be achieved relatively easily by the infusion method. Those patients with high titers and without measurable factor level during the infusion have also been known to stop bleeding with an infusion technique, likely because complete inhibition of the factor only occurs after 1 to 2 hours. If the factor is continuously infused, some of it will always be circulating, unneutralized and hemostatically active.

Gordon EM, Mungo R, Goldsmith JG: Lingual hemorrhage in a patient with hemophilia A complicated by a high titer inhibitor. Am J Pediatr Hematol Oncol 15:107–110, 1993.

B.6. How much factor VIII activity is present in fresh-frozen plasma (FFP)?

What risks are associated with the administration of FFP?

Fresh-frozen plasma, which is prepared from a single donor, contains all plasma proteins, particularly factor VIII. As a result of the preparation process, factor VIII activity is between 0.7 and 0.9 U of clotting activity per milliliter of FFP. Normally, FFP is produced to include approximately 200 ml/bag.

The risks associated with the transfusion of FFP are the same as with any other single donor blood product: sensitization to foreign proteins and all infectious processes, including hepatitis and AIDS. The incidence of hepatitis B and hepatitis C transmission following transfusion is estimated to be 1:200,000 and 1:3,300, respectively, whereas the risk of transmission of acquired immune deficiency syndrome (AIDS) is felt to be between 1:450,000 and 1:660,000 per donor exposure.

ASA Task Force: Practice guideline for blood component therapy. Anesthesiology 84:732–747, 1996

Katz J, Steward DJ (eds): Anesthesia and Uncommon Pediatric Diseases, pp 503–505. Philadelphia, WB Saunders, 1987

Vander Wound JC, Milam JD, Walker WE et al: Cardiovascular surgery in patients with congenital plasma coagulopathies. Ann Thorac Surg 46(3):33–37, 1988

B.7. How much factor VIII activity is present in cryoprecipitate?

Cryoprecipitate is the fraction of plasma that precipitates when FFP is thawed. This solution contains high concentrations of factor VIII in a small volume, usually between 5 and 13 U of factor VIII clotting activity per milliliter of solution. Cryoprecipitate is a single-donor unit product that also contains fibrinogen, fibronectin, and von Willebrand's factor. Cryoprecipitate can also contain red cell fragments; therefore, it can sensitize Rh negative individuals to the Rh antigens if the donor is Rh positive.

Stoelting RK, Dierdorf SF (eds): Anesthesia and Co-existing Disease, 3rd ed, p 419. New York, Churchill Livingstone, 1993

Tetit CR, Klein HG: Hemophilia, hemophiliacs and the health care delivery system, p 31. Bethesda, MD, Department of HEW Publication No. (NIH) 76-871, 1976

B.8. Describe the products that are available for transfusion of factor VIII activity and their advantages and disadvantages.

See Table 40-3.

Schulman S, Varon D, Keller N et al: Monoclonal purified FVIII for continuous infusion: Stability, microbiological safety, and clinical experience. Thromb Haemost 72:403–407, 1994

White GC, McMillan CW, Kindon HS et al: The use of recombinant antihemophilic factor in the treatment of two patients with classic hemophilia. N Engl J Med 320:154, 1989

B.9. Would you use DDAVP (desmopressin) preoperatively for hemostatic management of this patient?

A synthetic analog of antidiuretic hormone, DDAVP can be used to prepare mild to moderate hemophiliacs for minor surgery. Factor VIII:C is released from endothelial cell storage sites in response to DDAVP. Unfortunately, elimination half-time of this released factor VIII:C is approximately 12 hours and repeated administration of desmopressin will deplete this storage capability. DDAVP releases tissue plasminogen activator; therefore, administration of epsilon-aminocaproic acid is recommended as well.

Stoelting RK, Dierdorf SF (eds): Anesthesia and Co-existing Disease, 3rd ed, p 412. New York, Churchill Livingstone, 1993

C. Intraoperative Management

C.1. Would you administer an intramuscular (IM) premedicant to this patient prior to surgery?

Intramuscular (IM) injections can be safely administered to any patient with factor VIII activity of 30% to 50% normal. Despite this, it is unlikely that an IM injection

Table 40-3.   The Advantages and Disadvantages of Factor VIII Products

COMPONENT	ADVANTAGE	DISADVANTAGE
Cryoprecipitate	Readily available, long shelf life, relatively low risk of hepatitis and AIDS.	Allergic reaction, hyperfibrinogenemia if large volumes are used.
Factor VIII concentrates	Easily stored and reconstituted, long life, known potency.	Multiple plasma product with high risk of infectious disease.
Monoclonal purified factor VIII	Stability, biological safety	Cost (?)

would be necessary for any such patient. If a sedative hypnotic or an anticholinergic drug needs to be administered to such a patient prior to anesthesia induction, it would be prudent to administer it through an intravenous (IV) route.

Sampson JF, Hamstra R, Aldrete JA: Management of hemophiliac patients undergoing surgical procedures. Anesth Analg 58:133–135, 1979

C.2. What type of anesthetic would you plan for this patient?

Clinicians have long considered regional anesthesia to be contraindicated in a patient with hemophilia owing to fear of hematoma formation. Successful axillary block technique has been reported in two hemophilic patients indicating that, with proper management of coagulation status, a regional technique is acceptable. In each case, the benefits of regional anesthesia must be weighed against a potential risk associated with it. In the absence of a full stomach and emergency procedure, it may be prudent to provide general anesthesia for this patient's procedure.

Sampson JF, Hamstra R, Aldrete JA: Management of hemophiliac patients undergoing surgical procedures. Anesth Analg 58:133–135, 1979

C.3. Is it safe to intubate this patient for general anesthesia?

Although protection of the airway is important for all patients, the hemophilic patient presents an unique challenge to the anesthesiologist. Hemorrhage in the tongue or neck could seriously impair the patency of the upper airway in such a patient. Absolute care must be used in placing the mask on such a patient to prevent trauma to the lips, tongue, or face. Laryngoscopy should be carried out following complete muscle relaxation by a skilled clinician to allow placement of a smaller than predicted, well-lubricated endotracheal tube. Nasal placement of an endotracheal tube is relatively contraindicated because of the potential for epistaxis. If at all possible, manipulation of the airway and the intubation should not be performed until the coagulation status of the patient has been corrected.

Hyderally H, Stark DCC: Hemophilia: Anesthetic implications. Mt. Sinai J Med 44(3):397–399, 1977

C.4. Would you use any special precautions for this patient who is HIV positive?

Universal precautions should be used for all patients regardless of their HIV status. This patient also presents a likely risk of hepatitis transmission because of a history of multiple transfusions, further reinforcing the need for universal precautions.

Stoelting RK, Dierdorf SF (eds): Anesthesia and Co-existing Disease, 3rd ed, p 412. New York, Churchill Livingstone, 1993

C.5. Are there special considerations in choosing anesthetic drugs for this patient?

The likely presence of co-existing liver disease secondary to hepatitis from prior blood or factor VIII transfusions would predispose this patient to sensitivity to those drugs that are metabolized or processed in the liver. As a result, use of such drugs should be avoided or the dose reduced in anticipation of hepatic metabolism. A balanced IV technique may be preferable to an inhaled anesthetic because of the effects of such drugs on hepatic blood flow.

Stoelting RK, Dierdorf SF (eds): Anesthesia and Co-existing Disease, 3rd ed, p 412. New York, Churchill Livingstone, 1993

C.6. During the operative procedure, the surgeon indicated that significant blood loss had occurred. Would you transfuse this patient with packed red blood cells or whole blood?

Blood banks generally fractionate approximately 80% of the units of whole blood that are donated into component parts, including red blood cells, platelets, fresh-frozen plasma, and cryoprecipitate. Following blood loss, packed red blood cells are transfused both to increase oxygen carrying capacity and for volume expansion. In a patient such as this the transfusion of packed red blood cells will dilute the circulating factor VIII levels; therefore, it would be prudent to transfuse whole blood in such a patient. In doing so, oxygen carrying capacity will be increased, as well as all necessary components of coagulation.

Ellison N: Hemostasis and hemotherapy. In: Miller RD (ed): Anesthesia, 4th ed, p 261. New York, Churchill Livingstone, 1994

C.7. During the transfusion of the first unit of whole blood, the patient's temperature rose from 36.8° to 37.9°C. What immediate steps should be taken by the anesthesiologist at this time?

The first step should be immediate discontinuation of the transfusion. Blood should be drawn from the patient and sent to the blood bank along with the questionable unit of blood, so that further crossmatching can be performed. One must first rule out an acute hemolytic transfusion reaction, which can be difficult in the anesthetized patient. The presence of free plasma hemoglobin, which will cause the plasma and urine to become red, may be diagnostic. If an acute hemolytic reaction has occurred, support of the blood pressure with vasopressors to maintain renal blood flow, and fluid and diuretic therapy to maintain urine flow, are the mainstays of treatment. After ruling out an acute hemolytic transfusion reaction, a febrile reaction (elevation of temperature of >1°C associated with transfusion) is the most common complication associated with blood transfusion; it is usually self-limited and need not be treated

Miller RD (ed): Anesthesia, 4th ed, p 262. New York, Churchill Livingstone, 1994

C.8. Does giving blood intraoperatively increase the potential for the development of factor VIII inhibitors?

Although 10% to 15% of all hemophilic patients will develop a circulating inhibitor of factor VIII, no evidence indicates that the development of such an inhibitor is related to the number of transfusions that the patient receives. As a result, the administration of blood products in this setting should not be withheld for fear of inducing an inhibitor response.

Behrman RE, Kliegman RM, Arvin AM (eds): Nelson Textbook of Pediatrics, 15th ed, pp 1426–1427. Philadelphia, WB Saunders, 1996

C.9. Can factor VIII be safely administered to patients who have developed circulating inhibitors?

Factor VIII inhibitors are IgG globulins, which are specifically active against factor VIII. The inhibitors can be of low titer and transient, or of extremely higher titer and very persistent. The Bethesda unit of inhibition is defined as the amount of inhibitory activity in 1 ml of plasma that decreases the factor VIII level in 1 ml of normal plasma from 1 to 0.5 U. It is almost impossible to overpower a high-titer inhibitor; however, when life-threatening hemorrhage occurs, massive doses of factor VIII concentrates or plasmapheresis with replacement with factor VIII should be given, which may be of temporary benefit. Immunosuppressive therapy is of no value.

Another approach at therapy of the hemophilic child with inhibitors involves the use of factor IX concentrates, which apparently contain amounts of activated factor VIII. These activated coagulants enter the coagulation cascade distal to the level of factor VIII and therefore bypass the effects of the inhibitor. However, thrombosis is a possible complication.

Porcine factor VIII is effective in hemophilia A patients with inhibitors. Porcine factor VIII provides adequate factor VIII activity in patients with <50 Bethesda units of inhibitor. The usual starting dose is 100 to 150 porcine U/kg.

Behrman RE, Kliegman RM, Arvin AM (eds): Nelson Textbook of Pediatrics, 15th ed, pp 1426–1427. Philadelphia, WB Saunders, 1996

C.10. Is it appropriate to suction the endotracheal tube and oropharynx of this patient prior to extubation?

Removal of secretions that might be aspirated is essential prior to the extubation of any patient; however, suctioning of the hemophilic patient can trap mucosa in the suction catheter and result in the formation of an oral hematoma. In a hemophilic patient, gentle oral suctioning under direct vision is appropriate to remove all secretions.

Hyderally H, Stark DCC: Hemophilia: Anesthetic implications. Mt. Sinai J Med 44(3):397–399, 1977

D. Postoperative Management

D.1. If the patient is to be discharged 7 hours following the surgical procedure, should any special instructions be given regarding pain management or the use of over-the-counter medications?

Postoperative pain management is important for any postsurgical patient. It is important in the hemophilic patient to avoid any medicine that might produce a bleeding diathesis. As a result, any analgesic containing an aspirin product or nonsteroid anti-inflammatory drugs should be avoided. Medications using acetaminophen or narcotics such as codeine would be appropriate for postoperative pain management. Similarly, antihistamines and antitussives can inhibit platelet aggregation and prolong bleeding time; therefore, these should be avoided in the postoperative patient.

Hilgartner MW: Factor replacement. In: Hilgartner NW (ed): Hemophilia in the Child and Adult. p 78. New York, Masson Publishers, 1983

D.2. What steps should be taken to enhance the coagulation status of this patient in the postoperative period while at home?

Administration of factor VIII concentrate by continuous infusion is routinely used at medical centers for postoperative inpatient hemophiliacs. In the transition of many surgical procedures to the outpatient arena, home infusion of factor VIII can provide the same level of hemostatic protection. Home infusion of purified factor VIII concentrate, which has been shown to be safe, efficacious, and convenient for postoperative patients, should be used for this patient.

Varon D, Schulman S, Bashari D et al: Home therapy with continuous infusion of factor VIII after minor surgery or serious hemorrhage. Hemophilia 2:207–210, 1996

Sickle Cell Disease

Vinod Malhotra

A 26-year-old African-American woman was admitted for bilateral tubal ligation. She had frequent joint and bone pain, a past history of abdominal pain, and jaundice. Hematocrit 22%, blood pressure 140/60 mm Hg, pulse 100 beats/min.

A. Medical Disease and Differential Diagnosis

1. What was the most likely medical problem in this patient?
2. What is sickle cell disease (SCD)?
3. What is sickle cell trait?
4. What does the term "heterozygote" imply in relation to sickle cell disease?
5. What are the clinical features of the disease?
6. What is sickle cell crisis?
7. What is the pathogenesis of sickle cell crisis?
8. What is acute chest syndrome?

B. Preoperative Evaluation and Preparation

1. What were the possible medically justifiable reasons for bilateral tubal ligation in this patient?
2. How would you evaluate this patient for anesthesia?
3. How would you prepare the patient for general anesthesia?
4. What is your opinion of preoperative exchange transfusion in this patient?
5. What are the indications for blood transfusion in sickle cell disease?

C. Intraoperative Management

1. What was the risk for anesthetic complications in this patient?
2. What anesthetic agents and techniques would you employ?
3. What special precautions should one take to prevent sickling in this patient?

D. Postoperative Management

1. How would you manage this patient in the immediate postoperative period?
2. What complications might occur in this patient in the immediate postoperative period?
3. What is the treatment of sickle cell crisis?

A. Medical Disease and Differential Diagnosis

A.1. What was the most likely medical problem in this patient?

In light of the fact that this young African-American patient presented with a history of joint pains, abdominal pain, jaundice, and anemia, sickle cell disease was the most likely diagnosis.

Katz J, Benumof J, Kadis LB (eds): Anesthesia and Uncommon Diseases: Pathophysiologic and Clinical Correlations, 3rd ed, pp 391–394. Philadelphia, WB Saunders, 1990

A.2. What is sickle cell disease (SCD)?

Sickle cell disease is a group of well-defined hemoglobinopathies involving abnormal alteration of the globin moiety. Under certain conditions, especially hypoxia, the hemoglobin aggregates to give the red blood cells a crescent shape (sickle) and hence the name.

Sickle hemoglobin (HbS) is a result of a mutation in the beta-globulin gene where valine substitutes glutamic acid in the amino acid chain of hemoglobin. Nearly 1 of 350 African-Americans have some type of SCD. Common genotypes include homozygous S mutation (sickle cell anemia, Hb SS disease), and heterozygous combinations such as HbS and HbC (Hb SC disease), HbS, and beta-thalassemia mutation (HbS-beta-thalassemia).

Lane PA: Sickle cell disease. Pediatr Clin North Am 43(3):639–664, 1996

Steinberg MH: Review: Sickle cell disease: Present and future treatment. Am J Med Sci 312(4): 166–174, 1996

A.3. What is sickle cell trait?

Sickle cell trait occurs in about 8% of African-Americans, and it is used to describe a person who is a heterozygote for a normal hemoglobin gene (A) with an abnormal gene (S). Persons with sickle cell trait lead a normal life and do not present with symptoms, morbidity, or mortality associated with SCD.

Lane PA: Sickle cell disease. Pediatr Clin North Am 43(3):639–664, 1996

McGoldrick KE (ed): Ambulatory Anesthesiology: A Problem-Oriented Approach, pp 68–69. Baltimore, Williams & Wilkins, 1995

Steinberg MH: Review: Sickle cell disease: Present and future treatment. Am J Med Sci 312(4): 166–174, 1996

A.4. What does the term "heterozygote" imply in relation to sickle cell disease?

The term "heterozygote" only describes the genotype of the individual and should not automatically be associated with sickle cell trait. Sickle cell trait is that heterozygous state in which is found one normal hemoglobin (A) gene and one abnormal hemoglobin (S) gene. If both the genes in the heterozygote are abnormal (e.g., SC, S Thal, SD), a disease state is evident. Classic SCD is homozygous for hemoglobin S and presents with the most severe form of the disease.

Lane PA: Sickle cell disease. Pediatr Clin North Am 43(3):639–664, 1996

McGoldrick KE (ed): Ambulatory Anesthesiology: A Problem-Oriented Approach, pp 68–69. Baltimore, Williams & Wilkins, 1995

Steinberg MH: Review: Sickle cell disease: Present and future treatment. Am J Med Sci 312(4): 166–174, 1996

A.5. What are the clinical features of the disease?

Sickle cell disease is most common among African-Americans, although it has also been observed in persons native to the Mediterranean area. The patients are young and present with the clinical picture of anemia, obstructive or hemolytic jaundice, joint and bone pains, abdominal and chest pains, lymphadenopathy, chronic leg ulcers, hematuria, epistaxis, priapism, finger clubbing, and skeletal deformities. The disease is characterized by periodic exaggeration of symptoms or sickle cell crisis.

A recent survey of 205 hospitalizations of 171 children with sickle cell disease revealed the main causes of hospitalization to be acute anemia, painful crises, and pulmonary and bone infections. The frequency of painful crises increased with age. Another 131 outpatients were found to have frequent fevers, anemia, hepatomegaly, splenomegaly, and growth disorders.

Lane PA: Sickle cell disease. Pediatr Clin North Am 43(3):639–664, 1996

McGoldrick KE (ed): Ambulatory Anesthesiology: A Problem-Oriented Approach, pp 68–69. Baltimore, Williams & Wilkins, 1995

Steinberg MH: Review: Sickle cell disease: Present and future treatment. Am J Med Sci 312(4):166–174, 1996

Thuillez V, Distambou V, Mba JR et al: Current aspects of sickle cell disease in children in Gabon. Arch Pediatr 3(7):668–674, 1996

A.6. What is sickle cell crisis?

Sickle cell crisis refers to the acute clinical picture generally caused by sickling of red blood cells in vivo. Four main clinical types of crises have been described. They are as follows:

- Vascular occlusion crises with organ infarction and pain
- Hemolytic crises with hematologic features of sudden hemolysis
- Sequestration syndrome with sequestration of red blood cells in liver and spleen causing their massive, sudden enlargement and an acute fall in peripheral hematocrit
- Aplastic crises with bone marrow suppression

Patients in painful crisis present with fever, anemia, limb pain, and abdominal pain. They are tachypneic and may have enlarged liver and spleen in addition to abdominal tenderness. Peripheral blood smear shows sickle cells, and radiologic changes in the bones are evident.

Katz J, Benumof J, Kadis LB (eds): Anesthesia and Uncommon Diseases: Pathophysiologic and Clinical Correlations, 3rd ed, p 393. Philadelphia, WB Saunders, 1990

Lane PA: Sickle cell disease. Pediatr Clin North Am 43(3):639-664, 1996

A.7. What is the pathogenesis of sickle cell crisis?

The pathogenesis of cell sickling involves the various factors that contribute to local hypoxia and acidosis. The pathogenesis is shown in Figure 41-1. Once sickling is initiated, it becomes a vicious cycle that causes more sickling unless proper remedial measures are undertaken.

Katz J, Benumof J, Kadis LB (eds): Anesthesia and Uncommon Diseases: Pathophysiologic and Clinical Correlations, 3rd ed, p 395. Philadelphia, WB Saunders, 1990

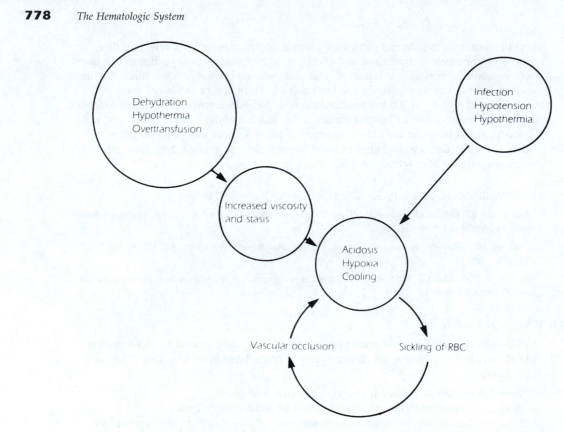

Figure 41-1. Pathogenesis of sickle cell crisis.

A.8. What is acute chest syndrome?

Acute chest syndrome is a term used to describe a constellation of pulmonary symptoms and signs in a patient with sickle cell disease. These include fever, cough, tachypnea, chest pain, and hypoxemia. Pulmonary infiltrates and pleural effusions are commonly seen on chest radiographs. Acute chest syndrome frequently follows vaso-occlusive crises and, therefore, vaso-occlusive pulmonary infarction may be a precipitating cause. Other causes include infection and pulmonary fat embolism due to bone marrow necrosis.

Acute chest syndrome is a potentially serious complication of vaso-occlusive painful crises and should be avoided by judicious hydration, effective analgesia, and avoiding even mild hypoxemia during the crises. Acute chest syndrome should be treated with antibiotics and exchange transfusion may be necessary.

Acute chest pain syndrome is a common postoperative complication following general anesthesia for surgery in these patients.

Castro O, Brambilla DJ, Thorington B: The acute chest syndrome in sickle cell disease: Incidence and risk factors. Blood 84:643, 1994

Emre U, Miller ST, Gutierez M et al: Effect of transfusion in acute chest syndrome of sickle cell disease. J Pediatr 125:901–904, 1995

Lane PA: Sickle cell disease. Pediatr Clin North Am 43(3):639–664, 1996

Vichinsky EP, Haberkern CM, Neumayo L: A comparison of conservative and aggressive transfusion regimens in the perioperative management of sickle cell disease. N Engl J Med 333:206–213, 1995

B. Preoperative Evaluation and Preparation

B.1. What were the possible medically justifiable reasons for bilateral tubal ligation in this patient?

In the past, in patients with sickle cell disease, the fetal and maternal mortality rate has been reported between 20% and 40%. Postpartum shock was reported due to sudden sequestration syndrome. Because each pregnancy was fraught with danger regardless of previous pregnancies, family planning was medically indicated.

Recent experience, however, indicates otherwise. In a multicenter study of 286 pregnancies in patients with SCD, non-sickle cell-related complications were no greater than those in patients who did not have SCD. One death was attributable to SCD. Furthermore, the morbidity due to SCD was not increased in pregnancy when compared with the nonpregnant state.

It has also been shown that prophylactic blood transfusion in the management of pregnant patients with SCD does not decrease perinatal morbidity or mortality when compared with restricted transfusion policy.

El-Shafei AM, Kaur DJ, Kaur SA: Indication for blood transfusion in pregnancy with sickle cell disease. Aust N Z J Obstet Gynecol 35:405–408, 1995

Smith JA, Espeland M, Bellevue R et al: Pregnancy in sickle cell disease: Experience of the cooperative study of sickle cell disease. Obstet Gynecol 87:199–204, 1996

B.2. How would you evaluate this patient for anesthesia?

A careful history and physical examination should be done and cardiopulmonary status should be thoroughly investigated in view of cardiac and pulmonary complications in these patients. One should correct dehydration or infection in the preoperative evaluation. Laboratory tests that should be carried out are complete blood count, blood urea nitrogen (BUN), serum creatinine, urinalysis, electrocardiogram (ECG), and chest x-ray film. In addition, the following specific tests should be carried out:

- Peripheral smear for evidence of sickle cells
- Sickle cell preparation
- Hemoglobin electrophoresis to determine hemoglobin S, quantitatively
- Reticulocyte count

Lane PA: Sickle cell disease. Pediatr Clin North Am 43(3):639–664, 1996

Uppington J: Coagulation disorders and the hemoglobinopathies. Int Anesthiol Clin 23:197–211, 1985

B.3. How would you prepare the patient for general anesthesia?

The patient's general condition should be improved and she should be well hydrated. Any infection should be treated promptly. Anemia should be treated with packed red blood cell transfusion if hemoglobin is <7 g/100 ml. A hematocrit of between 25% and 30% seems to be best tolerated by these patients. Make no attempt to increase the hematocrit to normal values because increased viscosity will predispose the patient to sickling.

Lane PA: Sickle cell disease. Pediatr Clin North Am 43(3):639–664, 1996

Ware RE, Wilston HC: Surgical management of children with hemoglobinopathies. Surg Clin North Am 72:1223–1236, 1992

B.4. What is your opinion of preoperative exchange transfusion in this patient?

Controversy exists to whether these patients should be exchange transfused preoperatively. For high risk surgical procedures, the exchange transfusion should be carried out with buffy-coat free packed red blood cells (RBCs) to reduce the hemoglobin S fraction to <40%. Data support the safety of preoperative transfusion of packed RBCs in children to suppress endogenous erythropoiesis and to reduce the concentration of sickle cell hemoglobin.

Growing evidence, however, indicates that most surgical procedures can be safely performed in patients with SCD. For example, it has been shown that a packed cell transfusion done simply to increase the hemoglobin level to 10 g/100 ml is as effective in decreasing perioperative morbidity as is aggressive exchange transfusions to reduce the HbS levels to 30%. It has also been shown that children can undergo most minor elective surgery safely without any preoperative blood transfusion. Preoperative transfusions have been proposed to be beneficial in thoracotomy, laparotomy, and tonsillectomy patients.

Derkay CS, Bray G, Milmol GJ et al: Adenotonsillectomy in children with sickle cell disease. South Med J 84(2):205–208, 1991

Griffin TC, Buchanan GR: Elective surgery in children with sickle cell disease without preoperative blood transfusion. J Pediatr Surg 28:681–685, 1993

Koshy M, Weiner SJ, Miller ST et al: Surgery and anesthesia in sickle cell disease. Cooperative study of sickle cell diseases. Blood 86:3676–3684, 1995

Vichinsky EP, Haberkern CM, Neumayo L: A comparison of conservative and aggressive transfusion regimens in the perioperative management of sickle cell disease. N Engl J Med 333:206–213, 1995

B.5. What are the indications for blood transfusion in sickle cell disease?

The indications for blood transfusion in sickle cell disease include the following:

Acute Conditions
- Vaso-occlusive crises with organ infarction and dysfunction
- Sequestration syndrome
- Acute hemolysin with exacerbation of anemia
- Aplastic crisis
- Acute chest syndrome
- Acute multiorgan failure
- Severe unresponsive priapism
- Protracted painful crisis
- High risk surgery (e.g., cardiovascular, thoracic)

Chronic Conditions
- Intractable leg ulcers
- Complicated pregnancy
- Stroke
- Recurrent painful syndrome
- Recurrent acute chest syndrome

Embury SH, Hebbel RP, Mohandas N (eds): Transfusion Therapy in Sickle Cell Disease: Basic Principles and Clinical Practice, pp 781–798. New York, Raven Press, 1994

Lane PA: Sickle cell disease. Pediatr Clin North Am 43(3):639–664, 1996

Steinberg MH: Review: Sickle cell disease: Present and future treatment. Am J Med Sci 312(4): 166–174, 1996

Wayne AS, Kevy SV, Nathan DG: Transfusion management of sickle cell disease. Blood 81: 1109–1115, 1993

C. Intraoperative Management

C.1. What was the risk for anesthetic complications in this patient?

This patient was anemic and might be debilitated with cardiopulmonary complications and ischemic damage to various organs. Patients with SCD often present with cardiomegaly, pulmonary hypertension, and heart failure. Pulmonary infarcts and infection are common. A significant percentage of these patients also have renal and hepatic dysfunction. All these problems, in addition to the potential for sickling crisis and sequestration syndrome, pose a greater risk than normal of complications from anesthesia. The patients at greater risk include those with homozygous state, sickle cell C disease, and sickle thalassemia. In contrast, patients with sickle cell trait do not present an increased risk for anesthesia.

Covitz W, Espeland M, Gallagher D et al: The heart in sickle cell anemia. The cooperative study of sickle cell disease. Chest 108:1214–1219, 1995

Koshy M, Weiner SJ, Miller ST et al: Surgery and anesthesia in sickle cell disease. Cooperative study of sickle cell diseases. Blood 86:3676–3684, 1995

Lane PA: Sickle cell disease. Pediatr Clin North Am 43(3):639–664, 1996

C.2. What anesthetic agents and techniques would you employ?

A general inhalation anesthetic technique with the trachea intubated following adequate preoxygenation is a suitable technique. We prefer to hyperventilate these patients moderately to avoid acidosis. We use at least 40% inspired oxygen in lower abdominal and limb surgery; higher concentrations are used for upper abdominal and thoracic surgery and if cardiopulmonary disease is evident. If the pathophysiology of this disease is understood and adequate precautions are taken to avoid complications, almost any anesthetic technique can be employed.

Katz J, Benumof J, Kadis LB (eds): Anesthesia and Uncommon Diseases: Pathophysiologic and Clinical Correlations, 3rd ed, p 396. Philadelphia, WB Saunders, 1990

Miller RD (ed): Anesthesia, 4th ed, pp 981–982. New York, Churchill Livingstone, 1994

C.3. What special precautions should one take to prevent sickling in this patient?

One should avoid or correct the factors that precipitate sickling. Special precautions include the following:

- Avoid hypoxia by preoxygenating the patient and employing higher than usual concentrations of inspired oxygen. A pulse oximeter should be used to monitor oxygen saturation of hemoglobin in the perioperative period and even mild hypoxemia should be avoided.
- Prevent acidosis by maintaining adequate oxygenation and cardiac output. Prevent respiratory acidosis by hyperventilation. Administration of alkaline buffer solutions has been recommended, although we have found them rarely necessary.
- Prevent stasis. This requires proper hydration and good regional blood flow. Blood viscosity should be maintained at a low level by limiting the rise in hematocrit to 30% and by avoiding overtransfusion. Low molecular weight dextran infusion may be helpful, too. Some advise against the use of tourniquets although they have been used without ill effects by others. If a tourniquet is used, it should only be used when absolutely necessary and for as short a period as possible. Special attention should be paid to maintain adequate oxygenation and to prevent respiratory or metabolic acidosis at the time of tourniquet release.
- Prevent dehydration. Patients should be well hydrated and we are generous with fluids in these patients. However, the cardiopulmonary complications should be kept in mind and cardiac overload should be avoided. In view of possible renal dysfunction, proper electrolyte balance should be maintained.
- Prevent hypothermia. All of these patients are monitored for body temperature and should be kept warm with a body warming device both in the operating room and postoperatively.
- Replace blood loss accurately to prevent anemia or overtransfusion, which can lead to increased viscosity and cardiac failure. Fresh blood is preferred to stored blood and all blood should be given through a blood warmer.

Adu-Gyamfi Y, Sankarankutty M, Marrwa S: Use of a tourniquet in patients with sickle-cell disease. Can J Anaesth 40:24–27, 1993

Lane PA: Sickle cell disease. Pediatr Clin North Am 43(3):639–664, 1996

Miller RD (ed): Anesthesia, 4th ed, pp 981–982. New York, Churchill Livingstone, 1994

D. Postoperative Management

D.1. How would you manage this patient in the immediate postoperative period?

All the prophylactic steps instituted in the preoperative period and carried on intraoperatively should be followed through in the immediate postoperative period—namely, prevention of hypoxia, acidosis, hypotension, stasis, and hypothermia. Respiratory depression should be avoided and supplemental oxygen should be given during the first 24 hours after anesthesia.

Katz J, Benumof J, Kadis LB (eds): Anesthesia and Uncommon Diseases: Pathophysiologic and Clinical Correlations, 3rd ed, p 396. Philadelphia, WB Saunders, 1990

Koshy M, Weiner SJ, Miller ST et al: Surgery and anesthesia in sickle cell disease. Cooperative study of sickle cell diseases. Blood 86:3676–3684, 1995

Lane PA: Sickle cell disease. Pediatr Clin North Am 43(3):639–664, 1996

Miller RD (ed): Anesthesia, 4th ed, pp 981–982. New York, Churchill Livingstone, 1994

D.2. What complications might occur in this patient in the immediate postoperative period?

The incidence of postoperative respiratory infection is high, and it is a leading cause of morbidity. Hypoxemic episodes are always a threat in that they might precipitate a sickling crisis. Acute chest syndrome is a potentially lethal postoperative complication in SCD patients who undergo general anesthesia for major surgery. Sequestration syndrome with shock is another potentially lethal complication, especially in the obstetric patient immediately postpartum. Patients with cardiomegaly and pulmonary hypertension are susceptible to heart failure. Renal and hepatic dysfunction can result in prolongation of the effects of certain drugs.

Katz J, Benumof J, Kadis LB (eds): Anesthesia and Uncommon Diseases: Pathophysiologic and Clinical Correlations, 3rd ed, p 396. Philadelphia, WB Saunders, 1990

Lane PA: Sickle cell disease. Pediatr Clin North Am 43(3):639–664, 1996

Vichinsky EP, Haberkern CM, Neumayo L: A comparison of conservative and aggressive transfusion regimens in the perioperative management of sickle cell disease. N Engl J Med 333:206–213, 1995

D.3. What is the treatment of sickle cell crisis?

The principles of treatment of painful sickle cell crisis include the following:

- Bed rest.
- Sedation.
- Hydration—oral or parenteral.
- Sodium bicarbonate—to treat or prevent acidosis.
- Oxygen therapy if hypoxemia is suspected.
- Treatment of infection and prophylactic antibiotics.
- Analgesics—preferably non-narcotics to avoid respiratory depression.
- Narcotics may be necessary in severe cases. Adequate analgesia must be obtained. Patient-controlled analgesia is useful in achieving this goal.
- Transfusion—partial exchange transfusions are helpful in reducing the amount of hemoglobin S and thus ameliorating the symptoms.

Lane PA: Sickle cell disease. Pediatr Clin North Am 43(3):639–664, 1996

Miller RD (ed): Anesthesia, 4th ed, pp 981–982. New York, Churchill Livingstone, 1994

Steinberg MH: Review: Sickle cell disease: Present and future treatment. Am J Med Sci 312(4): 166–174, 1996

Eye, Ear, Nose, and Throat   VIII

Open-Eye Injury

Theresa T. Kudlak

42

A 35-year-old carpenter presented to the emergency room after removing a nail that had struck and embedded itself in his right eye. He had eaten a full meal 1 hour prior to the accident.

A. Medical Disease and Differential Diagnosis

1. Why was this patient a particular challenge to the anesthesiologist?
2. What are the determinants of intraocular pressure (IOP) under normal circumstances? What is the normal range? What was the IOP in our patient's injured eye?
3. How is aqueous humor formed and eliminated?
4. How is IOP affected by arterial P_{CO_2}, systemic blood pressure, coughing and vomiting, deep inspiration, and hypoxemia?
5. What is the role of the central nervous system (CNS) on IOP?
6. What is glaucoma?
7. Is atropine premedication contraindicated in patients with glaucoma?
8. How do carbonic anhydrase inhibitors work to decrease IOP? By what mechanism can osmotic agents decrease IOP?
9. Are carbonic anhydrase inhibitors or osmotic diuretics indicated in open-globe injuries?
10. Are topically applied ophthalmic medications absorbed systemically? How can this absorption be reduced? Which eyedrops may have effects that are of concern to the anesthesiologist?

B. Preoperative Evaluation and Preparation

1. Is an open-globe injury always a surgical emergency?
2. What preoperative evaluation would you require?
3. The patient had eaten lunch 1 hour prior to the accident. Would you attempt to pass a nasogastric tube or to administer emetics to empty the stomach?
4. How would you premedicate this patient?

C. Intraoperative Management

1. What are some factors that can increase the risk of vitreous herniation during induction and maintenance of anesthesia?
2. Will you intubate this patient? Would you consider a laryngeal mask airway? How does intubation affect intraocular pressure? How can this effect be minimized?
3. Would you consider an awake intubation?
4. Is succinylcholine contraindicated in open-globe injuries? How does succinylcholine affect IOP?

787

5. Does pretreatment with nondepolarizing muscle relaxants prevent the succinylcholine-induced elevation in IOP?
6. How do nondepolarizing muscle relaxants affect intraocular pressure?
7. How will you perform a rapid-sequence induction and intubation without using succinylcholine?
8. What are the effects of ketamine on the eye?
9. Would you consider using etomidate as an induction agent? What about propofol?
10. How do inhalation agents affect intraocular pressure, and by what mechanism?
11. During the procedure, the patient's pulse suddenly dropped to 40 per minute. What do you think was happening? What is the oculocardiac reflex?
12. What are the afferent and efferent pathways of the oculocardiac reflex?
13. What factors contribute to the incidence of the oculocardiac reflex?
14. How do you diagnose and treat the oculocardiac reflex?
15. Is atropine useful?
16. Can retrobulbar block prevent the oculocardiac reflex? Is it appropriate in this patient?

D. Postoperative Management

1. Would you reverse the neuromuscular blockade in this patient?
2. Do reversal doses of atropine affect intraocular pressure?
3. What would you do prior to extubating this patient?
4. When would you extubate this patient?
5. The patient awakened in the recovery room and complained of pain and tearing in the opposite eye. The conjunctiva was inflamed. What was the likely cause?
6. Will taping the eyes shut or applying ointment prevent corneal abrasions? Are there any contributing factors?
7. What should you do when you suspect your patient might have a corneal abrasion?

A. Medical Disease and Differential Diagnosis

A.1. Why was this patient a particular challenge to the anesthesiologist?

The combination of a full stomach and an open-globe injury, both of which conditions may be problematic for the anesthesiologist, presents a unique challenge. Besides the increased risk of aspiration of gastric contents, any drug or maneuver that raises intraocular pressure (IOP) in the intact eye can cause extrusion of the vitreous humor and loss of vision when the globe is opened.

Cunningham AJ, Barry P: Intraocular pressure: Physiology and implications for anesthetic management. Can Anaesth Soc J 33:195, 1986

Holloway KB: Control of the eye during general anaesthesia for intraocular surgery. Br J Anaesth 52:671, 1980

Miller R (ed): Anesthesia, 4th ed, 2179–2180. New York, Churchill Livingstone, 1994

A.2. What are the determinants of intraocular pressure (IOP) under normal circumstances? What is the normal range? What was the IOP in our patient's injured eye?

Intraocular pressure is determined by the balance between production and drainage of aqueous humor, by changes in choroidal blood volume, and by vitreous volume and extraocular muscle tone. Resistance to outflow of aqueous humor in the trabecular tissue is probably the factor that maintains IOP within physiologic range, but the mechanism of homeostasis is unknown.

Normal IOP is 12 to 16 mm Hg in the upright posture and increases by 2 to 4 mm Hg in the supine position.

When the globe is open, the IOP is equal to ambient pressure. Our concern with this patient is not for IOP, but for the relative volume of choroid and vitreous humor within the eye. If this volume should increase while the eye is opened, the vitreous humor may be lost. Any deformation of the eye by external pressure in the globe will cause an apparent increase in intraocular volume.

Cunningham AJ, Barry P: Intraocular pressure: Physiology and implications for anaesthetic management. Can Anaesth Soc J 33:195–208, 1986

Jay JL: Functional organization of the human eye. Br J Anaesth 52:649, 1980

LeMay M: Aspects of measurement in ophthalmology. Br J Anaesth 52:655, 1980

Smith GB: Ophthalmic Anaesthesia, pp 1–13. Baltimore, University Park Press, 1983

A.3. How is aqueous humor formed and eliminated?

Aqueous humor is a clear fluid that occupies the anterior and posterior chambers of the eye. Its total volume is 0.3 ml. Aqueous humor is produced primarily in the posterior chamber, circulates through the pupil to the anterior chamber, passes through the trabeculated Fontana's spaces, and enters Schlemm's canal. From here, the fluid drains into the episcleral veins and finally into the cavernous sinus or jugular venous systems (Fig. 42-1).

Cunningham AJ, Barry P: Intraocular pressure: Physiology and implications for anaesthetic management. Can Anaesth Soc J 33:195–208, 1986

Jay JL: Functional organization of the human eye. Br J Anaesth 52:649, 1980

LeMay M: Aspects of measurement in ophthalmology. Br J Anaesth 52:655, 1980

Speth GL (ed): Ophthalmic Surgery: Principles and Practice, 2nd ed, pp 89–90. Philadelphia, WB Saunders, 1990

A.4. How is IOP affected by arterial P_{CO_2}, systemic blood pressure, coughing and vomiting, deep inspiration, and hypoxemia?

The choroidal arterioles vasodilate in response to hypercapnia and constrict during hypocapnia, thereby changing intraocular volume and pressure. However, the effect is minimal within the normal physiologic range of P_{CO_2}.

Minor fluctuations in arterial blood pressure also have minimal effects on IOP, although IOP may be seen to increase when hypertension is sustained and can fall to atmospheric levels with induced hypotension. Changes in venous pressure, on the other hand, have a major impact on IOP. Vomiting, coughing, and bucking on the endotracheal tube cause a dramatic increase in IOP by 30 to 40 mm Hg. These actions, resembling Valsalva's maneuver, cause congestion in the venous system, which impedes outflow of aqueous humor and increases the volume of choroidal blood. Also the globe is directly compressed by dilated episcleral veins.

A deep inspiration may reduce IOP by 5 mm Hg. Hypoxemia may increase IOP through choroidal vasodilatation.

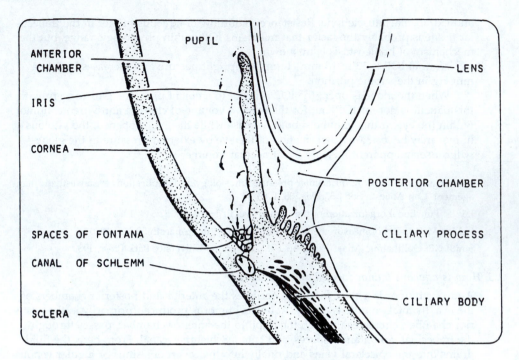

Figure 42-1.   Sites of formation, circulation, and drainage of aqueous humor. (Reprinted with permission from Cunningham AJ, Barry B: Intraocular pressure: physiology and implications for anesthetic management. Can Anaesth Soc J 33:197, 1986)

Calobrisi BL, Lebowitz P: Muscle relaxants and the open globe. Int Anesth Clin 28(2):83–88, 1990

Cunningham AJ, Barry P: Intraocular pressure: Physiology and implications for anaesthetic management. Can Anaesth Soc J 33:195, 1986

Miller R (ed): Anesthesia, 4th ed, pp 2177–2178. New York, Churchill Livingstone, 1994

Murphy DF: Anesthesia and intraocular pressure. Anesth Analg 64:520, 1985

Smith RB, Aass AA, Nemoto EM: Intraocular and intracranial pressure during respiratory alkalosis and acidosis. Br J Anaesth 53:967, 1981

Spaeth GL (ed): Ophthalmic Surgery: Principles and Practice, 2nd ed, pp 89–90. Philadelphia, WB Saunders, 1990

A.5. *What is the role of the central nervous system (CNS) on IOP?*

The CNS influences IOP through alterations in extraocular muscle tone or, indirectly, by hormonal or hemodynamic changes.

Cunningham AJ, Barry P: Intraocular pressure: Physiology and implications for anaesthetic management. Can Anaesth Soc J 33:195, 1986

Miller R (ed): Anesthesia, 4th ed, pp 2177–2178. New York, Churchill Livingstone, 1994

A.6. *What is glaucoma?*

Glaucoma is a pathologic elevation of IOP caused by increased resistance to outflow of aqueous humor from the eye. It is classified as either open or closed-angle glaucoma, depending on the anatomy and pathophysiology. Chronic elevation of IOP interferes with the intraocular blood supply and normal metabolism of the cornea. It can result in corneal opacities or decreased retinal blood flow.

The pathophysiology in glaucoma involves increased resistance to the flow of aqueous humor through Fontana's spaces as a result of scarring of the trabecular network or thickening of the endothelial covering of these channels. In closed-angle glaucoma the iris bulges forward, blocking the access of aqueous humor to the trabecular network. This can occur with pupillary dilation or with an acutely swollen lens.

Johnson DH, Brubaker RF: Glaucoma: An overview. Mayo Clin Proc 61:59, 1986

LeMay M: Aspects of measurement in ophthalmology. Br J Anaesth 52:655, 1980

A.7. Is atropine premedication contraindicated in patients with glaucoma?

It was previously thought by some clinicians that atropine is contraindicated in patients with glaucoma, especially narrow-angle glaucoma. However, this claim is true only when atropine is given intravenously (IV) or topically. Atropine in a standard premedication dose of 0.4 mg, intramuscularly (IM), causes no increase in intraocular pressure in either open or closed-angle glaucoma because only about 0.0001 mg is absorbed by the eye. Therefore, IM atropine for premedication is acceptable. However, scopolamine has a greater mydriatic effect than atropine. Therefore, scopolamine is not recommended for premedication in patients with known or suspected narrow-angle glaucoma.

Adams AK, Jones RM: Anaesthesia for eye surgery: General considerations. Br J Anaesth 52:663, 1980

Barash PG, Cullen BF, Stoelting RK (eds): Clinical Anesthesia, 3rd ed, p 914. Philadelphia, Lippincott-Raven, 1997

Miller RD (ed): Anesthesia, 4th ed, p 2178. New York, Churchill Livingstone, 1994

Rosen DA: Anesthesia in ophthalmology. Can Anaesth Soc J 9:545, 1962

Schwartz H, deRoeth A, Papper EM: Preanesthetic use of atropine in patients with glaucoma. JAMA 165:144, 1957

Smith RB (ed): Anesthesia in Opthamology, p 21. Boston, Little, Brown, 1973

Stoelting RK, Dierdorf SF: Anesthesia and Co-Existing Disease, 3rd ed, p 242. New York, Churchill Livingstone, 1993

A.8. How do carbonic anhydrase inhibitors work to decrease IOP? By what mechanism can osmotic agents decrease IOP?

Carbonic anhydrase inhibitors, such as acetazolamide, interfere with the sodium pump mechanism necessary for secretion of aqueous humor. An intravenous dose acts in 5 minutes, with maximal effect in 20 to 30 minutes. Chronic acetazolamide therapy can result in potassium depletion.

Osmotic agents, such as mannitol, increase plasma oncotic pressure relative to that of aqueous humor and produce an acute, transient drop in IOP. The maximal reduction in IOP occurs after 30 to 45 minutes and the effect lasts 5 to 6 hours.

Barash PG, Cullen BF, Stoelting RK (eds): Clinical Anesthesia, 3rd ed, p 915. Philadelphia, Lippincott-Raven, 1997

McGoldrick KE: Ocular drugs and anesthesia. Int Anesth Clin 28(2):72–77, 1990

A.9. Are carbonic anhydrase inhibitors or osmotic diuretics indicated in open-globe injuries?

No. If the globe is open, the IOP equals atmospheric pressure, and these agents are not useful. In addition, they can cause transient choroidal congestion, which could lead to loss of ocular contents.

Smith GB: Ophthalmic Anaesthesia. Baltimore, University Park Press, 1983

A.10. Are topically applied ophthalmic medications absorbed systemically? How can this absorption be reduced? Which eyedrops can have effects that are of concern to the anesthesiologist?

Topical ophthalmic drugs can be absorbed through the conjunctiva, or they may drain through the nasolacrimal duct and be absorbed through the nasal mucosa. Absorption is increased when the eye is instrumented, diseased, or traumatized. Finger pressure on the inner canthus for a few minutes after instillation of eyedrops will impede absorption by occluding the nasolacrimal duct.

Usage of the following topical medications can have implications for the anesthesiologist.

Atropine
- Used to produce mydriasis and cycloplegia. The 1% solution contains 0.2 to 0.5 mg of atropine per drop. Systemic reactions, seen primarily in children and the elderly, include tachycardia, flushing, thirst, dry skin, and agitation. Atropine is contraindicated in closed-angle glaucoma.

Scopolamine
- One drop of the 0.5% solution has 0.2 mg of scopolamine. CNS excitement can be treated with physostigmine, 0.015 mg/kg IV, repeated one or two times in a 15-minute period. It is contraindicated in closed-angle glaucoma.

Cyclopentolate (Cyclogel)
- Cyclopentolate is a short-acting mydriatic and cycloplegic that can cause transient neurotoxic effects, such as incoherence, visual hallucinations, slurred speech, ataxia, and seizures. It is contraindicated in closed-angle glaucoma.

Tropicamide (Midriacil)
- Tropicamide is used to produce mydriasis for refraction or fundoscopic examination. It can have CNS effects and can elevate IOP in closed-angle glaucoma.

Phenylephrine Hydrochloride (Neo-Synephrine)
- Phenylephrine hydrochloride is used to produce capillary decongestion and pupillary dilatation. Applied to the cornea, it can cause palpitations, nervousness, tachycardia, headache, nausea and vomiting, severe hypertension, reflex bradycardia, and subarachnoid hemorrhage. Solutions of 2.5%, 5%, and 10% (6.25 mg phenylephrine per drop) are available. The dose is 1 drop per eye per hour of the 2.5% solution (children) or the 5% solution (adults).

Epinephrine
- Topical 2% epinephrine will decrease aqueous secretion, improve outflow, and lower intraocular pressure in open-angle glaucoma. Side-effects include hyperten-

sion, palpitations, fainting, pallor, and tachycardia. The effects last about 15 minutes. One drop of 2% solution contains 0.5 to 1 mg of epinephrine. Epinephrine 1: 200,000 in a balanced salt solution is sometimes continuously infused into the anterior chamber during cataract surgery. Systemic effects can occur.

Timolol Maleate (Timoptic)
- Timolol maleate is a beta-blocker used in the treatment of chronic glaucoma. Side-effects include light-headedness, fatigue, disorientation, depressed CNS function, and exacerbation of asthma. Bradycardia, bronchospasm, and potentiation of systemic beta-blockers can occur.

Betaxolol HCl (Betoptic)
- Betaxolol HCl is a cardioselective (beta$_1$) blocking agent used to treat glaucoma. It can be hazardous in patients with sinus bradycardia, heart block, or heart failure.

Acetylcholine
- Acetylcholine can be injected intraoperatively into the anterior chamber to produce miosis. Side-effects are due to its parasympathetic action; they include hypotension, bradycardia, and bronchospasm. Intravenous atropine is an effective treatment.

Echothiophate Iodide (Phospholine Iodide)
- A cholinesterase inhibitor, echothiophate iodide is used as a miotic agent. It can prolong the effect of both succinylcholine and ester-type local anesthetics. Levels of pseudocholinesterase decrease by 80% after 2 weeks on the drug. It takes 3 to 6 weeks for return to normal pseudocholinesterase activity after stopping the drug (4 weeks for return to 75% activity). Succinylcholine and ester-type local anesthetics should be avoided. Demecarium is another such cholinesterase inhibitor.

Cocaine
- Cocaine is used to produce vasoconstriction and to shrink mucous membranes during dacryocystorhinostomy. One drop of 4% solution contains about 1.5 mg of cocaine, and the maximal dose is about 3 mg/kg. Systemic effects may be seen with a dose as low as 20 mg and involve the CNS, respiratory, and cardiovascular systems.

Ballin N, Becker B, Goldman ML: Systemic effects of epinephrine applied topically to the eye. Invest Ophthalmol 5:125, 1966

Barash PG, Cullen BF, Stoelting RK (eds): Clinical Anesthesia, 3rd ed, pp 917–918. Philadelphia, Lippincott-Raven, 1997

deRoeth A, Bettbar WD, Rosenberg P: Effect of phospholine iodine on blood cholinesterase levels. Am J Ophthalmol 49:586, 1963

Fraundfelder FT, Scafidi AF: Possible adverse effects from topical ocular 10 percent phenylephrine. Am J Ophthalno 84:447, 1978

Johnson DH: Glaucoma: An overview. Mayo Clin Proc 61:59, 1986

Lansche RK: Systemic reactions to topical epinephrine and phenylephrine. Am J Ophthalmol 49: 95, 1966

McGoldrick KE: Ocular drugs and anesthesia. Int Anesth Clin 28(2):72–77, 1990

Miller RD (ed): Anesthesia, 4th ed, p 2183. New York, Churchill Livingstone, 1994

Speth GL (ed): Ophthalmic Surgery: Principles and Practice, 2nd ed, pp 90–91. Philadelphia, WB Saunders, 1990

B. Preoperative Evaluation and Preparation

B.1. Is an open-globe injury always a surgical emergency?

No. In most cases surgery is not required immediately, and some time may be spent in adequately preparing the patient for anesthesia and surgery. However, the surgery should probably be performed within 12 hours to minimize the possibility of infection and other complications.

Arthur DS, Dewar KMS: Anaesthesia for eye surgery in children. Br J Anaesth 52:681, 1980

Smith GB: Ophthalmic Anaesthesia, pp 44–49. Baltimore, University Park Press, 1983

B.2. What preoperative evaluation would you require?

An accurate, thorough history and physical examination are the best means of evaluating this patient preoperatively, and they should reveal any existing medical problems that will guide selection of preoperative laboratory tests.

In this otherwise healthy young patient, no routine laboratory tests are indicated, unless they are required by the institution in which you are practicing. In cases where more extensive trauma is suspected, other injuries (e.g., fractures to the skull and orbit), intracranial hemorrhage, and other injuries as suggested by the history and physical examination must also be addressed.

Barash PG, Cullen BF, Stoelting RK (eds): Clinical Anesthesia, 3rd ed, pp 921–922. Philadelphia, Lippincott-Raven, 1997

Miller RD (ed): Anesthesia, 4th ed, pp 827–829. New York, Churchill Livingstone, 1994

B.3. The patient had eaten lunch 1 hour prior to the accident. Would you attempt to pass a nasogastric tube or to administer emetics to empty the stomach?

Absolutely not. These procedures are contraindicated when the eye has been perforated. Gagging, vomiting, and straining could cause a potentially disastrous increase in intraocular pressure. A cough can increase central venous pressure and choroidal blood volume, and it may raise IOP by 34 to 40 mm Hg.

Adams AK, Jones RM: Anaesthesia for eye surgery: General considerations. Br J Anaesth 52:663, 1980

Arthur DS, Dewar KMS: Anaesthesia for eye surgery in children. Br J Anaesth 52:681, 1980

Cunningham AJ, Barry P: Intraocular pressure: Physiology and implications for anaesthetic management. Can Anaesth Soc J 33:195, 1986

B.4. How would you premedicate this patient?

Premedications should be given parenterally because gastrointestinal absorption is unreliable. Sedatives and anxiolytics can be given as necessary. Metoclopramide (0.15 mg/kg IM) may be used to facilitate gastric emptying and to increase the tone of the cardiac sphincter. Narcotics should be avoided because they can cause nausea and vomiting. Nonparticulate antacids and H_2-receptor antagonists (cimetidine 2 mg/kg IM) should be considered to reduce the risk of aspiration pneumonitis. Intravenous droperidol or ondansetron can be given for antiemesis.

Atropine or glycopyrrolate are useful in reducing secretions and gastric acidity, and they may also inhibit the oculocardiac reflex.

Barash PG, Cullen BF, Stoelting RK (eds): Clinical Anesthesia, 3rd ed, pp 921–922. Philadelphia, Lippincott-Raven, 1997

Cunningham AJ, Barry P: Intraocular pressure: Physiology and implications for anaesthetic management. Can Anaesth Soc J 33:195, 1986

Smith GB: Ophthalmic Anaesthesia, pp 44–49. Baltimore, University Park Press, 1983

C. Intraoperative Management

C.1. What are some factors that can increase the risk of vitreous herniation during induction and maintenance of anesthesia?

- Face mask pressing on the eyeball
- Increased pressure from coughing, straining, bucking, head-down position
- Extraocular muscle spasm induced by depolarizing muscle relaxants or surgical stimulation during light anesthesia
- Poorly applied cricoid pressure, which blocks venous drainage from the eye
- Choroidal congestion from hypercarbia, hypoxia, osmotic diuretics, intubation, or increases in blood pressure

Cunningham AJ, Barry P: Intraocular pressure: Physiology and implications for anaesthetic management. Can Anaesth Soc J 33:195–208, 1986

Holloway KB: Control of the eye during general anaesthesia for intraocular surgery. Br J Anaesth 52:671, 1980

Libonati MM, Leahy JJ, Ellison N: The use of succinylcholine in open-eye surgery. Anesthesiology 62:637–640, 1985

C.2. Will you intubate this patient? Would you consider a laryngeal mask airway? How does intubation affect intraocular pressure? How can this effect be minimized?

It is imperative that this patient be intubated, not only to maintain the airway, which is close to the surgical field, but to avoid pressure by a face mask on the eyeball and to minimize the risk of aspiration. Although the laryngeal mask airway has been used successfully in opthalmologic anesthesia, it is not appropriate in this case because it does not protect the airway from aspiration. Many studies have demonstrated a significant increase in IOP caused by laryngoscopy and intubation under varying states of anesthetic depth and muscle relaxation. IOP can increase even with no visible reaction to intubation. This increase in IOP can be attenuated by topical laryngeal anesthesia and by increased depth of anesthesia to reduce coughing, straining, and blood pressure. The cardiovascular response to intubation can also be reduced by lidocaine (1.5 mg/kg IV), or beta-blockers.

Akhtar TM, McMurray P, Kerr WJ et al: A comparison of laryngeal mask airway with tracheal tube for intra-ocular ophthalmic surgery. Anaesthesia 47:668–671, 1992

Barash PG, Cullen BF, Stoelting RK (eds): Clinical Anesthesia, 3rd ed, p 921–922. Philadelphia, JB Lippincott 1997

Cook JH: The effect of suxamethonium on intraocular pressure. Anaesthesia 36:359, 1981

Gefke K, Anderson LW, Friesel H: Intravenous lidocaine as a suppressant of cough and laryngo-spasm with extubation after tonsillectomy. Acta Anaesth Scand 27:112, 1983.

Libonati MM, Leahy JJ, Ellison N: The use of succinylcholine in open-eye surgery. Anesthesiology 62:637–640, 1985

Miller RD (ed): Anesthesia, 4th ed, pp 2170–2180. New York, Churchill Livingstone, 1994

Smith RB, Aass AA, Nernoto EM: Intraocular and intracranial pressure during respiratory alkalosis and acidosis. Br J Anaesth 53:967, 1981

C.3. Would you consider an awake intubation?

Awake intubation is frequently accompanied by coughing and bucking. It is risky in an open-globe injury and other available safe methods of intubation should be used.

Calobrisi BL, Lebowitz P: Muscle relaxants and the open globe. Int Anesth Clin 28(2):83–88, 1990

C.4. Is succinylcholine contraindicated in open-globe injuries? How does succinylcholine affect IOP?

The use of succinylcholine in open-globe injuries is controversial. In the intact eye, following thiopental induction, succinylcholine has been shown to increase intraocular pressure by 6 to 8 mm Hg between 1 and 4 minutes after administration. Tracheal intubation further increases IOP. IOP returns to baseline in 5 to 7 minutes. In open-globe injuries, succinylcholine use has been associated with loss of ocular contents. The increase in IOP can be mediated by prolonged tonic contraction of the extraocular muscles, although IOP has been shown to rise after succinylcholine, even when the extraocular muscles have been severed. Other factors that may be contributory include choroidal blood flow, increased central venous pressure, and increased resistance to outflow of aqueous humor due to the cycloplegic effects of succinylcholine.

In fact, the hemodynamic response to laryngoscopy or intubation may have a much more significant effect on IOP than succinylcholine alone. Simply blinking will raise the IOP in a normal eye by 10 to 15 mm Hg, similar to the effect of succinylcholine. Pretreating with nifedipine or lidocaine, deepening the anesthesia, or using topical laryngeal anesthesia may attenuate the increase in IOP following succinylcholine and intubation.

Calobrisi BL, Lebowitz P: Muscle relaxants and the open globe. Int Anesth Clin 38(2):83–88, 1990

Cook JH: The effect of suxamethonium on intraocular pressure. Anaesthesia 36:359, 1981

Cunningham AJ, Barry P: Intraocular pressure: Physiology and implications for anaesthetic management. Can Anaesth Soc J 33:195–208, 1986

Holloway KG: Control of the eye during general anaesthesia for intraocular surgery. Br J Anaesth 52:671, 1980

Kelly RE, Dinner M, Turner LS et al: Succinylcholine increases intraocular pressure in the human eye with the extraocular muscles detached. Anesthesiology 79:948–952, 1993

Lincoff HA: The effect of succinylcholine on intraocular pressure. Am J Ophthalmol 40:501, 1955

Moreno RJ, Kloess P, Carlson DW: Effect of succinylcholine on the intraocular contents of open globes. Ophthalmology 98:636–638, 1991

Murphy DS, Davis MJ: Succinylcholine use in emergency eye operation. Can J Anaesth 34:101, 1987

Smith RB, Babinski M, Leano N: The effect of lidocaine on succinylcholine-induced rise in intraocular pressure. Can Anaesth Soc J 26:482, 1979

C.5. Does pretreatment with nondepolarizing muscle relaxants prevent the succinylcholine-induced elevation in IOP?

Available data are contradictory on this question, probably reflecting different methods of IOP measurement under varying depths of anesthesia, with a variety of anesthetic adjuvant agents. Many techniques have been tried to prevent succinylcholine-induced elevation of IOP, and none has been consistently effective. However, no reports have been published on loss of ocular contents when succinylcholine use has been preceded by pretreatment with a nondepolarizing relaxant and barbiturate for induction. Many anesthesiologists, therefore, feel this is a safe combination for rapid-sequence induction in the open-eye, full-stomach situation.

Bourke DL: Open-eye injuries. Anesthesiology 63:727, 1985

Bruce RA, McGoldrick DE, Oppenheimer P: Anesthesia for Ophthalmology, pp 74–75. Birmingham, Aesculapius, 1982

Calobrisi BL, Lebowitz P: Muscle relaxants and the open globe. Int Anesth Clin 28(2):83–88, 1990

Cunningham AJ, Barry P: Intraocular pressure: Physiology and implications for anaesthetic management. Can Anaesth Soc J 33:195–208, 1986

Hartman GS, Fiamengo SA, Riker WF Jr: Succinylcholine: Mechanism of fasciculations and their prevention by *d*-tubocurarine or diphenylhydantoin. Anesthesiology 65:405, 1986

Holloway KB: Control of the eye during general anaesthesia for intraocular surgery. Br J Anaesth 52:671, 1980

Konchigeri HN, Lee YE, Venugopal K: Effect of pancuronium on intraocular pressure changes induced by succinylcholine. Can Anaesth Soc J 26:479, 1979

Libonati MM, Leahy JJ, Ellison N: The use of succinylcholine in open-eye surgery. Anesthesiology 62:637–640, 1985

McGoldrick KE: The open globe: Is an alternative to succinylcholine necessary? J Clin Anesth 5:1, 1993

Meyers EF, Krupin T, Johnson M et al: Failure of nondepolarizing neuromuscular blockers to inhibit succinylcholine-induced increased intraocular pressure: A controlled study. Anesthesiology 48:149, 1978

Miller RD, Way WL, Hickey RF: Inhibition of succinylcholine-induced increased intraocular pressure by nondepolarizing muscle relaxants. Anesthesiology 29:123, 1968

Murphy DF: Anesthesia and intraocular pressure. Anesth Analg 64:520, 1985

C.6. How do nondepolarizing muscle relaxants affect intraocular pressure?

Non-depolarizing muscle relaxants either decrease or have no effect on intraocular pressure.

Abbott MA: The control of intraocular pressure during the induction of anaesthesia for emergency eye surgery. A high-dose vecuronium technique. Anaesthesia 42:1008, 1987

Agarwal LP, Mathur SP: Curare in ocular surgery. Br J Ophthalmol 36:603, 1952

Calobrisi BL, Lebowitz P: Muscle relaxants and the open globe. Int Anesth Clin 28(2):83–88, 1990

Cunningham AJ, Kelly CP, Farmer J et al: The effect of metocurine and pancuronium combination in intraocular pressure. Can Anaesth Soc J 29:617, 1982

Litwiller RW, Di Fazio CA, Rushia EL: Pancuronium and intraocular pressure. Anesthesiology 42: 750, 1975

Maharaj RJ, Humphrey D, Kaplan N et al: Effects of atracurium on intraocular pressure. Br J Anaesth 56:459, 1984

Miller RD (ed): Anesthesia, 4th ed, p 2179. New York, Churchill Livingstone, 1994

Schneider MJ, Stirt JA, Finholt DA: Atracurium, vecuronium, and intraocular pressure in humans. Anesth Analg 65:877, 1986

C.7. How will you perform a rapid-sequence induction and intubation without using succinylcholine?

The safety of the patient must always be the primary concern; the preservation of the injured eye is secondary. Measures must be taken to guarantee adequate anesthetic depth and to blunt the hemodynamic responses to laryngoscopy and endotracheal intubation. Pretreatment measures such as beta-blockers, calcium channel blockers, lidocaine, or diazepam should be considered. Prior to induction, the patient should breathe 100% oxygen for several minutes, administered by a gently applied face mask. Anesthesia can then be induced using carefully applied cricoid pressure with sodium thiopental (5 mg/kg IV) or propofol (2 to 3 mg/kg IV) and a nondepolarizing muscle relaxant. Several options exist:

- Pancuronium (0.15 to 0.2 mg/kg) provides intubation condition in 90 seconds. Tachycardia and prolonged muscle relaxation may be a problem.
- Atracurium (0.5 mg/kg) allows safe intubation in 3 minutes. A larger bolus (1.5 mg/kg) permits intubation in 60 to 90 seconds, but can cause hypotension and tachycardia.
- Cisatracurium (0.4 mg/kg) allows intubation in 60 to 90 seconds without histamine release.
- Vecuronium (0.2 to 0.25 mg/kg) permits intubation in 60 to 90 seconds.
- Rocuronium (0.45 to 0.6 mg/kg) gives excellent intubating conditions at 60 to 70 seconds. Time to recovery is rapid.
- An alternative is to pretreat the patient with a small dose of the nondepolarizing relaxant several minutes before induction, which may shorten the onset of action and lessen the dose required of subsequently administered relaxant. This has been referred to as a "priming" dose. Its use is controversial in that it can lead to diplopia, muscle weakness, respiratory distress, and aspiration while offering no definite advantage over a larger initial dosage of nondepolarizing muscle relaxants. The dosages for rapid tracheal intubation with succinylcholine or various nondepolarizing relaxants are listed in Chapter 19, Intestinal Obstruction, Table 19-4.

Whatever technique is selected, it is essential to monitor the degree of muscle relaxation with a neuromuscular blockade monitor. It is also possible to intubate the patient without any muscle relaxant at all after a deep level of anesthesia has been reached, but this is not a recommended technique. Not only is the airway unprotected for a long period of time, but prevention of bucking cannot be guaranteed and positive pressure ventilation by face mask may exert pressure on the eye.

Abbott MA: The control of intraocular pressure during the induction of anaesthesia for emergency eye surgery. A high-dose vecuronium technique. Anaesthesia 42:1008, 1987

Barash PG, Cullen BF, Stoelting RK (eds): Clinical Anesthesia, 3rd ed, pp 921–922. Philadelphia, Lippincott-Raven, 1997

Brown EM, Krishnaprasad D, Smiller BG: Pancuronium for rapid-induction technique for tracheal intubation. Can Anaesth Soc J 26:489, 1979

Foldes F: Rapid tracheal intubation with nondepolarizing neuromuscular blocking drugs. The priming principle. Br J Anaesth 56:663, 1984

Lennon RL, Olson RA, Gronert GA: Atracurium or vecuronium for rapid sequence endotracheal intubation. Anesthesiology 64:510, 1986

Mehta MP, Choi WW, Geris SD et al: Facilitation of rapid endotracheal intubations with divided doses of nondepolarizing neuromuscular blocking drugs. Anesthesiology 62:392, 1985

Musich J, Walts LF: Pulmonary aspiration after a priming dose of vecuronium. Anesthesiology 64: 517, 1986

Rich AL, Witherspoon CD, Morris RE et al: Use of nondepolarizing anesthetic agents in penetrating ocular injuries. Anesthesiology 65:108, 1986

Schneider MJ, Stirt JA, Finholt DA: Atracurium, vecuronium, and intraocular pressure in humans. Anesth Analg 65:87, 1986

Sosis MB: On use of priming with vecuronium in a patient with an open globe and a full stomach. Anesth Analg 70:336, 1990

C.8. What are the effects of ketamine on the eye?

Ketamine can cause nystagmus and blepharospasm, and it is therefore not suitable for ophthalmic surgery. Studies with respect to the effect of ketamine on IOP have shown both increased and decreased IOP in children, and no change in IOP in adults premedicated with diazepam and meperidine.

Antal M: Ketamine anesthesia and intraocular pressure. Ann Ophthalmol 10:1281, 1978

Ausinch E, Rayborn RL, Munsen ES, Levy NS: Ketamine and intraocular pressure in children. Anesth Analg 55:73, 1976

Cunningham AJ, Barry P: Intraocular pressure: Physiology and implication for anaesthetic management. Can Anaesth Soc J 33:195, 1986

Peuler M, Glass DD, Arens JF: Ketamine and intraocular pressure. Anesthesiology 5:575, 1975

Yoshikawa K, Murai Y: The effect of ketamine on intraocular pressure in children. Anesth Analg 50:199, 1971

C.9. Would you consider using etomidate as an induction agent? What about propofol?

Although etomidate has been associated with a decrease in IOP when used as an induction agent, the unpredictable incidence of generalized myoclonus seen with etomidate usage and resultant elevation of IOP may preclude its use in open-globe injuries, unless rapid and complete prior muscle relaxation can be guaranteed. Propofol, with its antiemetic properties and ability to decrease IOP, would be an excellent choice for induction.

Berry JM, Merin RG: Etomidate myoclonus and the open globe. Anesth Analg 69:256–259, 1989

Calla S, Gupta A, Sen N et al: Comparison of the effects of etomidate and thiopentone on intraocular pressure. Br J Anaesth 59:437, 1987

Ferrari LR, Donlon JV: A comparison of propofol, midazolam and methohexital for sedation during retrobulbar and peribulbar block. J Clin Anesth 4(2):93, 1992

C.10. How do inhalation agents affect intraocular pressure, and by what mechanism?

Inhalation agents cause dose-related decreases in intraocular pressure as a consequence of the following:

- Reduced aqueous humor production
- Depression of the central nervous system control center
- Facilitation of aqueous humor outflow
- Decreased extraocular muscle tension
- Lowered arterial blood pressure

The degree of intraocular pressure reduction is proportional to the depth of anesthesia.

Cunningham AJ, Barry P: Intraocular pressure: Physiology and implications for anaesthetic management. Can Anaesth Soc J 33:195, 1986

Miller RD (ed): Anesthesia, 4th ed, p 2178. New York, Churchill Livingstone, 1994

C.11. During the procedure, the patient's pulse suddenly dropped to 40 per minute. What do you think was happening? What is the oculocardiac reflex?

The oculocardiac reflex (OCR) is manifested by bradycardia, bigeminy, ectopy, nodal rhythms, atrioventricular block, and cardiac arrest. It is caused by traction on the extraocular muscles (medial rectus), ocular manipulation, or manual pressure on the globe. The OCR is commonly seen during eye muscle surgery, detached retina repair, enucleation, or whenever there is extensive traction or rotation of the eyeball.

Barash PG, Cullen BF, Stoelting RK (eds): Clinical Anesthesia, 3rd ed, p 916. Philadelphia, Lippincott-Raven, 1997

Miller RD (ed): Anesthesia, 4th ed, p 2182. New York, Churchill Livingstone, 1994

Speth GL (ed): Ophthalmic Surgery: Principles and Practice, 2nd ed, pp 89–90. Philadelphia, WB Saunders, 1990

C.12. What are the afferent and efferent pathways of the oculocardiac reflex?

The oculocardiac reflex is trigeminovagal. The afferent pathway is by way of the ciliary ganglion to the ophthalmic division of the trigeminal nerve, and through the gasserian ganglion to the main sensory nucleus in the fourth ventricle. The efferent pathway is through the vagus nerve.

Adams AK, Jones RM: Anaesthesia for eye surgery: General considerations. Br J Anaesth 52:663, 1980

Barash PG, Cullen BF, Stoelting RK (eds): Clinical Anesthesia, 3rd ed, p 916. Philadelphia, Lippincott-Raven, 1997

Smith GB: Ophthalmic Anesthesia, pp 66–72. Baltimore, University Park Press, 1983

C.13. What factors contribute to the incidence of the oculocardiac reflex?

Preoperative anxiety, light general anesthesia, hypoxia, hypercarbia, and increased vagal tone owing to age or drugs contribute to the incidence of OCR. The reported incidence of cardiac rhythm changes during eye muscle surgery is 32% to 82%. The incidence is higher in children.

Miller RD (ed): Anesthesia, 4th ed, p 2182. New York, Churchill Livingstone, 1994

Smith GB: Ophthalmic Anesthesia, pp 66–72. Baltimore, University Park Press, 1983

C.14. How do you diagnose and treat the oculocardiac reflex?

- Monitor the electrocardiogram intraoperatively and during any eye manipulation.
- Stop the surgical stimulus immediately.
- Ensure that ventilation is adequate.
- Ensure sufficient anesthetic depth.

The oculocardiac reflex may fatigue with repeated stimulation.

Miller RD (ed): Anesthesia, 4th ed, p 2182. New York, Churchill Livingstone, 1994

Smith GB: Ophthalmic Anesthesia, pp 66–72. Baltimore, University Park Press, 1983

C.15. Is atropine useful?

Atropine use is controversial. Atropine (0.4 mg IM) as a premedicant has no vagolytic effect after 60 minutes and is of no value in preventing or treating the OCR. Atropine (0.4 mg IV) is effective for 30 minutes in preventing bradycardia associated with the oculocardiac reflex. Doses >0.5 mg intravenously can cause tachycardia, which can be detrimental in certain patients with heart disease. At least 2 to 3 mg is required to ensure a total vagal block.

Blanc VF: Anticholinergic premedication for infants and children on the oculocardiac reflex [Letter]. Can Anaesth Soc J 30:683, 1983

Miller RD (ed): Anesthesia, 4th ed, p 2182. New York, Churchill Livingstone, 1994

Steward DJ: Anticholinergic premedication in infants and children on the oculocardiac reflex [Reply]. Can Anaesth Soc J 30:684, 1983

C.16. Can retrobulbar block prevent the oculocardiac reflex? Is it appropriate in this patient?

Retrobulbar block is not only unreliable in preventing the OCR, but may itself cause OCR, cardiac arrest, or retrobulbar hemorrhage.

Local infiltration of the recti muscles and a delicate operating technique may decrease the incidence of OCR. In this patient, retrobulbar block is contraindicated because it may increase intraocular pressure.

Allen ED, Elkington AR: Local anesthesia and the eye. Br J Anaesth 52:689, 1980

McGoldrick KE: Complications of regional anesthesia for ophthalmic surgery. Yale J Biol Med 66:443, 1993

Miller RD (ed): Anesthesia, 4th ed, pp 2176–2177. New York, Churchill Livingstone, 1994

D. Postoperative Management

D.1. Would you reverse the neuromuscular blockade in this patient?

No contraindication is seen to reversal, provided that efforts are made to minimize coughing or bucking on the tube.

D.2. Do reversal doses of atropine affect intraocular pressure?

Reversal doses of atropine, when given in conjunction with neostigmine, do not significantly alter intraocular pressure and this combination may be safely used, even in patients with glaucoma.

Barash PG, Cullen BF, Stoelting RK (eds): Clinical Anesthesia, 3rd ed, pp 923–924. Philadelphia, Lippincott-Raven, 1997

Cunningham AJ, Barry P: Intraocular pressure: Physiology and implications for anaesthetic management. Can Anaesth Soc J 33:195, 1986

D.3. What would you do prior to extubating this patient?

- Empty the stomach with an orogastric tube while the patient is still paralyzed.
- Suction the pharynx with the patient still paralyzed or deeply anesthetized.
- Give an antiemetic, such as droperidol (0.02 mg/kg IV) 20 to 30 minutes before the end of surgery.
- Give lidocaine (1.5 mg/kg IV) to prevent coughing during emergency.

Gefke K, Anderson LW, Friesel E: Intravenous lidocaine as a suppressant of cough and laryngospasm with extubation after tonsillectomy. Acta Anaesth Scand 27:112, 1983

Miller RD (ed): Anesthesia, 4th ed, p 2180. New York, Churchill Livingstone, 1994

D.4. When would you extubate this patient?

A conflict may be found between the desire to extubate the patient awake because of the full stomach and the desire to extubate the patient deep to prevent coughing and bucking. Because modern techniques of eye repair involve minimal risk of suture disruption with coughing, one may extubate light, thereby protecting the airway.

D.5. The patient awakened in the recovery room and complained of pain and tearing in the opposite eye. The conjunctiva was inflamed. What was the likely cause?

General anesthesia decreases tear production and reduces normal mechanical eyelid closure. Corneal abrasions are the most common perioperative ocular injury, and this patient's complaints are consistent with that diagnosis.

Barash PG, Cullen BF, Stoelting RK (eds): Clinical Anesthesia, 3rd ed, p 924. Philadelphia, Lippincott-Raven, 1997

Miller RD (ed): Anesthesia, 4th ed, p 2183. New York, Churchill Livingstone, 1994

D.6. Will taping the eyes shut or applying ointment prevent corneal abrasions? Are there any contributing factors?

There is no guarantee that an eye that has been taped shut or lubricated will not sustain a corneal abrasion. Most anesthesiologists protect the eyes in some way, yet abrasions still occur. Corneal abrasions represent the most common ophthalmic complication associated with general anesthesia. The incidence may be as high as 44% when no preventative measures have been taken and the cornea is exposed. The mechanism is thought to be drying of or direct trauma to exposed cornea. Possible contributing actors may be mask anesthesia, prone position, or having the face in the surgical field.

Barash PG, Cullen BF, Stoelting RK (eds): Clinical Anesthesia, 3rd ed, pp 924–925. Philadelphia, Lippincott-Raven, 1997

Bronheim D Abel M, Neustein S: Corneal abrasions following non-ophthalmic surgery: A retrospective view of 35,253 general anesthetics. Anesthesiology 83(3A):A1071, 1995

Gild WM, Posner KL, Caplan RA, Cheny FW: Eye injuries associated with anesthesia. Anesthesiology 76:204–208, 1992

D.7. What should you do when you suspect your patient might have a corneal abrasion?

Prompt consultation with an opthalmologist should be solicited for precise diagnosis and treatment. The patient should be reassured that corneal abrasions usually heal, and relief of pain occurs within 24 to 48 hours. Possible treatments include eye patching and topical administration of antibiotics, short-acting cycloplegics or anti-inflammatory agents. Eye patch use is controversial.

A topical anesthetic should never be given to a patient for self-administration. Misuse may cause delayed wound healing and keratopathy.

Hulbert MFG: Efficacy of eye pad in corneal healing after corneal foreign body removal. Lancet 337:643, 1991

Jampal HD: Patching for corneal abrasions. JAMA 274:1504, 1995

Kaiser PK: The corneal Abrasion Patching Study Group: A comparison of pressure patching versus no patching for corneal abrasions due to trauma or foreign body removal. Opthalmology 102: 1936–1942, 1995

Spaeth GL (ed): Ophthalmic Surgery: Principles & Practice, 2nd ed, pp 178–179. Philadelphia, WB Saunders, 1990

43 Laser Treatment of Recurrent Respiratory Papillomatosis

Matthew C. Gomillion

A 5-year-old girl with a past history of laryngeal papillomas was admitted because of having had progressive hoarseness for 2 months. Her mother reported that she had been "breathing funny" for several days. Inspiratory stridor was noted on examination. She was scheduled for direct laryngoscopy and laser excision of a suspected recurrent laryngeal papilloma.

A. Medical Disease and Differential Diagnosis

1. What is the cause of recurrent respiratory papillomatosis?
2. What is the clinical course of recurrent respiratory papillomatosis?
3. What are the available treatments for recurrent respiratory papillomatosis?
4. What is the differential diagnosis of hoarseness in this child?

B. Preoperative Evaluation and Preparation

1. How would you evaluate this patient's airway preoperatively?
2. What preoperative laboratory tests are necessary?
3. How would you premedicate this child before surgery?
4. What are the special considerations for anesthetic set-up in this case?

C. Intraoperative Management

1. What is a laser and how does it work?
2. What are the characteristics of laser radiation?
3. Discuss some advantages associated with laser use in laryngeal surgery.
4. What are the hazards of laser surgery?
5. What safety precautions must be taken?
6. What is the significance of laser plume?
7. What are the surgical requirements of laryngeal laser surgery?
8. How would you plan to monitor this patient?
9. How would you induce anesthesia?
10. What modifications of standard anesthetic techniques are necessary?
11. How would you protect the external surface of a conventional endotracheal tube for use during laser microlaryngoscopy?
12. What are the disadvantages of foil-wrapped tubes?
13. What special endotracheal tubes are available for laser surgery?
14. What is Venturi jet ventilation?
15. How would you institute and conduct manual jet ventilation?
16. What are the advantages of Venturi jet ventilation for microlaryngeal laser surgery?
17. What are the complications of jet ventilation?

18. What are the contraindications to the use of jet ventilation?
19. How is anesthesia maintained when using jet ventilation?
20. How would you manage an airway fire?

D. Postoperative Management

1. After uneventful laser microlaryngeal surgery using jet ventilation, this patient was extubated in the operating room and then transferred to the recovery room. What are the common postoperative complications?

A. Medical Disease and Differential Diagnosis

A.1. What is the cause of recurrent respiratory papillomatosis?

Recurrent respiratory papillomatosis (RRP) is caused by human papillomavirus (HPV), a DNA virus that is also responsible for condyloma acuminatum. Many authors have noted an association between RRP and maternal condyloma acuminatum present during childbirth. Evidence supporting this association is that a high percentage of children with RRP are born to women with active condylomata during pregnancy. Furthermore, DNA sequencing of the two types of HPV (HPV-6 and HPV-11), which are responsible for most RRP and genital warts, has shown papillomaviruses from the larynx and genital tract to be identical. However, maternal transmission of HPV is not the sole explanation for RRP as not all patients have such a history of maternal infection, and others do not develop the disease until many decades after birth. Furthermore, not all individuals born to mothers infected with genital papillomavirus develop RRP.

Bluestone CD, Stool SE, Kenna MA (eds): Pediatric Otolaryngology, 3rd ed, pp 1402–1403. Philadelphia, WB Saunders, 1996

Hartley C, Hamilton J, Birzgalis AR et al: Recurrent respiratory papillomatosis—The Manchester experience, 1974–1992. J Laryngol Otol 108:227–228, 1994

A.2. What is the clinical course of recurrent respiratory papillomatosis?

Recurrent respiratory papillomatosis, or juvenile laryngeal papillomatosis, is the most common benign tumor of the pediatric larynx. Papillomas in children are most commonly discovered before the child is 3 years of age and they can cause symptoms during the first year of life. The larynx is the region usually affected, but tracheal and bronchial involvement can occur.

Children with laryngeal papillomas usually present with symptoms related to airway obstruction. Early symptoms of hoarseness or voice change may progress to aphonia and respiratory distress, and stridor is a frequent finding. Severe laryngeal involvement can cause chronic airway obstruction and hypoventilation, eventually leading to pulmonary hypertension, right ventricular hypertrophy, and cor pulmonale. The rate of papilloma growth in RRP is variable, necessitating repeated airway evaluations and interval surgical removal of papilloma as needed to maintain a clear airway.

Bluestone CD, Stool SE, Kenna MA (eds): Pediatric Otolaryngology, 3rd ed, pp 1402–1403. Philadelphia, WB Saunders, 1996

Werkhaven J: Laser applications in pediatric laryngeal surgery. Otolaryng Clin North Am 29:1007, 1996

A.3. What are the available treatments for recurrent respiratory papillomatosis?

Because it has a tendency to recur and spread throughout the respiratory tract, RRP can often be a frustrating disease to treat. Numerous attempts at medical control, including antibiotics, interferon, steroids, hormones, podophyllin (a topical antiviral agent), antimetabolites (5-fluorouracil and methotrexate), and even radiation therapy, have had varying degrees of success. For relentless and recurrent papillomatosis the most effective treatment is surgical removal, most commonly by laser vaporization. The goal of laser therapy is not to cure the disease but to remove papilloma while preserving normal tissue, and thus maintain a patent airway and an acceptable voice.

Bluestone CD, Stool SE, Kenna MA (eds): Pediatric Otolaryngology, 3rd ed, pp 1404–1405. Philadelphia, WB Saunders, 1996

Crockett DM, Reynolds BN: Laryngeal laser surgery. Otolaryngol Clin North Am 23:55, 1990

Werkhaven J: Laser applications in pediatric laryngeal surgery. Otolaryngol Clin North Am 29:1007, 1996

A.4. What is the differential diagnosis of hoarseness in this child?

Hoarseness always indicates some abnormality of laryngeal structure or function. The list of possible causes of hoarseness in children is extensive but can be summarized by the following groupings:

Congenital
- Laryngeal anomalies—laryngomalacia, glottic webs, subglottic stenosis
- Cystic lesions—laryngocele, thyroglossal duct cyst
- Angiomas—lymphangioma, hemangioma
- Cri du chat syndrome (mental retardation, catlike cry, microcephaly, round face, and hypertelorism)

Neurogenic (Congenital and Acquired)
- Supranuclear—hydrocephalus, subdural hematoma, meningocele
- Nuclear—brain stem compression, Guillain-Barré syndrome
- Peripheral—neuropathies, recurrent laryngeal nerve trauma, mediastinal cysts and tumors, cardiovascular anomalies

Inflammatory
- Infectious—simple laryngitis, diphtheria, supraglottitis
- Noninfectious—chronic and allergic laryngitis, rheumatoid arthritis, angioneurotic edema

Neoplasia
- Recurrent respiratory papillomatosis
- Squamous cell carcinoma

Traumatic
- Hematoma
- Impacted foreign body
- Laryngeal cartilage fracture
- Arytenoid dislocation

- Postoperative—thyroidectomy, tracheoesophageal fistula repair, tracheotomy, cardiac surgery, postintubation granuloma
- Physical voice change of puberty
- Vocal abuse

Bluestone CD, Stool SE, Kenna MA (eds): Pediatric Otolaryngology, 3rd ed, p 1254. Philadelphia, WB Saunders, 1996

B. Preoperative Evaluation and Preparation

B.1. How would you evaluate this patient's airway preoperatively?

In addition to a thorough general medical assessment, the degree of obstruction, adequacy of ventilation, and feasibility of laryngoscopic examination and tracheal intubation must be carefully assessed in patients with airway lesions prior to laser microsurgery. Lesions in or near the airway can cause life-threatening airway obstruction during anesthesia induction. Furthermore, manipulation of airway lesions can result in bleeding or edema, which can rapidly convert partial obstruction to total airway occlusion, particularly in children.

During the preoperative evaluation it is important to pay careful attention to a parent's description of the child's respiratory pattern during sleep, noting particularly historical information suggestive of airway obstruction such as noisy breathing, snoring, or periods of silence followed by gasping. Useful clinical indicators of respiratory obstruction include the general appearance of the patient, the quality of the patient's voice, and the ventilatory pattern (observe the patient for use of accessory muscles of respiration, stridor, dyspnea and tachypnea). Examination of the mouth and neck may provide essential clues to potentially difficult airway management and intubation problems. Similarly, it is important to determine the external anatomy and range of motion of the head and neck. Indirect laryngoscopy performed by the otolaryngologist may also provide useful information about upper airway anatomy. The patient's medical records should be examined for techniques and equipment used successfully, as well as any problems encountered in the management of previous anesthetics. Finally, additional information on anatomic changes can be provided by x-rays, computed tomography (CT), magnetic resonance imaging (MRI) scans, and tomograms of the larynx.

Gregory GA (ed): Pediatric Anesthesia, 3rd ed, pp 675–676. New York, Churchill Livingstone, 1994

Sosis M: Anesthesia for laser surgery. Anesthesiol Clin North Am 11:579–580, 1993

B.2. What preoperative laboratory tests are necessary?

The preoperative laboratory evaluation in this patient is not different from what would normally be done for any pediatric patient scheduled for airway surgery. For a surgical procedure not associated with significant intraoperative blood loss in a child who is not at risk for severe and physiologically important anemia, no laboratory tests are required.

The need for further studies (e.g., x-rays, spirometry, arterial blood gases, CT and MRI scans, or tomograms) depends on the patient's respiratory status.

Gregory GA (ed): Pediatric Anesthesia, 3rd ed, p 187. New York, Churchill Livingstone, 1994

B.3. How would you premedicate this child before surgery?

Children who have experienced many trips to the operating room in the course of therapy for laryngeal papillomas may be very frightened and anxious about yet another procedure. In this situation the most important tool to allay fears is a reassuring preoperative visit by the anesthesiologist. One must avoid the temptation to heavily premedicate these "difficult" patients. Patients with severe airway compromise should not receive preoperative tranquilizers or narcotics because sedation may cause total airway obstruction. Anxious patients not at risk for airway obstruction may benefit from the careful use of tranquilizers or mild sedatives. Anticholinergic premedication can be used to reduce oral secretions.

Gregory GA (ed): Pediatric Anesthesia, 3rd ed, p 680. New York, Churchill Livingstone, 1994

B.4. What are the special considerations for anesthetic set-up in this case?

Careful preoperative planning and proper anesthetic set-up are essential before laryngeal laser surgery. As in any surgery involving the airway, the availability of certain equipment and personnel must be ensured before induction. A variety of laryngoscope blades, airways, and endotracheal tubes must be readily at hand. If the patient has a compromised airway or if intubation is likely to be difficult, a fiberoptic bronchoscope or laryngoscope should also be available. Before induction, the surgeon should ascertain that the laser is functional and that all laryngoscopes and bronchoscopes are operational. A tracheostomy set should be open and a skilled otolaryngologist should be ready to perform an emergency tracheostomy in the event of total airway obstruction.

The special considerations for airway surgery involving the use of a laser center around the prevention and treatment of an airway fire. Careful attention must be directed toward decreasing the combustibility of materials in the airway, including special selection and preparation of the endotracheal tube if one is to be used. If jet ventilation is planned, all necessary equipment must be assembled and ready. Finally, it is important that the anesthesiologist and all operating room personnel have a specific plan of action in case of an airway ignition so that rapid action can be taken.

Brown BR (ed): Anesthesia and ENT Surgery, pp 130–133. Philadelphia, FA Davis, 1987

Sosis M: Anesthesia for laser surgery. Anesthesiol Clin North Am 11:580, 1993

C. Intraoperative Management

C.1. What is a laser and how does it work?

The word "laser" is an acronym for **L**ight **A**mplification by **S**timulated **E**mission of **R**adiation. The basis of laser energy is the excitation of atoms. By absorbing energy, such as light, heat, or electricity, the electrons orbiting the nucleus of an atom can move to higher (excited) energy levels. An atom in the excited state tends to spontaneously decay to its original lower energy state, and in doing so emits energy in the form of a photon. The amount of energy absorbed or emitted by an electron as it moves from one energy level to another is related to the energy difference of the two states according to the Bohr formula: $E = hV$, where E is the energy difference between two energy levels, h is Planck's constant, and V is frequency.

During stimulated emission, an atom in an excited state is exposed to a photon whose energy is precisely the difference between two energy levels. The collision causes the atom to decay to a lower energy level, and when this occurs two photons are emitted—the injected photon plus the photon emitted by the electron returning to the lower energy level. Photons released in this manner have the same energy (hV), frequency, wavelength, phase, and direction. Thus, the stimulated radiation has the same frequency, wavelength, phase, and direction as the stimulating radiation. The result is that the stimulating radiation is amplified in a coherent pattern.

Three radiative processes are necessary for a laser to operate: absorption, spontaneous emission, and stimulated emission. A laser consists of a lasing medium, an optical cavity with two parallel mirrors, and an energy source. When the energy source is activated, absorption of this energy by the lasing medium causes the electrons to move to higher energy levels. Spontaneous emission then occurs as the atoms decay to lower energy levels, thus emitting photons. The parallel mirrors reflect those photons traveling along the axis of the laser back through the lasing medium, causing the stimulated emission of photons of the same energy, phase, and direction and, thereby, amplifying the intensity of the light. One of the mirrors is partially transmitting and allows a small amount of the coherent monochromatic laser beam to emerge.

Sosis M: Anesthesia for laser surgery. Int Anesthesiol Clin 11:573–575, 1993

Van Der Speck AFL, Spargo PM, Norton ML: The physics of lasers and implications for their use during airway surgery. Br J Anaesth 60:709–711, 1988

C.2. What are the characteristics of laser radiation?

Laser radiation has the following properties:

- Monochromaticity—all photons have the same wavelength.
- Coherence—all photons are in phase in both time and space.
- Collimation—all photons travel in parallel directions and do not diverge.

The coherent monochromatic light of a laser can be focused into an extremely small spot of very high power density (the energy delivered per unit area of cross section), which is capable of cutting and vaporizing tissue.

Pashayan AG: Anesthesia for laser surgery. ASA Annual Refresher Course Lectures #276, 1995

Sosis M: Anesthesia for laser surgery. Int Anesthesiol Clin 28:119, 1990

C.3. Discuss some advantages associated with laser use in laryngeal surgery.

Several characteristics of the interaction between laser light and tissues make lasers ideal for laryngeal surgery, especially in the pediatric patient. These include good hemostasis of small blood vessels, minimal production of postoperative edema, rapid healing, and minimal scar formation. The surgical precision and the preservation of normal tissues made possible by lasers are additional benefits.

The carbon dioxide (CO_2) laser is the laser of choice for most pediatric laryngeal lesions because of its more precise soft tissue interaction (shallower thermal effect and tissue penetration) than other available medical lasers, such as the potassium titanyl phosphate (KTP) and the neodymium:yttrium-aluminum-garnet (Nd:YAG) lasers.

Crockett DM, Reynolds BN: Laryngeal laser surgery. Otolaryngol Clin North Am 23:51, 1990

Werkhaven J: Laser applications in pediatric laryngeal surgery. Otolaryngol Clin North Am 29: 1005–1006, 1996

C.4. What are the hazards of laser surgery?

Because of the very high intensity of laser beams and the potential for tissue damage and combustion, significant hazards are associated with their use. Both the patient and all operating room personnel working in the vicinity of a laser are at risk for injury by a laser. Airway fire remains the most threatening hazard of airway laser surgery. The patient's eyes and skin are also at risk for damage, as are normal tissues adjacent to the operative field with the potential for tracheobronchial perforation of a major pulmonary blood vessel. Hypoxemia from inadequate ventilation and from distal collection of secretions, blood, debris, and smoke is a major cause of morbidity and mortality during and after laser resection. The major risks for operating room personnel are damage to the eyes and cutaneous burns.

Rebeiz EE, Shapsay SM, Ingrams DR: Laser applications in the tracheobronchal tree. Otolaryngol Clin North Am 29:987–1003, 1996

Sosis M: Anesthesia for laser surgery. Anesthesiol Clin North Am 11:578, 1993

C.5. What safety precautions must be taken?

All operating room personnel must wear safety glasses appropriate for the laser in use to protect their eyes. The patient's eyes should be closed during surgery and covered with wet eye pads or gauze. A conspicuous warning sign should be placed on the outside of the operating room door whenever the laser is being used, along with extra safety glasses for anyone entering the room. Because of the potential for direct, high-intensity contact with the laser beam, the patient's skin, teeth, and normal tissue adjacent to the operative field must be protected by wet gauze pads or surgical sponges. Water-based lubricants and flame-resistant surgical drapes should be used. Surgical instruments should be matte finished or ebonized rather than polished to prevent reflection and inadvertent misdirection of the laser beam.

Steps that can be taken to decrease the risk of fire in the patient's airway include minimizing the risk of endotracheal tube ignition by eliminating it, modifying a standard polyvinylchloride (PVC) or red rubber endotracheal tube, using a specially designed endotracheal tube, and decreasing the concentration of gases in the airway that will support combustion. In addition, the surgeon must have a thorough understanding of laser physics and an appreciation of its effects on tissue so that the minimum power, smallest spot size, and shortest exposure time possible are used to minimize the thermal effect and tissue penetration of the laser.

Courey MS, Osshoff RH: Laser applications in adult laryngeal surgery. Otolaryngol Clin North Am 29:973–977, 1996

Sosis M: Anesthesia for laser surgery. Int Anesthesiol Clin 28:578–579, 1990

Werkhaven J: Laser applications in pediatric laryngeal surgery. Otolaryngol Clin North Am 29: 1005–1006, 1996

C.6. What is the significance of laser plume?

Laser plume is the vapor and cellular debris produced during laser use. Concern has been raised recently about the safety of patient and personnel exposure to laser plume, because it is known to have detrimental effects on pulmonary airway resistance, gas exchange, and mucociliary function. In addition, viable bacteria have been shown by at least one author to be present in laser plume. It is not certain whether or not viral particles, including human immunodeficiency virus, papillomavirus, and hepatitis B virus, can be aerosolized by the laser. In addition, whether laser plume is harmful to operating room personnel or is infectious is not known. Therefore, it is recommended that laser plume be suctioned as adequately as possible.

Courey MS, Osshoff RH: Laser applications in adult laryngeal surgery. Otolaryngol Clin North Am 29:973, 1996

Miller RD (ed): Anesthesia, 4th ed, p 2203. New York, Churchill Livingstone, 1994

C.7. What are the surgical requirements of laryngeal laser surgery?

Surgical requirements include neck hyperextension combined with suspension laryngoscopy, a surgical field free of motion, and rapid return of consciousness and protective airway reflexes at the end of surgery.

Gregory GA (ed): Pediatric anesthesia, 2nd ed, p 1120. New York, Churchill Livingstone, 1989

C.8. How would you plan to monitor this patient?

Basic monitoring would include a pulse oximeter, a blood pressure cuff, an electrocardiograph, a precordial stethoscope, an oxygen analyzer, and a neuromuscular blockade monitor. Continuous end-tidal carbon dioxide analysis would be required if an endotracheal tube were used.

American Society of Anesthesiologists: Standards for basic anesthetic monitoring. American society of anesthesiologists: 1997 Directory of Members, 62nd ed, p 394, 1997

Sosis M: Anesthesia for laser surgery. Anesthesiol Clin North Am 11:580, 1993

C.9. How would you induce anesthesia?

The primary considerations during the induction of anesthesia are those of good anesthetic technique for airway surgery. If the patient has no airway compromise, any standard inhalation or intravenous induction technique can be used. However, if airway compromise exists, special care must be taken to ensure a safe induction. As mentioned, all necessary equipment and personnel must be assembled and ready in case the airway is lost or intubation is difficult (refer to question B.4.). An inhalation induction using halothane or sevoflurane and oxygen with spontaneous ventilation is usually the technique of choice in children and in adults unable to cooperate with an awake intubation. Constant vigilance to the airway and the degree of airway obstruction is essential. Slow induction should be anticipated because the compromised laryngeal inlet limits gas exchange. The ability to ventilate with positive pressure by mask should be demonstrated before muscle relaxants are administered. In cases of significant obstruction it may be preferable to perform laryngoscopy and intubation with the patient breathing spontaneously after an adequate depth of anesthesia has been established. Ketamine has been reported to be unsatisfactory because it tends to increase airway reflexes and may predispose to laryngospasm and obstruction.

In an adult patient with a compromised airway, an awake intubation under direct visualization, often aided by fiberoptic laryngoscopy using topical anesthesia, is a safe way to proceed in a cooperative patient. Blind oral or nasal intubations are not recommended because they carry the risk of trauma to the lesions and could result in complete airway obstruction. If upper airway obstruction is severe, an awake tracheostomy under local anesthesia may be the safest means of managing the airway. After verification by chest auscultation and capnography that the airway is secure, an intravenous or inhalation induction of general anesthesia may proceed.

Gregory GA (ed): Pediatric Anesthesia, 3rd ed, pp 680–681. New York, Churchill Livingstone, 1994

Miller RD (Ed): Anesthesia, 4th ed, p 2188. New York, Churchill Livingstone, 1994

Sosis M: Anesthesia for laser surgery. Int Anesthesiol Clin 28:124, 1990

C.10. What modifications of standard anesthetic techniques are necessary?

The first special consideration concerns the choice of endotracheal tube and the ventilation technique. With regard to the endotracheal tube, three options exist: use of a specially protected conventional tube, use of a noncombustible tube, or no tube in the airway. If the patient's trachea is to be intubated, ventilation will not be significantly affected by the laser surgery, and anesthesia can be maintained adequately by any combination of volatile and intravenous agents. An important consideration in this anesthetic technique is the gas mixture and its fire hazard. Because oxygen and nitrous oxide both have the ability to support combustion, it is necessary to modify their use during laser surgery. Oxygen should be diluted with nitrogen, helium, or air to reduce its concentration to <30%, or to the minimal fraction that provides satisfactory oxygen saturation, as determined by a pulse oximeter. Nitrous oxide should not be used during laser endoscopic surgery. The concentration of the volatile anesthetics normally used during clinical anesthesia is not flammable.

A popular technique for laryngeal laser surgery eliminates the presence of any type of endotracheal tube in the airway. The most commonly used mode of ventilation in these cases is Venturi jet ventilation, performed either manually or by a high frequency jet ventilation apparatus. Alternatively, the endotracheal tube can be removed intermittently and the patient rendered apneic during the periods of laser use. The patent is periodically re-intubated and manually ventilated with pure oxygen with or without a volatile agent to maintain an acceptable oxygen saturation and eliminate carbon dioxide. For lesions below the vocal cords, laser surgery is routinely performed through a rigid bronchoscope with either conventional or jet ventilation through the side arm of the bronchoscope.

Because it is essential that the surgical field be motionless, all patients undergoing laser surgery should be paralyzed. This can be accomplished with either a succinylcholine infusion or a nondepolarizing muscle relaxant of short or intermediate duration.

McGoldrick K: Anesthesia for Ophthalmic and Otolaryngologic surgery, pp 46–47. Philadelphia, WB Saunders, 1992

Miller RD (ed): Anesthesia, 4th ed, p 2190. New York, Churchill Livingstone, 1994

Sosis M: Anesthesia for laser surgery. Anesthesiol Clin North Am 11:584, 1993

C.11. How would you protect the external surface of a conventional endotracheal tube for use during laser microlaryngoscopy?

With the exception of metal tubes, all types of endotracheal tubes can be ignited by a laser beam. If one chooses to use a conventional endotracheal tube, such as a polyvinylchloride or red rubber tube, then special precautions must be taken. Because PVC tubes produce hydrochloric acid and other toxic compounds if they are ignited, red rubber endotracheal tubes are preferred as they are considered safer. A tube 1 to 2 mm smaller than usual can be wrapped with reflective metal tape, such as aluminum or copper foil adhesive-backed tapes. The protective foil is wrapped in an overlapping spiral manner beginning near the tip or cuff of the tube and ending at the level of the uvula. All tape edges should be smoothed, and the foil at the tip should be trimmed to decrease soft tissue trauma. Some authors advocate the use of wet muslin wrapping as an alternative to metallic foil tape. An additional alternative in older children and adults is the use of the Merocel Laser-Guard (Americal Corp., Mystic, CT), composed of a laminate of sponge backed with corrugated silver foil. In all cases, if a cuffed endotracheal tube is employed, the cuff should be filled with saline instead of air and covered with wet gauze or wet neurosurgical sponges to minimize the chance of ignition. Tinting the saline with methylene blue allows early visual detection of injury to the cuff.

Courey MS, Osshoff RH: Laser applications in adult laryngeal surgery. Otolaryngol Clin North Am 29:976, 1996

Hermens JM, Bennett MJ, Hirshman CA: Anesthesia for laser surgery. Anesth Analg 62:224–225, 1983

Sosis M: Anesthesia for laser surgery. Int Anesthesiol Clin 28:582, 1990

C.12. What are the disadvantages of foil-wrapped tubes?

Disadvantages of metallic foil-wrapped tubes include trauma to pharyngeal and laryngeal tissues by sharp edges of the foil, kinking of the tube, deflection of the laser beam by the reflective surface of the tape, airway obstruction from aspiration of detached pieces of foil, and ignition of the unprotected distal portion of the tube. In addition, foil wrapping increases the external diameter of the endotracheal tube and reduces its flexibility, limiting its usefulness in the small pediatric airway.

Gregory GA (ed): Pediatric Anesthesia, 3rd ed, p 679. New York, Churchill Livingstone, 1994

Van Der Speck AFL, Spargo PM, Norton ML: The physics of lasers and implications for their use during airway surgery. Br J Anaesth 60:719, 1988

C.13. What special endotracheal tubes are available for laser surgery?

Several manufacturers produce endotracheal tubes especially designed to minimize the chance of ignition during laser microlaryngoscopy. Laser-resistant tubes have larger outer diameters for a given inner diameter than conventional endotracheal tubes. They are not available in small pediatric size, however, precluding their use in small airways, such as pediatric patients and patients with tracheal stenosis or obstructing lesions. In addition, they tend to have decreased flexibility and more difficult cuff inflation and deflation properties. Tubes containing metal are potentially more abrasive, and all tubes are considerably more expensive than conventional PVC or red rubber tubes. Finally, all tubes have been shown to ignite if enough laser energy is applied. Commonly available laser-resistant endotracheal tubes include the Mallinckrodt Laser-Flex (airtight stainless steel with double PVC cuff), the Sheridan Laser-Trach (red rubber with copper foil tape and covered with polyester sleeve), the Xomed Laser Shield II (silicone wrapped with Teflon-coated aluminum tape), and the Bivona Torre-Cuf (aluminum covered with silicone and a unique, self-inflating foam cuff).

Miller RD (ed): Anesthesia, 4th ed, p 2207. New York, Churchill Livingstone, 1994

Sosis M: Anesthesia for laser surgery. Anesthesiol Clin North Am 11:584-588, 1993

C.14. What is Venturi jet ventilation?

The jet injector technique of ventilation for upper airway surgery was introduced by Sanders in 1967. A high velocity jet of oxygen exits from a needle or a nozzle placed within the lumen of a laryngoscope, causing a propulsive effect on the resting gas column. In addition, ambient gas is entrained through the open proximal end of the laryngoscope as the pressure around the needle and behind the jet exit point becomes negative with respect to the pressure in the rapidly moving mainstream gas flow (the Venturi effect). The result is a large volume of an oxygen-air mixture ventilating the lungs.

Van Der Speck AFL, Spargo PM, Norton ML: The physics of lasers and implications for their use during airway surgery. Br J Anaesth 60:720, 1988

C.15. How would you institute and conduct manual jet ventilation?

Before effective jet ventilation can begin, the operating laryngoscope must be inserted, the larynx adequately exposed and evaluated for appropriateness for jet ventilation, the suspension system installed, and the jet injector needle attached to the laryngoscope and properly aligned with the axis of the trachea. All of this takes time in an anesthetized, apneic patient. Therefore, it is our preference at the New York Hospital-Cornell Medical Center to begin with laryngoscopy and intubation using a standard PVC endotracheal tube if the airway appears appropriate for jet ventilation. Uninterrupted ventilation can now be performed while the operating laryngoscope and jet injector are positioned. When ready, the endotracheal tube is removed and jet ventilation begun. Alternatively, following anesthesia induction and demonstration of an adequate mask airway, the patient is paralyzed and the operating laryngoscope and jet injection are inserted and positioned while the patient is apneic.

Ventilation begins with a jet pressure of 5 to 10 psi in infants and children and 15 to 20 psi in adults. The jet pressure is gradually increased until adequate chest rise and fall is noted. Jet ventilation should produce good clinical expansion of the chest at a rate appropriate for the patient's age. The inspiratory:expiratory (I:E) ratio should allow for adequate passive exhalation. Arterial oxygen saturation should be monitored continuously by pulse oximetry. Constant vigilance is important, and chest excursion should be monitored both by palpation and auscultation of breath sounds to prevent airway complications.

Shikowitz MJ, Abramson AL, Liberatore L: Endolaryngeal jet ventilation: A 10-year review. Laryngoscope 101:457, 1991

C.16. What are the advantages of Venturi jet ventilation for microlaryngeal laser surgery?

The advantages of the Venturi jet ventilation system are avoidance of combustible material in the airway, an unobstructed view, a motionless field, adequate ventilation, clearing of smoke, and suitability for use in all age groups, including the smallest neonate.

Gregory GA (ed): Pediatric Anesthesia, 3rd ed, p 680. New York, Churchill Livingstone, 1994

Shikowitz MJ, Abramson AL, Liberatore L: Endolaryngeal jet ventilation: A 10-year review. Laryngoscope 101:455, 1991

Sosis M: Anesthesia for laser surgery. Int Anesthesiol Clin 11:589–590, 1993

C.17. What are the complications of jet ventilation?

Complications associated with the use of jet ventilation include barotrauma (pneumothorax, pneumomediastinum, or subcutaneous emphysema), gastric dilation with possible regurgitation, drying of mucosal surfaces, aspiration of resected material, and complete respiratory obstruction.

Shikowitz MJ, Abramson AL, Liberatore L: Endolaryngeal jet ventilation: A 10-year review. Laryngoscope 101:457–458, 1991

Sosis M: Anesthesia for laser surgery. Int Anesthesiol Clin 11: 590, 1993

C.18. What are the contraindications to the use of jet ventilation?

Jet ventilation is most suited for patients with unobstructed airways and normal lung and chest wall compliance. The presence of airway obstruction without a tracheostomy tube, obesity, increased risk for aspiration, or advanced chronic obstructive pulmonary disease represent contraindications to the use of jet ventilation. In addition, jet ventilation is not appropriate for removal of a foreign body.

Miller RD (ed): Anesthesia, 4th ed, p 2189. New York, Churchill, Livingstone, 1994

Sosis M: Anesthesia for laser surgery. Int Anesthiol Clin 11: 590, 1993

C.19. How is anesthesia maintained when using jet ventilation?

Most authors recommend a totally intravenous anesthetic technique during jet ventilation. A combination of a barbiturate, a benzodiazepine, or propofol with a short-acting opioid (alfentanil, fentanyl, or sufentanil) provides for the requirements of hypnosis, amnesia, and analgesia. In addition, muscle relaxation is essential to prevent patient movement and laryngospasm. Inhalation anesthetics are avoided because they pollute the operating room and because their concentration cannot be regulated in a jet ventilation system.

Gussack GS, Evans RF, Tacchi EJ: Intravenous anesthesia and jet ventilation for laser microlaryngeal surgery. Ann Otol Rhinol Laryngol 96:32, 1987

Sosis M: Anesthesia for laser surgery. Int Anesthesiol Clin 11:590, 1993

C.20. How would you manage an airway fire?

Whenever a laser is used, all operating room personnel must be prepared for the possibility of a fire and should have a plan of action rehearsed so that rapid action can be taken if a fire occurs. In the event of an airway fire, the anesthesiologist should immediately stop ventilation and disconnect the oxygen supply from the airway. If an endotracheal tube is being used, this is most easily accomplished by removing the tube. Discontinuing oxygen delivery will most likely extinguish the fire, but if the flame persists, the surgical field should be flooded with saline immediately. Once the fire has been completely extinguished, then ventilation with 100% oxygen is resumed by mask, or the trachea can be reintubated if the mask airway is inadequate. Before the patient is awakened, the extent of airway damage must be assessed. Fiberoptic or rigid bronchoscopy can be used to evaluate the extent of lower airway damage and edema, and it permits removal of burned debris. Direct laryngoscopic examination of the pharynx and larynx permits evaluation of the rostral limits of injury. The decision to extubate the patient should be based on bronchoscopic and laryngoscopic findings, as well as pulse oximetry readings and/or arterial blood gas analysis. Controlled ventilation by an endotracheal tube or tracheostomy will be necessary to manage extensive burns.

The patient should be monitored for at least 24 hours after the injury with serial chest examinations and oximetry. Inspired gases should be humidified. If the burns are severe, consider steroid use to minimize airway edema and antibiotics to treat superimposed infection. Prolonged mechanical ventilation and intensive supportive care may be necessary after severe injury.

Pashayan AG: Anesthesia for laser surgery. ASA Refresher Courses in Anesthesiology 17:224–225, 1989

Sosis M: Anesthesia for laser surgery. Int Anesthesiol Clin 11:588–589, 1993

D.   Postoperative Management

D.1. After uneventful laser microlaryngeal surgery using jet ventilation, this patient was extubated in the operating room and then transferred to the recovery room. What are the common postoperative complications?

Laryngeal edema can occur in the early postoperative period, and it is usually manifested by retractions and inspiratory stridor in the recovery room. After microlaryngeal surgery, children may benefit from humidified oxygen, intravenous steroids (e.g., dexamethasone), and racemic epinephrine inhalation. Laryngospasm can develop because of laryngeal hyperactivity. To reduce the incidence of laryngospasm, topical anesthesia may be applied to the larynx. If laryngospasm develops postoperatively, it is treated initially with positive pressure mask ventilation with 100% oxygen. More severe cases of laryngospasm may require the use of a small, subapneic dose of succinylcholine (0.1 to 0.2 mg/kg IV). The possibility of a pneumothorax should be considered after all cases involving jet ventilation. Pulmonary complications as a result of retained secretions and subsequent atelectasis have been reported.

Gregory GA (ed): Pediatric Anesthesia, 3rd ed, p 680. New York, Churchill Livingstone, 1994

Rebeiz EE, Shapsay SM, Ingrams DR: Laser applications in the tracheobronchal tree. Otolaryngol Clin North Am 29:996, 1996

44 Acute Epiglottitis and the Croup Syndrome

Miles Dinner

A 3-year-old boy was brought to the emergency room with a fever of 39.5°C. He was noted to be breathing quickly with substernal retractions. He complained of a sore throat.

A. Medical Disease and Differential Diagnosis

1. What is epiglottitis? What are its common causes?
2. What is the croup syndrome? What is the clinical presentation of laryngotracheobron-chitis?
3. What are the clinical manifestations of epiglottitis?
4. How has the incidence of epiglottitis changed over the decade?
5. Has there been a change in the pattern of *Haemophilius influenzae* in recent years?
6. How is the diagnosis of epiglottitis made?
7. What is the medical management of croup? Does this have applications for the anes-thesiologist?
8. What is postextubation croup? How is it managed?
9. What are some other causes of partial airway obstruction in children?

B. Preoperative Evaluation and Preparation

1. Why is general anesthesia administered to a child with epiglottitis?
2. How would you prepare the patient for anesthesia?

C. Intraoperative Management

1. How is the airway of the child with epiglottitis best secured?
2. How would you induce anesthesia?
3. Should a child with epiglottitis undergo a rapid-sequence induction?
4. Is awake intubation a practical alternative to secure this patient's airway?
5. Should this patient have a nasotracheal or ortotracheal tube placed?
6. Shortly after intubation, frothy secretions were obtained on suctioning the endotra-cheal tube. What is the reason for this? How can this be treated?

D. Postoperative Management

1. How long should this patient remain intubated? What criteria determine extubation time?
2. How would you make this patient comfortable during the period of intubation?

A. Medical Disease and Differential Diagnosis

A.1. What is epiglottitis? What are its common causes?

Epiglottitis is an inflammation of the epiglottis secondary to an infectious process. It can involve other supraglottic structures such as the arytenoid, false cords, and posterior tongue leading to obstruction of the airway. Progression of swelling can rapidly lead to complete airway occlusion and death. Epiglottitis is bacterial in origin. The causative agent is usually *Haemophilius influenzae* type B. *Streptococcus pneumoniae* has also been infrequently associated with epiglottitis.

Balkany TJ, Pashley N: Clinical Pediatric Otolaryngology, p 351. St. Louis, CV Mosby, 1986

Behrman RE, Kliegman RM, Arvin AM (eds): Nelson Textbook of Pediatrics, 15th ed, pp 1201–1205. Philadelphia, WB Saunders, 1996

Diaz JH: Croup and epiglottitis in children. Anesthesiology 64:621, 1985

Fauci AS, Braunwald Z, Isselbacher KJ et al: Harrison's Principles of Internal Medicine, 14th ed, pp 183-184. New York, McGraw-Hill, 1998

A.2. What is the croup syndrome? What is the clinical presentation of laryngotracheobronchitis?

Croup is a generalized term referring to infections of the upper respiratory tract with a characteristic cough, inspiratory stridor, and possible respiratory distress. Most cases occur during the colder months. Also known as laryngotracheobronchitis because of the structures involved, croup is usually caused by the *H. parainfluenzae* virus, and it affects children between 1 and 3 years of age. It manifests subacutely as a exacerbation of cold symptoms with low fever, barking cough, and hoarseness. If the swelling in the subglottic area progresses, stridor retractions may be noted. Exudative inflammation of the upper airway may cause dyspnea and in extreme cases can lead to exhaustion and frank hypoxia. In the vast majority of cases it is self-limited and benign. Table 44-1 contrasts the croup syndrome with epiglottitis.

Behrman RE, Kliegman RM, Arvin AM (eds): Nelson Textbook of Pediatrics, 15th ed, pp 1201–1205. Philadelphia, WB Saunders, 1996

Davis HW, Gartner JC, Galvis AG et al: Acute upper airway obstruction: Croup and epiglottitis. Pediatr Clin North Am 28: 859, 1981

Table 44-1. Characteristics of Croup and Epiglottitis

	CROUP	**EPIGLOTTITIS**
Etiology	Parainfluenza virus	*Haemophilus influenzae*
Age	Infancy 4 months–2 years	2–5 years
Onset	Subacute—exacerbation of preexistent URI	Acute
Temperature	Low-grade fever	High fever
Course	Usually mild, stridor may worsen at night	Rapid progress of symptoms
Symptomatology	Barky cough, stridor	Dysphagia, sore throat, respiratory distress, dysphonia

A.3. What are the clinical manifestations of epiglottitis?

This illness presents acutely in the otherwise healthy child between 2 and 5 years of age with fever as high as 40°C. Within a few hours the epiglottic inflammation progresses and the child becomes dyspneic. The child sits forward to use the accessory muscles of respiration and complains of a fullness and pain in the throat. Salivation is often characteristic and swallowing is difficult. The child appearing anxious and toxic concentrates only on breathing. As the child fatigues, cyanosis leading to complete asphyxia may ensue without intervention. Inspiratory effort is maximal with severe airway compromise, and negative pressure pulmonary edema can occur. Chest auscultation may reveal decreased breath sounds.

Balkany TJ, Pashley N: Clinical Pediatric Otolaryngology, p 351. St. Louis: CV Mosby, 1986

Behrman RE, Kliegman RM, Arvin AM (eds): Nelson Textbook of Pediatrics, 15th ed, pp 1201–1205. Philadelphia, WB Saunders, 1996

Diaz JH: Croup and epiglottitis in children: The anesthesiologist as diagnostician. Anesthes Analg 64:621, 1985

A.4. How has the incidence of epiglottitis changed over the decade?

The incidence of this disease is on a rapid decline. This is because of the Hib *(H. influenzae* type B) vaccine. Although many vaccination failures were reported before 1992, the introduction of new vaccines has had a major impact in virtually wiping out the infection. However, many poorer urban centers still have a high lack of compliance to vaccination and one cannot assume that this infection will be wiped out.

Wurtele P: Acute epiglottitis in children: Results of a large-scale anti-Hemophilius type B immunization program. J Otolaryngol 24:92,1995

A.5. Has there been a change in the pattern of **Haemophilius influenzae** *infection in recent years?*

In a recent study in the city of Philadelphia, it was found that a sharp decline in *H. influenzae* epiglottitis occurred. Nonetheless, 36% of those infected had ampicillin resistant *H. influenzae*, whereas no resistance had been found previously. In addition, nearly a 30% incidence of vaccination failure was seen before 1990. The anesthesiologist should be aware that this disease will still be seen and not to think of it as a totally extinct entity.

Kessler A, Wetmore RF, Marsh RR: Childhood epiglottitis in recent years. Int J Pediatr Otorhinolaryngol 25:155–162, 1993

A.6. How is the diagnosis of epiglottitis made?

Any child whose clinical presentation warrants the diagnosis of epiglottitis must be evaluated promptly in a hospital. Pharyngoscopy to visualize an inflamed epiglottis should not be attempted in an office setting, as this can stimulate upper airway reflexes and lead to increasing dyspnea. All medical centers should have in place a management protocol that standardizes the approach to this rapidly progressive and fatal disease, and which involves a team of physicians and nurses from the specialties of pediatrics, otolaryngology, and anesthesia. A logical approach is as follows:

- The child is kept calm with a parent in attendance at all times. Supplementary oxygen, maintaining a sitting position, and reassurance are essential.
- If the patient clinically conforms to a classical presentation of epiglottitis, the operating room is alerted and the child is taken there immediately for intubation.
- With other diagnostic considerations, such as a foreign body in the upper airway, retropharyngeal abscess, congenital anomalies, and croup, the child may be escorted to x-ray. The time taken for the x-rays should obviously be avoided in the critically ill child. In any event, a physician skilled in airway management should accompany the child with all necessary resuscitation equipment available.
- The classic thumb sign on a lateral film is an aptly named shape seen with epiglottic enlargement. However, the absence of this sign does not eliminate the diagnosis of epiglottitis. Croup is distinguished by the steeple sign representing a uniform narrowing of the subglottic airway by inflammation. Recently, magnetic resonance imaging has demonstrated the standard measurements for the hypopharyngeal space in various age groups, and it has correlated this measurement with the change produced by epiglottic inflammation. This may be a useful tool in the future to asses the severity of airway involvement.
- Laboratory evidence is nonspecific, although a high white count with bands and polymorphonuclear leukocytes is more suggestive of epiglottitis than of croup.
- Fiberoptic pharyngoscopy can be most effective if performed gently by a skilled examiner; it immediately confirms or eliminates the diagnosis.

Davis HW, Gartner JC, Galvis AG, et al: Acute upper airway obstruction: Croup and epiglottitis. Pediatr Clin North Am 28:859, 1981

Diaz JH: Croup and epiglottitis in children: The anesthesiologist as diagnostician. Anesth Anal 64: 621, 1985

Shorten GD, Opie NJ, Graziotti P et al: Assessment of upper airway anatomy in awake, sedated and anaesthetized patients using magnetic resonance imaging. Anaesth Intensive Care 22:165, 1994

A.7. What is the medical management of croup? Does this have applications for the anesthesiologist?

Once the diagnosis of croup has been established, the child is given a croup score, which helps determine therapy. Mild croup is treated with inspired gas humidification, hydration, and oxygen to improve the attendant hypoxemia. If the patient has moderate retractions and appears dyspneic, 0.5 ml of a 2.25% racemic epinephrine solution in 2.5 ml of normal saline can be administered via a nebulizer.

Airway resistance can be high with the reactive transudation and resultant intraluminal narrowing. By vasoconstricting the mucosal vasculature, racemic epinephrine relieves edema. The epinephrine is prepared as a mixture of the L and D isomers to limit cardiac stimulation. Patients improve markedly, but the clinician should be cautioned that the relief may be short lived and rebound airway compromise may occur after the epinephrine wears off.

Dexamethosone when given early in viral croup can be beneficial in reducing inflammation and alleviating symptoms.

Behrman RE, Kliegman RM, Arvin AM (eds): Nelson Textbook of Pediatrics, 15th ed, pp 1201–1205. Philadelphia, WB Saunders, 1996

Davis HW, Gartner JC, Galvis AG et al: Acute upper airway obstruction: Croup and epiglottitis. Pediatr Clin North Am 28:859, 1981

Ferrari LR: Anesthesia for Pediatric Ear, Nose and Throat Surgery. American Society of Anesthesiologists Refresher Courses in Anesthesiology 24:66, 1996

A.8. What is postextubation croup? How is it managed?

Anesthesiologists are often in the position of treating patients with postextubation airway edema, which resembles croup in its symptomatology.

Pediatric patients undergoing general endotracheal anesthesia can and may mimic many of the physical signs of the croup syndrome following extubation. The tracheal and subglottal mucosa have become irritated by the plastic tube, which initiates an inflammatory response causing airway luminal narrowing. As airway resistance is inversely proportional to the fourth power of the tracheal radius, the pediatric airway is especially compromised by edema. Halving the lumen will increase laminar airflow resistance 16 times.

Postextubation croup may be manifest more frequently in a patient who has received large quantities of fluid or transfusions, maintained unusual or strained lateral head positioning, a history of smoke inhalation, restrictive congenital anomalies such as a tracheoesophageal fistulas, acquired subglottic stenosis secondary to prolonged intubation as a neonate, co-existent upper respiratory infection, especially bronchitis, or has a cuffed endotracheal tube under high pressure.

Management involves reducing airway constriction by administering nebulized racemic epinephrine, steroids, and humidifications of inspired gases. On occasion, re-intubating with a soft endotracheal tube one half to one size smaller than previously used is necessary until the inflammation subsides. Note that topical lidocaine ointment can have vasodilatory actions, and should not be used in patients with postextubation croup.

Davis HW, Gartner JC, Galvis AG et al: Acute upper airway obstruction: Croup and epiglottitis. Pediatr Clin North Am 28:859, 1981

Ferrari LR: Anesthesia for Pediatric Ear, Nose and Throat Surgery. American Society of Anesthesiologists Refresher Courses in Anesthesiology 24:66, 1996

A.9. What are come other causes of partial airway obstruction in children?

Several congenital anomalies are associated with respiratory difficulties. These can be subdivided into intrinsic and extrinsic pathologies as follows:

Extrinsic Pathologies
- Cystic hygroma—a proliferation or expansion of lymphatic channels, usually in the cervical region, which can compress the airway and lead to enlargement of the tongue.
- Vascular anomalies—abnormalities of the aortic arch usually caused by aberrant vessels leads to compression of the airway. This is often position dependent and may be responsible for coughing and wheezing when the patient is supine.
- Neoplastic compression of the trachea by lymphoma, hemangioma, neurofibromatosis or rhabdomyosarcoma, and other neural tumors in the mediastinum may occur and enlarge or compress airway structures.

Intrinsic Pathologies

- Subglottic stenosis—especially as acquired in previously intubated neonates. This form of airway narrowing occurs below the vocal cords, and it can lead to marked airway obstruction with respiratory infections. The congenital form may not be appreciated till an upper respiratory infection is present, at which point stridor may occur.
- Vocal cord paralysis—considered the second most common laryngeal anomaly in children, it is associated with the Arnold-Chiari malformation.
- Laryngeal structural anomalies—webs, laryngoceles, and cysts.

Badgewell JM, McLead ME, Friedberg BA: Airway obstruction in infants and children. Can J Anaesth 341:90, 1987

B. Preoperative Evaluation and Preparation

B.1. Why is general anesthesia administered to a child with epiglottitis?

General anesthesia facilitates several activities. It gives the examiner a thorough look at the supraglottic area, which would be impossible and dangerous in the awake child. In addition, endotracheal intubation can be accomplished under controlled, relaxed conditions without trauma and laryngospasm. Intubation can be difficult because of the swelling and deformation of the paraepiglottic tissues. Clinicians who have no experience with this unusual appearance will find it easier to visualize landmarks and secure the airway when the patient is in a surgical plane of anesthesia.

Diaz JH: Croup and epiglottitis in children. Anesthesiology 64:628, 1985

B.2. How would you prepare the patient for anesthesia?

Expedience is crucial. Once the diagnosis is made and the operating room alerted, the child is transported accompanied by his parents and a physician with supportive equipment. It is not necessary to place an intravenous line, as this can be done more easily under anesthesia without upsetting the child. Any maneuver that causes the child to cry will potentially interfere with breathing. The child should therefore be kept calm and constantly reassured. Nasal prong or face tent oxygen should be provided and portable pulse oximetry should be used.

Equipment, which is prepared in the operating room, includes a suitable mask and endotracheal tube, sized two gauges (1 mm diameter) smaller than normally expected. Lidocaine, succinylcholine, atropine and ketamine in convenient dilutions should be readily available. A cricothyrotomy tray should be available as a precaution.

The parent is dressed in operating room attire to accompany the child into the operating room. Prior to induction, the parent is instructed on his or her role in comforting the child, encouraging complicity with mask breathing, and gently holding the child when the inhalation induction commences. The parent should also be told that as the child begins to fall asleep he or she will be asked to leave the room. For anesthesiologists unaccustomed to the presence of parents in the operating room, the extra anxiety created by parental presence can by attenuated by having them depart just as the patient begins to get sleepy. When parents can provide their assistance in an emotionally controlled, supportive way, a smooth, safe anesthetic induction can usually be well facilitated.

Berry FA: Management of the Pediatric Patient with Croup or Epiglottitis. ASA Annual Refresher Course Lectures #261, 1990

Davis HW, Gartner JC, Galvis AC et al: Acute upper airway obstruction: Croup and epiglottitis. Pediatr Clin North Am 28:859, 1981

C. Intraoperative Management

C.1. How is the airway of the child with epiglottitis best secured?

Little debate occurs over the safety and efficacy of endotracheal intubation provided supportive staff is readily available. In the smaller hospital without a pediatric intensive care facility or experienced personnel, a tracheotomy may be the safest route. Placing a smaller caliber endotracheal tube, which will remain for up to 2 days, mandates close scrutiny. Thick, copious secretions must be cleared frequently to prevent obstruction, and the child must be sedated properly to prevent the tube from dislodging and to allow for its toleration.

C.2. How would you induce anesthesia?

The child is seated on the parent's lap in the operating room and is preoxygenated. Gentle verbal assurance is constantly given. A low concentration of halothane (0.25%) is introduced and the child is encouraged to breathe normally. Sevoflurane or halothane are the most suitable inhalational agents as they lack the pungency of isoflurane or desflurane. They should be initiated slowly and increased in concentration as tolerated. As the child tires, the supine position is assumed and cricoid pressure applied as a safeguard against aspiration. The patient may undergo a brief period of excitement during which care is taken not to be overly zealous with ventilatory assistance. Spontaneous, unassisted ventilation continues and an intravenous line is started. Atropine (0.01 to 0.02 mg/kg) is given intravenously as a vagolytic and antisialogogue. Halothane is increased to 3% or 4% (sevoflurane to 6% to 7%) as hemodynamically tolerated. Ventilatory assistance but not control is provided to limit hypercarbia. End-tidal gas analysis is continually monitored and the airway is adjusted to provide maximal tidal exchange. If there is airway obstruction, anesthetic uptake may be delayed. Therefore, as long as 15 minutes may be necessary to achieve a deeply anesthetized patient with a slow inhalation induction. When the patient is in a deep plane of surgical anesthesia (remember that the minimal alveolar capacity [MAC] value of halothane in children is higher than that in adults), a careful laryngoscopy is carried out. Paralysis is unnecessary in this deep plane of anesthesia. However, if several attempts are required with the possibility of the patient becoming light and reactive, atracurium (0.5 mg/kg) or mivacurium (0.2 mg/kg) will serve to maintain stable intubating conditions. This should be given only after it has been shown that the patient can be ventilated with a bag and mask.

Berry FA: Management of the Pediatric Patient with Croup or Epiglottitis. ASA Annual Refresher course Lectures, #261, 1990

Gerber AC, Pfenninger J: Acute epiglottitis: Management by short duration of intubation and hospitalization. Intensive Care Med 12:407, 1986

C.3. Should a child with epiglottitis undergo a rapid-sequence induction?

In the child with a full stomach a mask induction leaves the airway unprotected from aspiration of gastric contents. However, a rapid-sequence induction may predispose the patient to severe hypoxia and hypoventilation should the clinician not be able to intubate expediently. Because the supraglottic landmarks are distorted by erythema and edema, recognition of the glottic inlet is obscured. In the spontaneously breathing patient, small air movements and the resultant secretional bubbling may highlight the glottic opening. In addition, paralysis in no way secures ventilatability.

If the patient needs to be manually ventilated, it is possible to meet with complete obstruction secondary to invagination of the swollen supraglottic tissues into the laryngeal introitus. In such a case positive end-expiratory pressure (PEEP) or the jaw thrust maneuver may fail to correct the airway obstruction.

Should the child be too agitated to cooperate with an inhalational induction, an intramuscular dose of ketamine (2 to 3 mg/kg) will accomplish sedation and preserve ventilation. However, it may accentuate airway reflexes, and the clinician should be wary of laryngospasm.

Berry FA: Management of the Pediatric Patient with Croup or Epiglottitis. ASA Annual Refresher Course Lectures, #261, 1990

C.4. Is awake intubation a practical alternative for securing this patient's airway?

Some authors suggest awake intubation with topical anesthesia. In such cases the anesthesiologist should be alerted to the possibility of adenoidal bleeding, difficult visualization, agitation, trauma, and compromised ventilation. Unless one has acquired great skill at awake pediatric intubation in the child with a normal airway, this technique should be avoided in these patients.

Diaz JH: Croup and epiglottitis in children. Anesthesiology 64:628, 1985

C.5. Should this patient have a nasotracheal or orotracheal tube placed?

The patient will better tolerate a nasal tube for prolonged intubation. Oropharyngeal toilet is also easier. However, because the intubation can be difficult with epiglottitis and may predispose the patient to the problems listed in question C.4, the orotracheal route is easier and thus safer. Once the airway is secured orally, a nasotracheal tube can be inserted with laryngoscopic guidance. The Magill forceps may be necessary to facilitate insertion of the nasal tube.

C.6. Shortly after intubation, frothy secretions were obtained on suctioning the endotracheal tube. What is the reason for this? How can this be treated?

Davis describes 7% of these patients as having pulmonary edema after intubation. This phenomenon relates to the transudation into the alveoli during periods of increased transpulmonary pressure. This occurs especially during obstructed inspiration. If the obstruction is complete, it is referred to as the "Müller" maneuver. The high negative pressures are buffered by the decreased venous return during exhalation. However, relief of the airway obstruction facilitates the extravasation of fluid for an increased venous return.

Treatment of this negative pressure pulmonary edema requires PEEP. Diuretics and fluid restriction are not required as this condition is generally self-correcting.

Davis HW, Gartener JC, Galvis AG et al: Acute upper airway obstruction: Croup and epiglottitis. Pediatr Clin North Am 28:859, 1981

D. Postoperative Management

D.1. How long should this patient remain intubated? What criteria determine extubation time?

Rothstein reported a mean intubation duration of 36 hours in 23 patients with a range of 19 to 67 hours. These patients were treated with ampicillin or chloramphenicol and the epiglottis was visualized prior to extubation. Hopkins recommended that the flexible fiberoptic laryngoscope be used to visualize the epiglottis and determine extubation time. Vernon and Sarnaik, however, feel that instrumentation and examination of the child is unnecessary and extubation at 36 to 48 hours can easily be accomplished in all patients.

Hopkins RL: Extubation in epiglottitis. Anesth Analg 63:468, 1984

Rothstein P, Lister G: Epiglottitis: Duration of intubation and fever. Anesthes Analg 62:795, 1983

Vernon DD, Sarnaik AP: Extubation in epiglottitis. Anesth Analg 63:469, 1984

D.2. How would you make this patient comfortable during the course of intubation?

The child must be kept sedated to minimize movement, prevent deliberate extubation, and provide anxiolysis. Midazolam (0.075 mg/kg) as a starting dose titrated upward to effect followed by a continuous infusion of 0.04 mg/kg/h will be effective in this regard. If necessary a fentanyl drip (2 µg/kg/h) can be supplemented. A bilateral superior laryngeal nerve block in experienced hands allows for better endotracheal tube toleration.

Of course respiratory care, humidification, suctioning, and secretion mobilization must receive attention.

Davis HW, Gartner JC, Galvis AG et al: Acute upper airway obstruction: Croup and epiglottitis. Pediatr Clin North Am 28:859, 1981

Cleft Palate

45

Marjorie J. Topkins

A newborn male was noted at birth to have a cleft lip and palate. Birth weight was 2960 g. Apgar score was 7 at 1 minute and 9 at 5 minutes. Mild icterus was noted on the second day.

A. Medical Disease and Differential Diagnosis

1. What are a cleft lip and a cleft palate?
2. What is the cause of a cleft lip or a cleft palate?
3. What is the incidence of a cleft lip with or without a cleft palate? Is there a sex difference in the incidence of cleft lip and palate? Are there racial differences in the incidence of cleft lip and cleft palate?
4. Discuss the pathophysiology of the cleft lip and cleft palate in the neonate and the older child (i.e., age >5 years).
5. What other conditions are associated with a cleft lip and palate?
6. What is Pierre Robin sequence?
7. What is Treacher Collins syndrome?
8. Why are Robin's and Treacher Collins syndromes mentioned at this time?
9. What surgical procedures are anticipated for this child? Discuss indications, timing, and complications of closure of the lip and palate.

B. Preoperative Evaluation and Preparation

1. What information do you need prior to closure of a cleft lip and a cleft palate?
2. What preoperative orders are needed?

C. Intraoperative Management

1. What monitors will you need for cheiloplasty and palatoplasty?
2. Discuss anesthetic agents for cheiloplasty and palatoplasty. Discuss epinephrine and halothane use.
3. Discuss the induction and anesthetic management for cheiloplasty and palatoplasty.
4. What are the reported complications of this type of surgery and anesthesia?
5. Discuss hemostasis during this procedure.
6. What is velopharyngeal incompetence?
7. How can velopharyngeal incompetence be diagnosed?
8. What is the relationship of tonsillectomy and adenoidectomy to velopharyngeal incompetence?
9. Briefly describe the operation known as push-back and pharyngeal flap.
10. How does a pharyngeal flap affect your anesthetic management or any subsequent anesthetic administered to this patient?
11. What is an Abbe flap? What are its anesthetic consequences?

12. **What is the crucial problem of anesthesia for cleft palate? Enumerate the consequences of failure.**

D. Postoperative Management

1. **What complications of cleft lip and cleft palate surgery may be seen in the recovery room?**
2. **How do you protect the airway postoperatively?**

A. Medical Disease and Differential Diagnosis

A.1. What are a cleft lip and a cleft palate?

Simply, a cleft lip or cleft palate is a defect in the lip or palate. These two entities can occur separately or together. The cleft lip can be classified anatomically by inspection. The cleft can be unilateral or bilateral. It can be complete or incomplete. The cleft can be associated with nasal deformity, most commonly columellar shortening or deformity, absence of the nasal floor, and deformity of the ala nasi.

The cleft palate is divided into prepalatal clefts and postpalatal clefts. The incisive foramen marks the boundary between these two. Prepalatal and postpalatal clefts develop differently embryologically. Prepalatal clefts involve the anterior palate, alveolus, lip, nostril floor, and ala nasi. They can be complete or incomplete. Postpalatal clefts are posterior to the incisive foramen. They can be complete or incomplete depending on whether or not they extend all the way through the soft and hard palates to the incisive foramen. The third type of palatal cleft is the submucosal cleft in which a bone defect exists without a mucosal defect. The most common cleft of the palate is a left complete cleft of the prepalatal and palatal structures. The second most common is a midline cleft of all the soft palate and part of the hard palate without a cleft in the prepalatal area. Various degrees of cleft palate and lip are shown in Figure 45-1.

Aston SJ, Beasley RW, Thorne CHM (eds): Grabb and Smith's Plastic Surgery, 5th ed, pp 245–263. Philadelphia, Lippincott–Raven, 1997

Gregory GA (ed): Pediatric Anesthesia, 3rd ed, p 710. New York, Churchill Livingstone, 1994

McCarthy JG (ed): Cleft lip and palate and craniofacial anomalies. Vol. 4. Plastic Surgery. Philadelphia, WB Saunders, 1990

A.2. What is the cause of a cleft lip or a cleft palate?

Prepalatal clefts are caused by a lack of mesodermal development. Three mesodermal islands, one central and two lateral, are described. When these mesodermal elements fail to develop and fuse, prepalatal clefts result. Palatal clefts are caused when the palatal ridges fail to migrate medially, contact, and fuse. The palatal ridges are vertical in the 7-week embryo and lie lateral to the tongue. The tongue drops down and the shelves rotate upward to the horizontal position and fuse from anterior to posterior to form an intact palate in the 12-week embryo.

Grabb WC, Rosenstein SW, Bzock KR: Cleft Lip and Palate, pp 54–65. Boston, Little, Brown, 1971

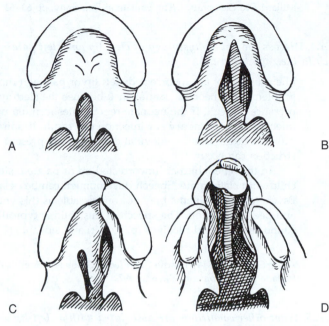

Figure 45-1. Various degrees of cleft palate and lip. **(A)** Cleft of the soft palate only. **(B)** Cleft of the soft and hard palate as far forward as the incisive foramen. **(C)** Complete unilateral alveolar cleft, usually involving the lip. **(D)** Complete bilateral alveolar cleft, usually associated with bilateral clefts of the lip. (Reprinted with permission from McCarthy JG [ed]: Cleft lip and palate and craniofacial abnormalities. Plastic Surgery. Vol 4. Philadelphia, WB Saunders, 1990)

Aston SJ, Beasley RW, Thorne CHM (eds): Grabb and Smith's Plastic Surgery, 5th ed, pp 230–234. Philadelphia, Lippincott–Raven, 1997

A.3. What is the incidence of a cleft lip with or without a cleft palate? Is there a sex difference in the incidence of cleft lip and palate? Are there racial differences in the incidence of cleft lip and cleft palate?

Considerable variation is seen in the reported incidence of a cleft lip with or without a cleft palate and less variation in the reported incidence of a cleft palate alone. In general, the incidence of a cleft lip varies according to race and sex. The highest incidence occurs in Asians (1.61/1000 births), whereas the lowest incidence is in the African-Americans (0.3/1000 births). The incidence in whites is intermediate (0.9/1000 births). The incidence among Native Americans probably exceeds that of Asians. Considerably less variation is seen in the incidence of isolated cleft palate. The incidence ranges from 0.2/1000 live births for African-Americans to 0.5/1000 live births in Asians, and it is approximately 0.4/1000 live births in whites. The incidence among Native Americans is again somewhat higher than among Asians. More males are born with a cleft lip with or without cleft palate, and the severity of the defect is greater in males. More females are born with isolated cleft palate. The male:female ratio of incidence of a cleft lip with or without a cleft palate is 62:38 and 43:57 for isolated cleft palate. Approximately 25% of affected patients have an isolated cleft lip, 50% have a cleft lip and palate, and 25% have only a cleft palate.

Aston SJ, Beasley RW, Thorne CHM (eds): Grabb and Smith's Plastic Surgery, 5th ed, pp 245–255. Philadelphia, Lippincott–Raven, 1997

Cooper HK (ed): Cleft Palate and Cleft Lip: A Team Approach, pp 116–119. Philadelphia, WB Saunders, 1979

Gregory GA (ed): Pediatric Anesthesia, 3rd ed, p 708. New York, Churchill Livingstone, 1994

Millard DR: Cleft craft. I. The Unilateral Deformity, pp 63–64. Boston, Little, Brown, 1976

A.4. Discuss the pathophysiology of cleft lip and cleft palate in the neonate and the older child (i.e., age >5 years).

The presence of an uncorrected cleft lip or palate in the neonate results in feeding problems. The neonate cannot suck because the cleft makes the creation of a negative pressure difficult. If the neonate regurgitates formula up into the nose, nasopharynx infection and secondary ear infection can result. Respiratory effects are not usually a problem unless other congenital anomalies are present. However, upper airway obstruction can occur.

In the older child an uncorrected lip or palate results in the typical speech of the child with cleft palate. Speech development can be delayed because of frustration. Psychological problems may be considerable as this youngster approaches school age and peer association. The speech of this child is typically nasal with an inability to sound the so-called plosives (p/k/d/t) and sibilants (s/sh).

Aston SJ, Beasley RW, Thorne CHM (eds): Grabb and Smith's Plastic Surgery, 5th ed, pp 238–239. Philadelphia, Lippincott–Raven, 1997

A.5. What other conditions are associated with a cleft lip and palate?

A child with one congenital anomaly may have other anomalies, which should be ruled out in the neonatal period. Associated abnormalities occur 30 times more frequently in the patient with an isolated cleft palate than in the noncleft population. Between 10% and 25% of patients with cleft lip and palate have abnormalities of other organs. Robin's syndrome is frequently associated with a cleft palate, as is Treacher Collins syndrome and first and second branchial-arch syndrome (hemifacial microsomia).

Cooper HK (ed): Cleft Palate and Cleft Lip: A Team Approach, pp 110–117. Philadelphia, WB Saunders, 1979

Curtis EJ: Genetic and environmental factors in the etiology of cleft lip and cleft palate. Can Dent Assoc J 23:576, 1957

Gorlin RJ, Cervenka J, Pruzansky D: Facial clefting and its syndromes. Birth Defects 7(7):3–39, 1971

Gregory GA (ed): Pediatric Anesthesia, 3rd ed, pp 704–706; 718. New York, Churchill Livingstone, 1994

A.6. What is Pierre Robin sequence?

Pierre Robin sequence is one of the few life-threatening congenital conditions of the neonatal period. The elements of this syndrome are limited to the jaw, tongue, and palate. There is retrognathia or micrognathia. The chin is displaced posteriorly owing either to hypoplasia of the mandible (micrognathia) or to posterior positioning of a normal mandible (retrognathia). Glossoptosis owing to retroposition of the mandible is found. The tongue falls back, obstructing the airway in a ball-valve fashion. The tongue may be either large or relatively small when compared with the micrognathia. A cleft palate is frequently present, most commonly incomplete. The lip is not usually involved. Occasionally, a high-arched palate is present without a cleft. The cause of the syndrome is divided between external pressure in utero on the anterior mandible with subsequent retardation of growth, and lack of growth potential in the mandible itself.

Aston SJ, Beasley RW, Thorne CHM (eds): Grabb and Smith's Plastic Surgery, 5th ed, p 234. Philadelphia, Lippincott–Raven, 1997

A.7. What is Treacher Collins syndrome?

Treacher Collins syndrome or mandibulofacial dysostosis is a congenital genetic anomaly that is autosomal dominant with variable penetrance and expressivity. It occurs in approximately 1/10,000 live births. The common features of this syndrome are notching of the lower eyelids and underdevelopment of the malar bones. The complete form of the syndrome is manifested by antimongoloid slant of the eyelids; hypoplasia of the facial, malar, and mandibular bones; notching of the outer portion of the lower eyelid (coloboma); malformation of the external ear, occasionally involving the middle and inner ear; macrostomia with a high palate; abnormal hair at the sideburn area; blind dimples or fistulae at the corner of the mouth; and skeletal defects, especially clefts of the face and palate. An incomplete form was described consisting of notching of the eyelid and hypoplasia of the malar bones. The third form, described as abortive, shows only the eyelid defect.

Pozwilla D: Pathogenesis of Treacher-Collins syndrome: Mandibular facial dysostosis. Br J Oral Surg 13:1, 1975

A.8. Why are Robin's and Treacher Collins syndromes mentioned at this time?

Because of the small size and retrognathic position of the mandible with or without a large tongue, Robin's syndrome can cause considerable difficulty in intubation. Treacher Collins syndrome produces even greater difficulty. However, anticipation of problems can prevent catastrophe.

Gregory GA (ed): Pediatric Anesthesia, 3rd ed, pp 719–720. New York, Churchill Livingstone, 1994

Miyabe M, Dohi S, Homma E: Tracheal intubation in an infant with Treacher-Collins syndrome: Pulling out the tongue by a forceps. Anesthesiology 62:213–241, 1985

Motoyama EK, Davis PS (eds): Smith's Anesthesia for Infants and Children, 6th ed, p 595. St. Louis, CV Mosby, 1996

A.9. What surgical procedures are anticipated for this child? Discuss indications, timing, and complications of closure of the lip and palate.

Care of this child will require multiple operations and a multidisciplinary approach to the problem. He will need a pediatrician to maintain his overall health, a surgeon and anesthesiologist to accomplish the various surgeries, a speech therapist to prevent or overcome the speech deficiencies associated with clefts of the palate, and an orthodontist to develop and maintain a relatively normal bite and dentition. The help of a psychologist or psychiatrist may be needed by the patient or his family.

The lip can be closed in the first week of life with no complicating associated conditions present. This permits the parents to take home a relatively normal-looking infant. Complications include breakdown of the closure with scarring of the tissues, bleeding, and infection. The "rule of ten" has been accepted by many plastic surgeons for timing the closure of the lip—hemoglobin 10 g/dl or greater, 10 weeks of age, and weighing 4.5 kg. The hard palate can be closed anytime up to 4 or 5 years, but the soft palate should be closed prior to speech development. Therefore, the usual age has been 12 to 15 months. Others report closure of the soft palate as early as 3 to 6 months. Complications of palatal closure include bleeding, obstruction to respiration, breakdown of the sutured tissues, scarring, and persistent palatal openings. Secondary procedures may be required in later years for cosmetic purposes. These may involve the columella, the nasal tip and alae, and include revision of the vermilion border. Additional procedures on the palate include the push back and pharyngeal flap operation.

Aston SJ, Beasley RW, Thorne CHM (eds): Grabb and Smith's Plastic Surgery, 5th ed, pp 241–244, 263–265. Philadelphia, Lippincott–Raven, 1997

Cooper HK (ed): Cleft Palate and Cleft Lip: A Team Approach, pp 145–150. Philadelphia, WB Saunders, 1979

Gregory GA (ed): Pediatric Anesthesia, 3rd ed, p 718. New York, Churchill Livingstone, 1994

Kaplan I, Dresner J: The simultaneous repair of cleft lip and palate in early infancy. Br J Plast Surg 27:134, 1974

Stark RB: Cleft lip: A timetable. Ann Plast Surg 8:107–117, 1982

B. Preoperative Evaluation and Preparation

B.1. *What information do you need prior to closure of a cleft lip and a cleft palate?*

General care of the patient with cleft lip and palate includes feeding; maintaining the airway, especially in the patient with a small or retropositioned mandible (Robin's syndrome); preventing or treating middle ear disease because eustachian tube function is impaired; and searching for and investigating associated anomalies, which are 30 times more frequent than in the noncleft population.

Preoperative anesthetic evaluation includes the history and physical examination plus suitable laboratory data. The hemoglobin and white blood count and hematocrit plus urinalysis are minimal requirements. If Treacher Collins or Pierre Robin syndrome is suspected, an x-ray film of the mandible may be helpful. Examination of the mouth may indicate potential intubation problems. The infant should be free of acute infection, gaining weight, have a hemoglobin 10 g/dl or better, and have a white blood count <10,000. With an open cleft palate, however, it is common to have crusting and low-grade infection of the nasopharynx owing to food and fluid regurgitation through the cleft. It is nearly impossible to eliminate this completely. Unless an acute inflammatory process is present, this has not led to complications.

Aston SJ, Beasley RW, Thorne CHM (eds): Grabb and Smith's Plastic Surgery, 5th ed, p 247. Philadelphia, Lippincott–Raven, 1997

Mladic R, Pickrell K, Gingrass K: Blood volume determination in cleft lip: Palate infant surgery. Plast Reconstr Surg 39:71, 1967

B.2. What preoperative orders are needed?

A trend is seen toward a more liberal policy concerning fluid restriction prior to surgery. Previously our policy was to give clear fluids to infants 6 months or younger up until 4 hours before surgery. Children <3 years of age were allowed fluids until 2 A.M. if surgery was scheduled for 8 A.M., and for those >3 years of age nothing was given past midnight. No solid foods or milk were permitted after midnight. Our policy now permits clear fluid up until 3 hours prior to surgery for infants, children, and adolescents. Solid foods and nonclear fluids should not be given within 6 hours of surgery. If the youngster is hospitalized the night before surgery, an intravenous (IV) infusion decreases the need for orally administered fluids. For children ≥6 months of age, a sedative and atropine should be ordered. Pentobarbitol (5 mg/kg) and atropine (0.01 to 0.02 mg/kg) are given. For infants <6 months of age, atropine alone is sufficient. The use of atropine for its vagolytic action is important to prevent the bradycardia produced by using halothane, mechanical stimulation, and succinylcholine for intubation. Because multiple operations may be required, the emotional trauma of each hospital experience must be minimized. Special orders include antibiotics if the infant or child has associated congenital heart disease, and the typing and crossmatching of a unit of blood for palatal surgery. Cheiloplasty rarely requires blood transfusion, but blood loss has been reported as high as 200 to 300 ml in palate surgery. A unit of blood should be available, although it is rarely administered.

Crawford M, Lerman J, Christensen S et al: Effects of duration of fasting on gastric fluid *p*H and volume in healthy children. Anesth Analg 71:400–402, 1990

Maltby JR, Sutherland AD, Sale JP et al: Preoperative oral fluids: Is a five-hour fast justified prior to elective surgery? Anesth Analg 65:1112–1116, 1986

Mladic R, Pickrell K, Gingrass R: Blood volume determinations in cleft lip: Palate infant surgery. Plast Reconstr Surg 39:71, 1967

Motoyama EK, Davis PS (eds): Smith's Anesthesia for Infants and Children, 5th ed, p 211. St Louis, CV Mosby, 1990

Splinter WM, Schaefer JD: Ingestion of clear fluids is safe for adolescents up to 3 hours before surgery. Br J Anaesth 66:48–52, 1991

C. Intraoperative Management

C.1. What monitors will you need for cheiloplasty and palatoplasty?

A suitable technique for measuring blood pressure is mandatory. Temperature should be monitored per rectum or axilla and a heating-cooling blanket should be placed under the patient for use if necessary or the Baer Hugger™ can be used. A precordial stethoscope monitors both heart and respiratory sounds. It is particularly important in this patient because once surgery is begun, the anesthesiologist no longer has easy direct access to the airway. An electrocardiogram provides visual and audible evidence of the electrical activity of the heart. Blood loss should be measured accurately. The use of pulse oximetry is mandatory. The position used for repair usually places the anesthesiologist at the side of a heavily draped patient. Therefore, it is difficult to observe the color of the patient. The pulse oximeter may alert the anesthesiologist to a problem earlier than might otherwise be possible. End-tidal CO_2 is advisable and mandated in some states.

C.2. Discuss anesthetic agents for cheiloplasty and palatoplasty. Discuss epinephrine and halothane use.

Halothane, nitrous oxide, and oxygen can be used for both cheiloplasty and palatoplasty. To avoid the possibility of retrolental fibroplasia, the inspired-oxygen concentration (F_IO_2) should not exceed 40% to 50% in normal full-term infants <2 weeks of age, and in premature infants until 3 months of age. Enflurane and isoflurane offer little advantage over halothane except that the myocardium is less sensitive to exogenous epinephrine. Recommended maximal dosage of lidocaine for palate or lip surgery is 5 mg/kg and of epinephrine 10 µg/kg. This epinephrine dose is for hypocarbic or normocarbic children. In practice, because the structures are very small, the total dose of epinephrine is far lower than these recommendations.

Ketamine, used without an endotracheal tube for cheiloplasty repair, is contraindicated because of the high incidence of severe laryngospasm, cardiac arrest, and vomiting followed by aspiration. Small infants react unpredictably to ketamine. Local anesthesia with sedation has been used for cheiloplasty in the past, but distortion of the structures by the injected local anesthetics is unsatisfactory for some surgeons. Endotracheal anesthesia offers safe airway management.

Godinez RI (ed): Special problems in pediatric anesthesia. Int Anesthesiol Clin 23(4):87–117, 1985

Karl HW, Swedlow DB, Lee KW: Epinephrine-halothane interaction in children. Anesthesiology 58:142, 1983

Motoyama EK, Davis PS (ed): Smith's Anesthesia for Infants and Children, 6th ed, pp 599–601. St. Louis, CV Mosby, 1996

Smith NT, Corbascio AN (eds): Drug Interactions in Anesthesia, 2nd ed, pp 354–355. Philadelphia, Lea & Febiger, 1986

Weda W, Hirakawa M, Mae D: Appraisal of epinephrine administration to patients under halothane for closure of cleft palate. Anesthesiology 58:574–576, 1983

C.3. Discuss the induction and anesthetic management for cheiloplasty and palatoplasty.

For cheiloplasty, after suitable monitors are attached, the infant is induced with nitrous oxide, oxygen, and halothane. An intravenous route is established as soon as the patient is asleep. Dextrose, 5% in one-quarter-strength normal saline, is a suitable infusate. Intubation can be facilitated with a nondepolarizing muscle relaxant, or succinylcholine (1 mg/kg). Muscle relaxants should not be given if any possibility of difficulty with intubation exists. Prepalatal clefts are most frequently on the left and the laryngoscope tends to fall into the cleft. Bilateral clefts often have a freely mobile premaxilla associated with them. Care must be taken to avoid traumatizing these structures. The endotracheal tube must not distort the anatomy. The tube curves over the lower lip where it is fastened in the midline. The RAE tube for oral intubation fulfills the requirement. Because it has a fixed length, care must be taken to ensure that it does not enter the right or left bronchus. A thermistor probe is placed either in the rectum or axilla. Rectal stimulation is postponed until after intubation to decrease the possibility of laryngeal reflexes. Care is taken to prevent heat loss. Cheiloplasty requires only a minimal depth of anesthesia and no muscle relaxation. The anesthesiologist sits or stands at the side of the table. The breath and heart sounds are monitored with the precordial stethoscope. It is necessary to have great cooperation between the surgeon and the anesthesiologist because the surgeon's tools and hands and the anesthesiologist's endotracheal tube and apparatus all occupy the same very small space.

Pediatric circle systems can be used, or the Mapleson systems may be satisfactory. The Mapleson A requires a fresh gas flow equal to the minute volume; the Mapleson D requires a fresh gas flow of 1.5 times minute volume. The minute volume equals tidal volume times respiratory rate, and tidal volume equals 7 ml/kg of body weight or three times the body weight in pounds.

For palatoplasty, halothane, nitrous oxide, and oxygen are satisfactory. A muscle relaxant can also be used, but if intubation difficulty is suspected, as might be expected with Robin's or Treacher Collins syndrome, it is best omitted. Dextrose 5% in one-quarter-strength normal saline at a rate of 4 ml/kg/h can be administered once an IV route is available. This is a conservative fluid allowance. Total fluid replacement should include the hours when the patient was not permitted anything orally and approximately 2 hours postoperative at which time clear oral feeding can usually be started. Blood is rarely required. If blood losses exceed 15% to 20% of the estimated blood volume, a transfusion should be started. During the palate repair a mouth gag (Dingman or Dott) is used, and the endotracheal tube is held under the tongue blade of the gag. Again, the RAE oral tube can be used. Others prefer the anode or armored tube. Great care must be taken as the gag is inserted and opened. The endotracheal tube is pushed caudad, where it can impinge on the carina or enter either main bronchus. Breath sounds are monitored as the gag is opened; if any change occurs, the gag is closed and the endotracheal tube repositioned. This is repeated as often as necessary until the breath sounds are normal with the gag fully open. Relaxants are not necessary and the patient should be almost awake when extubated. The infant is turned on the side and when awake extubated in this position.

Suture removal following cheiloplasty is usually accomplished with anesthesia. Rectal methohexital (30 mg/kg), inhalation agents, or ketamine (4 to 6 mg/kg IM or 2 mg/kg IV) can be used.

Abadir AR, Humayun SG (eds): Anesthesia for Plastic and Reconstructive Surgery, pp 210–216. St. Louis, Mosby-Year Book, 1991

Furman EB: Specific therapy in water, electrolyte and blood volume replacements in pediatric surgery. Anesthesiology 42:187, 1975

Gregory GA (ed): Pediatric Anesthesia, 3rd ed, p 726–727. New York, Churchill Livingstone, 1994

Morgan GA, Steward DJ: Airway dimensions in children with and without a cleft palate. Can Anaesth Soc J 28:500, 1981

Sklar GS, King BD: Endotracheal intubation and Treacher-Collins syndrome. Anesthesiology 44:247, 1976

C.4. What are the reported complications of this type of surgery and anesthesia?

Anesthetic complications include obstruction of the endotracheal tube, inadvertent extubation during the procedure, and cardiac arrest. Postanesthetic complications include airway obstruction, bleeding with or without aspiration, and pneumonia. Complications not related to anesthetic management are wound healing, diarrhea, and otitis media. The mortality rate has been reported to be <0.5%.

Grabb WC, Rosenstein SW, Bzock KR: Cleft Lip and Palate, pp 385–386. Boston, Little, Brown, 1971

Gregory GA (ed): Pediatric Anesthesia, 3rd ed, pp 726–727. New York, Churchill Livingstone, 1994

C.5. Discuss hemostasis during this procedure.

Epinephrine injected into the operative site decreases bleeding. As mentioned, the total dose should not exceed 10 µg/kg. During palatoplasty, large areas of denuded palate are left after mobilization of the flaps for closure. Frequently these tissues ooze postoperatively. Bleeding can jeopardize the airway unless care is taken to prevent aspiration. Induced hypotensive techniques have been tried in the past in an attempt to reduce operative bleeding. Although a good operative field resulted, more postoperative bleeding was noted. In a comparative study of anesthetic agents and blood loss, methoxyflurane appeared to produce less bleeding than other agents. However, methoxyflurane is no longer used.

Abadir AR, Humayun SG (eds): Anesthesia for Plastic and Reconstructive Surgery, p 216. St. Louis, Mosby-Year Book, 1991

Black GW, Coppel MB, Hugh NC et al: Anesthesia for cleft palate repair: A comparative study of anesthetic methods. Br J Plast Surg 22:343, 1969

Herbert KJ, Eartley R, Milward TM: Assessing blood loss in cleft lip and palate surgery. Br J Plast Surg 43:497–498, 1990

Katz RL, Epstein RA: Interaction of anesthetic agents and adrenergic drugs to produce cardiac arrhythmias. Anesthesiology 29:763, 1968

Tempest MN: Some observations on blood loss and harelip and cleft palate surgery. Br J Plast Surg 11:34, 1958

C.6. What is velopharyngeal incompetence?

To produce the plosive sounds, p/k/t/d, or the sibilants, s/sh, the soft palate must touch the posterior pharyngeal wall to close the nose. Failure of closure results in the typical hypernasal speech. The most common cause of this is the cleft palate, but patients with congenitally short palates and no cleft can also have this typical speech. Treatment consists of surgical lengthening of the palate by the push-back operation with or without a pharyngeal flap.

Aston SJ, Beasley RW, Thorne CHM (eds): Grabb and Smith's Plastic Surgery, 5th ed, pp 265–266. Philadelphia, Lippincott–Raven, 1997

C.7. How can velopharyngeal incompetence be diagnosed?

The diagnosis of velopharyngeal incompetence can be suggested by the child's speech. More objective evidence can be obtained by direct vision of the soft palate while the child is pronouncing certain key words (kah, kah), by the fogging of a hand mirror placed under the nose during speech, and from cinefluorographic x-ray films.

Aston SJ, Beasley RW, Thorne CHM (eds): Grabb and Smith's Plastic Surgery, 5th ed, pp 265–267. Philadelphia, Lippincott–Raven, 1997

C.8. What is the relationship of tonsillectomy and adenoidectomy to velopharyngeal incompetence?

Because the adenoids and tonsils tend to close the nasopharynx, they prevent or decrease velopharyngeal incompetence. A youngster who had normal speech may suddenly develop hypernasality after tonsillectomy and adenoidectomy. The tonsils and adenoids, therefore, are preserved if at all possible. A cleft palate constitutes a relative contraindication to removal of tonsils and adenoids.

Shirkey HC: Pediatric Surgery, p 1046. St. Louis, CV Mosby, 1975

C.9. Briefly describe the operation known as push-back and pharyngeal flap.

The palate is incised in an inverted U or W fashion laterally and anteriorly. It is mobilized and displaced posteriorly, and a flap from the posterior pharyngeal wall is elevated and attached to the free border of the palate. This results in partial closure of the nasopharynx. Breathing can take place through lateral openings left on either side of the pharyngeal flap.

Aston SJ, Beasley RW, Thorne CHM (eds): Grabb and Smith's Plastic Surgery, 5th ed, pp 267–268. Philadelphia, Lippincott–Raven, 1997

Gregory GA (ed): Pediatric Anesthesia, 3rd ed, pp 718–719. New York, Churchill Livingstone, 1994

C.10. How does a pharyngeal flap affect your anesthetic management or any subsequent anesthetic administered to this patient?

The presence of this flap prohibits nasoendotracheal intubation and makes many nasal techniques difficult (e.g., insertion of nasogastric tube). The degree of obstruction is related to the width of the flap. Traumatic rupture of this flap secondary to attempted nasotracheal intubation could produce bleeding, aspiration, and laryngospasm. Knowledge of prior surgery is essential to good anesthetic management. Following the push-back and pharyngeal flap operation (pharyngoplasty) significant airway obstruction has been noted in the early postoperative period. Sleeping pulse oximetry has demonstrated obstruction and desaturation in the first 48 to 72 hours.

Brown TCK, Fisk GC (eds): Anesthesia for Children, 3rd ed, p 254. Oxford, Blackwell Scientific Publications, 1992

C.11. What is an Abbe flap? What are its anesthetic consequences?

An Abbe flap is a full-thickness pedicle flap taken from the lower lip and swung on its own artery to a position in the upper lip to replace a tissue deficit resulting from any cause, such as surgical excision of malignancy or loss of tissue in a bilateral cleft lip. The lips must remain closed until the flap "takes," when it can be detached from its blood supply. Usually this operation is performed in children of an older age under local anesthesia, but it occasionally requires general anesthesia if the patient is young. All the problems of a closed mouth, such as the possibility of vomiting and aspirating, are encountered in addition to those associated with preservation of the flap.

Momma WG, Kobes W, Mai W: Indications for and results of the Abbe flap operation. Scand J Plast Reconstr Surg 8:142–147, 1974

C.12. What is the crucial problem of anesthesia for cleft palate? Enumerate the consequences of failure.

The establishment, maintenance, and protection of the airway comprise the crucial problem of anesthesia for palate surgery. Failure to establish, maintain, and protect the airway results in tachypnea, CO_2 retention, hypoxemia, increased bleeding, hypovolemia, arrhythmia, cardiac arrest, and death. The major cause of cardiac arrest in infants and children is hypoxia. The fear of retinopathy of prematurity (ROP) should not cloud judgment in the operating room. Hypoxemia is life threatening, hyperoxia is not. The pediatric anesthesiologist does not want to relearn this lesson in the operating room.

Collins V: Principles of Anesthesia, pp 1347, 1351. Philadelphia, Lea & Febiger, 1976

Coté CJ, Ryan JF, Todres ID et al (eds): A Practice of Anesthesia for Infants and Children, pp 116–117; 212; 225–241. Philadelphia, WB Saunders, 1993

Healy TJ, Cohen PJ (eds): Wylie and Churchill Davidson's A Practice of Anaesthesia, 6th ed, pp 306–311. London, Edward Arnold, 1995

D. Postoperative Management

D.1. What complications of cleft lip and cleft palate surgery may be seen in the recovery room?

Complications include airway obstruction, bleeding, and hypothermia. Airway obstruction is the result of closure of the cleft structures plus some edema secondary to trauma. In the case of the push-back procedure with or without a pharyngeal flap, the obstruction is due to the new posterior position of the palate and the pharyngeal flap. Blood loss is not an anesthetic complication but replacement is the anesthesiologist's responsibility, as is prevention of aspiration. Hypothermia delays emergence and produces metabolic acidosis and respiratory and myocardial depression. The most important problem for the anesthesiologist is maintenance of the airway.

Motoyama EK, Davis PS (eds): Smith's Anesthesia for Infants and Children, 6th ed, pp 599–601. St. Louis, CV Mosby, 1996

Stehling LC, Zauder HL (eds): Anesthetic Implications of Congenital Anomalies in Children, p 136. New York, Appleton-Century-Crofts, 1980

D.2. How do you protect the airway postoperatively?

Following palatoplasty, the pharynx and nasopharynx are suctioned prior to extubation. Some anesthesiologists advocate that this be done with the aid of the laryngoscope to ensure removal of any mucus, blood, or clots. If suctioning is done prior to removing the Dingman gag, the laryngoscope may not be necessary. The infant should be as awake as possible. A long traction suture is placed through the tongue and tied loosely. Traction on the suture stimulates respiration and clears the airway. Neither an oral nor nasal airway should be inserted; either one could disrupt the sutures and undo all the surgical work. The traction suture is removed when the infant leaves the recovery room.

Following palate surgery, the infant is placed in the prone or lateral position with the head dependent, turned to the side, and hyperextended. This position can be achieved with a jack placed under the foot of the crib or by placing a bulky bath blanket under the hips of the infant. Any blood or mucus will accumulate in the dependent cheek or roll out the mouth.

Following cleft lip surgery, a Logan bow is frequently used to take tension off the newly sutured lip. The infant can still be placed in the lateral position. Elbow restraints are essential, and they are placed on the infant or child before leaving the operating room. A high-humidity atmosphere is recommended postoperatively to reduce the incidence of postoperative tracheitis, but others have failed to show any correlation between the use of humidity and the incidence of tracheitis.

Aston SJ, Beasley RW, Thorne CHM (eds): Grabb and Smith's Plastic Surgery, 5th ed, p 247. Philadelphia, Lippincott–Raven, 1997

Koka B, Jeon IS, Andre JM et al: Postintubation croup in children. Anesth Analg 56:501, 1977

Motoyama EK, Davis PS (eds): Smith's Anesthesia for Infants and Children, 6th ed, pp 599–601. St. Louis, CV Mosby, 1996

46 Cervical Mass in Infancy

Miles Dinner

A 1-week-old male infant was brought to the operating room for resection of a large cervical mass. The infant was diagnosed shortly after birth with DiGeorge syndrome and had an interrupted aortic arch.

A. Medical Disease and Differential Diagnosis

1. What is DiGeorge syndrome?
2. What are the associated cardiovascular defects in DiGeorge syndrome?
3. What are the metabolic consequences of DiGeorge syndrome and the attendant manifestations?
4. What are the immunologic findings in DiGeorge syndrome?
5. What is the differential diagnosis of cervical masses in infancy?
6. What is a cystic hygroma? What are the complications? What is the treatment?
7. What is the interrupted aortic arch anomaly?
8. What is the pathophysiology of the interrupted aortic arch syndrome?
9. How is ductal patency maintained?
10. What are the side-effects of prostaglandin infusion?

B. Preoperative Evaluation and Preparation

1. What preoperative studies should be obtained to evaluate the neck mass?
2. What features of the difficult airway can be noted on physical examination?
3. How would you optimize preoperatively, the ability to secure the airway in the operating room?
4. What laboratory studies are necessary prior to surgery?
5. What are the causes of congestive heart failure (CHF) in the infant? How would you assess this infant on your preoperative evaluation for signs of CHF?
6. How would you optimize the preoperative treatment of congestive heart failure?
7. How would you premedicate this infant?
8. When is premedication useful in infants and children?
9. Prior to the planned surgery, the infant is scheduled for a magnetic resonance imaging (MRI) scan. You are asked to assure that the baby remains immobile for a period of 20 minutes to perform the scan adequately. How would you accomplish this?

C. Intraoperative Management

1. What anesthesia equipment, circuit, and monitors would you use?
2. Describe techniques other than direct laryngoscopy that would be useful for securing the airway in this baby?
3. How would you monitor blood loss in this patient?

4. What anesthetic technique should be used in a patient who may experience severe loss of blood intraoperatively?
5. How would you induce anesthesia in this infant?
6. Would you use nitrous oxide?
7. Intraoperatively, the surgeon needs to dissect the tumor in the anterior mediastinum and wishes to have a quiet surgical field. How would you accomplish this in the infant?

D. Postoperative Management

1. How would you manage this patient postoperatively?

A. Medical Disease and Differential Diagnosis

A.1. What is DiGeorge syndrome?

The DiGeorge anomaly is characterized by thymic and parathyroid aplasia or hypoplasia, cardiovascular defects, and dysmorphic facies. It arises as a consequence of a developmental defect in the embryology of the third and fourth pharyngeal pouches. It is currently thought to be caused by inadequate neural crest migration into the pharyngeal pouches with the subsequent limitation in growth of the derivative structures. The condition arises either from Mendelian disorders, teratogen exposure, or cytogenetic abnormalities.

Hong R: The DiGeorge anomaly. Immunodefic Rev 3(1):1–14, 1991

A.2. What are the associated cardiovascular defects in DiGeorge syndrome?

Most patients with the DiGeorge syndrome have associated anatomic cardiovascular anomalies involving the aortic arch system. Of these, the most common abnormality is an interrupted aortic arch seen in nearly half of the neonates with this condition. Persistent truncus arteriosus is seen in about one third and the remainder have tetralogy of Fallot or an isolated ventricular septal defect (VSD). These defects arise during the crucial developmental stages of the truncoconal parts of the heart from the pharyngeal pouch derivatives.

Van Mierop LH, Kutsche LM: Cardiovascular anomalies in DiGeorge syndrome and importance of neural crest as a possible pathogenetic factor. Am J Cardiol 58:133–137, 1986

A.3. What are the metabolic consequences of DiGeorge syndrome and the attendant manifestations?

Because of the inadequate development of the parathyroid glands, patients with DiGeorge syndrome fail to make parathyroid hormone or they are severely deficient in its production. Subsequently, hypocalcemia occurs. Hypocalcemia in the neonate is often difficult to detect clinically, but it can lead to irritability, jitteriness, twitching or frank seizure activity, failure to thrive, tachycardia, and hypotension.

A.4. What are the immunologic findings in DiGeorge syndrome?

Patients with DiGeorge syndrome demonstrate marked variability in the degree of involvement of the immune system. Total lymphocyte counts, percent of T cells, and T-lymphocyte function ranges from normal to severely depressed. The most consistent abnormality is a decrease in total T cells. Spontaneous resolution of immunodeficiency occurs in some patients, but progressive loss of function can be seen in others. Patients with the partial DiGeorge anomalad can be immunized and generate good antibody responses; therefore, humoral immunity is often intact.

Junker AK, Driscoll DA: Humoral immunity in DiGeorge syndrome. J Pediatr 127:231–237, 1986

A.5. What is the differential diagnosis of cervical masses in infancy?

Neck masses can originate from a congenital anatomic anomaly, neoplasm, or infection. In the first category are branchial cysts, thyroglossal duct cysts, and failed thymic descent. Branchial cysts arise in the embryo from the thymic stalk or the pharyngeal pouch. They may be present at birth or arise later. They lie beneath the sternomastoid muscle and may bulge out from the anterior border. They can become infected and thus enlarge with pus. When this occurs the airway or upper esophagus may be compressed.

Thyroglossal duct cysts are spherical, midline masses that may extend back to the base of the tongue and may represent all the thyroid tissue that the baby has. The thymus gland arises high in the neck and must descend in the embryo to the anterior mediastinum. If this caudad movement becomes arrested, the thymus can appear as a soft, compressible mass along the anterior border of the sternocleidomastoid muscle.

Neoplastic masses in the cervical region can be teratomas, hemangiomas, neurofibromas, lymphomas, goiters, or cystic hygromas. Teratomas are firm, midline masses arising adjacent to the thyroid isthmus. Hemangiomas may be extensive and compress vital structures. Neurofibromas may arise individually or as a consequence of neurofibromatosis (von Recklinghausen's syndrome), and they can be very large. A goiter represents an enlarged thyroid gland, which may be hypothyroid, hyperthyroid, or euthyroid.

Rudolph AM, Kamei RA: Rudolph's Fundamentals of Pediatrics, p 240. Norwalk, CT, Appleton & Lange, 1994

A.6. What is a cystic hygroma? What are the complications? What is the treatment?

Cystic hygroma is a developmental malformation of the lymphatic system that is found most often in the posterior triangle of the neck and axilla of children. They are divided into supra- and subhyoid masses. They are compressible masses that are most often found in infants aged <1 year, and they intermittently enlarge. Suprahyoid masses can be extremely difficult to manage due to the obstructive symptoms and feeding difficulties, and they may become infected, producing rapid compromise of breathing.

Complete surgical removal of these masses is often impossible and repeat debulking is sometimes the only treatment. Facial paresis may be a consequence of resection. The mortality of obstructing cystic hygroma diagnosed prenatally exceeds 20% following delivery. Intubation of the neonate during delivery under uninterrupted maternal-fetal circulation has been performed to prevent the fatal consequences of immediate postpartum airway obstruction. Bleomycin has also been used as a sclerosant agent with favorable results.

Orford J, Barker A, Thonell S et al: Bleomycin therapy for cystic hygroma. J Pediatr Surg 30: 1282–1287, 1995

Ricciardelli EJ, Richardson MA: Cervicofacial cystic hygroma. Patterns of recurrence and management of the difficult case. Arch Otolaryngol Head Neck Surg 117:546–553, 1991

Tanaka M, Sato S, Naito H et al: Anesthetic management of a neonate with prenatally diagnosed cervical tumour and upper airway obstruction. Can J Anaesth 41: 236–240, 1994

A.7. What is the interrupted aortic arch anomaly?

Interrupted aortic arch is a group of three anatomic abnormalities in which the aorta has a complete atresia at a site somewhere along the arch. In type A, which accounts for 43%, the aorta is interrupted between the left subclavian artery and the aortic isthmus. Type B, the most common (53%) has the lack of continuity between the left carotid and the left subclavian arteries. The defect in type C (4%) is between the right and left carotid arteries. A VSD is present in most patients with this anomaly.

Matsumoto M, Okamoto Y, Knoishi Y et al: Isolated interruption of the aortic arch. J Cardiovasc Surg 29:574–576, 1988

A.8. What is the pathophysiology of the interrupted aortic arch syndrome?

Because of the discontinuity between the descending aorta and the arch, no blood flow can go to the descending aorta unless a patent ductus arteriosus exists. If the ductus is inadequate to provide perfusion to the lower body due to its closure, severe metabolic acidosis and renal insufficiency develops. With a VSD, most of the cardiac output will be directed into the pulmonary vascular bed as the ductus closes. Unless ductal patency can be maintained, death will occur.

A.9. How is ductal patency maintained?

Ductal patency is maintained by the infusion of prostaglandin E_1. Both PGE_1 and PGE_2 are produced endogenously in the ductus, metabolized in the lungs, and achieve high levels in the fetus relative to adults. Postnatally, the levels fall associated with increased metabolism due to the increase in pulmonary blood flow. An infusion of prostaglandin will delay the natural closure of the ductus and improve systemic arterial oxygenation. In the case of an interrupted aortic arch, circulation to the lower body is totally dependent on the patency of the ductus and, therefore, continual infusion of PGE_1 is critical to keep the infant alive. The infusion is titrated at a rate of 0.05–0.1 µg/kg/min. Because of its relatively long half-life, discontinuation of the drip will not acutely cause ductal closure in the event of inadvertent stoppage.

Freed MD, Heymann MA, Lewis AB et al: Prostaglandin E_1 in infants with ductus arteriosus-dependent congenital heart disease. Circulation 64:889–905, 1981

A.10. What are the side-effects of prostaglandin infusion?

Prostaglandin infusion has a variety of side-effects ranging from fever to hypotension, seizures, flushing, and edema. Apnea is noted in premature infants and those <2 kg. Thus mechanical ventilation may be necessary in these babies.

Lake CL: Pediatric Cardiac Anesthesia, 2nd ed, p 332. Norwalk, CT, Appleton & Lange, 1993

B. Preoperative Evaluation and Preparation

B.1. What preoperative studies should be obtained to evaluate the neck mass?

Because of the extremely variable nature, invasiveness, and potential for airway compression, MRI studies and a sonogram should be obtained prior to surgery. These studies will better define the nature of the cystic hygroma and highlight the region of airway compression. These cysts are known to invade the anterior mediastinum and can thus cause extrinsic distortion of the lower airway anywhere from the cricoid ring to the carina. Cyst fluid can be aspirated under sonography to reduce the size of the mass and potentially relieve compressive symptoms.

On rare occasion, there may be in-growth of the pericardium and displacement of the lung. For suprahyoid masses, radiologic studies will define the scope of laryngeal compression and retropharyngeal involvement, which will obviously impact on the ability to intubate the trachea.

B.2. What features of the difficult airway can be noted on physical examination?

Many anatomic abnormalities can be discerned prior to direct laryngoscopy. Starting at the mouth and working caudally, we can examine a host of physical features that can challenge the clinician. Conditions that result in a constricted oral opening, such as scleroderma, epidermolysis bullosa, burn cicatrization, or congenital microstomia, prevent insertion of the laryngoscope. A small lower jaw and maxillary protrusion often accompany the anterior larynx, making laryngeal inlet exposure during laryngoscopy impossible. This is seen with Robin's, Apert's, Crouzon's, Treacher Collins, and many other craniofacial syndromes.

Macroglossia as a consequence of certain metabolic storage diseases, cystic abnormalities, and hamartomatous tumors of the tongue (Goltz syndrome) can make effective laryngoscopy impossible.

Temporomandibular ankylosis as seen in patients with juvenile rheumatoid arthritis and other rheumatic processes may prevent mouth opening. A narrow, high arched palate may suggest a problematic intubation. Neck extension problems may accompany some neuromuscular disorders, trauma, arthritis, or Goldenhar's syndrome.

Berry FA (ed): Anesthetic Management of Difficult and Routine Pediatric Patients, p 167. New York, Churchill Livingstone, 1986

B.3. How would you optimize preoperatively, the ability to secure the airway in the operating room?

Because of the risk inherent in inducing anesthesia in this infant, plan for a fiberoptic laryngoscopy. The infant bronchoscope is of such small diameter that it does not have a suction port and visualization is especially impaired because of secretions. An antisialogogue is a must to permit proper anatomic recognition through the fiberoptic scope. Glycopyrrolate (0.01 mg/kg) given one half hour prior to anesthesia will limit secretions without the excessive tachycardia which may occur with atropine. In this infant with cardiac compromise, any unnecessary stress on the heart should be avoided.

B.4. What laboratory studies are necessary prior to surgery?

Because of the strong association of DiGeorge syndrome with hypocalcemia, serum calcium should be measured. In addition, because of the inherent dsyphagia with a cystic hygroma, the infant will not have been feeding. To assure that adequate parenteral nutrition and hydration were provided, serum glucose and sodium levels should be noted. Because of the potential for severe metabolic acidosis secondary to underperfusion of the lower body through the interrupted descending aorta, a serum pH and bicarbonate concentrations must be obtained. A $PaCO_2$ will indicate the adequacy of ventilation in the face of a potentially obstructing mass and a baseline PaO_2 will serve as a guideline to the infant's degree of congestive heart failure, pulmonary insufficiency, and central shunting.

Because the surgery can be extensive with a significant loss of blood, a baseline complete blood count with hematocrit should be drawn. In addition, the prothrombin time (PT) and partial thromboplastin time (PTT) should be obtained prior to surgery of this magnitude because of the possibility of baseline immaturity in coagulation factor production and the inherent bleeding potential from the large dissection that will be done. Specific gravity of the urine will suggest the diagnosis of dehydration, although urinary concentrating ability does not mature until the infant is 3 months of age. A chest x-ray will define the state of the lungs and indicate whether there is tracheal deviation.

B.5. What are the causes of congestive heart failure (CHF) in the infant? How would you assess this infant on your preoperative evaluation for signs of CHF?

CHF occurs either in response to an excessive volume or pressure load or as a consequence of myocardial muscle impairment. Volume overload is due to factors causing a large increase in cardiac output (e.g., large VSD or ductus arteriosus). In these circumstances, there must be a sufficiently large enough left-to-right shunt to cause a severe strain on the heart. In the normal newborn, these lesions do not usually produce heart failure until 1 to 2 months of age because it takes longer than usual for the pulmonary vascular resistance (PVR) to fall. The elevated PVR protects the left ventricle from the stress of overcirculation. This is not true in premature infants who do not manifest the same degree of pulmonary arteriolar constriction. Thus they are susceptible to large left-to-right shunts early and show CHF more easily.

Regurgitant valvular lesions can lead to CHF. In complex congenital heart disease such as truncus arteriosus or tricuspid atresia with transposition, the additional stress of hypoxemia or univentricular overload may herald the early onset of CHF. Large arteriovenous malformations may occur intracranially and cause CHF. Excessive pressure loads are seen in obstruction to cardiac output from aortic stenosis, aortic coarctation, and aortic interruption. In the immediate newborn period, right-sided CHF is seen with greater frequency due to severe pulmonary hypertension. Pulmonary hypertension has many causes: intrinsic lung parenchymal insufficiency or pathology as in diaphragmatic hernia, meconium aspiration or hyaline membrane disease, chronic hypoxemia, hypervolemia, and polycythemia.

Primary myocardial failure is unusual in the newborn; it occurs with endocardial fibroelastosis or anomalous coronary circulation. However, the myocardium in the infant is susceptible to depression from metabolic derangements such as hypoglycemia, hypocalcemia, or birth asphyxia. Certainly severe anemia with the associated decrease in systemic and myocardial oxygen supply forces an increase in myocardial work which can lead to CHF.

Infants are different from adults in their manifestations of CHF. Because of possible coexisting lung disease in many premature infants, signs of cardiac dilation may be absent due to the decreased systemic venous return from elevated intrathoracic pressure. Although immature, the carotid baroreceptors still initiate an increase in sympathetic outflow in response to reduced perfusion. The increased alpha-adrenergic stimulation impairs blood flow to the systemic arteriolar beds, resulting in cold, underperfused extremities and diminished splanchnic perfusion. Fatigue, loss of appetite, and failure to thrive follow. Tachycardia from beta-receptor stimulation occurs. Generalized sweating results from sympathetic cholinergic fiber stimulation. Extracellular water increases due to decreased renal excretion of sodium from a lowered glomerular filtration rate. Peripheral pitting edema is much less common in infants than older children and adults. The venous system in infants is extremely distensible and thus raised right atrial pressure may not show large jugular venous engorgement. The most prominent manifestation of CHF in the infant is tachypnea. As pulmonary venous pressure is elevated from left ventricular failure, the lung compliance falls due to the augmented interstitial fluid. Breathing becomes rapid and shallow and the resultant increase in oxygen requirement causes a cyclic dependency to maintain both tachycardia and tachypnea. Subcostal retractions are seen due to the increase in respiratory effort.

Infants have a greater lymphatic drainage capacity than adults and thus can clear interstitial accumulations more readily. Therefore, rales are not as frequent a manifestation of CHF in infants as in adults. The bronchial mucosa may be swollen because of the engorgement of the bronchial venous system. The lumen of the airway is narrowed, resulting in wheezing that is often seen in infantile CHF. Hepatomegaly is a cardinal sign of right ventricular failure in infants.

Nadas A, Hauck A: Pediatric aspects of congestive heart failure. Anesth Analg 39:466–472, 1960

B.6. How would you optimize the preoperative treatment of congestive heart failure?

The typical manifestations of CHF in infants, namely tachycardia, tachypnea, subcostal retractions, and rhonchi, are also cardinal signs of pulmonary infection in this age group. They are hard to distinguish. Often, they coexist and treatment must address both conditions. Here the structural abnormality, namely the interrupted aortic arch, needs surgical correction which must be deferred until the neck mass is resected. In this infant, the congestive heart failure is caused by pressure overload from the interrupted aortic arch and the hypocalcemia is due to parathyroid hormone insufficiency. Calcium must be normalized by intravenous infusion. If glucose is low as would be expected in undernourishment, glycogen depletion from the stress of illness, or increased utilization, it should be supplemented by slow intravenous administration. Myocardial work is compromised by the presence of metabolic acidosis, which occurs as a consequence of the increased lactic acid production during anaerobic metabolism. The *p*H should be normalized with sodium bicarbonate. Because of the attendant sodium load, tromethamine (THAM) may be an alternative.

   Myocardial function should be optimized with digitalis in most infants with congestive heart failure. However, in the interrupted aortic arch syndrome, there may be decreased renal perfusion. As a consequence the digoxin levels may rise and toxicity may occur. Catecholamine (e.g., dopamine or dobutamine) should be infused to boost contractility. Pulmonary symptoms should be treated with antibiotics and positive pressure ventilation with oxygen carefully adjusted to arterial blood gas measurements. Intubation and mechanical ventilation may be necessary in many infants with CHF. Diuresis with furosemide will promote restoration of pulmonary compliance by decreasing lung water in conjunction with fluid restriction.

Kambam J: Cardiac Anesthesia for Infants and Children, pp 117–118. St. Louis, Mosby, 1994

B.7. How would you premedicate this infant?

Infants <2 years of age do not routinely require preoperative anxiolytics or narcotics. Premedicants such as midazolam have no place in this scenario. An infant with a compromised airway and circulation cannot tolerate any degree of respiratory depression. Therefore no sedatives should be given at all. As mentioned, because a fiberoptic intubation is planned, glycopyrrolate should be given for its antisecretory activity.

B.8. When is premedication useful in infants and children?

Patients with dynamically responsive cyanotic congenital heart disease (i.e., tetralogy of Fallot) benefit from premedication prior to coming to the operating room. In these children, the inherent anxiety of transfer to unfamiliar surroundings, change in temperature, and parental separation may trigger infundibular spasm and reduce pulmonary blood flow thus leading to a blue spell. Acute hypoxemia is not an optimal state in which to initiate an anesthetic induction. Thus sedation with oral midazolam or rectal pentobarbital is useful to allay the child's impending state of panic and reduce the risk of provoking a hypoxemic spell. Of course premedication is always helpful to make the overall experience of the operating room seem less imposing to the young child. In producing variable degrees of amnesia and reducing the potential for physical agitation, premedication offers a real benefit for those children who are intensely frightened of the operating room.

B.9. Prior to the planned surgery, the infant is scheduled for a magnetic resonance imaging (MRI) scan. You are asked to assure that the baby remains immobile for a period of 20 minutes to perform the scan adequately. How would you accomplish this?

Given this infant's extreme risk of complete airway occlusion, there is no safe method other than endotracheal intubation which will guarantee immobility on demand and assure a patent airway. The more routine method of sedating an infant for a MRI scan, namely chloral hydrate, oral midazolam, or a lytic cocktail such as the "DPT" (demerol, phenergan, thorazine) shot cannot be used here. Establishing an airway emergently in this infant may be impossible even with a laryngeal mask airway (LMA) and thus sedation can proceed only after the trachea is intubated. See question C.2 for details on fiberoptic intubation in infants.

C. Intraoperative Management

C.1. What anesthesia equipment, circuit, and monitors would you use?

Because of the depressed cellular immunity, this patient is susceptible to infection. Thus particularly strict attention must be paid to sterile technique during line placement and instrumentation of the patient. The anesthesiologist must wear gowns and gloves to protect the infant. Sterility of the disposable circle system, mask, endotracheal tube, fiberoptic bronchoscope, and laryngoscope should be assured. Routine monitors for all surgery on infants include a precordial stethoscope, rectal temperature probe, electrocardiogram, blood pressure, capnograph, and spirometer. Multiple pulse oximeters should be used to offer flexibility in the event of dysfunction. In this case the interrupted aortic arch prevents saturation data from the lower body and left arm. End-tidal expired gas concentrations should be recorded of anesthetic gases, nitrogen, and oxygen. Accurate capnography in small infants may be hampered by the side-arm gas sampling type due to the relatively high gas flows relative to the expired gas flow from the infant.

In this procedure an arterial line should be inserted in the right radial site, as the aortic arch interruption will not allow for pressure determination on the left side. Because of the potential for significant blood loss, a central line should be placed either through the femoral vein or subclavian vein if possible. Keep in mind the distorted anatomy and the potential for difficulty in cannulation with the subclavian site. If the subclavian site is elected, before proceeding with this complicated case, a chest x-ray should be obtained to document the absence of a pneumothorax and good line position. The femoral vein may be chosen as an alternate site. Catheter length is important, and it is easy in an infant to inadvertently place the central line across the tricuspid valve, in which case misleading values of the right ventricular pressure would be obtained. Remember in setting the transducer height that small variances in the alignment of the zero point can result in relatively large central venous pressure value (CVP) discrepancies. Therefore, the transducer should be placed with great care to approximate the right atrial level and be moved accordingly as the table height is changed.

The neuromuscular junction should be monitored with electrodes on a readily visible extremity.

C.2. Describe techniques other than direct laryngoscopy that would be useful for securing the airway in this baby?

It is highly unlikely that laryngeal visualization could be accomplished in this infant with direct visualization. On the computed tomography (CT) scan the mass is seen to elevate the tongue and deviate the larynx to the side. Because of this limitation in direct visualization, the clinician should be well acquainted with alternative methods before emergently instituting them. The following techniques can be useful when laryngoscopy cannot be accomplished easily.

Retrograde Cricothyroid Wire
Although technically difficult, the retrograde cricothyroid wire technique can be successful, and it is best for oral intubation. A guidewire is inserted through a large-gauge needle used to puncture the cricothyroid membrane and is threaded cephalad to be retrieved out the mouth. This wire then serves as a stent for placement of the endotracheal tube.

Blind Nasal Intubation

Although very successful in the adult patient, the blind nasal intubation technique
can be difficult in infants or small children. Certainly, performing an awake, sedated
intubation in this fashion mandates giving adequate topical anesthesia to a less than
cooperative infant. In addition, the smaller endotracheal tubes used in pediatrics are
far more compliant than others, especially when warmed with nasopharyngeal respiratory gases, which makes it difficult to maintain the anterior curve on the tube to
enter the larynx. Styleted nasal tubes should be used only by clinicians skilled in this
specialized technique.

Nasal Intubation with Laryngoscope and Magill Forceps

If the larynx cannot be visualized by laryngoscopy, an anesthetized spontaneously
breathing nasal intubation with laryngoscopic assistance can be carried out in some
patients. In this case, great care is taken to ensure that the patient maintains adequate
ventilatory exchange during the inhalational induction. Halothane or sevoflurane is
initiated, because either is less pungent and more easily tolerated than the halogenated ethers, and the anesthesiologist should be ever mindful that total obstruction is
possible in some of these infants because of their airway abnormalities. If spontaneous breathing can be maintained, the intubation should be attempted after a surgical plane of anesthesia is achieved. The laryngoscope is used to visualize the epiglottis, and the tip of the endotracheal tube is aligned with the help of a Magill forceps
and then advanced in the subepiglottic region. Capnographic monitoring during this
maneuver can help verify the direction of the endotracheal tube tip.

Fiberoptic Intubation

Fiberoptic intubation is most successful when carried out as the initial maneuver. It
may be impossible to use after several unsuccessful attempts with conventional laryngoscopy because the upper airway is then often traumatized and hypersecretory. Fiberoptic technology is still not widely disseminated to the infant population. Most
centers do not have the smallest, "ultrathin" bronchoscopes, which come as small as
2.2 mm in diameter. Limitations are found in their use because of the size and lack of
a suction port. The endotracheal tube requires good lubrication prior to threading
over the scope.

In older patients three specialized fiberoptic methods are available that may be
useful in intubating difficult infants. First, the clinician can pass a guidewire through
the suction port of the larger instrument to serve as a stylet for the endotracheal
tube. Second, the scope can be used to visualize and guide a nasal endotracheal tube
inserted into the opposite nostril. Finally, a 4.5 mm tube can be placed at the laryngeal orifice to be used as a stint for inserting a small guidewire which can in turn be
used to place a smaller endotracheal tube.

Another useful technique is the application of a laryngeal mask airway as a
guide for the endotracheal tube.

Of course, safety is the foremost consideration in any technique for inserting an
artificial airway. If the anesthesiologist cannot perform a cricothyrotomy, personnel
capable of an accurate and quick cricothyrotomy should be on hand in case of a life-
threatening loss of airway control. In an emergency cricothyrotomy, a longitudinal incision is made in the skin and fascia above the cricothyroid membrane, after which
the cricothyroid membrane is punctured and entered with a small endotracheal tube.
Another technique utilizes a 14 gauge angiocatheter, which is inserted into the cricothyroid membrane. Intratracheal location is verified by the loss of resistance with an

attached syringe and the aspiration of air. The catheter is attached to a 3 ml syringe (without plunger), which is then connected to the Y-piece of the anesthesia circuit by an adapter from a 7.0 mm internal diameter (ID) endotracheal tube.

Berry FA (ed): Anesthetic Management of Difficult and Routine Pediatric Patients, p. 137. New York, Churchill Livingstone, 1986

DeSoto H: The Child with A Difficult Airway, Recognition and Management. ASA Annual Refresher Course Lectures #236, 1996

C.3 How would you monitor blood loss in this patient?

In many of these procedures, blood loss can be significant, often exceeding the patient's calculated blood volume. Often much of this loss is not measurable because blood is either lost under the drapes or irrigated away. Certainly meticulous weighing of sponges and observation of suction canisters are important, but blood loss can be continuous from the time of skin incision and be seemingly relentless for an inexperienced clinician. Absolute changes in the CVP are a relative guide to the volume in the central compartment, but no one isolated value correlates with a known blood volume. A falling CVP in association with a downward trend in blood pressure during periods of surgical intervention known to produce significant bleeding should be treated aggressively with brisk transfusion. If blood loss is allowed to continue, severe hypotension can rapidly ensue.

C.4. What anesthetic technique should be used in a patient who may experience severe loss of blood intraoperatively?

Blood loss should be replaced milliliter for milliliter to prevent falling behind in volume. It is wise to choose an anesthetic technique that produces a relatively stable blood pressure throughout the surgery so that new downward trends in blood pressure can be attributable to blood loss and not to pharmacologic action. For instance, if a steady level of forane and nitrous oxide anesthesia is given at 1.25 minimal alveolar concentration (MAC) with a resultant mean arterial pressure (MAP) 15% lower than awake, further dips in MAP during surgical intervention can be taken as intravascular volume depletion secondary to bleeding and replaced accordingly. This interpretation would be obscured if there were frequent anesthetic interventions associated with MAP changes (e.g., intermittent narcotization, pancuronium bolusing, droperidol or other alpha-blockade administration) or up and down titration of hypotension-inducing agents.

An important clue to the blood volume loss of the patient is the blood pressure at a MAC of anesthesia. If a stable pressure is established at a given MAC of inhalational agent, a lower than expected blood pressure at this MAC is almost always indicative of hypovolemia and thus calls for fluid or blood replacement. Frequent hematocrit determinations drawn with the arterial blood gases are important. Remember it is most unusual in an otherwise healthy infant to produce hypotension with intravascular overload.

C.5 How would you induce anesthesia in this infant?

After securing the airway with fiberoptic intubation or awake tracheotomy and checking for bilateral breath sounds, narcotic titration with fentanyl should be given in repeated doses of 2 μg/kg. Remember, this infant may behave quite sensitively to any anesthetic agent due to the cardiovascular anomalies. Thus, beat-to-beat monitoring of the blood pressure with an arterial line as the fentanyl is administered ensures inadvertent drops in pressure. As this patient is not going to be extubated, fentanyl can be given in the range of 50 μg/kg or higher to allow for dense analgesia. Because this will be a long procedure, pancuronium can be administered slowly to mitigate against the tachycardia. If tolerated, small concentrations of about 0.5% to 2% desflurane can be administered to synergize with the narcotic and assist with amnesia and unconsciousness. The prostaglandin infusion should be maintained throughout the entire surgery.

C.6 Would you use nitrous oxide?

The adult experience suggests that nitrous oxide may have augmenting effects on PVR, especially in patients with already elevated PVR. It may also decrease cardiac index in conjunction with narcotics. In infants, however, little consequence is seen in administering nitrous oxide unless there is a profound myocardial disturbance. It is avoided by some anesthesiologists because of the potential of expanding intravascular air bubbles.

Kambam J: Cardiac Anesthesia for Infants and Children, p 130. St. Louis, Mosby, 1994

C.7. Intraoperatively, the surgeon needs to dissect the tumor in the anterior mediastinum and wishes to have a quiet surgical field. How would you accomplish this in the infant?

Double lumen tubes are not used in the neonatal age group because of the exceedingly small lumen and the technical difficulties of securing both lungs. Instead a single lumen endotracheal tube can be advanced to the right or left main stem bronchus to allow for one-lung ventilation. This may be fraught with consequences in this infant with interrupted aortic arch, but it can still be attempted. Keep in mind that hypoxic pulmonary vasoconstriction may not occur readily in the neonate and excessive shunting may be in evidence. In addition, having an infant on one-lung ventilation may lead to an elevated $PaCO_2$ from pulmonary insufficiency. During thoracotomies in infants for pulmonary banding or Blalock-Taussig shunts it is not uncommon to see extremely elevated $PaCO_2$ values from retraction of the lung, especially the right side, which has almost 60% of the total lung surface area.

D. Postoperative Management

D.1. How would you manage this patient postoperatively?

This procedure, involving extensive dissection around the neck and upper thorax, warrants that the patient stay intubated or have a tracheostomy placed. A tremendous amount of upper airway and neck edema will surely ensue, which would make extubation life-threatening. To facilitate care over the next day, the patient should be well narcotized and paralyzed if necessary to coordinate effective mechanical ventilation. Artificial ventilation and oxygen supplementation should be titrated to arterial blood gas determinations. In addition, the prostaglandin drip must be continued to assure ductal patency. Generous narcotic supplementation will ensure that the pulmonary vascular resistance stays in a state of relative quiescence. If an endotracheal tube is maintained, fiberoptic visualization of the laryngeal inlet after 24 hours will enable a more educated decision to the suitability of extubation. Anatomic airway factors aside, the interrupted aortic arch and associated congestive heart failure will make extubation of this baby more challenging. Assuming all other factors are under control, the following ventilatory parameters should be met prior to extubation: normal arterial blood gases with satisfactory oxygenation on 28% O_2, spontaneous tidal volume >5 ml/kg, and inspiratory force >12 cm H_2O. One should always be on the alert for airway obstruction and ready to intercede with reintubation or tracheostomy if prompt deterioration occurs.

Airway Trauma

47

Alexander W. Gotta
Colleen A. Sullivan
Rita Donovan

A 20-year-old man was attacked. His face was beaten with a blunt weapon and he was shot in the chest with a handgun. He was unable to open his mouth and had bruises on the anterior part of his neck. He appeared intoxicated and confused, and admitted to the use of cocaine.

A. Medical Disease and Differential Diagnosis

1. Are handguns protective?
2. How would you evaluate the patient's mental status?
3. What other significant trauma might be present?
4. How would you evaluate the airway?
5. Why could the patient not open his mouth?
6. What are the common points of fracture in the mandible?
7. What is the significance of a bimandibular fracture?
8. How can the airway be restored in the presence of a bimandibular fracture?
9. What are LeFort I, II, and III fractures?
10. When should one suspect a basal skull fracture in association with a fractured mandible?
11. What are the signs and symptoms of airway penetration?
12. What immediate treatment is necessary?

B. Preoperative Evaluation and Preparation

1. What laboratory tests would you want?
2. What x-ray studies would you want?
3. Could injury to the cervical spine be determined definitely?
4. Was an electrocardiogram (ECG) necessary?
5. Should a nasogastric tube be placed to empty the stomach?
6. Would you premedicate this patient?

C. Intraoperative Management

1. What monitors would you use? Was invasive monitoring necessary? Was the patient's temperature important?
2. How would you secure the airway?
3. How would you perform superior laryngeal and translaryngeal nerve blocks?
4. Was a double lumen tube necessary?
5. Was fiberoptic intubation necessary?
6. What problems might arise during ventilation and intubation?

853

7. If the patient could not be ventilated, what options are available?
8. How would you secure the airway after a penetrating injury to the airway?
9. What are the indications for tracheostomy in patients with upper airway trauma?
10. What are the complications of cricothyrotomy?
11. Would you use the laryngeal mask airway in this patient?
12. How would you induce anesthesia?
13. What maintenance anesthetics were indicated or contraindicated in this patient?

D. Postoperative Management

1. What are the criteria for extubation?
2. What techniques might be used during extubation?
3. How does alcohol abuse and use of illicit drugs affect postoperative management?
4. What pain medication would you use?

A. Medical Disease and Differential Diagnosis

A.1. Are handguns protective?

In the United States trauma is the leading cause of death among young people, and each year it accounts for the waste of thousands of potentially productive years of life. The rate of homicide in the United States exceeds that of all other developed countries and is exceeded only by rates in developing areas. Guns in the household are not protective, but rather increase the risk for violent death.

Kassirer JP: Guns in the household. N Engl J Med 329:1117–1119, 1993

Kellerman AL, Rivara FP, Rushforth NB et al: Gun ownership as a risk factor for homicide in the home. N Engl J Med 329:1084–1091, 1993

Kellerman AL, Rivara FP, Somes G et al: Suicide in the home in relation to gun ownership. N Engl J Med 327:467–472, 1992

A.2. How would you evaluate the patient's mental status?

The patient's mental status may be altered by his injury and by his drug and alcohol use. Questions should be directed to determine the patient's orientation of time, place, and person. Inquiry should be made to the time of food and alcohol ingestion and latest drug use. He should be asked to specify the drugs he commonly uses. Does he remember the attack? Failure to remember is indicative of amnesia and may point to intracranial injury.

A.3. What other significant trauma might be present?

Injuries to the face are associated with fracture or dislocation of the cervical spine in 1% to 6% of patients. Significant intracranial injury has been reported in up to 15% of patients. The obvious distortion of the face should not distract the physician from searching for potentially life-threatening injuries within the abdomen or chest. The abdomen must be palpated. A ruptured spleen or liver with resulting hemorrhage may present a greater threat than the facial injury. Chest and heart auscultation is essential. Hypotension and muffled heart sounds should lead one to suspect cardiac tamponade. A careful neurologic examination must be performed to aid in determining if the spinal cord is intact.

Haug RH, Wible RT, Likavec MJ et al: Cervical spine fractures and maxillofacial trauma. J Oral Maxillofac Surg 49:725–729, 1991

A.4. How would you evaluate the airway?

If endotracheal intubation is to be accomplished under direct vision the patient must be able to open his mouth and extend his tongue beyond the incisors. Can he extend, rotate, and flex his head voluntarily? Forced movements are contraindicated because of the possibility of cervical spine injury. With extension of the head, the distance between the hyoid bone and the mentum should accommodate at least three finger breadths. The mouth must be examined for loose teeth and an edematous, obstructing tongue. Auscultation of the larynx may reveal stridor. The nasal passages must be evaluated for fracture and patency. If nasotracheal intubation is chosen it must be remembered that the posterior nares vary in size. It is useful to close each nostril serially and use the force of expiration through each nostril as an index of patency.

Gotta AW: Management of the traumatized airway. ASA Refresher Course in Anesthesiology 23: 103–115, 1995

A.5. Why could the patient not open his mouth?

Motion of the jaw may be limited by any one or more of several factors (Table 47-1). Trismus is spasm of the masseter muscles binding the jaw closed. Trismus will respond to an anesthetic and muscle relaxant unless it has been present for 2 weeks or longer. Pain, which is the most common cause of immobility of the jaw, will be relieved by an anesthetic. However, mechanical disruption of the jaw can cause unyielding immobility. A fracture of the condyle in its articulation within the temporomandibular joint may interfere with normal function of the joint.

A fracture of the zygomatic arch of the temporal bone always limits jaw motion, and it also limits the anesthesiologist's ability to intubate the patient. It is difficult to fracture the zygomatic arch, which is protected by the temporal fascia. It splits into lateral and medial sheets enveloping the bone. A blow from above and from the side may rupture the fascia and break the bone, driving fractured segments onto the coronoid process of the mandible. The mandible has two motions: a hingelike action on an axis passing through the condyles and an anterior-posterior motion (translation). Translation is limited by the fracture fragments impinging on the coronoid, and the mouth will not open completely. The anesthesiologist may be deceived when perceiv-

Table 47-1. Factors Limiting Mobility of the Jaw After Trauma

Trismus
Edema
Pain
Mechanical Disruption
   fracture of the condyle
   fracture of the zygomatic arch of the temporal bone
   fracture of the zygoma

ing motion in the jaw, not realizing that further opening may not occur after the administration of an anesthetic and muscle relaxant. A fracture of the zygoma may also impinge on the coronoid and limit translation.

Bermejo A, Gonzalez O, Gonzalez JM: The pig as an animal model for experimentation on the temporomandibular articular complex. Oral Surg Oral Med Oral Pathol Oral Radiol 75:19–23, 1993

Mathog RH: Atlas of Craniofacial Trauma, p 263. Philadelphia, WB Saunders, 1992

Rees LA: The structure and function of the mandibular joint. Br Dent J 96:125–133, 1954

A.6. What are the common points of fracture in the mandible?

Because the mandible is a tubular bone, it derives its strength from the cortex. It will be strongest and least vulnerable to fracture where the cortex is thickest (i.e. at the anteroinferior border). The cortex at the posterior of the mandible, near the angle, is considerably thinner. With high speed, high impact injuries, such as result from an automobile crash, the most common points of fracture are the ramus, condyle, and angle of the mandible. With low speed, low impact injuries, such as those occurring with the blow from a fist, or a fall, most fractures will occur within the body of the mandible, symphysis, and parasymphyseal region. The different sites of fracture location are probably due to the kinetics of applied forces but also to the fact that a low impact blow to the face is usually anticipated, allowing the victim to turn the face away and take the impact on the lateral side of the body of the mandible.

Halazonetis JA: The ''weak'' regions of the mandible. Br J Oral Surg 6:37–48, 1968

Huelke DF: Mechanics in the production of mandibular fractures: A study of the ''stresscoat'' technique. I. Symphyseal impacts. J Dent Res 40:1042–1056, 1961

Huelke DF, Patrick LM: Mechanics in the production of mandibular fractures: Strain-gauge measurements of impacts to the chin. J Dent Res 43:437–446, 1964

Nahum AM: The biomechanics of facial bone fracture. Laryngoscope 85:140–156, 1975

Rowe NL, Williams JL (eds): Maxillo Facial Injuries, pp 3–4. Edinburgh, Churchill Livingstone, 1985

A.7. What is the significance of a bimandibular fracture?

One of the common points of fracture within the mandible is in the body at the level of the first or second molar. A fracture at this point on both sides of the mandible can lead to distraction of the anterior fracture segment and posteroinferior displacement of the segment, taking with it the tongue and associated soft tissues. Impaction into the upper airway can cause partial or complete closure of the airway and an airway management emergency. This fracture causes a characteristic foreshortening of the mandible, and it is sometimes called an ''Andy Gump'' fracture after a comic strip character popular many years ago.

Seshul MB, Sinn DP, Gerlock AJ: The Andy Gump fracture of the mandible: A cause of respiratory obstruction or distress. J Trauma 18:611–612, 1978

A.8. How can the airway be restored in the presence of a bimandibular fracture?

If the airway is stable, and the patient has no respiratory distress, it may be possible to intubate him either awake or after anesthesia has been induced. If the soft tissue impaction into the upper airway, together with developing edema, blood, and secretions threaten the patient's ability to breathe, he may require tracheostomy or cricothyrotomy emergently. In a truly emergent situation the anesthesiologist should grasp the mandible in the midline and gently, but forcefully, draw it forward, reducing the fracture and disimpacting the soft tissue lodged in the oropharynx.

Gotta AW: Management of the traumatized airway. ASA Refresher Course in Anesthesiology 23: 103–115, 1995

A.9. What are LeFort I, II, and III fractures?

The LeFort I fracture is also known as Guérin or transverse maxillary fracture. It is a dental-alveolar fracture of the maxilla, passing above the floor of the nose, involving the lower third of the nasal septum, and mobilizing the palate, maxillary alveolar process, the lower third of the pterygoid plates, and part of the palatine bone. The fracture segment can be displaced posteriorly or laterally, rotated about an axis, or any such combination. Little airway compromise is seen, and the patient may be intubated orally or nasally, usually without great difficulty (Fig. 47-1).

Also known as pyramidal fracture of the maxilla, the LeFort II fracture involves the thick upper part of the nasal bone and the thinner portion forming the upper margin of the anterior nasal aperture. The fracture crosses the medial wall of the orbit, including the lacrimal bone, runs beneath the zygomaticomaxillary suture, crossing the lateral wall of the antrum, and then continues posteriorly through the pterygoid plates. The segment can be displaced posteriorly or rotated about an axis. Nasotracheal intubation is relatively contraindicated because of the presence of a fractured nose (see Fig. 47-1).

A LeFort III fracture is also called craniofacial disjunction. The line of fracture runs parallel to the base of the skull, separating the midfacial skeleton from the cranial base. The zygomatic arch of the temporal bone is fractured. The fracture line extends through the base of the nose and the ethmoid bone in its depth. The cribriform plate of the ethmoid may be fractured, thus disrupting the integrity of the base of the skull and opening into the subarachnoid space. The midface is separated from the

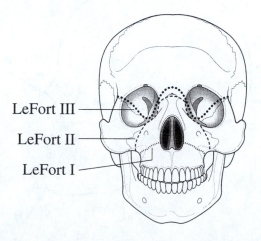

Figure 47-1. The usual lines of LeFort fractures of the midface. (Reprinted with permission from Gotta AW: Management of the traumatized airway, ASA Refresher Course in Anesthesiology 23:103–115, 1995)

LeFort III

LeFort II

LeFort I

cranial skeleton; it is usually distracted posteriorly, creating the characteristic "dish face deformity." Awake tracheostomy is usually used to secure the airway, thus obviating the risks associated with possible fracture of the base of the skull, and leaving the operative field to the surgeon (see Fig. 47-1).

LeFort R: Etude experimentale sur les fractures de la machoire supérieure. Rev Chir 23:208–227; 360–379; 479–507, 1901

A.10. When should one suspect a basal skull fracture in association with a fractured mandible?

The craniofacial skeleton is actually two skeletons approximated to each other (i.e., the cranial skeleton and the facial skeleton). To protect one skeleton against trauma committed on the other a series of bony buttresses is built into the craniofacial configuration, and several arches serve to disperse applied forces, thus creating a normal vector of force dispersion and redistribution. A blow to the mandible along the normal vector can fracture the mandible at the point of impact or elsewhere, but it will not extend into the skull. A blow to the midface, however, tends to create an abnormal shearing force, which can tear the facial skeleton from the cranial skeleton and extend the fracture line into the base of the skull. Basal skull fracture should always be considered a possibility in the presence of severe midfacial trauma (Fig. 47-2).

Haug RH, Adams JM, Conforti PJ et al: Cranial fractures associated with facial fractures: A review of mechanism, type and severity of injury. J Oral Maxillofac Surg 52:729–735, 1994

A.11. What are the signs and symptoms of airway penetration?

The signs and symptoms of airway penetrance are indicative of entry into an air transport system that is highly vascular. They include hemoptysis, stridor, hoarseness, and subcutaneous and/or mediastinal emphysema (Table 47-2).

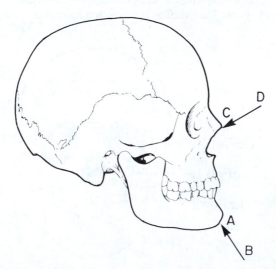

Figure 47-2. The normal vectors of force dispersion of facial trauma. A blow along the line *(A-B)* follows a normal vector of force dispersion. The force may be sufficient to fracture the mandible at the point of impact or elsewhere, but it will not extend the fracture into the base of the skull. A blow along the line *(C-D)* creates an abnormal shearing force tending to tear the facial skeleton from the cranial skeleton and extending the fracture line into the base of the skull. (Reprinted with permission from Gotta AW: Management of the traumatized airway. ASA Refresher Course in Anesthesiology 23:103–115, 1995)

Table 47-2.   Signs and Symptoms of Airway Penetrance

Hemoptysis
Stridor
Hoarseness
Emphysema
   subcutaneous
   mediastinal

A.12. What immediate treatment is necessary?

Oxygen should be administered via face mask or nasal prongs. If the patient has a pneumothorax or a hemothorax, a chest tube must be placed. Intravenous infusion must be started using large bore ($\geq$16 gauge) catheters and crystalloid solution infused.

B.   Preoperative Evaluation and Preparation

B.1. What laboratory tests would you want?

Hemoglobin or hematocrit is an imprecise but rough index of blood loss; changes may be followed in the perioperative period. A drug screen to include alcohol is useful for perioperative management. Urinalysis may indicate renal damage. Blood should be sent for typing and screening. Laboratory tests should never delay instituting necessary therapy.

B.2. What x-ray studies would you want?

Radiographs of the facial bones and chest are necessary. Computed tomography (CT) of the skull, especially of the base of the skull is indicated, as are x-rays of the cervical spine. It may be necessary to obtain a CT of the cervical spine if the plain films are inconclusive.

B.3. Could injury to the cervical spine be determined definitely?

Radiographs of the cervical spine may not reveal damage to C1 to C2 or C7; clinical correlation is essential. CT may be of value in establishing the diagnosis.

B.4. Was an electrocardiogram (ECG) necessary?

Although usually of little value in a young person, ECG is indicated when there is chest trauma to aid in diagnosing myocardial damage.

B.5. Should a nasogastric tube be placed to empty the stomach?

The presence of a full stomach, coupled with a compromised airway, increases the risk of vomiting and aspiration. However, passing a nasogastric tube is hazardous if basal skull fracture is present. Placing a nasogastric tube does not guarantee an empty stomach because the tube cannot remove large solid particles, and it may act as a wick, facilitating aspiration.

Seebacher J, Rozik D, Mathieu A: Inadvertent intracranial introduction of a nasogastric tube, a complication of severe maxillofacial trauma. Anesthesiology 42:100–102, 1975

B.6. Would you premedicate this patient?

If awake intubation is planned in a hemodynamically stable patient, small intravenous incremental doses of midazolam (0.25 mg, up to 4 to 5 mg) may be used to sedate the patient. Careful monitoring is essential, because midazolam, even in small doses, may unmask hypovolemia.

C. Intraoperative Management

C.1. What monitors would you use? Was invasive monitoring necessary? Was the patient's temperature important?

Blood pressure, electrocardiography, capnography, and pulse oximetry should be employed as with any patient. A Foley catheter should be inserted. Measurement of urine output is indicative of renal and other organ perfusion.

An arterial line is useful for moment-to-moment measurement of blood pressure, and in determining blood gases and the adequacy of ventilation. More invasive monitoring, via pulmonary artery catheter or a central venous pressure catheter, is necessary only in the presence of hemodynamic instability.

Cooling is a natural and important process in the traumatized patient and even mild hypothermia can lead to coagulopathy, cardiac arrhythmias, cardiac arrest, delayed metabolism of many drugs, and delayed awakening from anesthesia. Normothermia should be maintained using warming devices such as the Bair warmer and fluid warmers, and inspired gas humidifiers. It may be useful to increase the temperature in the operating room.

Karlin A: Hemodynamic monitoring of trauma patients during anesthesia. Anesthesiol Clin North Am 14(1):85–99, 1996

Schmied H, Kurz A, Sessler DI et al: Mild hypothermia increases blood loss and transfusion requirements during total hip arthroplasty. Lancet 347:289–292, 1996

C.2. How would you secure the airway?

If the jaw immobility was caused only by trismus or pain, intubation might be effected in the usual manner with intravenous induction and muscle relaxant. However, if awake intubation was indicated it might be necessary to anesthetize the airway using bilateral superior laryngeal nerve blocks and transtracheal installation of local anesthetic. Fracture of the base of the skull contraindicates nasotracheal intubation because of the possibility of introducing the nasotracheal tube, foreign material, or air into the skull.

Seebacher J, Rozik D, Mathieu A: Inadvertent intracranial introduction of a nasogastric tube, a complication of severe maxillofacial trauma. Anesthesiology 42:100–102, 1975

C.3. How would you perform superior laryngeal and translaryngeal nerve blocks?

Superior laryngeal nerve block: with the patient lying supine, a 22 gauge needle attached to a syringe containing 2 ml of 2% lidocaine is directed at the most posterior palpable part of the hyoid bone, near the greater cornu, and anterior to the carotid sheath. The needle must be parallel to the table, and never directed posteriorly for fear of penetrating the carotid sheath. When the needle strikes the hyoid, it is carefully walked caudad until it just slips off the hyoid, and then advanced a short distance through the hyothyroid membrane. Aspiration should produce nothing. The 2 ml of lidocaine is injected, and the block repeated on the opposite side.

Translaryngeal nerve block: a 22 gauge needle, attached to a syringe containing 4 ml of 2% to 4% lidocaine is thrust through the cricothyroid membrane in the midline and air freely aspirated. The patient is asked to inhale deeply, and then to exhale fully. At the end of expiration the lidocaine is injected rapidly and the needle quickly removed. The resultant coughing will ensure a wide distribution of local anesthetic droplets throughout the airway.

Gotta AW: Management of the traumatized airway. ASA Refresher Course in Anesthesiology 23: 103–115, 1995

Gotta AW, Sullivan CA: Anaesthesia of the upper airway using topical anaesthetic and laryngeal nerve block. Br J Anaesth 53:1055–1058, 1981

Gotta AW, Sullivan CA: Superior laryngeal nerve block: An aid to intubating the patient with fractured mandible. J Trauma 24:83–85, 1984

C.4. Was a double lumen tube necessary?

A double lumen tube is useful in isolating the wounded lung. If only one side of the thorax is injured the double lumen tube may isolate this side and allow for adequate ventilation of the uninjured side. If both sides are injured it may be possible to ventilate the least injured side while the other is repaired, and then to switch the ventilated side from one to the other. However, if nasal intubation is necessary, the double lumen tube is of no value because its large size would not allow passage through the posterior nares.

C.5. Was fiberoptic intubation necessary?

Fiberoptic intubation might be a useful option when the larynx could not be adequately visualized because of the traumatized face. However, fiberoptic intubation is often of little value in the presence of anatomic distortion, hemorrhage, and edema.

C.6. What problems might arise during ventilation and intubation?

In the presence of a basal skull fracture manual ventilation via bag and mask may force air or foreign material into the skull, increasing intracranial pressure (ICP) and risking meningitis. Passing a nasotracheal tube risks mechanical damage to the intracranial contents.

Dacosta A, Billard J, Gery P et al: Posttraumatic intracerebral pneumatocele after ventilation with a mask: Case report. J Trauma 36:255–257, 1994

Kitahata LM, Collins WF: Meningitis as a complication of anesthesia in a patient with basal skull fracture. Anesthesiology 32:282–283, 1970

C.7. If the patient could not be ventilated what options are available?

Cricothyrotomy is the most expedient method of gaining access to the airway. This procedure can be accomplished by surgical opening of the cricothyroid membrane and placing an endotracheal tube into the trachea. An alternate technique involves placing a 14 gauge catheter over a needle through the cricothyroid membrane, removing the needle, and using the catheter for jet ventilation.

Benumof JL, Scheller MS: The importance of transtracheal jet ventilation in the management of the difficult airway. Anesthesiology 71:769–778, 1989

C.8. How would you secure the airway after a penetrating injury to the airway?

If the larynx or cervical trachea had been penetrated, a long uncut endotracheal tube should be positioned so that the tube cuff is below the penetrance site. The airway would thus be protected and the surgeon might repair the disruption without interfering with ventilation. Because of the rich blood supply in the neck and the enveloping layers of the cervical fascia, injuries to the neck carry the risk of bleeding into a confined space, with consequent increases in volume and pressure. The larynx may be angulated on the trachea, and the trachea itself may be deviated and compressed. It is possible for the airway to close completely within as little as 15 minutes. Early intubation is preferable. Laryngeal injuries are usually best treated with tracheostomy as opposed to fiberoptic intubation.

C.9. What are the indications for tracheostomy in patients with upper airway trauma?

The indications for tracheostomy are:

- Inability to intubate
- Unrelieved airway obstruction
- Basal skull fracture if orotracheal intubation is impossible or unacceptable
  - LeFort III most usual
  - Cerebrospinal fluid rhinorrhea, an absolute contraindication to nasotracheal intubation
  - Associated mandibular trauma requiring internal fixation
- Severe nasal fracture if orotracheal intubation is impossible or unacceptable

Gotta AW: Management of the traumatized airway. ASA Refresher Courses in Anesthesiology 23: 103–115, 1995

C.10. What are the complications of cricothyrotomy?

If the endotracheal tube or laryngeal jet ventilation catheter is not properly placed within the larynx and trachea, attempts at ventilation will produce subcutaneous emphysema, which may extend through the fascial planes of the neck and thorax and become mediastinal emphysema and pneumothorax.

Gotta AW: Management of the traumatized airway. ASA Refresher Courses in Anesthesiology 23: 103–115, 1995

C.11. Would you use the laryngeal mask airway in this patient?

The laryngeal mask airway (LMA) has little role to play in the management of the traumatized airway. It will not protect against aspiration of vomitus and does not offer the security of a properly placed endotracheal tube. However, if the upper airway is severely compromised and endotracheal intubation is impossible and ventilation is inadequate, the LMA may prove to be a life-saving expedient technique of last resource.

Maltby JR, Loken RG, Watson NC: The laryngeal mask airway: Clinical appraisal in 250 patients. Can J Anaesth 37:509–513, 1990

Roberts JT (ed): Clinical Management of the Airway, pp 219–227, Philadelphia, WB Saunders, 1994

C.12. How would you induce anesthesia?

If the patient were hemodynamically stable, anesthesia might be induced with a barbiturate such as thiopental. With hemodynamic instability etomidate is preferred. Ketamine is contraindicated in cases of head injury because it increases ICP and causes focal alterations in cerebral metabolism. Evidence of a protective effect of ketamine is controversial. No evidence indicates that ketamine is useful in maintaining blood pressure in the traumatized patient.

Gardner AE, Olson BE, Lichtiger M: Cerebrospinal-fluid pressure during dissociative anesthesia with ketamine. Anesthesiology 35:226–228, 1971

Hoffman WE, Pelligrino D, Werner C et al: Ketamine decreases plasma catecholamines and improves outcome from incomplete cerebral ischemia in rats. Anesthesiology 76:755–762, 1992

Takeshita H, Okuda Y, Sari A: The effects of ketamine on cerebral circulation and metabolism in man. Anesthesiology 36:69–75, 1972

Zsigman EK, Matsuki A, Kothafy SP: Arterial hypoxemia caused by intravenous ketamine. Anesth Analg 55:311–314, 1976

C.13. What maintenance anesthetics are indicated or contraindicated in this patient?

Nitrous oxide is contraindicated in the presence of pneumothorax or intracranial injury. Inhalation anesthetics increase ICP, but this adverse effect can be moderated by hyperventilation. Narcotics are useful, especially in the narcotic addict, and they may delay the withdrawal phenomenon. During airway surgery halothane is contraindicated because of its ability to cause abnormal conduction and ventricular arrhythmias. Any muscle relaxant can be used, but pancuronium often causes tachycardia which may limit the clinician's ability to evaluate anesthetic depth and hemodynamic stability.

Gotta AW, Sullivan CA, Pelkofski J et al: Aberrant conduction as a precursor to cardiac arrhythmias during anesthesia for oral surgery. J Oral Surg 34:421–427, 1976

D. Postoperative Management

D.1. What are the criteria for extubation?

The patient must have complete return of neuromuscular function as determined by a nerve stimulator. He should be able to lift his head and keep it elevated for at least 5 seconds. Negative airway pressure of 20 cm H_2O is a useful indicator of adequate respiratory ability. The patient should follow simple commands such as opening his eyes. Significant edema may occur with airway trauma and surgery, making immediate postoperative extubation inappropriate. The endotracheal tube must be maintained in place and secured until edema has subsided. Although it may be impossible to visualize the interior of the airway, external edema is indicative of internal edema. A particularly useful sign is an edematous tongue that extends beyond the incisors. In the presence of this sign the patient must not be extubated.

Barash PG, Cullen BF, Stoelting RK (eds): Clinical Anesthesia, 3rd ed, pp 929–943. Philadelphia, Lippincott-Raven, 1997

Kirby RR, Gravenstein N (eds): Clinical Anesthesia Practice, pp 1268–1282. Philadelphia, WB Saunders, 1994

D.2. What techniques might be used during extubation?

After airway trauma the airway is in jeopardy immediately after extubation because edema may compromise the patient's ability to breathe. It is useful to place a ventilating tube changer through the endotracheal tube as it is removed. A fiberoptic bronchoscope may also be placed through a nasotracheal tube and the tube removed over it, ready for immediate replacement. It is imprudent to use narcotics to blunt airway reflexes at the time of extubation because of the respiratory depressant effects of this class of drugs. However, 3 to 4 ml of 2% lidocaine may be directly injected into the endotracheal tube prior to its removal, thus providing partial anesthesia of the airway without the hazard of respiratory depression. The airway remains in its tenuous condition for as long as 1 hour after extubation. Auscultation of the larynx must be performed frequently, searching for stridor.

Barash PG, Cullen BF, Stoelting RK (eds): Clinical Anesthesia, 3rd ed, pp 929–943. Philadelphia, Lippincott-Raven, 1997

Kirby RR, Gravenstein N (eds): Clinical Anesthesia Practice, pp 1268–1282. Philadelphia, WB Saunders, 1994

D.3. How does alcohol abuse and use of illicit drugs affect postoperative management?

Symptomatic withdrawal from alcohol usually occurs within 24 hours. Delirium tremens usually develops in approximately 72 hours after cessation of alcohol. Withdrawal from narcotics will occur in 4 to 6 hours. The use of narcotics in anesthetic management will delay or prevent occurrence of withdrawal phenomena.

Wyngaarden JB, Smith LH, Bennett JC (eds): Cecil Textbook of Medicine, 19th ed, pp 44–52. Philadelphia, WB Saunders, 1992

D.4. What pain medication would you use?

If pain is moderate, ketorolac is useful, especially because it has no respiratory depressant effect. If the patient is still intubated and mechanically ventilated narcotics can be used.

Brown CR, Moodie JE, Phillips E: Different responses to postoperative analgesics by inpatients and outpatients. Clin Pharmacol Ther 49:183, 1991

Vaslef SN, Vender JS: Postoperative care of the trauma patient. Anesthesiol Clin North Am 14(1): 239–256, 1996

Miscellaneous

IX

Myasthenia Gravis

48

Cynthia A. Lien
Alan Van Poznak

A 43-year-old woman presented for a thymectomy. Her history was significant for diplopia and dysphagia, which worsened as the day progressed.

A. Medical Disease and Differential Diagnosis

1. What should be included in this patient's differential diagnosis?
2. What is the incidence of myasthenia gravis?
3. Describe the clinical classification of myasthenia gravis.
4. What is the clinical course of myasthenia gravis?
5. What treatment regimens are available for patients with myasthenia gravis?
6. What is the role of surgery in the treatment of myasthenia gravis?
7. What are the electrical and humoral events that take place during normal neuromuscular transmission? How are these altered in patients with myasthenia gravis?
8. What is the cause of myasthenia gravis? How is the diagnosis of myasthenia gravis made?

B. Preoperative Evaluation and Preparation

1. How should you assess this patient preoperatively?
2. What preoperative laboratory data are required?
3. Should this patient be premedicated?

C. Intraoperative Management

1. What intraoperative monitors should be used?
2. What anesthetic regimen would you choose for this patient?
3. Can muscle relaxants be used in patients with myasthenia gravis?

D. Postoperative Management

1. Will this patient require prolonged postoperative ventilatory support?
2. How should this patient's postoperative pain be treated?
3. This patient was extubated in the operating room without difficulty. Forty minutes later, in the recovery room, she suddenly complained of feeling weak and being unable to breathe. Why?

A. Medical Disease and Differential Diagnosis

A.1. What should be included in this patient's differential diagnosis?

Although this patient's presentation is consistent with a diagnosis of myasthenia gravis, other disorders should be included in the initial differential diagnosis, including thyrotoxicosis, neurasthenia, progressive external ophthalmoplegia, other restricted myopathies, muscular dystrophies, brain tumors, Eaton-Lambert syndrome, amyotrophic lateral sclerosis, D-penicillinamine administration, illnesses with dysarthria and dysphagia but without ptosis or strabismus, and myasthenic polymyopathy with hypersensitivity to neostigmine.

Adams RD, Victor MV: Principles of Neurology, pp 1074–1089. New York, McGraw-Hill, 1985

Drachman DB: Myasthenia gravis. N Engl J Med 330(25):1797–1810, 1994

Eisenkraft JB: Anesthetic considerations in patients with myasthenia gravis. Cardiothorac Vasc Anesth Update 1:1, 1990

Osserman KE, Genkins G: Studies in myasthenia gravis: Review of a twenty-year experience in over 1200 patients. Mt Sinai J Med 38:497–538, 1971

Rakel RE (ed): Saunders Manual of Medical Practice, pp 1056–1057. Philadelphia, WB Saunders, 1996

A.2. What is the incidence of myasthenia gravis?

Myasthenia gravis is a relatively rare disease with an incidence of approximately 1 in 30,000. Two thirds of patients with myasthenia gravis are women.

The age at which the disease manifests varies with the gender of the patient. Women most commonly present between the ages of 10 and 40 years. Men develop the disease after 40 years of age. Patients younger than 16 years of age account for approximately 10% of all cases.

Drachman DB: Myasthenia gravis. N Engl J Med 330(25):1797–1810, 1994

Harvard CWH, Scadding GK: Myasthenia gravis: Pathogenesis and current concepts in management. Drugs 26:174, 1983

Kurtzke JF: Epidemiology of myasthenia gravis. In: Advances in Neurology, pp 545–566. New York, Raven Press, 1978

A.3. Describe the clinical classification of myasthenia gravis.

Many systems of clinical classification are found for myasthenia gravis. In the system described by Osserman and Genkins, patients are differentiated on the basis of their symptoms as follows:

- Class I—ocular symptoms only
- Class IA—ocular symptoms with electromyographic evidence of peripheral muscle involvement
- Class IIA—mild generalized symptoms
- Class IIB—more severe and rapidly progressive symptoms
- Class III—acute, presenting in weeks to months with severe bulbar symptoms
- Class IV—late in the course of the disease with severe bulbar symptoms and marked generalized weakness

Osserman KE, Genkins G: Studies in myasthenia gravis: Review of a twenty-year experience in over 1200 patients. Mt. Sinai J Med 38:497–538, 1971

A.4. What is the clinical course of myasthenia gravis?

Myasthenia gravis is typically insidious in onset and presents as a fluctuating weakness of voluntary muscles that is exacerbated by exercise and is improved after a period of rest. The characteristic distribution of weakness includes the extraocular, bulbar, neck, limb girdle, distal limb, and trunk muscles in decreasing order of involvement. In fact, diplopia is the most common chief complaint. Ptosis, which is the second most common presenting problem, may be unilateral or bilateral and characteristically it alternates between the right and left side. Dysarthria and difficulties in chewing and swallowing are early symptoms of bulbar involvement. Only 15% to 20% of patients present with extremity weakness. Respiratory muscle weakness is an even rarer presenting symptom. Disease progression is slow if symptoms remain localized to the eyes for >2 years.

The disease is exacerbated by infection, physical or emotional stress, hyperthyroidism, or drugs such as quinidine, procainamide, and aminoglycoside antibiotics.

Drachman DB: Myasthenia gravis. N Engl J Med 330(25):1797–1810, 1994

Grob D, Arsura El, Brunner NG, Namba T: Part IV. Diagnosis and treatment of myasthenia gravis. The course of myasthenia gravis and therapies affecting outcome. Ann NY Acad Sci 505:472, 1987

Kennedy FS, Moersch FP: Myasthenia gravis: A clinical review of 87 cases observed between 1915 and the early part of 1932. Can Med Assoc J 37:216, 1937

Oosterhuis H (ed): Myasthenia Gravis, pp 21–50. New York, Churchill Livingstone, 1984

Rakel RE (ed): Saunders Manual of Medical Practice, pp 1056–1057. Philadelphia, WB Saunders, 1996

A.5. What treatment regimens are available for patients with myasthenia gravis?

A number of different forms of medical treatment for myasthenia gravis are available.

Anticholinesterases

Anticholinesterases have been used in the treatment of myasthenia gravis since 1934. These agents prolong the duration of acetylcholine at the postsynaptic membrane of the neuromuscular junction. Because patient response to these agents is tremendously variable, varying from patient to patient and within a patient over the course of a day, patient education and maximal patient involvement are required for their optimal use. Anticholinesterases are frequently combined with corticotropin (ACTH) or immunosuppressive drugs in the treatment of myasthenia gravis.

Pyridostigmine (Mestinon) is the most commonly used drug because it has fewer muscarinic side-effects than neostigmine. Its onset of action is within 15 to 30 minutes after oral administration, its peak effect is within 1 to 2 hours, and its duration of action is 3 to 4 hours. It is available in three doses: 10, 60, and 180 mg. Common daily doses are from 30 to 120 mg, divided into three to six administrations per day. Although a long-acting form (Mestinon Timespan) is available, its use is generally discouraged except for patients with profound morning weakness or nocturnal respiratory distress because of the increased potential for overdose.

Neostigmine bromide (Prostigmin) lasts 1 to 2 hours and may be given parenterally. Its muscarinic side-effects are greater than those of pyridostigmine.

Ambenonium (Mytelase) is the least widely used of the anticholinesterase compounds.

Edrophonium (Tensilon), in doses of 5 to 10 mg intravenously, has been used between regularly scheduled doses of anticholinesterase to determine if the patient has received too much or too little medication.

Immunosuppression

Corticosteroid therapy is used to complement rather than replace anticholinesterase therapy. Treatment with steroids can lead to marked improvement or remission. The risks of this therapy are high, however; they include generalized immunosuppression, infection, cataracts, metabolic bone disease, and myopathy. Although the mechanism of steroid action is not entirely clear, steroids appear to cause a reduction in the number of antibodies to the acetylcholine receptors. Clinical improvement after initiation of therapy is slow and may take weeks. Initial deterioration in a patient's condition can be minimized by starting with small doses of steroids and increasing them gradually. A number of dosing schedules have been suggested, although scant evidence is available to recommend one over the other.

Azathioprine, methotrexate, actinomycin C, or cyclophosphamide may be used with steroids to treat severe cases of myasthenia gravis. Onset of improvement takes anywhere from 6 months to 1 year. Eleven percent remission and 50% clinical improvement have been reported with the use of these medications.

ACTH

ACTH has been used in the treatment of severe myasthenia gravis. Although it has been found to be useful when previous therapy with steroids has failed, the number of patients receiving ACTH has decreased. This form of treatment is being replaced with plasmapheresis.

Plasmapheresis

Plasmapheresis has been found to alleviate the symptoms of myasthenia gravis, but the degree and duration of induced remission are unpredictable. The actual role of plasmapheresis in the treatment of myasthenia gravis has yet to be determined. Although no linear relationship is seen between decreasing antibody levels and clinical improvement, the plasma removed from patients with myasthenia gravis will cause some of the symptoms to appear in laboratory animals.

Drachman DB: Myasthenia gravis. N Engl J Med 330(25):1797–1810, 1994

Grob D, Arsura El, Brunner NG, Namba T: The course of myasthenia gravis and therapies affecting outcome. Ann NY Acad Sci 505:472, 1987

Rakel RE (ed): Saunders Manual of Medical Practice, pp 1056–1057. Philadelphia, WB Saunders, 1996

Simpson JA, Thomaides T: Treatment of myasthenia gravis. Q J Med 64 (244):693, 1987

A.6. What is the role of surgery in the treatment of myasthenia gravis?

Thymectomy has been used as a treatment for myasthenia gravis since 1939, when the removal of a cyst from the area of the thymus of a myasthenic patient, described by Blalock, resulted in remission of the patient's disease. Although the role of the thymus in the pathogenesis of myasthenia gravis remains unclear, 75% of patients with myasthenia have thymic abnormalities that include thymoma and thymic hyperplasia. Only 30% of patients with a thymoma have symptoms of myasthenia gravis. Approximately 50% of patients with myasthenia will demonstrate clinical improvement after thymectomy, and 21% to 38% will go into complete remission (compared with 13% of those treated medically). Exacerbations of the disease, however, can occur in these patients several years after surgery. For all patients with myasthenia, therefore, except for those with only ocular symptoms and those who are prepubertal children with medically manageable disease, thymectomy is the treatment of choice.

Disagreement is found on whether a trans-sternal or transcervical approach should be used for thymectomy. In Blalock's 1941 series, he reported that a total thymectomy should be performed. The trans-sternal approach allows a more complete search for the thymic gland, which can be found adjacent to the phrenic nerves and in the pericardial fat, as well as in the neck near the thyroid. The transcervical approach, because of its less invasive nature, causes less morbidity and mortality than the trans-sternal approach. The rates of remission with the two surgical approaches are comparable.

Buchinghan JM, Howard FM, Bernaty PE et al: The value of thymectomy in myasthenia gravis. Ann Surg 184:453, 1976

Drachman DB: Myasthenia gravis. N Engl J Med 330(25):1797–1810, 1994

Papatestas AE, Genhins G, Kornfeld P et al: Comparison of the results of transcervical and transsternal thymectomy in myasthenia gravis. Ann NY Acad Sci 377:766, 1981

Rakel RE (ed): Saunders Manual of Medical Practice, pp 1056–1057. Philadelphia, WB Saunders, 1996

A.7. What are the electrical and humoral events that take place during normal neuromuscular transmission? How are these altered in patients with myasthenia gravis?

Normal electrochemical equilibria are such that the inside of the cell is kept negative with respect to the outside by a potential difference of 70 to 90 mV. When an action potential occurs, ionic fluxes are such that the interior of the cell becomes positive by approximately 40 mV. Quanta of acetylcholine are liberated from nerve terminals by the arrival of nerve action potentials. The acetylcholine crosses the synaptic cleft and attaches to receptor sites on the sarcolemma, causing the depolarization known as the "end-plate potential." If the threshold for excitation is exceeded by the summation of many action potentials, an action potential invades the muscle cell membrane and spreads along its surface, causing muscle contraction.

In myasthenia gravis, the amount of acetylcholine released presynaptically is normal or even increased. Histologic alterations are found at the neuromuscular junction. There is a widening of the synaptic space at the neuromuscular junction and a degeneration of the junctional folds. Most importantly, the concentration of available acetylcholine receptors on the postsynaptic membrane is reduced. This reduction in the number of available acetylcholine receptors, typically by >70%, is caused by receptor antibodies.

Adams RD, Victor MV: Principles of Neurology, pp 883–994. New York, McGraw-Hill, 1985

Drachman DB: Myasthenia gravis. N Engl J Med 330:1797–1810, 1994

Drachman DB, Kao J, Pestronk A et al: Myasthenia gravis as a receptor disorder. Ann NY Acad Sci 274:226, 1976

Harvard CWH, Scadding GK: Myasthenia gravis: Pathogenesis and current concepts in management. Drugs 26:174, 1983

A.8. What is the cause of myasthenia gravis? How is the diagnosis of myasthenia gravis made?

Myasthenia gravis is an autoimmune disease caused by antibody and T-cell attack on the nicotinic acetylcholine receptors (AChR) of the muscle endplate. Between 85%

and 95% of myasthenia gravis patients have antibodies to their AChRs. T-cell immunity is theorized to occur after sensitization in the thymus to a protein similar or identical to the embryonic AChR.

Diagnosis of myasthenia gravis is made primarily by history and then confirmed with any of several diagnostic tests. These tests may be either electrophysiologic, pharmacologic, or serologic.

Electrophysiologic testing involves testing a peripheral nerve, usually the circumflex humoral, median, or ulnar nerve, by stimulating it with a supramaximal stimulus of 2 Hz four times over 2 seconds in a train-of-four pattern. A decrease in twitch response to stimuli of >10% when the fourth response is compared with the first is diagnostic of myasthenia gravis. Myasthenia gravis patients also show less post-tetanic facilitation during this examination than their healthy counterparts.

Pharmacologic testing involves administering edrophonium (2.5 to 5 mg) intravenously. Patients will show an immediate dramatic improvement in their muscle strength in response to administration of this small dose of anticholinesterase.

The curare test is rarely used because of the morbidity and mortality that is associated with it. Because myasthenia gravis patients can have up to 70% of their acetylcholine receptors blocked, their margin of safety of impulse transmission at the neuromuscular junction is markedly diminished. Therefore, they may develop profound neuromuscular blockade and respiratory arrest after the administration of even a small dose of parenteral *d*-tubocurarine. The curare test can be done as either a regional or a systemic test. With the regional curare test a tourniquet is applied to each arm and inflated. In one arm a dose of 0.2 mg *d*-tubocurarine in 20 ml of normal saline is given intravenously. In the other arm 20 ml of normal saline alone is given intravenously. Muscle function is tested before, during, and every few minutes with electromyography until 16 minutes after administration of the curare-saline or saline mixture. In myasthenia gravis patients a marked decrease in muscle response is seen in the arm receiving the curare. During a systemic curare test, 0.5 to 1 mg increments of tubocurarine to a maximal dose of 0.03 mg/kg are administered intravenously to exacerbate myasthenic symptoms. In myasthenia gravis patients, marked weakness is seen with <10% of the normal curarizing dose. Muscle function is assessed 5 minutes after each dose. The test is stopped as soon as exacerbation of weakness is observed. Because the regional curare test examines only select muscle groups that may not be as severely affected by myasthenia gravis as other muscle groups, the systemic curare test is more sensitive than the regional one. The regional curare test, however, is the safer of the tests because of less potential for respiratory arrest.

In generalized myasthenia gravis, AChR antibody is elevated up to 95% of the time, but is less with ocular myasthenia gravis. Other tests that have been described as being useful in the diagnosis of myasthenia gravis include single-fiber electromyography, stapedius reflexometry, and nystagraphy.

Davies DW, Steward DJ: Myasthenia gravis in children and anesthetic management for thymectomy. Can Anaesth Soc J 20:253, 1973

Drachman DB: Myasthenia gravis. N Engl J Med 330(25):1797–1810, 1994

Foldes FF, Klonymus DH, Maisel W et al: A new curare test for the diagnosis of myasthenia gravis. JAMA 203:649, 1968

Rakel RE (ed): Saunders Manual of Medical Practice, pp 1056–1057. Philadelphia, WB Saunders, 1996

Samaha FJ: Electrodiagnostic studies in neuromuscular disease. N Engl J Med 285:1244, 1971

Viets HR (ed): Myasthenia Gravis, pp 411–434. Springfield, IL, CC Thomas, 1961

B. Preoperative Evaluation and Preparation

B.1. How should you assess this patient preoperatively?

The preoperative interview must be extensive in these patients. Factors that may be indicative of the need for postoperative ventilation include duration and severity of the disease, and the total daily dose of pyridostigmine or other medication. This information will guide the anesthesiologist in choosing preoperative medication and in making arrangements for postoperative care. The patient's medication requirements need to be detailed. Myasthenic patients are usually knowledgeable about their medication; they can adjust their own regimen on the basis of their clinical status.

Whether to alter a patient's anticholinesterase medication preoperatively is much debated. In patients with only mild weakness, discontinuation of the anticholinesterase would seem to be preferable. Its continued use can complicate anesthesia by rendering patients more susceptible to vagal arrhythmias. Furthermore, anticholinesterase inhibits plasma cholinesterase as well as acetylcholinesterase, and it can slow the metabolism of ester local anesthetics, succinylcholine, and mivacurium. Certainly, patients who are dependent on their medication should continue it. In this case, however, the anesthesiologist needs to be aware that postoperative requirements may be markedly reduced. Whether the patient is taking or has taken steroids in the past year needs to be determined.

Because other autoimmune diseases occur with increased frequency in myasthenic patients, evidence of hypothyroidism, pernicious anemia, systemic lupus erythematosus, and rheumatoid arthritis should be sought.

Katz J, Benumof J, Kadis L (eds): Anesthesia and Uncommon Diseases, 3rd ed, p 619. Philadelphia, WB Saunders, 1990

Stoelting RK, Dierdorf SF (eds): Anesthesia and Co-Existing Disease, 3rd ed, pp 441–442. New York, Churchill Livingstone, 1993

B.2. What preoperative laboratory data are required?

In addition to routine preoperative laboratory data, myasthenic patients should have their sodium and potassium measured, because electrolyte abnormalities can exacerbate weakness. If prolonged postoperative ventilation is anticipated, arterial blood gas and pulmonary function tests may be helpful in determining a baseline at which the patient can be extubated.

B.3. Should this patient be premedicated?

For the patient who is taking steroids preoperatively, stress doses should be given in the perioperative period.

Patients should not be overly sedated preoperatively, but they should also not arrive in the operating room extremely anxious. A thorough preoperative interview with a full explanation of what to expect in the perioperative period, including monitors and the possibility of postoperative ventilation, often decreases the need for preoperative sedation. If medication is required, patients should be given an anxiolytic.

Miscellaneous

Medication that causes respiratory depression is not suitable. An antisialagogue such as 0.2 mg glycopyrrolate may be given intramuscularly 1 hour preoperatively.

Barash PG, Cullen BF, Stoelting RK (eds): Clinical Anesthesia, 3rd ed, pp 463–465. Philadelphia, JB Lippincott, 1997

Stoelting RK, Dierdorf SF (eds): Anesthesia and Co-Existing Disease, 3rd ed, pp 441–443. New York, Churchill Livingstone, 1993

C. Intraoperative Management

C.1. What intraoperative monitors should be used?

These patients should be monitored with an electrocardiogram, blood pressure cuff, pulse oximeter, esophageal temperature, and end-tidal capnometry. After anesthesia induction, if they are undergoing an intrathoracic procedure or are expected to remain intubated postoperatively, they should also be monitored with an arterial line.

A nerve stimulator should be used to monitor muscle strength whether or not they are going to receive muscle relaxants intraoperatively. This is because inhalational anesthetics have been shown to cause twitch suppression in the absence of muscle relaxants. Patients with myasthenia gravis are extremely sensitive to the neuromuscular depressing properties of the volatile anesthetics.

Wahlin A, Havermark KG: Enflurane (Ethrane) anaesthesia on patients with myasthenia gravis. Acta Anaesth Belg 2:215, 1974

C.2. What anesthetic regimen would you choose for this patient?

The anesthetic regimen should be planned to provide the least and briefest interference with both ventilatory and neuromuscular function. After preoxygenation, anesthesia can be induced with thiopental, etomidate, propofol, or ketamine. Because patients with myasthenia gravis exhibit increased sensitivity to the ventilatory depressant effects of opioids, their use during induction and maintenance of anesthesia should be done sparingly and cautiously. Ventilation with 100% oxygen should be assisted and then controlled as necessary. Once an adequate airway is established, a volatile anesthetic should be added to the gas mixture. Muscle relaxants are rarely required for laryngoscopy and intubation if the patient's level of anesthesia is deep enough. Once the vocal cords have been visualized during laryngoscopy, they should be sprayed with 4% topical lidocaine before the trachea is intubated. Respiration should then be controlled to ensure adequate ventilation, and anesthesia should be maintained with oxygen, nitrous oxide, a volatile anesthetic, a continuous infusion of a short-acting intravenous anesthetic, or a combination of a volatile anesthetic and a short-acting intravenous anesthetic.

As the surgery is completed, the anesthesia is tapered to allow for prompt emergence. The patient should not be extubated until she is awake, responsive, strong, and able to generate a negative inspiratory force of at least negative 20 cm H_2O. She should be able to maintain normal oxygenation and normocapnea prior to extubation.

Katz J, Benumof J, Kadis LB (eds): Anesthesia and Uncommon Diseases, pp 615–621. Philadelphia, WB Saunders, 1990

Stoelting RK, Dierdorf SF (eds): Anesthesia and Co-Existing Disease, 3rd ed, pp 442–443. New York, Churchill Livingstone, 1993

C.3. Can muscle relaxants be used in patients with myasthenia gravis?

The myasthenic patient's response to muscle relaxants is altered because of his or her inherent disease process and because of the treatment of the disease.

Succinylcholine has been used to facilitate endotracheal intubation. However, myasthenic patients appear to be relatively resistant to the effects of succinylcholine. Furthermore, phase II block has been shown to occur with a single intubating dose of succinylcholine, and recovery may be slower than in patients without myasthenia. Further complicating the picture is whether or not the patient is being treated with anticholinesterases, which interfere with the metabolism of the depolarizing muscle relaxant. Patients treated with anticholinesterases can show a prolonged response to succinylcholine. Although the use of succinylcholine is not contraindicated in these patients, many clinicians prefer not to use it because of the possibility of prolonged neuromuscular blockade.

The myasthenia gravis patient's response to nondepolarizing neuromuscular blockade is, on the other hand, extremely predictable. They can be exquisitely sensitive to the nondepolarizing neuromuscular blocking agents and can demonstrate a profound weakness with a precurarizing dose of muscle relaxant. This sensitivity is due to the fact that the number of acetylcholine receptors may be decreased by up to 70% in patients with myasthenia gravis. The number of available receptors in these patients is just sufficient to produce end-plate potentials that are above the threshold required for neuromuscular transmission and muscle contraction. This reduced receptor concentration reduces the plasma concentration and the dose of relaxant required for muscle relaxation. Blockade of 70% of acetylcholine receptors, or an effective decrease in the number of receptors by this same amount, will cause fade in the mechanomyographic response to a train-of-four stimulus in patients without myasthenia gravis.

However, despite this increased sensitivity to nondepolarizing muscle relaxants, they can be used safely in patients with myasthenia gravis, but markedly decreased doses should be used and the degree of neuromuscular blockade should be carefully monitored. Pancuronium has been reported to cause 95% neuromuscular blockade with only one fourth of the usual dose (0.005 to 0.01 mg/kg). Therefore, the intermediate-acting muscle relaxants, atracurium and vecuronium, can be more suitable for patients with myasthenia gravis because of their shorter duration of action. Because of mivacurium's metabolism by plasma cholinesterase, it may not be well-suited for use in patients with myasthenia gravis.

A number of case reports have described the safe use of intermediate-acting muscle relaxants in myasthenic patients. Doses ranging from 10% to 50% of those required in nonmyasthenic patients were used, and prompt extubation was done after either spontaneous or pharmacologic reversal.

Barash PG, Cullen BF, Stoelting RK (eds): Clinical Anesthesia, 3rd ed, pp 463–465. Philadelphia, JB Lippincott, 1997

Blitt CD, Wright WA, Peat J: Pancuronium and the patient with myasthenia gravis. Anesthesiology 42:624, 1975

Buzello W, Noeldge G, Krieg N et al: Vecuronium for muscle relaxation in patients with myasthenia gravis. Anesthesiology 64:507, 1986

Foldes FF, McNall PG: Myasthenia gravis: A guide for anesthesiologists. Anesthesiology 23:837, 1962

Katz J, Benumof J, Kadis LB (eds): Anesthesia and Uncommon Diseases, pp 615–623. Philadelphia, WB Saunders, 1990

Lake CL: Curare sensitivity in steroid-treated myasthenia gravis: A case report. Anesth Analg 57:132, 1978

Nilsson E, Meretoja OA: Vecuronium dose-response and maintenance requirements in patients with myasthenia gravis. Anesthesiology 73:28, 1990

Vacanti CA, Ali HH, Schweiss JF et al: The response of myasthenia gravis to atracurium. Anesthesiology 62:692, 1985

D. Postoperative Management

D.1. Will this patient require prolonged postoperative ventilatory support?

A number of predictive criteria for the need for prolonged postoperative ventilatory support have been proposed. Leventhal et al. assigned a scoring system to four factors they found to be predictive:

- Duration of >6 years   12 points
- History of chronic obstructive pulmonary disease   10 points
- >750 mg/d pyridostigmine   8 points
- Vital capacity <2.9 liters   4 points

Patients scoring <10 points in their series could be extubated immediately postoperatively; those scoring >12 points required postoperative ventilatory support. This system of predicting whether a patient will require prolonged intubation and ventilation has not proved to be universally applicable. Patients undergoing trans-sternal thymectomy require postoperative ventilatory support more frequently than those undergoing transcervical thymectomy, perhaps because the less invasive procedure has less of an effect on respiratory function. Similarly, one could predict that the patient with myasthenia gravis undergoing an upper abdominal procedure would be more likely to require postoperative ventilation than the patient undergoing a more peripheral procedure. Obviously, one must consider each patient individually when assessing the need for postoperative ventilatory support.

Barash PG, Cullen BF, Stoelting RK (eds): Clinical Anesthesia, 3rd ed, pp 463–465. Philadelphia, JB Lippincott, 1997

Eisenkraft JB, Papatestas AE, Kahn CH et al: Predicting the need for postoperative mechanical ventilation in myasthenia gravis. Anesthesiology 65:79, 1986

Eisenkraft JB, Papatestas AE, Posner JN et al: Prediction of ventilatory failure following transcervical thymectomy in myasthenia gravis. Ann NY Acad Sci 505:888, 1987

Grant RP, Jenkins LC: Prediction of the need for postoperative mechanical ventilation in myasthenia gravis: A dose response study. Anesthesiology 69:760, 1988

Leventhal SR, Orkin FK, Hirsch RA: Prediction of the need for postoperative mechanical ventilation in myasthenia gravis. Anesthesiology 53:26, 1980

Stoelting RK, Dierdorf SF, McCammon RL (eds): Anesthesia and Co-Existing Disease, 3rd ed, pp 442–443. New York, Churchill Livingstone, 1993

D.2. How should this patient's postoperative pain be treated?

The postoperative analgesic regimen should be designed to provide adequate pain relief with minimal interference with ventilatory function. These patients are extremely sensitive to the ventilatory depressant effects of parenteral narcotics, and they should be used in the smallest doses possible to relieve postoperative pain. Epidural administration of narcotics could be considered as an alternative way to provide postoperative pain relief. This form of medication provides better pain relief with less ventilatory depression than parenteral administration.

Smith CA: Postoperative management after thymectomy. Br Med J 1:309, 1975

D.3. This patient was extubated in the operating room without difficulty. Forty minutes later, in the recovery room, she suddenly complained of feeling weak and being unable to breathe. Why?

The anesthesiologist needs to determine whether this exacerbation of weakness is due to a cholinergic crisis or a myasthenic crisis. During a myasthenic crisis patients have a decreased response to anticholinesterases; a cholinergic crisis is caused by an overdose of anticholinesterases. Either can be suspected in the immediate postoperative period, when the stress of surgery can cause an exacerbation of myasthenic weakness and when anticholinergic requirements may be altered. In either case increased muscle weakness may require ventilatory support.

With both myasthenic and cholinergic crisis increase in muscle weakness, salivation, and sweating occur. It has been recommended that the two crises be differentiated from each other on the basis of the patient's response to an intravenously administered dose of 10 mg of edrophonium. The patient in a myasthenic crisis should show some improvement in muscle strength; the patient in cholinergic crisis will show either no increase in muscle strength or a worsening of respiratory distress.

Katz J, Benumof J, Kadis LB (eds): Anesthesia and Uncommon Diseases, 3rd ed, pp 615–621. Philadelphia, WB Saunders, 1990

49 Malignant Hyperthermia

Vinod Malhotra

A 5-year-old boy with kyphoscoliosis was scheduled in ambulatory surgery for repair of strabismus under general anesthesia. Previous anesthetic history included an uneventful halothane and nitrous oxide anesthesia for bilateral myringotomy. However, the mother was very nervous because a first cousin of the boy had died under anesthesia in Wisconsin the previous year.

A. Medical Disease and Differential Diagnosis

1. What was the problem of concern in this case?
2. What is malignant hyperthermia?
3. What are the clinical features of a susceptible patient?
4. Does the history of previous uneventful halothane anesthesia reasonably exclude the patient's susceptibility to malignant hyperthermia?
5. What are the clinical features of the syndrome?
6. What are the laboratory findings during an acute crisis of malignant hyperthermia?
7. What are the two clinical types of the syndrome?
8. What is the incidence of this syndrome?
9. What is the mode of inheritance of the disease?
10. What genetic disorder results in malignant hyperthermia susceptibility?
11. What is the etiopathology of the syndrome?
12. What laboratory tests can further substantiate the susceptibility of the patient to malignant hyperthermia?
13. What is neurolept malignant syndrome?

B. Preoperative Evaluation and Preparation

1. How would you prepare this patient for anesthesia and surgery?
2. Is dantrolene prophylaxis indicated?
3. What laboratory tests would you wish to obtain prior to surgery?
4. Is outpatient surgery appropriate for this patient?
5. In anticipation of general anesthesia, what preparations would you make?

C. Intraoperative Management

1. What anesthetic techniques and agents would you employ?
2. What anesthetic agents are contraindicated?
3. If the surgeon wishes to use local anesthesia for a procedure, what agents will you recommend?
4. What is the significance of masseter muscle spasm following succinylcholine administration?
5. Twenty minutes into the procedure, the patient developed increasing tachycardia

with ventricular premature beats and mottled skin. What emergency measures would you take?
6. What modalities would you monitor closely during management of the crisis?

D. Postoperative Management

1. **What complications may follow this syndrome?**
2. **What would be your follow-up on this case?**
3. **What would you advise the patient and the family?**

A. Medical Disease and Differential Diagnosis

A.1. What was the problem of concern in this case?

The patient was a 5-year-old child with kyphoscoliosis and strabismus. There was a history of an anesthetic-related death in the family in Wisconsin. Therefore, in addition to the respiratory problems associated with kyphoscoliosis, he presented a likelihood of susceptibility to malignant hyperpyrexia syndrome. The supporting factors for strong suspicion were the musculoskeletal disease, the family history, and the geographic location indicated.

In a recent review of 503 reported cases of malignant hyperthermia (MH), 52% of patients were <15 years of age and 66% were male. Congenital defects and musculoskeletal surgical procedures were clearly associated with malignant hyperthermia. Family history was positive in 25% of the cases.

Miller RD (ed): Anesthesia, 4th ed, pp 1075–1093. New York, Churchill Livingstone, 1994

Rosenberg H: Malignant hyperthermia and other anesthesia induced myodystrophies. ASA Annual Refresher Course Lectures #126, 1997

Strazis KP, Fox AW: Malignant hyperthermia: A review of published cases. Anesth Analg 77(2): 297–304, 1993

Wedel DJ: Malignant hyperthermia and neuromuscular disease. Neuromuscul Disord 2(3):157–164, 1992

A.2. What is malignant hyperthermia?

Malignant hyperthermia, first described by Denborough and Lorell in 1960, is a clinical syndrome of markedly accelerated metabolic state characterized by fever, tachycardia, tachypnea, cyanosis, and hypercarbia. The clinical syndrome occurs in a susceptible patient when a triggering agent is employed.

Denborough MA, Lorell RRH: Anesthetic deaths in a family. Lancet 2:45, 1960

Miller RD (ed): Anesthesia, 4th ed, pp 1075–1093. New York, Churchill Livingstone, 1994

Rosenberg H: Malignant hyperthermia and other anesthesia induced myodystrophies. ASA Annual Refresher Course Lectures #126, 1997

Table 49-1. Associated Musculoskeletal Disorders in Patients Susceptible to Malignant Hyperthermia

---

Short, stocky stature
Bulky muscles and rounded belly
Muscle hypertrophy
Atrophied muscle groups
Muscle cramps
Kyphoscoliosis
Strabismus
Joint hypermobility with spontaneous dislocation
Hernias
Clubfoot
Pectus carinatum
Hypoplastic mandible
Poor dental enamel
Central-core disease
Osteogenesis imperfecta
Neuroleptic malignant heat syndrome
Myotonia congenita
Arthrogryposis
King syndrome

A.3. What are the clinical features of a susceptible patient?

Those patients who are susceptible to developing MH usually present with musculoskeletal disorders (Table 49-1). A close association of central core disease and MH underscores this relationship. Genetic studies of central core disease have identified an abnormal locus on chromosome 19, which is located close to a similar locus linked to abnormality of the ryanodine receptor responsible for MH syndrome in approximately 5% of humans. A family history, if present, is a strong indicator of malignant hyperthermia susceptibility. However, as indicated, a review of 503 reported cases was notable for lack of family history in 75% of cases.

Haan EA, Freemantle CJ, McCure JA: Assignment of the gene for central core disease to chromosome 19. Hum Genet 86:187, 1990

Levitt RC: Prospects for the diagnosis of malignant hyperthermia susceptibility using molecular genetic approaches. Anesthesiology 76:1039, 1992

Rosenberg H: Malignant hyperthermia and other anesthesia induced myodystrophies. ASA Annual Refresher Course Lectures #126, 1997

Strazis KP, Fox AW: Malignant hyperthermia: A review of published cases. Anesth Analg 77(2): 297–304, 1993

Wedel DJ: Malignant hyperthermia and neuromuscular disease. Neuromuscul Disord 2(3):157–164, 1992

A.4. Does the history of previous uneventful halothane anesthesia reasonably exclude the patient's susceptibility to malignant hyperthermia?

No, it does not. About one third of the cases occur during a second or subsequent anesthetic course.

Miller RD (ed): Anesthesia, 4th ed, pp 1075–1093. New York, Churchill Livingstone, 1994

Rosenberg H: Malignant hyperthermia and other anesthesia induced myodystrophies. ASA Annual Refresher Course Lectures #126, 1997

Strazis KP, Fox AW: Malignant hyperthermia: A review of published cases. Anesth Analg 77(2): 297–304, 1993

A.5. What are the clinical features of the syndrome?

The clinical features of this malignant hyperthermia essentially represent an uncontrolled, exaggerated, hypermetabolic state triggered by the use of certain drugs. The common early manifestations include the following:

- Increase in end-tidal CO_2 during constant ventilation (the most sensitive sign)
- Tachycardia—96% of patients (the most consistent clinical sign)
- Tachypnea—85% of patients
- Arrythmias
- Increased temperature—30% of patients (not uncommonly >43°C)
- Cyanosis—70% of patients
- Skin mottling
- Profuse sweating
- Overheated CO_2 absorber
- Rigidity—80% of patients (the most specific sign)
- Altered blood pressure—85% of patients

Larach MG, Localio AR, Allen GC et al: A clinical grading scale to predict malignant hyperthermia susceptibility. Anesthesiology 80:(4):771–779, 1994

Malignant Hyperthermia Association of the United States (MHAUS): Clinical Update 1995/1996: Managing Malignant Hyperthermia. Sherburne, NY, 1995

Miller RD (ed): Anesthesia, 4th ed, pp 1075–1093. New York, Churchill Livingstone, 1994

A.6. What are the laboratory findings during an acute crisis of malignant hyperthermia?

The laboratory values, once again, reflect changes of a hypermetabolic state and muscle tissue damage (Table 49-2).

Table 49-2.   The Laboratory Findings of Acute Malignant Hyperthermia

Metabolic and respiratory acidosis
ABG
$\downarrow\downarrow$ pH
$\downarrow\downarrow$ Po_2
$\uparrow\uparrow\uparrow$ Pco_2
Electrolytes
$\uparrow$ K
$\uparrow$ Ca
$\uparrow$ Mg
$\downarrow$ Na
Serum
$\uparrow$ Lactate
$\uparrow$ Pyruvate
$\uparrow$ CPK
$\uparrow$ LDH
$\uparrow$ Aldolase
$\uparrow$ Myoglobin

Miller RD (ed): Anesthesia, 4th ed, pp 1075–1093. New York, Churchill Livingstone, 1994

A.7. What are the two clinical types of the syndrome?

The syndrome has been classified as the rigid or the nonrigid type, depending on the development or absence of muscle contractures, respectively. The rigid type of MH is seen in approximately 75% of affected patients, and the nonrigid type in 25%.

Gronert GA: Malignant hyperthermia. Anesthesiology 53:396, 1980

A.8. What is the incidence of this syndrome?

Previously, estimated incidences were about 1 in 15,000 among children and 1 in 50,000 among adults. Data from Denmark report the incidence of fulminant, classic malignant hyperthermia to be 1 in 260,000 when general anesthetics were used and 1 in 60,000 when succinylcholine was used. A 10% mortality rate was observed. In this study, the overall incidence of suspected MH (masseter muscle rigidity, unexplained tachycardia, unexplained fever) was approximately 1 in 15,000 with general anesthetics and 1 in 5000 when inhalation agents and succinylcholine were used in combination.

The incidence of MH is lower in children <3 years of age and in geriatric patients. The age groups most likely to be affected are the older children and adults up to the third decade. Both sexes are affected equally up to puberty, but after puberty males are affected more frequently.

Miller RD (ed): Anesthesia, 4th ed, pp 1075–1093. New York, Churchill Livingstone, 1994

Ording H: Incidence of malignant hyperthermia in Denmark. Anesth Analg 64:700–704, 1985

Strazis KP, Fox AW: Malignant hyperthermia: A review of published cases. Anesth Analg 77(2): 297–304, 1993

A.9. What is the mode of inheritance of the disease?

The familial nature of the disease is well known, although most cases are nonfamilial. The genetic inheritance is autosomal dominant with reduced penetrance and variable expressivity. Recently, it has been suggested to be polygenic in origin. A gene for malignant hyperthermia has also been tentatively localized to chromosome 19 in humans.

McCarthy TV, Sandra Healey JM, Jeffron JA et al: Localization of the malignant hyperthermia susceptibility locus to human chromosome 19q. 12–13.2. Nature 343:562–563, 1990

McPherson EW, Taylor CA: The genetics of malignant hyperthermia: Evidence for heterogeneity. Am J Med Genet 11:273, 1982

Miller RD (ed): Anesthesia, 4th ed, pp 1075–1093. New York, Churchill Livingstone, 1994

A.10 What genetic disorder results in malignant hyperthermia susceptibility?

Porcine MH is inherited in an autosomal recessive pattern. MH susceptibility in swine is carried on the chromosomal locus for the ryanodine receptor due to a single point mutation for all breeds. The mutation consists of substitution of thymidine for cytosine in DNA with resultant substitution of cysteine for arginine at the ryanodine receptor.

Ryanodine is a plant alkaloid that has been shown to bind to calcium release channels of the sarcoplasmic reticulum. The binding site is termed the "ryanodine receptor." The ryanodine receptor locus in humans is on chromosome 19. In contrast to animal models, ryanodine receptor abnormality resulting from a chromosome 19 disorder has only been linked with 3% to 7% of MH susceptible patients. Evidence for chromosome 17 and other gene abnormalities in these patients exists as well. Hence, MH is a heterogeneous polygenic disorder.

Fagerlund TH, Islander G, Twetman ER et al: A search for three known gene mutations in 41 Swedish families with predisposition to malignant hyperthermia. Clin Genet 48(1):12–16, 1995

Fletcher JE, Tripolitis L, Hubert M et al: Genotype and phenotype relationships in the ryanodine receptor in patients referred for a diagnosis of malignant hyperthermia. Br J Anaesth 75(3):307–310, 1995

Levitt RC, Noun N: Evidence for genetic heterogeneity in malignant hyperthermia susceptibility. Genomics 11:543–547, 1991

A.11. *What is the etiopathology of the syndrome?*

In the normal skeletal muscle, depolarization induces release of calcium (DIRC) from sarcoplasmic reticulum. This increase in intracellular concentration activates cross bridges between actin and myosin filaments causing them to interdigitate resulting in contraction. Muscle relaxation follows because of calcium reuptake by the sarcoplasmic reticulum. In the cardiac muscle small amounts of calcium flux across the sarcolemma causes quantum release of calcium-induced release of calcium (CIRC). Whereas DIRC is the generally accepted process in skeletal muscle, CIRC may become operative once MH has set in. Because calcium channel blockers exert more effect on cardiac muscle than skeletal muscle, their reported effects on MH muscle are contradictory.

According to the best accepted theory of pathophysiology of malignant hyperthermia, the defect lies in excitation-contraction coupling of calcium to the sarcolemma in the muscle. The basic defect lies in the muscle fiber involving subcellular membrane permeability of the sarcolemma and reuptake of calcium by the sarcoplasmic reticulum, which results in an inability to control calcium concentrations within the fiber. The resultant events are heat production and muscle contracture secondary to enhanced glycolysis, uncoupling of oxidative phosphorylation and sustained activation of actin-myosin filaments.

Adnet PJ, Krivosic-Horber RM et al: Effects of calcium-free solution, calcium antagonists and the calcium agonist BAYK8644 on mechanical responses of skeletal muscle from patients susceptible to malignant hyperthermia. Anesthesiology 75:413–417, 1991

Foster PS, Hopkinson KC, Denborough MA: Effect of diltiazem, verapamil and dantrolene on the contractility of isolated malignant hyperpyrexia susceptible muscle. Clin Exp Pharmacol Physiol 16:799–803, 1989

Miller RD (ed): Anesthesia, 4th ed, pp 1075–1093. New York, Churchill Livingstone, 1994

A.12. What laboratory tests can further substantiate the susceptibility of the patient to malignant hyperthermia?

The two tests of importance are measurement of serum creatine phosphokinase (CPK) and a muscle biopsy. Serum CPK levels can be greatly elevated in these patients as well as in their relatives. Therefore, a markedly elevated CPK level is of diagnostic value, but a normal CPK level is of no value because one third of the susceptible patients have normal CPK levels. Besides, CPK levels can be altered by other factors, such as stress, injury, exercise, intramuscular injection, and certain drugs, as well as by collecting and measuring techniques.

With skeletal muscle biopsy, the caffeine-contracture test is the most diagnostic test for malignant hyperthermia-susceptible (MHS) patients. Strips of skeletal muscle are obtained from the quadriceps. These strips are then transported in Ringer's solution to the laboratory, where isometric tensions are recorded in a bath on a polygraph. Varying concentrations of caffeine are then added to the bath, with and without halothane, and contracture tension is recorded. The rigid MHS muscle shows contracture at much lower caffeine concentrations compared with the normal muscle, in both caffeine and caffeine-plus-halothane baths. In contrast, the nonrigid MHS muscle requires much higher concentrations of caffeine for the same effect when compared with the normal muscle. This test is sensitive and specific in diagnosing MHS patients because there is little overlap between normal and MHS muscle, and this abnormality is not shared by other myopathies. Although some doubts have been raised about the false-positive results in some myopathies, false-negative results have not been reported with the halothane-caffeine-contracture test. The other tests that may commonly show abnormality in MHS patients, but are not diagnostic of the syndrome, include electromyography (EMG), motor unit counting, microscopic examination of muscle, electrocardiogram (ECG), echocardiogram, myocardial scan, and adenosine diphosphate (ATP) depletion test. Genetic testing of DNA-containing tissue for ryanodine mutation, although feasible in porcine tissue, is only helpful in 3% to 7% of humans susceptible to MH. Magnetic resonance imaging of a stressed or ischemic muscle holds promise as a noninvasive test in the future, but it is far from any standardization.

Allen GC, Rosenberg H, Fletcher J: Safety of general anesthesia in patients tested negative for malignant hyperthermia susceptibility. Anesthesiology 72:619–622, 1990

Iaizzo PA, Wedel DJ, Gallagher WJ: In vitro contracture testing for determination of susceptibility to malignant hyperthermia: A methodologic update. Mayo Clin Proc 66:998–1001, 1991

Miller RD (ed): Anesthesia, 4th ed, pp 1075–1093. New York, Churchill Livingstone, 1994

A.13. What is neurolept malignant syndrome?

The neurolept malignant syndrome is characterized by fever, rhabdomyolysis, acidosis, and tachycardia, and its features mimic malignant hyperthermia. It is precipitated by haloperidol and phenothiazines. The caffeine-contracture test may be positive for malignant hyperthermia susceptibility.

This syndrome differs from malignant hyperthermia in that central dopamine depletion is responsible for the clinical picture and a dopamine agonist such as bromocriptine is effective treatment. Patients also respond to dantrolene therapy.

Miller RD (ed): Anesthesia, 4th ed, pp 1075–1093. New York, Churchill Livingstone, 1994

Rosenberg H: Malignant hyperthermia. ASA Annual Refresher Course Lectures 245, 1990

B. Preoperative Evaluation and Preparation

B.1. How would you prepare this patient for anesthesia and surgery?

Preoperative preparation should include assessment of the patient's physical status, evaluation of laboratory findings, and specific investigations to determine the susceptibility of the patient to malignant hyperthermia. Three possible scenarios include the following:

- The caffeine-contracture test is normal. The patient should be considered not susceptible to MH and the anesthetic should be nonrestrictive.
- The caffeine-contracture test is abnormal, implying MHS. In this case, trigger-free anesthetic agents should be employed and all preparation should be made to quickly treat the syndrome if it develops.
- The caffeine-contracture test is not available. This is frequently the case because this test is done in only 15 centers in the country. In such situations the patient should be treated as MHS and all appropriate steps should be followed.

Allen GC, Rosenberg H, Fletcher J: Safety of general anesthesia in patients tested negative for malignant hyperthermia susceptibility. Anesthesiology 72:619–622, 1990

Miller RD (ed): Anesthesia, 4th ed, pp 1075–1093. New York, Churchill Livingstone, 1994

Rosenberg H: Malignant hyperthermia and other anesthesia induced myodystrophies. ASA Annual Refresher Course Lectures #126, 1997

B.2. Is dantrolene prophylaxis indicated?

Oral dantrolene prophylaxis is no longer recommended. Cases of malignant hyperthermia have been reported in patients despite oral dantrolene prophylaxis. This prompted a recommendation of giving a dose of 2.5 mg/kg of dantrolene, administered over a 15- to 30-minute period shortly before surgery. Although various regimens have been recommended in the past for dantrolene prophylaxis, its worth as a routine prophylactic measure has not been proved.

Most recent data on 2214 malignant hyperthermia-susceptible patients (1082 biopsy-positive) reported five malignant hyperthermia reactions (incidence 0.46%). The five malignant hyperthermia reactions that did occur happened in the recovery room and were easily resolved. With the judicious use of trigger-free anesthetics, the incidence of malignant hyperthermia is small. The syndrome can be treated effectively if intravenous dantrolene is employed at the earliest manifestation of the malignant hyperthermia reaction. In addition, dantrolene can cause side-effects, such as nausea, vomiting, pain at the injection site, and depression of the twitch response, which can predispose the patient to respiratory insufficiency in the postoperative period. Because of these factors, the routine prophylactic use of dantrolene is questionable. It would seem prudent to reserve intravenous prophylactic dantrolene for patients with massive muscle trauma or sepsis or for other circumstances where the anesthesiologist feels that prophylaxis is necessary.

Carr AS, Lerman J, Cunliffe M et al: Incidence of malignant hyperthermia reactions in 2,214 patients undergoing muscle biopsy. Can J Anaesth 42(4):281–286, 1995

Ruhland G, Hinkle A: Malignant hyperthermia after oral and intravenous pretreatment with dantrolene in a patient susceptible to malignant hyperthermia. Anesthesiology 60:159–160, 1984

B.3. What laboratory tests would you wish to obtain prior to surgery?

Chest x-ray and ECG should be ordered if dictated by his kyphoscoliosis or any other associated medical illness. Otherwise, no routine laboratory testing is indicated for strabismus surgery in this child. Some may advocate obtaining serum CPK for baseline study. However, the diagnostic and prognostic value of a single CPK level is of limited value.

B.4. Is outpatient surgery appropriate for this patient?

With the use of trigger-free anesthetics and appropriate monitoring, outpatient eye surgery can be safely performed on this patient. Postoperative admission to the hospital solely on the basis of MHS is not warranted. Based on experience with MHS patients who received trigger-free anesthetics, the incidence of MH was extremely low (0.4%) for all surgery and practically nil for minor surgery. Furthermore, in all instances the MH occurred in the immediate postoperative period—usually not beyond 4 hours postoperatively. Therefore, it is prudent to keep the patient longer than usual in the postanesthesia care unit (PACU) in a monitored setting and also a little longer in the ambulatory discharge area.

Yentis SM, Levine MF, Hartley EJ: Should all children with suspected or confirmed malignant hyperthermia susceptibility be admitted after surgery? A 10-year review. Anesth Analg 75(3): 345–350, 1992

B.5. In anticipation of general anesthesia, what preparations would you make?

A satisfactory preparation for administering anesthesia to this patient should include measures to prevent and treat an acute crisis of malignant hyperthermia. The following should be available:

- Equipment
  - Vapor-free anesthesia machine (no vaporizers attached)
  - Fresh circuit and reservoir bag
  - Ventilator
  - Pulse oximeter
  - End-expiratory CO_2 monitor
  - ECG and blood pressure monitors
  - Temperature monitor
- Cooling aids
  - Hypothermia blanket
  - Crushed ice
  - Cold saline for irrigation and intravenous infusion
  - Tubes for cavity cooling
  - Bypass pump team
- Drugs
  - Anesthetic drugs, sodium bicarbonate, mannitol, furosemide, dantrolene (intravenous), procainamide, insulin, 50% dextrose, heparin, propranolol

Rosenberg H: Malignant hyperthermia and other anesthesia induced myodystrophies. ASA Annual Refresher Course Lectures #126, 1997

C. Intraoperative Management

C.1. What anesthetic techniques and agents would you employ?

No anesthetic is completely safe in these patients; however, one should adhere to the technique that is least likely to trigger an attack. Anesthesia should be induced with a barbiturate (e.g., thiopental sodium) and the patient should be ventilated with 100% oxygen. Fentanyl should be added to ensure adequate depth of anesthesia. Topical anesthesia of the larynx and vocal cords should be achieved with a local anesthetic spray. The trachea is then intubated with or without the use of a muscle relaxant. Cisatracurium or rocuronium can be used to facilitate intubation, if necessary. Other short-acting or intermediate-acting nondepolarizing muscle relaxants can be used too. Anesthetic maintenance is achieved by using oxygen and nitrous oxide, fentanyl, and cisatracurium as required. Vital signs are monitored with close attention to capnography.

Miller RD (ed): Anesthesia, 4th ed, pp 1075–1093. New York, Churchill Livingstone, 1994

Rosenberg H: Malignant hyperthermia and other anesthesia induced myodystrophies. ASA Annual Refresher Course Lectures #126, 1997

C.2. What anesthetic agents are contraindicated?

In general, the anesthetic agents best avoided include potent inhalation agents and muscle relaxants. Of the agents commonly employed today, the following have been implicated in triggering MH or increasing mortality:

- Inhalation agents—halothane (most commonly), enflurane, isoflurane, methoxyflurane, desflurane, sevoflurane
- Muscle relaxants—succinylcholine (most frequently), *d*-tubocurarine
- Premedications and other drugs—phenothiazines

Fu ES, Scharf JE, Mangar D et al: Malignant hyperthermia involving the administration of desflurane. Can J Anaesth 43(7):687–690, 1996

Miller RD (ed): Anesthesia, 4th ed, pp 1075–1093. New York, Churchill Livingstone, 1994

Otsuka H, Komura Y, Mayumi T et al: Malignant hyperthermia during sevoflurane anesthesia in a child with central core disease. Anesthesiology 75(4):699–701, 1991

Rosenberg H: Malignant hyperthermia and other anesthesia induced myodystrophies. ASA Annual Refresher Course Lectures #126, 1997

C.3. If the surgeon wishes to use local anesthesia for a procedure, what agents will you recommend?

Both ester and amide local anesthetics are now considered safe for use in malignant hyperthermia-susceptible patients.

Harrison GG, Morrell DF: Response of MHS swine to intravenous infusion of lignocaine and bupivacaine. Br J Anesth 52:385–387, 1980

Maccani RM, Wedel DJ, Melton A et al: Femoral and lateral femoral cutaneous nerve block for muscle biopsies in children. Paediatr Anaesth 5(4):223–227, 1995

C.4. What is the significance of masseter muscle spasm following succinylcholine administration?

Masseter muscle rigidity has been reported in about 1% of children after halothane induction and succinylcholine administration. It has been observed that approximately half of the patients developing trismus after succinylcholine are malignant hyperthermia-susceptible. Therefore, some have recommended that if trismus is observed, the anesthetic should be discontinued and the patient followed up for MH susceptibility. However, controversy exists regarding the association of masseter muscle spasm following succinylcholine administration with MH. First, if the reported incidence of trismus and MHS is correct, then one can extrapolate that MHS should be prevalent in approximately 1 of every 200 children. That would be a much larger incidence than actually observed (1 of 15,000). Second, studies have shown that in normal children under halothane anesthesia, the skeletal muscle tone of the jaw increases following succinylcholine administration. Thus, we believe that if trismus is observed, then a possibility of MHS should be kept in mind and the anesthetic should proceed with careful monitoring of the patient for signs of MH. One should switch to trigger-free anesthetic agents. Others believe that the anesthetic should be discontinued and the procedure halted. Some agreement is found in that if the jaw is tight and impossible to open (so-called jaw of steel) or the tightness persists for several minutes, the procedure should be stopped and anesthetics discontinued.

Gronert GA, Rosenberg H: Management of patients in whom trismus occurs following succinylcholine. Anesthesiology 68:653–655, 1988

Miller RD (ed): Anesthesia, 4th ed, pp 1075–1093. New York, Churchill Livingstone, 1994

O'Flynn RP, Schutak JG, Rosenberg H: Masseter muscle rigidity and malignant hyperthermia susceptibility in pediatric patients. An update on management and diagnosis. Anesthesiology 80(6): 1228–1233, 1994

Rosenberg H, Fletcher JE: Masseter muscle rigidity and malignant hyperthermia susceptibility. Anesth Analg 65:161–164, 1985

Schwartz L, Rockoff MA, Koka BV: Masseter spasm with anesthesia incidence and implications. Anesthesiology 61:722–775, 1984

Van der Spek AFL, Fang WB, Ashton-Miller JA et al: Increased masticatory muscle stiffness during limb muscle flaccidity associated with succinylcholine administration. Anesthesiology 69:11–16, 1988

C.5. Twenty minutes into the procedure, the patient developed increasing tachycardia with ventricular premature beats and mottled skin. What emergency measures would you take?

Although tachycardia may arise from other more common causes (e.g., light plane of anesthesia and hypovolemia), its association with mottled skin in this patient—who is susceptible to the syndrome of malignant hyperthermia—is the first key to the onset of the syndrome. End-expiratory CO_2 should be monitored, and if rising, this constitutes a critical emergency. The following steps should be taken immediately:

• Stop all anesthetics and surgery.
• Administer 100% oxygen.

- Hyperventilate the patient.
- Check the machine and eliminate vaporizers and soda lime from the circuit. If possible, get another machine with a new circuit and no soda lime canister or vaporizer.
- Employ a non-rebreathing circuit.
- Establish lines—a wide-bore cannula for central venous pressure, arterial line (if not already in place), Foley catheter, nasogastric tube.
- Administer specific drug therapy—start dantrolene sodium early while muscle perfusion is still present. An initial intravenous dose of 2.5 mg/kg should be followed by repeated doses of 1 to 2 mg/kg to a total of 10 mg/kg depending on the patient's response.
- Initiate aggressive cooling immediately for rapidly increasing temperatures and for those above 40°C—methods for cooling include the following: surface cooling with the patient on a cooling blanket and packed in ice; gastric, rectal, or peritoneal lavage with iced saline; iced intravenous fluids; and pump bypass with a heat exchanger. Cooling should be stopped when the patient's temperature falls below 38°C to prevent inadvertent hypothermia.
- Treat acidosis with sodium bicarbonate (2 mEq/kg initial dose) and titrate as necessary).
- Treat hyperkalemia with sodium bicarbonate, insulin, and 20% dextrose.
- Treat arrhythmias with procainamide (15 mg/kg), avoid calcium channel blockers if dantrolene has been given.
- Maintain urine output with mannitol or furosemide.
- Provide energy substrate with 20% to 50% dextrose with insulin.
- Provide cardiorespiratory support.
- Seek help in conducting the regimen.
- Monitor the pertinent signs very closely.
- The Malignant Hyperthermia Association of the United States (MHAUS) can be contacted: MHAUS, P.O. Box 3231, Darien, CT 06820. Hotline: 1-800-MH-HYPER; ask for Index Zero.

Miller RD (ed): Anesthesia, 4th ed, pp 1075–1093. New York, Churchill Livingstone, 1994

Rosenberg H: Malignant hyperthermia and other anesthesia induced myodystrophies. ASA Annual Refresher Course Lectures #126, 1997

C.6. What modalities would you monitor closely during management of the crisis?

The modalities that should be monitored closely include the following:

- Pulse oximetry
- Electrocardiogram
- Temperature
- Arterial blood pressure
- Urine output
- Central venous pressure
- Arterial blood gases
- Capnography

Miller RD (ed): Anesthesia, 4th ed, pp 1075–1093. New York, Churchill Livingstone, 1994

Rosenberg H: Malignant hyperthermia and other anesthesia induced myodystrophies. ASA Annual Refresher Course Lectures #126, 1997

D. Postoperative Management

D.1. What complications may follow this syndrome?

One should be alert to possible late complications of malignant hyperthermia, which include consumption coagulopathy, acute renal failure, hypothermia, hyperkalemia, pulmonary edema, muscle edema and necrosis, neurologic sequelae, and syndrome recurrence.

Gronert GA: Malignant hyperthermia. ASA Refresher Courses in Anesthesiology 17:107–115, 1989

Miller RD (ed): Anesthesia, 4th ed, pp 1075–1093. New York, Churchill Livingstone, 1994

Rosenberg H: Malignant hyperthermia and other anesthesia induced myodystrophies. ASA Annual Refresher Course Lectures #126, 1997

D.2. What would be your follow-up on this case?

The vigorous therapy started in the operating room should be continued in the immediate postoperative period. This includes maintaining the following:

- Cardiovascular stability
- Body temperature below 38°C
- Urine output
- Normal coagulation
- Acid-base and electrolyte balance
- Along with the above measures, dantrolene sodium should be administered for at least 3 days after successful treatment of the syndrome.

Gronert GA: Malignant hyperthermia. ASA Refresher Courses in Anesthesiology 17:107–115, 1989

D.3. What would you advise the patient and the family?

The patient should be warned of the dangerous nature of this syndrome and should be advised to carry an identification band at all times. The pedigree of the family should be prepared and the members should be investigated for susceptibility to this syndrome and issued Medic Alert bands accordingly.

Malignant Hyperthermia Association of United States (MHAUS) has been active since 1981 and offers current information and advice on patient management. The following are some useful contact numbers:

Emergency Hotline: 1-800-MH-HYPER (1-800-644-9737)
Outside U.S. call: 1(315) 428-7924.
Address: MHAUS, 32 South Main Street, P.O. Box 1609, Sherburne, NY 13815
Phone: 1-800-98-MHAUS
FAX-on-demand: 1-800-440-9990
Internet: through Gasnet http://www.gasnet.med.Yale.edu

Gronert GA: Malignant hyperthermia. ASA Refresher Courses in Anesthesiology 17:107–115, 1989

Miller RD (ed): Anesthesia, 4th ed, pp 1075–1093. New York, Churchill Livingstone, 1994

Rosenberg H: Malignant hyperthermia and other anesthesia induced myodystrophies. ASA Annual Refresher Course Lectures #126, 1997

Prolonged Apnea

50

Alan Van Poznak

After eating a large meal, a young woman in the first trimester of pregnancy experienced severe lower abdominal pain, vaginal bleeding, and great weakness. In getting to the hospital, she fell down stairs and struck her head. On arrival, she was unresponsive and in frank shock. A pelvic mass was found and emergency laparotomy was proposed for presumed ruptured ectopic pregnancy.

Anesthesia was induced with a rapid-sequence technique including succinylcholine. The patient remained apneic, not only throughout the procedure, but also in the recovery room. Her husband arrived and stated that several other members of her family had had similar difficulty.

A. Medical Disease and Differential Diagnosis

This case is presented to stimulate a review of several other conditions that are treated elsewhere in this book and to which the reader is referred. These include anesthesia for the patient with a full stomach, anesthesia for the patient in shock, and anesthesia for the patient with head trauma. The reader is also referred to the parts of this book that discuss the normal mechanism of neuromuscular transmission, particularly with respect to the acetylcholine theory.

1. Describe the humoral events in normal neuromuscular transmission.
2. What is acetylcholinesterase?
3. What is serum cholinesterase?
4. How does succinylcholine resemble acetylcholine?
5. How does succinylcholine differ from acetylcholine?
6. What is the incidence of atypical cholinesterase activity?
7. How many genes are known to be involved in the determination of serum cholinesterase?
8. What is the significance of cholinesterase units?
9. What is the significance of the dibucaine number?
10. Discuss possible cardiovascular effects of succinylcholine. What patients are especially at risk?
11. What are some factors that can lower pseudocholinesterase levels?
12. Should succinylcholine be routinely used in pediatric anesthesia?

B. Preoperative Preparation

The reader is referred to the sections on anesthesia for patients with full stomach, in shock, and with head trauma. In this emergency situation there was no opportunity to be aware of the atypical cholinesterase variant.

C. Intraoperative Management

The reader is again referred to the sections mentioned above. However, the anesthesiologist should have made some attempt to have the patient regain spontaneous respiration and should be concerned that breathing has not returned.

D. Postoperative Management

1. What is the differential diagnosis for postoperative apnea? How would you treat it?

A. Medical Disease and Differential Diagnosis

A.1. Describe the humoral events in normal neuromuscular transmission.

Quanta of acetylcholine are liberated from nerve terminals by the arrival of nerve action potentials. The acetylcholine crosses the synaptic cleft and attaches to the receptor sites on the sarcolemma, thereby causing the depolarization known as the "end-plate potential." If the threshold is exceeded, an action potential invades the muscle cell membrane and spreads up and down its surface much like the nerve action potential. The liberated acetylcholine is hydrolyzed by cholinesterase and then resynthesized by choline acetylase.

Standaert FG: Release of transmitter at the neuromuscular junction. Br J Anaesth 54:131, 1982

A.2. What is acetylcholinesterase?

Acetylcholinesterase is a relatively specific enzyme that hydrolyzes acetylcholine faster than it does other choline esters. It is found in red blood cells, the central nervous system, and the neuromuscular junction. It is responsible for hydrolyzing and inactivating the acetylcholine produced during normal neuromuscular transmission. It does not hydrolyze succinylcholine and, in fact, is inhibited by the drug.

Stanbury JB, Wyngaarden JB, Fredrickson DS: The Metabolic Basis of Inherited Disease, 3rd ed, p 1730. New York, McGraw-Hill, 1972

Taylor P, Schumacher M, MacPhee-Quingley K et al: The structure of acetylcholinesterase: Relationship to its function and cellular disposition. Trends Neurosci 10:93, 1987

A.3. What is serum cholinesterase?

This enzyme, also called cholinesterase, pseudocholinesterase, butyrylcholinesterase, and nonspecific cholinesterase, hydrolyzes many choline esters, including succinylcholine. It is found in many human tissues, but not in the red blood cell. It is synthesized in the liver. Its physiologic function is unknown, but it may hydrolyze choline esters, such as propionylcholine and butyrylcholine, which may be formed by bacterial action in the gut and also by the enzyme systems responsible for the formation of acetylcholine.

Massoulie J, Bon S: Molecular forms of cholinesterase and acetylcholinesterase in vertebrates. Annu Rev Neurosci 5:57, 1982

Pantuck EJ: Plasma cholinesterase: Gene and variations. Anesth Analg 77:380–386, 1993

Stanbury JB, Wyngaarden JB, Fredrickson DS: The Metabolic Basis of Inherited Disease, 3rd ed, p 1730. New York, McGraw-Hill, 1972

Whittaker M: Plasma cholinesterase variants and the anesthetist. Anaesthesia 35:174, 1980

A.4. How does succinylcholine resemble acetylcholine?

Succinylcholine causes depolarization of the postsynaptic membrane.

Durant MW, Katz RI: Suxamethonium. Br J Anaesth 54:195, 1982

Hardman JG, Limbird LE, Molinoff PB et al (eds): Goodman and Gilman's The Pharmacological Basis of Therapeutics, 9th ed, pp 183–189. New York, McGraw-Hill, 1996

A.5. How does succinylcholine differ from acetylcholine?

Succinylcholine cannot be hydrolyzed by acetylcholinesterase. Instead, it must undergo much slower hydrolysis by the nonspecific plasma cholinesterase.

Albuquerque EX, Akaike A, Shaw KP et al: The interaction of anticholinesterase agents with the acetylcholine receptor-ionic channel complex. Fundam Appl Toxicol 14:S27, 1984

Stanbury JB, Wyngaarden JB, Fredrickson DS: The Metabolic Basis of Inherited Disease, 3rd ed, p 1730. New York, McGraw-Hill, 1972

Viby-Mogensen J: Correlation of succinylcholine duration of action with plasma cholinesterase activity in subjects with the genotypically normal enzyme. Anesthesiology 53:517, 1980

A.6. What is the incidence of atypical cholinesterase activity?

The incidence of atypical cholinesterase varies with the population studied, but it is approximately 1:2800 in the general population of the United States, with a 1:1 male:female ratio.

Kalow W, Genest K: A method for detection of atypical forms of human serum cholinesterase: Determination of dibucaine numbers. Can J Biochem 35:339, 1957

Stanbury JB, Wyngaarden JB, Fredrickson DS: The Metabolic Basis of Inherited Disease, 3rd ed, p 1730. New York, McGraw-Hill, 1972

A.7. How many genes are known to be involved in the determination of serum cholinesterase?

Four alleles have been identified as being involved in the determination of serum cholinesterase. They include the normal (N), dibucaine-resistant (D), fluoride-resistant (F), and the silent (S). These four genes can form ten genotypes, of which six produce a marked decrease in the hydrolysis of succinylcholine (D-D, F-F, S-S, D-F, D-S, F-S; see Table 50-1).

Pantuck EJ: Plasma cholinesterase: Gene and variations. Anesth Analg 77:380, 1993

A.8. What is the significance of cholinesterase units?

Cholinesterase units indicate the affinity of the enzyme for the substrate. Various test substrates have been used, among them benzylcholine and butyrylthiocholine. Unitage differs according to the laboratory method employed. The correlation between

Table 50-1. Human Plasma Cholinesterase Variants[a]

COMMON NAME	PHENOTYPIC DESCRIPTION	AMINO ACID ALTERATION	DNA ALTERATION
Usual	Normal	None	None
Atypical	Dibucaine resistant	70 Asp → Gly	nt 209 (GAT → GGT)
Silent-1	Silent, no activity	117 Gly → frameshift	nt 351 (GGT → GGAG)
Silent-2	Silent, no activity	6 Ile → frameshift	nt 16 (ATT → TT)
Silent-3	Silent, no activity	500 Tyr → stop	nt 1500 (TAT → TAA)
Fluoride-1	Fluoride resistant	243 Thr → Met	nt 728 (ACG → ATG)
Fluoride-2	Fluoride resistant	390 Gly → Val	nt 1169 (GGT → GTT)
K variant	K polymorphism	539 Ala → Thr	nt 1615 (GCA → ACA)
H variant	H polymorphism	142 Val → Met	nt 424 (GTG → ATG)
J variant	J polymorphism	497 Glu → Val	nt 1490 (GAA → GTA)
		539 Ala → Thr	nt 1615 (GCA → ACA)

nt, nucleotide.
[a] *Shown are variants whose structures were published before 1993.*
(Reprinted with permission from Pantuck EJ: Plasma cholinesterase: Gene and variations. Anesth Analg 77:380, 1993)

duration of succinylcholine neuromuscular blockade and plasma cholinesterase activity is shown in Figure 50-1.

Stanbury JB, Wyngaarden JB, Fredrickson DS: The Metabolic Basis of Inherited Disease, 3rd ed, p 1734. New York, McGraw-Hill, 1972

Viby-Mogensen J: Correlation of succinylcholine duration of action with plasma cholinesterase activity in subjects with the genotypically normal enzyme. Anesthesiology 53:517, 1980

A.9. What is the significance of the dibucaine number?

The dibucaine number is used to identify the heterozygote. Dibucaine in 10^{-5} M concentration produces the maximal difference in inhibition between the usual and the atypical forms of serum cholinesterase. The term "dibucaine number" has been applied to the percentage of inhibition of serum cholinesterase. The usual homozygote has a dibucaine number of approximately 80, the atypical homozygote has a value below 30, and the heterozygote has a value between 45 and 69. The relationship between dibucaine number and duration of succinylcholine neuromuscular blockade is shown in Table 50-2.

Kalow W, Genest K: A method of detection of atypical forms of human serum cholinesterase: Determination of dibucaine numbers. Can J Biochem 35:339–353, 1957

Table 50-2. Relationship Between Dibucaine Number and Duration of Succinylcholine Neuromuscular Blockade

TYPE OF PSEUDO-CHOLINESTERASE	GENOTYPE	FREQUENCY	DIBUCAINE NUMBER[a]	RESPONSE TO SUCCINYLCHOLINE OR MIVACURIUM
Homozygous typical	$E^u E^u$	Normal	70–80	Normal
Heterozygous	$E^u E^a$	1/480	50–60	Slightly prolonged
Homozygous atypical	$E^a E^a$	1/3,200	20–30	Markedly prolonged

[a] The dibucaine number indicates the percentage of enzyme inhibited.

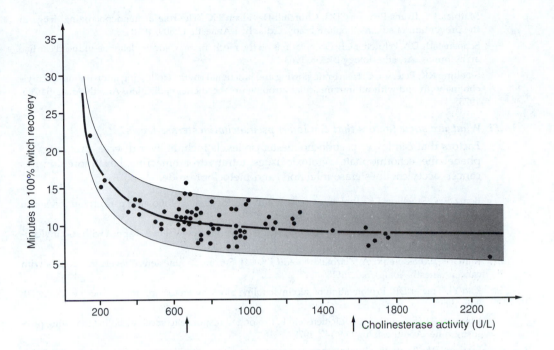

Figure 50-1. Relationship between enzymatic activity and times to 100% recovery of control twitch height following administration of succinylcholine. 1 mg/kg IV to 70 patients with the normal plasma cholinesterase genotype. The fitted regression line and 95% prediction region are given. Arrows indicate the normal range of plasma cholinesterase activity. (Reprinted with permission from Viby-Mogensen J: Correlation of succinylcholine duration of action with plasma cholinesterase activity in subjects with the genotypically normal enzyme. Anesthesiology 53:517, 1980)

A.10. Discuss possible cardiovascular effects of succinylcholine. What patients are especially at risk?

Succinylcholine stimulates all cholinergic autonomic receptors, including nicotinic receptors in both sympathetic and parasympathetic ganglia as well as muscarinic receptors in the sinus node of the heart. Cardiac arrhythmias may easily arise as a result of this generalized autonomic stimulation. These arrhythmias include sinus bradycardia, nodal (junctional) rhythms, and ventricular arrhythmias.

Craythorne NWB, Turndorf H, Dripps RD: Changes in pulse rate and rhythm associated with the use of succinylcholine in anesthetized patients. Anesthesiology 21:465, 1960

Galindo AHF, Davis TB: Succinylcholine and cardiac excitability. Anesthesiology 23:32, 1962

Goat VA, Feldman SA: The dual action of suxamethonium on the isolated rabbit heart. Anaesthesia 27:149, 1972

Leigh MD, McCoy DD, Belton KM et al: Bradycardia following intravenous administration of succinylcholine chloride to infants and children. Anesthesiology 18:698, 1957

Leiman BC, Katz J, Butler BD: Mechanisms of succinylcholine-induced arrhythmias in hypoxic or hypoxic:hypercarbic dogs. Anesth Analg 66:1292, 1987

Mathias JA, Evans-Prosser CDG, Churchill-Davidson HC: The role of nondepolarizing drugs in the prevention of suxamethonium bradycardia. Br J Anaesth 42:609, 1970

Schoenstadt DA, Whitcher CE: Observations on the mechanism of succinylcholine-induced cardiac arrhythmias. Anesthesiology 24:358, 1963

Stoelting RK, Peterson C: Heart-rate slowing and junctional rhythm following intravenous succinylcholine with and without intramuscular atropine preanesthetic medication. Anesth Analg 54:705, 1975

A.11. What are some factors that can lower pseudocholinesterase levels?

Factors that can lower pseudocholinesterase levels include liver disease, pregnancy, phenelzine, echothiophate, cytotoxic drugs, tetrahydroaminacrine, hexafluorenium, cancer, acetylcholinesterase inhibitors, and metoclopramide.

Bentz EW, Stoelting RK: Prolonged response to succinylcholine following pancuronium reversal with pyridostigmine. Anesthesiology 44:258, 1976

Foldes FF, Rendell-Baker L, Birch JH: Causes and prevention of prolonged apnea with succinylcholine. Anesth Analg 35:609, 1956

Kaniaris P, Fassoulaki A, Tiarmakopoulou K et al: Serum cholinesterase levels in patients with cancer. Anesth Analg 58:82, 1979

Kao YJ, Turner DR: Prolongation of succinylcholine block by metoclopramide. Anesthesiology 70:905, 1989

Kopman AF, Strachovsky G, Lichtenstein L: Prolonged response to succinylcholine following physostigmine. Anesthesiology 49:142, 1978

Lindsay PA, Tumley J: Suxamethonium apnoea mask by tetrahydroaminacrine. Anaesthesia 33:620, 1978

Pantuck EJ, Pantuck CB: Cholinesterases and anticholinesterases, p 143. In: Katz RL (ed): Muscle Relaxants. Amsterdam, Excerpta Medica, 1975

A.12. Should succinylcholine be routinely used in pediatric anesthesia?

Succinylcholine should probably not be routinely used in pediatric anesthesia unless an urgent need is seen to secure the airway rapidly. The increasing number of reports of adverse cardiovascular reactions and the introduction of new shorter acting nondepolarizing muscle relaxants have decreased the need for the routine use of succinylcholine, and have caused a modification of the package insert as promulgated by the Food and Drug Administration.

Delphin E, Jackson D, Rothstein P: Use of succinylcholine during elective pediatric anesthesia should be re-evaluated. Anesth Analg 66:1190, 1987

Rosenberg H, Gronert GA: Intractable cardiac arrest in children given succinylcholine. Anesthesiology 77:1054, 1992

Schulte-Sasse VU, Eberlein HJ, Schumucker I et al: Should the use of succinylcholine during pediatric anesthesia be reevaluated? Anesteziol Reanimatol 18:13, 1993

D. Postoperative Management

D.1. What is the differential diagnosis for postoperative apnea? How would you treat it?

The differential diagnosis for postoperative apnea includes the following:
- Residual anesthetic agent

- Residual narcotic
- Residual muscle relaxant
- Hypocarbia
- Results of head trauma
- Occurrence of some medical complication during anesthesia, such as stroke or embolism

Treatment of the patient would include discontinuance of anesthetics, reversal of narcotics with naloxone, reversal of nondepolarizing relaxants with atropine and neostigmine, determination of arterial blood gases and appropriate adjustment of ventilation, and such other treatment as might be appropriate for the head trauma, including steroids and hyperosmotic solutions to lessen brain swelling. Ventilatory and circulatory support should be continued while arrangements are made to determine cholinesterase unitage. Should these indicate an atypical cholinesterase, the patient and her family should be so informed. She should also be given a letter to be transmitted to any anesthesiologist who might provide care for her in the future.

51 Burns

Gregg S. Hartman

A 48-year-old man presented in the emergency room after being transported from the scene of a house fire. He sustained 50% second- and third-degree burns over his face, neck, chest, abdomen, and upper extremities. Blood pressure (BP), 160/100 mm Hg; pulse rate (PR), 140/min sinus rhythm respiratory rate (RR), 35/min; weight, 75 kg.

A. Medical Disease and Differential Diagnosis

1. How are burns classified?
2. What functions does the skin perform?
3. How is the severity of a burn injury quantitated?
4. What modifications in these calculations of burn size need to be made for children versus adults?
5. What is the prognosis for this patient, and how is it determined?
6. What pathophysiologic changes characterize the acute and subacute phases of the burn injury?
7. This patient exhibited stridor, dyspnea, and wheezing. What are the most likely causes? What further evaluation is indicated?
8. What is an inhalation injury? What effects do toxic metabolites have on the tracheo-bronchial tree?
9. How is an inhalation injury diagnosed and treated?
10. This patient required intubation. How would you proceed?
11. What is carbon monoxide poisoning? How is it treated?
12. How is the oxygen content of the blood calculated?
13. What cardiovascular changes typify the burn injury?
14. How are fluids managed during the acute and subacute phases of a burn injury?
15. What other organ systems are affected by a burn injury?
16. How is the immune system altered by a burn injury?
17. What hematologic changes can be anticipated in a burn injury?
18. What changes in liver function occur? What are the anesthetic implications of such changes?
19. What are Curling's ulcers? How are they prevented?

B. Preoperative Evaluation and Preparation

1. What are the various operative and management options?
2. What is tangential excision/split-thickness skin grafting (TE/STSG)? What are the principles of this grafting technique?
3. What is the advantage of early TE/STSG?
4. What are the particular concerns in the preoperative evaluation of a burned patient?
5. On the fifth postburn day, this patient was intubated and monitored with an arterial line and a pulmonary artery (PA) catheter. Vital signs were BP 80/45, PR 140/min, car-

diac output 9 liters/min, pulmonary artery (PA) pressure 20/10 mm Hg. What hemody-namic derangement did this patient exhibit? What was the cause? What were the therapeutic options?

6. Why did this deterioration occur?
7. What information can be obtained from an arterial line and a PA catheter? How are these calculations performed?
8. What is the definition of shock? What are the different classifications of shock?
9. Describe an algorithm for treating shock.
10. What are the different adrenergic receptors? What are the different adrenergic ago-nists?
11. What are amrinone and milrinone? Discuss their pharmacology.
12. The patient's arterial blood gases (ABGs) on ventilator settings of tidal volume (TV) 1000 (ml), RR 16/min, F_IO_2 50%, and positive end-expiratory pressure (PEEP) 5 cm H_2O were as follows: pH 7.32; P_{CO_2}, 48 mm Hg; P_{O_2}, 56 mm Hg; O_2 saturation, 88%. What are the most likely causes of the hypoxemia in this patient?

C. Intraoperative Management

1. What monitors would you employ?
2. This patient was already intubated. If he had not been intubated, how should you have proceeded with the anesthetic induction?
3. What is the innervation of the larynx and trachea?
4. What is the anesthetic choice for this patient? Why?
5. What is normothermia for a burned patient?
6. How is temperature best maintained?
7. Why is a heated-humidified circuit used?
8. What derangements occur with hypothermia?
9. What forms of intravenous (IV) access are required?
10. What is Poiseuille's equation for resistance during laminar flow? What is its signifi-cance?
11. What relaxant would you choose and why?
12. How are the neuromuscular blockers pancuronium, curare, metocurine, atracurium, vecuronium, doxacurium, and pipecuronium metabolized and eliminated? Which of them has significant histamine release?
13. What is the difference between metabolism and elimination of drugs?
14. Why is succinylcholine contraindicated for patients with a burn injury? For how long is it contraindicated?
15. How are the doses of nondepolarizing muscle relaxants affected by a burn injury?
16. What additional complications are associated with electrical burns?
17. What is myoglobinuria? What are common causes? What therapy is indicated?

D. Postoperative Management

1. How would you monitor this patient during transport?
2. This patient was anesthetized with a narcotic–nitrous oxide–relaxant technique. How could hypoxemia occur when nitrous oxide is discontinued and the patient is breathing room air?
3. The patient was shivering in the recovery room on emergence from anesthesia. What are the problems associated with this situation?

A. Medical Disease and Differential Diagnosis

A.1. How are burns classified?

Burns are classified in three categories by the depth of destruction of the cellular layers of the skin. Superficial or first-degree burns consist of destruction of the epidermal tissues. Partial-thickness or second-degree burns exhibit both epidermal and dermal destruction. Although thermal damage has occurred to the deeper dermal structures, the basement membrane is intact and hence architectural integrity of the skin is preserved. Blisters and bullae are common. Regeneration from epithelial cells lining the sweat ducts and hair follicles often occurs early in the course of healing. Full-thickness or third-degree burns result in destruction of all the layers of the skin: epidermis, dermis, and the dermal appendages. Because these epithelial elements are destroyed, third-degree burns will not heal spontaneously, and they will require skin grafting. Coagulation and thrombosis of deep veins may also be present.

Fourth-degree burns refer to deep thermal injuries involving bony tendon plus muscle: treatment may require elaborate debridement or even amputation.

Schwartz SI, Shives GT, Spencer FC (eds): Principles of Surgery, 6th ed, pp 230–232. New York, McGraw Hill, 1994

A.2. What functions does the skin perform?

The skin is the largest organ of the body with surface area ranging from 1.5 to 2.0 m² in the adult. It performs the important functions of protection from microorganism invasion, thermal regulation, fluid and electrolyte homeostasis, and sensation (touch, temperature, pain). The pathophysiology seen with thermal injury results from the destruction of the skin and the derangements in the performance of these functions. The skin also has metabolic functions including vitamin D metabolism.

Herndon DN (ed): Total Burn Care, pp 63–64. Philadelphia, WB Saunders, 1996

Hollinshead WH: Textbook of Anatomy, pp 141–142. Hagerstown, MD, Harper & Row, 1974

A.3. How is the severity of a burn injury quantitated?

The severity of a burn injury is based on the amount of surface area burned. In the "rule of nines" method of estimation, the major body parts are portioned as follows:

Head and neck	9%
Upper extremities	9% each
Chest (anterior and posterior)	9% each
Abdomen	9%
Lower back	9%
Lower extremities	18% each
Perineum	1%

Herndon DN (ed): Total Burn Care, pp 35–37. Philadelphia, WB Saunders, 1996

Table 51-1. Percentage of Total Body Surface Area by Age

AREA	BIRTH–1 YEAR	1–4 YEARS	5–9 YEARS	10–14 YEARS	15 YEARS	ADULT
Head	19	17	13	11	9	7
Neck	2	2	2	2	2	2
Anterior trunk	13	13	13	13	13	13
Posterior trunk	13	13	13	13	13	13
Right buttock	2.5	2.5	2.5	2.5	2.5	2.5
Left buttock	2.5	2.5	2.5	2.5	2.5	2.5
Genitalia	1	1	1	1	1	1
Right upper arm	4	4	4	4	4	4
Left upper arm	4	4	4	4	4	4
Right lower arm	3	3	3	3	3	3
Left lower arm	3	3	3	3	3	3
Right hand	2.5	2.5	2.5	2.5	2.5	2.5
Left hand	2.5	2.5	2.5	2.5	2.5	2.5
Right thigh	5.5	6.5	8	8.5	9	9.5
Left thigh	5.5	6.5	8	8.5	9	9.5
Right leg	5	5	5.5	6	6.5	7
Left leg	5	5	5.5	6	6.5	7
Right foot	3.5	3.5	3.5	3.5	3.5	3.5
Left foot	3.5	3.5	3.5	3.5	3.5	3.5

Note how the percentage of the total body surface area, represented by the head and lower extremity, changes with age.

A.4. What modifications in these calculations of burn size need to be made for children versus adults?

The "rule of nines" is modified in children because the head and neck are proportionately larger than in adults. Age-adjusted nomograms are a better method because they reflect the gradual change in relative body surface areas with age (Table 51-1).

Davis JH (ed): Clinical Surgery, pp 2840–2841. St. Louis, CV Mosby, 1987

A.5. What is the prognosis for this patient, and how is it determined?

The prognosis for this patient is poor. Statistical survival based on total body surface area (TBSA) alone would predict a <50% chance of survival. Additional factors play a role in this determination. These include age, size and depth of burn, associated pulmonary injury, general medical condition prior to injury, and other injuries sustained. The major early cause of death is asphyxia. If the patient survives the fire itself, prognosis depends on early cardiovascular resuscitation. The most common cause of long-term mortality, however, is septic complications.

A.6. What pathophysiologic changes characterize the acute and subacute phases of the burn injury?

Burn shock is a complex process of circulatory and microcirculatory dysfunction. Acute changes result directly from destruction of the skin and related elements. Destruction of capillary beds surrounding the wound results in leakage of protein-rich fluid and its sequestration in the interstitial spaces. Cellular insults result in membrane alteration and cellular swelling. The fluid sequestration results in hemoconcentration and decreased circulating blood volume. Increased secretion of antidiuretic hormone (ADH) stimulates renal conservation mechanisms; urine output drops markedly or can even cease. Alteration in vascular beds occurs in areas distant to the burn injury as well. Membranes throughout the vascular tree exhibit increased permeability. This increased permeability has its most morbid manifestation in the lungs, where resultant pulmonary edema can be fatal.

Herndon DN (ed): Total Burn Care, pp 44–52. Philadelphia, WB Saunders, 1996

A.7. This patient exhibited stridor, dyspnea, and wheezing. What are the most likely causes? What further evaluation is indicated?

This patient probably sustained an inhalation injury. Until proved otherwise, a respiratory injury should be assumed to have occurred in any patient with respiratory difficulty or if the burn was sustained in a closed space. The presence of carbonaceous sputum, perioral soot, burns to the face and neck, or respiratory distress (e.g., stridor, dyspnea, or wheezing) are indications for further examination of the airway. The pharynx and upper trachea have a large capacity for cooling gases. Therefore, direct thermal injury below the cords is uncommon except with steam injuries. Because the thermal capacity of water is 4000 times that of air, thermal injury to structures deep in the tracheobronchial tree is possible with steam inhalation. Definitive examination is achieved with either direct or fiberoptic examination of the upper airway, vocal cords, and tracheobronchial tree.

Herndon DN (ed): Total Burn Care, pp 184–192. Philadelphia, WB Saunders, 1996

Rue LW III, Cioff WG Jr, Mason ADJR et al: Improved survival of burned patients with inhalation injury. Arch Surg 128:772–780, 1993

A.8. What is an inhalation injury? What effects do toxic metabolites have on the tracheobronchial tree?

An inhalation injury occurs when hot gases and reactive particles are conducted into the tracheobronchial tree. Airborne toxins react rapidly with the mucus of the airway to form strong acids and alkalis. Either directly or from subsequent tissue reaction, these substances result in wheezing, bronchospasm, corrosion, and airway edema. In addition, particulate matter interferes with mucociliary function, impairing bacterial clearance.

Herndon DN (ed): Total Burn Care, pp 184–185. Philadelphia, WB Saunders, 1996

A.9. How is an inhalation injury diagnosed and treated?

Diagnosis depends on a high degree of suspicion, critical examination, and laboratory testing. Often the early signs and symptoms are minimal. The pharynx and vocal cords may be erythematous and edematous or simply soot stained. Typical x-rays early after the injury are normal; this is the "clear or lucid interval." Arterial blood gases and carbon monoxide levels may be useful in determining the current degree of insult. A low threshold is found for elective intubation of a suspicious airway. With fluid resuscitation, swelling can increase dramatically, with the potential for complete airway obstruction. Intubation in this setting may be extremely difficult or impossible. Conversely, little morbidity is associated with several days of elective intubation in the setting of appropriate sedation.

Herndon DN (ed): Total Burn Care, pp 186–189. Philadelphia, WB Saunders, 1996

A.10. *This patient required intubation. How would you proceed?*

First, all equipment should be ready and checked. In this elective setting, nasotracheal intubation is preferred because it is often better tolerated for longer periods and somewhat more easily secured in place. Topical anesthesia with either lidocaine ointment-coated nasal airways or 4% cocaine-soaked pledgets may be used. Cocaine has the added advantage of being a vasoconstrictor. Vasoconstriction can be achieved, however, through the use of phenylephrine drops. Topical anesthesia of the airway is achieved with either Cetacaine or lidocaine spray. Further blockade may be attained by superior laryngeal nerve and transtracheal blocks. Topical anesthesia for a nasal intubation can also be achieved by the rapid injection of 4 ml of 4% lidocaine mixed with 3 mg phenylephrine directed at the superior or posterior aspect of the nasal canal. The patient is preoxygenated and then sedated with small incremental doses of midazolam (1 mg IV) or diazepam (2.5 mg IV) until mild slurring of speech is observed. Fiberoptic-assisted intubation is then performed.

Ovassapian A: Fiberoptic Airway Endoscopy in Anesthesia and Critical Care, pp 45–49. New York, Raven Press, 1990

A.11. *What is carbon monoxide poisoning? How is it treated?*

Carbon monoxide is the leading cause of hypoxia in survivors of burn injuries. Carbon monoxide has a 200 times greater affinity for hemoglobin than does oxygen and therefore displaces oxygen from its hemoglobin binding sites. Fortunately, this reaction is a competitive, reversible one, so oxygen therapy should be instituted immediately. The half-life for carbon monoxide elimination from hemoglobin can be shortened from 4 hours to 45 minutes with an inspired oxygen concentration of 100%. It should be remembered that, although the PaO_2 may be normal, the actual content of oxygen in the blood is markedly reduced.

Fein A, Leffa, Hopewell PC: Pathophysiology and management of the complications resulting from fire and the inhaled products of combustion: Review of the literature. Crit Care Med 94:98, 1980

Herndon DN (ed): Total Burn Care, p 187. Philadelphia, WB Saunders, 1996

A.12. *How is the oxygen content of the blood calculated?*

Oxygen is transported in the blood, either bound to hemoglobin or dissolved in solution. The equation is as follows:

$$\{1.34 \times Hb \ (g \ \%) \times \% \ sat\} + \{0.003 \times Pa \ O_2\} = O_2 \ content, \ ml/dl$$

Nunn JF: Nunn's Applied Respiratory Physiology, 4th ed, p 283. Boston, Butterworth Heinemann, 1993

A.13. *What cardiovascular changes typify the burn injury?*

Damage to the cardiovascular system develops in several phases. Acutely, fluid sequestration in the burned area and from capillary leak caused by direct thermal destruction of the capillary membranes result in massive shifts of fluid and proteins from the intravascular to interstitial spaces. This derangement accounts for the marked acute decrease in circulating blood volume with a corresponding fall in cardiac filling pressures (preload). This is the syndrome of burn shock. Cardiac output is depressed as much as 50% from baseline because of the fall in preload. Intense vasoconstriction from catecholamine release may further compromise forward flow. In animal models, a myocardial depressant protein has been isolated that may be a mediator for additional depression of cardiac output through a direct action of myocardial contractility. Similar molecules have been found in the serum of burn patients.

Herndon DN (ed): Total Burn Care, pp 44–52. Philadelphia, WB Saunders, 1996

Sugi K, Theissen J, Traber LD et al: Impact of carbon monoxide on cardiopulmonary dysfunction after smoke inhalation injury. Circ Res 66:69–75, 1990

A.14. How are fluids managed during the acute and subacute phases of a burn injury?

Rapid restoration of blood volume is essential for improving survival and limiting renal damage from hypoperfusion. The amount of fluid shift from the intravascular to the extravascular space will be roughly proportional to the extent of the burn and the patient's size. Numerous formulae exist for calculating fluid requirements, varying with respect to their crystalloid versus colloid content. The Parkland or Baxter formula is commonly followed. The initial resuscitation is performed with isotonic crystalloid fluids, with colloid solutions being added only after the first day. Most investigators feel that the increased capillary permeability of the early burn wound would result in leaking of any exogenously administered colloids. Proteins leaked into the interstitial spaces through these fragile membranes would remain sequestered there and exert their oncotic effect for a long time. Following resuscitation, fluid administration is divided between maintenance of water and glucose, some colloid to maintain plasma volume, and additional fluid as needed to support hemodynamics and diuresis. Data suggest that children require more fluid for burn shock than adults with similar injury. In both adults and children the adequacy of fluid resuscitation must be constantly assessed by the quantitation of urine output through a Foley catheter and through the use of invasive cardiac monitoring if indicated.

Parkland Formula
Initial (first 24 hours)
- 4 ml/kg/% total body surface area (TBSA) burned
- Composition—isotonic crystalloid (e.g., lactated Ringer's solution, Normosol, normal saline)
- 50% over first 8 hours with 25% over each next 8 hours
- Maintain urine output at 0.5 to 1.0 ml/kg/h

Second 24 hours
- D_5W to maintain urinary output (adults); in children, add 50% to 25% normal saline to avoid hyponatremia
- Colloid solutions (e.g., albumin) amount proportional to burn
  - 30% to 50% burn—0.3 ml/kg/% burn
  - 50% to 70% burn—0.4 ml/kg/% burn

- >70% burn—0.5 ml/kg/% burn

Grareo TA, Cioffi WG, McManus WF et al: Fluid resuscitation of infants and children with massive thermal injury. J. Trauma 28:1656–1659, 1988

Herndon DN (ed): Total Burn Care, pp 53–60. Philadelphia, WB Saunders, 1996

A.15. *What other organ systems are affected by a burn injury?*

A burn injury has effects on many organ systems, including the immune, hematologic, hepatic, and renal systems. It also affects metabolism.

A.16. *How is the immune system altered by a burn injury?*

Infection is the major cause of morbidity and mortality in burn patients who survive the initial insult. Burned skin is a perfect culture medium; organisms colonizing the eschar rapidly gain access to the blood stream. Endotoxins mediate changes in cell integrity. The loss of skin represents an easy route of entry of microorganisms into the body. The presence of many invasive catheters further increases exposure. Compounding these insults, burn patients have an altered immune response, and thus are more susceptible to sepsis. Alterations in phagocytic and chemotactic properties of white cells have been demonstrated. Strict antiseptic precautions must be observed in handling these patients because of their altered immune status and also to minimize cross contamination between patients. Quantitative wound biopsies are used to assess degree of colonization and to aid in determining and modifying antimicrobial therapy. Catheters are changed and cultured routinely every 3 days because they are potential septic foci. Infection also contributes to derangements in the hematologic system.

Herndon DN (ed): Total Burn Care, pp 98–135. Philadelphia, WB Saunders, 1996

A.17. *What hematologic changes can be anticipated in a burn injury?*

Ongoing infection can result in subacute activation of the coagulation cascade. Consumption of circulating procoagulants results in various degrees of coagulopathy. Platelet function is both qualitatively and quantitatively depressed. Red cells are also affected, and they exhibit decreased survival times. Peripheral blood smears show many fragmented and deformed erythrocytes. In addition, burn patients commonly show changes consistent with an inflammatory response of the whole organ including hyperthermia, tachycardia, hyperventilation, and leukocytosis.

Herndon DN (ed): Total Burn Care, p 207. Philadelphia, WB Saunders, 1996

A.18 *What changes in liver function occur? What are the anesthetic implications of such changes?*

Hypoperfusion during burn shock can result in decreased hepatic function, severely depressing the detoxification capacity of the liver. Decreased levels of albumin may result in greater free fractions of bound drugs such as benzodiazepines and phenytoin. In contrast, the injury-stimulated rise in the acute-phase reactant alpha-1-acid-glycoprotein increases the binding of basic drugs such as muscle relaxants, lidocaine, and propranolol.

Herndon DN (ed): Total Burn Care, pp 150–151. Philadelphia, WB Saunders, 1996

Martyn JAJ: The use of neuromuscular relaxants in burn patients. In: Rupp SM (ed): Problems in Anesthesia 3(3):482. Philadelphia, JB Lippincott, 1989

A.19. What are Curling's ulcers? How are they prevented?

Curling's ulcer is an ulcer (stress ulcer) of the duodenum following a severe burn on the surface of the body. Gastric ulceration may also occur. The frequency and severity of both correlate with the size of the injury and without treatment can approach an incidence of 86%. Prophylaxis with antacids and H_2 antagonists greatly lowers the incidence of bleeding from these lesions.

Herndon DN (ed): Total Burn Care, pp 362–363. Philadelphia, WB Saunders, 1996

Pruitt A, Goodwin CW: Stress ulcer disease in the burned patient. World J Surg 5:209–222, 1981

B. Preoperative Evaluation and Preparation

B.1. What are the various operative and management options?

Following initial resuscitation, the burn patient is monitored closely for several days. Areas of full-thickness injury will require grafting for healing. In addition, the burned skin or eschar is a perfect culture medium for bacteria. Initial attempts at controlling infection are through topical antibiotic creams such as silver sulfadiazine (Silvadene). This is painless, has good microbial activity, and is easily applied. No acid-base disturbance occurs with its use; however, prolonged exposure can lead to neutropenia and the development of resistant organisms. Other solutions, such as silver nitrate and mafenide acetate (Sulfamylon) are used, but these have their own complicating side-effects. Silver nitrate can cause deficits in sodium, potassium, and chloride, and it can potentially cause methemoglobinemia. Its staining of the equipment and environment is also problematic. Mafenide acetate is painful on partial-thickness burns, and it causes acidosis secondary to inhibition of carbonic anhydrase. Definitive treatment is excision of the dead eschar.

The exact timing of surgical excision and grafting varies from center to center. Some favor early excision (<24 hours from burn). At The New York Hospital–Cornell Medical Center Burn Unit, the goal is to excise and graft in the first 4 to 7 days following injury.

Herndon DN (ed): Total Burn Care, pp 136–147. Philadelphia, WB Saunders, 1996

B.2. What is tangential excision/split-thickness skin grafting (TE/STSG)? What are the principles of this grafting technique?

Tangential excision/split-thickness skin grafting is a procedure to debride the dead skin and graft on new layers. The burn eschar is sharply excised from the underlying subcutaneous tissue. Brisk capillary bleeding signifies that adequate excision has been achieved and viable tissue uncovered. Skin grafts may be either full thickness or split (partial) thickness. Full-thickness grafts include all layers of epidermis and dermis in their sample. Therefore, the donor site must be closed primarily. Suitable donor sites are the skin folds of the axilla and groin. A tissue expander is commonly used to increase the available donor skin. Full-thickness grafts have the advantage of better cosmesis and durability, and they are also useful when tissue bulk is desired. More commonly, split-thickness skin grafts are used. These grafts are obtained by slicing the superficial layers of the skin through the level of the dermal pegs. Because maturation of skin cells occurs as they migrate superficially, the graft has many viable layers of dermal cells. When placed on a viable bed of subcutaneous tissue, ingrowth of vessels occurs and the graft remains viable. In addition, because the excision of donor skin is through the dermis, the deep basement membrane and skin appendages remain intact. Hence, the donor site will heal on its own, architecturally normal, usually with only mild discoloration.

Herndon DN (ed): Total Burn Care, pp 142–147. Philadelphia, WB Saunders, 1996

B.3. What is the advantage of early TE/STSG?

By excising the burn eschar early (within 7 to 10 days), one can remove the bacterial load quickly and achieve prompt skin coverage, with resultant lessening of septic complications; the hospital and recovery phases are thus shortened. Very early excision, however, has the disadvantage of the patient undergoing a major operation during the resuscitative phase of the injury.

Cultured epithelial autografts are an exacting new technique that can be of great utility in patients with large TBSA burns in which donor sites are few in number.

Davis JH (ed): Clinical Surgery, pp 2869–2875. St. Louis, CV Mosby, 1987

Herndon DN (ed): Total Burn Care, pp 136–147. Philadelphia, WB Saunders, 1996

Herndon DN, Barrow RE, Rutan TC et al: A comparison of conservative versus early excision. Ann Surg 209 (5):547–553, 1989

Munster AM, Weiner SH, Spence RJ: Cultured epidermis for the coverage of massive burn wounds: A single center experience. Ann Surg 211:676–680, 1990

B.4. What are the particular concerns in the preoperative evaluation of a burned patient?

As with any preoperative evaluation, a medical history should be taken and a physical examination performed. In addition to the usual concerns regarding cardiac disease, renal function, anesthetic history, and so forth, several areas require special attention. The adequacy of resuscitation should be assessed. Hemodynamic stability should have been achieved. The adequacy of urine output should be assessed. It is useful to note which measures and monitors were required to stabilize the patient. A patient who had trouble handling the resuscitation volume will probably require additional monitoring in the operating room during TE/STSG. The pulmonary status of the patient should be evaluated. Wheezing or rhonchi may indicate a pneumonia. Aggressive pulmonary toilet facilitates the clearing of secretions. Some patients may benefit from bronchodilator therapy. If the patient is already intubated, it is important to note the ventilator settings. Often, high minute volumes and peak airway pressures are required. Often this is due to decreased compliance from an inhalation injury or pneumonia or because of chest wall tightness from a contracting eschar. Many older anesthesia ventilators cannot generate sufficient pressures or volumes to ventilate these patients adequately. In this setting, a floor-type ventilator (e.g., MA-2, Siemens Servo, PB 7200) is required. Anticipation of this is most helpful in facilitating coordination between the respiratory therapy and operating room personnel. During transfer from the unit to the operating room, attention should also be paid to temperature maintenance. Wet, bulky dressings can result in tremendous evaporative heat loss. These dressings should be changed and the patient shrouded in thermal reflective plastic, often called "space blankets," to minimize evaporation and heat loss.

Hartman GS: Anesthetic considerations for the burn patient. In: Wellcome Trends in Anesthesiology 9(1):11. New York, F & M Projects, December 1990

Herndon DN (ed): Total Burn Care, pp 148–153. Philadelphia, WB Saunders, 1996

B.5. On the fifth postburn day, this patient was intubated and monitored with an arterial line and a pulmonary artery (PA) catheter. Vital signs were BP 80/45 mm Hg, PR 140/min, cardiac output 9 liters/min, pulmonary artery PA pressure 20/10 mm Hg. What hemodynamic derangement did this patient exhibit? What was the cause? What were the therapeutic options?

This patient was in hyperdynamic septic shock. This hemodynamic picture is typical of patients who are adequately hydrated at the time of exposure to an endotoxin insult. This syndrome is characterized by hypotension, high pulse pressure and cardiac output, normal filling pressures, and low peripheral resistance. Shock is defined as perfusion inadequate to meet the demands of tissues. Despite the high cardiac output, tissue acidosis may occur from arteriovenous shunting and from primary cellular defects in oxygen use. Metabolic acidosis with a bicarbonate <20 mEq/liter is typical. In patients who are hypovolemic or in whom sepsis is persistent, the hemodynamic pattern changes to that of hypodynamic septic shock. Then hypotension in conjunction with low cardiac output, high peripheral resistance, and low filling pressures is typical. Hypodynamic septic shock often represents a premorbid condition.

The cause of septic shock is most commonly both gram-positive and gram-negative bacteria. Other organisms include fungi, viruses, and parasites. Circulating endotoxin from gram-negative bacteria accounts for most of the hemodynamic derangements. The most effective treatment of septic shock is to remove the source of sepsis. Both human and animal studies of burn injury have demonstrated that early excision of the eschar with grafting reverses many of the septic effects. Prompt treatment of the septic source is required, and supportive measures to maximize tissue perfusion should be instituted. Preload, afterload, and contractility determine cardiac output. Hypovolemia as indicated by low central venous pressure (CVP) or pulmonary capillary wedge pressure (PCWP) should be treated promptly. Volume expansion may be achieved through crystalloid and colloid infusions. Blood replacement is also helpful because it is the most efficient way to increase oxygen delivery. Following adequate hydration, no increase in cardiac output is an indication for inotropic support. Concurrent optimization of afterload is also indicated. Hypotension with a low peripheral resistance is an indication for vasopressor therapy.

Chernow B, Nguyen JPM: Shock: Pathophysiology and Pharmacotherapy. ASA Refresher Course in Anesthesiology 22:87–99, 1994

B.6. Why did this deterioration occur?

The deterioration occurred as the dead skin became colonized by bacteria. Endotoxin from the bacteria along with mediators from the devitalized tissue itself have widespread effects throughout the body, including vasodilation, alteration in local vascular regulation, pulmonary insufficiency, and myocardial depression.

Herndon DN (ed): Total Burn Care, pp 44–52. Philadelphia, WB Saunders, 1996

B.7. What information may be obtained from an arterial line and a PA catheter? How are these calculations performed?

The arterial line provides beat-to-beat information on blood pressure. This is most useful in low pressure states or in conditions such as atrial fibrillation with an irregular ventricular response where marked variations in perfusion pressure occur. In addition, it serves as ready vascular access for blood sampling.

Pulmonary artery catheter information is helpful for guiding therapy in septic patients. The PCWP parallels left atrial (LA) pressures. LA pressures reflect left ventricular diastolic pressures, which are helpful in assessing the preload status of the left ventricle. CVP, although potentially useful as a rough estimate of preload, does not correlate with left ventricular end-diastolic pressure when either isolated right or left-sided cardiac dysfunction occurs. The PA catheter also permits determination of cardiac output through the thermodilution method. The proximal port also permits sampling of mixed venous blood. These different measurements permit the following calculations:

$$\text{Cardiac index (CI)} = \frac{\text{CO}}{\text{body surface area}} \text{ (liter/min/m}^2\text{)}$$

$$\text{Stroke volume (SV)} = \frac{\text{CO}}{\text{heart rate}} \text{ (ml/beat)}$$

$$\text{Stroke index (SI)} = \frac{\text{CI}}{\text{heart rate}} \text{ (ml/beat/m}^2\text{)}$$

$$\text{Systemic vascular resistance (SVR)} = \frac{\text{mean BP} - \text{CVP}}{\text{CO}} \times 80 \text{ (dynes} \cdot \text{sec} \cdot \text{cm}^{-5}\text{)}$$

$$\text{Pulmonary vascular resistance (PVR)} = \frac{\text{mean PAP} - \text{PCWP}}{\text{CO}} \times 80 \text{ (dynes} \cdot \text{sec} \cdot \text{cm}^{-5}\text{)}$$

Cardiac output = SV times heart rate; SV is determined by preload, afterload, and contractility. Four of these variables can be either measured or calculated, and therefore contractility can be determined.

Mixed venous blood samples are needed for shunt calculations:

$$\frac{\text{Qs}}{\text{QT}} = \frac{\text{CcO}_2 - \text{CaO}_2}{\text{CcO}_2 - \text{C}\bar{\text{v}} - \text{O}_2}$$

A low mixed venous oxygen level (<30 mm Hg) is suggestive of inadequate tissue perfusion.

Kaplan JA (ed): Cardiac Anesthesia, 3rd ed, pp 209–234. Philadelphia, WB Saunders, 1993

B.8. What is the definition of shock? What are the different classifications of shock?

Shock, which is a clinical state in which tissue blood flow is inadequate for tissue needs, is caused by many factors. In 1934, Blalock classified four categories of shock:

- Hematogenic (hemorrhagic, hypovolemic)
- Neurogenic (loss of central autonomic input)
- Cardiogenic (primary pump failure)
- Vasogenic (septic)

A more modern classification system is as follows:

- Distributive shock (abnormal vascular volume)
- Hypovolemic shock (decreased blood volume)
- Obstructive shock (obstruction to blood flow, e.g., pulmonary embolism)
- Cardiogenic shock (abnormal pump function)

Chernow B, Nguyen JPM: Shock: Pathophysiology and Pharmacotherapy. ASA Refresher Course in Anesthesiology 22:87–99, 1994

Donegan J (ed): Anesthesia for Emergency Surgery, pp 259–289. New York, Churchill Livingstone, 1987

B.9. Describe an algorithm for treating shock.

The appropriate therapy depends on the cause of the shock state. Hypovolemic shock is treated with aggressive fluid replacement. Initially, this may be isotonic crystalloid solutions, but blood product therapy may be appropriate for hemorrhagic hypovolemia or following the dilutional effects of massive crystalloid resuscitation.

Vasogenic shock falls into two therapeutic schemes. In moderate to low cardiac output states volume therapy is indicated if the PCWP is <15 mm Hg. Adequate filling pressures indicate the need for inotropic support. With high cardiac output, low filling pressure should be treated with volume replacement. Adequate filling pressures in this setting indicate the need for vasopressor therapy to improve perfusion pressures.

Cardiogenic shock therapy should proceed in the following order:

- Optimize preload
- Provide inotropic support (low CO)
- Reduce afterload (if adequate BP)
- Correct acid-base disturbances
- Use intra-aortic balloon counterpulsation or vasopressors

Donegan J (ed): Anesthesia for Emergency Surgery, pp 259–289. New York, Churchill Livingstone, 1987

B.10. What are the different adrenergic receptors? What are the different adrenergic agonists?

Adrenergic receptors are categorized into four subsets:

- alpha-1—contraction of vascular and nonvascular smooth muscle
- alpha-2—prejunctional sympathetics inhibiting sympathetic outflow
- beta-1—myocardial inotropy, myocardial chronotropy
- beta-2—mediate smooth muscle relaxation in bronchi, vasculature, uterus

Table 51-2 lists the commonly used sympathomimetics.

Kaplan JA (ed): Cardiac Anesthesia, 3rd ed, p 1062. Philadelphia, WB Saunders, 1993

B.11. What are amrinone and milrinone? Discuss their pharmacology.

Amrinone is the first phosphodiesterase fraction III (PDE-III) inhibitor for intravenous use in the treatment of acute heart failure. Milrinone, a second generation PDE-III inhibitor, has largely replaced amrinone at our institution. Both relative cost and some platelet-sparing qualities have driven this change. Catecholamines stimulate

Table 51-2. Sympathomimetics

DRUG	DOSAGE Intravenous	DOSAGE Infusion	SITE OF ACTION alpha	SITE OF ACTION beta	MECHANISM OF ACTION
Methoxamine (Vasoxyl)	2–10 mg	—	+ + + +		Direct
Phenylephrine (Neo-Synephrine)	50–500 μg	10 mg/500 ml 20 μg/ml 10–50 μg/min	+ + + +	±	Direct
Norepinephrine (Levarterenol)	—	8 mg/500 ml 16 μg/ml 2–16 μg/min	+ + + +	+ + +	Direct
Metaraminol (Aramine)	100 μg	20–200 mg/500 ml 40–400 μg/ml 40–500 μg/min	+ + + +	+	Direct and indirect
Epinephrine (Adrenalin)	2–16 μg	4 mg/500 ml 8 μg/ml 2–10 μg/min	+ + +	+ + +	Direct
Ephedrine	5–25 mg	—	+	+ +	Direct and indirect
Dopamine (Intropin)	—	400 mg/500 ml 800 μg/ml 2–30 μg/kg/min	+ +	+ + +	Direct and indirect
Dobutamine (Dobutrex)	—	250 mg/500 ml 500 μg/ml 2–20 μg/kg/min	+	+ + + +	Direct
Isoproterenol (Isuprel)	1–4 μg	2 mg/500 ml 4 μg/ml 1–5 μg/min		+ + + +	Direct

Reprinted with permission from Kaplan JA (ed): Cardiac Anesthesia, 3rd ed, p. 1062. Philadelphia, WB Saunders, 1993

beta-1 receptors on the surface of myocardial cells, which in turn causes intracellular activation of adenylate cyclase. Adenylate cyclase catalyzes the reaction leading to the formation of cyclic adenosine monophosphate (cAMP), which plays a pivotal role in promoting myocardial contraction and relaxation by altering the movement of calcium within myocardial cells. PDE-III degrades cAMP. Therefore, inhibition of PDE-III results in increased myocardial contractility. When calcium reuptake into the sarcoplasmic reticulum is facilitated, relaxation of myocardial tissue is also improved (lusitropic effect). Both also have effects on vascular smooth muscle, causing vasodilatation in arterial and capacitance vessel beds.

Typical loading doses for milrinone are 50 μg/kg followed by a maintenance infusion of 0.5 to 0.75 μg/kg/min. Vasodilation may be pronounced, and the concomitant use of a vasopressor (e.g., epinephrine, dopamine, norepinephrine) may be required, especially during the administration of the loading bolus.

Hines R: New Cardiotonic Agents. ASA Refresher Courses in Anesthesiology 22:156–168, 1994

Levy JH, Ramsey J, Bailey JM: Pharmacokinetics and pharmacodynamics of phosphodiesterase-III inhibitors. J Cardiothorac Anesth 4(6)(Suppl 5):7–11, 1990.

B.12. The patient's arterial blood gases (ABGs) on ventilator settings of tidal volume (TV) 1000 ml, RR 16/min, F_1O_2 50%, and positive end-expiratory pressure (PEEP) 5 cm H_2O were as follows: pH 7.32, P_{CO_2} 48 mm Hg, P_{O_2} 56 mm Hg, O_2 saturation 88%. What are the most likely causes of the hypoxemia in this patient?

Ventilation-to-perfusion ($\dot{V}/\dot{Q}$) mismatch is the most common cause of hypoxemia. This is especially true of hypoxemia unresponsive to increased inspired oxygen concentrations. $\dot{V}/\dot{Q}$ mismatches range from dead space to shunt ($\dot{V}/\dot{Q} = \infty$ to 0). Shunt is caused by ineffective ventilation to perfused areas of the lung. Common causes include atelectasis, mucus plugging, pneumonia, and pulmonary edema.

Herndon DN (ed): Total Burn Care, pp 175–183. Philadelphia, WB Saunders, 1996

C. Intraoperative Management

C.1. *What monitors would you employ?*

Such routinely used monitors as electrocardiogram (ECG), blood pressure, temperature, inspired oxygen, pulse oximetry, and capnography would be used in this patient. A Foley catheter is essential to assess urine output. Frequently, the standard ECG electrodes are difficult to secure. Lipolysis from the burn injury and the antibiotic creams often render the adhesive of the ECG pads ineffective. Alternatives include needle electrodes and esophageal leads. We have used foam electrodes secured to the burn eschar with a skin stapler. This has proved effective, and it lessens the possibility of needle stick exposure in both staff and patients. The need for invasive monitors is dictated by the severity of the burn wound, the general medical condition of the patient, and the areas to be grafted and harvested. How well a given patient handles the acute-phase resuscitative volumes serves as a good indication of operative outcome.

This patient was in septic shock. Adequate fluid, vasopressor, and inotropic therapy is best guided by invasive arterial and PA catheters. On occasion, when both upper extremities are being excised and the thighs are being used as donor sites, an arterial line may be required to obtain routine blood pressure measurements.

Hartman GS: Anesthetic considerations for the burn patient. In: Wellcome Trends in Anesthesiology 9(1):9–11. New York, F & M Projects, December 1990

Herndon DN (ed): Total Burn Care, pp 151–152. Philadelphia, WB Saunders, 1996

C.2. *This patient was already intubated. If he had not been intubated, how should you have proceeded with the anesthetic induction?*

This patient had burns over his face and neck. A thorough examination of the mouth opening, throat, and airway should be performed, and one should expect a difficult intubation. In this setting, the safest way to proceed is with an awake intubation. This is best achieved with mild sedation, topical anesthesia, and either direct or fiberoptic-guided intubation. If prolonged postoperative intubation is anticipated, the nasotracheal route may be advantageous; it is more easily secured in place, better tolerated by patients, and permits better oral hygienic care. Vasoconstriction of the nasal mucosa may be achieved by either phenylephrine drops or the application of cocaine-soaked pledgets.

Ovassapian A: Fiberoptic Airway Endoscopy in Anesthesia and Critical Care, pp 45–79. New York, Raven Press, 1990

C.3. *What is the innervation of the larynx and trachea?*

The motor and sensory innervation of the larynx is supplied by the two branches of the vagus nerve, the superior and recurrent laryngeal nerves. The superior laryngeal nerve divides into the internal and external divisions, with the external division accounting for sensory innervation to the anterior subglottic mucosa and motor to the cricothyroid muscle (the adductor and tensor of the vocal cords). The internal branch is entirely sensory, with innervation to the epiglottis, base of the tongue, supraglottic mucosa, and thyroepiglottic and cricothyroid joints. The recurrent laryngeal nerve is sensory to the subglottic mucosa and motor to the remaining laryngeal musculature, including the thyroarytenoids, the lateral cricoarytenoid, the interarytenoid (adductors), and the posterior arytenoid (abductors).

Innervation of the trachea via the vagus includes both mechanical and chemical receptors. Stretch receptors, which are also located in the posterior tracheal wall, are involved in regulating the rate and depth of breathing. Receptors in the tracheal circumference are involved with detecting irritating substances, and they play a role in initiating the cough reflex.

Miller RD (ed): Anesthesia, 4th ed, p 1404. New York, Churchill Livingstone, 1994

Ovassapian A: Fiberoptic Airway Endoscopy in Anesthesia and Critical Care, pp 45–79. New York, Raven Press, 1990

C.4. What is the anesthetic choice for this patient? Why?

This patient was critically ill and in septic shock. Further, he was already on mechanical ventilation. The anesthetic chosen should provide adequate sedation, amnesia, analgesia, lack of movement, and muscle relaxation with minimal derangement in hemodynamic performance. An anesthetic technique that best fulfills these goals is a high-dose narcotic–amnestic–relaxant combination. At The New York Hospital–Cornell Medical Center, a useful scheme for categorizing TE/STSG procedures has been devised, and it is presented in Table 51-3. Patients in group I are relatively straightforward, and with a few caveats can be anesthetized as nonburn patients. Patients in group II require an anesthetic that affords hemodynamic stability during the hemorrhagic excision portion of the procedure, permits smooth emergence and extubation, and provides a high level of postoperative analgesia. Although these requirements may be met with inhalational-based anesthetic techniques, the nitrous oxide–narcotic–amnestic–relaxant combination is highly successful. Good intraoperative hemodynamic stability coupled with excellent postoperative analgesia highlights this technique. Group III patients, as in this case, have numerous medical problems. Because the prolonged respiratory depression from high-dose narcotic technique is not a disadvantage, this technique, with its hemodynamic stability, is the best choice.

Hartman GS: Anesthetic considerations for the burn patient. In: Wellcome Trends in Anesthesiology 9(1):9–11. New York, F & M Projects, December 1990

Table 51-3. *Categorization of Grafting Procedures*

GROUP	TBSA %	DURATION (min)	EBL (mL)	OMP	ANESTHESIA
I	<10	30–90	<500	few	
II	10–30	60–240	500–2500	+/−	Fentanyl, sufentanil, or alfentanil in combination with N_2O and a relaxant or inhalation-based anesthesia
III	>30	>120	>3000	yes	High-dose narcotic-relaxant technique

TBSA%, % total body surface area; EBL, estimated blood loss; OMP, other medical problems

C.5. What is normothermia for a burned patient?

Because burned patients have a resetting of the centrally mediated thermostat, normothermia is about 38.5°C.

Herndon DN (ed): Total Burn Care, p 140. Philadelphia, WB Saunders, 1996

C.6. How is temperature best maintained?

Hypothermia is an ever present problem. Burned patients have lost much of their natural insulation of the skin. Heat loss can occur through convection, conduction, and evaporation. It is important to remember that it is much easier to cool a patient than to warm one. The gradient for cooling can be relatively large (e.g., a room temperature of 20°C gives a gradient of 18°C). Warming from mild hypothermia of 35°C at best can be achieved with a temperature of 39° to 40°C, a 4° to 5°C gradient. In addition, during normothermia, cutaneous blood flow is normal. During a period of hypothermia, peripheral vasoconstriction occurs, which limits the effectiveness of surface rewarming efforts. Heat conservation should take many forms. A warming blanket minimizes loss to the operating room table. All fluids should be warmed to at least 37°C. An in-line humidifier is effective in minimizing the heat loss required to vaporize and humidify anesthetic gases. The time in which the patient is exposed should also be minimized. Warming the operating room is particularly effective when large surface areas are exposed for extended periods of time.

Hartman GS: Anesthetic considerations for the burn patient. In: Wellcome Trends in Anesthesiology 9(1):9–11. New York, F & M Projects, December 1990

Herndon DN (ed): Total Burn Care, pp 139–142. Philadelphia, WB Saunders, 1996

C.7. Why is a heated-humidified circuit used?

A heated-humidified circuit is most effective because in conserving and providing humidity, total body energy is conserved. Because airway gases must be 100% humidified, there is a tremendous vaporization demand on the airways. The latent heat of vaporization is 570 cal/ml of water. Thus, evaporation of tissue water consumes a tremendous amount of energy, and a significant heat sink can occur to patients at risk for hypothermia.

Miller RD (ed): Anesthesia, 4th ed, pp 219–224. New York, Churchill Livingstone, 1994

C.8. What derangements occur with hypothermia?

Hypothermia decreases the rate of metabolism, which can prolong the duration of many anesthetic drugs. In addition, hepatic blood flow itself is lowered, thus slowing delivery of drugs to the site of metabolism. Postoperative shivering can increase metabolic demands several times. Hypothermia decreases heart rate, cardiac output, and blood pressure. At temperatures <28°C, atrial pacing becomes irregular and ventricular ectopy increases. Ventricular fibrillation occurs between 25° and 30°C.

Miller RD (ed): Anesthesia, 4th ed, pp 1369–1373. New York, Churchill Livingstone, 1994

C.9. What forms of intravenous (IV) access are required?

Because the need for large fluid volume replacements is anticipated, adequate intravenous access is essential. One or two short, large-bore catheters are far better than many small-gauge ones. Intravenous access can be achieved through cannulation of large peripheral veins in the arms and legs. The femoral vein is a site often used for placement of large 7 French Cordis introducers as a means of access. Central sites for intravenous access may be used when needed. They have the added advantage of providing a measurement of central venous pressures but may also constitute a portal for infection.

C.10. What is Poiseuille's equation for resistance during laminar flow? What is its significance?

Under laminar flow, resistance is equal to 8 times the length times the viscosity divided by *P* times the radius to the 4th power. The significance of this is that doubling the radius of an intravenous catheter decreases resistance to flow 16 times.

Miller RD (ed): Anesthesia, 4th ed, p 586. New York, Churchill Livingstone, 1994

C.11. What relaxant would you choose and why?

A nondepolarizing relaxant should be used. For cases of short to moderate duration (<2 hours), either vecuronium or atracurium should be used. For cases of longer duration, pancuronium, doxacurium, or pipecuronium is indicated. In general, the choice of muscle relaxant should be based on the duration of the case and the presence of any co-existing diseases that might affect metabolism of the drug.

C.12. How are the neuromuscular blockers pancuronium, curare, metocurine, atracurium, vecuronium, doxacurium, and pipecuronium metabolized and eliminated? Which of them has significant histamine release?

See Table 51-4.

C.13. What is the difference between metabolism and elimination of drugs?

Drug metabolism is the chemical modification of a substance and drug elimination includes all processes that are responsible for the termination of a drug in the body.

In drug metabolism, the two most important processes are phase I and phase II

Table 51-4. The Metabolism, Elimination, and Histamine Release of Muscle Relaxants

RELAXANT	% HEPATIC METABOLISM	% RENAL ELIMINATION	% PLASMA METABOLISM	HISTAMINE RELEASE
Curare	?	40–60	None	Moderate
Metocurine	?	80–100	None	Slight
Pancuronium	15–40	60–80	None	None
Atracurium	?	<5	80–95	Slight
Vecuronium	15–40	10–20	None	None
Pipecuronium	?	60–90	None	None
Doxacurium	?	60–90	None	None

Reprinted with permission from Miller RD (ed): Anesthesia, 3rd ed, pp 398–407. New York, Churchill Livingstone, 1990 metabolism. Phase I metabolism consists of chemical reactions of oxidation, reduction, and hydrolysis. Many of these involve catalysis by the cytochrome P-450 system predominantly in the liver. Phase II reactions consist of conjugations, or the combining of endogenous substances with drugs. This is also called "the synthetic mode of biotransformation."

Drug elimination processes include not only metabolism but also renal and hepatobiliary excretion and pulmonary excretion (CO_2, anesthetics).

Miller RD (ed): Anesthesia, 4th ed, p 65. New York, Churchill Livingstone, 1994

C.14. Why is succinylcholine contraindicated for patients with a burn injury? For how long is it contraindicated?

The hyperkalemic response to succinylcholine in burn patients is well documented. Increases in serum potassium of >10 mEq/liter with resultant cardiac arrest have been reported. The exact mechanism of this phenomenon is not known, but most likely it is related to the release of potassium from hypersensitive muscle membranes. Increased acetylcholine receptor sites are found on the muscle membranes of burn victims; these may mediate the potentially lethal efflux of potassium when the acetylcholine agonist succinylcholine is administered.

The exact time period for this hypersensitivity is unclear. Most authors recommend the avoidance of succinylcholine from 24 to 48 hours following the burn injury and extending well until complete healing has occurred. A hyperkalemic response has been reported in a patient after 480 days. The recommended limit now is extended to about 2 years following the burn injury.

Gronert GA, Theye RA: Pathophysiology of hyperkalemia induced by succinylcholine. Anesthesiology 43:89–99, 1975

Rupp SM (ed): Problems in Anesthesia 3(3):482. Philadelphia, JB Lippincott, 1989

C.15. How are the doses of nondepolarizing muscle relaxants affected by a burn injury?

The burn patient usually shows a resistance to the blocking effects of neuromuscular relaxants. Although these patients have altered pharmacokinetics and increased plasma protein binding of these drugs, most of the increased requirements (documented for *d*-tubocurarine, pancuronium, atracurium, and vecuronium) are best explained by alterations in the number and affinity of junctional receptors.

It is most important to remember that this alteration is quite variable. In burn patients it becomes particularly important to use a peripheral nerve stimulator to assess the adequacy of both neuromuscular blockade and antagonism and the reversal with anticholinesterases.

Hartman GS: Anesthetic considerations for the burn patient. In: Wellcome Trends in Anesthesiology 9(1):11. New York: F & M Projects, December 1990

Rupp SM (ed): Problems in Anesthesia 3(3):482. Philadelphia, JB Lippincott, 1989

Wood M: Plasma drug binding: Implications for anesthesiologists. Anesth Analg 65:786–804, 1986

C.16. What additional complications are associated with electrical burns?

The burn from electrical current results from the conversion of high-voltage electrical energy to thermal energy. Determinants of damage include the area of contact, the duration of current flow, and the varying resistances of the body. Often the current path through the body is unclear because the electrical current may flow beneath the level of the skin. Often only the surface entrance and exit sites show immediate visible injury because of the high current concentration at these points. Large viscera are most often spared because their large volume permits dissipation of the thermal insult. Conversely, extremities are vulnerable because of the limited volume for diffusion of current. The extent of the injury may often be unclear for several days. Conduction of the electrical current through the blood vessels results in damage to their endothelium. Vascular complications such as thrombosis can be a late complication. The heart is particularly susceptible to electrical damage. Ectopy and congestive heart failure are signs of injury. Elevations in serial creatine phosphokinase (CPK)-MB isoenzymes are useful in quantitating any myocardial damage. These patients should be monitored closely for dysrhythmias for several days.

Herndon DN (ed): Total Burn Care, pp 401–407. Philadelphia, WB Saunders, 1996

Vassallo SA, Martyn JAJ: Pathophysiology and anesthetic management of burn injury. In: Katz RL (ed): Seminars in Anesthesia 8(4):275–284. Philadelphia, WB Saunders, 1989

C.17. *What is myoglobinuria? What are common causes? What therapy is indicated?*

Myoglobin and hemoglobin may be released into the circulation following massive burns (especially electrical burns involving muscle destruction) and crush injuries. Other causes include strenuous exercise in the setting of hypovolemia, transfusion reactions, and malignant hyperpyrexia. Renal obstruction leading to ischemia and acute renal failure (ARF) may follow. Aggressive volume expansion and diuresis is the mainstay of therapy. Osmotic diuretics (mannitol) are advantageous in that they may prevent intratubular precipitation of pigments. Unfortunately, in experiments mannitol has been useful only when given prior to the insult. Overall mortality from ARF has not improved significantly in the past several decades; thus prevention is essential.

Miller RD (ed): Anesthesia, 4th ed, pp 685–686. New York, Churchill Livingstone, 1994

D. Postoperative Management

D.1. *How would you monitor this patient during transport?*

This patient was critically ill and still under a general anesthetic. Standard monitors must include assessment of heart rate and rhythm, blood pressure, and respirations. These can be achieved by a transport monitor with ECG, BP (either cuff or invasive), oximetry, and controlled ventilation with an Ambu-bag with oxygen supply.

D.2. *This patient was anesthetized with a narcotic–nitrous oxide–relaxant technique. How could hypoxemia occur when nitrous oxide is discontined and the patient is breathing room air?*

Patients anesthetized with a nitrous oxide-oxygen mixture are at risk for diffusion hypoxia. This may occur during the first 5 to 10 minutes following discontinuation of anesthesia if the patient is allowed to breathe or is ventilated with room air. As described by Fink and associates in 1954, this occurs when the more soluble nitrous oxide is eliminated rapidly through the lungs (nitrous oxide is 35 times more soluble in blood than nitrogen). The nitrous oxide diffuses in much greater quantities into the alveoli than the nitrogen diffuses from the alveoli into the blood. Therefore, the remaining alveolar oxygen concentration (room air 21%) is diluted by the nitrous oxide, and a hypoxic mixture results. Diffusion hypoxia of this sort can be avoided by the use of high inspired oxygen concentrations during emergence and transportation on oxygen for patients previously anesthetized with a nitrous oxide-oxygen anesthetic.

Fink R, Carpenter SL, Holiday DA et al: Diffusion anoxia during recovery from nitrous oxide-oxygen anesthesia. Fed Proc 13:354, 1954

D.3. *The patient was shivering in the recovery room on emergence from anesthesia. What are the problems associated with this situation?*

Postoperative shivering can be a common phenomenon. It is more common following inhalational general anesthetics, and it may be related to alteration in the descending control of spinal reflexes following general anesthesia. Shivering, however, increases the metabolic rate, causing demand for increased cardiac output and respiratory effort. The mechanism is not always caused by hypothermia because many patients who shiver are normothermic, but it is important to prevent hypothermia as a cause of shivering. These measures include warm blankets and radiant heaters, warmed intravenous solutions, and humidified gases. Supplemental oxygen should be administered to counter the increased ventilatory requirements. Although many drugs are purported to be effective, meperidine in doses of 25 to 50 mg intravenously is recommended.

Macintyre PE, Paulin EG, Dworsteg JF: Effect of meperidine on oxygen consumption, carbon dioxide production and respiratory gas exchange in postanesthesia shivering. Anesth Analg 66:751, 1987

Miller RD (ed): Anesthesia, 4th ed, p 2322. New York, Churchill Livingstone, 1994

Trauma

52

Ralph L. Slepian

A 31-year-old man sustained a gunshot wound to the left upper quadrant of his abdomen. Vital signs were blood pressure (BP) 85/60 mm Hg, heart rate (HR) 130/min, respiratory rate (RR) 32/min, temperature 34.5°C. Hematocrit (Hct) was 27%. He was emergently brought to the operating room for an exploratory laparotomy.

A. Medical Disease and Differential Diagnosis

1. How is trauma classified?
2. What are the most commonly injured organs in blunt abdominal trauma?
3. What is peritoneal lavage?
4. Why was peritoneal lavage not performed for this patient?
5. Define shock.
6. What are the four types of shock?
7. List the signs and symptoms of shock.
8. What is the pathophysiology of hypovolemic shock?
9. How would you classify hemorrhage?
10. What is the initial treatment of hemorrhagic shock?
11. Would you choose crystalloid or colloid therapy to treat hypovolemic shock?
12. Is there a place for dextran or hetastarch (Hespan) in treating hypovolemic shock?
13. Is there a place for hypertonic saline in the treatment of hypovolemic shock?

B. Preoperative Evaluation and Preparation

1. What premedication would you order?

C. Intraoperative Management

1. How would you monitor this patient?
2. How would you induce anesthesia?
3. What agents would you choose to maintain anesthesia?
4. What muscle relaxant would you choose?
5. Five minutes after intubation, the peak airway pressure increased from 20 cm H_2O to 40 cm H_2O. What are the possible causes?
6. How would you make a diagnosis of tension pneumothorax?
7. What is the treatment for tension pneumothorax?
8. The patient's blood loss was continuing and the hematocrit was 18%. What type of blood would you give if the type and crossmatch are not completed?
9. What precautions should be taken if > 2 U of type O Rh negative uncrossmatched whole blood is given?
10. What are the complications associated with any blood transfusion?
11. What is considered a massive transfusion?

12. What are the complications associated with a massive transfusion?
13. Can the shift of the oxygen-hemoglobin dissociation curve be quantitated?
14. How is hypothermia defined?
15. What are the adverse effects of hypothermia?
16. What is the treatment of hypothermia?
17. What are the effects of blood transfusion on the immune system?
18. What are the guidelines for transfusion of blood products?
19. If the patient were a member of the Jehovah's Witness religious sect, would you give a blood transfusion?
20. If a child is a Jehovah's Witness and suffered from hemorrhagic shock, what would you do?
21. Are there artificial blood substitutes available?

D. Postoperative Management

1. What is adult respiratory distress syndrome (ARDS)?
2. How is ARDS treated?
3. In the recovery room, you are called to see this patient because of oliguria. How would you evaluate and treat this patient?

A. Medical Disease and Differential Diagnosis

A.1. How is trauma classified?

Trauma is usually separated into two distinct categories: penetrating and blunt trauma. Both can wreak havoc on the body's vascular, visceral, musculoskeletal, and nervous systems.

A.2. What are the most commonly injured organs in blunt abdominal trauma?

In blunt abdominal trauma, the most commonly injured organs are the spleen, liver, kidneys, and bowel. Generally, blunt abdominal trauma leads to higher mortality rates than penetrating trauma. The reason is multifactorial and includes greater difficulty in diagnosis and frequent association with other injuries, such as head injury, chest trauma, and fractures.

Schwartz SI (ed): Principles of Surgery, 6th ed, p 193. New York, McGraw-Hill, 1994

Siegel JH (ed): Trauma: Emergency Surgery and Critical Care, p 889. New York, Churchill Livingstone, 1987

A.3. What is peritoneal lavage?

Peritoneal lavage is a procedure performed in the emergency room to help determine if a patient has internal bleeding that requires an exploratory laparotomy. It is done by performing a minilaparotomy under local anesthesia. A catheter is then placed into the abdomen and is aspirated for gross blood. If <20 ml of blood is aspirated, then 1 liter of lactated Ringer's solution or normal saline is allowed to drain into the abdomen. The lavage fluid is then allowed to return by gravity, and it is sent to the laboratory for analysis. Criteria for a positive peritoneal lavage are an erythrocyte count of $\geq$100,000/mm^3, a white blood cell count of $\geq$500/mm^3, the presence of bile or food particles, and a fluid amylase concentration of ≥175 U/dl. If the peritoneal lavage meets one or more of these criteria, then the patient comes to the operating room for an exploratory laparotomy.

Feliciano DV, Moore EE, Mattox KL (eds): Trauma, 3rd ed, p 133. Stamford, CT, Appleton & Lange, 1996

Schwartz SI (ed): Principles of Surgery, 6th ed, pp 195–196. New York, McGraw-Hill, 1994

A.4. Why was peritoneal lavage not performed for this patient?

Peritoneal lavage was not done for two reasons. First, it is felt that all gunshot wounds to the abdomen need to be surgically explored. Second, this patient was exhibiting signs of shock and obviously needed to be sent to the operating room without delay.

Moylan JA (ed): Trauma Surgery, pp 22–24. Philadelphia, JB Lippincott, 1988

Schwartz SI (ed): Principles of Surgery, 6th ed, pp 197–198. New York, McGraw-Hill, 1994

A.5. Define shock.

Shock can be defined as "a clinical condition characterized by signs and symptoms which arise when the cardiac output is insufficient to fill the arterial tree with blood under sufficient pressure to provide organs and tissues with adequate blood flow." Shock of all forms appears to be invariably related to inadequate tissue perfusion. The low-flow state in vital organs seems to be the final common denominator in all forms of shock.

Schwartz SI (ed): Principles of Surgery, 6th ed, p 119. New York, McGraw-Hill, 1994

A.6. What are the four types of shock?

For a working classification of shock, the following classification offered by Blalock in 1934 is still useful and functional:

- Hematogenic (hypovolemic, hemorrhagic) shock—characterized by a loss of circulatory blood volume
- Cardiogenic shock—characterized by an inability of the myocardium to pump blood
- Vasogenic (septic) shock—characterized by an infection that causes a decrease in peripheral vascular resistance
- Neurogenic shock—characterized by an impairment of the central nervous system-mediated control of vascular tone

Moylan JA (ed): Trauma Surgery, pp 27–42. Philadelphia, JB Lippincott, 1988

Schwartz SI (ed): Principles of Surgery, 6th ed, p 119. New York, McGraw-Hill, 1994

A.7. List the signs and symptoms of shock.

Tachycardia, hypotension, cool extremities, pallor, oliguria, tachypnea, decreased capillary refill, anxiety, restlessness, and loss of consciousness are signs and symptoms of shock.

Moylan JA: Trauma Surgery, p 30. Philadelphia, JB Lippincott, 1988

A.8. What is the pathophysiology of hypovolemic shock?

Cardiovascular Derangement

An acute decrease in circulating blood volume leads to an increase in sympathetic activity with an outpouring of epinephrine and norepinephrine from the adrenal gland. The alpha-adrenergic response causes vasoconstriction, which shunts blood from the skin, viscera, and muscle, thereby preserving the coronary and cerebral circulation. With constriction of both pre- and postcapillary sphincters, a reduction occurs in hydrostatic pressure of the capillary bed, which allows the osmotic pressure to draw fluid back into the vascular space from the interstitial space. This process of hemodilution tends to expand the patient's blood volume. In addition to the vasoconstriction and hemodilution, a tachycardic response may also be noted.

Myocardial depressant factor (MDF) is a peptide thought to be released from the pancreas during low-flow states. This peptide is thought to be responsible for some of the decreased cardiac performance seen in trauma patients.

Acid-Base Disturbances

Metabolic acidosis is almost always seen in association with a shock state. As a result of decreased blood flow or low rate of perfusion, oxygen delivery to vital organs is reduced and consequently a mandatory change occurs from aerobic to anaerobic metabolism. This shift will lead to the production of lactic acid instead of carbon dioxide as the end product of metabolism. The increase in lactic acid leads to a metabolic acidosis.

Capan LM, Miller SM, Turndorf H (eds): Anesthesia and Intensive Care, pp 84–89. Philadelphia, JB Lippincott, 1991

Schwartz SI (ed): Principles of Surgery, 6th ed, p 120. New York, McGraw-Hill, 1994

Stene JK, Gerarde CM (eds): Trauma: Anesthesia, pp 100–110. Baltimore, Williams & Wilkins, 1991

A.9. How would you classify hemorrhage?

The American College of Surgeons has classified hemorrhage based on blood loss, as shown in Table 52-1.

Experience has shown that in young healthy patients, crystalloid therapy can be

Table 52-1. Classification of Hemorrhage Based on Blood Loss

CLASS	BLOOD LOSS	SIGNS & SYMPTOMS	TREATMENT
I	<15%	Mild tachycardia, vasoconstriction	1–2 liters of fluid
II	15%–30%	Tachycardia, decreased pulse pressure, anxiety, restlessness	2 liters of fluid
III	30%–40%	Marked tachycardia, tachypnea, hypotension, altered mental status	3× fluid loss check hematocrit PRBC to maintain O_2 transport
IV	>40%	Life-threatening, extreme tachycardia, tachypnea, hypotension, low urine output, depressed mental status	PRBC, crystalloid and colloid to maintain O_2 transport

used to treat blood loss of up to 30%. Oxygen delivery is believed to be adequate when a hemoglobin level is down to as low as 7 g/dl.

American College of Surgeons, Committee on Trauma: Advanced Trauma Life Support Course Manual. Chicago, American College of Surgeons, 1989.

Grande CM: Textbook of Trauma, Anesthesiology and Critical Care, pp 400–401. St. Louis, Mosby, 1993

Practice guidelines for blood component therapy: A report by the ASA Task Force on Blood Component Therapy. Anesthesiology 84:732–747, 1996.

A.10. What is the initial treatment of hemorrhagic shock?

The initial treatment of hemorrhagic shock is to attempt to stabilize hemodynamics by administering fluids and blood products as required to maintain tissue perfusion and oxygen delivery.

Kruskall MS, Mintz PD, Bergin JJ et al: Transfusion therapy in emergency room medicine. Ann Emerg Med 17:327–335, 1988

A.11. Would you choose crystalloid or colloid therapy to treat hypovolemic shock?

Hemoglobin-free solutions can sustain hemodynamics and deliver adequate oxygenation in healthy patients who have lost as much as 30% of their total blood volume. At present, some controversy exists to the use of crystalloid versus colloid therapy.

Proponents of crystalloid therapy state that both intravascular and interstitial fluid losses occur in hypovolemic shock, and that these can be readily replaced with crystalloids. Another benefit of crystalloids is the decrease in blood viscosity, which may enhance perfusion. A particular advantage of lactated Ringer's solution is that lactate is metabolized to bicarbonate, which may help to buffer the patient's acidosis. Finally, in this age of medical economics, the cost of crystalloid is much less than that of colloid. Because crystalloid leaves the intravascular space and enters the interstitial space, large quantities are needed, and some fear that these quantities may lead to both pulmonary and peripheral edema, although studies have not confirmed this fear.

Proponents of colloid therapy state that much less volume of fluid is needed to counteract hypovolemic shock. Colloids maintain the oncotic pressure, and they will hold the interstitial fluids in the intravascular space, which is felt may prevent pulmonary edema. However, if leaky alveolar capillary membranes are seen within the lung, then colloids may worsen pulmonary edema. Another disadvantage is the possible link to renal tubular dysfunction after colloid resuscitation.

In summary, the benefits of crystalloid therapy outweigh the benefits of colloid therapy, and therefore we resuscitate with crystalloids.

Churchill WH, Kaitz SR (eds): Transfusion Medicine, pp 172–175. Boston, Blackwell Scientific, 1988

Kruskall MS, Mintz PD, Bergin JJ et al: Transfusion therapy in emergency room medicine. Ann Emerg Med 17:327–335, 1988

Miller RD (ed): Anesthesia, 4th ed, p 1642. New York, Churchill-Livingstone, 1994

Richardson JD (ed): Trauma: Clinical Care and Pathophysiology, pp 29–34. Chicago, Year Book Medical Publishers, 1987

Rossi EC, Simon TL, Moss GS et al (eds): Principles of Transfusion Medicine, pp 617; 627–633. Baltimore, Williams & Wilkins, 1996

A.12. Is there a place for dextran or hetastarch (Hespan) in treating hypovolemic shock?

Dextran and hetastarch are synthetic polysaccharide solutions with varying mean molecular weights. Dextran 40, dextran 70, and hetastarch have all been used as volume expanders. Dextrans are relatively inexpensive, increase effective blood volume, and decrease blood viscosity. However, their negative aspects are considerable. They impair coagulation by coating platelets, and they impair typing and crossmatching by coating red blood cells. In addition, the incidence of anaphylatic reactions has been reported to be from 0.07% to 1.1%. At present, they would appear to be of little use in the treatment of hypovolemic shock.

Churchill WH, Kaitz SR (eds): Transfusion Medicine, pp 175–179. Boston, Blackwell Scientific, 1988

Richardson JD (ed): Trauma; Clinical Care and Pathophysiology, p 30. Chicago, Year Book Medical Publishers, 1987

Rossi EC, Simon TL, Moss GS et al (eds): Principles of Transfusion Medicine, pp 628–629. Baltimore, Williams & Wilkins, 1996

A.13. Is there a place for hypertonic saline in the treatment of hypovolemic shock?

Hypertonic saline is now being used for resuscitation at some major centers. Its effects tend to be of short duration, and therefore it is not used alone. However, if one combines hypertonic saline 7.5% and dextran 70, the effective resuscitation will be prolonged. The optimal doses are thought to be 4 ml/kg of 7.5% saline in 12% dextran 70.

The potential advantage is that the greater the sodium concentration, the less total volume will be required for resuscitation. A serious potential danger exists in that patients may become hypernatremic, which can lead to brain dehydration. In patients with high intracranial pressure (ICP), it is possible that this brain dehydration may have a potential benefit in lowering the ICP.

At this time, too much controversy appears to exist to recommend a switch to this regimen. Further clinical trials need to be performed to delineate the role of hypertonic saline in resuscitative measures.

Miller RD (ed): Anesthesia, 4th ed, pp 1643; 2166. New York, Churchill Livingstone, 1994

Rossi EC, Simon TL, Moss GS, Gould SA (eds): Principles of Transfusion Medicine, p 632. Baltimore, Williams & Williams, 1996

B. Preoperative Evaluation and Preparation

B.1. What premedication would you order?

None. This is a critically ill patient who is coming to the operating room for emergency surgery. Narcotics and sedatives would be contraindicated because they could worsen his already tenuous hemodynamic state.

C. Intraoperative Management

C.1. How would you monitor this patient?

Routine noninvasive monitors would include electrocardiogram (ECG), BP cuff, O_2 monitor, pulse oximeter, end-tidal CO_2, esophageal stethoscope, temperature probe, and Foley catheter.

Invasive monitors for this patient would include an arterial line and a central venous catheter. An arterial line would be useful for blood samplings and direct blood pressure monitoring. The central venous line would be helpful in determining the patient's volume status. A Swan-Ganz catheter would be indicated if the patient were showing signs of heart failure.

C.2. How would you induce anesthesia?

Because all trauma patients are considered to have a full stomach, the best way to protect the patient's airway would be an awake intubation. For an uncooperative patient, one would do a rapid-sequence induction. First, the patient should be preoxygenated for 3 to 5 minutes. Then one would give a defasciculation dose of a nondepolarizing muscle relaxant such as curare (3 mg). Next, ketamine (0.5 to 1.0 mg/kg) might be given, followed by succinylcholine (1.5 mg/kg) while maintaining cricoid pressure. Ketamine was chosen in this case because of its cardiovascular stimulating effects and the patient's unstable hemodynamics. If the patient was adequately resuscitated in the emergency room, then one could possibly use a small dose of thiopental or midazolam for induction.

C.3. What agents would you choose to maintain anesthesia?

As the patient stabilizes and the hemodynamics improve, other anesthetic agents can be carefully titrated to prevent hypotension as listed below.

- Sedatives or amnestics should be added to the anesthetic as soon as tolerated. Remember to start with small doses and to check the patient's response between doses.
- Narcotics should be titrated to control the hemodynamic response to surgery.
- Nitrous oxide must be carefully considered, because it has the capacity to accumulate in closed air spaces (e.g., pleura, bowel).
- Inhalational anesthetics may be used in low concentrations as not to compromise the patient's hemodynamics. The inhalational agents are adjuvants to the sedatives and narcotics.

C.4. What muscle relaxant would you choose?

One would want a long-acting drug with no cardiovascular side-effects, such as doxacurium or pipecuronium. Vecuronium, rocuronium or cisatracurium which is free of cardiovascular side-effects and has an intermediate duration of action, would also be an acceptable choice.

Pancuronium is a long-acting muscle relaxant with vagolytic properties that may be deleterious to the patient.

Curare, metocurine, and atracurium all have the potential to cause hypotension, and therefore would not be chosen for this case.

C.5. Five minutes after intubation, the peak airway pressure increased from 20 cm H₂O to 40 cm H₂O. What were the possible causes?

- Tension pneumothorax
- Bronchospasm
- Endobronchial intubation
- Pulmonary edema
- Secretions
- Kink in the anesthesia circuit or endotracheal tube

Capan LM, Miller SM, Turndorf H (eds): Trauma: Anesthesia and Intensive Care, p 71. Philadelphia, JB Lippincott, 1991

Stene JK, Gerarde CM (eds): Trauma: Anesthesia, pp 79–81. Baltimore, Williams & Wilkins, 1991

C.6. How would you make a diagnosis of tension pneumothorax?

A tension pneumothorax can be defined by the absence of breath sounds on the affected side. The chest movement may be asymmetric. Neck veins will be full, and systemic hypotension can occur if the tension pneumothorax is severe. It should be emphasized that any patient who deteriorates under anesthesia and has wounds to the upper abdomen, lower neck, or ribs should be assumed to have a tension pneumothorax until proved otherwise.

Capan LM, Miller SM, Turndorf H (eds): Trauma: Anesthesia and Intensive Care, p 32. Philadelphia, JB Lippincott, 1991

Moylan JA (ed): Trauma Surgery, p 103. Philadelphia, JB Lippincott, 1988

Stene JK, Gerarde CM (eds): Trauma Anesthesia, p 209. Baltimore, Williams & Wilkins, 1991

C.7. What is the treatment for tension pneumothorax?

Immediate decompression of the chest is mandatory for tension pneumothorax because this patient's hemodynamics have deteriorated. An 18-gauge angiocatheter is placed in the second intercostal space at the mid-clavicular plane. After the air escapes and the lung is decompressed, a formal chest tube can be inserted.

Remember that a tension pneumothorax is potentially lethal and must always be of concern when caring for trauma patients.

Capan LM, Miller SM, Turndorf H (eds): Trauma: Anesthesia and Intensive Care, p 32. Philadelphia, JB Lippincott, 1991

Stene JK, Gerarde CM (eds): Trauma Anesthesia, p 210. Baltimore, Williams & Wilkins, 1991

C.8. The patient's blood loss was continuing and the hematocrit was 18%. What type of blood would you give if the type and crossmatch are not completed?

This patient should have blood transfused as soon as possible. Type O Rh negative packed cells is the universal donor. This should be started while type-specific blood is being made available. Whenever the type-specific blood is ready, one can switch over to it. However, if the transfusion begins with type O Rh negative whole blood and >2 U has been infused, only type O Rh negative blood should continue to be used. Usually by the time a patient reaches the operating room from the emergency room a partial crossmatch can be done. This usually takes 5 to 10 minutes, after which type-specific blood can be transfused.

Huestis DW, Bove JR, Case J: Practical Blood Transfusion, 4th ed, pp 218–220. Boston, Little, Brown, 1988

Kruskall MS, Mintz PD, Bergin JJ et al: Transfusion therapy in emergency room medicine. Ann Emerg Med 17:331–333, 1988

C.9. What precautions should be taken if > 2 U of type O Rh negative uncrossmatched whole blood are given?

The plasma from type O Rh negative whole blood contains anti-A and anti-B antibodies, which can cause hemolytic reactions with type A and type B blood cells if given in significant quantities. Therefore, only type O Rh negative blood should continue to be transfused, although this will lead to minor hemolysis of the patient's own red cells. The patient should not receive his type-specific blood until the blood bank determines that the transfused anti-A and anti-B antibody levels have fallen sufficiently low to permit safe transfusion of type-specific blood. This usually requires a 2-week waiting period.

Churchill WH, Kaitz SR (eds): Transfusion Medicine, pp 212–214. Boston, Blackwell Scientific, 1988

Huestis DW, Bove JR, Case J: Practical Blood Transfusion, 4th ed, pp 218–220. Boston, Little, Brown, 1988

Kruskall MS, Mintz PD, Bergin JJ et al: Transfusion therapy in emergency room medicine. Ann Emerg Med 17:331–333, 1988

Miller RD (ed): Anesthesia, 4th ed, p 1623. New York, Churchill Livingstone, 1994

C.10. What are the complications associated with any blood transfusion?

The following discussion covers complications that can be seen with the transfusion of just 1 U of blood. They include transfusion reactions, transmission of diseases, and microembolization.

Transfusion Reactions
- Febrile reactions occur in approximately 1.0% of all transfusions. In an awake patient this is usually no more than an annoyance that requires decreasing the infusion rate.
- Allergic reactions to properly crossmatched blood will manifest as an increase in temperature, pruritus, and urticaria. This may be hard to diagnose in the anesthetized patient. Treatment consists of administration of antihistamines and discontinuation of the transfusion.
- Hemolytic reactions occur when incompatible blood is administered. Caused by activation of the complement system, they can be life-threatening. In the awake patient fever, chills, dyspnea, and substernal and lumbar pain are seen in addition to hypotension. Under general anesthesia the only sign that is not masked is hypotension. Also, if free hemoglobin cannot be documented in the plasma or urine, this too would be indicative of a transfusion reaction. Substances released by the hemolyzed cells can lead to disseminated intravascular coagulation and acute renal failure. Treatment consists of immediate discontinuation of the transfusion. Hypotension should be treated with hydration, vasopressors, and inotropes if needed.

Urinary output must be maintained by hydration, loop diuretics, and/or mannitol. Although its value is uncertain, sodium bicarbonate has been used to alkalinize the urine to improve the solubility of the hemoglobin degradation products. This risk of an ABO-incompatible transfusion is 1:33,000 red cell transfusions. The probability of a fatal hemolytic transfusion reaction is uncertain, but estimates range from 1:500,000 to 1:800,000.

Transmission of Diseases

• Transmission of disease can be a serious problem. Human immunodeficiency virus (HIV), hepatitis B virus, hepatitis C (non-A, non-B) virus, and cytomegalovirus can all be transmitted by transfusion. Because the risk of disease transmission increases with each unit of blood or its components given, they must be carefully scrutinized before they are administered. The incidence of post-transfusion HIV infection is between 1:450,000 and 1:600,000 per transfused unit of blood. The risk of post-transfusion hepatitis B transmission is approximately 1:200,000 units. The risk of post-transfusion hepatitis C seroconversion is 0.03% (1:3,300) per unit transfused. Malaria, syphilis, Lyme disease, Chagas' disease, and other diseases may also be transmitted through transfusion. As new nonhemoglobin solutions appear on the market, less blood will be transfused and disease transmission will diminish.

Microembolization

• Microembolization can occur from the transfusion of blood or its components. Stored blood forms microaggregates that are too small to be removed by the standard 170 μ blood filters. Smaller filters have been developed to remove these particles. However, when using blood filters of the 20 to 40 μ range, the rate of transfusion is dramatically decreased because of the increased resistance of the filters. Some early reports suggested that these microaggregates may lead to pulmonary dysfunction, but this has never been proved.

Churchill WH, Kaitz SR (eds): Transfusion Medicine, pp 91–126. Boston, Blackwell Scientific, 1988

The Greater New York Blood Program Pamphlet, May 1990

Kruskall MS, Mintz PD, Bergin JJ et al: Transfusion therapy in emergency room medicine. Ann Emerg Med 17:329–331, 1988

Miller RD (ed): Anesthesia 4th ed, p 1633. New York, Churchill Livingstone, 1994

Practice guidelines for blood component therapy: A report by the ASA Task Force on Blood Component Therapy. Anesthesiology 84:732–734, 1996

C.11. What is considered a massive transfusion?

A massive transfusion is defined as the replacement of the patient's total blood volume in a 24-hour time period. This is usually between 8 to 10 U of packed red blood cells (PRBC). Many trauma cases far exceed this amount and may require other blood components in addition to the red blood cells.

Churchill WH, Kaitz SR (eds): Transfusion Medicine, p 211. Boston, Blackwell Scientific, 1988

Kruskall MS, Mintz PD, Bergin JJ et al: Transfusion therapy in emergency room medicine. Ann Emerg Med 17:329, 1988

C.12. *What are the complications associated with a massive transfusion?*

Complications of a massive transfusion include dilutional coagulopathy, disseminated intravascular coagulation (DIC), fibrinolysis, citrate toxicity, hyperkalemia, hypokalemia, acid-base imbalance, impaired hemoglobin function, and hypothermia.

Dilutional coagulopathy usually becomes a problem during massive transfusions. Both platelets and coagulation factors are markedly decreased and need to be replaced. They should be administered after laboratory documentation of the deficiency. It is no longer accepted practice to give fresh-frozen plasma (FFP) routinely after 5 U of PRBC, nor is it proper to give platelets after 10 U of PRBC. At present, dilutional coagulopathies appear to be rare, even with the transfusion of one blood volume. Approximately 40% of the coagulation factors remain after one blood volume replacement, and this should be sufficient to allow normal coagulation. Platelets can be reduced to 30% to 40% of normal after one blood volume transfusion. This decrease will usually represent a platelet count $<100,000/mm^3$ and may lead to a prolonged bleeding time.

Disseminated intravascular coagulation (DIC) and fibrinolysis may occur following massive transfusions. An important triggering event of DIC and fibrinolysis is shock, with its accompanying tissue ischemia, acidemia, and waste product accumulation. Therefore, early and prompt treatment of hypoperfusion is mandatory.

Citrate toxicity is frequently discussed, but it is rarely a problem. Citrate is added to stored blood to bind calcium and therefore prevent clotting. The citrate anticoagulant stays with the plasma, and obviously fresh-frozen plasma (FFP) would contain much more citrate than packed cells. Citrate binds calcium and decreases the patient's ionized calcium level. Hypocalcemia may present as a prolongation of the QT interval with little effect on cardiac performance. In some cases ventricular performance may be compromised. However, cardiac performance may also be decreased by acidemia, hyperkalemia, and hypothermia, which all accompany the shock state. Therefore, the routine administration of supplemental calcium is not indicated. A point worth noting is that citrate is metabolized to bicarbonate, and it can contribute to post-transfusion metabolic alkalosis.

Hyperkalemia can be a rare occurrence in the massively transfused patient. Plasma potassium levels of stored whole blood range between 12 and 32 mEq/liter. The potassium level increases approximately 1 mEq/liter per day in stored blood. A unit of whole blood would contain between 4 and 8 mEq of potassium, which is hardly enough to cause hyperkalemia. A unit of PRBC contains insignificant amounts of potassium because most plasma is removed. However, in the shock state with hypoperfusion and acidemia, hyperkalemia may become evident.

Hypokalemia is also a possibility following a massive transfusion. Citrate is metabolized to bicarbonate, resulting in a metabolic alkalosis that can cause hypokalemia. In addition, the transfused red blood cells take up potassium, which can also result in hypokalemia.

Acid-base imbalance is a problem following massive transfusion. Banked blood with a *p*H of 6.8 is acidotic and may worsen the acidosis that accompanies shock. However, this acidosis is easily reversible with the restoration of normal perfusion. No need is seen to give supplemental bicarbonate based on an arbitrary number of units transfused. However, if a metabolic acidosis persists, then sodium bicarbonate is warranted. As stated, citrate from stored blood and lactate from lactated Ringer's solution are metabolized to bicarbonate, and this can cause a metabolic alkalosis.

Impaired hemoglobin function is a theoretic possibility after massive transfusions. The 2,3-diphosphoglycerate (2,3-DPG) level is decreased in banked blood. This will shift the oxygen-hemoglobin dissociation curve to the left, and oxygen will be held more tightly by the hemoglobin molecule. However, no studies have documented any adverse effects from this.

Hypothermia is an obvious consequence of infusing cold banked blood. Therefore, it is recommended that the blood be reconstituted with warm normal saline. In addition, all fluids should pass through a warming device to help prevent hypothermia.

Churchill WH, Kaitz SR (eds): Transfusion Medicine, pp 216–226. Boston, Blackwell Scientific, 1988

Kruskall MS, Mintz PD, Bergin JJ et al: Transfusion therapy in emergency room medicine. Ann Emerg Med 17:329–331, 1988

Miller RD (ed): Anesthesia, 4th ed, pp 1624–1632. New York, Churchill Livingstone, 1994

C.13. Can the shift of the oxygen-hemoglobin dissociation curve be quantitated?

Yes, the shift of the oxygen-hemoglobin dissociation curve is quantitated by means of the P 50 values. P 50 refers to the partial pressure of oxygen at which hemoglobin is 50% saturated with oxygen. A leftward shift of the curve indicates a low P 50 value. The normal P 50 of blood is 27 mm Hg, and the normal level of 2,3-DPG is 4.8 mmol/ml of erythrocytes.

Miller RD (ed): Anesthesia, 4th ed, p 1624. New York, Churchill Livingstone, 1994

C.14. How is hypothermia defined?

Hypothermia is defined as a body core temperature of <35°C. A trauma patient brought to the emergency room may already be hypothermic. In the emergency room, this patient will receive intravenous fluids and will be exposed to the ambient temperature of the emergency room, both of which will further decrease his core temperature. In the operating room this patient will lose heat by conduction, convection, and increased evaporative losses.

Feliciano DV, Moore EE, Mattox KL (eds): Trauma, 3rd ed, pp 717–718, 955. Stamford, CT, Appleton & Lange, 1996

Stene JK, Gerarde CM (eds): Trauma: Anesthesia, pp 340–341. Baltimore, Williams & Wilkins, 1991

C.15. What are the adverse effects of hypothermia?

- Shivering can increase O_2 consumption by as much as 400%.
- The oxygen-hemoglobin dissociation curve shifts to the left.
- Coagulation of blood decreases.
- Epinephrine and norepinephrine levels are increased, causing peripheral vasoconstriction.

As hypothermia becomes severe, both heart rate and blood pressure can decrease. Finally cardiac irritability leading to ventricular fibrillation can be seen.

Feliciano DV, Moore EE, Mattox KL (eds): Trauma, 2nd ed, p 954. Stamford, CT, Appleton & Lange, 1996

Stene JK, Gerarde CM (eds): Trauma: Anesthesia, pp 347–350. Baltimore, Williams & Wilkins, 1991

C.16. What is the treatment of hypothermia?

The normal response to hypothermia is shivering, which is blocked by general anesthesia. Therefore, it is of utmost importance to prevent and treat hypothermia. Recommendations include the following:

- Increase the temperature of the operating room.
- Use a warming blanket.
- Preheat intravenous fluids.
- Pass all fluids through a warming device.
- Use low-flow anesthesia.
- Add a heated humidifier or an artificial heat moisture exchanger (HME) to the anesthesia circuit.

Feliciano DV, Moore EE, Mattox KL (eds): Trauma, 3rd ed, pp 957–958. Stamford, CT, Appleton & Lange, 1996

Stene JK, Gerarde CM (eds): Trauma: Anesthesia, pp 343–347. Baltimore, Williams & Wilkins, 1991

C.17. What are the effects of blood transfusion on the immune system?

Blood transfusion will result in immunologic changes that can be harmful in some patients and helpful in other patients. This immunomodulation occurs from immune suppression. At a cellular level is seen stimulation of immunologic suppressor cells on inhibition of immunologic effector cells. The blood components crucial to these changes are thought to be the white cells or plasma.

An example of a beneficial effect is the increased survival of the renal allograft in patients who had received a prior transfusion. In cancer patients, a possible harmful effect of immunosuppression is the increased cancer recurrence rate seen in patients who have had prior transfusions. Finally, a number of clinical studies have demonstrated that perioperative transfusion is associated with an increased incidence of infection and sepsis.

Landers DF, Hill GE, Wong KC, Fox IJ: Blood transfusion-induced immunomodulation. Anesth Analg 82:187–204, 1996

C.18. What are the guidelines for transfusion of blood products?

The New York Hospital Guidelines for blood product usage are as follows:

Red Cell Transfusion Criteria
- Hemogloglobin (Hgb) <8 g/dl (Hct <26%) and mean red cell volume (MCV) within normal limit (WNL) (81–100 fl, 70–125 fl age ≤14 years)
- Hgb <8 g/dl (Hct <26%) and high risk/acute bleed[1]
- Hgb <11 g/dl (Hct <36%) and clinically symptomatic[2]
- Hgb <11 g/dl (Hct <36%) and bleed >1 U/24 h

---

[1]High risk: Patient with coronary artery disease, chronic pulmonary disease, cerebrovascular disease, or congenital or acquired anemia.
[2]Symptomatic: Patients with signs or symptoms of anemia, such as tachycardia, angina, ECG changes or of neonatal respiratory distress, known hemoglobinopathy, and so forth.

- Any Hgb and high risk[1] and acute bleed
- Any Hgb and symptomatic[2] and acute bleed
- Any Hgb and bleed >2 U/24 h, or >15% of blood volume/24 h

Platelet Transfusion Criteria
- Platelet count <20,000/mm³ without thrombotic thrombocytopenic purpura (TTP), idiopathic thrombocytopenic purpura (ITP), post-transfusion purpura, or hemolytic uremic syndrome
- Platelet count <50,000/mm³ with minor bleed, preoperative for a minor procedure or prematurity
- Platelet count <90,000/mm³ with bleed requiring red blood cell (RBC) transfusion or preoperative for a major procedure
- Massive RBC transfusion (>8 U/24 h)
- Bleeding time >10 minutes
- Open heart surgery transfusion of more than mean number of RBC units (6)/case

Fresh-Frozen Plasma Transfusion Criteria
- Massive transfusion >8 U RBC/24 h (>1 blood volume infants/children)
- Abnormal coagulation test result(s) (prothrombin time [PT] >15 seconds or partial thromboplastin time [PTT] >45 seconds) during prior 24 hours or known congenital coagulation factor disorder (factor II, V, VII, IX, X, XI, XII) and bleeding or prophylaxis for major procedures
- Clinical evidence of abnormal bleeding from venipuncture sites or generalized oozing
- Patients with diagnosis of TTP
- Open heart surgery transfusion of more than mean number RBC units (6)/case

Cryoprecipitate Transfusion Criteria
- Massive transfusion >8 U/24 h
- Open heart surgery transfusion of more than mean number RBC units (6)/case
- Bleeding or invasive procedure with hypofibrinogemia or DIC
- Deficient VIII or von Willebrand (VWD) factor or abnormal fibrinogen and presurgical or bleed

Practice guidelines for blood component therapy: A report by the ASA Task Force on Blood Component Therapy. Anesthesiology 84:732–747, 1996

New York Hospital Protocols, 1997

C.19. If a patient were a member of the Jehovah's Witness religious sect, would you give a blood transfusion?

Jehovah's Witnesses are best known for refusing the transfusion of blood and blood products. They believe all hope of eternal life is forfeited if they accept a transfusion. Therefore a blood transfusion is considered a physical violation. They will refuse transfusion of whole blood, packed red cells, white blood cells, plasma, and platelets. However, they will allow the use of cardiopulmonary bypass, dialysis, or similar equipment as well as intraoperative blood salvage where the extracorporeal circulation is uninterrupted. Their religious understanding does not absolutely prohibit albumin, immune globulins, or hemophiliac preparations; those products must be decided on an individual basis. They accept all nonblood replacements, including nonblood colloids, crystalloids, dextrans, or oxygen-carrying blood substitutes.

The right of a Jehovah's Witness to refuse a blood transfusion is absolute. The courts have upheld their rights to refuse a blood transfusion. Most witnesses take adequate legal steps to relieve the liability of the medical personnel. Most carry a medical alert card that states their wishes and they usually have made arrangements for proxy or surrogate decision makers. In addition, an open and honest avenue of communication must exist between the patient, surgeon, and anesthesiologist.

An anesthesiologist may refuse to care for any patient when a procedure is elective. In an emergency situation, legal and ethical requirements apply. Conversely, any competent adult also has the right to refuse any therapy, and to treat such a patient against that person's will is to commit battery.

C.20. If a child is a Jehovah's Witness and suffered from hemorrhagic shock what would you do?

Care of minors presents the greatest concern and often leads to legal action against the parents under child-neglect status. Such actions are questioned by Jehovah's Witnesses who do seek good medical care for their children, while claiming that consideration be given to their families' religious beliefs. Doctors can apply to the court for permission to transfuse blood to children of this sect who are under age. In an unforeseeable emergency, generally blood may be given without consulting a court.

DuBose ER (ed):The Jehovah's Witness Tradition: Religious Beliefs and Health Care Practices. 1995

C.21. Are there artificial blood substitutes available?

Three types of artificial blood are being investigated: hemoglobin solutions, liposome-encapsulated hemoglobin, and perflurocarbons.

Hemoglobin Solutions
Hemoglobin can now be prepared from outdated human blood. Intravascular free hemoglobin has a high affinity for oxygen and is quickly excreted. Hemoglobin can now be modified and dissolved in an isotonic medium that will decrease renal filtration, prolong intramuscular life, and restore a normal P 50 of oxygen. Hemoglobin solutions can restore circulating blood volume and provide adequate tissue oxygenation in animal models. Detrimental effects include renal toxicity and increased systemic and pulmonary vascular pressures. Of note, in 1992 a human recombinant hemoglobin substitute was designed. It functions like normal hemoglobin, but it does not require crossmatching nor does it transmit disease or become rapidly outdated.

Liposome-Encapsulated Hemoglobin
Hemoglobin can be membrane encapsulated for modification. It is then possible to add 2,3-DPG, or inositol hexaphosphate to the membrane thereby adjusting the P 50 to match the red blood cells. In theory, the encapsulated hemoglobin will have a longer intravascular duration and greater oxygen carrying capacity. The membrane is being further modified to try to decrease the deposition in the reticuloendothelial system, thus further increasing the intravascular duration.

Perflurocarbons
Perflurocarbons are synthetic substances that have a capacity for dissolved oxygen. It is unlikely these will be useful because a high PaO_2 is needed to allow the perflurocarbon to carry even small amounts of dissolved O_2.

Further direction of blood substitutes will increase oxygen carrying capacity while decreasing the side-effects. Then after benefits have been proved, they may become replacements for red blood cell transfusions. Currently, artificial blood substitute use is not indicated.

Biro GP: Perflurocarbon-based red blood cell substitutes. Transfusion Medicine Reviews 7:84–85, 1993

Dietz NM, Joyner MJ, Warner MA: Blood substitutes: Fluids, drugs, or miracle solutions? Anesth Analg 82:390–405, 1996

Miller RD (ed): Anesthesia, 4th ed, p 1643. New York, Churchill Livingstone, 1994

Rudolph AS: Encapsulated hemoglobin: current issues and future goals. Ant Cells Blood Subs Immobilization Biotechnol 2:347–360, 1994

D. Postoperative Management

D.1. What is adult respiratory distress syndrome (ARDS)?

Adult respiratory distress syndrome is an acute respiratory failure seen in patients with healthy lungs after being exposed to shock, trauma, sepsis, aspiration, transfusion, or some other rare conditions. Initially, when this lung injury was thought to be related to the shock state and its resuscitation, names such as "shock lung" and "traumatic wet lung" were applied to acute respiratory insufficiency following injury. It is now recognized that many types of lung insults will result in damage to the alveolar capillary membrane, resulting in leakage of proteinaceous fluid from the intravascular space into the interstitium and subsequently into the alveolar spaces.

This injury with its resulting interstitial and alveolar edema produces a clinical picture ranging from mild to severe pulmonary dysfunction that can actually be fatal.

Adult respiratory distress syndrome is characterized by the following:

- Hypoxemia—is relatively unresponsive to increasing inspired oxygen concentration
- Decreased pulmonary compliance—clinically appears as "stiff lungs"
- Initially normal chest x-ray progressing to diffuse infiltrates or even to areas of complete consolidation
- Decrease in resting lung volumes, specifically, functional residual capacity

Barash PG, Cullen BF, Stoelting RK (eds): Clinical Anesthesia, 3rd ed, pp 1371–1372. Philadelphia, JB Lippincott, 1997

Feliciano DV, Moore EE, Mattox KL (eds): Trauma, 3rd ed, pp 1107–1109. Stamford, CT, Appleton & Lange, 1996

Schwartz SI (ed): Principles of Surgery, 6th ed, pp 123–126. New York, Churchill Livingstone, 1994

D.2. How is ARDS treated?

The treatment of ARDS is primarily supportive and consists of the following:

- Correct the primary cause, such as sepsis.
- Use positive end-expiratory pressure (PEEP) and high-inspired oxygen concentration to maintain adequate oxygenation.
- Transfuse PRBC only as needed if the patient is severely anemic to increase hemoglobin concentration and therefore improve oxygen delivery.

- Use hemodynamic monitoring to guide fluid therapy and cardiovascular support.

These efforts comprise the current mainstay of treatment. ARDS is a time-related process and most patients can be supported through the respiratory failure. However, approximately 50% of the ARDS patients will die from sepsis or a complication of their initial injury.

Barash PG, Cullen BF, Stoelting RK (eds): Clinical Anesthesia, 3rd ed, pp 1372–1373. Philadelphia, JB Lippincott, 1997

Feliciano DV, Moore EE, Mattox KL (eds): Trauma, 3rd ed, pp 1117–1127. Stamford, CT, Appleton & Lange, 1996

Schwartz SI (ed): Principles of Surgery, 6th ed, pp 128–130. New York, McGraw-Hill, 1994

D.3. In the recovery room, you are called to see this patient because of oliguria. How would you evaluate and treat this patient?

Oliguria is a decrease in urinary output to <0.5 ml/kg/h. Renal failure can be divided into three categories:

Prerenal
Prerenal failure is usually caused by a low cardiac output due to hypovolemia or cardiac failure. It can be evaluated by checking the patient's heart rate, blood pressure, central venous pressure, pulmonary capillary wedge pressure, and cardiac output. If hypovolemia is the cause, then treatment would consist of a fluid bolus. If the patient is in cardiac failure, then inotropic support and diuretics could be administered.

Renal
Intrinsic renal failure is generally due to toxic injury or ischemia. Ischemic injury is caused by a decrease in perfusion pressure that can lead to renal cellular dysfunction. Toxic injury can be caused by substances that affect renal tubular function in addition to renal blood flow. Urinalysis may show cells and/or casts that are indicative of acute renal failure. Intrinsic renal failure can be minor and short-lived or it can progress to chronic renal failure, depending on the severity of the insult. Currently, dopamine (2 to 3 µg/kg/min) can be used to dilate the afferent renal arterioles. Diuretics are another class of drugs frequently used to help improve urinary output. Before administering a diuretic, it is important to ensure that the patient is adequately hydrated. Furosemide, a loop diuretic, and mannitol, an osmotic diuretic, are both well known for their ability to increase urinary output. In addition, studies have shown that these drugs may have another site of action that can cause dilation of the afferent renal arterioles. If the administration of diuretics is successful in increasing urinary output, all hope is not lost. However, if this patient is unable to produce urine, acute renal failure will ensue and dialysis will probably be needed.

Postrenal
Urinary tract obstruction must be sought and corrected to treat possible causes of postrenal oliguria. This usually requires irrigation and/or changing of the Foley catheter. Consider the possibility of an intraoperative mishap causing postrenal obstruction.

Barash PG, Cullen BF, Stoelting RK (eds): Clinical Anesthesia, 3rd ed, pp 1376–1378. Philadelphia, JB Lippincott, 1997

Feliciano DV, Moore EE, Mattox KL (eds): Trauma, 3rd ed, pp 1141–1145. Stamford, CT, Appleton & Lange, 1996

53 Scoliosis

Victor M. Zayas

A 14-year-old girl with scoliosis is scheduled for posterior spine fusion with Cotrel-Dubousset instrumentation. She has been told that her scoliosis is idiopathic. Her past medical history was unremarkable but her mother stated that she appeared to get short of breath more easily than her friends when she played basketball.

A. Medical Disease and Differential Diagnosis

1. What is scoliosis?
2. What is the most common type of scoliosis?
3. What are other types of scoliosis?
4. How is the severity of scoliosis assessed and why is the severity important?
5. What abnormalities in pulmonary function tests are most commonly seen in scoliosis? What is the cause of these abnormalities?
6. What is the most common arterial blood gas abnormality seen in scoliosis? What are possible causes for this abnormality?
7. What abnormalities of ventilatory drive can be associated with scoliosis?
8. How can the cardiovascular system be affected in patients with scoliosis?
9. What is the relationship between scoliosis and malignant hyperthermia?

B. Preoperative Evaluation and Preparation

1. What should the anesthesiologist know about the nature of the curve?
2. What aspects of the history are most important?
3. What aspects of the physical examination are most important?
4. Why is a preoperative neurologic assessment important?
5. What tests would you order preoperatively?
6. What preparation should the patient have preoperatively?
7. What should you consider in ordering preoperative medications?

C. Intraoperative Monitoring

1. What monitoring would you use?
2. What is the incidence of neurologic complications in scoliosis surgery and which patients are at highest risk? What monitoring techniques are used to minimize this complication?
3. What are somatosensory evoked potentials (SSEPs) and how are they used?
4. How reliable are SSEPs for predicting spinal injury?
5. How are SSEPs affected by anesthetic agents? What other factors affect SSEPs?
6. What should be done if the SSEPs become abnormal during surgery?
7. How is the "wake-up test" performed? What complications can occur during this test?

8. What is the optimal anesthetic technique for scoliosis surgery?
9. What complications occur related to positioning the patient?
10. How will the surgical procedure influence estimated blood loss and fluid requirements?
11. What techniques can be used to minimize transfusion requirements?
12. What techniques would you use to produce deliberate hypotension during scoliosis surgery? What is the major concern of using this technique?

D. Postoperative Management

1. When would you extubate the patient?
2. What should be done to optimize pulmonary status?
3. What laboratory tests should be ordered postoperatively?
4. What fluid therapy would you use postoperatively?
5. What complications may occur following scoliosis surgery?

A. Medical Disease and Differential Diagnosis

A.1. What is scoliosis?

The spine normally curves posteriorly in the thoracic region and anteriorly in the lumbar. These physiologic curves are the thoracic kyphosis and the lumbar lordosis, respectively. The spine is not normally curved when viewed from the front or back. Scoliosis refers to a lateral curvature of the spine. Curves are classified as structural or nonstructural. A nonstructural curve, such as lumbar scoliosis from a leg length discrepancy, will resolve when the patient is supine or uses a lift, and it does not require surgical correction. In contrast, structural scoliosis lacks normal flexibility and does not correct with bending or lying supine. In addition to the lateral curvature of the spine, the vertebrae are rotated and the rib cage may be markedly deformed (Fig. 53-1). As demonstrated in the computed tomography (CT) scan image in Figure 53-2, this thoracic deformity can lead to a significant decrease in total lung volume. Particularly note the decrease in left lung volume relative to the right.

A.2. What is the most common type of scoliosis?

Idiopathic scoliosis is the most common type of scoliosis (70% of all cases); it occurs in an infantile, a juvenile, or an adolescent form. As the name implies, the cause is unknown, but it appears to be multifactorial, including abnormalities of collagen, brain stem function, equilibrium, hormones, and growth. Genetic factors are important in its development as evidenced by an increased incidence of scoliosis in relatives of affected patients. The mode of inheritance is unclear but appears to be polygenic. The prevalence of idiopathic scoliosis in large screening studies depends on the definition of scoliosis and the population screened. The prevalence of curves >10 degrees is 1.5% to 3.0%, >20 degrees it is 0.3% to 0.5%, and >30 degrees it is 0.2% to 0.3%. The adolescent form of idiopathic scoliosis is by far the most common in the United States. The prevalence was 1.2% in a large screening study of 125 million students age 10 to 16. The male:female ratio depends in part on the age of the patient, but curves requiring surgical correction are more common in females.

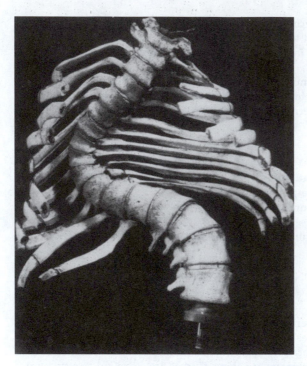

Figure 53-1. In addition to producing a lateral deformity of the spine, scoliosis also results in rotation of the vertebral bodies and significant rib cage deformity.

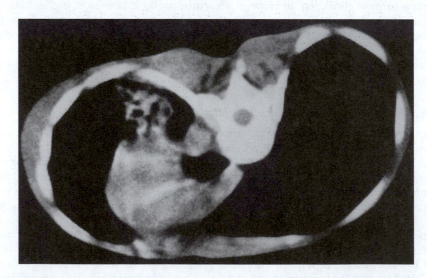

Figure 53-2. A computed tomography (CT) scan of the thorax, which demonstrates significant loss of lung volume due to the rib cage deformity.

Lonstein JE: Adolescent idiopathic scoliosis. Lancet 344(8934):1407–1412, 1994

Lonstein JE, Bjorklund S, Wanniger MH et al: Voluntary school screening for scoliosis in Minnesota. J Bone Joint Surg 64A:481–488, 1982

Weinstein SL (ed): The Pediatric Spine: Principles and Practice, pp 445–462. New York, Raven Press, 1994

A.3. What are other types of scoliosis?

Many etiologic classifications of structural scoliosis exist. Neuromuscular scoliosis (paralytic scoliosis) can occur as a result of diseases such as cerebral palsy, muscular dystrophy, poliomyelitis, familial dysautonomia, and so on. Congenital scoliosis is the result of congenital anomalies such as hemivertebrae, and fused vertebrae or ribs. Neurofibromatosis and Marfan's syndrome are also associated with scoliosis. These underlying conditions can have a major impact on the anesthetic plan. The classification of structural scoliosis is as follows:

Idiopathic
- Infantile
- Juvenile
- Adolescent

Neuromuscular (Paralytic)
- Neuropathic
  - Upper motor neuron (e.g. cerebral palsy, spinal cord injury)
  - Lower motor neuron (e.g., poliomyelitis, meningomyelocoele);
  - Familial dysautonomia
- Myopathic
  - Muscular dystrophy
  - Myotonic dystrophy

Congenital
- Hemivertebrae
- Congenitally fused ribs

Neurofibromatosis

Mesenchymal Disorders
- Marfan's syndrome
- Ehlers-Danlos syndrome

Trauma
- Vertebral fracture or surgery
- Post-thoracoplasty
- Postradiation

Bradford DS, Lonstein JE, Moe JH et al (eds): Moe's Textbook of Scoliosis and Other Spinal Deformities, pp 41–45. Philadelphia, WB Saunders, 1987

A.4. How is the severity of scoliosis assessed and why is the severity important?

In 1966, the Scoliosis Research Society standardized the method for assessing scoliosis severity. The most common measure of severity is Cobb's angle. Figure 53-3 illustrates how Cobb's angle is measured on a roentgenogram of the spine. A perpen-

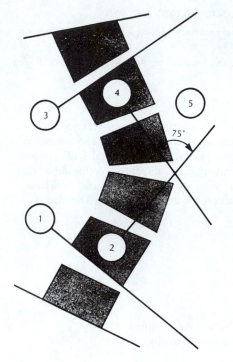

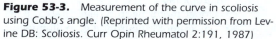

Figure 53-3. *Measurement of the curve in scoliosis using Cobb's angle. (Reprinted with permission from Levine DB: Scoliosis. Curr Opin Rheumatol 2:191, 1987)*

dicular (2) is constructed from the bottom of the lowest vertebrae (1) whose bottom tilts toward the concavity of the curve, and another perpendicular (4) from the top of the highest vertebrae (3) whose top tilts toward the concavity. The angle (5) at which these perpendiculars intersect is Cobb's angle. Numerous studies have documented that the more severe the thoracic curve (greater Cobb's angle), the more profound the disturbance in pulmonary function. Surgical treatment is usually recommended for curves > 45 to 50 degrees. Curves >60 degrees are usually associated with decreases in pulmonary function.

In a series of 79 patients with thoracic scoliosis, the mean Cobb's angle was 45 degrees and vital capacity was decreased by an average of 22%. Figure 53-4 demonstrates that forced vital capacity (FVC) and forced expiratory volume in 1 second (FEV_1) decrease with increasing thoracic curve severity.

Scoliosis severity and impairment of pulmonary function also increase with the greater number of vertebrae involved, more cephalad location of the curve, and loss of the normal thoracic kyphosis. Severe curves have a worse prognosis because they tend to progress and if they are long-standing can cause permanent damage of the lung parenchyma, respiratory failure, cor pulmonale, and death. It is important to note that patients with neuromuscular types of scoliosis may have a much more profound decrease in pulmonary function for any given curve severity.

Bradford DS, Lonstein JE, Moe JH et al (eds): Moe's Textbook of Scoliosis and Other Spinal Deformities, pp 586–587. Philadelphia, WB Saunders, 1987

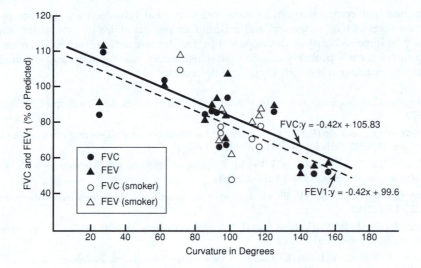

Figure 53-4. Relationship between forced vital capacity (FVC) and forced expiratory volume in one second (FEV$_1$), and size of the curve in 20 patients with thoracic scoliosis. (Reprinted with permission from Weinstein SL, Zavala DC, Ponseti IV: Idiopathic scoliosis: Long-term follow-up and prognosis in untreated patients. J Bone Joint Surg Am 63:701, 1981)

Kearon C, Viviani GR, Kirkley A et al: Factors determining pulmonary function in adolescent idiopathic thoracic scoliosis. Am Rev Respir Dis 148(2):288–294, 1993

Levine DB: Scoliosis. Curr Opin Rheumatol 2:190–195, 1990

Weinstein SL (ed): The Pediatric Spine: Principles and Practice, pp 463–477. New York, Raven Press, 1994

Weinstein SL, Zaval DC, Ponseti IV et al: Idiopathic scoliosis. Long-term follow-up and prognosis in untreated patients. J Bone Joint Surg Am 63:702–712, 1981

A.5. What abnormalities in pulmonary function tests are most commonly seen in scoliosis? What is the cause of these abnormalities?

A decrease in lung volumes, a restrictive pattern, is most commonly seen in thoracic scoliosis. The greatest reduction occurs in vital capacity that is typically reduced to 60% to 80% of predicted. Total lung capacity, functional residual capacity (FRC), inspiratory capacity, and expiratory reserve volume are also decreased. An increase in residual volume has been reported in patients with congenital scoliosis and in patients with idiopathic scoliosis 3 years following corrective spine fusion.

During exercise, ventilation is adequate but tidal volume is reduced and respiratory rate is increased. Maximal work capacity may also be decreased. Unless there is coexisting obstructive airway disease, the ratio of the FEV$_1$:FVC is normal. Impaired respiratory muscle function also occurs in scoliosis as evidenced by a decrease in inspiratory force to 70% of normal values.

These abnormalities in pulmonary function are usually the result of abnormal thoracic cage geometry producing a marked decrease in chest wall compliance rather than any abnormality in the lungs or respiratory muscles themselves. These changes in chest wall compliance can be mimicked in normal volunteers by chest strapping. Exceptions include congenital and infantile scoliosis in which growth of the lungs may be impaired early in development by the thoracic deformity. The decrease in inspiratory force is probably caused by the inspiratory muscles working at a mechanical disadvantage due to the chest wall deformity.

Bergofsky EH: Respiratory failure in disorders of the thoracic cage. Am Rev Respir Dis 119:643–669, 1979

Bradford DS, Lonstein JE, Moe JH et al (eds): Moe's textbook of scoliosis and other spinal deformities, pp 585–592. Philadelphia, WB Saunders, 1987

Cooper DM, Rojas JV, Mellins RB et al: Respiratory mechanics in adolescents with idiopathic scoliosis. Am Rev Respir Dis 130:16–22, 1984

Day GA, Upadhyay SS, Ho EK et al: Pulmonary functions in congenital scoliosis. Spine 19(9): 1027–1031, 1993

Jones RS, Kennedy JD, Hasham F et al: Mechanical inefficiency of the thoracic cage in scoliosis. Thorax 36:456–461, 1981

Kearon C, Viviani GR, Killian KJ: Factors influencing work capacity in adolescent idiopathic thoracic scoliosis. Am Rev Respir Dis 148(2):295–303, 1993

Weinstein SL, Zavala DC, Ponseti IV: Idiopathic scoliosis: Long-term follow-up and prognosis in untreated patients. J Bone Joint Surg Am 63:702–712, 1981

A.6. What is the most common arterial blood gas abnormality seen in scoliosis? What are possible causes for this abnormality?

It has been documented that patients with thoracic scoliosis have arterial oxygen desaturation compared with normal controls. Both arterial P_{CO_2} and *p*H are usually normal. Several studies have failed to show a correlation between the severity of the curve and the amount of desaturation.

Arterial hypoxemia is probably caused by ventilation-perfusion inequalities. Decreased diffusing capacity and alveolar hypoventilation may also play a role. However, the diffusing capacity is not decreased sufficiently to be the sole cause of the hypoxemia. Similarly, alveolar ventilation at rest and during exercise is usually normal because arterial P_{CO_2} is usually normal. It has been reported that some patients have a closing capacity higher than FRC resulting in premature airway closure during normal tidal breathing. This is probably not a common cause of hypoxemia because other studies have failed to demonstrate this finding. Some authors have reported an increase in the ratio of dead space to tidal volume (VD/VT), whereas other recent series have found VD/VT to be normal. This discrepancy may be related to the patient population studied, the severity of the scoliosis, or both. Severe curves and/or long-standing scoliosis can produce severe $\dot{V}/\dot{Q}$ abnormalities, alveolar hypoventilation, CO_2 retention, and more severe hypoxemia. Surgically untreated severe scoliosis increases the individual's risk of premature death from respiratory failure after 40 years of age. A survey of patients with respiratory failure in Sweden found that a vital capacity <50% of predicted and a Cobb's angle >100 degrees indicated an increased risk of respiratory failure.

Bergofsky EH: Respiratory failure in disorders of the thoracic cage. Am Rev Respir Dis 119:643–669, 1979

Kafer ER: Respiratory and cardiovascular functions in scoliosis and the principles of anesthetic management. Anesthesiology 32:339–351, 1980

Pehrsson K, Nachemson A, Olofson J et al: Respiratory failure in scoliosis and other thoracic deformities. Spine 17:714–718, 1992

Weber W, Smith JP, Briscoe WA, et al: Pulmonary function in asymptomatic adolescents with idiopathic scoliosis. Am Rev Respir Dis 111:389–397, 1975

A.7. What abnormalities of ventilatory drive can be associated with scoliosis?

The slope of the ventilatory response to CO_2 may be decreased in patients with scoliosis. This is probably not specific to scoliosis because this response is known to be reduced in situations in which the work of breathing is increased even in the absence of a chest wall deformity. Patients with mild scoliosis have been reported to exhibit abnormal ventilatory patterns in response to hypoxia and hypercarbia. This pattern tends to minimize the work of breathing (e.g., higher respiratory rate and lower tidal volume).

Kafer ER: Respiratory and cardiovascular functions in scoliosis and the principles of anesthetic management. Anesthesiology 32:339–351, 1980

Smyth RJ, Chapman KR, Wright TA et al: Ventilatory patterns during hypoxia, hypercapnia, and exercise in adolescents with mild scoliosis. Pediatrics 77(5):692–697, 1986

Weber W, Smith JP, Briscoe WA et al: Pulmonary function in asymptomatic adolescents with idiopathic scoliosis. Am Rev Respir Dis 111:389–397, 1975

A.8. How can the cardiovascular system be affected in patients with scoliosis?

Patients with scoliosis may develop elevated pulmonary vascular resistance and pulmonary hypertension. This can result in right ventricular hypertrophy and, eventually, right ventricular failure. A 50-year study of untreated scoliosis demonstrated that the mortality rate of these patients was twice that of the general population and respiratory failure or right ventricle failure accounted for 60% of the deaths.

The increase in pulmonary vascular resistance is probably due to several factors. First, hypoxemia results in pulmonary vasoconstriction, increasing pulmonary vascular resistance and hence an increase in pulmonary arterial pressure. If the hypoxemia is chronic, hypertensive vascular changes can occur and pulmonary hypertension may become irreversible. It has also been proposed that the chest wall deformity compresses some lung regions, increasing vascular resistance in them. Finally, if scoliosis develops in the first 6 years of life, the growth of the pulmonary vascular bed may be impaired by the chest wall deformity. Supporting this concept are reports of a decrease in the number of vascular units per lung volume in patients with scoliosis.

The most common cardiovascular abnormality in patients with scoliosis is mitral valve prolapse. Antibiotic prophylaxis should be administered prior to catheterization of the bladder and perhaps prior to laryngoscopy in these patients.

Some conditions associated with scoliosis also affect the cardiovascular system. Patients with Duchenne's muscular dystrophy develop a cardiomyopathy in the second decade of life that may not be appreciated on the basis of clinical symptoms because these patients lead a very sedentary life. The electrocardiogram may reveal tachycardia, prolonged PR and QRS intervals, ST abnormalities, bundle branch block,

Q waves in the left precordium, and tall R waves in the right precordium. Ejection fraction may be decreased on echocardiogram.

Patients with Marfan's syndrome may have mitral and aortic insufficiency, aneurysm of the proximal ascending aorta, and abnormalities of the conduction system.

The association of scoliosis and congenital heart disease has been well established. Although no specific cardiac lesion has been identified, some series have suggested that scoliosis is more common in patients with cyanotic heart disease.

Bradford DS, Lonstein JE, Moe JH et al (eds): Moe's Textbook of Scoliosis and Other Spinal Deformities, pp 609–611. Philadelphia, WB Saunders, 1987

Kafer ER: Respiratory and cardiovascular functions in scoliosis and the principles of anesthetic management. Anesthesiology 32:339–351, 1980

Kawakami N, Mimatsu K, Deguchi M et al: Scoliosis and congenital heart disease. Spine 20(11): 1252–1255, 1995

A.9. What is the relationship between scoliosis and malignant hyperthermia?

In 1970, a statistical, retrospective review of 89 patients who developed malignant hyperthermia reported that 6 of these patients had "idiopathic kyphoscoliosis." Although this report suggests an association between idiopathic scoliosis and malignant hyperthermia, data are not yet available regarding the incidence of this disorder in scoliosis patients. Certainly some scoliosis patients do have an increased risk of malignant hyperthermia because of their underlying disease. For example, patients with certain muscle disorders (e.g., Duchenne's muscular dystrophy) are at increased risk of developing both malignant hyperthermia and scoliosis.

Britt BA, Kalow W: Malignant hyperthermia: A statistical review. Can Anaesth Soc J 17:293–315, 1970

Brownell AKW: Malignant hyperthermia: Relationship to other diseases. Br J Anaesth 60:303–308, 1988

B. Preoperative Evaluation and Preparation

B.1. What should the anesthesiologist know about the nature of the curve?

It is important to identify the location of the curve, the age of onset, its severity, the direction of the curve, and the cause of the scoliosis. The location of the curve is important because thoracic scoliosis is associated with pulmonary function abnormalities. Cervical scoliosis can cause difficulties in airway management, and it may be associated with other congenital anomalies.

The single most important feature of the curve may be the age of onset. The lung continues to grow and develop from birth until 8 years of age. The number of alveoli increases from approximately 20 million at birth to 250 million at 4 years of age. The development of significant thoracic scoliosis during this phase of rapid growth impairs lung development. A significant reduction in alveolar number has been demonstrated in patients with early onset thoracic scoliosis, predisposing these patients to impaired gas exchange and pulmonary hypertension.

Severity of the curve is important because thoracic curves >60 degrees generally produce significant decreases in pulmonary function. Curves >100 degrees can be associated with significant impairment in gas exchange. Most curves in adolescent idio-pathic scoliosis are convex to the right just as most people are right-handed. A left thoracic convexity should raise the index of suspicion to look for underlying conditions and congenital anomalies. Finally, an understanding of the cause of the scoliosis is important because underlying conditions such as muscular dystrophy or cerebral palsy will influence anesthetic management.

Bradford DS, Lonstein JE et al (eds): Moe's textbook of scoliosis and other spinal deformities, pp 585–592. Philadelphia, WB Saunders, 1987

Weinstein SL (ed): The Pediatric Spine: Principles and Practice, pp 421–429. New York, Raven Press, 1994

B2. What aspects of the history are most important?

Cardiopulmonary reserve should be assessed by questioning the patient about shortness of breath, dyspnea on exertion, exercise tolerance, and so forth. As a general rule patients who can exercise normally and "keep up with friends" in vigorous activities will have good cardiopulmonary function. Pulmonary symptoms such as episodes of wheezing or cough can indicate parenchymal lung disease and alter perioperative management. Patients with muscular dystrophy, Marfan's syndrome, and neurofibromatosis should be questioned about symptoms suggestive of cardiac conduction abnormalities such as palpitations or syncope.

B.3. What aspects of the physical examination are most important?

Particular emphasis in the physical examination should be directed toward the heart and lungs. Auscultation of the lungs may reveal wheezing or rales suggesting obstructive airway disease or parenchymal lung disease. On examining the heart, check for signs of pulmonary hypertension and right ventricular hypertrophy in addition to auscultating for murmurs and gallops. Pulmonary hypertension causes accentuation of the pulmonic component of the second heart sound and a right ventricular lift indicates right ventricular enlargement. Signs of right ventricular failure include engorged neck veins, an enlarged liver due to passive liver congestion, and lower extremity edema. If neurofibromatosis is suspected, the skin should be examined for the presence of café au lait spots or cutaneous neurofibroma. The airway should be evaluated closely for abnormalities such as cervical scoliosis, neurofibroma, or high arched palate associated with Marfan's syndrome that may make endotracheal intubation difficult.

B.4. Why is a preoperative neurologic assessment important?

A preoperative neurologic assessment is important because patients who have preexisting neurologic deficits are at increased risk for developing spinal cord injury during scoliosis surgery. Furthermore, it is important to document preoperative neurologic function to avoid confusion about postoperative neurologic complications.

B.5. What tests would you order preoperatively?

It is probably best to tailor diagnostic testing based on the severity of the scoliosis and underlying conditions rather than ordering a standard battery of diagnostic tests. In the current climate emphasizing medical cost containment, each institution needs to critically reassess preoperative testing. This healthy 14-year-old may only need a complete blood count prior to surgery. If the history or physical examination suggests that pulmonary reserve is decreased, then standard pulmonary function testing should be considered. If vital capacity is significantly diminished, arterial blood gas assessment is indicated. If routine pulmonary function testing reveals evidence of obstructive airway disease (a decrease in the ratio of the FEV_1/FVC or a decrease in $FEF_{25\%-75\%}$) then a bronchodilator should be administered to determine if the airway obstruction is reversible.

Patients with onset of scoliosis in the first 8 years of life should have pulmonary function testing, arterial blood gas analysis, and an electrocardiogram. If the electrocardiogram reveals abnormalities such as right ventricular hypertrophy (large R in V_1 and V_2), right atrial enlargement ($P > 2.5$ mm), or evidence of a cardiomyopathy, an echocardiogram or even cardiac catheterization may be indicated.

Kafer ER: Respiratory and cardiovascular functions in scoliosis and the principles of anesthetic management. Anesthesiology 32:339–351, 1980

B.6. What preparation should the patient have preoperatively?

The patient should be prepared both physiologically and psychologically for surgery. First, preoperative teaching of coughing and incentive spirometry should be emphasized. Patients with evidence of parenchymal lung disease or obstructive airway disease should have aggressive pulmonary toilet and/or bronchodilator therapy preoperatively. Finally, if an intraoperative wake-up test is planned (see below), the patient should be informed and reassured that he or she will feel no pain or discomfort. It is helpful to rehearse the wake-up test during the preoperative visit.

B.7. What should you consider in ordering preoperative medications?

Heavy premedication and narcotics are probably best avoided in patients with neuromuscular disease, evidence of pulmonary hypertension, impaired gas exchange, or markedly decreased pulmonary function. Use of an antisialagogue may be desirable because many of these surgical procedures are performed in the prone position and copious secretions may wet the tape securing the endotracheal tube and cause it to slip.

C. Intraoperative management

C.1. What monitoring would you use?

Minimal monitoring for posterior spine fusion should include blood pressure, electrocardiogram, pulse oximetry, end-tidal CO_2, esophageal stethoscope, and core temperature. A radial artery catheter is used for continuous monitoring of blood pressure, particularly if deliberate hypotension is planned to reduce blood loss. This will also facilitate obtaining blood samples for blood gas and hematocrit determination. All patients should have a urinary catheter placed to document urine output during and particularly after the surgical procedure. Monitoring of central filling pressures may be indicated if the expected blood loss is large, or cardiovascular disease is present or suspected. A pulmonary artery catheter may be useful in patients with cardiomyopathy from Duchenne's muscular dystrophy and in those with pulmonary hypertension or right ventricular failure to optimize volume replacement therapy. When placing pulmonary artery catheters in patients with pulmonary hypertension, remember that the risk of pulmonary artery rupture, a complication with a mortality of 50%, is increased in such patients. Neuromuscular blockade should be monitored if a balanced anesthetic technique is used.

C.2. What is the incidence of neurologic complications in scoliosis surgery and which patients are at highest risk? What monitoring techniques are used to minimize this complication?

In the 1987 morbidity report of the Scoliosis Research Society the rate of complete or partial paraplegia was 0.26%. The highest rate was 0.86% with sublaminar wires, followed by a rate of 0.60% with Cotrel-Dubousset instrumentation, and the lowest rate (0.23%) with Harrington rods. It has been proposed that distraction of the cord and straightening of the deformity compresses the spinal cord and disrupts the arterial blood supply of the cord. The spinal cord and nerve roots can also be injured directly by hooks or instrumentation.

Prevention of neurologic complications begins with identification of the high risk group. Patients are at increased risk for developing paraplegia if they have a severe rigid deformity (>120 degrees), kyphosis, neurofibromatosis, congenital or postinfectious scoliosis, a preexisting neurologic deficit, or require instrumentation that includes sublaminar wires (e.g., Luque rods). Congenital scoliosis is associated with intraspinal anomalies including lipomas, tethered cord, cysts, and teratomas that also increase the risk of postoperative neurologic complications. A preoperative myelogram or magnetic resonance imaging (MRI) is indicated in these patients.

The two monitoring techniques commonly used in the United States to monitor spinal cord function during scoliosis surgery are somatosensory evoked potentials (SSEPs) and the intraoperative wake-up test. Monitoring of motor evoked responses by electrical or magnetic stimulation of the brain or spinal cord is still considered to be investigational by many neurophysiologists. Preoperative prophylaxis with high dose corticosteroids should be considered for patients with a preexisting neurologic deficit.

Bradford DS, Lonstein JE, Moe JH et al (eds): Moe's Textbook of Scoliosis and Other Spinal Deformities, pp 471–472. Philadelphia: WB Saunders, 1987

Lonstein JE: Adolescent idiopathic scoliosis. Lancet 344:1407–1412, 1994

Weinstein SL (ed): The Pediatric Spine: Principles and Practice, pp 1764–1765. New York, Raven Press, 1994

C.3. What are somatosensory evoked potentials (SSEPs) and how are they used?

Sensory information from the periphery passes through the posterior columns of the spinal cord on its way to the cerebral cortex. The functional integrity of this pathway can be continually assessed by intraoperative monitoring of SSEPs. This technique involves applying repeated electrical stimuli to a peripheral nerve (e.g. posterior tibial nerve) and measuring the evoked response over the cerebral cortex using standard electroencephalogram (EEG) scalp electrodes. Because these evoked potentials are of low amplitude, computer averaging or summation must be used to distinguish them

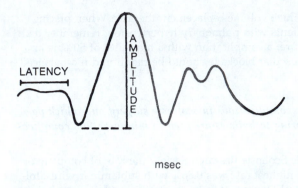

Figure 53-5. Typical somatosensory evoked potential trace. (Reprinted with permission from Cunningham JN Jr, Laschinger JC, Merkin HA, et al: Measurement of spinal cord ischemia during operations on the thoracic aorta: Initial clinical experience. Ann Surg 196:285–296, 1982)

from background noise and the patient's EEG. A typical evoked potential waveform is shown in Figure 53-5. The time interval between electrical stimulation of peripheral nerve to recording the evoked response over the cortex is defined as the latency. An increase in the latency (slower conduction), a decrease in the amplitude, or a complete loss of the evoked potential should be considered indicative of surgical injury or ischemia until proved otherwise. It is difficult to define standard values for latency and amplitude because of the differences in recording technique among laboratories; therefore, it is important to be familiar with the normal limits for the system that is in use. The consensus opinion appears to be that an increase in latency of 10% to 15% or more and a decrease in amplitude of >50% should be cause for serious concern.

Miller RD (ed): Anesthesia, 4th ed, pp 1329–1337. New York, Churchill Livingstone, 1994

Nash CL, Brown RH: Current concepts review—Spinal cord monitoring. J Bone Joint Surg 71A(4): 627–630, 1989

C.4. How reliable are SSEPs for predicting spinal injury?

Normal intraoperative SSEPs are good predictors of normal postoperative sensory function. Although posterior (sensory) and anterior (motor) spinal injuries tend to occur together during spine surgery or spinal trauma, there have been reports of postoperative paraplegia with normal intraoperative SSEPs. This probably represents ischemia in the distribution of the anterior spinal artery while monitoring the posterior columns that receive their blood supply from the posterior spinal arteries. For this reason, it is probably best to use both SSEPs and the intraoperative wake-up test to monitor spinal cord function during scoliosis surgery.

In a recent survey of 173 orthopedic spinal surgeons, it was found that experienced SSEP monitoring teams had fewer neurologic complications per 100 cases than teams with less experience. Neurologic defects with normal SSEPs (false-negative result) occurred in only 0.063% of cases.

Lesser RP, Raudzens P, Lueders H et al: Postoperative neurological deficits may occur despite unchanged intraoperative somatosensory evoked potentials. Ann Neurol 19:22–25, 1986

Nash CL, Brown RH: Current concepts review—Spinal cord monitoring. J Bone Joint Surg 71A(4): 627–630, 1989

Nuwer MR, Dawson EG, Carlson LG et al: SSEP spinal cord monitoring reduces neurologic deficits after scoliosis surgery: Results of a large multicenter study. Electroenceph Clin Neurophysiol 96: 6–11, 1995

Spielholz NI, Benjamin NV, Engler GL et al: Somatosensory evoked potentials during decompression and stabilization of the spine: Methods and findings. Spine 4:500, 1979

C.5. How are SSEPs affected by anesthetic agents? What other factors affect SSEPs?

All anesthetic agents except muscle relaxants affect SSEPs to a varying degree. This has been documented for potent inhalation agents, nitrous oxide, diazepam, droperidol, etomidate, thiopental, and even narcotics. Of all these, narcotics probably have the least effect on SSEPs. Nitrous oxide produces a decrease in amplitude without an increase in latency. The addition of nitrous oxide appears to produce a larger decrease in amplitude than addition of 1% isoflurane or enflurane to a fentanyl-based anesthetic.

Although it is important to realize that anesthetic agents can depress evoked potentials, excellent results can be obtained if anesthetic depth is stable. For example, it is preferable to administer narcotics by continuous infusion rather than by intermittent doses. Adequate SSEPs can be recorded using 50% nitrous oxide with up to 0.5% halothane or 1.0% isoflurane. It is most important to maintain a stable anesthetic before and during periods when monitoring of SSEPs is critical (i.e., during spine distraction or instrumentation).

A decrease in arterial pressure below levels of cerebral autoregulation produces a decrease in amplitude with no change in latency. Hypothermia will produce an increase in latency and a decrease in amplitude. Changes in oxygen delivery to neural tissues will also alter SSEPs. Isovolumic hemodilution at hematocrits below 15% and hypoxemia have been shown to alter SSEPs.

Miller RD (ed): Anesthesia, 4th ed, pp 1329–1337. New York, Churchill Livingstone, 1994

C.6. What should be done if the SSEPs become abnormal during surgery?

When SSEPs become abnormal, the anesthesiologist should ensure that oxygen delivery and spinal cord perfusion are adequate. Hypovolemia and anemia should be corrected. Arterial oxygen tension should be optimized and arterial P_{CO_2} should be normalized if the patient is being hyperventilated. It has been reported that normalizing arterial pressure if deliberate hypotension is being used, or raising arterial pressure above normal, can improve spinal cord perfusion and restore SSEPs to normal. The surgeon should seek a surgical cause such as too much distraction or surgical trespass with instrumentation and correct the problem as quickly as possible. If SSEPs are persistently abnormal despite corrective action, a wake-up test should be performed to determine if the instrumentation should be adjusted or removed. Evidence indicates that the shorter the interval between detection of injury and removal of instrumentation, the better the neurologic outcome.

Grundy BL, Nash CL, Brown CR: Arterial pressure manipulation alters spinal cord function during correction of scoliosis. Anesthesiology 54:249–253, 1981

C.7. How is the "wake-up" test performed? What complications can occur during this test?

The wake-up test is used to assess the integrity of the spinal motor pathways. It is performed by "lightening" the depth of anesthesia sufficiently to allow the patient to follow commands. This is usually done as soon as all instrumentation is in place. The patient is first instructed to squeeze the anesthesiologist's hand, confirming responsiveness, and then asked to move the feet and toes. In patients who are able to squeeze the anesthesiologist's hands but unable to move their feet, the amount of spine distraction must be reduced until a safe degree of correction is achieved. When the patient can move his or her feet, anesthesia is quickly deepened with small doses of benzodiazepine (e.g., midazolam 2 mg/70 kg) or thiopental (1 to 1.5 mg/kg) and a muscle relaxant. Recall of intraoperative events is very unusual with this technique.

The anesthesiologist should have one or two assistants available in the event the patient moves excessively during the wake-up test. Although this occurs rarely when a nitrous oxide-narcotic-relaxant technique is used, it is best to be prepared. I do not recommend the use of narcotic antagonists because of the potential for the patient to experience pain and become agitated in the prone position. If naloxone is deemed necessary to arouse the patient, a small dose (0.3 to 0.5 µg/kg) should be administered and repeated every 2 to 3 minutes until the respiratory depression of the narcotic is reversed. In our experience, it is not necessary to reverse neuromuscular blockade if at least three twitches are present on train-of-four stimulation.

Complications of this technique include extubation in the prone position, recall of intraoperative events, myocardial ischemia, self-injury, and dislodgement of instrumentation. Air embolus from open venous sinuses can occur if the patient is breathing spontaneously and inhales vigorously.

C.8. What is the optimal anesthetic technique for scoliosis surgery?

No simple answer is found for the optimal anesthetic technique. Most patients with idiopathic scoliosis are healthy adolescents who tolerate anesthesia and surgery well, and a wide variety of techniques have been used successfully. I favor a nitrous oxide-narcotic infusion-relaxant technique. The advantages of this technique are that it interferes minimally with detection of SSEPs, provides a stable depth of anesthesia, and reliably provides a rapid, pain-free awakening for the intraoperative wake-up test. If a potent inhalation agent is used, it must be discontinued at least 10 to 15 minutes before the wake-up. However, this produces a changing depth of anesthesia at precisely the time monitoring of SSEPs is critical (i.e., during instrumentation of the spine).

Succinylcholine should be avoided in patients with muscle disorders. Its administration in patients with Duchenne's muscular dystrophy can produce hyperkalemia, cardiac arrythmias, and myoglobinuria or precipitate malignant hyperthermia. Patients with myotonic muscular dystrophy may exhibit sustained skeletal muscle contractions in response to succinylcholine. This may produce difficulty in ventilation and intubation. A variety of nondepolarizing muscle relaxants have been used successfully during scoliosis surgery. My preference is use of an intermediate-acting muscle relaxant such as vecuronium or atracurium rather than a longer acting relaxant such as pancuronium. This is because a high degree of neuromuscular blockade can be maintained with an intermediate-acting relaxant, yet recovery is rapid enough that it is usually not necessary to reverse the block for the wake-up test.

C.9. What complications occur related to positioning the patient?

If the head is not positioned carefully, pressure on the eyes can cause thrombosis of the central retinal artery producing loss of vision or blindness. The horseshoe-type

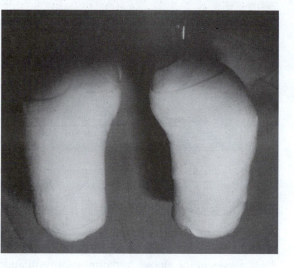

Figure 53-6. *This horseshoe-type head rest has been associated with unilateral eye blindness because of pressure on the eye during surgery. The forehead rests on the upper portion with the chin free in the wider, open portion.*

head rest (Fig. 53-6) has been implicated in a number of reports of unilateral eye blindness and should be used with great caution if at all. The head should be positioned without excessive flexion or extension and in such a way that face and eyes can be inspected easily. The position of the head and neck will move during surgical manipulation of the spine and should be frequently checked during the procedure. Patients with Marfan's syndrome and neurofibromatosis may have abnormalities of the cervical spine and must be turned and positioned with great caution.

The upper extremities should be positioned at no more than 90 degrees of abduction to the trunk as illustrated in Figure 53-7A. Figure 53-7B demonstrates improper arm positioning because the arms are abducted above the head. This stretches the brachial plexus and may result in a brachial plexus palsy. Both axillae should be inspected to ensure that the frame does not compress the axillary sheath. Figure 53-8B demonstrates improper positioning on the frame resulting in pressure on the axilla. Proper positioning is shown in Figure 53-8A. Note that ample space exists between

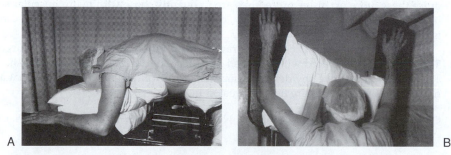

A   B

Figure 53-7. **(A)** Proper positioning of the arms at 90 degrees of abduction (relative to the trunk). **(B)** Improper arm positioning with the arms abducted above the head, which results in stretching of the brachial plexus.

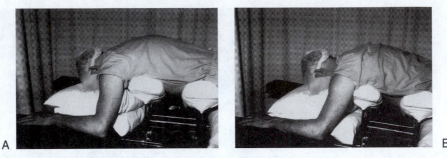

A   B

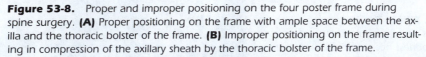

Figure 53-8. Proper and improper positioning on the four poster frame during spine surgery. **(A)** Proper positioning on the frame with ample space between the axilla and the thoracic bolster of the frame. **(B)** Improper positioning on the frame resulting in compression of the axillary sheath by the thoracic bolster of the frame.

the thoracic bolster of the frame and the axilla. Care should be taken to pad the ulnar nerves at the elbow. Impairment of ventilation and increased bleeding from increased venous pressure can occur if the abdomen is compressed by the operating frame.

C.10. How will the surgical procedure influence estimated blood loss and fluid requirements?

A variety of surgical procedures are commonly performed for posterior spine fusion. The blood lost during these procedures can be considerable, and it varies according to the procedure, the operative time, the number of segments fused, whether deliberate hypotension is used, and other factors. Even when deliberate hypotension is used, blood loss in the range of 15 to 25 ml/kg is not uncommon during uncomplicated spine fusion with Harrington rods or Cotrel-Dubousset instrumentation. This represents a blood loss of 1 to 2 liters for a 70 kg patient. Postoperative bleeding may equal or exceed this, which emphasizes the need for continued monitoring of these patients in the postoperative period. More extensive procedures (e.g., combined anterior-posterior spine fusion, instrumentation with Luque rods into the pelvis, or, especially, osteotomy of the spine to correct rigid deformities) may be associated with blood loss exceeding the patient's own blood volume (75 ml/kg). Patients who require these more extensive procedures are frequently those with neuromuscular scoliosis (Duchenne's muscular dystrophy, cerebral palsy) who may already have diminished reserves.

Moderate third space losses of intravascular fluid occur during scoliosis surgery. These should be replaced with balanced salt solution at a rate of 5 to 7 ml/kg/h. This is over and above any deficit or maintenance requirements. Procedures that are more extensive may require higher infusion rates.

Guay J, Haig M, Lortie L et al: Predicting blood loss in surgery for idiopathic scoliosis. Can J Anaesth 41(9):775–781, 1994

C.11. What techniques can be used to minimize transfusion requirements?

Several techniques are available to minimize homologous blood transfusion requirements. A simple and important way to minimize bleeding is to minimize intra-abdominal pressure, because any increase in abdominal pressure is transmitted to the vertebral venous plexus, increasing venous bleeding. Careful positioning avoids external pressure on the abdomen, and muscle relaxants or deeper levels of anesthesia have been used to prevent a rise in abdominal wall tension.

A method that has gained popularity is preoperative banking of blood by the patient over a period of several weeks prior to surgery. Most patients are able to bank 2 to 3 U of their own (autologous) red cells using this technique. The autologous blood program minimizes transfusion risks because patients then receive their own blood and that blood is subject to stringent standards for collection and storage.

Isovolumic hemodilution may also be used to minimize red cell loss during surgery. Prior to incision the hematocrit is lowered to 20% to 25% by removing blood aseptically and storing it in anticoagulated bags. Intravascular volume is maintained by replacing the blood with three times the volume of a balanced saline solution or an equal volume of 5% albumin. Intraoperatively, the previously withdrawn blood is replaced as needed. Obviously this technique requires careful monitoring of intravascular volume status, hemoglobin level, and probably mixed venous oxygen saturation. Some patients who are members of the Jehovah's Witness sect and will not accept blood tranfusions may accept this type of blood conservation method because the blood can be kept in continuity with the circulation.

Blood salvaging during the surgical procedure can play an important role as an adjunct to an autologous blood program. In our experience, 50% to 60% of the red blood cells lost can be recovered, concentrated, washed, and returned to the patient using commercially available autotransfusion devices. These red cells are obviously lacking in platelets and plasma. Some Jehovah's Witness patients may also accept this technique if the autotranfusion device is kept in continuity with the circulation.

Deliberate hypotension has been used widely to decrease blood loss and improve operating conditions during spine fusion surgery. It has been shown to decrease blood loss 30% to 50% when mean arterial pressure is maintained at 50 to 60 mm Hg.

Fontana JL, Welborn L, Mongan P et al: Oxygen consumption and cardiovascular function in children during profound intraoperative hemodilution. Anesth Analg 80:219–225, 1995

Miller RD (ed): Anesthesia, 4th ed, pp 1481–1483. New York, Churchill Livingstone, 1994

C.12. What techniques would you use to produce deliberate hypotension during scoliosis surgery? What is the major concern of using this technique?

Many techniques have been used to produce deliberate hypotension. These include using high doses of potent inhalation anesthetic agents, vasodilators (sodium nitroprusside, nitroglycerin, adenosine), ganglionic blocking agents (trimethaphan), beta-adrenergic blocking agents (propranolol, esmolol), angiotensin converting enzyme inhibitors (captopril), and combinations of these agents. Because high doses of potent anesthetics interfere with monitoring of somatosensory evoked potentials and make it more difficult to perform an intraoperative wake-up test, this technique is not commonly used during scoliosis surgery. Recent animal experiments have suggested that deliberate hypotension with trimethaphan may be associated with a decrease in spinal cord blood flow compared with sodium nitroprusside or nitroglycerin. The technique that we favor employs a short-acting vasodilator (e.g., sodium nitroprusside) and a short-acting beta-adrenergic blocker (e.g., such as esmolol). Mean arterial pressure can be rapidly stabilized at 50 to 65 mm Hg and will return to normal within minutes of discontinuing these agents.

The major concern of using deliberate hypotension during scoliosis surgery is the potential for spinal cord blood flow to be compromised with resultant spinal cord injury. This is of particular concern when the spine is distracted because levels of hypotension that are considered safe under normal conditions may compromise spinal cord blood flow after spine distraction. A study in dogs demonstrated that spinal cord blood flow decreases with deliberate hypotension but returns to baseline levels after about 35 minutes. Therefore, it has been recommended that the spine should not be distracted until 35 minutes after the start of deliberate hypotension.

In high risk patients (see question C.2), it is important to balance the potential benefits of deliberate hypotension with the potential risks, and if deliberate hypotension is used it is probably prudent to maintain mean arterial pressure no lower than 60 or 65 mm Hg.

Grundy BL, Nash CL, Brown CR: Arterial pressure manipulation alters spinal cord function during correction of scoliosis. Anesthesiology 54:249–253, 1981

Kling TF, Ferguson NV, Leach AB et al: The influence of induced hypotension and spine distraction on canine spinal cord blood flow. Spine 10:878–883, 1985

Miller RD (ed): Anesthesia, 4th ed, pp 1483–1490. New York, Churchill Livingstone, 1994

D. Postoperative Management

D.1. When would you extubate the patient?

The decision to continue mechanical ventilation in the postoperative period is usually made preoperatively. Most patients with adolescent idiopathic scoliosis have mild to moderate pulmonary function abnormalities and may be extubated in the operating room. Mechanical ventilation should be continued in patients with severe restrictive lung defects (vital capacity <30% of predicted) or severe gas exchange abnormalities such as CO_2 retention. Postoperative mechanical ventilation should be considered for patients with Duchenne's muscular dystrophy, familial dysautonomia, or severe cerebral palsy.

The parameters for extubation given below are the same as for other respiratory disorders:

- Vital capacity >10 ml/kg
- Tidal volume >3 ml/kg
- Spontaneous respiratory rate <30 per minute
- Negative inspiratory force > -30 cm H_2O

Bradford DS, Lonstein JE, Moe JH et al (eds): Moe's Textbook of Scoliosis and Other Spinal Deformities, p 590. Philadelphia, WB Saunders, 1987

D.2. What should be done to optimize pulmonary status?

Incentive spirometry should be taught preoperatively and should be used aggressively in the postoperative period. Coughing and deep breathing should be encouraged. Patients with obstructive or reactive airway disease will benefit from bronchodilators. Theophylline may be useful in neuromuscular scoliosis because it may improve diaphragmatic contractility. Narcotics should be used judiciously with the goal of providing adequate analgesia to allow coughing and incentive spirometry without excessive respiratory depression.

D.3. What laboratory tests should be ordered postoperatively?

On arrival in the recovery room, blood should be sent for analysis of arterial blood gases, hematocrit, electrolytes, blood urea nitrogen (BUN), and creatinine; if blood loss has been great, platelet count, prothrombin, and partial thromboplastin time should be evaluated as well. Determination of arterial blood gases should be repeated if clinically indicated. Hyponatremia with high urinary sodium excretion has been reported following scoliosis surgery, and it has been attributed to the syndrome of inappropriate antidiuretic hormone secretion. Therefore, electrolytes should be followed at least every 12 hours for the first 24 hours and then daily for the first 2 days. These patients produce small amounts of concentrated urine and excrete large amounts of urinary sodium, and efforts to increase their urine output by fluid administration are unsuccessful and worsen the hyponatremia. Rapid decreases in serum sodium concentration or sodium concentrations <125 mEq/liter may produce swelling of brain cells (intracellular "edema") and convulsions.

Brenner BM, Rector FC (eds): The Kidney, p 418. Philadelphia, WB Saunders, 1986

Burrows FA, Shutack JG, Crone RK: Inappropriate secretion of antidiuretic hormone in a postsurgical pediatric population. Crit Care Med 11(7):527–531, 1983

D.4. What fluid therapy would you use postoperatively?

Significant losses of intravascular fluid continue to occur in the postoperative period. These should be replaced with balanced salt solution such as lactated Ringer's solution to maintain urine output at a minimum of 0.5 to 1.0 ml/kg/h. Hypotonic fluids should be avoided in the first 24 to 36 hours postoperatively. The risk of postoperative hyponatremia can be increased if fluid replacement is excessive or hypotonic in nature. Some authors recommend the use of colloid replacement solutions because serum albumin is often decreased following scoliosis surgery.

Brenner BM, Rector FC (eds): The Kidney, p 418. Philadelphia, WB Saunders, 1986

Burrows FA, Shutack JG, Crone RK: Inappropriate secretion of antidiuretic hormone in a postsurgical pediatric population. Crit Care Med 11(7):527–531, 1983

D.5. What complications may occur following scoliosis surgery?

Complications that have been reported in the postoperative period include pneumothorax, atelectasis, pleural effusion, hemothorax, thoracic duct injury, and neurologic injury. Pneumothorax can occur because of both anterior and posterior surgical dissections, as well as secondary to central venous line placement. A chest x-ray should be obtained on arrival in the postanesthesia care unit. Atelectasis can occur because of prolonged supine positioning and narcotic use. Anterior spine fusion via thoracotomy poses the greatest risk of pulmonary complications. Almost 100% of patients undergoing these procedures will develop some degree of atelectasis. Incentive spirometry and deep breathing should be emphasized and may require specialized nursing care.

In addition to intraoperative neurologic complications during instrumentation or distraction of the spine, a number of reports are found of delayed neurologic complications in the first few days postoperatively. This emphasizes the need for continuing to monitor the patient's neurologic status postoperatively.

Postoperative adynamic ileus can occur and some authors recommend placement of nasogastric tubes in all patients.

Kahanowitz N, Levine DB: Iatrogenic complications of spinal surgery. Contemporary Orthopaedics 9(2):23–39, 1984

Weinstein SL (ed): The Pediatric Spine: Principles and Practice, pp 1761–1784. New York, Raven Press, 1994

Hypoxia and Equipment Failure

54

Alan D. Kestenbaum

A 59-year-old woman had a cataract of her left eye. The cataract was to be removed and an intraocular lens implanated under monitored anesthesia care with sedation. She had a 50-pack-a-year history of smoking and peripheral vascular disease. Her arterial blood gas on room air showed pH 7.38, P_{CO_2} 45 mm Hg, P_{O_2} 60 mm Hg, and O_2 saturation 90%.

A. Medical Disease and Differential Diagnosis

1. What is hypoxia, and what is hypoxemia?
2. Is there a relationship between P_{O_2} and age?
3. Was this patient hypoxemic?
4. What are the common causes of hypoxemia?
5. What is venous admixture?
6. What is a pulse oximeter?
7. How does a pulse oximeter work?
8. What interferes with the use of a pulse oximeter?
9. How can one tell when the reading on the pulse oximeter is probably correct?
10. What is meant by capnometry and capnography? What value are they in gas monitoring?
11. What is meant by end-tidal CO_2 concentration?
12. What does a normal capnogram look like, and what does it mean?
13. Has capnography been shown to correlate with other quantitative methods of respiratory function?
14. What are mainstream and sidestream end-tidal CO_2 monitors?
15. Illustrate some common capnograms and give a differential diagnosis of each event.
16. What is the arterial to alveolar difference for carbon dioxide (a-ADCO$_2$)?
17. What are some of the important safety features of anesthesia machines?
18. What are common sites where gas leaks occur?
19. How can we test for leaks?
20. What are some of the important alarm conditions built into the anesthesia machine?

B. Preoperative Evaluation and Preparation

1. What should be included in the equipment checkout in preparation for anesthesia?
2. What emergency equipment should be easily available to the anesthesiologist?
3. How should this patient be premedicated?

C. Intraoperative Management

1. How would you monitor this patient?
2. After the eye had been opened, the patient became agitated and restless. What would you do?

3. Anesthesia was induced and the patient was intubated. You squeezed the ventilation bag and there was a huge leak. Where might the leak be, and what should you do now?

D. Postoperative Management

1. What criteria would you use for extubation?
2. What are the causes of postoperative hypoxemia?
3. How would you administer oxygen postoperatively?

A. Medical Disease and Differential Diagnosis

A.1. What is hypoxia, and what is hypoxemia?

Although these terms are often used interchangeably, they are not the same. According to *Stedman's Medical Dictionary*, hypoxia refers to subnormal levels of oxygen in air, blood, or tissue, whereas hypoxemia refers specifically to decreased levels of oxygen in arterial blood.

Stedman's Medical Dictionary, 25th ed, p 685. Baltimore, Williams & Wilkins, 1990

A.2. Is there a relationship between Po_2 and age?

Yes. The arterial Po_2 shows a progressive decline with age. In 1972, Marshall and Whyche analyzed 12 studies in healthy human subjects and arrived at the following relationship:

$$\text{Mean arterial } Po_2 = 102 - 0.33 \text{ (age in years)}$$

This has 95% confidence limits (2 standard deviations) of 10 mm Hg.

For a more practical approach, Shapiro et al. suggest subtracting 1 mm Hg from the minimal 80 mm Hg (which they say is the minimal Po_2 for a normal adult) for every year over 60 years of age. For example:

- If a person is 60 years old, the Po_2 should be >80 mm Hg.
- If a person is 70 years old, the Po_2 should be >70 mm Hg.
- If a person is 80 years old, the Po_2 should be >60 mm Hg.

Marshall BE, Whyche MQ: Hypoxemia during and after anesthesia. Anesthesiology 37:178, 1972

Nunn JF: Nunn's Applied Respiratory Physiology, 4th ed, p 268. Philadelphia, Butterworth-Heinemann, 1993

Shapiro BA, Harrison RA, Walton JR: Clinical Application of Blood Gases, 4th ed, p 82. Chicago, Year Book Medical Publishers, 1989

A.3. Was this patient hypoxemic?

Yes. For a patient 60 years of age, the mean arterial should be >80 mm Hg.

Nunn JF: Nunn's Applied Respiratory Physiology, 4th ed, p 268. Philadelphia, Butterworth-Heinemann, 1993

A.4. What are the common causes of hypoxemia?

From the shunt equation, arterial oxygen content is related to the change in pulmonary capillary oxygen tension, venous oxygen content, and venous admixture. It is easier to classify hypoxemia into the following three categories:

Decreased Pulmonary Capillary Oxygen Tension
- Hypoventilation
- Low F_IO_2
- Ventilation/perfusion abnormalities from pulmonary parenchymal change
- Diffusion abnormality (rare)

Increased Shunting, Either Intrapulmonary or Cardiac

Reduced Venous Oxygen Content
- Congestive heart failure—low cardiac output
- Increased metabolism—fever, hyperthyroidism, shivering
- Decreased arterial oxygen content

Shapiro BA, Harrison RA, Walton JR: Clinical Application of Blood Gases, 4th ed, pp 71–72. Chicago, Year Book Medical Publishers, 1989

A.5. What is venous admixture?

In discussing hypoxemia, the concept of venous admixture, more commonly known as shunt, must be considered. Venous admixture is that amount of venous blood that combines with pulmonary end-capillary blood to produce the observed difference between arterial and pulmonary end-capillary oxygen tensions. Causes of venous admixture are as follows:

Anatomic Shunt
- Venae cordis minimae (thebesian veins)
- Bronchial veins
- Pleural veins

Physiologic Shunt
- Areas of low ventilation:perfusion ratio (low $\dot{V}/\dot{Q}$)

Pathologic Shunt
- Congenital heart disease
- Pneumonia
- Pulmonary edema
- Pneumothorax
- Pulmonary tumor
- Pulmonary arteriovenous shunts

Nunn JF: Nunn's Applied Respiratory Physiology, 4th ed, pp 178–197. Philadelphia, Butterworth-Heinemann, 1993

A.6. What is a pulse oximeter?

Pulse oximeters noninvasively monitor the oxygen saturation of arterial hemoglobin. There are transmissive oximeters and reflectant oximeters. Transmissive oximeters measure the absorption of light passed through an arteriolar bed, and reflectant oximeters measure reflected light. In the more commonly used transmissive oximetry, light must pass through a tissue bed, such as a finger or an earlobe, to reach the photodetector in opposition to the light source. Reflectant oximeter probes can be placed on a flat surface such as the forearm where the light source and the photodetector are in the same plane.

Barash PG, Cullen BF, Stoelting RF (eds): Clinical Anesthesia, 3rd ed, pp 624–625. Philadelphia, Lippincott-Raven, 1997

A.7. How does a pulse oximeter work?

The pulse oximeter transmits two wavelengths of light, red (660 nm) and infrared (940 nm), through a tissue bed. After the light passes through the tissue bed, the photodetector in the probe converts the transmitted light energy into an electronic signal proportional to the absorbance. If we measure the ratio of the red to the infrared absorbances during pulsatile and nonpulsatile flow, then we can relate the ratio of the red to the infrared "pulse-added" (AC/DC) absorbances to a nonlinear function of arterial oxygen saturation. The "pulse-added" absorbance is the ratio of the pulsatile (AC) component to the nonpulsatile (DC) component of absorbance at each wavelength.

Barash PG, Cullen BF, Stoelting RF (eds): Clinical Anesthesia, 3rd ed, pp 624–625. Philadelphia, Lippincott-Raven, 1997

Tremper KK, Barker SJ: Pulse oximetry. Anesthesiology 70:98–108, 1989

A.8. What interferes with the use of a pulse oximeter?

Many things can interfere with the proper functioning of the pulse oximeter. These include motion artifact, electrical noise from the electrocautery, intravenous dyes (methylene blue and indocyanine green), increased carboxyhemoglobin and methemoglobin levels, ambient light, nail polish, and poor extremity blood flow from hypotension and vasoconstrictors.

Barash PG, Cullen BF, Stoelting RF (eds): Clinical Anesthesia, 3rd ed, pp 624–625. Philadelphia, Lippincott-Raven, 1997

Severinghaus JW: Pulse oximetry: Uses and limitations. ASA Annual Refresher Course Lectures #122, 1990

A.9. How can one tell when the reading on the pulse oximeter is probably correct?

Some oximeters have displays that indicate signal strength. Other oximeters can be incorporated into larger monitors that display pulsatile waveforms according to signal strength and heart rate. Those signals that show good strength and closely approximate the pulse rate readings, such as that of the electrocardiogram (ECG) monitor, are probably indicating correct readings of oxygen saturation.

Severinghaus JW: Pulse oximetry: Uses and limitations. ASA Annual Refresher Course Lectures #122, 1990

A.10. What is meant by capnometry and capnography? What value are they in gas monitoring?

Capnometry is the measurement of the concentration of carbon dioxide during the respiratory cycle, and capnography is the graphic representation of this information.

The capnograph is a front-line monitor for esophageal intubation, ventilation failure, gas embolism, sudden circulatory collapse, malignant hypothermia, and anesthesia circuit disconnects. It is a valuable back-up monitor when other monitors (low pressure alarm, pulse oximeter) are not in use, are being used incorrectly, or fail.

Dorsch JA, Dorsch SE: Understanding Anesthesia Equipment, 3rd ed, p 581. Baltimore, Williams & Wilkins, 1994

Williamson J, Webb R, Cockings J: The Australian Incident Monitoring Study. The capnograph: Applications and limitations—An analysis of 2000 incident reports. Anesth Intensive Care 21(5): 551–557, 1993

A.11. What is meant by end-tidal CO₂ concentration?

End-tidal CO_2 ($P_{ET}CO_2$) is the partial pressure of CO_2 at the end of an exhaled breath, normally reflecting the alveolar partial pressure of carbon dioxide, or $PaCO_2$. The measurement of end-tidal CO_2 is important for determining optimal minute ventilation, hypoventilation or lack of ventilation secondary to ventilator malfunction, circuit leak, airway disconnect, or airway obstruction. It is also helpful for identifying esophageal intubations, inspiratory and expiratory valve malfunction, and exhausted soda-lime canisters.

Barash PG, Cullen BF, Stoelting RF (eds): Clinical Anesthesia, 3rd ed, pp 622–623. Philadelphia, Lippincott-Raven, 1997

Dorsch JA, Dorsch SE: Understanding Anesthesia Equipment, 3rd ed, p 584. Baltimore, Williams & Wilkins, 1994

A.12. What does a normal capnogram look like, and what does it mean?

A normal capnogram is represented in Figure 54-1. We can identify four distinct phases of the capnogram:

Phase I
The expiratory baseline. This is traced as CO_2-free gas from the airways flows past the CO_2 sensor during expiration. This represents anatomic dead space; gas from those parts of the airway do not contribute to gas exchange.

Phase II
The Expiratory upstroke. This represents the arrival of CO_2 at the sensor just after exhalation begins. It is normally very steep. Dead space gas mixes with alveolar gas.

Figure 54-1. Phases of the normal capnogram. *(I)* inspiratory baseline, *(II)* expiratory upstroke, *(III)* expiratory plateau, and *(IV)* inspiratory downstroke. (Reprinted with permission from Good ML: Capnography: Uses, interpretation, and pitfalls. ASA Refresher Courses in Anesthesiology 18:179, 1990)

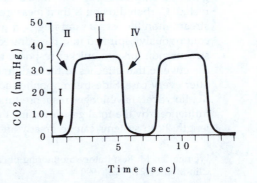

Phase III

The expiratory or alveolar plateau. This represents mixed alveolar CO_2. It usually has a very slight upward rise and in patients with normal lungs appears nearly horizontal. The peak expired CO_2 is taken as the end-tidal CO_2 level.

Phase IV

The inspiratory downstroke. This is the beginning of mechanical inspiration, where fresh gas is inhaled and the curve steeply falls to zero.

Barash PG, Cullen BF, Stoelting RF (eds): Clinical Anesthesia, 3rd ed, pp 622–623. Philadelphia, Lippincott-Raven, 1997

Bhavani-Shankar K, Kumar A, Moseley H et al: Terminology and the current limitations of time capnography: A brief review. J Clin Monit 11(3):175–182, 1995

Good ML: Capnography: Uses, interpretation and pitfalls. ASA Refresher courses in Anesthesiology 18:175–193, 1990

A.13. Has capnography been shown to correlate with other quantitative methods of respiratory function?

Yes. Capnography has been shown to significantly correlate with spirometric function, especially the angle between phase II and phase III of the capnogram. This is sometimes referred to as the "alpha angle" and may offer a quantitative way of evaluating the severity of airway obstruction, such as in bronchospasm. In addition, capnography may offer other advantages such as noninvasiveness and effort-independence during tidal breathing, and may therefore be useful in children.

Bhavani-Shankar K, Kumar A, Moseley H et al: Terminology and the current limitations of time capnography: A brief review. J Clin Monit 11(3):175–182, 1995

Good ML: Capnography: Uses, interpretation and pitfalls. ASA Refresher courses in Anesthesiology 18:175–193, 1990

You B, Peslin R, Duvivier C et al: Expiratory capnography in asthma: Evaluations of various shape indices. Eur Respir J 7(2):318–323, 1994

A.14. What are mainstream and sidestream end-tidal carbon dioxide monitors?

A mainstream monitor uses a cuvette which attaches to the endotracheal tube. The gases flow past a window in the cuvette through which an infrared light beam is directed. Carbon dioxide is then measured via its detection by infrared light. A sidestream monitor uses a sampling port with a long sampling line through which gas is continuously aspirated into the infrared analyzer. The main advantages of mainstream monitors are quicker response times and less waveform distortion. However, the cuvette that attaches to the endotracheal tube is heavy and needs to be sterilized after every case. Sidestream monitor adapters are lightweight and disposable. They do, however, have longer response times; they are more susceptible to leaks and are influenced by the total gas flow rate, the sampling rate, and the sample tubing length. Both systems can be greatly affected by bodily secretions and moisture.

Weingarten M: Respiratory monitoring of carbon dioxide and oxygen: A ten-year perspective. J Clin Monit 6:217–225, 1990

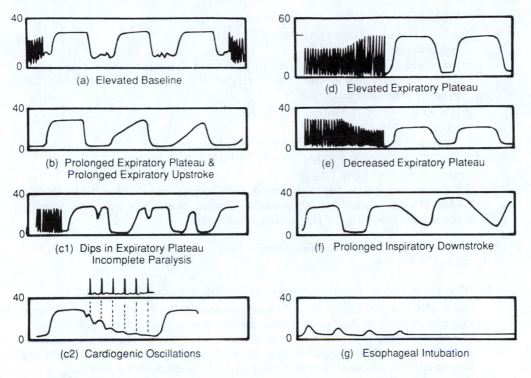

Figure 54-2. Abnormal capnograms.

A.15. Illustrate some common capnograms and give a differential diagnosis of each event.

Elevated Baseline (Fig. 54-2a)
- Incompetent expiratory valve
- Possibly incompetent inspiratory valve
- Exhausted soda-lime canister
- Channeling through partially exhausted soda-lime canister

Prolonged Expiratory Plateau and Prolonged Expiratory Upstroke (Fig. 54-2b)
- Mechanical obstruction (e.g., kinked endotracheal tube)
- Chronic obstructive pulmonary disease
- Bronchospasm

Dips in the Expiratory Plateau (Fig. 54-2c)
- Inspiratory effort (e.g., incomplete paralysis)
- Cardiogenic oscillations

Elevated Expiratory Plateau (Fig. 54-2d)
- Hypoventilation
- Leak
- Mechanical obstruction
- Inadequate ventilator settings
- CO_2 rebreathing

- Increasing CO_2 production (malignant hyperthermia, fever)

Decreased Expiratory Plateau (Fig. 54-2e)
- Hyperventilation
- Decreased CO_2 production delivery (hypothermia, decreased cardiac output)
- Increased a-ADCO$_2$ gradient (ventilation/perfusion inequality, endobronchial intubation, pulmonary embolism)

Prolonged Inspiratory Downstroke (Fig. 54-2f)
- Incompetent inspiratory valve
- Slow sampling flow rate in sidestream CO_2 analyzer
- Inspiratory obstruction to gas flow (kinked endotracheal tube)

Esophageal Intubation (Fig. 54-2g)
After an esophageal intubation, carbon dioxide may be found within the stomach, especially if mask ventilation has preceded intubation. Notice how the carbon dioxide concentration tends toward zero within a few breaths.

Good ML: Capnography: Uses, interpretation and pitfalls. ASA Refresher Courses in Anesthesiology 18:175–193, 1990

A.16. What is the arterial to alveolar difference for carbon dioxide (a-ADCO2)?

The a-ADCO$_2$ is defined as the difference between arterial PaCO$_2$, normally 40 mm Hg, and the alveolar P$_A$CO$_2$, commonly measured as the end-tidal CO_2 (P$_{ET}$CO$_2$). The ideal alveolar carbon dioxide concentration is also 40 mm Hg, which would make the ideal a-ADCO$_2$ equal to zero. However, dead-space ventilation results in a large a-ADCO$_2$, whereas shunt perfusion causes little effect on the a-ADCO$_2$. A small degree of ventilation perfusion inequality and dead-space ventilation occurs, which accounts for small a-ADCO$_2$ in the normal awake state. Under anesthesia, shunt perfusion and dead-space ventilation both increase, leading to increased arterial to alveolar carbon dioxide gradients.

Swedlow DB: Capnometry and capnography: The anesthesia disaster early warning system. Seminars in Anesthesiology 5(3):194–205, 1986

A.17. What are some of the important safety features of anesthesia machines?

The Pin Index Safety System (PISS) was adopted in 1952 to help ensure the correct delivery of anesthetic gases from E cylinders or smaller cylinders. The receiving yoke of each supply line has two pins that correspond to two holes drilled into the cylinder valve. The arrangement of this interlock system differs for each type of cylinder gas. However, because of breakage and bending of the pins and other PISS bypass methods, this system is not foolproof.

The pressure-sensor shut-off valve, or "fail-safe system," as it was formerly known, interconnects the oxygen and nitrous oxide supply lines to prevent the flow of nitrous oxide from the supply source to the flow control valve. As the new name infers, it senses oxygen pressure and shuts off nitrous oxide. When the oxygen supply pressure falls below 25 psig, nitrous oxide cannot flow to the outlet. Note that this is only a pressure valve and does not ensure delivery of oxygen to the patient. Therefore, the old "fail-safe system" was a misnomer, because it did not prevent hypoxic mixtures from being delivered to the patient.

The oxygen supply failure alarm system is an audible signal of oxygen failure. An equilibrium is reached between the oxygen pressure in the reservoir of the whistle and the oxygen pressure in the supply lines. When oxygen failure occurs, the pressure in the supply lines falls and the oxygen rushes out of the reservoir past a metal reed, giving a loud whistle for approximately 7 seconds. The end of the alarm, however, does not signify the restoration of oxygen pressure.

The oxygen flow control knob is designed to be different from the other flow control knobs. It is fluted, larger in diameter, and color and symbol coded to help prevent oxygen control mishaps by the clinician.

The position of the oxygen flowmeter relative to the other flowmeters is important in preventing hypoxic gas mixtures. By convention in the United States, the oxygen flowmeter is located to the right or downstream of the other flowmeters. If the oxygen flowmeter were positioned upstream, a leak would cause loss of oxygen and a possible hypoxic gas mixture downstream. When the oxygen flowmeter is downstream, upstream leaks cause loss of anesthetic gases and do not create a hypoxic situation.

The flow of nitrous oxide and oxygen can be linked mechanically with a chain-link mechanism. Each gas can be operated independently as long as the oxygen level is maintained above the factory preset level, usually 25% to 28%. If the clinician attempts to increase the nitrous oxide concentration above 75%, the oxygen flow increases automatically. Again, this does not prevent the delivery of hypoxic gas mixtures.

Bowie E, Huffman LM: The Anesthesia Machine: Essentials for Understanding, pp 65–71. Madison, Ohmeda, 1985

Dorsch JA, Dorsch SE: Understanding Anesthesia Equipment, 3rd ed, pp 66–88. Baltimore, Williams & Wilkins, 1994

A.18. *What are common sites where gas leaks occur?*

Gas leaks can occur at almost any point within the machine. Some of the more common leaks occur at the seating of the vaporizers or the carbon dioxide absorber head. The inspiratory and expiratory valves atop the carbon dioxide absorber head may be unseated, loose, or cracked. Cracks can also occur in the flowmeters, the breathing bags, hoses, and Y-pieces. Leaks in the ventilator or humidifier are also common.

Dorsch JA, Dorsch SE: Understanding Anesthesia Equipment, 3rd ed, pp 331–332. Baltimore, Williams & Wilkins, 1994

A.19. *How can we test for leaks?*

A positive pressure leak test is used to test for integrity of the external elements up to the check valve within the common gas outlet of the machine. A negative pressure leak test is used to check for generally smaller leaks within the machine beyond the outlet check valve.

Positive Pressure Test

Close the adjustable pressure limit (APL) valve, pressurize the system to 30 cm H_2O, and set the oxygen flow to 100 ml per minute. If the pressure continues to increase, the leakage is within an acceptable range. A one-way check valve as shown in Figure 54-3 prevents backflow into the anesthesia machine with the positive pressure test.

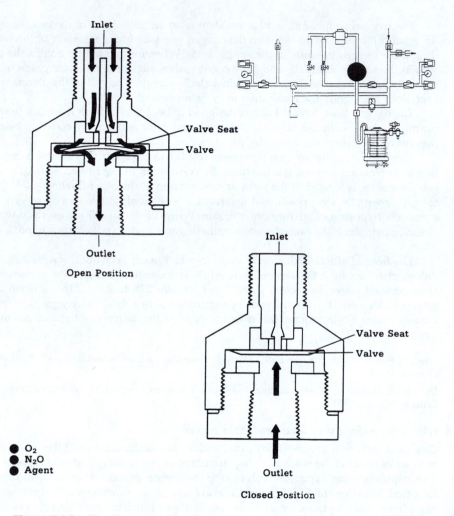

Figure 54-3. The check valve located between the vaporizer outlet and the machine outlet. (Reprinted with permission from Bowie E, Huffman L: The Anesthesia Machine: Essentials for Understanding, pp 65–71. Madison, Ohmeda, 1985)

Negative Pressure Test
Insert a deflated suction bulb supplied by the manufacturer into the common gas outlet and note the rate of bulb expansion. If the bulb takes longer than 30 seconds to fill, the leakage is acceptable.

Bowie E, Huffman L: The Anesthesia Machine: Essentials for Understanding, pp 65–71. Madison, Ohmeda, 1985

Dorsch JA, Dorsch SE: Understanding Anesthesia Equipment, 3rd ed, pp 700–703. Baltimore, Williams & Wilkins, 1994

Modulus II Plus anesthesia system. In: Operation and Maintenance Manual, p 4-2. Madison, Ohmeda, 1989

A.20. What are some of the important alarm conditions built into the anesthesia machine?

Alarms will sound for conditions such as apnea, low oxygen concentration, high oxygen concentration, high airway pressure, low airway pressure, sustained airway pressure, subatmospheric pressure, and low minute volume.

Bowie E, Huffman L: The Anesthesia Machine: Essentials for Understanding, pp 65–71. Madison, Ohmeda, 1985

Modulus II Plus anesthesia system. In: Operation and Maintenance Manual, pp 3–25. Madison, Ohmeda, 1989

B. Preoperative Evaluation and Preparation

B.1. What should be included in the equipment checkout in preparation for anesthesia?

Sources vary on equipment checkout in preparation for anesthesia, but the basics should include the following:

- Inspect the machine for a complete and undamaged breathing system with fresh CO_2 absorbant. Make sure that all of the hoses are present and intact and that the machine is undamaged.
- Turn on all of the monitors and make sure they are functioning properly.
- Make sure the waste gas scavenging system is connected and functioning.
- Check the oxygen and nitrous oxide pipeline supplies. Make sure the oxygen and nitrous oxide cylinders are filled.
- Test the oxygen supply failure system.
- Check the flowmeters and the integrity of the oxygen-nitrous oxide proportioning system.
- Calibrate the oxygen monitors and set alarms.
- Test for leaks in the circle system and the machine.
- Check the inspiratory and expiratory valves for proper function.
- Make sure the ventilator is functioning properly.
- Check for the presence of emergency ventilatory equipment.

Bowie E, Huffman LM: The Anesthesia Machine: Essentials for Understanding, p 69. Madison, Ohmeda, 1985

B.2. What emergency equipment should be easily available to the anesthesiologist?

It is essential that all anesthetic locations be equipped with an Ambu bag for emergency ventilation and some means for performing an emergency cricothyroidotomy. Many kits are commercially available for performing this procedure that can be placed in or taped to the side of the anesthesia machine.

Bowie E, Huffman LM: The Anesthesia Machine: Essentials for Understanding, p 69. Madison, Ohmeda, 1985

B.3. How should this patient be premedicated?

Narcotics should be avoided in this patient in view of her pulmonary disease. Hypoventilation with hypoxemia and hypercarbia could lead to increased intraocular pressure. A better choice would be a light benzodiazepine premedicant to help relieve anxiety.

Miller RD (ed): Anesthesia, 4th ed, pp 2004–2006. New York, Churchill Livingstone, 1994

C. Intraoperative Management

C.1. How would you monitor this patient?

An ECG, noninvasive blood pressure cuff, pulse oximeter, and precordial stethoscope should be used to monitor this patient. Nasal oxygen should be used in light of the sedatives that the patient may receive.

C.2. After the eye had been opened, the patient became agitated and restless. What would you do?

Agitation is the hallmark sign of hypoxemia and should be ruled out initially. If the patient has received intraoperative sedatives, she may become confused and restless. Check the patient's ventilation, color, and oxygen saturation. General anesthesia may need to be performed. Induction and intubation may be facilitated with sodium thiopental and one of the short or intermediate-acting nondepolarizing muscle relaxants.

C.3. Anesthesia was induced and the patient was intubated. You squeezed the ventilation bag and there was a huge leak. Where might the leak be, and what should you do now?

Check the common gas outlet, because the nasal cannula is commonly connected here. If the hose to the common gas outlet is properly connected, check the seating of the carbon dioxide absorber canisters and the vaporizers. In addition, check for cracks in ventilation hoses, ventilation bags, and Y-pieces. If the source of the leak cannot be located quickly, ventilate with an ambu bag and continue to remedy the problem.

Dorsch JA, Dorsch SE: Understanding Anesthesia Equipment, 3rd ed, pp 331–332. Baltimore, Williams & Wilkins, 1994

D. Postoperative Management

D.1. What criteria would you use for extubation?

Commonly accepted guidelines for extubation include the following:

- A vital capacity >15 ml/kg
- A negative inspiratory force > -20 cm H_2O
- Arterial partial pressures of oxygen > 60 mm Hg at an inspired oxygen concentration of <50%
- A dead space to tidal volume ratio <0.6

Stoelting RK, Dierdorf SF, McCammon RL (eds): Anesthesia and Co-Existing Disease, 3rd ed, p 177. New York, Churchill Livingstone, 1993

D.2. What are the causes of postoperative hypoxemia?

Postoperative hypoxemia can be caused by the following:

- A low inspired oxygen concentration.
- Hypoventilation.
- Ventilation/perfusion ($\dot{V}/\dot{Q}$) inequality.
- Increased intrapulmonary right-to-left shunt. This is the most common cause of hypoxemia, of which atelectasis is the main contributor.

Other causes of postoperative hypoxemia include pneumothorax, pulmonary edema (adult respiratory distress syndrome, congestive heart failure), and pulmonary embolism.

Miller RD (ed): Anesthesia, 4th ed, pp 2118–2119. New York, Churchill Livingstone, 1994

D.3. How would you administer oxygen postoperatively?

Mild to moderate hypoxemia can usually be corrected with oxygen via nasal cannula or face mask. Many patients, especially those with upper abdominal or chest incisions, will have marked decreases in their functional residual capacity and will need supplemental oxygen postoperatively. Those with severe hypoxemia may be candidates for continuous positive airway pressure (CPAP) by face mask or will need endotracheal intubation and mechanical ventilation. The adequacy of the chosen therapy can be monitored by pulse oximetry or arterial blood gases.

Miller RD (ed): Anesthesia, 4th ed, p 2121. New York, Churchill Livingstone, 1994

55 Ambulatory Surgery

Matthew C. Gomillion

A 37-year-old woman with endometriosis was scheduled for laparoscopy in the ambulatory surgical suite. Her preoperative outpatient questionnaire indicated a long history of depression with two prior hospitalizations for attempted suicide. She had taken a dose of phenelzine 4 hours previously with a small cup of water.

A. Medical Disease and Differential Diagnosis

1. What is phenelzine? How do monoamine oxidase (MAO) inhibitors work?
2. What are the side-effects associated with MAO inhibitors?
3. What are the important interactions seen with MAO inhibitors and other drugs?
4. Should MAO inhibitors be discontinued before elective surgery?

B. Preoperative Evaluation and Preparation

1. What advantages does outpatient surgery offer?
2. What are the goals of the preoperative evaluation of the surgical outpatient?
3. To ensure thorough screening for disease, should one put all outpatients through a full battery of laboratory testing?
4. What preoperative laboratory testing is necessary for the surgical outpatient?
5. Which outpatients should receive a preoperative chest roentgenogram?
6. In which patients is an electrocardiogram necessary before outpatient anesthesia and surgery?
7. Would a patient's age or physical status influence the decision to perform outpatient surgery?
8. What patients would be considered inappropriate for ambulatory surgery?
9. How would you premedicate this patient?
10. Should every surgical outpatient receive prophylaxis against acid aspiration pneumonitis?
11. Is an overnight fast justified for all outpatients?
12. Would you proceed with elective surgery in the pediatric outpatient with an upper respiratory tract infection (URI)?

C. Intraoperative Management

1. What are the important considerations in choosing an anesthetic technique for outpatient surgery?
2. What are the anesthetic implications of MAO inhibitor therapy?
3. How would you monitor this patient?
4. What are the anesthetic options for laparoscopy?
5. What anesthetic agents would you use to induce and maintain general anesthesia in this patient?

6. What muscle relaxant would you choose for this patient?
7. Would you avoid the use of nitrous oxide in this ambulatory patient?
8. Discuss the physiologic changes induced by laparoscopy.
9. In addition to the physiologic changes described above, what other intraoperative complications are associated with laparoscopy?

D. Postoperative Management

1. What are the common causes of nausea and vomiting in outpatients?
2. How are postoperative nausea and vomiting treated in the ambulatory patient?
3. How is postoperative pain treated?
4. What criteria would you use to establish that a patient can be safely discharged after ambulatory surgery?
5. How would you decide when to discharge a patient after regional anesthesia?
6. What instructions would be given to an ambulatory surgical patient at discharge?

A. Medical Disease and Differential Diagnosis

A.1. What is phenelzine? How do monoamine oxidase (MAO) inhibitors work?

Phenelzine is one of the MAO inhibitors. Monoamine oxidase is the principal intra-neuronal enzyme responsible for the inactivation of nonmethylated biogenic amines, including dopamine, norepinephrine, epinephrine, and serotonin. Inhibition of MAO, often irreversible, leads to the accumulation of these amines in the cytoplasm of nerve terminals, the liver, and other organs. Increase in cerebral neuronal neurotransmitters is believed to be the mechanism by which MAO inhibitors produce their anti-depressant effects.

Bluestone CD, Stool SE, Kenna MA (eds): Pediatric Otolarygnology, 3rd ed, p 1403. Philadelphia, WB Saunders, 1996

Hartley C, Hamilton J, Birzgalis AR et al: Recurrent respiratory papillomatosis—the Manchester experience, 1974–1992. J Laryngol Otol 108:227–228, 1994

Stack CG, Rogers P, Linter SPK: Monoamine oxidase inhibitors and anaesthesia: A review. Br J Anaesth 60:222–227, 1988

Stoelting RK (ed): Pharmacology and Physiology in Anesthestic Practice, 2nd ed, pp 379–380. Philadelphia, JB Lippincott, 1991

A.2. What are the side-effects associated with MAO inhibitors?

Hepatotoxicity can result when MAO inhibitors hinder the activity of monoamine oxidase in the liver. Excessive central stimulation manifesting as tremors, insomnia, and hyperhidrosis can occur. Agitation and hypomanic behavior and, rarely, hallucinations and confusion are observed. In addition, convulsions have been reported. Peripheral neuropathy following the use of MAO inhibitors may possibly be related to a pyridoxine deficiency. Orthostatic hypotension occurs with all the MAO inhibitors currently being used, possibly reflecting the cytoplasmic accumulation of the false neurotransmitter octopamine in sympathetic nerve terminals. Constipation is common with the use of MAO inhibitors.

Hardman JG, Limberd LE (eds): Goodman and Gilman's The Pharmacological Basis of Therapeutics, 9th ed, pp 442–443. New York, McGraw-Hill, 1996

Stoelting RK (ed): Pharmacology and Physiology in Anesthetic Practice, 2nd ed, p 380. Philadelphia, JB Lippincott, 1991

A.3. What are the important interactions seen with MAO inhibitors and other drugs?

Because of the widespread inhibition of monoamine oxidase, MAO inhibitors have considerable potential for interference with the pharmacodynamics and biotransformation of other drugs. Severe reactions have been reported between MAO inhibitors and several drugs, although it should be pointed out that these reported adverse drug reactions occurred in only a few patients.

Narcotic Analgesics/MAO Inhibitor Interactions
The administration of meperidine to a patient receiving MAO inhibitors can produce hyperpyrexia, most likely from an increase in cerebral serotonin caused by MAO inhibitors. Other reactions seen with the combination of meperidine and MAO inhibitors include hypertension, hypotension, respiratory depression, skeletal muscle rigidity, seizures, coma, and even death. Reactions to other narcotics seem to be much less likely. Experimental and clinical studies involving morphine and fentanyl use with MAO inhibitors have failed to implicate them in causing the severe reactions seen with meperidine. Morphine and fentanyl are currently thought to be safe to use in a patient taking MAO inhibitors.

Sympathomimetic Amines/MAO Inhibitor Interactions
The so-called "cheese reaction" involves hypertensive crises associated with the ingestion of cheese in patients receiving MAO inhibitors, and it is the most feared toxic effect associated with MAO inhibitor therapy. Tyramine present in cheese is the agent responsible for precipitating episodes of life-threatening hypertension in a dose-related fashion. Inhibition of monoamine oxidase prevents the breakdown of tyramine in the liver and gastrointestinal tract, allowing tyramine to cause the release of endogenous catecholamines that are present in supranormal amounts. Other foods capable of producing this syndrome include beer, wine, chicken liver, pickled herring, snails, yeast, large quantities of coffee, citrus fruits, canned figs, and chocolate and cream and their products.

The actions of indirect-acting and, to a lesser extent, direct-acting sympathomimetic amines are potentiated following the use of MAO inhibitors. Because MAO inhibitors act primarily intraneuronally, more catecholamines stored in nerve endings become available for release by indirect-acting sympathomimetics (e.g., ephedrine and amphetamine), and severe hypertension can result. No significant cardiovascular problems have been reported with direct-acting agents.

Barbiturates/MAO Inhibitor Interactions
A nonspecific inhibitory effect of MAO inhibitors on hepatic microsomal enzymes has been suggested in animals, raising the possibility that potentiation of barbiturates can be expected. Indeed, several animal studies have reported prolonged sleeping times after barbiturates, causing some authors to advocate reduced doses in patients on MAO inhibitor therapy. However, no clear relationship has been established in humans.

Neuromuscular Blocking Agents/MAO Inhibitor Interactions
Decreased pseudocholinesterase levels have been demonstrated in some patients receiving phenelzine, and a few cases of prolonged succinylcholine effect in patients on

phenelzine therapy have been reported. No problem has been reported with other MAO inhibitors or with the use of nondepolarizing relaxants.

Hardman JG, Limberd LE (eds): Goodman and Gilman's The Pharmacological Basis of Therapeutics, 9th ed, pp 444–445. New York, McGraw-Hill, 1996

Stack CG, Rogers P, Linter SPK: Monoamine oxidase inhibitors and anaesthesia: A review. Br J Anaesth 60:222–227, 1988

Stoelting RK, Dierdorf SF (eds): Anesthesia and Co-Existing Disease, 3rd ed, pp 520–521. New York, Churchill Livingstone, 1993

Wells DG, Bjorksten AR: Monoamine oxidase inhibitors revisited. Can J Anaesth 36:67–70, 1989

A.4. Should MAO inhibitors be discontinued before elective surgery?

Because inhibition of monoamine oxidase is often irreversible, it has been widespread practice to recommend that MAO inhibitors be discontinued at least 2 weeks before elective surgery to allow for new synthesis of the enzyme. This recommendation came as a result of case reports in the anesthesia literature suggesting the potential for serious adverse drug interactions during anesthesia. However, this practice has been questioned by many authorities. As long as certain drugs are avoided (namely, meperidine and indirect-acting sympathomimetic amines) and careful attention is paid to patient monitoring, elective surgery can be safely performed in patients maintained on MAO inhibitor therapy. Patients on MAO inhibitors often have severe depressive illnesses that pose a major risk of suicide. Discontinuance of these drugs, therefore, can be life-threatening.

Rogers MC, Tinker JH, Covino BG et al (eds): Principles and Practice of Anesthesiology, p 570. St. Louis, Mosby-Year Book, 1993

Stoelting RK, Dierdorf SF (eds): Anesthesia and Co-Existing Disease, 3rd ed, p 520. New York, Churchill Livingstone, 1993

B. Preoperative Evaluation and Preparation

B.1. What advantages does outpatient surgery offer?

- Significant reductions in medical care costs
- More efficient use of operating rooms
- Convenience to the patient (decreased time away from home, family, and work)
- Reduced stress and emotional disturbance to patients
- Reduced risk of infection, particularly in the immunosuppressed patient and the pediatric patient

White PF: Ambulatory Anesthesia and Surgery, pp 5–6. Philadelphia, WB Saunders, 1997

B.2. What are the goals of the preoperative evaluation of the surgical outpatient?

The purpose of the preoperative evaluation is threefold:

- To perform medical assessments, obtain data, arrange for laboratory tests and consultations, and prescreen for disease in order to optimize perioperative outcome
- To obtain informed consent

- To provide information and instructions to reduce patient anxiety and improve perioperative management

Organization of the preoperative screening varies among ambulatory surgical facilities throughout the country. The screening process can be organized with an office or facility visit prior to the day of surgery, by a telephone interview or review of health questionnaire without a visit, or by preoperative screening and visit on the morning of surgery. Each of these systems has its own advantages and disadvantages. Nevertheless, the system for preoperative evaluation of ambulatory surgical patients should ensure that screening is performed far enough in advance so that preexisting disease can be evaluated, treatment optimized, and laboratory data recorded before the patient presents for anesthesia. Written instructions should be supplied to the patient in advance describing the preoperative work-up, admission, and recovery periods.

Twersky RS (ed): The Ambulatory Anesthesia Handbook, pp 21–27. St. Louis, Mosby-Year Book, 1995

White PF: Ambulatory Anesthesia and Surgery, pp 8–9. Philadelphia, WB Saunders, 1997

B.3. To ensure thorough screening for disease, should one put all outpatients through a full battery of laboratory testing?

No. The practice of preoperative "shotgun" laboratory screening for outpatient surgery has received much criticism. In addition to unnecessarily adding several billion dollars annually to the cost of health care, laboratory screening tests in asymptomatic patients have been shown to be of dubious value. A combined history and physical examination is a better means of screening for disease, and it should serve to reduce expensive, potentially harmful, and inappropriate tests.

Twersky RS (ed): The Ambulatory Anesthesia Handbook, p 14. St. Louis, Mosby-Year Book, 1995

White PF: Ambulatory Anesthesia and Surgery, pp 158–161. Philadelphia, WB Saunders, 1997

B.4. What preoperative laboratory testing is necessary for the surgical outpatient?

Most outpatient surgical facilities determine requisite preoperative tests by considering the operative procedure; the patient's age, medical condition, and medication history; and state and local regulations. For instance, no laboratory testing may be necessary for healthy ambulatory patients between the ages of 1 and 40 years having a minor surgical procedure. Hemoglobin or hematocrit determination is appropriate for surgical procedures associated with blood loss, and for patients at risk for anemia or polycythemia, such as children <1 year of age or with suspected sickle cell disease; patients with a history of anemia, blood dyscrasia, or malignancy; patients with congenital heart disease or chronic disease; menstruating females; and patients >60 years of age. Additional testing depends on an individual's preexisting condition. For example, serum electrolyte testing would be indicated for a patient with a history of hypertension, diabetes mellitus, renal disease, or for a patient using a diuretic, digoxin, steroid, or angiotension-converting enzyme inhibitor. Likewise, measurement of the partial thromboplastin time (PTT) and the prothrombin time (PT) would be necessary in the presence of a bleeding disorder, anticoagulant use, liver disease, or poor nutritional status. Preoperative urinalysis has not been shown to be useful as a screening test, and is no longer required in a routine anesthetic evaluation.

In view of the possibility of MAO inhibitor-induced abnormalities, it is recommended that this patient should have a preoperative evaluation of her liver function.

Twersky RS (ed): The Ambulatory Anesthesia Handbook, pp 15–19. St. Louis, Mosby-Year Book, 1995

Wells DG, Bjorksten AR: Monoamine oxidase inhibitors revisited. Can J Anaesth 36:70, 1989

White PF (ed): Ambulatory Anesthesia and Surgery, pp 163–165. Philadelphia, WB Saunders, 1997

B.5. Which outpatients should receive a preoperative chest roentgenogram?

Patients who are >75 years of age should routinely have a chest x-ray before outpatient surgery. Abnormalities in the chest x-ray in asymptomatic patients <75 years of age are rare, and the risks to the patient probably exceed the benefits. A preoperative chest x-ray would also be indicated in patients with a history of pulmonary or cardiovascular disease, malignancy, radiation therapy, and a smoking history of 20 pack-years or more.

Twersky RS (ed): The Ambulatory Anesthesia Handbook, pp 20–21. St. Louis, Mosby-Year Book, 1995

White PF (ed): Ambulatory Anesthesia and Surgery, p 164. Philadelphia, WB Saunders

B.6. In which patients is an electrocardiogram necessary before outpatient anesthesia and surgery?

A preoperative electrocardiogram should be routine for all patients >40 years of age, and for all women >50 years of age. In addition, an electrocardiogram would be indicated for patients <40 years of age with cardiovascular or pulmonary disease, history of hypertension, diabetes mellitus, morbid obesity, or a history of digoxin use or cocaine abuse.

Twersky RS (ed): The Ambulatory Anesthesia Handbook, pp 20–21. St. Louis, Mosby-Year Book, 1995

White PF (ed): Ambulatory Anesthesia and Surgery, p 164. Philadelphia, WB Saunders, 1997

B.7. Would a patient's age or physical status influence the decision to perform outpatient surgery?

Even patients at the extremes of age (e.g., <6 months and >70 years) have been managed successfully at ambulatory centers throughout the country. With the exception of the preterm infant, age alone should not be considered a deterrent in the selection of patients for outpatient surgery. In infants born prematurely, an increase in the incidence of apnea for 12 hours after anesthesia has been well documented. Several studies have attempted to determine the postconceptual age at which the former premature infant no longer represents an increased risk for postoperative apnea and therefore would be considered an acceptable candidate for an ambulatory surgical procedure. The recommended age at which former premature infants no longer require inpatient apnea monitoring for at least 12 hours postoperatively varies from 44 (Welborn et al.) to 60 (Kurth et al.) postconceptual weeks.

For the geriatric patient, recent clinical experience has not demonstrated an age-related effect on the duration of recovery or the incidence of postoperative complications after outpatient surgery. However, in determining the acceptability of a geriatric patient for an ambulatory surgical procedure, one must consider the patient's physiologic age and physical status, the surgical procedure, the anesthetic technique, and the quality of care that will be provided at home after surgery.

No longer is outpatient surgery restricted to patients of the American Society of Anesthesiologists (ASA) physical status I and II. ASA physical status III and IV patients whose diseases are well controlled preoperatively are at no higher risk for postoperative complications, and may be considered acceptable candidates for outpatient surgery.

Apfelbaum JL: Current concepts in outpatient anesthesia. International Anesthesia Research Society Review Course Lectures, p 104, 1989

Kurth CD, Spitzer AR, Broennle MD et al: Postoperative apnea in former premature infants. Anesthesiology 63:A475, 1985

Welborn LG, Ramirez N, Oh TH et al: Postanesthetic apnea and periodic breathing in infants. Anesthesiology 65:658, 1986

Wetchler BV: Outpatient Anesthesia. II. Problems in Anesthesia, p 128. Philadelphia, JB Lippincott, 1988

White PF (ed): Ambulatory Anesthesia and Surgery, pp 133–137, 620. Philadelphia, WB Saunders, 1997

B.8. What patients would be considered inappropriate for ambulatory surgery?

An individual may be classified as an inappropriate ambulatory surgery patient for the following reasons:

- The existence of a condition that places an infant at risk:
  - History of prematurity in an infant <44 to 60 weeks postconceptual age
  - Apneic episodes, feeding difficulty, or failure to thrive
  - Respiratory distress syndrome (RDS) which has required intubation and ventilatory support (may take up to a year for symptoms to resolve)
  - Bronchopulmonary dysplasia (BPD) with any degree of significant decrease in pulmonary function or requirement for supplemental oxygen
  - Family history (sibling) of sudden infant death syndrome (SIDS) in an infant <6 months of age
- Acute concurrent illness
- Malignant hyperthermia (MH) or susceptibility to malignant hyperthermia (MHS)
- ASA physical status III or IV with poorly controlled disease
- Acute substance abuse
- Morbid obesity with other systemic diseases
- No available adult at home
- Refusal to have surgical procedure done as an outpatient
- Unwilling to follow instructions

The appropriateness of each patient for outpatient surgery must be evaluated on an individual basis, taking into account a combination of several factors, such as the patient, surgical procedure, anesthetic technique, and comfort level of the anesthesiologist.

Barash PG, Cullen BF, Stoelting RK (eds): Clinical Anesthesia, 3rd ed, pp 1137–1138. Philadelphia, Lippincott-Raven, 1997

Twersky RS (ed): The Ambulatory Anesthesia Handbook, p 4. St. Louis, Mosby-Year Book, 1995

White PF (ed): Ambulatory Anesthesia and Surgery, pp 133–137. Philadelphia, WB Saunders, 1997

B.9. How would you premedicate this patient?

Whether the ambulatory surgical patient should receive premedication has been the subject of much interest and debate. Keeping in mind that a prompt recovery is an important consideration in outpatient anesthesia, many authors have recommended that little or no premedication (especially the centrally active depressant premedicants) be given to surgical outpatients so that recovery is not prolonged. Interestingly, most prospective clinical studies have failed to demonstrate a prolonged recovery following premedication with sedative-anxiolytic and analgesic drugs. However, narcotic premedicants have been shown to increase the incidence of postoperative nausea, which could prolong recovery time, and they are not recommended unless the patient is in pain preoperatively.

In view of the goals one might want to achieve with outpatient preoperative medication, including anxiety relief, sedation, amnesia, analgesia, vagolysis, prophylaxis against aspiration pneumonia, and prevention of postoperative nausea, premedicant drugs can be safely used if needed by the patient provided the drug and the dosage are carefully chosen. Drugs commonly used as premedicants for outpatients include sedative-hypnotics, opioids, anticholinergics, antacids, gastrokinetics, H_2-receptor antagonists, and antiemetics.

It is commonly recommended that premedication should be administered to patients on MAO inhibitor therapy prior to elective surgery to alleviate anxiety and its accompanying sympathetic discharge. In this ambulatory patient, the preoperative use of a benzodiazepine, either midazolam or diazepam, could provide adequate anxiety relief without prolonging recovery or time to discharge. Lorazepam's long duration of action makes it unsuitable for use in the ambulatory surgical patient.

Barash PG, Cullen BF, Stoelting RK (eds): Clinical Anesthesia, 3rd ed, pp 1140–1145. Philadelphia, Lippincott-Raven, 1997

Miller RD (ed): Anesthesia, 4th ed, pp 2218–2224. New York, Churchill Livingstone, 1994

Wells DG, Bjorksten AR: Monoamine oxidase inhibitors revisited. Can J Anaesth 36:70, 1989

White PF (ed): Ambulatory Anesthesia and Surgery, pp 173–182. Philadelphia, WB Saunders, 1997

B.10. Should every surgical outpatient receive prophylaxis against acid aspiration pneumonitis?

Surgical outpatient surgery has been shown to have a high percentage of patients "at risk" (gastric pH <2.5 and gastric volume >25 ml) for acid aspiration. The possibility that they have a greater potential for acid aspiration than the inpatient, although controversial, has prompted several authors to recommend some form of aspiration prophylaxis for all patients scheduled for outpatient surgery. However, the incidence of pulmonary aspiration in ambulatory surgical patients is in fact low (1.7 per 10,000) with a very low mortality rate. Although individual ambulatory surgery centers must determine their own policies, many authors recommend that only high-risk patients (e.g., those with hiatal hernia, diabetes mellitus, morbid obesity, second trimester termination of pregnancy) should receive prophylaxis against acid aspiration.

Miller RD (ed): Anesthesia, 4th ed, pp 2223–2224. New York, Churchill Livingstone, 1994

White PF (ed): Ambulatory Anesthesia and Surgery, pp 180–182. Philadelphia, WB Saunders, 1997

B.11. Is an overnight fast justified for all outpatients?

The value of the traditional overnight fast for surgical outpatients, particularly pediatric outpatients, has been questioned by several investigators. Prolonged fasting does not guarantee an empty stomach at the time of induction. It does, however, cause patient discomfort and can produce significant physiologic disturbances in infants and young children. Studies in children and in adults have shown no increase in volume or decrease in pH of gastric fluid when clear liquids were administered as late as 2 hours before anesthesia induction. Therefore, arbitrary restrictions on the preoperative fast for surgical outpatients, such as "NPO (nothing orally) after midnight," appear to be unwarranted. Infants <2 years of age may safely be given clear fluids until 3 hours before surgery. Feedings of solid food and nonclear liquids should be discontinued at least 6 hours before anesthesia induction. Patients >3 years of age should have no solid food on the day of surgery, but can be allowed clear fluids in reasonable amounts up to 3 hours preoperatively.

Stoelting RK: NPO—Facts and Fictions. International Anesthesia Research Society Review Course Lectures, pp 4–7, 1995

Twersky RS (ed): The Ambulatory Anesthesia Handbook, p 4. St. Louis, Mosby-Year Book, 1995

White PF (ed): Ambulatory Anesthesia and Surgery, pp 9–10. Philadelphia, WB Saunders, 1997

B.12. Would you proceed with elective surgery in the pediatric outpatient with an upper respiratory tract infection (URI)?

Anesthesiologists are traditionally taught to avoid anesthetizing patients for elective procedures who harbor viral infections. This is a result of a belief that respiratory tract infections can be exacerbated by general anesthesia, and that the potential for perioperative complications is increased. The incidence of runny nose and respiratory infection in infants and children, particularly in the preschool group, is high.

Several authors have investigated this issue recently. In a prospective study of 489 pediatric patients, Tait and Knight reported no increased incidence of complications in patients with an active viral infection of the upper respiratory tract, who were anesthetized for myringotomy and the placement of tympanostomy tubes, where there was no endotracheal tube and the anesthetic course was approximately 20 minutes. A large retrospective survey by Tait and Knight suggested that increase in intraoperative respiratory complications is associated with patients presenting with uncomplicated upper respiratory tract infections. However, patients in their survey who were asymptomatic at the time of surgery but who had a history of symptoms associated with a URI within the 2 weeks preceding surgery had a small but statistically significant increase in the incidence of intraoperative respiratory complications. Tait and Knight found no significant differences in intraoperative respiratory complications between patients managed with and without endotracheal intubation. More recently, the study by Cohen and Cameron examined 22,159 children and reported a two- to sevenfold increase in the incidence of respiratory-related adverse events during the intraoperative, recovery room, and postoperative phases of the surgical experience for children with a URI. More importantly, if a child had endotracheal anesthesia in the presence of a URI, the risk of a respiratory complication was increased 11 times. From these and other authors some suggestions have emerged:

- In a child with a URI of the nasopharynx, it is probably safe to proceed with surgery if the operative procedure is of short duration and an endotracheal tube is not required.
- In a child with a URI, if the surgical procedure is anticipated to last >20 minutes or if intubation is likely, it would be advisable to cancel surgery.
- If an infant or child presents for outpatient surgery with a runny nose and cough that has developed within the last 24 hours, and if the parents say that this is the usual state for their child, current opinion would be to proceed with elective surgery, even if endotracheal intubation and surgery of long duration are involved.
- If a significant respiratory infection exists (arbitrarily defined as one that lasts 3 to 7 days and that is associated with fever, cough, and malaise), it would be prudent to wait until 4 weeks after the last day of acute illness to perform elective surgery.

Cohen MM, Cameron CB: Should you cancel the operation when a child has an upper respiratory tract infection? Anesth Analg 72:282–288, 1991

Gregory GA (ed): Pediatric Anesthesia, 3rd ed, pp 664–665. New York, Churchill Livingstone, 1994

Tait AR, Knight PR: The effects of general anesthesia on upper respiratory tract infections in children. Anesthesiology 67:930–935, 1987

Tait AR, Knight PR: Intraoperative respiratory complications in patients with upper respiratory tract infections. Can J Anaesth 34:300–303, 1987

White PF (ed): Ambulatory Anesthesia and Surgery, pp 793–794. Philadelphia, WB Saunders, 1997

C. Intraoperative Management

C.1. What are the important considerations in choosing an anesthetic technique for outpatient surgery?

- Smooth and rapid onset of action
- Intraoperative amnesia and analgesia
- Good operating conditions
- Rapid recovery period without side-effects

To date, no "ideal" anesthetic drug or technique has been identified for outpatients. No single agent or combination of agents, either inhaled or intravenous (IV), has been clearly demonstrated to reduce recovery time and allow faster discharge of the ambulatory surgical patient. However, with its smooth induction and short elimination half-life, propofol may prove to be the induction and maintenance agent of choice for outpatient anesthesia. The newer halogenated ether compounds, sevoflurane and desflurane, have become increasingly popular in ambulatory anesthesia because of their rapid onset and speedy termination of clinical effects. Currently, desirable anesthetic conditions with an acceptable recovery profile can be produced by a large array of pharmacologically active drugs and general, regional, and local anesthesia techniques combined in a rational manner and carefully titrated.

Kapur PA: Controversy: What are the best drugs for ambulatory surgery? International Anesthesia Research Society Review Course Lectures, pp 98–102, 1995

White PF (ed): Ambulatory Anesthesia and Surgery, pp 11–13. Philadelphia, WB Saunders, 1997

C.2. What are the anesthetic implications of MAO inhibitor therapy?

Anesthesia and surgery can be safely undertaken in patients maintained on chronic MAO inhibitor therapy. Guidelines to follow in these patients include:

- Preoperative examination of liver function
- Generous premedication
- Careful heart rate and blood pressure monitoring (beat-to-beat monitoring via an arterial cannula might be considered in all patients)
- Anesthetic techniques which tend to avoid sympathetic stimulation
- Maintenance of intravascular volume
- Avoidance of meperidine
- Careful titration of direct-acting sympathomimetic drugs as needed for treatment of hypotension
- Avoidance of cocaine if topical anesthesia is needed

Stoelting RK, Dierdorf SF (eds): Anesthesia and Co-Existing Disease, 3rd ed, pp 520–521. New York, Churchill Livingstone, 1993

Wells DG, Bjorksten AR: Monoamine oxidase inhibitors revisited. Can J Anaesth 36:71, 1989

C.3. How would you monitor this patient?

The effects of anesthesia during ambulatory procedures should be monitored using the same standards applicable to inpatient procedures. Standard monitoring in this patient would include a blood pressure cuff, electrocardiogram, pulse oximeter, precordial or esophageal stethoscope, temperature probe, and measurement of inspired oxygen and end-tidal carbon dioxide. With the history of MAO inhibitor use in this patient, heart rate and blood pressure should be closely monitored. The potential for hypoxia and hypercarbia during laparoscopy requires careful monitoring of oxygen saturation and expired carbon dioxide tension. In addition, intra-abdominal pressure must be measured during gas insufflation into the peritoneal cavity.

Miller RD (ed): Anesthesia, 4th ed, pp 2022–2023. New York, Churchill Livingstone, 1994

Wells DG, Bjorksten AR: Monoamine oxidase inhibitors revisited. Can J Anaesth 36:70–71, 1989

White PF (ed): Ambulatory Anesthesia and Surgery, pp 218–219. Philadelphia, WB Saunders, 1997

C.4. What are the anesthetic options for laparoscopy?

In recent years anesthesiologists have successfully employed local, regional, and general anesthesia for laparoscopy. Local and regional anesthesia offer the potential advantages of faster postoperative recovery and reduced postoperative complications. They also avoid the postoperative discomforts of general anesthesia, such as sore throat, muscle pains, and airway trauma. However, steep Trendelenburg position, pneumoperitoneum, and surgical manipulation often make spontaneous ventilation difficult during local or regional anesthesia. In addition, the potential for postspinal headache may detract from the use of regional anesthesia in the outpatient. Most laparoscopic procedures continue to be performed under general anesthesia. General anesthesia offers the advantages of elimination of patient anxiety, complete amnesia and analgesia, the ability to control ventilation, muscle relaxation, and a motionless operative field.

In this patient, concurrent MAO inhibitor therapy tends to make general anesthesia the preferred technique because it would eliminate intraoperative anxiety, provide for prevention of hypercarbia with controlled ventilation, and blunt sympathetic responses to stimulation. Although epidural and spinal anesthesia have been used successfully in these patients, their potential for hypotension and consequent need for vasopressors seem to favor general anesthesia use.

Palahniuk RJ: Clinical Pearls—The patient for oscopy surgery. International Anesthesia Research Society Review Course Lectures, p 104, 1995

Wells DG, Bjorksten AR: Monoamine oxidase inhibitors revisited. Can J Anaesth 36:71, 1989

C.5. What anesthetic agents would you use to induce and maintain general anesthesia in this patient?

In planning the anesthetic for this patient, one must keep in mind the important considerations in choosing an anesthetic technique for the surgical outpatient as well as the anesthetic implications of MAO inhibitor therapy (discussed previously). A number of anesthetic agents in a variety of combinations can be used successfully to provide general anesthesia in this patient. A reasonable approach would be to induce anesthesia with propofol or a short-acting barbiturate (e.g., sodium thiopental) after a preinduction dose of a short-acting narcotic (e.g., alfentanil or fentanyl). After intubation, anesthesia is maintained with a volatile anesthetic (e.g., sevoflurane or desflurane), given the patient's history of MAO inhibitor use, in a nitrous oxide–oxygen mixture, supplemented with a short-acting narcotic as needed and a muscle relaxant. In addition, a small dose of droperidol (e.g., 0.625 to 1.25 mg) can be given to decrease the incidence of postoperative nausea and vomiting.

C.6. What muscle relaxant would you choose for this patient?

Adequate muscle relaxation with an acceptable recovery profile can be provided to the surgical outpatient by several muscle relaxants, namely, succinylcholine, cisatracurium, mivacurium, rocuronium, and vecuronium. Personal preference and the anticipated short duration of the surgical procedure influences selection of a muscle relaxant. In addition, consideration should be given to the fact that phenelzine use has been associated with decreased pseudocholinesterase levels in some patients, and a few cases of prolonged succinylcholine effect in patients on phenelzine therapy have been reported.

At the New York Hospital we would choose either mivacurium, cisatracurium, rocuronium, or vecuronium to provide the muscle relaxation necessary during intubation and surgery in this patient. At the completion of the procedure, any residual neuromuscular block should be antagonized with an anticholinesterase.

Use of an intermediate-acting nondepolarizing relaxant has been recommended to decrease the incidence of postoperative myalgias in patients undergoing outpatient laparoscopy. However, work by several authors has demonstrated that substitution of a nondepolarizer for succinylcholine does not decrease postoperative muscle pain.

Barash PG, Cullen BF, Stoelting RK (eds): Clinical Anesthesia, 3rd ed, pp 1151–1152. Philadelphia, Lippincott-Raven, 1997

Wells DG, Bjorksten AR: Monoamine oxidase inhibitors revisited. Can J Anaesth 36:71, 1989

White PF (ed): Ambulatory Anesthesia and Surgery, pp 395–405. Philadelphia, WB Saunders, 1997

Zahl K, Apfelbaum JL: Muscle pain occurs after outpatient laparoscopy despite the substitution of vecuronium for succinylcholine. Anesthesiology 70:408–411, 1989

C.7. Would you avoid the use of nitrous oxide in this ambulatory patient?

The controversy surrounding the use of nitrous oxide in outpatient anesthesia centers around the still unresolved question of its role in producing postoperative nausea and vomiting. Reports by several authors of a significantly higher incidence of nausea and vomiting in patients who received nitrous oxide as part of their anesthetic have caused many anesthesiologists to advocate the elimination of nitrous oxide from outpatient anesthesia. Studies demonstrating no increase in the incidence or severity of postoperative emesis after nitrous oxide have challenged this conclusion. In a recent review of 27 studies in the literature, Hartung concluded that nitrous oxide did, in fact, increase the incidence of emesis. Despite any potential drawbacks, nitrous oxide continues to be the inhalational anesthetic most frequently administered in the ambulatory setting.

Barash PG, Cullen BF, Stoelting RK (eds): Clinical Anesthesia, 3rd ed, p 1151. Philadelphia, Lippincott-Raven 1997

Hartung J: Twenty-four of twenty-seven studies show a greater incidence of emesis associated with nitrous oxide than with alternative anesthetics. Anesth Analg 83:114–116, 1996

White PF (ed): Ambulatory Anesthesia and Surgery, p 378. Philadelphia, WB Saunders, 1997

C.8. Discuss the physiologic changes induced by laparoscopy.

Physiologic changes occur as a result of the pneumoperitoneum and the Trendelenburg position that are required during laparoscopy. Carbon dioxide or nitrous oxide can be used to produce the pneumoperitoneum. Insufflation of gas into the peritoneal cavity elevates intra-abdominal pressure and impairs venous return. As intra-abdominal pressure rises above 20 mm Hg, central venous pressure, arterial pressure, pulse pressure, and cardiac output all decrease. Although rare, severe hypotension and cardiac arrest have been reported. The pneumoperitoneum also sequesters blood in the legs, thus decreasing the circulating blood volume. Vital capacity is significantly reduced as the diaphragm is displaced cephalad by the Trendelenburg position and pneumoperitoneum. Pulmonary compliance is decreased, functional residual capacity is diminished, and aeration of the lower lobes is compromised, predisposing the patient to the development of hypoxia and atelectasis. As the intraperitoneal gas is released and intra-abdominal pressure decreases, all cardiovascular and respiratory parameters return to normal.

Miller RD (ed): Anesthesia, 4th ed, pp 2016–2020. New York, Churchill Livingstone, 1994

Palahniuk RJ: Clinical Pearls—The patient for oscopy surgery. International Anesthesia Research Society Review Course Lectures, pp 104–105, 1995

C.9. In addition to the physiologic changes described above, what other intraoperative complications are associated with laparoscopy?

Absorption of carbon dioxide used for peritoneal insufflation can produce hypercarbia, resulting in hypertension, hypotension, catecholamine stimulation, cardiac arrhythmias, and acidosis. Arrhythmias can also be produced by vasovagal reflexes. Hemorrhage accounts for nearly half of the complications from laparoscopy. A cephalad shift of the mediastinum may cause the endotracheal tube to pass into a bronchus after the Trendelenburg position is assumed. Other complications include gas embolization, tension pneumothorax, pneumomediastinum, perforation and electrical injury of organs, and passive regurgitation and aspiration.

Miller RD (ed): Anesthesia, 4th ed, pp 2012–2020. New York, Churchill Livingstone, 1994

Palahniuk RJ: Clinical Pearls—The patient for oscopy surgery. International Anesthesia Research Society Review Course Lectures, pp 104–105, 1995

D. Postoperative Management

D.1. What are the common causes of nausea and vomiting in outpatients?

Nausea and vomiting are significant problems following ambulatory surgery, and they are some of the most frequent causes of unexpected hospital admission from the ambulatory surgical facility. A number of different factors affect the incidence of postoperative nausea and vomiting. Patients who have a history of motion sickness and a previous experience of postoperative nausea and vomiting are more likely to develop postoperative emetic symptoms, as are patients who are obese or pregnant or have diabetes mellitus. Postoperative nausea and vomiting are common in children; the incidence decreases with age. Males and females are equally affected until puberty, when the incidence becomes higher in females. Excessive anxiety and noncompliance with fasting can increase gastric volume and predispose patients to postoperative nausea and vomiting.

Narcotic analgesics, particularly morphine and meperidine, used as premedication or as part of the anesthetic technique, increase the incidence of nausea and vomiting following outpatient anesthesia. Methohexital is less likely than either thiopental or etomidate to cause postoperative nausea. Recently, propofol was shown to have a low incidence of emetic symptoms postoperatively.

Surgical procedures such as laparoscopy, dilatation and curettage, strabismus correction, myringotomy and tympanostomy tube placement, and orchiopexy are associated with more postoperative nausea and vomiting, with the incidence increasing with increasing surgical and anesthesia time. Assisted mask ventilation also causes nausea and vomiting.

Pain, hypotension, and early ambulation are postoperative factors demonstrated to increase nausea and vomiting. Relief of pain often relieves concomitant nausea.

White PF (ed): Ambulatory Anesthesia and Surgery, pp 490–491. Philadelphia, WB Saunders, 1997

D.2. How are postoperative nausea and vomiting treated in the ambulatory patient?

General measures such as reassurance and adequate preoperative explanation of the procedure to allay anxiety help reduce nausea and vomiting. Many different medications have been used to control postanesthetic nausea and vomiting in the outpatient, some with only limited success. Droperidol has proved to be effective in the prevention and treatment of postoperative nausea and vomiting. Low doses, such as 0.625 to 1.25 mg and even as low as 10 to 20 μg/kg, have been shown to be useful without an increase in postoperative sedation. In fact, by decreasing nausea and vomiting, droperidol may decrease the time for patients to meet discharge criteria, and thus may shorten the hospital stay. A maximal dose of 75 μg/kg or 2.5 mg has been recommended for the surgical outpatient to avoid drowsiness. Metoclopramide (10 to 20 mg IV) has also been used successfully in the treatment of postoperative nausea and vomiting without prolonging hospital stay. Ondansetron (4 to 8 mg IV) is also highly effective, but its high cost may limit its use to patients who are at increased risk for developing nausea and vomiting postoperatively. Transdermal scopolamine effectively reduces nausea and vomiting if given as a premedicant well in advance of the surgery, but the high incidence of anticholinergic side-effects and prolonged residual effects of cognitive performance detract from its usefulness in the ambulatory patient.

Twersky RS (ed): The Ambulatory Anesthesia Handbook, pp 414–416. St. Louis, Mosby, 1995

White PF (ed): Ambulatory Anesthesia and Surgery, pp 22–23. Philadelphia, WB Saunders, 1997

D.3. How is postoperative pain treated?

Pain control is one of the most important factors in determining when a surgical outpatient can be discharged. Pain should be treated rapidly and effectively to minimize postoperative symptoms so that ambulation and discharge are not delayed. Begin controlling postoperative pain intraoperatively by supplementing the anesthetic technique with a short-acting narcotic analgesic or a regional block. Intravenous fentanyl is usually the drug of choice for postoperative pain relief. It may be given in small doses of 12.5 μg at 5-minute intervals and titrated to relief of pain. Ketorolac, a nonsteroidal anti-inflammatory drug, has become increasingly popular in the management of postoperative pain in the ambulatory patient because of its lack of opioid-related side-effects (e.g., sedation, nausea, vomiting, respiratory depression). It is available for oral and parenteral administration, and its use may decrease a patient's requirement for opioid analgesics. Controversy still surrounds the perioperative use of ketorolac because of the potential for bleeding complications and renal dysfunction. Local and regional anesthetic techniques can be used to provide effective postoperative analgesia, and when used to supplement general anesthesia, facilitate a pleasant emergence and minimize the need for opioids. Commonly used techniques include local infiltration of the incision site, intra-articular injection, nerve blockade (e.g., dorsal nerve penile block for circumcision, and ilioinguinal and iliohypogastric nerve blocks for inguinal hernia repair), and caudal blocks. When the patient has resumed intake of oral fluids, oral analgesics (e.g., acetaminophen, nonsteroidal anti-inflammatory drugs, and codeine and other opioid analgesics) can be administered to control pain after discharge.

Twersky RS (ed): The Ambulatory Anesthesia Handbook, p 439. St. Louis, Mosby, 1995

White PF (ed): Ambulatory Anesthesia and Surgery, pp 459–461. Philadelphia, WB Saunders, 1997

D.4. What criteria would you use to establish that a patient can be safely discharged after ambulatory surgery?

For patients to be discharged from an ambulatory facility, they must satisfy specific criteria that are usually summarized on simplified checklists. Although each ambulatory surgical facility must determine its own set of criteria, generally accepted guidelines for safe discharge after ambulatory surgery include:

- Stable vital signs for at least 1 hour.
- No evidence of respiratory depression.
- Oriented to person, place, and time.
- Able to walk unassisted.
- Able to dress unassisted.
- Minimal nausea or vomiting.
- No active bleeding or oozing.
- Pain controllable with oral analgesics.
- Responsible adult to escort patient home.
- Discharge by both the person who administered anesthesia and the person who performed surgery, or their designees. Written instructions for the postoperative period at home must be supplied to the patient before discharge.

Two additional variables commonly used include ability both to void and to tolerate orally administered fluids; however, the role of these variables as criteria for discharge has not been established.

Twersky RS (ed): The Ambulatory Anesthesia Handbook, p 439. St. Louis, Mosby, 1995

White PF (ed): Ambulatory Anesthesia and Surgery, pp 459–461. Philadelphia, WB Saunders, 1997

D.5. How would you decide when to discharge a patient after regional anesthesia?

Patients recovering from regional anesthesia must satisfy the discharge criteria listed above. In addition, if spinal or epidural anesthesia has been used for outpatients, it is important to ensure recovery from the sympathetic and the motor blocks. Hypotension and syncope on standing may be signs that the sympathetic nervous system is still blocked. An indication that the motor block is no longer functioning is the ability to move the legs and feet freely. A simple test is to have the patient run each heel up and down the opposite leg from the big toe to the knee. A patient's ability to walk to the bathroom and void are excellent recovery tests after epidural or spinal anesthesia, because these abilities reflect recovery of both the motor and the sympathetic functions.

Twersky RS (ed): The Ambulatory Anesthesia Handbook, p 441. St. Louis, Mosby, 1995

White PF (ed): Ambulatory Anesthesia and Surgery, pp 521–522. Philadelphia, WB Saunders, 1997

D.6. What instructions would be given to an ambulatory surgical patient at discharge?

Patients should be instructed that after surgery they should not ingest an alcoholic beverage or depressant medication unknown to their surgeon or anesthesiologist, nor should they drive a car or operate complex machinery for at least 24 hours. In addition, the discharge instructions should provide a list of possible problems that require immediate notification of the surgeon (e.g., bleeding that does not stop and persistent nausea and vomiting).

White PF (ed): Ambulatory Anesthesia and Surgery, pp 522–524. Philadelphia, WB Saunders, 1997

56 Magnetic Resonance Imaging

Matthew C. Gomillion

A 5-year-old boy weighing 24 kg is scheduled for an outpatient magnetic resonance imaging (MRI) scan for evaluation of a pelvic tumor. The MRI technician reports that an attempt to obtain a scan last week was unsuccessful due to patient movement despite adequate sedation by the pediatrician. The child's past medical history is unremarkable, and NPO (nothing orally) status has been maintained for at least 6 hours.

A. Medical Disease and Differential Diagnosis

1. What is magnetic resonance imaging, and how does it work?
2. What are some advantages of MRI scanning?
3. What are some disadvantages associated with MRI?
4. What are the contraindications to MRI scanning?
5. What are the biologic effects of clinical MRI scanning?
6. What are the anesthetic considerations for this procedure?

B. Preoperative Evaluation and Preparation

1. What type of patients may require sedation or general anesthesia for a magnetic resonance examination?
2. What preoperative laboratory testing would you require for this patient?
3. How would you premedicate this patient?

C. Intraoperative Management

1. What are some of the anesthetic options for this patient?
2. How is an MRI scan conducted?
3. How would you monitor this patient?
4. What special considerations apply to the monitoring equipment used during MRI scanning?
5. How would you induce and maintain anesthesia in this patient?
6. How would you maintain the airway during the scan?
7. What is the laryngeal mask airway (LMA)?
8. What are advantages of the LMA compared with the face mask?
9. What are advantages of the LMA compared with the endotracheal tube?
10. What are complications associated with the use of the LMA?
11. What are contraindications to the use of the LMA?
12. What can be done to minimize the risk of aspiration when using the LMA?
13. What are indications for the use of the LMA?
14. What size LMA is appropriate for this child, and how much air would routinely be required to properly inflate the cuff?
15. How is the LMA inserted?

16. What are the common causes of poor LMA placement?
17. Examination of the patient before the table is fed into the MRI scanner reveals wheezing. What most likely is happening, and what do you do?
18. Discuss how the LMA can be used as a conduit for tracheal intubation.
19. Discuss the uses of the LMA in the patient with a difficult airway.

D. Postoperative Management

1. When is the LMA removed?
2. How will you have the patient recover from anesthesia?

A. Medical Disease and Differential Diagnosis

A.1. What is magnetic resonance imaging, and how does it work?

Magnetic resonance imaging (MRI) is a noninvasive diagnostic technique that uses magnetic properties of atomic nuclei to produce high-resolution, multiplane cross-sectional images of the body. Atoms having an odd number of protons and/or neutrons in their nuclei have an associated electrical charge, and the net rotation of protons or neutrons produces a local magnetic field similar to the electromagnetic field produced by the flow of electrons in a wire loop. Normally, the magnetic fields surrounding these nuclei are randomly oriented. When placed in the powerful static magnetic field of the MRI scanner, the nuclei align themselves longitudinally so that they lie parallel to the magnetic field.

Within the MRI a specific radio frequency pulse (a second magnetic field) is directed toward the patient at right angles to the static magnetic field, thus displacing the orientation of the aligned nuclei from the longitudinal magnetic field. As the radio frequency pulse is removed, the nuclei return to their magnetic alignment positions. This is termed "relaxation." The energy released as the nuclei relax is detected by the receiver coil of the scanner and used to produce the magnetic resonance image. The time it takes for relaxation to occur varies for specific body tissues, especially water and fat, allowing for differentiation of body structures, as well as normal and pathologic tissue. Different atoms respond to different radio frequencies, with the response being proportional to the strength of the static magnetic field. Hydrogen is the atom most often used for imaging. Resolution of the image requires a strong magnetic field. Most MRI scanners in use today have a magnetic field of 0.5 to 2.0 T (the magnetic field of the earth is 5×10^{-5} T). The magnetic field of an MRI takes several days to establish. Therefore, it is constantly applied even in the absence of a patient, and it is deactivated only in an emergency.

Menon DK, Peden CJ, Hall AS: Magnetic resonance for the anaesthetist. Part I. Physical principles, applications, safety aspects. Anaesthesia 47:241–242, 1992

Patteson SK, Chesney JT: Anesthetic management for magnetic resonance imaging: Problems and solutions. Anesth Analg 74:121–122, 1992

A.2. What are some advantages of MRI scanning?

Advantages of MRI include the lack of ionizing radiation, excellent contrast between normal tissues (e.g., gray and white matter) and between normal and pathologic tissue, multiplanar imaging capacity, lack of image artifact from bone, and the ability to use a noniodinated intravenous (IV) contrast agent.

Rawson JV, Siegel MJ: Techniques and strategies in pediatric body MR imaging. Magn Reson Imaging Clin North Am 4:589, 1996

A.3. What are some disadvantages associated with MRI?

The most significant disadvantage is the attraction of ferromagnetic objects to the magnetic field of an MRI. In addition to the risk to the patient of dislodgement of implanted metallic objects, a potential exists for injury to patients, personnel, and equipment from propelled ferromagnetic objects brought into the magnetic field, such as pens, keys, laryngoscopes, scissors, stethoscopes, paper clips, vials, and needles. Therefore, everyone coming near an MRI scanner should be carefully screened for ferromagnetic objects. The peripheral field of the magnet can be responsible for malfunction of electronic equipment (such as monitors and infusion pumps) and it can erase computer discs or the magnetic tape on credit cards.

Additional disadvantages of MRI are the relatively long time necessary to obtain the images (as much as 15 minutes per image, with a total scanning period of 1 to 3 hours), and the fact that any motion (e.g., cardiac contractions, respirations, cerebrospinal fluid [CSF] flow, and bowel peristalsis) can produce image artifacts. Furthermore, the relatively small bore of the magnet makes examination of obese patients impossible, and creates a feeling of claustrophobia in some patients.

Menon DK, Peden CJ, Hall AS et al: Magnetic resonance for the anaesthetist. Part I. Physical principles, applications, safety aspects. Anaesthesia 47:248, 1992

Miller RD (ed): Anesthesia, 4th ed, p 2259. New York, Churchill Livingstone, 1994

Patteson SK, Chesney JT: Anesthetic management for magnetic resonance imaging: Problems and solutions. Anesth Analg 74:122, 1992

A.4. What are the contraindications to MRI scanning?

Patients with cardiac pacemakers should be excluded from MRI studies because of the possibility of pacemaker malfunction or inactivation in the magnetic field. Other implanted metallic materials that might be dislodged by the magnetic field (e.g., vascular clips, wires, cochlear implants) and interventional radiology devices (e.g., coils, filters, and stents), also preclude MRI examination. Artificial heart valves other than the pre-6000 Starr Edwards valve do not cause a problem during MRI. The electronic control circuitry of implantable infusion pumps, neurostimulators, and automatic implantable cardiac defibrillators can dysfunction in the magnetic field; therefore, patients with these devices should not undergo MRI. Orthodontic braces and dentures, and tattoos or cosmetics that contain metallic dyes, although safe, can degrade the image quality significantly.

Menon DK, Peden CJ, Hall AS et al: Magnetic resonance for the anaesthetist. Part I. Physical principles, applications, safety aspects. Anaesthesia 47:249, 1992

Miller RD (ed): Anesthesia, 4th ed, p 2259. New York, Churchill Livingstone, 1994

Patteson SK, Chesney JT: Anesthetic management for magnetic resonance imaging: Problems and solutions. Anesth Analg 74:122, 1992

A.5. What are the biologic effects of clinical MRI scanning?

Although an area of controversy and ongoing investigation, no significant deleterious effects have been shown to occur to patients or health care professionals from exposure to the static magnetic field of an MRI according to the vast volume of human data available. Also controversial is the use of MR imaging during pregnancy, as the effects of magnetic fields on the human fetus cannot be easily determined. However, current evidence does not support the suggestion that routine clinical exposure of the pregnant patient to MRI can cause developmental abnormalities in the fetus. Pregnant patients have undergone MRI safely during all stages of pregnancy. Nevertheless, caution is advised. The appropriateness of MRI examination and the acuteness of the diagnostic need must be considered. Ultrasonography use is preferred if it can provide equivalent diagnostic information, and consideration should be given to postponing the MRI until late in the pregnancy or until after delivery.

Colletti PM, Sylvestre PB: Magnetic resonance imaging in pregnancy. Magn Reson Imaging Clin North Am 2:291, 1994

Kanal E, Shellock FG, Talagala L: Safety considerations in MR imaging. Radiology 176:593–594; 602, 1990

Menon DK, Peden CJ, Hall AS, et al: Magnetic resonance for the anaesthetist. Part I. Physical principles, applications, safety aspects. Anaesthesia 47:250–251, 1992

A.6. What are the anesthetic considerations for this procedure?

The problems that complicate the anesthetic management of any patient outside the operating room environment exist for patients requiring sedation or general anesthesia for MRI. The MRI unit is often located some distance from the operating room and anesthesia department, limiting the availability of backup assistance and supplies. Frequently, the MRI suite has been designed without consideration for anesthetic needs, such as pipeline gases, and suctioning or waste anesthetic exhaust systems. As with other remote anesthetizing locations, personnel may not be familiar with the requirements of anesthetized patients, decreasing their ability to provide assistance. In addition, an area suitable for recovery after anesthesia may not be available, making a trip to the main recovery room necessary.

In addition to these problems there are anesthetic challenges unique to the MRI suite. Because the physical structure of the unit is bulky and the patient is often far removed from the anesthesiologist, access to the airway is limited, and intravenous lines, anesthesia circuits, oxygen tubings, and monitor cables must be of sufficient length to reach the patient deep inside the scanner. The strong magnetic field generated by the imager necessitates the exclusion of all ferromagnetic objects and equipment. The displays of standard monitoring devices can be distorted or displaced by the magnetic field, and the monitors themselves can degrade the MRI image by disturbing the signal:noise ratio of the MRI.

Patteson SK, Chesney JT: Anesthetic management for magnetic resonance imaging: Problems and solutions. Anesth Analg 74:123, 1992

Rogers MC, Tinker JH, Covino BG (eds): Principles and Practice of Anesthesiology, p 2345. St. Louis, Mosby-Year Book, 1993

B. Preoperative Evaluation and Preparation

B.1. What type of patients may require sedation or general anesthesia for a magnetic resonance examination?

Although MRI is painless, patients must remain still throughout the time required to make each cut (as much as 15 minutes) to obtain images free of movement artifacts. Patients who are unable to cooperate adequately (e.g., infants, young children, and adults who are confused, mentally ill or intellectually subnormal) usually require the services of an anesthesiologist to reduce movement during the examination. In addition, anesthesiologists frequently care for claustrophobic or anxious adults, as well as for patients who require either airway protection (unconscious or critically ill patients) or control of ventilation (patients with head injuries or elevated intracranial pressure) during MRI to ensure that an adequate examination is obtained safely and efficiently.

Peden CJ, Menon DK, Hall AS et al: Magnetic resonance for the anaesthetist. Part II. Anaesthesia and monitoring in MR units. Anaesthesia 47:509, 1992

Rogers MC, Tinker JH, Covino BG et al (eds): Principles and Practice of Anesthesiology, pp 2345–2346. St. Louis, Mosby-Year Book, 1993

B.2. What preoperative laboratory testing would you require for this patient?

In this healthy child without systemic disease for a procedure not associated with blood loss, no preoperative laboratory tests would be required.

White PF: Ambulatory Anesthesia and Surgery, pp 163–165. Philadelphia, WB Saunders, 1997

B.3. How would you premedicate this patient?

The goals of premedication for this child would be to produce sedation and facilitate the induction of anesthesia. At The New York Hospital-Cornell Medical Center pediatric patients (especially outpatients) are not routinely given pharmacologic premedicants for this purpose. Rather it is our practice to allow one parent to be present at the induction of anesthesia, and in this way help to allay the child's anxiety and ease the induction. If one elects to administer a sedative drug to this child, a logical choice would be oral midazolam (0.5 mg/kg) in a small amount of cherry or strawberry syrup.

Gregory GA (ed): Pediatric Anesthesia, 3rd ed, pp 188–193. New York, Churchill Livingstone, 1994

C. Intraoperative Management

C.1. What are some of the anesthetic options for this patient?

Many different anesthetic techniques have been used for anesthetizing children undergoing MRI or other painless radiologic procedures. These range from simple sedation with oral chloral hydrate, rectal barbiturates, or intramuscular meperidine/promethazine/thorazine, to general anesthesia with ketamine, propofol, or inhaled anesthetics. Because conscious sedation of children is frequently insufficient to prevent patient movement, deeper levels of sedation or general anesthesia are frequently required to successfully anesthetize the pediatric patient for MRI scan. The ideal anesthetic should allow the anesthesiologist the ability to titrate and maintain stable drug concentrations, prevent undesired patient movement during the scan, provide rapid rates of induction and recovery with minimal side-effects, and have minimal requirement for special MRI-compatible equipment.

Intravenous anesthesia with propofol meets several of the above criteria, and it is an excellent technique for MRI. Continuous intravenous infusion of propofol allows for a precise, rapid titration to the desired effect, and provides for a rapid recovery. Propofol use eliminates the need for a special nonferromagnetic, MRI-compatible anesthesia machine and the necessity of scavenging waste anesthetic gases—two drawbacks to an inhalational anesthetic. Ketamine has the disadvantages of myoclonic movements that are not desirable during MRI, increased intracranial pressure, depressed laryngeal reflexes, and hallucinations.

Frankville DD, Spear RM, Dyck JB: The dose of propofol required to prevent children from moving during magnetic resonance imaging. Anesthesiology 79:953–958, 1993

Martin LD, Pasternak R, Pudimat MA: Total intravenous anesthesia with propofol in pediatric patients outside the operating room. Anesth Analg 74:611, 1992

C.2. How is an MRI scan conducted?

The patient is placed on a long, thin table outside the scanner. After obtaining an adequate level of anesthesia, the patient is positioned. If the head is to be examined it is often enclosed within a small coil or tube. Next, the table with the patient is fed into the long tube of the MRI magnet. The portion of the body to be examined is usually centered in the magnet approximately 1 m from the end of the tube. During the examination the delivery of the radio frequency pulses produces a loud thumping noise which can average 95 dB in a 1.5 T scanner. To obtain a high quality scan, the patient must refrain from moving during the acquisition of an individual cut or from changing position at any time during the entire examination. An individual cut can take several minutes, and the total scanning time may be from 1 to 3 hours.

Menon DK, Peden CJ, Hall AS et al: Magnetic resonance for the anaesthetist. Part I. Physical principles, applications, safety aspects. Anaesthesia 47:246–247, 1992

Peden CJ, Menon DK, Hall AS et al: Magnetic resonance for the anaesthetist. Part II. Anaesthesia and monitoring in MR units. Anaesthesia 47:508, 1992

C.3. How would you monitor this patient?

Reliable and accurate monitoring of an unconscious individual during an MRI scan is essential for a safe examination, because the patient cannot be seen adequately and is not readily accessible to the anesthesiologist (two unique aspects of providing anesthesia for an MRI scan). For sedation techniques standard monitoring would include a blood pressure cuff, pulse oximeter, and an electrocardiogram. Assessment of ventilation in the spontaneously breathing sedated patient may be difficult if the patient is far inside the magnet and out of view. Use of a precordial stethoscope may be unsatisfactory because of the length of tubing required and the difficulty hearing breath (or heart) sounds due to the loud noise of the MRI scanner. Monitoring end-tidal carbon dioxide from one limb of the nasal oxygen prongs or via a nasal catheter is frequently successful, and it is highly recommended. Additional monitors during general anesthesia would include measurement of inspired oxygen and end-tidal carbon dioxide. Temperature should also be monitored in all patients, as air flow through the scanner cavity increases heat loss, making hypothermia a potential problem, especially in the pediatric patient. This can be accomplished by using nonferromagnetic temperature strips, axillary probes, or esophageal or rectal probes where feasible.

Jorgensen NH, Messiak JM, Gray J et al: ASA monitoring standards and magnetic resonance imaging. Anesth Analg 79:1141–1147, 1994

Peden CJ, Menon DK, Hall AS, et al: Magnetic resonance for the anaesthetist. Part II. Anaesthesia and monitoring in MR units. Anaesthesia 47:513–516, 1992

C.4. What special considerations apply to the monitoring equipment used during MRI scanning?

Unshielded ferromagnetic materials in monitors or their cables can interfere with imaging signals, causing a distortion of MRI results. Similarly, the radiofrequency signals of the scanner can induce currents in ferromagnetic elements of the monitors, causing a distortion of the monitoring signal, and making the monitor unusable. Fortunately, MRI-compatible monitors and equipment (e.g., electrocardiographic [ECG] electrodes), which use shielding, non-ferromagnetic components, and filters to produce satisfactory functioning without a distortion of signal, are readily available. Their use is preferred. To avoid magnetic pull monitors should be placed at least 5 to 8 feet from the magnet bore, or permanently mounted.

The ECG may show significant changes within a static magnetic field, particularly in the T waves and the late ST segments, mimicking the ECG changes of conditions such as hyperkalemia and pericarditis. This is due to an induced voltage in blood (a conducting fluid) flowing through the magnetic field. These changes are directly related to field strength, but they do not appear to represent any significant physiologic alteration.

The high radiofrequency power used in MRI scanning poses the risk of excessive heat at the monitoring sites and thus the risk of thermal injury. To minimize the risk of burns from monitoring cables one should:

- Inspect the insulation on all monitoring wires to ensure that it is intact
- Place cables and lead wires in straight alignment (do not allow monitoring wires to form loops)
- Remove all leads or wires not in use
- Separate cables from patient's skin
- Keep the cable and sensor out of the scanning area (e.g., place a pulse oximeter probe on the toe of a patient whose chest is being examined)
- Avoid excessive power

Menon DK, Peden CJ, Hall AS et al: Magnetic resonance for the anaesthetist. Part I. Physical principles, applications, safety aspects. Anaesthesia 47:249, 1992

Patteson SK, Chesney JT: Anesthetic management for magnetic resonance imaging: Problems and solutions. Anesth Analg 74:122–123, 1992

Peden CJ, Menon DK, Hall AS et al: Magnetic resonance for the anaesthetist. Part II. Anaesthesia and monitoring in MR units. Anaesthesia 47:513–514, 1992

C.5. How would you induce and maintain anesthesia in this patient?

Anesthesia induction can be accomplished with inhalation of sevoflurane or halothane in nitrous oxide and oxygen via face mask in a room adjacent to the MRI scanner. It is the practice at The New York Hospital-Cornell Medical Center to allow one parent to be present during induction of anesthesia in pediatric patients. After the child has lost consciousness the parent is escorted back to the waiting room while intravenous access is established. The anesthetic level is deepened with a loading dose of propofol (e.g., 1 to 2 mg/kg), and the airway is secured. The child is then moved into the scanner room, placed on the MRI table, and positioned for the scan. Anesthesia is maintained with a continuous intravenous infusion of propofol, combined with nitrous oxide in oxygen.

Alternatively, an intravenous catheter can be inserted under local anesthesia and anesthesia induced with intravenous propofol (3 mg/kg).

Frankville DD, Spear RM, Dyck JB: The dose of propofol required to prevent children from moving during magnetic resonance imaging. Anesthesiology 79:954, 1993

C.6. How would you maintain the airway during the scan?

Limitation of access to the patient's airway is one of the greatest challenges for the anesthesiologist during an MRI scan. Because the patient is not visible in the magnet bore and the head is inaccessible, the airways of unconscious or anesthetized patients should be secured with either an endotracheal tube or a laryngeal mask airway to avoid difficulty with airway control that can result in airway obstruction and hypoventilation during anesthesia. Respiration can be spontaneous or controlled depending on personal preference and the needs of the patient.

Peden CJ, Menon DK, Hall AS et al: Magnetic resonance for the anaesthetist. Part II. Anaesthesia and monitoring in MR units. Anaesthesia 47:511, 1992

C.7. What is the laryngeal mask airway (LMA)?

The laryngeal mask airway (LMA) is a device introduced by a British anesthesiologist, Dr. Archie Brain. It fills the gap in airway management between use of the face mask and tracheal intubation. Constructed of soft medical-grade silicone rubber, the LMA consists of an elliptical spoonshaped mask with an inflatable rim fused at a 30 degree angle to an internally ridged tube with a standard 15 mm proximal connector. On the concavity of the laryngeal mask is a fenestrated aperture with three orifices through which the distal end of the tube opens. The cuff of the mask is inflated through a pilot balloon. On the posterior curvature of the tube is a black line running longitudinally to assist in orientating the tube in situ. The standard LMA is latex-free and contains no ferromagnetic components except a small metal spring in the pilot-tube valve mechanism. It is nondisposable, and with repeated autoclaving, it is designed to be used numerous times (as many as 40).

The small amount of metal in the spring valve is not sufficient to be attracted by the magnetic field and dislodge the LMA. However, if the valve lies within close proximity of the area being scanned, the scan's image can be distorted. Also available is a flexible LMA that is reinforced with a stainless steel wire coil, but its use during MRI is not recommended.

Pennant JH, White PF: The laryngeal mask airway. Its uses in anesthesiology. Anesthesiology 79: 145–146, 1993

C.8. What are advantages of the LMA compared with the face mask?

When used as an alternative to the face mask, the LMA gives the anesthesiologist more freedom to perform other tasks (e.g., record keeping, monitoring, and drug administration), and decreases the incidence of operator hand fatigue. Capnography is more reliably performed with an LMA by the use of sideport monitoring. In addition, LMA use has been shown to be superior to that of the face mask for maintaining higher hemoglobin oxygen saturations. The LMA also requires less repositioning of the head and/or jaw to maintain a patent airway, and it seems to be less affected by the position of the mandible, tongue, or neck. Furthermore, injury to the eyes and facial nerves may be reduced by avoidance of a face mask.

Brimacombe J: The advantages of the LMA over the tracheal tube or facemask: A meta-analysis. Can J Anaesth 42:1020, 1995

Pennant JH, White PF: The laryngeal mask airway. Its uses in anesthesiology. Anesthesiology 79: 157, 1993

Smith I, White PF: Use of the laryngeal mask airway as an alternative to a face mask during outpatient arthroscopy. Anesthesiology 77:853–854, 1992

Springer DK, Jahr JS: The laryngeal mask airway. Safety, efficacy, and current use. Am J Anesthesiol 12:67, 1995

C.9. What are advantages of the LMA compared with the endotracheal tube?

Although the LMA does not replace the endotracheal tube (especially in longer cases and when protection from aspiration is important), it has some advantages. One of the advantages of the LMA is that its placement and presence cause less stimulation (i.e., less coughing, gagging, swallowing, breath holding, and bronchospasm, and minimal cardiovascular response) than an endotracheal tube. Therefore, lighter levels of anesthesia are usually tolerated when an LMA is used. Placement of the LMA is associated with less of a rise in intraocular pressure, and presence of the device on emergence causes less coughing than an endotracheal tube. Also, the LMA can be inserted without visualization of the larynx or administration of muscle relaxants. In inexperienced hands the LMA is more rapidly and reliably placed than an endotracheal tube, suggesting a potential role in resuscitation. Trauma to the vocal cords is limited, because the LMA does not pass through this area. In adults the incidence of sore throat after LMA use is reduced compared with the tracheal tube.

Brimacombe J: The advantages of the LMA over the tracheal tube or facemask: A meta-analysis. Can J Anaesth 42:1019, 1995

Pennant JH, White PF: The laryngeal mask airway. Its uses in anesthesiology. Anesthesiology 79: 157, 1993

Springer DK, Jahr JS: The laryngeal mask airway. Safety, efficacy, and current use. Am J Anesthesiol 12:67, 1995

Wilkins CJ, Cramp PGW, Staples J et al: Comparison of the anesthetic requirement for tolerance of laryngeal mask airway and endotracheal tube. Anesth Analg 75:796, 1992

C.10. What are complications associated with the use of the LMA?

The most serious potential problem of the LMA device is that it does not protect the trachea from aspiration of gastric contents. Although no study has yet determined the incidence of aspiration with the LMA, most authors recommend that it not be used in patients at high risk for regurgitation. Conversely, aspiration of pharyngeal contents has not been shown to be a problem with the LMA, and its use has been reported to be suitable during ear nose and throat and dental procedures. When positive pressure ventilation is employed and airway pressures exceed 20 cm H_2O, inflation of the stomach has occurred. Sore throat occurs in 4% to 12% of patients after LMA use, an incidence comparable to use of a face mask and oropharyngeal airway. The frequency of coughing and laryngospasm is also similar with the LMA and the oropharyngeal airway. Although not clinically important in most instances, partial airway obstruction occurs in 25% to 50% of pediatric and 10% of adult cases (usually resulting from a downfolding of the epiglottis). Herniation or rupture of the cuff can occur after repeated autoclaving of the device. Other problems include failure to insert or function properly (incidence of 0.4% to 6%), overt trauma, and complete displacement of the LMA from the pharynx.

Benumof JL: Laryngeal mask airway and the ASA difficult airway algorithm. Anesthesiology 84: 689, 1996

Nair I, Bailay PM: Review of uses of the laryngeal mask in ENT anaesthesia. Anaesthesiology 50: 898–900, 1995

Pennant JH, White PF: The laryngeal mask airway. Its uses in anesthesiology. Anesthesiology 79: 158, 1993

C.11. What are contraindications to the use of the LMA?

The following conditions contraindicate the use of the LMA:
- Increased risk of gastric regurgitation
- Limited ability to open the mouth or extend the neck (e.g., severe rheumatoid arthritis, ankylosing spondylitis) such that advancement of the LMA into the hypopharynx is difficult
- Low pulmonary compliance or high airway resistance
- Airway obstruction at or below the level of the larynx
- Oropharyngeal pathology (e.g., hematoma, abscess, tissue disruption)
- One-lung ventilation

Pennant JH, White PF: The laryngeal mask airway. Its uses in anesthesiology. Anesthesiology 79: 158–159, 1993

C.12. What can be done to minimize the risk of aspiration when using the LMA?

The inflatable cuff of the LMA does not guarantee a protective barrier to the larynx from vomitus, and the LMA is not an alternative to the cuffed endotracheal tube for reliably isolating the airway. Although regurgitation and aspiration have been shown to occur with the LMA, the overall incidence of these events is unknown. The single most important factor in decreasing the risk of aspiration is proper patient selection. In addition, the cuff should be routinely tested for defects before use. Lubricant should be applied only to the posterior surface of the mask, as lubricant from the anterior surface may be aspirated. An adequate anesthetic depth must be obtained before insertion of the LMA and maintained throughout its use to decrease retching and coughing in response to the device. As patients emerge from anesthesia, they should not be disturbed and the cuff should remain inflated until they are awake.

Pennant JH, White PF: The laryngeal mask airway. Its uses in anesthesiology. Anesthesiology 79: 150, 1993

C.13. What are indications for the use of the LMA?

The LMA is best suited for use in any patient in whom anesthesia can be safely maintained through a face mask (except in a patient with pathology of the oropharynx). It has been used routinely in a variety of surgical procedures such as minor gynecologic and urologic procedures, operations on the extremities, and bronchoscopic and endoscopic diagnostic procedures. In addition, the device may be useful in surgery around the face where tracheal intubation is required only because maintenance of the airway through a face mask would interfere with the surgery. Other types of surgery where the LMA has been used successfully include dental extraction, adenotonsillectomy, repair of cleft palate, myringotomy and placement of tympanostomy tubes, and eye surgery. Furthermore, use of the LMA in the management of the difficult airway is increasing.

Asai T, Morris S: The laryngeal mask airway: Its features, effects and role. Can J Anaesth 41:944–945, 1994

Nair I, Bailey PM: Review of uses of the laryngeal mask in ENT anaesthesia. Anaesth 50:898–899, 1995

C.14. What size LMA is appropriate for this child, and how much air would routinely be required to properly inflate the cuff?

In this patient weighing 24 kg a size 2.5 LMA with a cuff volume of 14 ml would be appropriate. A guide to selecting the appropriate LMA based on patient weight, and the cuff volumes of the different LMAs is shown in Table 56-1.

Benumof JL: Laryngeal mask airway and the ASA difficult airway algorithm. Anesthesiology 84: 694, 1996

Pennant JH, White PF: The laryngeal mask airway. Its uses in anesthesiology. Anesthesiology 79: 145, 1993

Table 56-1. The Selection of LMA Size and Cuff Volume According to Patient's Weight

LMA SIZE	PATIENT WEIGHT (kg)	CUFF VOLUME (ml)
1	<6.5	2–5
2	6.5–20	7–10
2.5	20–30	14
3	30–70	15–20
4	>70	25–30
5	>90	40

C.15. How is the LMA inserted?

Before insertion, the cuff of the LMA should be completely deflated and the posterior surface of the cuff lubricated. Care should be taken to avoid lubricating the anterior surface, as the lubricant may obstruct the distal aperture or be accidentally aspirated into the larynx. After induction of anesthesia the patient's head is positioned as for tracheal intubation with flexion of the neck, and the mouth is opened. Holding the device like a pen with the index finger of the dominant hand positioned at the junction of the tube and the mask, the posterior surface of the lubricated, deflated cuff is firmly applied against the hard palate as the LMA is guided over the back of the tongue and advanced into the hypopharynx until the upper esophageal sphincter is engaged (at this point a characteristic resistance is felt). If difficulty is encountered on advancing the LMA, rotating the tube, thrusting the jaw, or using a laryngoscope may be helpful. The cuff is then inflated with air. The longitudinal black line on the surface of the tube should lie against the upper lip in the midline. Tape is used to secure the LMA in position in a manner similar to that used to secure an endotracheal tube.

When correctly positioned the bowl of the LMA mask lies over the laryngeal inlet with the tip of the LMA cuff resting against the upper esophageal sphincter in the hypopharynx, and the sides of the cuff resting in the piriform fossae. Although the epiglottis often lies within the bowl of the LMA mask, the device usually creates a satisfactory airway even when the epiglottis assumes an awkward position (e.g., downfolded).

Pennant JH, White PF: The laryngeal mask airway. Its uses in anesthesiology. Anesthesiology 79: 146–149, 1993

Springer DK, Jahr JS: The laryngeal mask airway. Safety, efficacy, and current use. Am J Anesthesiol 12:66, 1995

C.16. What are the common causes of poor LMA placement?

The three most common conditions which result in failure to achieve proper placement of the LMA are inadequate depth of anesthesia or muscle relaxation, inability to negotiate the 90 degree turn from the posterior pharynx to the hypopharynx, and use of the wrong LMA size. In addition, patients with a small mouth, a large tongue, large tonsils, or a posteriorly located larynx present more of a challenge to proper LMA placement. In 2% to 33% of all patients, more than one attempt at LMA placement is necessary.

Benumof JL: Laryngeal mask airway and the ASA difficult airway algorithm. Anesthesiology 84: 689, 1996

C.17. Examination of the patient before the table is fed into the MRI scanner reveals wheezing. What most likely is happening, and what do you do?

The most common causes of wheezing with the use of the LMA are partial closure of the vocal cords due to light anesthesia or inadequate muscle relaxation and malpositioning of the device with the tip of the mask being against the glottis. One should deepen the anesthetic in the spontaneously breathing patient, or administer muscle relaxant in the patient whose ventilation is being controlled as an initial treatment. If the problem is not relieved despite an adequate level of anesthesia and/or paralysis, the device should be reinserted.

Asai T, Morris S: The laryngeal mask airway: Its features, effects and role. Can J Anaesth 41:935, 1994

C.18. Discuss how the LMA can be used as a conduit for tracheal intubation.

The LMA has been used successfully as a conduit for blind tracheal intubation with an endotracheal tube or intubating tracheal stylet or for the passage of a fiberoptic bronchoscope (FOB) under direct vision (an endotracheal tube can then be passed over the FOB). Blind techniques at intubation through the LMA have the greatest chance of success when the LMA has a perfect central position around the larynx (45% to 60% of the time); they are less likely to succeed with greater degrees of noncentral location of the LMA. Furthermore, the chance of passing an endotracheal tube blindly through the LMA into the trachea is decreased with the use of cricoid pressure. Obviously, attempting to pass a semirigid object blindly through the laryngeal aperture can result in laryngopharyngeal injury.

On the other hand, passage of an FOB through the LMA is successful nearly 100% of the time. With an appropriately sized endotracheal tube (see below) threaded on the proximal end of the FOB, the scope is passed down the lumen of the LMA and under direct visualization into the trachea. The endotracheal tube is then passed over the shaft of the FOB and the trachea is intubated. Three problems occur with this technique. First, the endotracheal tube may not be long enough to ensure that the cuff is situated below the vocal cords when the LMA is left in situ in patients with long incisor-to-glottis distances. Second, the internal diameter of the LMA limits the size of endotracheal tube used, and may not allow passage of a tube large enough to provide for effective ventilation. Third, removal of the LMA over the endotracheal tube risks extubation of the patient. A variety of solutions to these problems have been proposed, including using a tube exchanger to replace the LMA and endotracheal tube with a larger diameter and longer endotracheal tube, and deflating the LMA cuff to gain 1.0 to 1.5 cm of depth in which to advance the LMA and endotracheal tube together. However, if the endotracheal tube that has been passed through the LMA is of adequate size, the LMA should be left in place with its cuff deflated. Table 56-2 lists the LMA size that can accommodate the size of endotracheal tube and fiberoptic bronchoscope.

Benumof JL: Laryngeal mask airway and the ASA difficult airway algorithm. Anesthesiology 84: 690–693, 1996

Table 56-2. The LMA Size That Can Accommodate the Size of Endotracheal Tube and Fiberoptic Bronchoscope (FOB)

LMA SIZE	LARGEST ENDOTRACHEAL TUBE (ID, mm)	FOB SIZE (mm)
1	3.5	2.7
2	4.5	3.5
2.5	5.0	4.0
3	6.0 cuffed	5.0
4	6.0 cuffed	5.0
5	7.0 cuffed	6.0

Pennant JH, White PF: The laryngeal mask airway. Its uses in anesthesiology. Anesthesiology 79: 151–153, 1993

C.19. Discuss the uses of the LMA in the patient with a difficult airway.

In addition to serving as a routine airway during general anesthesia, the LMA has proved to be valuable in supporting airways that are difficult to manage, as well as useful as a conduit for tracheal intubation. Uses of the LMA in the patient with a difficult airway include:

As a Conduit for Fiberoptic Tracheal Intubation in the Awake Patient
When the preoperative evaluation indicates that the patient should be tracheally intubated awake, the LMA can be placed in the properly prepared awake patient and used as a conduit for fiberoptic intubation. Insertion of an LMA is a relatively moderate stimulus that may be better tolerated in the awake patient than the very stimulating methods of conventional rigid laryngoscopy and bronchoscopy. Visualization of the laryngeal inlet with a fiberoptic bronchoscope is usually easy through the shaft of a properly positioned LMA. In patients whose airways are potentially difficult but who do not require endotracheal intubation, an LMA can be placed when they are awake and used as the primary means of airway control.

As an Airway in the Anesthetized Patient Who Cannot Be Tracheally Intubated
The LMA is an alternative to the face mask in the patient under general anesthesia who cannot be tracheally intubated but whose lungs can be ventilated via mask. An exception to this is the patient in whom cricoid pressure must be continuously applied (e.g., the patient at risk for regurgitation). In this situation, placement of the LMA might induce vomiting and aspiration, and would have little benefit over a conventional mask. As noted previously in question C.9, the LMA has several advantages over the face mask. An additional advantage of the LMA is that it can be used as a conduit for FOB intubation.

As a Conduit for FOB Tracheal Intubation in the Anesthetized Patient Who Cannot Be Intubated, But Whose Lungs Can Be Ventilated
Refer to question C.18.

As an Emergency Airway in the Patient Who Cannot Be Ventilated or Intubated
Insertion of the LMA has provided a life-saving emergency airway in this situation, and is a reasonable maneuver to try before transtracheal jet ventilation provided that there is no known periglottic pathology. The LMA works well as a routine airway device in most patients, and it is usually easily placed in patients whose airways are Mallampati class 3 or 4 and/or grade III or IV laryngoscopic view. Most anesthesiologists are familiar with placement of an LMA, and can effectively insert one with little trauma (as compared to transtracheal ventilation).

As a Conduit for Tracheal Intubation in the Patient Who Cannot Be Ventilated or Intubated
If the airway is successfully established with an LMA in this situation, precious time has been obtained to subsequently use the LMA as a conduit for tracheal intubation. If the LMA provides for adequate ventilation, it is likely that the glottic opening lies within the bowl of the LMA and FOB-guided intubation through the LMA will be successful. If ventilation is poor after LMA insertion, the LMA may not be adequately aligned with the laryngeal inlet or there may be periglottic pathology. In both these situations FOB-guided tracheal intubation may be difficult and transtracheal jet ventilation or tracheostomy may be necessary.

Benumof JL: Laryngeal mask airway and the ASA difficult airway algorithm. Anesthesiology 84: 694–696, 1996

Briacombe J, Berry A: Mallampati classification and laryngeal mask airway insertion. Anesthesiology 48:347, 1993

D. Postoperative Management

D.1. When is the LMA removed?

Because the LMA serves to protect the larynx from pharyngeal secretions, it should remain in place with the cuff inflated until protective airway reflexes have returned. At the completion of the procedure, the anesthetic is discontinued and the patient is allowed to spontaneously recover without stimulation. If the patient is to be transferred from the MRI table or moved in any way, anesthesia should be maintained at a depth adequate to prevent reflex responses to the stimulus of being moved. With the bite block in place the patient is allowed to awaken, and the LMA cuff is deflated and the device removed when the patient opens the mouth on command. Suctioning of secretions from the pharynx is usually not necessary because they do not enter the larynx provided that the cuff is not deflated until just prior to removal. If the hypopharynx is to be suctioned before removal of the LMA, it is important to ensure that an adequate level of anesthesia is present to avoid unnecessary airway stimulation. As with extubation of the trachea, equipment for managing airway emergencies must be immediately available.

Asai T, Morris S: The laryngeal mask airway: Its features, effects and role. Can J Anaesth 41:935, 1994

Pennant JH, White PF: The laryngeal mask airway. Its uses in anesthesiology. Anesthesiology 79: 149, 1993

D.2. How will you have the patient recover from anesthesia?

Postanesthesia recovery care after an MRI is the same as that required after an anesthetic in the operating room. This can be accomplished in a designated area of the MRI suite provided that adequate facilities and trained personnel are available. However, this is frequently not the case and the patient will require transport to the main recovery room, a trip which may be of considerable distance. To transport the patient quickly and safely, it is important to have adequate personnel and the proper equipment organized in advance. It is useful to have the location of recovery and logistics of transport (if necessary) planned before the procedure begins.

At The New York Hospital-Cornell Medical Center patients who receive conscious sedation are routinely recovered in the MRI suite by a member of the anesthesia team. Patients who required deep sedation or general anesthesia are usually transported to the main recovery room after return of consciousness and protective airway reflexes.

Rogers MC, Tinker JH, Covino BG et al: Principles and Practice of Anesthesiology, p 2347. St. Louis, Mosby-Year Book, 1993

Morbid Obesity

57

Fun-Sun F. Yao
John J. Savarese

A 30-year-old Caucasian woman with cholelithiasis was scheduled for cholecystectomy and possible common bile duct exploration. She weighed 150 kg and was 150 cm tall. She was found somnolent during the preoperative visit. Her blood pressure was 150/90 mm Hg; pulse 80/min; respiration 6 to 8/min.

A. Medical Disease and Differential Diagnosis

1. What problems exist with this patient? Define the terms overweight, obesity, morbid obesity, and normal weight.
2. What is the pickwickian syndrome?
3. What kind of metabolic problems would you expect to find in morbidly obese patients?
4. Describe the changes that occur in the following respiratory functions in morbidly obese patients:
   - Lung volumes—tidal volume, functional residual capacity (FRC), residual volume, vital capacity, inspiratory and expiratory reserve volumes, and total lung capacity
   - Compliances—lung, chest wall, total
   - Work of breathing
5. What changes occur in PaO_2 and $PaCO_2$?
6. What changes occur in QS/QT and VD/VT? Describe the equations.
7. What changes occur in the cardiovascular system of the obese patient? Discuss cardiac output, blood volume, blood pressure, and pulmonary arterial pressure.
8. Are there any other disease entities usually associated with obesity?
9. What anatomic changes that affect the airway are associated with morbid obesity?
10. What derangements of the gastrointestinal system are associated with morbid obesity?

B. Preoperative Evaluation and Preparation

1. How would you evaluate the patient preoperatively?
2. Interpret the following arterial blood gases: pH, 7.25; P_{CO_2}, 50 mm Hg; P_{O_2}, 58 mm Hg; HCO_3^-, 25 mEq/liter on room air.
3. What is the equation for blood pH?
4. What are the normal values of blood pKa, dCO_2, HCO_3^-, and H_2CO_3?
5. Interpret the following spirometry screening test: vital capacity (VC), 2360 ml (expected 3375 ml); forced expiratory volume in 1 second/forced vital capacity (FEV_1/FVC), 82%; VC, 70% of expected value.
6. How would you premedicate the patient? Why?
7. What are the side-effects of cimetidine?

C. Intraoperative Management

1. How would you monitor the patient?
2. How would you induce anesthesia? Describe the intubation technique.
3. Why is it important to preoxygenate the obese patient? How would you do it? Compare the effectiveness of the 4-maximal-breath and 3-minute techniques.
4. How would you maintain the anesthesia? What is your choice of agents?
5. What kind of muscle relaxants would you use?
6. Can regional anesthesia be used? What are the advantages and disadvantages of regional anesthesia?
7. What is the effect of narcotics on Oddi's sphincter?
8. During surgery, arterial blood gases showed pH, 7.35; PaO_2, 57 mm Hg; $PaCO_2$, 52 mm Hg; F_IO_2, 0.6; respirator tidal volume, 1000 ml, and rate, 15/min. To the circuit was added 10 cm H_2O positive end-expiratory pressure (PEEP), and the tidal volume was increased to 1200 ml. Twenty minutes later, the arterial blood gases showed pH, 7.32; PaO_2, 55 mm Hg; $PaCO_2$, 55 mm Hg. What is the explanation for these changes?

D. Postoperative Management

1. When are you going to extubate the patient? What are the criteria for extubation?
2. What are the major early postoperative complications in the morbidly obese patient?
3. How does position affect respiratory function in obese patients?
4. How would you prevent postoperative atelectasis?
5. How long would you give supplementary oxygen postoperatively?
6. How would you control postoperative pain?

A. Medical Disease and Differential Diagnosis

A.1. What problems exist with this patient? Define the terms overweight, obesity, morbid obesity, and normal weight.

Obesity and cholelithiasis are the main problems. Overweight is defined as body weight as much as 20% greater than predicted ideal weight. Obesity is defined as excess adipose tissue or body weight >20% greater than ideal weight. Morbid obesity is defined as body weight more than twice ideal weight. Ideal body weight is difficult to define. It is generally based on American life insurance statistics on height, build, sex, and age. The so-called "body mass index" (BMI), body weight in kilograms divided by height in meters squared, appears to be useful. The normal BMI is 22 for men and 20 for women. Obesity is defined as a BMI of >27 for men and >25 for women (Table 57-1). On the basis of population studies, a triceps skin-fold thick-

Table 57-1. Severity of Obesity

SEVERITY	BODY MASS INDEX (kg/m²)	PERCENTAGE OVERWEIGHT
Normal	<24–25	<10
Mild	27–30	20–40
Moderate	31–35	41–100
Morbid (severe)	>35	>100

ness >23 mm in men and >30 mm in women should be defined as obesity. In practice we use the Broca index, height in centimeters less 100 for males and less 105 for females, as ideal body weight in kilograms. The ideal body weight for a man 170 cm tall is 70 kg.

- For men: Ideal weight (kg) = height (cm) − 100
- For women: Ideal weight (kg) = height (cm) − 105

Brodsky JB: Anesthetic management of the morbidly obese patient. Int Anesthesiol Clin 24(1): 93–103, 1986

Buckley FP: Anesthetizing the morbidly obese patient. ASA Refresher Courses in Anesthesiology 18:53–68, 1990

Fauci AS, Braunwald E, Isselbacher KJ et al (eds): Harrison's Principles of Internal Medicine, 14th ed, p 454. New York, McGraw-Hill, 1998

Rakel RZ (ed): Saunders Manual of Medical Practice, pp 683–695. Philadelphia, WB Saunders, 1996

Shenkman Z, Shir Y, Brodsky JB: Perioperative management of the morbidly obese patient. Br J Anaesth 70:349, 1993

Vaughan RW: Obesity: Implications in anesthetic management and toxicity. ASA Refresher Courses in Anesthesiology 9:184, 1981

A.2. What is the pickwickian syndrome?

The pickwickian syndrome was named by Burwell in 1956. He felt that the first adequate description of this syndrome had been made in 1837 by Charles Dickens in the *Posthumous Papers of the Pickwick Club* in which he described an obese, somnolent boy named Joe. The complete pickwickian syndrome consists of massive obesity, somnolence, alveolar hypoventilation, periodic respiration, hypoxemia, secondary polycythemia, right heart failure, and right ventricular hypertrophy. The hypersomnolence is a manifestation of nighttime sleep apnea. In these individuals, once sleep begins, upper airway obstruction leads to hypoxemia and hypercapnia, causing arousal with return of normal respiration. Many such episodes occur each night, leading to chronic sleep deprivation and daytime somnolence. Progestational agents have been used therapeutically in the obesity-hypoventilation syndrome because they stimulate the ventilatory response to hypercapnia and hypoxia in normal subjects. Medroxyprogesterone increases ventilation and improves heart function and erythrocytosis in these patients, although obstructive sleep apnea continues.

Burwell CB, Robin ED, Whaley RD et al: Extreme obesity associated with alveolar hypoventilation: A pickwickian syndrome. Am J Med 21:811–818, 1956

Fauci AS, Braunwald E, Isselbacher KJ et al (eds): Harrison's Principles of Internal Medicine, 14th ed, pp 1343, 1479, 1481. New York, McGraw-Hill, 1998

A.3. What kind of metabolic problems would you expect to find in morbidly obese patients?

The basic problem in morbid obesity is the increase in total absolute oxygen consumption and in carbon dioxide production associated with the increase in total tissue mass. The increases in metabolism show a linear relationship to body weight and body surface area. However, the basal metabolic rate in obesity is within normal limits.

Buckley FP: Anesthetizing the morbidly obese patient. ASA Refresher Courses in Anesthesiology 18:53–68, 1990

White RL Jr, Alexander JK: Body oxygen consumption and pulmonary ventilation in obese subjects. J Appl Physiol 20:197–201, 1965

A.4. Describe the changes that occur in the following respiratory functions in morbidly obese patients:

- **Lung volumes—tidal volume, functional residual capacity (FRC), residual volume, vital capacity, inspiratory and expiratory reserve volumes, and total lung capacity**
- **Compliances—lung, chest wall, total**
- **Work of breathing**

Tidal volume (VT) is normal or increased in nonpickwickian obesity and decreased in pickwickian obesity. Inspiratory reserve volume (IRV) is decreased. Expiratory reserve volume (ERV) is most markedly decreased, because the heavy weight of the torso decreases the normal expansive tendency of the rib cage. Residual volume (RV) is normal. Functional residual capacity (FRC) is markedly decreased because of a decrease in the expiratory reserve volume (FRC = RV + ERV). Vital capacity is decreased because of markedly decreased ERV (VC = IRV + VT + ERV). Total lung capacity is decreased. Lung compliance is often normal, but it is decreased when pulmonary and circulatory complications are present. Chest wall compliance is always decreased because of the weight of the torso and the abdominal contents against the diaphragm. Total compliance is always decreased. The work of breathing is always increased because of low compliance.

Alexander JK, Buthrie AE, Sakaguch H et al: Lung volume changes with extreme obesity. Clin Res 7:171, 1959

Barash PG, Cullen BF, Stoelting RK (eds): Clinical Anesthesia, 3rd ed, pp 975–982. Phildelphia, Lippincott-Raven, 1997

Buckley FP: Anesthetizing the morbidly obese patient. ASA Refresher Courses in Anesthesiology 18:53–68, 1990

Pasulka PS, Bistrian BR, Benotti PN et al: The risks of surgery in obese patients. Ann Intern Med 104:540–546, 1986

Vaughan RW: Obesity: Implications in anesthetic management and toxicity. ASA Refresher Courses in Anesthesiology 9:183–202, 1981

Vaughan RW: Pulmonary and cardiovascular derangements in the obese patients. Cont Anesth Pract 5:19–39, 1982

Zerah F, Hart A, Perlwmuter L et al: Effects of obesity on respiratory resistance. Chest 103:1470, 1993

A.5. What changes occur in PaO$_2$ and PaCO$_2$?

The most common abnormal blood gas finding in the obese patient is hypoxemia. Although hypoxemia can occur as a result of hypoventilation, most often it is due to a low ventilation:perfusion ratio. The pulmonary perfusion is increased in obese patients because of increased cardiac output, increased circulating blood volume, and pulmonary hypertension. The alveolar ventilation is decreased, secondary to airway closure, as a result of a markedly decreased expiratory reserve volume, which is often lower than the closing volume. The changes in PaCO$_2$ are variable depending on the alveolar ventilation. The following three types of alveolar ventilation are found among the morbidly obese:

- Alveolar hyperventilation in response to hypoxic drives—This is usually seen in young, active, obese patients with a $PaCO_2$ of about 35 mm Hg.
- Alveolar hypoventilation in older or more obese patients with pickwickian syndrome—The $PaCO_2$ is always >40 mm Hg.
- Periodic hypoventilation—The patients maintain normal or below normal $PaCO_2$ values during the daytime but retain CO_2 at night or at rest.

Bendixen HH: Morbid obesity. ASA Refresher Courses in Anesthesiology 6:1–14, 1978

Buckley FP: Anesthetizing the morbidly obese patient. ASA Refresher Courses in Anesthesiology 18:53–68, 1990

A.6. What changes occur in QS/QT and VD/VT? Describe the equations.

The intrapulmonary shunt QS/QT is always increased because of a low ventilation:perfusion ratio and as a result of airway closure, decreased FRC, hypoventilation, and increased pulmonary circulation. (Normal QS/QT is <5%.)

$$\text{Shunt equation: } QS/QT = \frac{CcO_2 - CaO_2}{CcO_2 - C\bar{v}O_2}$$

CcO_2: pulmonary capillary oxygen content

CaO_2: arterial oxygen content

$C\bar{v}O_2$: mixed venous oxygen content

In the absence of complications, VD/VT is often less than normal because of increased tidal volume and unchanged dead space.

$$\text{Bohr equation: } VD/VT = \frac{PaCO_2 - P\bar{e}CO_2}{PaCO_2}$$

$P\bar{e}CO_2$: mixed expired CO_2 tension

Bendixen HH: Morbid obesity. ASA Refresher Courses in Anesthesiology 6:1–14, 1978

Buckley FP: Anesthetizing the morbidly obese patient. ASA Refresher Courses in Anesthesiology 18:53–68, 1990

Nunn JF: Nunn's Applied Respiratory Physiology, 4th ed, pp 172–179. Boston, Butterworth-Heinemann, 1993

A.7. What changes occur in the cardiovascular system of the obese patient? Discuss cardiac output, blood volume, blood pressure, and pulmonary arterial pressure.

Cardiac output and stroke volume increase in proportion to oxygen consumption and the degree of obesity. Blood volume is expanded when it is expressed in absolute values. However, it is contracted when calculated in terms of body weight of adipose tissue compared with lean body mass. Hypertension is more prevalent in obese people because of increased cardiac output and blood volume. The relationship between body weight and arterial pressure is greater for systolic than for diastolic pressure. Pulmonary hypertension is usually present in pickwickian obesity as a result of hypoxic pulmonary vasoconstriction and increased cardiac output. However, pulmonary arterial pressure is normal in nonpickwickian obese patients without heart or lung disease. Because of hypertension and increased cardiac output, congestive heart failure occurs in about 10% of obese patients. Two mechanisms appear to operate in the pathogenesis of heart failure. In one group of obese patients, pulmonary and systemic vascular congestion develops as a consequence of chronic volume overload superimposed on the effect of diminished diastolic ventricular compliance caused by ventricular hypertrophy. In the other group, chronic volume overload and high cardiac output result in myocardial hypertrophy, which is inadequate, such that the wall thickness:cavity radius ratio is reduced and left ventricular systolic dysfunction is superimposed. Despite gross anatomic involvement, electrocardiographic (ECG) evidences of left ventricular hypertrophy are absent. Conduction defects secondary to fatty infiltration of the conduction system are probably implicated in the predisposition to sudden death. The contribution of obesity per se to coronary artery disease is small or nonexistent, whereas serum cholesterol and systolic blood pressure are potent risk factors. At present the principal link between coronary disease and marked obesity is the extent to which the latter predisposes to hypertension.

Braunwald E (ed): Heart Disease, 5th ed, pp 1905–1907. Philadelphia, WB Saunders, 1997

Hurst JW (ed): The Heart, 8th ed, pp 1937–1942. New York, McGraw-Hill, 1994

Reisin E, Frohlich ED: Obesity: Cardiovascular and respiratory pathophysiological alterations. Arch Intern Med 141:431–434, 1981

Shenkman Z, Shir Y, Brodsky JB: Perioperative management of the morbidly obese patient. Br J Anaesth 70:349, 1993

A.8. Are there any other disease entities usually associated with obesity?

Secondary obesity can be associated with hypothyroidism, Cushing's disease, insulinoma, hypogonadism, and hypothalamic disorders. Although only a minority of obese patients are diabetic, 80% to 90% of nonketotic diabetics are obese. Increased insulin secretion and insulin resistance owing to tissue insensitivity are well-characterized features of obesity. Obesity exacerbates the diabetic state. Osteoarthritis, sciatica, varicose veins, thromboembolism, ventral and hiatal hernias, fatty liver, and cholelithiasis are more common in obese patients.

Fauci AS,, Braunwald E, Isselbacher KJ et al (eds): Harrison's Principles of Internal Medicine, 14th ed, pp 458–459. New York, McGraw-Hill, 1998

A.9. What anatomic changes that affect the airway are assoiated with morbid obesity?

Because of the numerous chins and low cervical and upper thoracic fat pads, flexion and extension of the neck and the atlantoaxial joint are often markedly restricted. Mouth opening can be limited by submental fat. The airway may be narrowed by fleshy cheeks, a large tongue, and copious flaps of palatal, pharyngeal, and supralaryngeal soft tissue. Moreover, a high and anterior infantile laryngeal position may be present in the obese patient.

Barash PG, Cullen BF, Stoelting RK (eds): Clinical Anesthesia, 3rd ed, pp 975–982. Philadelphia, Lippincott-Raven, 1997

A.10. What derangements of the gastrointestinal system are associated with morbid obesity?

Morbidly obese patients have a high incidence of gastroesophageal reflux and hiatal hernia, and a linear increase in intra-abdominal pressure with increasing body weight. During induction of anesthesia, 90% of fasted morbidly obese patients have a dangerous combination of gastric juice volume >25 ml and gastric juice *p*H <2.5. Therefore, morbidly obese patients are at a high risk for acid aspiration pneumonitis.

The incidence of liver diseases is greater in obese patients, mainly fatty liver, cholelithiasis, hepatitis, fibrosis, and cirrhosis.

Barash PG, Cullen BF, Stoelting RK (eds): Clinical Anesthesia, 3rd ed, pp 975–982. Phildelphia, Lippincott-Raven, 1997

Shenkman Z, Shir Y, Brodsky JB: Perioperative management of the morbidly obese patient. Br J Anaesth 70:349, 1993

Vaughn RW, Bauer S, Wise L: Volume and pH of gastric juice in obese patients. Anesthesiology 43:686, 1975

B. Preoperative Evaluation and Preparation

B.1. How would you evaluate the patient preoperatively?

Preoperative evaluation should include a detailed history, physical examination, and laboratory tests. Special attention should be paid to circulatory, pulmonary, and hepatic functions. Circulatory evaluation includes symptoms and signs of right or left ventricular failure, history of hypertension, and electrocardiogram. Respiratory evaluation should include smoking history, exercise tolerance, history of hypoventilation and somnolence, pulmonary function tests with spirometry and baseline arterial blood gases, and chest x-ray film. Hepatic function tests should include serum albumin and globulin, serum glutamic oxaloacetic transaminase (SGOT), serum glutamic pyruvic transaminase (SGPT), bilirubin, alkaline phosphatase, prothrombin time, and cholesterol levels. Upper airway assessment should be emphasized. Evaluation should include checking the full range of motion at the atlanto-occipital and temporomandibular joints with the head maximally extended, checking the adequacy of the distance between the thyroid promontory and the mentum of the mandible, and, finally, subjectively assessing the ease of performing laryngoscopy and intubation.

Barash PG, Cullen BF, Stoelting RK (eds): Clinnical Anesthesia, 3rd ed, pp 975–982. Phildelphia, Lippincott-Raven, 1997

Buckley FP: Anesthetizing the morbidly obese patient. ASA Refresher Courses in Anesthesiology 18:53–68, 1990

Katz J, Benumof J, Kadis LB (eds): Anesthesia and Uncommon Diseases: Pathophysiologic and Clinical Correlations, 3rd ed, pp 496–498. Philadelphia, WB Saunders, 1990

Vaughan RW: Obesity: Implications in anesthetic management and toxicity. ASA Refresher Courses in Anesthesiology 9:183–202, 1981

B.2. Interpret the following arterial blood gases: *p*H, 7.25; PCO_2, 50 mm Hg; PO_2, 58 mm Hg; HCO_3^-, 25 mEq/liter on room air.

These blood gases indicate respiratory acidosis and metabolic acidosis with hypoxemia. HCO_3^-, 25 mEq/liter is a laboratory error. A *p*H of 7.25 suggests acidosis, which may be respiratory or metabolic or a combination of both. If no metabolic ab-

Table 57-2. Predicted *p*H at Different PaCO$_2$ Levels in the Absence of Metabolic Acid-Base Abnormality

PaCO$_2$	*p*H (APPROXIMATE)
80	7.20
60	7.30
40	7.40
30	7.50
20	7.60

Note: Each 10-mm Hg decrease in PaCO$_2$ from normal increases the *p*H 0.1 unit. Each 20-mm Hg increase in PaCO$_2$ from normal decreases the *p*H 0.1 unit.

normality is present, a Pco$_2$ of 50 mm Hg should produce a *p*H of 7.35 (Table 57-2). The difference in *p*H (7.35 − 7.25 = 0.10 unit) is due to metabolic acidosis. For each 7 mEq/liter of acid or base excess, *p*H changes 0.10 unit in the appropriate direction. A metabolic acidosis of 0.1 unit *p*H means a 7 mEq/liter base deficit. The HCO$_3$⁻ is expected to be 17 mEq/liter (24 − 7 = 17), but a change in Pco$_2$ itself will change the HCO$_3$⁻ from chemical equilibrium. Each 10-mm Hg increase in PaCO$_2$ from normal increases the HCO$_3$⁻ by 1 mEq in acute CO$_2$ retention and by 4 mEq in a chronic situation. Therefore, we expect the HCO$_3$⁻ to be 17 + 1 = 18 mEq in acute CO$_2$ retention or 17 + 4 = 21 mEq in chronic CO$_2$ retention. The blood gas machine provides direct measurement of the *p*H, Pco$_2$, and Po$_2$. The HCO$_3$⁻ is usually derived from an equation or from a nomogram. If a discrepancy is found between the *p*H, Pco$_2$, and HCO$_3$⁻, the technical error is usually in the HCO$_3$⁻. It is important to recheck the blood gases according to clinical conditions. A PaCO$_2$ of 50 mm Hg means alveolar hypoventilation owing to decreased minute volume or increased dead space. To interpret PaO$_2$, the F$_1$O$_2$ should always be available. A PaO$_2$ of 100 mm Hg may mean severe pulmonary failure if the F$_1$O$_2$ is 1.0. Hypoxemia in obese patients usually is caused by increased venous admixture from decreased ventilation:perfusion ratio as a result of low FRC and hypoventilation. Metabolic acidosis with hypoxemia indicates lactic acidosis from anaerobic metabolism.

Dripps RD, Eckenhoff JE, Vandam LD (eds): Introduction to Anesthesia: The Principles of Safe Practice, 7th ed, pp 267–268. Philadelphia, WB Saunders, 1988

Shapiro BA, Harrison RA, Cane RD et al: Clinical Application of Blood Gases, 3rd ed, pp 80–85. Chicago, Year Book Medical Publishers, 1989

B.3. *What is the equation for blood* **pH***?*

The Henderson-Hasselbalch equation is:

$$pH = pK + \log \frac{(HCO_3^-)}{(H_2CO_3)}$$

The H$_2$CO$_3$ concentration is low and cannot be measured directly. Normal blood H$_2$CO$_3$ concentration is 0.0017 mMol/liter. H$_2$CO$_3$ is proportional and not equal to dissolved CO$_2$. Clinically dissolved CO$_2$ is used to replace H$_2$CO$_3$. Therefore, pK is changed to pKa. Dissolved CO$_2$ is calculated as a Pco$_2$; a, being the solubility coefficient for carbon dioxide in body fluids, is 0.031 mMol/liter/mm Hg Pco$_2$. For a normal Pco$_2$ of 40 mm Hg, dissolved CO$_2$ is calculated to be 40 × 0.031 = 1.2 mMol/

liter. The pKa is 6.1, but this is variable with temperature and pH. The modified Henderson-Hasselbalch equation is as follows:

$$pH = pKa + \log \frac{(HCO_3^-)}{(dCO_2)} \text{ or } pH = pKa + \log \frac{(HCO_3^-)}{(0.031 \times P_{CO_2})}$$

Nunn JF: Nunn's Applied Respiratory Physiology, 4th ed, pp 219–222. Boston, Butterworth-Heinemann, 1993

B.4. What are the normal values of blood pKa, dCO₂, HCO₃⁻, and H₂CO₃?

The normal values are pKa, 6.1; dCO_2, 1.2 mMol/liter; HCO_3^-, 24 mEq/liter; and H_2CO_3, 0.0017 mMol/liter.

Nunn JF: Nunn's Applied Respiratory Physiology, 4th ed, p 220. Boston, Butterworth-Heinemann, 1993

B.5. Interpret the following spirometry screening test: vital capacity (VC), 2360 ml (expected 3375 ml); forced expiratory volume in 1 second/forced vital capacity (FEV₁/FVC), 82%; VC, 70% of expected value.

The spirometry shows mild restrictive lung disease and no evidence of obstructive lung disease. Normal vital capacity depends on sex, age, and height. The normal FEV_1/FVC is >80%. In restrictive lung disease, vital capacity is <75% of expected value. In obstructive lung disease, the FEV_1/FVC is <75%. The expected vital capacity in liters in young adult males is approximately equal to (height in meters)^2. The residual volume equals approximately 30% of vital capacity. Vital capacity can also be estimated at 65 ml/in. or 25 ml/cm height for males and 52 ml/in. or 20 ml/cm height for females.

Ayers LN, Whipp BJ, Ziment I: A Guide to the Interpretation of Pulmonary Function Tests, 2nd ed. New York, Roerig, 1978

Fauci AS, Braunwald E, Isselbacher KJ et al (eds): Harrison's Principles of Internal Medicine, 14th ed, pp 1410–1412. New York, McGraw-Hill, 1998

Hand Book of Physiology, Section 3, Respiration, p 388. Washington DC, American Physiological Society, 1964

Macklem PT: Tests of lung mechanics. N Engl J Med 293:339, 1975

B.6. How would you premedicate the patient? Why?

No sedatives or narcotics should be given as premedication to a pickwickian obese patient. Light sedation may be given to an obese nonpickwickian patient. Once sedative drugs have been given, supplementary oxygen should be provided to prevent hypoxia from respiratory depression. We believe that a well-conducted preoperative visit is more important than sedation. It is important to explain to the patient the possibility of postoperative intubation and ventilator support. Because markedly obese patients have an increased incidence of hiatus hernia and increased volume and acidity of gastric juice, there is increased risk of aspiration pneumonitis (also see question A.10). Therefore, an H_2-receptor antagonist, such as cimetidine or ranitidine, is recommended for premedication. Cimetidine 300 mg orally the night before surgery plus 300 mg intravenously 1 hour prior to surgery, appears to be effective and widely used. Ranitidine 150 mg orally the night before surgery and 50 to 100 mg intravenously (IV) given 1 to 2 hours prior to surgery, appears to be equally effective. However, ranitidine has several advantages over cimetidine, such as longer duration of action, fewer adverse reactions, and less interference with metabolism of other drugs. Metoclopramide 10 mg IV and nonparticulate antacids, such as 30 ml of 0.3-M sodium citrate, can also be given to prevent aspiration pneumonitis. Anticholinergic agents should be given to dry airway secretions if a difficult intubation is anticipated. Premedication, if any, should be given intravenously or orally, because intramuscular injection usually results in an intrafat injection, leading to unpredictable absorption.

Barash PG, Cullen BF, Stoelting RK (eds): Clinical Anesthesia, 3rd ed, pp 975–982. Phildelphia, Lipincott-Raven, 1997

Bendixen HH: Morbid obesity. ASA Refresher Courses in Anesthesiology 6:1–14, 1978

Buckley FP: Anesthetizing the morbidly obese patient. ASA Refresher Courses in Anesthesiology 18:53–68, 1990

Lam AM, Grace DM, Penny FJ et al: Prophylactic IV cimetidine reduces the risk of acid aspiration in morbidly obese patients. Anesthesiology 65:684–687, 1986

Manchikanti L, Roush JR, Colliver JR: Effect of pre-anesthetic ranitidine and metoclopramide on gastric contents of morbidly obese patients. Anesth Analg 65:195–199, 1986

Miller RD (ed): Anesthesia, 3rd ed, p 801. New York, Churchill Livingstone, 1990

Shenkman Z, Shir Y, Brodsky JB: Perioperative management of the morbidly obese patient. Br J Anaesth 70:349, 1993

Vaughan RW, Bauer S, Wise L: Volume and pH of gastric juice in obese patients. Anesthesiology 43:686–689, 1975

B.7. What are the side-effects of cimetidine?

Cardiovascular Effects
Rapid intravenous administration of cimetidine occasionally can produce bradycardia, hypotension, arrhythmias, and even cardiac arrest in seriously ill patients. Cimetidine blocks the H_2 receptors in the myocardium and peripheral blood vessels, resulting in negative inotropic and chronotropic responses.

Respiratory Effects
Cimetidine blocks the bronchodilatory effects of H_2 receptors and can potentiate histamine-induced bronchospasm.

Hematologic Effects
The incidence of leukopenia is reported as 1 in 100,000 patients, whereas agranulocytosis and thrombocytopenia are reported as 3 in 1,000,000 patients.

Metabolic Effects
Cimetidine inhibits hepatic microsomal drug metabolism, resulting in slow clearing of warfarin, diazepam, phenytoin, theophylline, and propranolol. Cimetidine also decreases liver blood flow and slows elimination of propranolol and lidocaine.

Neurologic Effects
Infrequent reports indicate agitation, mental confusion, and coma have been associated with cimetidine therapy in critically ill patients.

Freston JW: Cimetidine. II. Adverse reactions and patterns of use. Ann Intern Med 97:728, 1982

Manchikanti L, Kraus JW, Edds SP: Cimetidine and related drugs in anesthesia. Anesth Analg 61: 595–608, 1982

Miller RD (ed): Anesthesia, 4th ed, pp 1452–1454. New York, Churchill Livingstone, 1994

C. Intraoperative Management

C.1. How would you monitor the patient?

In addition to the routine monitors of ECG, blood pressure, esophageal stethoscope, end-tidal CO_2, pulse oximetry, and temperature, an arterial line is inserted for frequent assessment of blood gases and for continuous blood pressure tracing. A pulse oximeter is used for continuous monitoring of arterial oxygen saturation. Central venous pressure and hourly urine output are monitored to evaluate fluid balance and cardiac function. A Swan-Ganz catheter is not routinely placed for this kind of surgical patient without documented pulmonary hypertension or left ventricular failure. The advantages of invasive monitoring have to be weighed against the possible complications. A peripheral nerve stimulator should be used to monitor the effects of muscle relaxants.

Barash PG, Cullen BF, Stoelting RK (eds): Clinical Anesthesia, 3rd ed, pp 975–982. Philadelphia, Lippincott-Raven, 1997

Buckley FP: Anesthetizing the morbidly obese patient. ASA Refresher Courses in Anesthesiology 18:53–68, 1990

Shenkman Z, Shir Y, Brodsky JB: Perioperative management of the morbidly obese patient. Br J Anaesth 70:349, 1993

C.2. How would you induce anesthesia? Describe the intubation technique.

Difficult intubation is common in obese patients because of suprasternal pads of fat, short neck, and poor extension of the head (also see question A.9). All of the appropriate airway management equipment should be available. They include endotracheal tubes of different types and sizes, intubation stylets, oropharyngeal and nasopharyngeal airways, and different types of laryngoscopes. Fiberoptic endoscopes and equipment for transtracheal ventilation and cricothyrotomy (Fig. 57-1) also should be available. Because of increased risk of aspiration and possible difficult intubation, awake intubation is the technique of choice. Awake intubation can be done after adequate sedation with fentanyl, droperidol, or diazepam and topical use of local anesthetics, such as 4% lidocaine or benzocaine (Cetacaine) spray around the mouth and pharynx. Oral intubation under direct laryngoscopy can be attempted first. If it is difficult to expose the larynx, a fiberoptic bronchoscope can be used to facilitate intubation. Blind nasal intubation, which has been advocated by some, often causes epistaxis and should be avoided. After awake intubation, anesthesia can be induced with thiopental sodium.

If the patient is not cooperative, a rapid-sequence induction can be used with cricoid compression (Sellick maneuver). After pretreatment with 6 mg of *d*-tubocurarine and preoxygenation for 3 to 5 minutes, anesthesia is induced with thiopental sodium (3 to 4 mg/kg), followed immediately by succinylcholine (1.5 mg/kg) to facilitate intubation. Morbidly obese patients have higher pseudocholinesterase activity than nonobese subjects, therefore dosages of succinylcholine should be increased to 1.2 to 1.5 mg/kg.

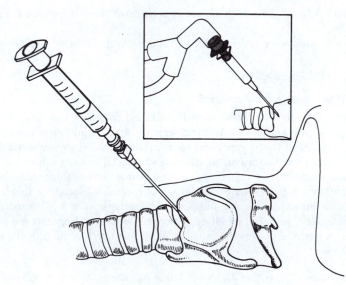

Figure 57-1. An emergency cricothyrotomy may be performed by passing a 14 gauge IV catheter through the cricothyroid membrane into the trachea. A 3 ml syringe with the plunger removed will accept a 15 mm endotracheal tube adapter that allows attachment of an oxygen delivery system. (Reprinted with permission from Barash PG, Cullen BF, Stoelting RK [eds]: Clinical Anesthesia, 3rd ed, p 592. Philadelphia, Lippincott-Raven, 1997)

If both awake intubation and rapid-sequence induction are unsuccessful, a breathing induction with a potent inhalation agent (e.g., isoflurane or halothane) can be used with oxygen to keep the patient breathing spontaneously. Then, intubation is accomplished with a fiberoptic bronchoscope. To ensure adequate oxygenation during a difficult intubation, nitrous oxide should not be added to the circuit before intubation.

Barash PG, Cullen BF, Stoelting RK (eds): Clinical Anesthesia, 3rd ed, pp 975–982. Phildelphia, Lippincott-Raven, 1997

Benumof JL: Management of the difficult adult airway, with special emphasis on awake tracheal intubation. Anesthesiology 75:1087–1110, 1991

Brodsky JB: Anesthetic management of the morbidly obese patient. Int Anesthesiol Clin 24(1): 93–103, 1986

Buckley FP: Anesthetizing the morbidly obese patient. ASA Refresher Courses in Anesthesiology 18:53–68, 1990

Hamm CW, Koehler LS: The implications of morbid obesity for anesthesia: Report of a series. Anesth Rev 6:29–35, 1979

Shenkman Z, Shir Y, Brodsky JB: Perioperative management of the morbidly obese patient. Br J Anaesth 70:349, 1993

Vaughan RW: Anesthetic management of the morbidly obese patient. Cont Anesth Pract 5:71–94, 1982

C.3. Why is it important to preoxygenate the obese patient? How would you do it? Compare the effectiveness of the 4-maximal-breath and 3-minute techniques.

Thorough preoxygenation is important because intubation may take longer in the morbidly obese than in the nonobese; moreover, because the obese have a small intrapulmonary store of oxygen (FRC) which is rapidly depleted (high VO_2), they are at particular risk of hypoxemia.

We recommend that the obese patient be preoxygenated with 100% oxygen for at least 3 minutes to obtain SaO_2 99% to 100%. Drummond and Park have shown that obesity is related to the rapidity of desaturation after induction of anesthesia. They suggest that three vital capacity breaths of 100% oxygen will allow for a 3-minute period of apnea before the onset of hypoxemia. In their study, without preoxygenation, only 1 minute elapsed before significant desaturation occurred. Valentine et al. compared the effectiveness of the 4-maximal-breath and 3-minute techniques in elderly patients. They found similar peak oxygen saturation values after preoxygenation with these two techniques. However, a significantly shorter time to all levels of desaturation was associated with the 4-maximal-breath method when the patients were kept apneic and exposed to room air. The average times to 90% saturation were 3.5 minutes in the 4-breath group and 6.5 minutes in the 3-minute group. Therefore, we suggest that preoxygenation with 3-minute breathing of 100% oxygen offers more protection against hypoxia due to prolonged apnea after induction of anesthesia than does the 4-maximal-breath technique. Recently Nakatsuka and McVey recommended using both oxygraphy and pulse oximetry to acheive SaO_2 99% to 100% during induction to ensure maximal oxygen availability and safe duration of apnea (159 ± 60 minutes) in morbidly obese patients.

Drummond GB, Park GR: Arterial oxygen saturation before intubation of the trachea: An assessment of oxygenation techniques. Br J Anaesth 56:987–992, 1984

Gambee AM, Hertzka RE, Fisher DM: Preoxygenation techniques: Comparison of three-minutes and four-breaths. Anesth Analg 66:468–470, 1987

Jense HG, Dubin SA, Silverstein PL et al: Effect of obesity on safe duration of apnea in anesthetized humans. Anesth Analg 2:89–93, 1991

Nakatsuka M, McVey F: Oxygen disaturation during rapid sequence induction in morbidly obese patients. Am J Anesthesiol 23:273–276, 1996

Valentine SJ, Marjot R, Monk CR: Preoxygenation in the elderly: A comparison of the four-maximal-breath and three-minute techniques. Anesth Analg 71:516–519, 1990

C.4. How would you maintain the anesthesia? What is your choice of agents?

We use isoflurane and N_2O-O_2 (3:2) for maintenance. Almost all anesthetic techniques and agents have been used successfully. We prefer inhalation agents because they provide for easy control of the depth of anesthesia, potentiation of muscle relaxants, and the use of high oxygen concentration when needed. Neuroleptic anesthesia may require a large amount of relaxant for adequate surgical exposure and large doses of narcotics to achieve adequate analgesia. Both of these can create postoperative respiratory difficulty. The morbidly obese patient may need a very high F_IO_2 to achieve adequate oxygenation, and a balanced technique usually depends on 50% to 70% N_2O to keep the patient unconscious.

Among the currently available inhalation agents, isoflurane, sevoflurane, and desflurane may be the best choice because of their low biotransformation rates. Obesity itself increases the biotransformation rate of methoxyflurane, enflurane, and halothane, resulting in increased serum fluoride-ion levels. Methoxyflurane should be avoided in surgery for this kind of patient. Because of the frequent presence of coexisting liver dysfunction due to fatty infiltration, halothane should probably also be avoided. In addition, the combination of hypoxia and halothane can result in postoperative jaundice, which is occasionally reported in the obese patients.

Bently JB, Vaughn RW, Millern MS et al: Serum inorganic fluoride levels in obese patients during and after enflurane anesthesia. Anesth Analg 58:409–412, 1979

Frink EJ, Malan TP, Brown RA et al: Plasma inorganic fluoride levels with sevoflurane anesthesia in morbidly obese patients. Anesth Analg 76:1333, 1993

Samuelson PN, Merin RG, Tabes DR et al: Toxicity following methoxyflurane anesthesia. IV. The role of obesity and effect of low-dose anesthesia on fluoride metabolism and renal function. Can Anaesth Soc J 23:465–479, 1976

Strube PJ, Hulands GM, Halsey MJ: Serum fluoride levels in morbidly obese patients: Enflurane compared with isoflurane. Anaesthesiology 42:685–689, 1987

Sutton TSS, Hoblin DD, Gruenke LD et al: Fluoride metabolites after prolonged exposure of patients and volunteers to desflurane. Anesth Analg 73:180, 1991

Young SR, Stoelting RK, Peterson C et al: Anesthesia biotransformation and renal function in obese patients during and after methoxyflurane and halothane anesthesia. Anesthesiology 42:451–457, 1975

C.5. What kind of muscle relaxants would you use?

Nondepolarizing relaxants, such as vecuronium, cisatracurium, atracurium, rocuronium, doxacurium, pipecuronium, pancuronium, or *d*-tubocurarine would be used. Pancuronium is preferred when hypotension or bradycardia is present. Curare is preferred when there is hypertension or tachycardia. Succinylcholine, IV drip, should be avoided because of the possibility of dual block from prolonged use of a high dose of succinylcholine. If an infusion technique is desired, mivacurium (half-life 2 minutes) provides easily controllable depth of relaxation with fast, spontaneous recovery and no change in the blockade mechanism.

When mivacurium is administered on a milligram per kilogram (mg/kg) body weight basis, it has similar pharmacodynamics in normal weight and morbidly obese patients. To produce a given degree of neuromuscular blockade, a larger dose of pancuronium must be given to morbidly obese patients than to normal-weight patients. However, if the dose is related to body surface area, it is similar to the dose in normal-weight patients. When vecuronium and metocurine are given on a mg/kg body weight basis, recovery in the morbidly obese is slower than in normal-weight patents. In contrast, when atracurium is given on a mg/kg body weight basis, its duration of action is similar in both populations. Therefore, atracurium or cisatracurium may be the muscle relaxants of choice.

A peripheral nerve stimulator should be used to monitor the extent of relaxation and to avoid overdose of relaxants to correct inadequate surgical exposure. Dosage should be based on ideal rather than actual body weight.

Schwartz AE, Matteo RS, Ornstein E et al: Pharmacokinetics and dynamics of metocurine in the obese. Anesthesiology 65:A295, 1986

Tseueda K, Warren JE, McCafferty LA: Pancuronium bromide requirement during anesthesia for the morbidly obese. Anesthesiology 48:483, 1978

Tuchy GK, Tuchy E, Bleyberg M et al: Pharmacodynamics of mivacurium in obese patients. Anesthesiology 81:A1069, 1994

Varin F, Ducharme J, Thoret Y et al: The influence of extreme obesity on body disposition and neuromuscular blocking effect at atracurium. Clin Pharmacol Ther 48:18, 1990

Weinstein JE, Matteo RS, Ornstein E et al: Pharmacodynamics of vecuronium and atracurium in the obese surgical patient. Anesth Analg 65:684, 1986

C.6. Can regional anesthesia be used? What are the advantages and disadvantages of regional anesthesia?

Continuous spinal anesthesia has been reported as an anesthetic approach. This approach demands that patients remain on their side during surgery to maintain adequate spontaneous ventilation. One disadvantage of regional anesthesia is that it is both technically difficult and time consuming to use with the obese patient because of poor landmarks and enormous distances from skin to spinal canal. Another disadvantage is inadequate spontaneous ventilation when an obese patient is in the supine position and has paralyzed abdominal muscles. Psychological stress can be another disadvantage.

In an effort to control respiration during surgery, Hamm and Koehler used continuous thoracic epidural anesthesia combined with light endotracheal general anesthesia. Several advantages have been seen in combining epidural analgesia and light general anesthesia. This technique minimized stress to the cardiovascular system during surgery. It provided stable hemodynamic conditions, with decreased blood pressure and heart rate, decreased left ventricular stroke work, and decreased peripheral vascular resistance and oxygen consumption. It avoided using narcotics and potent inhalation agents. Postoperative emergence was rapid, which permitted early extubation. Epidural analgesia provided postoperative pain relief without respiratory depression. Although these minor advantages were reported, routine use of the technique was not recommended by the authors of that article. We feel that general anesthesia can be easily and successfully administered, as long as the anesthetics are titrated to the needs of surgery and the patients are carefully monitored.

Gelman S, Laws HL, Potzick J et al: Thoracic epidural vs balanced anesthesia in morbid obesity: An intraoperative and postoperative hemodynamic study. Anesth Analg 59:902–908, 1980

Hamm CW, Koehler LS: The implications of morbid obesity for anesthesia: Report of a series. Anesth Rev 6:29–35, 1979

Shenkman Z, Shir Y, Brodsky JB: Perioperative management of the morbidly obese patient. Br J Anaesth 70:349, 1993

C.7. What is the effect of narcotics on Oddi's sphincter?

Subcutaneous morphine (10 mg) increases the pressure in common bile duct more than tenfold within 15 minutes; this effect can be present for 2 hours or more. Morphine causes spasm of Oddi's sphincter, which can interfere with intraoperative cholangiography. Demerol and fentanyl have minimal effects on the sphincter. Morphine is not a good choice for biliary tract surgery. Atropine only partially prevents morphine-induced biliary spasm, but opioid antagonists, such as naloxone, can prevent or relieve it.

Hardman JG, Limbird LG, Molinoff PB et al (eds): Goodman and Gilman's The Pharmacological Basis of Therapeutics, 8th ed, p 532. New York, Macmillan, 1996

C.8. During surgery, arterial blood gases showed pH, 7.35; PaO$_2$, 57 mm Hg; PaCO$_2$, 52 mm Hg; F$_I$O$_2$, 0.6; respirator tidal volume, 1000 ml, and rate, 15/min. To the circuit was added 10 cm H$_2$O positive end-expiratory pressure (PEEP), and the tidal volume was increased to 1200 ml. Twenty minutes later, the arterial blood gases showed pH, 7.32; PaO$_2$, 55 mm Hg; PaCO$_2$, 55 mm Hg. What is the explanation for these changes?

Usually, PEEP increases PaO$_2$, and increasing the tidal volume decreases PaCO$_2$. Occasionally, PEEP and hyperventilation will paradoxically decrease PaO$_2$ and increase PaCO$_2$, especially in morbidly obese patients, mainly because of excessively high airway pressure, whether from the use of PEEP or because of a high tidal volume. High airway pressure can interrupt pulmonary small-vessel blood flow in the uppermost parts of the lungs at peak inspiration. Interrupting the pulmonary blood flow in these ventilated alveoli results in an increase in VD/VT and increased PaCO$_2$. Meanwhile, the impeded blood flow will be redistributed to the areas of shunting that are not affected by the high airway pressure, resulting in an increase in QS/QT. High airway pressure also decreases venous return and cardiac output. This will further decrease PaO$_2$ and increase PaCO$_2$.

Bendixen HH: Morbid obesity. ASA Refresher Courses in Anesthesiology 6:1–14, 1978

In-amani M, Kiduta Y, Nagai H et al: The increase in pulmonary venous admixture by hypocapnia is enhanced in obese patients. Anesthesiology 63:A520, 1985

Salem MR, Dalal FY, Zygmunt MP et al: Does PEEP improve intraoperative arterial oxygenation in grossly obese patients? Anesthesiology 48:280–281, 1978

Salem MR, Joseph N, Lim R et al: Respiratory and hemodynamic response to PEEP in grossly obese patients. Anesthesiology 61:A511, 1984

D. Postoperative Management

D.1. When are you going to extubate the patient? What are the criteria for extubation?

Prophylactic ventilatory support throughout the first postoperative night may be indicated for the obese pickwickian patient. However, the obese nonpickwickian patient can be extubated as soon as the following extubation criteria are met:

- The patient is alert and awake.
- Muscle relaxants are adequately reversed.
- Acceptable blood gases are found on 40% inspired oxygen—*p*H, 7.35 to 7.45; PaO$_2$, >80 mm Hg; PaCO$_2$, <50 mm Hg.
- Acceptable respiratory mechanics are present—A maximal inspiratory force of at least 25 to 30 cm H$_2$O; a vital capacity of >10 ml/kg; tidal volume >5 ml/kg.
- A stable circulatory status has been reached.

Barash PG, Cullen BF, Stoelting RK (eds): Clinical Anesthesia, 3rd ed, pp 975–982. Philadelphia, Lippincott-Raven, 1997

Buckley FP, Robinson NB, Simonowitz DA et al: Anaesthesia in the morbidly obese. Anaesthesia 38:840–851, 1983

D.2. What are the major early postoperative complications in the morbidly obese patient?

Most morbidity is related to thromboembolism, wound infection, and pulmonary failure. Early ambulation is encouraged.

Fauci AS, Braunwald E, Isselbacher KJ et al (eds): Harrison's Principles of Internal Medicine, 14th ed, pp 459–461. New York, McGraw-Hill, 1998

Shenkman Z, Shir Y, Brodsky JB: Perioperative management in the morbidly obese patient. Br J Anaesth 70:349, 1993

D.3. How does position affect respiratory function in obese patients?

In the supine position, intra-abdominal contents elevate the diaphragm, and FRC is decreased. Reduced FRC is associated with increases in airway closure and in volume of trapped gas, resulting in an increase in venous admixture (QS/QT) and a decrease in PaO_2. Therefore, the patient should be nursed in a sitting or semisitting position as soon as the circulatory condition is stable. FRC increases 30% by changing from the supine position to the sitting position, both in normal humans and in post-laparotomy patients. FRC decreases about 25% in both the sitting and supine positions on the first postoperative day after laparotomy.

Hsu HO, Hickey RF: Effect of posture on functional residual capacity postoperatively. Anesthesiology 44:520–521, 1976

Paul DR, Hoyt JL, Boutros AR: Cardiovascular and respiratory changes in response to change of posture in the very obese. Anesthesiology 45:73–78, 1976

Shenkman Z, Shir Y, Brodsky JB: Perioperative management of the morbidly obese patient. Br J Anaesth 70:349, 1993

Tucker DH, Sieker HO: The effect of change in body position on lung volume and intrapulmonary gas mixing in patients with obesity, heart failure and emphysema. Am Rev Respir Dis 82:787–791, 1960

Vaughan RW, Bauer S, Wise L: Effect of position of postoperative oxygenation in markedly obese subjects. Anesth Analg 55:37–41, 1976

D.4. How would you prevent postoperative atelectasis?

Early ambulation, chest physical therapy with incentive spirometry, and effective coughing and deep breathing are encouraged to improve respiration. Prolonged recumbency is avoided because of its adverse effects on the ventilation:perfusion ratio. Careful titration of postoperative pain medication should be emphasized to prevent splinting owing to pain and hypoventilation from excessive narcotics.

Barash PG, Cullen BF, Stoelting RK (eds): Clinical Anesthesia, 3rd ed, pp 975–982. Philadelphia, Lippincott-Raven, 1997

Shenkman Z, Shir Y, Brodsky JB: Perioperative management of the morbidly obese patient. Br J Anaesth 70:349, 1993

D.5. How long would you give supplementary oxygen postoperatively?

Hypoxemia is a universal hazard in morbidly obese patients. Following abdominal surgery, hypoxemia can persist for 4 to 6 days. Therefore, nasal or mask oxygen should be given for several days postoperatively to prevent dangerous hypoxemia.

Barash PG, Cullen BF, Stoelting RK (eds): Clinical Anesthesia, 3rd ed, pp 975–982. Philadelphia, Lippincott-Raven, 1997

Vaughan RW, Engelhart RC, Wise L: Postoperative hypoxemia in obese patients. Ann Surg 180: 872–877, 1974

D.6. How would you control postoperative pain?

Postoperative analgesia may be achieved by parenteral narcotics or epidural analgesia.

Narcotics should be used cautiously in obese patients because of their respiratory depression. The routine use of intramuscular narcotics probably will result in unpredictable and subanalgesic blood levels of narcotics because of an enlarged volume of distribution and poor absorption of narcotics due to intrafat deposition. If narcotics are used, they should probably be administered intravenously by careful titration or by the use of patient-controlled analgesia (PCA) machines.

Epidural analgesia with either local anesthetics or narcotics is associated with a faster speed of recovery and a lower incidence of respiratory complications than conventional narcotic regimens. The epidural doses of either local anesthetics or narcotics necessary to provide analgesia appear to be similar to those for nonobese patients. However, epidural narcotics have the potential to produce delayed respiratory depression, and because morbidly obese patients have the potential for airway difficulties, they probably should be nursed in an intensive care unit or recovery room.

Barash PG, Cullen BF, Stoelting RK (eds): Clinical Anesthesia, 3rd ed, pp 975–982. Philadelphia, Lippincott-Raven, 1997

Rawal N, Sjostrand V, Christofferson E et al: Comparison of intramuscular and epidural morphine for postoperative analgesia in the grossly obese: Influence on postoperative ambulation and pulmonary function. Anesth Analg 63:583–593, 1984

Shenkman Z, Shir Y, Brodsky JB: Perioperative management of the morbidly obese patient. Br J Anaesth 70:349, 1993

Index

Page numbers followed by f indicate a figure; t following a page number indicates tabular material